ADVANCED RECONSTRUCTION

Knee

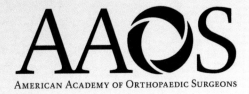

AAOS

AMERICAN ACADEMY OF ORTHOPAEDIC SURGEONS

ADVANCED RECONSTRUCTION
Knee

Edited by

Jay R. Lieberman, MD
Director, New England Musculoskeletal Institute
Professor and Chairman, Department of Orthopaedic Surgery
University of Connecticut Health Center
Farmington, Connecticut

Daniel J. Berry, MD
Chair, Department of Orthopedic Surgery
Professor of Orthopedics
Mayo Clinic College of Medicine
Mayo Clinic
Rochester, Minnesota

Frederick M. Azar, MD
Professor and Sports Medicine Fellowship Director
University of Tennessee—Campbell Clinic
Department of Orthopaedic Surgery
Chief of Staff, Campbell Clinic
Memphis, Tennessee

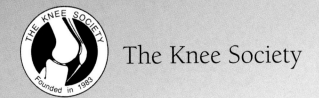

The Knee Society

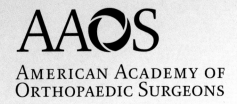

AAOS
AMERICAN ACADEMY OF
ORTHOPAEDIC SURGEONS

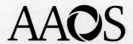

AAOS
AMERICAN ACADEMY OF ORTHOPAEDIC SURGEONS

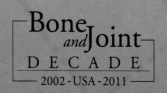

Bone and Joint
DECADE
— 2002 - USA - 2011 —

Acknowledgments

**Advanced Reconstruction Knee
Editorial Board**

Jay R. Lieberman, MD

Daniel J. Berry, MD

Frederick M. Azar, MD

**The Knee Society
Executive Board 2010-2011**

Arlen D. Hanssen, MD
President

Robert B. Bourne, MD
1st Vice President

Giles R. Scuderi, MD
2nd Vice President

Steven J. MacDonald, MD
3rd Vice President

Thomas K. Fehring, MD
Treasurer

Robert T. Trousdale, MD
Secretary

William L. Healy, MD
Douglas A. Dennis, MD
Past Presidents

James P. McAuley, MD
Membership Committee Chair

Jess H. Lonner, MD
Membership Committee Chair-Elect

Mark W. Pagnano, MD
Education Committee Chair

Michael D. Ries, MD
Education Committee Chair-Elect

Thomas P. Vail, MD
E. Michael Keating, MD
Members-at-Large

Contributors

Ayesha Abdeen, MD, FRCSC
Instructor, Orthopaedic Surgery
Harvard Medical School
Department of Orthopaedic Surgery
Beth Israel Deaconess Medical Center
Boston, Massachusetts

Joseph B. Aderinto, MD, FRCS (Tr & Orth)
Consultant Orthopaedic Surgeon
Department of Orthopaedic Surgery
Chapel Allerton Orthopaedic Centre
Leeds, West Yorkshire, England

Sam Akhavan, MD

Muhyeddine Al-Taki, MD
Clinical Fellow in Lower Limb Reconstruction and Oncology
Department of Orthopaedics
University of British Columbia
Vancouver, British Columbia, Canada

Annunziato Amendola, MD
Professor and Callaghan Chair
Director, UI Sports Medicine Center
Department of Orthopaedics
University of Iowa
Iowa City, Iowa

Allen F. Anderson, MD
Director, Lipscomb Foundation for Research and Education
Tennessee Orthopaedic Alliance
St. Thomas Hospital
Nashville, Tennessee

Christian N. Anderson, MD
Department of Orthopaedic Surgery
Vanderbilt University Medical Center
Nashville, Tennessee

James R. Andrews, MD
Medical Director, Andrews Sports Medicine and
   Orthopaedic Center
Birmingham, Alabama

Robert A. Arciero, MD
Professor of Orthopaedics
Department of Orthopaedics
University of Connecticut
Farmington, Connecticut

Keegan P. Au, MD, FRCSC
Clinical Fellow
Adult Hip and Knee Reconstruction
University of Western Ontario
London Health Sciences Centre
London, Ontario, Canada

Douglas K. Ayres, MD, MBA
Vice Chief of Department of Orthopaedic Surgery
Chief of Adult Arthroplasty
Beth Israel Deaconess Medical Center
Boston, Massachusetts

Frederick M. Azar, MD
Professor and Sports Medicine Fellowship Director
University of Tennessee—Campbell Clinic
Department of Orthopaedic Surgery
Chief of Staff, Campbell Clinic
Memphis, Tennessee

Bernard R. Bach, Jr, MD
Professor, The Claude N. Lambert, MD—Helen S. Thomson
   Endowed Chair of Orthopaedics
Director, Division of Sports Medicine
Department of Orthopaedic Surgery
Rush University Medical Center
Chicago, Illinois

David Backstein, MD, MEd, FRCSC
Associate Professor, Department of Surgery
Mount Sinai Hospital
University of Toronto
Toronto, Ontario, Canada

Champ L. Baker, Jr, MD
Staff Physician
The Hughston Clinic
Columbus, Georgia

Champ L. Baker III, MD
Staff Physician
The Hughston Clinic
Columbus, Georgia

C. Lowry Barnes, MD
Managing Partner
Arkansas Specialty Orthopaedics
Little Rock, Arkansas

Robert L. Barrack, MD
Charles F. and Joanne Knight Distinguished Professor
Chief of Service
Department of Orthopaedic Surgery
Washington University School of Medicine
St. Louis, Missouri

James Benjamin, MD
University Orthopedic Specialists
Tucson, Arizona

Keith R. Berend, MD
Clinical Assistant Professor
Department of Orthopaedics
The Ohio State University
Mount Carmel Health System
Columbus, Ohio

Michael E. Berend, MD
Fellowship Director
Center for Hip and Knee Surgery
Joint Replacement Surgeons of Indiana
Mooresville, Indiana

Daniel J. Berry, MD
Chair, Department of Orthopedic Surgery
Professor of Orthopedics
Mayo Clinic College of Medicine
Mayo Clinic
Rochester, Minnesota

Anil Bhave, PT
Director
Rehabilitation Services
Rubin Institute for Advanced Orthopedics
Sinai Hospital of Baltimore
Baltimore, Maryland

Yossef C. Blum, MD
Fellow, Arthroplasty Service
Hospital for Special Surgery
New York, New York

Davide Edoardo Bonasia, MD
Sports Medicine Fellow
Department of Orthopaedics
Sports Medicine Center
University of Iowa
Iowa City, Iowa

Robert E. Booth, Jr, MD
Chief of Orthopaedic Surgery
Pennsylvania Hospital
Clinical Professor
Department of Orthopaedic Surgery
University of Pennsylvania
Philadelphia, Pennsylvania

Michael H. Bourne, MD
Chairman, Department of Surgery
Salt Lake Orthopaedic Clinic
St. Mark's Hospital
Salt Lake City, Utah

Karen K. Briggs, MPH
Director of Clinical Research
Steadman Philippon Research Institute
Vail, Colorado

William Bugbee, MD
Associate Professor
Department of Orthopaedics
University of California
San Diego, California

R. Stephen J. Burnett, MD, FRCSC
Adult Reconstructive Surgery Academic Program Director
Division of Orthopaedic Surgery
Vancouver Island Health, Royal Jubilee Hospital
Victoria, British Columbia, Canada

E. Lyle Cain, Jr, MD
Fellowship Director
American Sports Medicine Institute
Andrews Sports Medicine and Orthopaedic Center
Birmingham, Alabama

John J. Callaghan, MD
Lawrence and Marilyn Dorr Chair
Department of Orthopaedics
University of Iowa and VA Medical Center
Iowa City, Iowa

Thomas Carter, MD
Emeritus Head of Orthopaedic Surgery
Arizona State University
Tempe, Arizona

Yoowang Choi, MD
Clinical Research Fellow
Orthopaedic Adult Knee and Hip
Hospital for Special Surgery
New York, New York

Clifford D. Clark, MD
Total Joint Fellow
Visiting Instructor
Department of Orthopaedics
University of Utah
Salt Lake City, Utah

Henry D. Clarke, MD
Assistant Professor of Orthopedics
Mayo Clinic College of Medicine
Department of Orthopedics
Mayo Clinic
Phoenix, Arizona

Brian J. Cole, MD, MBA
Section Head, Rush Cartilage Restoration Center
Departments of Orthopaedic Surgery and Anatomy
  Cell Biology
Rush University Medical Center
Chicago, Illinois

Alexis Chiang Colvin, MD
Assistant Professor
Department of Orthopaedics
Mount Sinai School of Medicine
New York, New York

Clifford W. Colwell, Jr, MD
Medical Director
Shiley Chair for Orthopaedic Research
Shiley Center for Orthopaedic Research and Education
Scripps Health
La Jolla, California

Jack Conoley, MD
Sports Medicine Fellow
Department of Orthopaedic Surgery
University of Tennessee—Campbell Clinic
Memphis, Tennessee

Fred Cushner, MD
Director
Insall Scott Kelly Institute
Orthopaedic Surgery
New York, New York

David F. Dalury, MD
Towson Orthopaedic Associates
Towson, Maryland

Michael R. Dayton, MD
Assistant Professor
Department of Orthopaedics
University of Colorado Denver
Aurora, Colorado

Joseph P. DeAngelis, MD
Instructor
Department of Orthopaedic Surgery
Harvard Medical School
Beth Israel Deaconess Medical Center
Boston, Massachusetts

Thomas M. DeBerardino, MD
Director, John A. Feagin, Jr, Sports Medicine Fellowship
Department of Orthopaedic Surgery
Keller Army Community Hospital
West Point, New York

Craig J. Della Valle, MD
Associate Professor
Department of Orthopaedic Surgery
Rush University Medical Center
Chicago, Illinois

Douglas A. Dennis, MD
Assistant Clinical Professor
University of Colorado Health Sciences Center
Colorado Joint Replacement
Denver, Colorado

John P. Dunleavy, MD
Clinical Fellow
Adult Reconstruction
Department of Orthopaedic Surgery
Brigham and Women's Hospital
Boston, Massachusetts

Gerard A. Engh, MD
Director, Knee Research
Anderson Orthopaedic Research Institute
Alexandria, Virginia

Jesse James F. Exaltacion, MD
Fellow, Adult Reconstructive Surgery
Center for Orthopaedic Surgery
The Methodist Hospital
Houston, Texas

Gregory C. Fanelli, MD
Orthopaedic Surgery
Danville, Pennsylvania

Thomas K. Fehring, MD
OrthoCarolina Hip and Knee Center
Charlotte, North Carolina

Drew Fehsenfeld, MD, PhD
Department of Orthopaedic Surgery
University of Connecticut
Farmington, Connecticut

David C. Flanigan, MD
Assistant Professor
Team Physician, Athletic Department
Department of Orthopaedic Surgery
The Ohio State University
Columbus, Ohio

Freddie H. Fu, MD, DSc (Hon), DPs (Hon)
David Silver Professor and Chairman
Department of Orthopaedic Surgery
University of Pittsburgh Medical Center
Pittsburgh, Pennsylvania

John P. Fulkerson, MD
Clinical Professor of Orthopedic Surgery
University of Connecticut
Orthopedic Associates of Hartford, PC
Farmington, Connecticut

Donald S. Garbuz, MD

Kevin L. Garvin, MD
L. Thomas Hood, MD, Professor and Chair
Orthopaedic Surgery and Rehabilitation
University of Nebraska Medical Center
Omaha, Nebraska

Brett Gibson, MD
Attending Physician
Orthopaedic Surgery
CHS Professional Practice
Coordinated Health
Bethlehem, Pennsylvania

Terence J. Gioe, MD
Adjunct Professor of Orthopaedic Surgery
Department of Orthopaedic Surgery
University of Minnesota Medical School
Minneapolis, Minnesota

Andreas H. Gomoll, MD
Assistant Professor of Orthopaedic Surgery
Orthopaedic Surgery/Cartilage Repair Center
Brigham and Women's Hospital
Harvard Medical School
Boston, Massachusetts

Simon Görtz, MD
Research Fellow
Department of Orthopaedic Surgery
University of California San Diego
La Jolla, California

William L. Griffin, MD
Hip and Knee Center
OrthoCarolina
Charlotte, North Carolina

Allan E. Gross, MD, FRCSC
Professor, Faculty of Medicine
University of Toronto
Orthopaedic Surgeon
Division of Orthopaedic Surgery
Mount Sinai Hospital
Toronto, Ontario, Canada

Robert C. Grumet, MD
Fellow, Sports Medicine
Department of Orthopaedic Surgery
Rush University Medical Center
Chicago, Illinois

George J. Haidukewych, MD
Orthopedic Trauma and Adult Reconstruction
Florida Orthopedic Institute
University of South Florida
Tampa, Florida

William G. Hamilton, MD
Senior Technical Advisor
Anderson Orthopaedic Research Institute
Alexandria, Virginia

Arlen D. Hanssen, MD
Professor of Orthopedic Surgery
Mayo Clinic and Mayo Foundation
Rochester, Minnesota

Mary E. Hardwick, MSN, RN
Manager, Research Publications
Shiley Center for Orthopaedic Research and Education
Scripps Health
La Jolla, California

Christopher D. Harner, MD
Professor and Medical Director
Department of Orthopaedics
University of Pittsburgh
Pittsburgh, Pennsylvania

Jennifer A. Hart, MPAS, PA-C
Physician Assistant
Orthopaedic Surgery
Division Sports Medicine
University of Virginia
Charlottesville, Virginia

David C. Hay, MD
Resident
Department of Orthopaedics
Stanford University
Stanford, California

William L. Healy, MD
Chairman, Orthopaedic Surgery
Lahey Clinic
Burlington, Massachusetts

Sherwin S.W. Ho, MD
Associate Professor of Surgery
Section of Orthopaedic Surgery
University of Chicago
Chicago, Illinois

Aaron A. Hofmann, MD
Professor
Department of Orthopaedics
University of Utah
Salt Lake City, Utah

Carl Imhauser, PhD
Biomechanics Department
Hospital for Special Surgery
New York, New York

Stephen J. Incavo, MD
Section Head, Adult Reconstructive Surgery
Department of Orthopaedics
The Methodist Hospital
Houston, Texas

Richard Iorio, MD
Associate Professor
Orthopaedic Surgery
Lahey Clinic
Burlington, Massachusetts

Joshua J. Jacobs, MD
Professor and Chairman
Department of Orthopaedic Surgery
Rush University Medical Center
Chicago, Illinois

William A. Jiranek, MD
Associate Professor
Chief, Adult Reconstruction
Department of Orthopaedic Surgery
VCU Health Systems
Richmond, Virginia

Derek R. Johnson, MD
Total Joint Fellow
Colorado Joint Replacement
Denver, Colorado

Christopher Kaeding, MD
Judson Wilson Professor
Medical Director, Sports Medicine Center
Head Team Physician
Department of Orthopaedics
The Ohio State University
Columbus, Ohio

E. Michael Keating, MD
Center for Hip and Knee Surgery
Mooresville, Indiana

Peter A. Keblish, MD
Past Chief
Division of Orthopedic Surgery
Allentown, Pennsylvania

Keith Kenter, MD
Director of Orthopaedic Resident Program
Team Orthopaedic Surgeon
Department of Orthopaedic Surgery
University of Cincinnati
Cincinnati, Ohio

Raymond H. Kim, MD
Orthopaedic Surgeon
Colorado Joint Replacement
Denver, Colorado

Dukhwan Ko, MD
Assistant Professor
Department of Orthopaedic Surgery
Konkuk University
Chungju, Chungbuk, Korea

Mininder S. Kocher, MD, MPH
Associate Director, Division of Sports Medicine
Department of Orthopaedic Surgery
Children's Hospital Boston
Boston, Massachusetts

Jason L. Koh, MD
Associate Professor
Department of Orthopaedic Surgery
Northwestern University
Chicago, Illinois

Richard D. Komistek, PhD
Fred M. Roddy Endowed Professorship
Co-Center Director, Center for Musculoskeletal Research
Mechanical, Aerospace and Biomedical Engineering
The University of Tennessee
Knoxville, Tennessee

Kenneth A. Krackow, MD
Clinical Director
Department of Orthopaedic Surgery
Kaleida Health–Buffalo General Hospital
Buffalo, New York

Aaron J. Krych, MD
Orthopedic Surgery Resident
Mayo Clinic
Rochester, Minnesota

Sharat K. Kusuma, MD, MBA
Associate Director
Hip and Knee Reconstruction
Grant Medical Center
Columbus, Ohio

Robert F. LaPrade, MD, PhD
The Steadman Clinic
Vail, Colorado

Bruce A. Levy, MD
Assistant Professor
Orthopedic Surgery
Mayo Clinic
Rochester, Minnesota

Jay R. Lieberman, MD
Director, New England Musculoskeletal Institute
Professor and Chairman, Department of Orthopaedic Surgery
University of Connecticut Health Center
Farmington, Connecticut

Steve S. Liu, MD
Associate Research Scientist
Orthopaedics
University of Iowa
Iowa City, Iowa

Adolph V. Lombardi, Jr, MD, FACS
Clinical Assistant Professor
Department of Orthopaedics
Department of Biomedical Engineering
The Ohio State University
Mount Carmel Health System
Columbus, Ohio

William J. Long, MD, FRCSC
Attending Orthopaedic Surgeon
Insall Scott Kelly Institute
North Shore–LIJ Health System
New York, New York

Jess H. Lonner, MD
Director, Knee Replacement Surgery
Department of Orthopaedic Surgery
Pennsylvania Hospital
Philadelphia, Pennsylvania

Tad M. Mabry, MD
Instructor of Orthopedic Surgery
Department of Orthopedic Surgery
Division of Orthopedic Trauma and Adult Reconstruction
Mayo Clinic
Rochester, Minnesota

Steven J. MacDonald, MD, FRCSC
Professor of Orthopaedic Surgery
Chief of Surgery, Chief of Orthopaedics
University of Western Ontario
London Health Sciences Centre
London, Ontario, Canada

Bert Mandelbaum, MD

E. Marc Mariani, MD
Salt Lake Orthopaedic Clinic
St. Mark's Hospital
Salt Lake City, Utah

Bassam A. Masri, MD, FRCSC
Professor and Chairman
Department of Orthopaedics
University of British Columbia
Vancouver, British Columbia, Canada

Wadih Y. Matar, MD, MSc, FRCSC
Orthopaedic Surgeon
Adult Reconstruction
Rothman Institute
Philadelphia, Pennsylvania

Matthew J. Matava, MD
Associate Professor
Orthopaedic Surgery
Washington University
St. Louis, Missouri

David R. McAllister, MD
Associate Professor
Chief, Sports Medicine Service
Department of Orthopaedic Surgery
University of California, Los Angeles
Los Angeles, California

Eric C. McCarty, MD
Associate Professor
Chief of Sports Medicine and Shoulder Surgery
Department of Orthopaedic Surgery
University of Colorado Denver School of Medicine
Denver, Colorado

Mike S. McGrath, MD
Fellow
Center for Joint Preservation and Replacement
Rubin Institute for Advanced Orthopedics
Sinai Hospital of Baltimore
Baltimore, Maryland

John B. Meding, MD
Orthopaedic Surgeon
Center for Hip and Knee Surgery
Mooresville, Indiana

Steven W. Meisterling, MD
St. Croix Orthopaedics
Stillwater, Minnesota

Mark D. Miller, MD
S. Ward Casscells Professor of Orthopaedic Surgery
Head, Division of Sports Medicine
University of Virginia
Charlottesville, Virginia

Robert H. Miller III, MD
Associate Professor
University of Tennessee
Campbell Clinic
Department or Orthopaedic Surgery
Memphis, Tennessee

Tom Minas, MD, MS
Cartilage Repair Center
Department of Orthopaedics
Brigham and Women's Hospital
Harvard Medical School
Boston, Massachusetts

Michael A. Mont, MD
Director
Center for Joint Preservation and Replacement
Rubin Institute for Advanced Orthopedics
Sinai Hospital of Baltimore
Baltimore, Maryland

Claude T. Moorman III, MD
Associate Professor, Orthopaedic Surgery
Director, Sports Medicine
Division of Orthopaedic Surgery
Duke University Medical Center
Durham, North Carolina

Patrick Morgan, MD
Assistant Professor
Orthopaedic Surgery
University of Minnesota
Minneapolis, Minnesota

Charles L. Nelson, MD
Associate Professor of Orthopaedic Surgery
Department of Orthopaedic Surgery
University of Pennsylvania
Philadelphia, Pennsylvania

Michael Nett, MD
Attending Physician
Department of Orthopaedic Surgery
Insall Scott Kelly Institute
Bayshore, New York

Gregg T. Nicandri, MD
Sports Medicine Fellow
Division of Orthopaedic Surgery
Duke University Medical Center
Durham, North Carolina

Mark W. Pagnano, MD
Professor of Orthopedics
Consultant Orthopedic Surgery
Department of Orthopedics
Mayo Clinic
Rochester, Minnesota

Richard D. Parker, MD
Professor and Chairman
Department of Orthopaedics
Orthopaedic Rheumatology Institute
Cleveland Clinic Foundation
Cleveland, Ohio

Cecilia Pascual-Garrido, MD
Research Fellow
Department of Orthopedic Surgery
Rush University Medical Center
Chicago, Illinois

Dana P. Piasecki, MD
Fellow
Division of Sports Medicine
Rush University Medical Center
Chicago, Illinois

Trevor R. Pickering, MD
Orthopaedic Surgeon
Center for Hip and Knee Surgery
Mooresville, Indiana

Tony Quach, MD
Orthopedic Surgery Sports Medicine Fellow
Department of Orthopaedic Surgery
University of California, Los Angeles
Los Angeles, California

Amar S. Ranawat, MD
Attending Orthopaedic Surgeon
Hospital for Special Surgery
New York, New York

Chitranjan S. Ranawat, MD
Clinical Professor of Orthopaedic Surgery
Weill Cornell Medical College
Hospital for Special Surgery
New York, New York

James A. Rand, MD
Professor Emeritus
Department of Orthopedics
Mayo Clinic, Arizona
Scottsdale, Arizona

Michael D. Ries, MD
Professor of Orthopaedic Surgery
Department of Orthopaedic Surgery
University of California, San Francisco
San Francisco, California

Samuel P. Robinson, MD
Department of Orthopaedic Surgery, Sports Medicine
Jordan-Young Institute
Virginia Beach, Virginia

Scott A. Rodeo, MD
Attending Orthopaedic Surgeon
Co-Chief, Sports Medicine and Shoulder Service
The Hospital for Special Surgery
Professor of Orthopaedic Surgery
Weill Cornell Medical College
New York, New York

William G. Rodkey, DVM
Chief Scientific Officer
Steadman Philippon Research Institute
Vail, Colorado

James R. Romanowski, MD
Fellow
Department of Orthopaedic Sports Medicine
University of Pittsburgh Medical Center
Pittsburgh, Pennsylvania

Aaron Rosenberg, MD
Professor of Surgery
Department of Orthopaedic Surgery
Rush University Medical Center
Chicago, Illinois

Seth Rosenzweig, MD
Sports Medicine Fellow
Department of Orthopaedic Surgery
University of Tennessee
Campbell Clinic
Memphis, Tennessee

Roberto Rossi, MD
Assistant Professor
Department of Orthopaedics and Traumatology
University of Turin
Turin, Italy

Oleg Safir, MD, MEd, FRCSC
Department of Surgery, Orthopaedic Division
University of Toronto
Mount Sinai Hospital
Toronto, Ontario, Canada

Marc R. Safran, MD
Professor
Associate Director, Sports Medicine
Department of Orthopaedic Surgery
Stanford University
Stanford, California

Alexander P. Sah, MD
Orthopedic Surgeon
Department of Orthopedics
Washington Hospital Healthcare System
Fremont, California

Richard D. Scott, MD
Professor of Orthopaedic Surgery
Harvard Medical School
Department of Orthopaedic Surgery
Brigham and Women's Hospital
New England Baptist Hospital
Boston, Massachusetts

Giles R. Scuderi, MD
Director
Insall Scott Kelly Institute for Orthopaedics and
    Sports Medicine
New York, New York

Thomas P. Sculco, MD
Surgeon-In-Chief
Hospital for Special Surgery
New York, New York

Peter F. Sharkey, MD
Professor
Department of Orthopaedic Surgery
Thomas Jefferson University Hospital
Rothman Institute
Philadelphia, Pennsylvania

Adrija Sharma, PhD
Department of Mechanical, Aerospace
    and Biomedical Engineering
The University of Tennessee
Knoxville, Tennessee

K. Donald Shelbourne, MD
Associate Clinical Professor
Indiana University School of Medicine
Department of Orthopaedics
Shelbourne Knee Center
Indianapolis, Indiana

Walter Shelton, MD
Mississippi Sports Medicine and Orthopaedic Center
Jackson, Mississippi

Joshua T. Snyder, MD
Orthopaedic Sports Medicine Fellow
Section of Orthopaedic Surgery
University of Chicago
Chicago, Illinois

Lawrence M. Specht, MD
Clinical Assistant Professor of Orthopaedic Surgery
Department of Orthopaedic Surgery
Lahey Clinic
Burlington, Massachusetts

Kurt P. Spindler, MD
Professor
Department of Orthopaedics and Rehabilitation
Vanderbilt University Medical Center
Nashville, Tennessee

Bryan D. Springer, MD
OrthoCarolina Hip and Knee Center
Charlotte, North Carolina

J. Richard Steadman, MD
Managing Partner
Founder and Chairman
Steadman Clinic
Steadman Philippon Research Institute
Vail, Colorado

James B. Stiehl, MD
Associate Clinical Professor
Department of Orthopaedic Surgery
Medical College of Wisconsin
Milwaukee, Wisconsin

Michael J. Stuart, MD
Professor and Vice-Chairman
Department of Orthopedic Surgery
Mayo Clinic
Rochester, Minnesota

Thomas S. Thornhill, MD

John F. Tilzey, MD, PhD
Department of Orthopaedic Surgery
Lahey Clinic
Burlington, Massachusetts

Robert T. Trousdale, MD
Professor, Orthopedic Surgery
Mayo Medical School
Department of Adult Reconstructive Orthopedic Surgery
Mayo Medical Center
Rochester, Minnesota

Kimberly K. Tucker, MD
Orthopaedic Surgeon
Department of Joint Replacement
Orthopaedic Associates
Towson, Maryland

Scott E. Urch, MD
Orthopaedic Surgeon
Shelbourne Knee Center
Indianapolis, Indiana

Thomas Parker Vail, MD
Professor and Chairman
Department of Orthopaedic Surgery
University of California, San Francisco
San Francisco, California

Kelly G. Vince, MD, FRCS(C)
Consultant Orthopedic Surgeon
Department of Orthopedic Surgery
The Wellington Hospital
Wellington, New Zealand

Ray C. Wasielewski, MS, MD
Director
Minimally Invasive Orthopedics
Grant Medical Center
Columbus, Ohio

Russell E. Windsor, MD
Attending Orthopaedic Surgeon
Professor of Orthopaedic Surgery
Hospital for Special Surgery
Weill Medical College of Cornell University
New York, New York

Rick W. Wright, MD
Associate Professor
Department of Orthopaedic Surgery
Washington University
St. Louis, Missouri

Timothy Wright, PhD
Director of Biomechanics
Department of Biomechanics
Hospital for Special Surgery
New York, New York

Michael G. Zywiel, MD
Fellow
Center for Joint Preservation and Replacement
Rubin Institute for Advanced Orthopedics
Sinai Hospital of Baltimore
Baltimore, Maryland

Preface

The American Academy of Orthopaedic Surgeons and The Knee Society decided to partner to develop a unique orthopaedic textbook that covers all aspects of reconstruction of the knee in adults. This comprehensive text focuses on joint preservation procedures, primary and revision total knee arthroplasty, and various arthroscopic and ligament repair procedures. This book is not just another reference text; it is intended to be used as a surgical guide. We envision that surgeons will use this text to help plan and carry out a specific surgical procedure or to manage a difficult clinical problem. The 6 sections contain 94 chapters that are organized to allow one to quickly locate and thoroughly prepare for a particular surgical procedure. Because of this emphasis on technique, it is not as heavily referenced as other textbooks, but each chapter contains numerous photographs, illustrations, diagrams, and radiographs to highlight specific management strategies and surgical techniques. In addition, 14 surgical videos are included to further enhance the learning experience.

The authors of this text were invited to contribute their work because of their special expertise related to each topic. In each chapter they describe the indications, contraindications, and the techniques that can be used when confronted with a particular problem related to the knee or when using a particular device or implant. Each chapter also reviews alternative management options and potential pitfalls. The chapters have been formatted to facilitate a rapid review of the surgical technique or a more detailed study of a specific problem related to the knee.

Advanced Reconstruction: Knee would not have been possible without the efforts of numerous individuals. First, we would like to thank the authors for dedicating their time and expertise in creating this outstanding reference. Extra effort was required to identify the photographs, illustrations, and radiographs that enhance this book, and the authors have clearly done a superb job in choosing these items. We also would like to give special thanks to Laurie Braun, Managing Editor, and Steven Kellert, Senior Editor, for both their editorial expertise and their hard work, and to Marilyn Fox, PhD, Director of Publications, for her leadership. This book would never have fulfilled its mission without their effort. Finally, we want to thank the American Academy of Orthopaedic Surgeons and The Knee Society for their support of this project. It is our hope that you find this book to be a valuable tool and that you will use it on a regular basis when dealing with problems of the adult knee.

Jay R. Lieberman, MD
Director, New England Musculoskeletal Institute
Professor and Chairman, Department of
*   Orthopaedic Surgery*
University of Connecticut Health Center
Farmington, Connecticut

Daniel J. Berry, MD
Chair, Department of Orthopedic Surgery
Professor of Orthopedics
Mayo Clinic College of Medicine
Mayo Clinic
Rochester, Minnesota

Frederick M. Azar, MD
Professor and Sports Medicine Fellowship Director
University of Tennessee—Campbell Clinic
Department of Orthopaedic Surgery
Chief of Staff, Campbell Clinic
Memphis, Tennessee

Table of Contents

Knee Dislocation

Meniscal Injuries

Patellofemoral Injuries

DVD

Chapter 1

Primary Total Knee Arthroplasty: Medial Parapatellar Approach

Stephen J. Incavo, MD
Michael R. Dayton, MD
Jesse James F. Exaltacion, MD

Indications

Many methods of surgical exposure allow successful total knee arthroplasty (TKA). Regardless of the method used, exposure that is sufficient to allow consistently successful total knee implant placement and alignment should be a primary concern. A standard anterior midline skin incision with a medial parapatellar arthrotomy continues to be the most widely used method of exposure for TKA. The extensor mechanism of the knee—composed of the quadriceps muscle and tendon, patella, and patellar tendon—comprises biomechanically and anatomically complex, interacting structures that work together to provide effective knee function. Proper preservation of the extensor mechanism is vital to successful recovery following TKA. The main advantage of the anterior approach to the knee is that it provides excellent visualization and access to the distal femur, proximal tibia, and patella. Although not extensile in the classic sense, it is more extensile than most TKA approaches.

The medial parapatellar approach is used for both primary and revision TKA. Variations in pathologic morphology may include varus or valgus deformity, patella alta or patella infera, and previous tibial or femoral osteotomy. The approach can be used regardless of preoperative range of motion. Patients of short stature, obese patients, and patients with muscular lower extremities are ideal candidates for this approach. The tissue along the medial course of the patella and knee capsule is sufficiently thick to provide a satisfactory closure following TKA. The approach is straightforward to perform and exposes the knee joint efficiently.

Additional indications for the medial parapatellar arthrotomy include the situation when lateral patellar subluxation is required, because this approach allows medial imbrication (advancement) of the arthrotomy. Furthermore, should the patellar tendon be excessively thin or compromised by the approach, a side-to-side repair of this structure can be achieved. In the setting of revision or a profoundly ankylosed knee, a modified anterior exposure may be necessary. Quadriceps snip, V-Y quadricepsplasty, and tibial tubercle osteotomy have all been used in conjunction with the medial parapatellar approach to enhance safe exposure.

The medial parapatellar approach has evolved over the past decade, largely due to the popularization of minimally invasive surgical techniques. In general, incisions have decreased in length from the traditional incision, which was made from one handbreadth proximal to the patella and extended distally past the tibial tubercle. Excellent exposure usually can be achieved by a shorter incision, from 4 cm proximal to the superior pole of the patella to 1 cm proximal to the tibial tubercle. Lateral eversion of the patella is no longer considered necessary in all cases of TKA and has been replaced frequently by simple lateral subluxation of the patella. En-

Dr. Incavo or an immediate family member is a board member, owner, officer, or committee member for The Knee Society, the American Association of Hip and Knee Surgeons, the American Academy of Orthopaedic Surgeons, and the Texas State Orthopaedic Society; has received royalties from Exactech; is a paid consultant for or is an employee of Stryker and Wright Medical; has received research or institutional support from Stryker; owns stock or stock options in Otismed; and has received nonincome support (such as equipment or services), commercially derived honoraria, or other non–research-related funding (such as paid travel) from Nimbic Systems. Dr. Dayton or an immediate family member is a member of a speakers' bureau or has made paid presentations on behalf of Smith & Nephew; serves as a paid consultant for or is an employee of Smith & Nephew; serves as an unpaid consultant to Smith & Nephew and DePuy; and has received research or institutional support from Exactech, DePuy, Stryker, and Smith & Nephew. Neither Dr. Exaltacion nor any immediate family member has received anything of value from or owns stock in a commercial company or institution related directly or indirectly to the subject of this chapter.

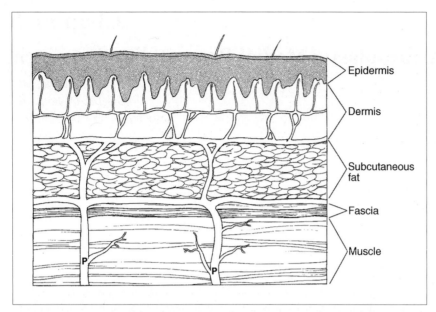

Figure 1 Soft-tissue microvascular anatomy. Note that the vessels just superficial to the deep fascia form a vascular anastomosis, which provides the skin's blood supply. Perforating arteries just superficial to the deep fascia supply this anastomosis. Because of this, dissection of the soft tissue just into the deep fascia is more protective of the skin blood supply than dissection of the dermis and subcutaneous fat from the deep fascia. P = perforating artery. (Reproduced from Younger AS, Duncan CD, Masri BA: Surgical exposures in revision total knee arthroplasty. *J Am Acad Orthop Surg* 1998;6:55-64.)

thusiasm for minimally invasive approaches to the knee has decreased considerably because of the belief that the limited surgical exposure achieved may result in less-than-optimal component placement or inadvertent soft-tissue damage.

Contraindications

Previous skin incisions oriented longitudinally and lateral to the line through which a medial parapatellar approach would be performed are a relative contraindication. Narrow skin bridges pose a considerable risk of skin necrosis; therefore, incisions 4 cm or less from a previous incision should be avoided. If skin bridges of 4 cm or less must be used for the TKA, close attention to wound healing is mandatory. If skin necrosis develops, soft-tissue coverage should be obtained expeditiously, before wound breakdown. The blood supply to the skin overlying the knee is supplied by perforating arteries located just superficial to the deep fascia. To minimize disruption of these vessels (and the skin blood supply), dissection of medial and lateral soft tissues should be deep to the fascia (**Figure 1**).

Specific circumstances may require alternative approaches to the medial parapatellar arthrotomy. Previous surgery using a lateral approach may compromise the blood supply to the patella. The patella is supplied by the midpatellar vessels in the middle third of the anterior surface. These vessels enter the patellar apex behind the tendon. Specifically, the upper half of the patella is supplied only by the midpatellar vessels. Cadaver studies have shown absence of vascular filling after medial arthrotomies performed too close to the patella, and also after radical fat pad excision, lateral release too close to the patella, and cautery of the prepatellar vessels. Although osteonecrosis of the patella is uncommon after a medial parapatellar surgical approach, unnecessary vascular disruption should be avoided.

Extensive scarring of the extensor mechanism prohibits a simple medial parapatellar approach. In patients with quadriceps contracture and limited flexion, modification of the standard medial parapatellar approach may be necessary to avoid compromise of the extensor mechanism and facilitate proper flexion and exposure for TKA.

Alternative Treatments

Any surgical approach for TKA must satisfactorily allow soft-tissue releases that correctly align the knee. In addition, the approach must avoid undesirable loosening or attenuation of tissue in areas already weakened by disease.

Subvastus Approach

Although the original description of the subvastus approach dates back to 1929, this approach as described by Hofmann and associates has gained popularity recently. Indications for this approach are similar to those for the medial parapatellar approach. Theoretical advantages include decreased patellar subluxation and vascular devitalization, but this remains a topic of considerable debate. Disadvantages include the potentially increased technical difficulty, particularly in muscular patients and in short individuals.

Midvastus Approach

The midvastus approach became popular in the 1990s. This technique, theoretically combining advantages of the medial parapatellar and subvastus approaches, divides the vastus medialis obliquus (VMO) in its midsubstance, in line with its fibers. A unique feature of this approach in contrast to the medial parapatellar approach is the lack of disruption of the VMO insertion into the quadriceps tendon. Another theoretical advantage of this muscle-splitting approach with regard to healing potential is that the quadriceps tendon receives its nutrition mainly from the overlying paratenon and soft tissue, and therefore it takes more time to heal than does a muscle incision. Medial capsular advancement may be difficult to perform with this approach at the time of closure. Compared with the subvastus approach, however, this option allows easier eversion and lateral displacement of the patella. Both of these techniques are relatively contraindicated in muscular and short patients and in patients with previous high tibial osteotomy, previous revision surgery, or aggressive ossific osteoarthritis.

Lateral Parapatellar Approach

This approach is most commonly used in the presence of valgus knee deformity, where lateral intra-articular adhesions or contractures may be present. This approach also may be useful when lateral retinacular release is necessary. Laterally based dissection avoids the attenuation of medial tissue that accompanies medial exposure. The lateral tissue, however, is considerably thinner in the capsule, potentially hampering the integrity of the capsular closure. This is a more technically demanding exposure, particularly given the inconsistent presentations with which valgus knees may present. Anatomy is reversed with this approach, and difficulty may be encountered with medial patellar reflection, even in the primary TKA setting. Medial patellar reflection also may be difficult in the setting of revision TKA.

■——

■ Results

A clinical study examining two consecutive groups using the subvastus (167 knees) or medial parapatellar (169 knees) approach showed no differences in clinical outcome parameters, including Knee Society scores, range of motion, or stair climbing.

Studies examining differences in vastus-splitting versus medial parapatellar approaches emerged in the late 1990s. Results are mixed and do not show a strong advantage to either approach; however, one study noted frequent abnormal postoperative electromyograms (43%) in the muscle-splitting group. All other outcome measures in the study were equal, including range of motion, postoperative strength, tourniquet time, and proprioception.

Data for the lateral approach are more scant. One clinical series of 53 knees noted improvement in motion from 85° to 115°. Intraoperative complications included three fractures and one failed patellar component. One malpositioned tibial component required revision, and two nerve palsies occurred, both of which resolved (**Table 1**).

■——

■ Technique

Setup/Exposure

The patient is placed supine, with a bump under the affected hip if excessive lower extremity external rotation is present. A device to hold the foot alternately in flexion and extension is helpful. Application of a proximal thigh tourniquet is standard, and routine preparation and draping should allow full exposure of relevant anatomy and landmarks, including the tibial tubercle, patella, and distal quadriceps.

Instruments/Equipment/ Implants Required

The medial parapatellar approach generally does not require specific instrumentation or equipment. Some retraction tools, however, may be very helpful. A bent Hohmann retractor is useful for lateral tissue distraction whether or not the patella is everted. A marking tool may be helpful to note the extent of the arthrotomy from the medial side of the quadriceps tendon, along the medial border of the patella (ensuring at least 5 mm from the medial patellar edge), distally to the medial border of the patellar tendon. This is to ensure reapproximation at identical points. In cases of a tight extensor mechanism, a pin through the patellar tendon and into the proximal tibia may be helpful to avoid avulsion of the former from its attachment into the tibial tubercle. If the extensor mechanism is extremely tight, however, the surgeon should not hesitate to decrease patellar ligament tension by using a quadriceps snip or tibial tubercle osteotomy.

Procedure

With the knee in extension, the anterior skin incision is marked from 4 cm proximal to the patella to 1 cm distal to the tibial tubercle (**Figure 2**, *A*). The knee is placed in the flexed position for the skin incision (**Figure 2**, *B*). Often the entire length of the marked skin incision is not needed because of the stretching of the skin with the knee flexed. The incision should be extended far enough proximally to provide exposure of at least 2 to 3 cm of the quadriceps tendon. The dissection should occur through the fat just deep to the muscle fascia to minimize disruption to the skin blood supply. Full-thickness skin flaps, one medial flap and one smaller lateral flap, are developed. The arthrotomy is then started 2 cm proximal to the patella, curving along the medial patella and then parallel to the patellar ligament to the tibial tubercle. The arthrotomy

Table 1 Results for Various Arthrotomy Techniques

Authors (Year)	Number of Knees	Procedure or Approach	Mean Patient Age in Years (Range)	Mean Follow-up	Results
Dalury and Jiranek (1999)	48 (24 knees in each group)	Bilateral TKA: midvastus vs paramedian	70	12 weeks	Midvastus: decreased early pain and time to SLR, increased strength No differences in releases, ROM
White et al (1999)	218 (109 knees in each group)	Bilateral TKA: midvastus vs medial parapatellar	68 (44-87)	6 months	Midvastus: decreased time to SLR at 8 days, decreased pain up to 6 weeks with midvastus; Medial parapatellar: increase in releases No differences in ROM, EBL, tourniquet time, SLR at 6 months
Parentis et al (1999)	51 (22 midvastus, 29 medial parapatellar)	Vastus-splitting (midvastus) vs medial parapatellar	68 for midvastus 65 for medial parapatellar	5.8 months	Medial parapatellar: increased lateral release, EBL Midvastus only: 43% abnormal electromyogram No differences in ROM, knee scores, tourniquet time, proprioception, or patellar tracking
Keating et al (1999)	200 (100 knees in each group)	Bilateral TKA: midvastus vs medial parapatellar	70 (42-86)	POD 3 (discharge)	No differences in lateral release, POD 2 ROM, discharge day ROM, day able to do SLR, leg circumference, extensor lag
Matsueda and Gustilo (2000)	336 (169 medial parapatellar [1988-1992], 167 subvastus [1992-1996])	Medial parapatellar vs subvastus	67 (30-88) for medial parapatellar 69 (32-86) for subvastus	6 months	Subvastus: decreased lateral release, increased central patellar tracking No difference in ROM, stair climbing, knee scores Groups done in different time periods
Lin et al (2009)	60 patients (80 knees, 40 in each group)	Minimal incision medial parapatellar vs QS	70.2 for medial parapatellar 69.6 for QS	2 months	QS: tourniquet and surgical times lengthened, varus postoperative alignment tended to increase No difference in muscle strength, postoperative pain, functional outcomes

TKA = total knee arthroplasty, SLR = straight-leg raise, ROM = range of motion, EBL = estimated blood loss, POD = postoperative day, QS = quadriceps-sparing.

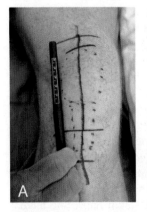 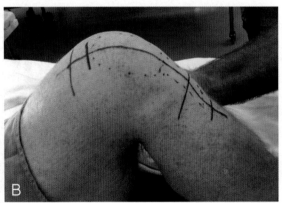

Figure 2 Skin incision for the medial parapatellar approach. **A,** The incision has been marked from 4 cm proximal to the superior pole of the patella to 2 cm distal to the tibial tubercle. The incision initially begins from the superior pole of the patella to 1 cm proximal to the tibial tubercle and is extended as needed to prevent skin tension during exposure. **B,** With the knee flexed, the incision stretches longitudinally to provide additional exposure without additional soft-tissue tension. This also aids in the dissection of the medial and lateral flaps deep to the muscular fascia.

should maintain a 5-mm cuff of soft tissue lateral to the vastus medialis insertion and medial to the patella and patellar ligament (**Figure 3**).

The knee is then extended and the proximal medial tibia is exposed. In most knees, this is done by elevating the medial capsular flap and deep medial collateral ligament from the bone to the midcoronal plane (**Figure 4**). If more medial release is required, this can be continued farther, to the posteromedial corner of the knee joint. In the case of a valgus knee with possible medial collateral ligament laxity, the medial capsular dissection should initially be limited and not carried all the way to the midcoronal plane. This can be released farther if needed later in

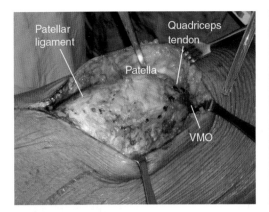

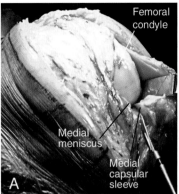

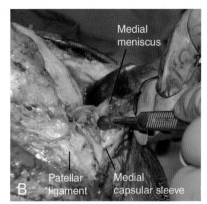

Figure 3 Medial patellar arthrotomy. This should leave a 5-mm cuff of soft-tissue attachment medial to the patella and to the patellar ligament. VMO = vastus medialis obliquus.

Figure 4 Deep dissection of the medial capsule and deep medial collateral ligament tissue. **A,** Initial release. **B,** Farther release to the midcoronal plane. In cases of severe deformity and difficult exposure, this can be performed farther to release the posteromedial capsule.

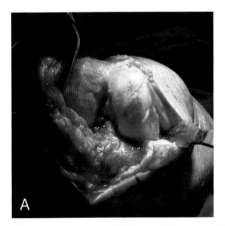

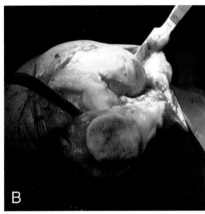

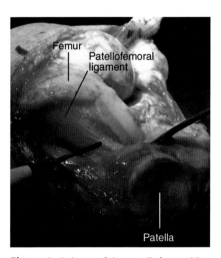

Figure 5 Exposure with the medial parapatellar approach. **A,** Exposure with lateral patellar subluxation. **B,** Additional exposure with eversion of the patella.

Figure 6 Release of the patellofemoral ligament for additional exposure is best performed with the patella everted, to place this structure in stretch.

the procedure. The anterolateral tibia is exposed by retracting the patellar ligament anteriorly. The patella can then be subluxed laterally (**Figure 5, A**) or everted (**Figure 5, B**) when the knee is flexed, with care being taken not to place undue tension on the patellar tendon insertion. A Hohmann retractor is placed under the lateral meniscus after the anterior portion has been cut. If additional lateral exposure is desired after patellar eversion, the patellofemoral ligament can be cut in its midsubstance, which is facilitated by gentle retraction with the lateral retractor (**Figure 6**). With retractors in place, the areas of the patellar fat pad that are limiting lateral visualization can be carefully resected.

The distal femoral or proximal tibial bone cuts can now be performed. With the knee manually flexed, a small posterior retractor is placed anterior to the posterior cruciate ligament to subluxate the tibia anteriorly to aid in instrumentation and resection of the proximal tibia (**Figure 7**). Proper tibial component rotation is critical to a successful TKA. After all bone cuts are made, the proximal tibia can be visualized completely by using a posterior retractor. We prefer a large posterior retractor for optimal visualization, but this can be difficult to place in an obese patient. A smaller posterior retractor can be used in this case (**Figure 8**).

Wound Closure

Side-to-side closure of the medial parapatellar arthrotomy is achieved by first securing the arthrotomy at the superior and inferior aspects of the patella. Once this is done, the wound can be closed further with interrupted or running absorbable sutures in a single layer (**Figure 9**). If medial advancement of the arthrotomy is desired, this can be performed in a "pants-over-vest" fashion; once this is secured and

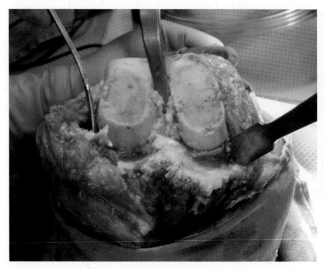

Figure 7 The distal femoral bone cut has been made and the tibia is subluxated anteriorly with maximal knee flexion and a small retractor placed just anterior to the posterior cruciate ligament.

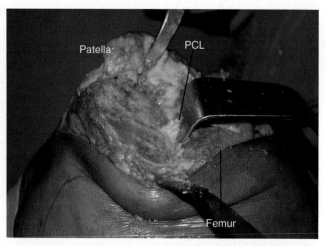

Figure 8 After all bone cuts are made, the proximal tibia can be completely visualized by placing a large posterior retractor. This greatly facilitates tibial component placement. PCL = posterior cruciate ligament.

stable with the knee in 90° of flexion, the free edge of the medial capsule can be oversewn. Care should be taken to realign the arthrotomy correctly to avoid advancing the patella inferiorly. Large suture knots should be avoided, even if using absorbable suture, particularly in patients with thin subcutaneous tissue or skin within overlying soft tissue, as dermal irritation may occur.

Variations

Although there is general consensus on the utility of the anterior midline incision, variations of the arthrotomy bear consideration. The most common variations include making the proximal limb of the arthrotomy 5 mm medial to the VMO insertion (von Langenbeck) or making the patellar portion of the arthrotomy in a straight line directly over the medial patellar bone (Insall). These small variations all can be performed using a standard anterior skin incision. For a true extensile approach of the distal femur and knee joint for a tumor-style prosthesis, a lateral knee arthrotomy (Kocher) continued proximally and laterally below the vastus lateralis is advisable.

Instead of an anterior skin incision, a medial parapatellar skin incision may be used. Although this incision has been shown to be better oriented in relation to cleavage lines about the knee and to be subject to less tension during flexion of the knee, it is not commonly used at present.

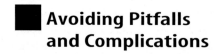

■ Postoperative Regimen

Full weight bearing is permissible postoperatively, with early range of motion. In cases where tight capsular closure is not achieved, a drain may be preferable to avoid hematoma communication between the joint and superficial structures.

■ Avoiding Pitfalls and Complications

The surgeon should avoid malalignment in extensor mechanism closure,

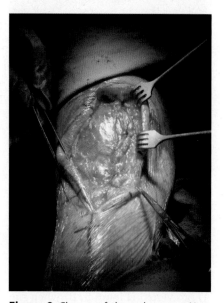

Figure 9 Closure of the arthrotomy. Note that it was not necessary to use the full extent of the planned skin incision.

a situation that may lead to patellar maltracking, pain, and poor range of motion. Inaccurate closure also may induce patella infera, with similar consequences. Excessive patellar eversion without proximal release may encourage tendon avulsion, particularly in revision TKA and patella infera. Surgical approaches, particularly those minimizing incision length, that limit full visualization of relevant anatomy may defeat the purpose of minimally invasive surgery. This can lead to a protracted recovery at best, and, at worst, revision of poorly aligned implants or extensor mechanism failure.

———■

■ Bibliography

Dalury DF, Dennis DA: Mini-incision total knee arthroplasty can increase risk of component malalignment. *Clin Orthop Relat Res* 2005;440:77-81.

Dalury DF, Jiranek WA: A comparison of the midvastus and paramedian approaches for total knee arthroplasty. *J Arthroplasty* 1999;14(1):33-37.

Dennis DA: A stepwise approach to revision total knee arthroplasty. *J Arthroplasty* 2007;22(4 Suppl 1):32-38.

Engh GA, Holt BT, Parks NL: A midvastus muscle-splitting approach for total knee arthroplasty. *J Arthroplasty* 1997; 12(3):322-331.

Hofmann AA, Plaster RL, Murdock LE: Subvastus (Southern) approach for primary total knee arthroplasty. *Clin Orthop Relat Res* 1991;269(269):70-77.

Johnson DP, Houghton TA, Radford P: Anterior midline or medial parapatellar incision for arthroplasty of the knee: A comparative study. *J Bone Joint Surg Br* 1986;68(5):812-814.

Keating EM, Faris PM, Meding JB, Ritter MA: Comparison of the midvastus muscle-splitting approach with the median parapatellar approach in total knee arthroplasty. *J Arthroplasty* 1999;14(1):29-32.

Lin WP, Lin J, Horng LC, Chang SM, Jiang CC: Quadriceps-sparing, minimal-incision total knee arthroplasty: A comparative study. *J Arthroplasty* 2009;24(7):1024-1032.

Matsueda M, Gustilo RB: Subvastus and medial parapatellar approaches in total knee arthroplasty. *Clin Orthop Relat Res* 2000;371(371):161-168.

Parentis MA, Rumi MN, Deol GS, Kothari M, Parrish WM, Pellegrini VD Jr: A comparison of the vastus splitting and median parapatellar approaches in total knee arthroplasty. *Clin Orthop Relat Res* 1999;367(367):107-116.

Scott RD: Primary total knee arthroplasty, in Scott RD, ed: *Surgical Technique in Total Knee Arthroplasty*. Philadelphia, PA, Saunders Elsevier, 2006, pp 20-38.

Stern SH: Surgical exposure in total knee arthroplasty, in Barrack RL, Booth RE Jr, Lonner JH, et al, eds: *Orthopaedic Knowledge Update: Hip & Knee Reconstruction 3*. Rosemont, IL, American Academy of Orthopaedic Surgeons, 2006, pp 3-15.

White RE Jr, Allman JK, Trauger JA, Dales BH: Clinical comparison of the midvastus and medial parapatellar surgical approaches. *Clin Orthop Relat Res* 1999;367(367):117-122.

	Coding		
CPT Code		**Corresponding ICD-9 Codes**	
27447	Arthroplasty, knee, condyle and plateau; medial AND lateral compartments with or without patella resurfacing (total knee arthroplasty)	715 715.80	715.16 715.89

CPT copyright ©2010 by the American Medical Association. All rights reserved.

Chapter 2

Primary Total Knee Arthroplasty: Lateral Approach

Peter A. Keblish, MD

Indications

The lateral approach for total knee arthroplasty (TKA) was developed by the author to address the significant technical challenges presented by the knee with fixed valgus. Surgical approaches in TKA should allow access to the knee in the safest, most direct manner that allows for correction of biomechanical alignment at the tibiofemoral joint and predictable patellofemoral stability. My initial surgical experience as well as published reports from other authors indicated that when a standard medial approach was used, a higher complication rate was seen in the knee with fixed, developmental valgus than in the more common varus knee. Major concerns were higher rates of patellar instability, soft-tissue skin necrosis, and peroneal nerve palsy, and less than optimal tibiofemoral stability, especially in type II valgus (medial cruciate ligament [MCL]–deficient) knees.

Developmental valgus deformity is often associated with tibiofemoral malrotation, deficiency of the lateral femoral condyle, and tight soft-tissue structures, including the posterolateral complex, iliotibial band (ITB), and lateral retinaculum. The Q angle is increased with the patellar tendon inserted laterally. The patella is fre-quently deformed, small, subluxated, or laterally oriented over the abnormally flattened anterolateral condyle. Patella alta is more common. The deformity is more common in females and in patients with rheumatoid arthritis. Osteopenia, therefore, often is a factor adding to the technical challenge.

Specific indications for the lateral approach are fixed valgus deformity with lateral patellar subluxation and nonyielding soft-tissue contractures; the multiply operated (often posttraumatic) knee with laterally placed incisions; the knee that has undergone postoperative tibial osteotomies that have failed in valgus; the knee that has undergone lateral unicompartmental knee arthroplasty; and the knee with rheumatoid arthritis, gross instability, and expanded soft tissues, where exposure is easy and the multiple advantages of the lateral approach are realized. Relative indications include the knee with neutral to slight varus with lateral patellar tendon and tibial tubercle orientation, a tight retinaculum and ITB, and a laterally oriented patella.

Using the standard medial approach in the valgus knee has several disadvantages, including the following: It is an indirect approach that is opposite to the pathology; it requires lateral patellar dislocation and/or translation, which increases the external tibial rotation, making the posterolateral corner less accessible for direct and sequential releases; soft-tissue vascularity is compromised, because lateral releases are still required; the deep lateral soft-tissue gap is often left uncovered with lack of joint seal; and the skin is at greater risk, especially in thin or tight-skinned knees, which are common in the rheumatoid arthritis population.

Advantages of the lateral approach include the following: It is a direct approach, which allows safe anatomic exposure of the concave side contractions; it preserves the medial side, including the vascular supply to the patella; it involves medial patellar displacement, which rotates the tibia internally, bringing the lateral corner forward for maximum exposure; it allows self-centering of the patellar tendon and tibial tubercle, which optimizes patellar tracking; and joint seal and gap coverage is ensured because the expanded soft-tissue exposure allows for closure without tension. Although the lateral approach is not currently chosen by most surgeons, the reconstructive TKA surgeon should consider becoming familiar with the lateral approach to the knee and should understand its advantages and technical aspects, because it may be the safest and most logical approach

Dr. Keblish or an immediate family member holds stock or stock options in Celgene.

when correcting a particular knee with severe valgus.

Although indications for the lateral approach are relatively broad, it has not been adopted or used extensively in the United States. The medial approach, with variations such as subvastus, midvastus, and, more recently, minimally invasive surgery techniques, is standard teaching in residency and fellowship training programs, and most surgeons gain little or no experience with the lateral approach for TKA during their training.

——————■

Contraindications

The relative complexity of the lateral approach and its significant technical difference from medial approaches leads to a steeper learning curve, which can be a major deterrent to adopting the approach. Therefore, inexperience with the approach is a contraindication, and if the surgeon is not willing to learn the approach, it will not become part of his or her armamentarium. Other contraindications to the lateral approach include the following: a severe varus knee with fixed contractures; a neutral and/or mild varus knee with normal patellar tracking and tubercle position; revision, previously operated, or posttraumatic valgus knees in which the safest incision with regard to skin vascularity is medially based; and the fully correctable valgus knee with normal patellar tracking.

The medial approach has been successful as described in the literature, usually with semiconstrained prostheses and sequential releases. Most literature reports and surgeons' personal experience emphasize that the knee with fixed valgus presents more problems and concerns, especially regarding stability and patellar tracking, when the standard medial approach is used.

——————■

Alternative Treatments

The universal medial parapatellar approach (or variants) allows for access to most knee deformities and has been used successfully in fixed valgus. When a medial approach is used, the subvastus variant is suggested because it allows relatively easy lateral patellar dislocation and it preserves the vastus medialis, which is often displaced laterally and stretched out medially. The medial approach should avoid any medial release. Lateral patellar dislocation increases tibial external rotation and decreases access to the posterolateral corner; therefore, when the medial approach is used, releases must be made after the prosthesis has been placed. Releases may be performed prospectively (as described in this chapter) with the lateral approach, which is considered to be a technical advantage.

When the medial approach is used, sequential soft-tissue releases must be made with care (after placement of the prosthesis), because they are performed from the opposite side with less than optimal exposure. Inadequate lateral extension space (after normal bone resection) is common in fixed valgus; therefore, lateral column release (retinaculum, ITB, and lateral collateral ligament [LCL]) is often required. Tibiofemoral malrotation is more common in valgus deformity; therefore, care must be taken to optimize femoral component rotation. Use of the tibial axis with conventional instrumentation or computer-assisted surgery (CAS) techniques will decrease errors in resection and prosthesis placement.

——————■

Results

Results in TKA are usually reported in relation to factors such as deformity, a specific implant, patellar manage-

ment, bone grafting, or osteotomy, rather than in relation to a specific approach. Most reports assume or simply describe the standard medial approach as part of the procedure. Alternate approaches such as the medial variants (midvastus, subvastus) and the lateral approach are less commonly used. Reports related to surgical exposure often represent specific issues such as the biomechanical rationale of a given approach or prosthesis or patellar issues, assuming that a standard medial approach was used.

The lateral approach in TKA is not used extensively; therefore, fewer results are reported in the literature. Although there are no reported prospective studies comparing medial and lateral approaches for TKA in the valgus knee, several studies (mostly from outside the United States) report comparable or improved results with the lateral approach, stressing the advantages previously listed, especially in regard to biomechanical rationale and patellar stability. All authors addressing the valgus knee emphasize that this deformity requires more complex soft-tissue and bone management than does the varus knee. Several authors who focus on evaluation of the lateral approach use technical variations, from a soft tissue–only exposure to the use of a tibial tubercle osteotomy in all cases. The basic principles of the approach, however, are the same.

In my early experience with the lateral approach, I encountered a small number of bearing failures, including one rotating platform spinout and two cases of early bearing wear. These failures were the result of inadequate deep soft-tissue column release (primarily the LCL) and resultant extension gap imbalance. Reoperation through the same lateral approach allowed direct access for proper balancing and bearing exchange. The failures motivated me to make changes in my technique and develop the approach described here.

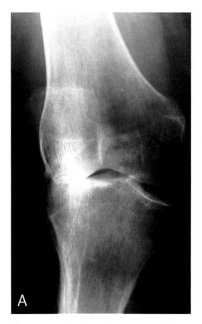
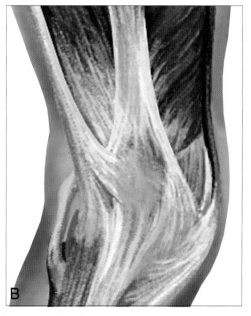
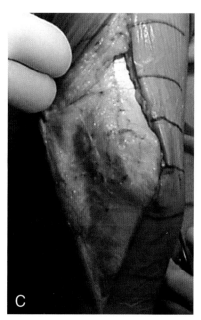

Figure 1 The lateral position of the patella in a moderately severe valgus knee is demonstrated in an AP radiograph (**A**) and an anatomic drawing (**B**). **C,** The skin incision for the lateral approach is slightly lateral and exposes the lateral soft tissues.

The lateral approach has been used (with good success) for both varus and valgus knees in some international centers. One large series stressed the ease and safety of the approach, the elimination of patella problems, and more rapid return of function.

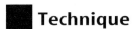

Technique

Setup/Exposure

The setup for surgery using the lateral approach is routine, with slight variations. A bolster under the ipsilateral pelvis is recommended because the extremity is more severely rotated. A tourniquet is used routinely unless there is a specific contraindication, such as vascular compromise or a very short, large extremity. I recommend releasing the tourniquet after the prosthesis is implanted.

The surgical technique for the direct lateral approach differs substantially from the standard medial parapatellar approach. Pitfalls include the fact that surgeons are less familiar with the

lateral side of the knee, orientation is reversed, and more careful handling of the soft tissues is required. In the knee with no previous surgical scars, the recommended skin incision follows the Q angle and is slightly lateral to the patella, the lateral border of the patellar tendon, and the tibial tubercle (**Figure 1**). The skin incision should be adequate to expose the distal quadriceps proximally and the proximal anterior compartment fascia distally. Longer incisions are necessary in very large legs. In previously operated knees, the existing incision should be incorporated and extended proximally and distally. If multiple incisions are present, either the most direct or most recent should be used. A sham incision may be performed and consultation with a plastic surgeon considered if skin necrosis is a major concern.

The surgical technique is described here in detail. I have modified the retinacular incision sequence and exposure since I originally reported it. Initially, I used a fat pad expansion without the coronal Z-plasty expansion technique. Other authors who have adopted this technique have de-

| Table 1 | Steps in Total Knee Arthroplasty Using a Lateral Approach |

1. Iliotibial band release and lengthening
2. Retinacular release and lateral arthrotomy
3. Patellar dislocation and joint exposure
4. Tibial sleeve release
   Posterior capsular exposure/release
   Lateral collateral ligament lengthening (if required)
5. Instrumentation and prosthesis insertion
   Fine-tune soft-tissue balance
6. Soft-tissue closure in flexion

scribed modifications, but the basic principles are similar. The sequence of exposure and release steps varies depending on surgeon preference and/or the nature of the deformity.

After the skin incision is made (anterior and slightly lateral), the lateral retinaculum is exposed. The rest of the procedure can be broken down into six major steps, as listed in Table 1 and described in detail below.

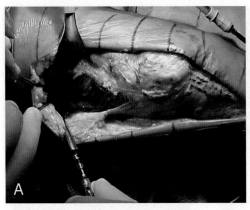
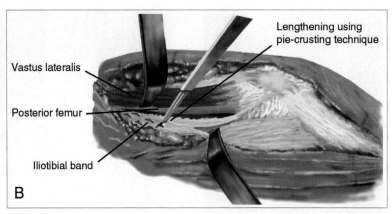

Figure 2 Iliotibial band release and lengthening. **A,** Posterior femoral release. **B,** Drawing shows lengthening of the iliotibial band using a multiple-puncture (pie-crusting) technique.

Step 1: ITB Release and Lengthening (if required)

If the ITB is tight ("bowstringing" with varus stress), it is exposed proximally by separating the inner fascial sleeve from the vastus lateralis muscle (**Figure 2**). The vastus lateralis is carefully retracted to the linea aspera approximately 10 cm proximal to the joint line. The fascial band is released from the posterior femur and "finger stripped" distally to the posterolateral corner. A varus stress in extension will bowstring the tight fascial bands, allowing for lengthening using a multiple-puncture ("pie-crusting") technique. This is performed under visual and digital control, while paying attention to the most posterior fibers and peroneal nerve. The peroneal nerve can be exposed, but this is seldom required. Fascial release/lengthening decreases the potential for peroneal nerve entrapment and/or stretching after correction of the valgus deformity.

Step 2: Retinacular Release and Lateral Arthrotomy

RETINACULAR RELEASE

The lateral retinacular incision is initiated 2 to 3 cm lateral to the patellar border proximally and through the anterior mid portion of the Gerdy tubercle (deep to bone) distally. A natural separation from the fat pad and

capsular structures will occur and should be preserved for subsequent soft-tissue closure. A hemostat placed distal to proximal helps define the interval before the retinacular release. Following the retinacular release, an immediate separation of retinacular fibers is noted and partial patellar correction occurs (**Figure 3**). The fat pad and lateral retinacular vessel are exposed. Lateral joint exposure is now approached with a goal of preserving and/or expanding lateral soft tissues.

LATERAL ARTHROTOMY

The goal of lateral joint exposure is to preserve and/or expand the lateral soft tissues. Proximally, the arthrotomy incision extends from superficial lateral to deep medial. The parallel fibers of the central quadriceps tendon allow for a natural separation. The vastus lateralis tendon insertion on the proximal lateral patella, however, is nonyielding. To gain soft-tissue length at this point, a coronal plane Z-plasty can be performed (**Figure 3**). The tendon is usually quite thick and allows for preservation of satisfactory tissue proximally (vastus lateralis tendon) and distally (extended patellar retinaculum) for the expansion closure. If soft tissues are not contracted, a standard proximal arthrotomy is adequate.

After the proximal exposure is completed, the fat pad/capsular layer is released from the lateral patellar border. Lateral geniculate vessels are cauterized. Distally, the capsule/fat pad layer is incised deep to the lateral patellar tendon border. Retention of approximately 50% of the fat pad and the lateral meniscal rim allows for mobilization of a stable, expanded soft-tissue sleeve. The expanded fat pad can be used for lateral joint closure if coronal Z-plasty is inadequate. If not required, the fat pad is replaced in the most anatomic position to preserve optimum blood supply and soft-tissue protection of the prosthetic components. As coronal plane Z-plasty expansion techniques have improved (**Figure 4**), the expanded fat pad, as originally described, is used less frequently. However, preservation of the fat pad is recommended, because soft-tissue gap closure requirements may be greater than initially anticipated.

The distal extension of the retinacular incision splits the Gerdy tubercle and continues distally into the anterior compartment fascia (**Figure 5**). An osteoperiosteal sleeve elevation (using a sharp osteotome) extends to, but stops short of, the tibial tubercle and patellar tendon attachment. As the osteoperiosteal sleeve is elevated, the anterior fascia and muscle fibers of

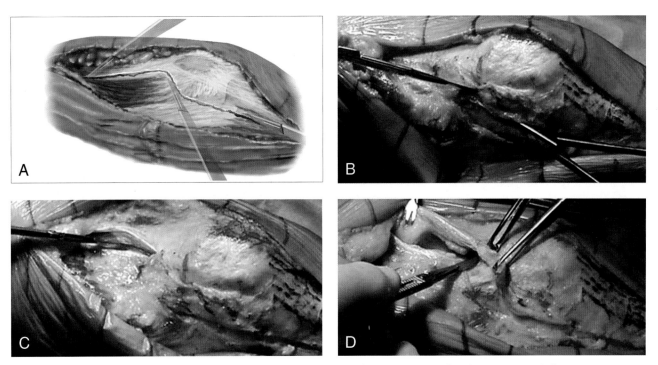

Figure 3 Retinacular release. **A,** Drawing showing the course of a lateral arthrotomy. **B,** Retinacular release. **C,** Method of expansion exposure and Z-plasty release of the central tendon. **D,** The vastus lateralis tendon release is accomplished from superficial (proximal) to deep (distal), through the midsubstance of the tendon.

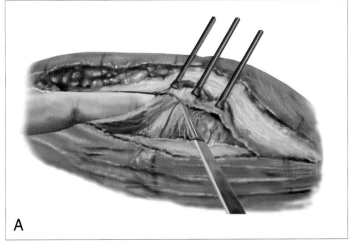

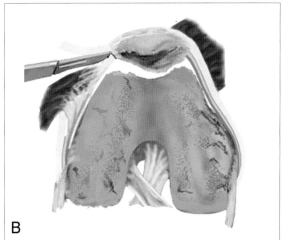

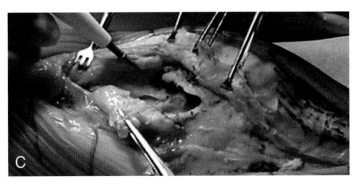

Figure 4 The coronal plane Z-plasty expansion technique. Drawings **A** and **B** show different views of the technique. **C,** Clinical photograph showing the natural separation of the superficial and deep layers. Following release from the patella, the deep layer of the vastus lateralis tendon remains in continuity with the lateral retinaculum. The fat pad incision is then made parallel and adjacent to the patellar tendon.

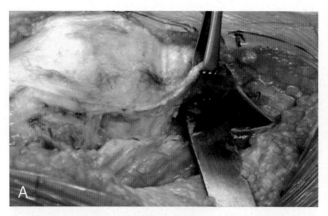
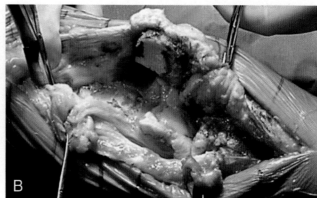
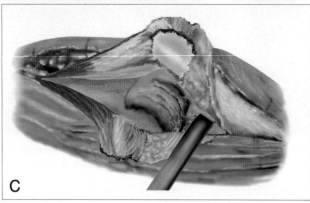

Figure 5 Distal tubercle elevation. **A,** Osteoperiosteal elevation from the middle of the Gerdy tubercle. **B,** Patellar eversion. **C,** Drawing shows the preserved patellar tendon insertion as the patella is dislocated.

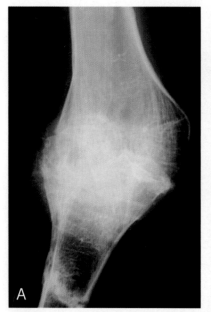
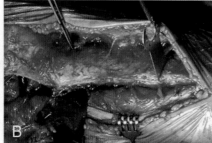
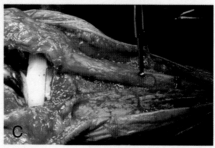

Figure 6 Tibial tubercle osteotomy. **A,** AP radiograph of an extreme valgus knee that required tibial tubercle osteotomy (**B**). **C,** Note the excellent anatomic fixation and excellent prosthetic stability.

the tibialis anterior are visualized and preserved in their natural plane. Because the elevation stops at the lateral border of the patellar tendon, the tendon insertion is protected and the tension stresses are dissipated to the an-terior compartment sleeve. A formal lateral-to-medial tibial tubercle osteotomy can be performed to enhance exposure in difficult cases or according to surgeon preference (**Figure 6**). The osteoperiosteal elevation *does not* compromise the osteotomy. If in doubt, and in difficult revisions, an osteotomy should be performed. Anatomic reduction and compression screw fixation of the osteotomy allow for excellent fixation.

Step 3: Patellar Dislocation and Joint Exposure

The patella is dislocated/everted medially, with varus stress applied as the leg is moved from extension to flexion. Grasping the patella with a towel clip is helpful. Following patellar eversion, a cobra-type retractor is placed medially through the periphery of the medial meniscus, over the medial cortical rim. Patellar dislocation can be performed during this step or after the tibial sleeve release. Joint exposure in flexion allows better access for the prospective deep lateral releases and subsequent bone resections.

Medial dislocation/eversion of the patella is often more difficult than lateral dislocation. Methods of enhancing exposure include a long proximal incision with a lateral-to-medial rectus snip (if indicated), osteophyte removal, planned resection of the patella, femoral downsizing to normal peripheral anatomy, and posterior cruciate ligament (PCL) release.

Step 4: Tibial Sleeve Release

The tibial sleeve release to the posterolateral corner is a key step. Osteoperiosteal release from the middle of the Gerdy tubercle to the posterolateral tibia is best completed in flexion following patellar dislocation (**Figure 7**). Medial patellar dislocation rotates the tibia internally, brings the tibia forward, and best exposes the posterolateral corner and posterior capsule. Tibial osteophytes are removed, and the posterior capsule is released. Preliminary medial-lateral balance correction in flexion and extension is checked initially with lamina spreaders (before bone resections) and/or following bone resections and spacer block evaluations. The PCL can be released at this time if required because of noncorrectable contractures or by

surgeon's choice. Surgeons who favor PCL-retaining prostheses should assess the status and value of PCL retention. If it is judged to be satisfactory, the PCL is preserved at this time. It can be released later if required. Surgeons who favor PCL-substituting prostheses should release the PCL at this step. PCL-substituting prostheses are required in most fixed valgus knees. If initial releases appear adequate, proceed with instrumentation and bone resection. In mild cases, the full tibial sleeve release may not be required; however, my experience favors using this step because it improves the exposure and rotational correction of the tibia, especially in knees with severe, long-standing posterolateral contractures.

LCL LENGTHENING (IF REQUIRED)

If soft-tissue releases (and bony osteophyte removal) do not provide satisfactory correction, a tight lateral space in extension is usually present and further lateral column release, specifically LCL release, will be required. Whatever method of LCL release is chosen, it should not create lateral instability and should maintain the integrity of the LCL. My preferred method is the distal LCL release (**Figure 8**). With this technique, the fibular head and LCL attachment are visualized and evaluated. The proximal tibia-fibular joint can be mobilized with periosteal elevators. The proximal fibula is enucleated using gouges or curved osteotomes, preserving the outer cortex. The outer fibular cortex,

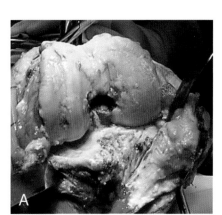
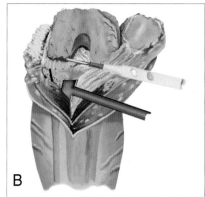

Figure 7 Tibial sleeve release. **A,** Knee exposure in flexion. **B,** Drawing of lateral tibial sleeve release and capsular release as required.

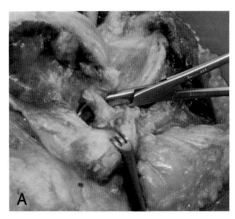
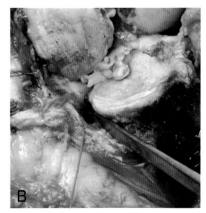
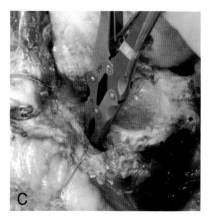

Figure 8 LCL lengthening. **A,** Exposure of contracted LCL. **B,** Fibular head mobilization. **C,** Fibular head decompression. The integrity of the lengthened LCL (suture) and lateral sleeve remains intact.

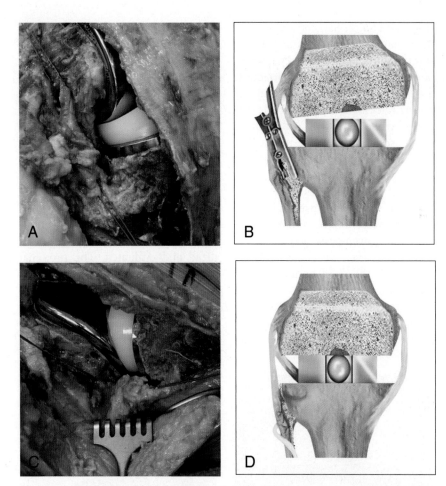

Figure 9 Intraoperative photograph **(A)** and drawing **(B)** demonstrating extension gap imbalance present after bone resections. Intraoperative photograph **(C)** and drawing **(D)** showing the knee after LCL lengthening was performed, resulting in extension gap balancing and prosthetic stability.

with the attached ligament sleeve, will translate anteriorly and medially, allowing for indirect LCL lengthening without weakening the lateral soft-tissue structures. LCL lengthening can be addressed before bone cuts, after bone cuts and gap balancing, or after trial prosthesis insertion (**Figure 9**).

Other methods of LCL lengthening include direct Z-plasty, the multiple-puncture (pie-crusting) technique, and femoral sleeve release of the LCL origin, all of which may weaken the LCL. Femoral condylar sliding osteotomy with screw fixation, which preserves LCL integrity, is reserved for more severe cases.

Step 5:   Instrumentation and Prosthesis Implantation

After adequate exposure and preliminary release have been achieved, instrumentation, bone resection, and trial insertion are accomplished, using the surgeon's preferred prosthesis. Remember that the reverse orientation encountered with the lateral approach may be confusing, especially the rotational and varus-valgus resections and subsequent prosthesis placement. Commonly used methods of determining the distal femoral rotation resection based on the transepicondylar axis may be less than accurate in the valgus knee because of the distorted anatomy. Prospective referencing to the tibial axis will decrease resection errors. Us-

ing a flexion-tension gap-balancing technique allows self-adjustment of the distal femur rotation and resection based on stable medial-lateral soft-tissue balance. CAS technology, if available, also is helpful. Standard-level bone resections are recommended; deeper tibial cuts may compromise stability. In lateral tibial bone deficiency, bone graft or lateral tibial metal augments may be required to achieve an optimally stable implant. Flexion-extension gap balance is then confirmed with spacer blocks and trial inserts.

Following relocation, the patella will track centrally as the tibial tubercle rotates medially, exerting a natural correction of the Q angle (**Figure 10, A**). The patella is evaluated and retained or resurfaced. When anatomic or conforming (non–central-domed) patellar replacements are used, rotational position checks should be made and double-checked because of the reverse orientation and risk of malpositioning the prosthesis. **Figure 10, B** shows a trial reduction using a rotating-platform prosthesis. Note the medial position of the tibial tubercle with correction of tibial rotation and natural patellar tracking.

Step 6:   Soft-Tissue Closure in Flexion

Lateral joint closure is completed in flexion (60° to 90°) to ensure that a vascularized tissue sleeve covers the prosthesis (**Figure 11**). The soft-tissue expansion exposure described previously in this chapter will optimize a tension-free closure. A distal-to-proximal closure is preferred. Distally, the previously elevated tibial sleeve (in continuity) is secured to the upper tibia with transosseous sutures to reestablish anterolateral stability. The closure continues to the midportion, which includes the fibro-fatty capsular synovial layer to the lateral border of the retinaculum. If required, the fat pad can be expanded and used to fill soft-tissue gaps. Proximally, the ex-

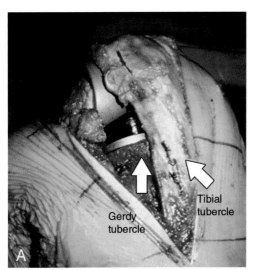
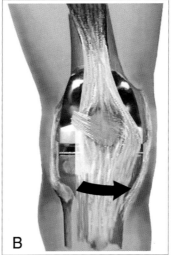

Figure 10 Prosthesis implantation. **A,** Natural patellar tracking occurs in flexion. **B,** Drawing of medial corrective force in extension. Note the central (rotational) correction of the tibial tubercle following prosthesis insertion.

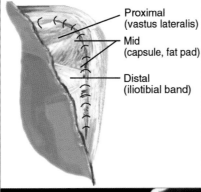
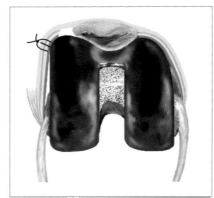
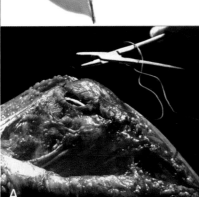
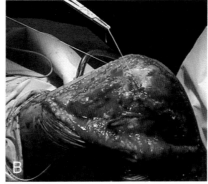

Figure 11 Soft-tissue closure in flexion. **A,** Drawing (top) and clinical photograph (bottom) show initiation of closure in flexion. The iliotibial band is reattached anatomically via transosseous sutures. **B,** Coronal plane drawing (top) and lateral intraoperative photograph (bottom) showing completion of the lengthening soft-tissue closure.

panded vastus lateralis tendon is sutured to the previously lengthened, expanded patellar retinaculum. The quadriceps central tendon closure is then completed in a tension-free manner.

Postoperative Regimen

The postoperative regimen is the same as our routine TKA protocol, which includes use of continuous passive motion to tolerance beginning in the recovery room, early mobilization as medical status allows, and heel-toe protective weight bearing to tolerance. Drains have been used routinely because soft-tissue release is more extensive. Ambulation begins with a walker and progresses to a cane in 2 to 3 weeks, and again is patient dependent. Full weight bearing at 4 to 6 weeks is the norm. Radiographs are obtained postoperatively (**Figure 12**) and at routine follow-up intervals (**Figure 13**).

Avoiding Pitfalls and Complications

The risk of complications increases when less common surgical approaches are used. This is true of the lateral approach, which requires exposure of soft-tissue structures that are less commonly manipulated in current orthopaedic practice. This was not the case before the advent of intra-articular anterior cruciate ligament surgery, when orthopaedic surgeons used the lateral side for extra-articular ligament reconstructive procedures and became more comfortable with the surgical anatomy. Today, surgeons beginning to use the lateral approach will experience a steep learning curve.

Approaching the difficult valgus knee from the lateral side presents challenges related to both soft-tissue and bony structures. First, the skin should be handled gently, to avoid undermining. Preparation of the deep soft-tissue sleeve requires careful planning and a plastic surgeon's thought

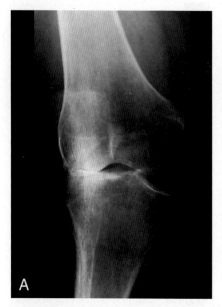
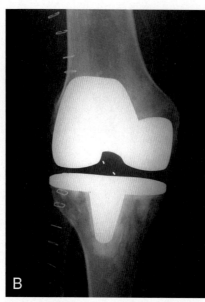

Figure 12 Preoperative (**A**) and immediate postoperative (**B**) radiographs of the knee of the patient whose procedure is shown in Figures 1 through 11.

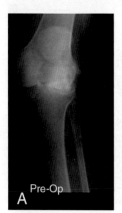
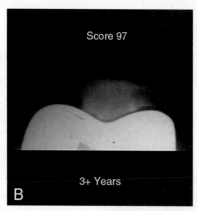
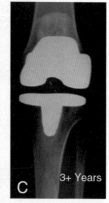

Figure 13 Preoperative AP view (**A**) and postoperative skyline (Merchant) (**B**) and AP (**C**) views obtained at 3-year follow-up in a patient who had a moderately severe valgus knee. The postoperative views show excellent patellar and tibiofemoral alignment.

process. To ensure soft-tissue closure and a joint seal, the approach needs to anticipate the soft-tissue expansion that will be required. Some knees are tight and rigid and require the maximum expansion release; others are more supple and require less soft-tissue expansion. Patients with thin, atrophic tissues (usually seen in women with rheumatoid arthritis) require especially gentle handling of the soft tissues and expanded fat pad coverage, as described earlier.

Release of the ITB from inside out minimizes skin undermining and protects the peroneal nerve. Stripping the fascia from the posterior femoral attachment enhances the exposure and fascial lengthening. A varus stress in extension allows for tensioning of the fascia and a multiple-puncture (pie-crusting) technique. However, Z-plasty or oblique release can be used. The release also may be performed with an outside-in technique through a small second incision.

To protect the patellar tendon attachment, the deep distal incision is best made 1 to 2 cm lateral to the lateral border of the patellar tendon attachment, through the Gerdy tubercle. This adds a protective sleeve and decreases the stress on the patellar tendon as it is subluxated or dislocated medially. Pinning the middle portion of the patellar tendon is recommended during bone preparation. If the tendon is at risk, proceed with a tubercle osteotomy, which can be hinged medially.

Joint exposure may present problems because medial patellar dislocation is often more difficult, primarily because the medial femoral condyle is larger. Joint exposure may be enhanced by initially subluxating rather than dislocating the patella, debulking a large patella, or making the permanent patellar resection for resurfacing before medial patellar dislocation. If this is not sufficient, conservative debulking of the larger medial, posterior, and/or distal femoral condyle is recommended. This maneuver does not affect the femoral resection if bone removal is minimal and the final prosthesis size is determined prospectively. These measures ensure safe access to the joint with medial patellar dislocation.

When distal LCS lengthening is performed, enucleation of the proximal fibula must be done carefully, because the peroneal nerve courses around the fibular neck. Preserving the outer cortex of the fibular head will avoid potential contact and/or stretch on the peroneal nerve. Fragmentation of the outer fibular cortex may occur and may be reported as a fracture on postoperative radiographs, so explanation to patients and radiologists may be in order.

Another method of increasing the lateral space for gap balancing is to increase the femoral valgus resection to 7° rather than the usual 4° to 5°. Patients with long-standing severe valgus will tolerate undercorrection and mild valgus. If adequate correction (lateral extension space) is not achieved by following all of the described methods, a sliding femoral condylar osteostomy should be considered.

A final note of caution is in order regarding the reverse orientation at all stages of the procedure, especially the significant internal rotation of the tibia. This *unusual* tibial positioning and the increased bulk at the tibial tubercle may distort extramedullary instruments and lead to incorrect resection. Therefore, intramedullary instrument checks or use of CAS is recommended. Minimal medial tibial plateau resection is the norm because some stretching of the medial structures is common. In type II valgus (medial side laxity), a more constrained implant is recommended.

Despite the multiple potential pitfalls and challenges associated with the lateral approach, it is a safe alternative to the standard medial approach and can become a valuable part of the knee surgeon's armamentarium for TKA. The lateral approach, with its sparing of medial soft-tissue anatomy, has many of the advantages of the currently favored medial minimally invasive surgery techniques. I believe that patients experience a more rapid recovery, earlier and better range of motion, improved healing, and fewer minor symptoms such as skin paresthesias when a lateral approach is used.

———————■

 ## Bibliography

Arnold MP, Friederich NF, Widmer H, Müller W: Patellar substitution in total knee prosthesis—is it important? *Orthopade* 1998;27:637-641.

Brilhault J, Lautman S, Favard L, Burdin P: Lateral femoral sliding osteotomy lateral release in total knee arthroplasty for a fixed valgus deformity. *J Bone Joint Surg Br* 2002;84:1131-1137.

Buechel FF: A sequential three-step lateral release for correcting fixed valgus knee deformities during total knee arthroplasty. *Clin Orthop Relat Res* 1990;260:170-175.

Burki H, von Knoch M, Heiss C, Drobny T, Munzinger U: Lateral approach with osteotomy of the tibial tubercle in primary total knee arthroplasty. *Clin Orthop Relat Res* 1999;362:156-161.

Favorito PJ, Mihalko WM, Krackow KA: Total knee arthroplasty in the valgus knee. *J Am Acad Orthop Surg* 2002;10:16-24.

Fiddian NJ, Blakeway C, Kumar A: Replacement arthroplasty of the valgus knee: A modified lateral capsular approach with repositioning of vastus lateralis. *J Bone Joint Surg Br* 1998;80:859-861.

Insall JN, Scott WN, Keblish PA, et al: Total knee arthroplasty exposures and soft tissue balancing, in Insall JN, Scott WN, eds: *Videobook of Knee Surgery*. Philadelphia, PA, Lippincott, 1994.

Keblish PA: Alternate surgical approaches in mobile-bearing total knee arthroplasty. *Orthopedics* 2002;25(2 Suppl):s257-s264.

Keblish PA: The lateral approach to the valgus knee: Surgical technique and analysis of 53 cases with over two-year follow-up evaluation. *Clin Orthop Relat Res* 1991;271:52-162.

Keblish PA: Valgus deformity in TKR: The lateral retinacular approach. *Orthop Trans* 1985;9:28.

Krackow KA, Mihalko WM: Flexion-extension joint gap changes after lateral structure release for valgus deformity correction in total knee arthroplasty: A cadaveric study. *J Arthroplasty* 1999;14:994-1004.

Lootvoet L, Blouard E, Himmer O, Ghosez JP: Complete knee prosthesis in severe genu valgum: Retrospective review of 90 knees surgically treated through the anterio-external approach. *Acta Orthop Belg* 1997;63:278-286.

Munsinger UK, Boldt JG, Keblish PA: *Primary Knee Arthoplasty*. Berlin, Heidelberg, Springer-Verlag, 2004, pp 160-168.

Peters CL, Mohr RA, Bachus KN: Primary total knee arthroplasty in the valgus knee: Creating a balanced soft tissue envelope. *J Arthroplasty* 2001;16:721-729.

Ranawat AS, Ranawat CS, Elkus M, Rasquinha VJ, Rossi R, Babhulkar S: Total knee arthroplasty for severe valgus deformity. *J Bone Joint Surg Am* 2005;87(Suppl 1 Pt 2):271-284.

Tsai CL, Chen CH, Liu TK: Lateral approach without ligament release in total knee arthroplasty: New concepts in the surgical technique. *Artif Organs* 2001;25:638-643.

Watanabe Y, Moriya H, Takahashi K, et al: Functional anatomy of the posterolateral structures of the knee. *Arthroscopy* 1993;9:57-62.

Zenz P, Huber M, Obenaus H, Schwäqerl W: Lengthening of the iliotibial band by femoral detachment and multiple puncture: A cadaver study. *Arch Orthop Trauma Surg* 2002;122:429-431.

Coding

CPT Codes		Corresponding ICD-9 Codes	
27447	Arthroplasty, knee, condyle and plateau; medial AND lateral compartments with or without patella resurfacing (total knee arthroplasty)	715 715.80	715.16 715.89

CPT copyright © 2010 by the American Medical Association. All rights reserved.

Chapter 3

Primary Total Knee Arthroplasty: Less Invasive Approaches

Mark W. Pagnano, MD
Aaron J. Krych, MD

■ Indications

Both patients and surgeons have shown considerable interest in the so-called minimally invasive surgery (MIS) approaches for total knee arthroplasty (TKA). The exact definition of MIS TKA continues to evolve, but most would agree that it involves a short skin incision, avoids eversion of the patella, and limits the amount of surgical dissection in the suprapatellar pouch, thus minimizing damage to that richly innervated region of the knee. Importantly, the introduction of MIS TKA also has been accompanied by substantial changes in perioperative anesthesia techniques. The goals of MIS, mainly rapid rehabilitation and improved patient function, cannot be achieved without excellent postoperative anesthesia.

The indications for a less invasive TKA are essentially the same as those for a standard TKA—specifically, the presence of disabling pain associated with advanced joint degeneration. The surgeon should be experienced and well-rehearsed with standard TKAs before endeavoring to undertake MIS techniques.

Several different MIS TKA approaches have been described, including the mini-subvastus, mini-midvastus, mini-medial parapatellar, and quadriceps-sparing approaches. The mini-subvastus approach can be used in most patients; it is indicated when earlier return to function of the quadriceps after primary TKA is desired. Historically, the standard subvastus approach was discouraged in obese or muscular patients because everting the patella was either difficult or caused damage to the vastus medialis obliquus (VMO) and the surrounding soft tissues. With the mini-subvastus approach, the patella is not everted, and with minimal release, the patella can be translated relatively easily into the lateral gutter. This makes the mini-subvastus approach applicable to a wider range of patients.

■ Contraindications

Although the indications for MIS TKA seem to be broad, the complexity of these surgical techniques demands that the contraindications be thoroughly considered. A mini-subvastus approach can be performed on the vast majority of patients undergoing standard TKAs; however, we do not use this approach in patients with substantial patella baja (patella infera) as demonstrated on lateral radiographs or in patients with marked knee stiffness, as it can be very difficult to translate the patella laterally in these situations. Patients with compromised skin (peripheral vascular disease, poorly controlled diabetes mellitus, or chronic corticosteroid use) are poor candidates for any small-incision approach to TKA because substantially more tension is placed on the skin edges during these approaches, and that places patients with compromised skin at risk for wound healing problems. Obesity or muscularity of the patient is not an absolute contraindication to using the mini-subvastus approach, although these conditions add some technical difficulty. Simple maneuvers such as extending the skin incision by 2 or 3 cm often can notably facilitate the mini-subvastus approach in these patients. The knee with inflammatory arthritis may have softer bone surfaces that will collapse slightly with retraction and should be carefully evaluated for suitability of these techniques. Most surgeons should pursue specialized cadaver training before using MIS approaches to TKA in clinical practice.

Dr. Pagnano or an immediate family member has received royalties from DePuy and Zimmer and has received research or institutional support from DePuy, Musculoskeletal Transplant Foundation, National Institutes of Health, Stryker, and Zimmer. Neither Dr. Krych nor any immediate family member has received anything of value from or owns stock in a commercial company or institution related directly or indirectly to the subject of this chapter.

Table 1 Results of Less Invasive Approaches for Total Knee Arthroplasty

Authors (Year)	Study Design	Number of Knees	Approach	Mean Patient Age in Years (Range)	Mean Follow-up	Results
Fauré et al (1993)	Prospective randomized	20	Subvastus vs medial parapatellar	70 (55-81)	3 months	Subvastus had greater strength at 1 week and 1 month; preferred by patients 4:1
Roysam and Oakley (2001)	Prospective randomized	89	Subvastus vs medial parapatellar	Subvastus: 69.8 Medial parapatellar: 70.2	3 months	Subvastus had greater knee flexion, used fewer narcotics at 1 week ($P < 0.001$), had earlier straight-leg raising
Boerger et al (2005)	Matched retrospective	120	Subvastus vs medial parapatellar	Subvastus: 69 (55-82) Medial parapatellar: 68 (59-83)	3 months	Subvastus had less blood loss, less postoperative pain, faster straight-leg raising, better early flexion
Dalury and Dennis (2005)	Retrospective comparative	60	Mini-midvastus vs medial parapatellar	Subvastus: 68.9 Medial parapatellar: 67.4	3 months	Varus malalignment more common in mini-midvastus knees
Aglietti et al (2006)	Prospective randomized	60	Subvastus vs quadriceps-sparing approach	Subvastus: 70 (59-80) Medial parapatellar: 71 (58-84)	3 months	Subvastus had earlier straight-leg raising, better flexion at 10 and 30 days
Schroer et al (2008)	Matched retrospective	300	Subvastus vs medial parapatellar	Subvastus: 70 (44-87) Medial parapatellar: 71 (42-90)	2 years	Subvastus had earlier straight-leg raising, shorter hospital stay, better knee flexion
Jackson et al (2008)	Prospective	209	Quadriceps-sparing	NA	6 months	Increased complication rates compared with standard TKA

NA = not available, TKA = total knee arthroplasty.

Alternative Treatments

The preoperative physical examination should be targeted to identify substantial patella baja, knee stiffness, or compromised skin. Most patients with one or more of these issues would be better served with a traditional medial parapatellar approach for the TKA.

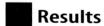

Results

Several prospective randomized trials have shown better results with the mini-subvastus approach over other TKA approaches (**Table 1**), including earlier straight-leg raising and better flexion. These studies confirm an added benefit to the subvastus approach in the early postoperative period. The long-term advantages of this approach have not yet been established. Some studies, however, demonstrate a higher complication rate with MIS TKA approaches. Because of the increased risk of complications and the learning curve associated with MIS, we recommend specialized training before incorporating minimally invasive approaches into clinical practice.

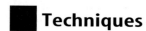

Techniques

Setup/Exposure

The patient is positioned supine with a nonsterile tourniquet placed as far proximal as possible. We prefer not to use any leg positioning devices. Rather, the amount of flexion or extension of the knee can be controlled easily and adjusted frequently throughout the surgery by supporting the foot against the surgeon's hip. The knee is prepared and draped in a standard fashion, with iodine-impregnated drapes on all exposed skin.

A straight, midline, or medially biased incision is made starting at the superior pole of the patella and extending distally to the top of the tibial

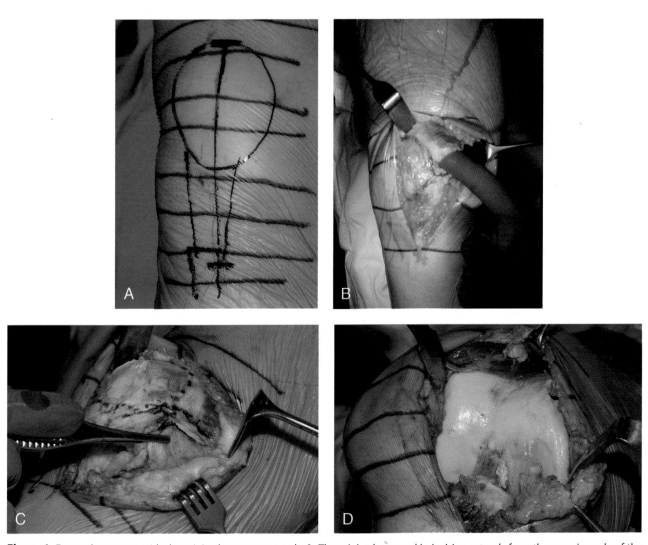

Figure 1 Femoral exposure with the mini-subvastus approach. **A,** The mini-subvastus skin incision extends from the superior pole of the patella to the top of the tibial tubercle. This shows the straight midline incision. **B,** The inferior border of the VMO muscle belly is identified. The surgeon can place a finger beneath this muscle belly, but on top of the synovial capsule and out of the knee joint, to facilitate leaving a thin edge of myofascial tissue attached to the inferior border of the VMO when making the arthrotomy. **C,** The arthrotomy for the mini-subvastus exposure follows the inferior border of the VMO, intersects the patella, and then turns distally to parallel the medial edge of the patellar tendon to the medial margin of the tibial tubercle. **D,** The patella is retracted into the gutter with relatively little tension on the VMO. A second 90° bent Hohmann retractor is placed medially to visualize the distal femur.

tubercle (**Figure 1,** *A*). A medial full-thickness skin flap is raised to clearly identify the distal border and insertion of the VMO while preserving its overlying fascia. It is helpful to establish a plane between the undersurface of the VMO and the capsule before making the arthrotomy. This can be accomplished by incising the overlying fascia of the VMO and bluntly freeing the muscle belly from the underlying synovial layer (**Figure 1,** *B*). This will preserve a myofascial band of tissue at

the inferior border of the VMO, which the retractor will rest against later in the procedure. If the tendon is not preserved, the retractor will move proximally and tear or macerate the VMO muscle fibers, causing unwanted damage and bleeding. The arthrotomy starts along the inferior border of the VMO, extends laterally to the midpole of the patella, and then turns distally to parallel the medial border of the patellar tendon to the level of the tibial tubercle (**Figure 1,** *C*).

After the arthrotomy is completed, the medial soft-tissue sleeve along the proximal tibia can be elevated in a standard fashion with subperiosteal elevation of the deep medial collateral ligament. A Kocher clamp can be placed on the capsule above the level of the medial meniscus to assist with medial tibial exposure throughout the surgery. After ensuring sufficient patellar mobility, a 90° bent Hohmann retractor is placed in the lateral gutter to rest against the tendon edge of the

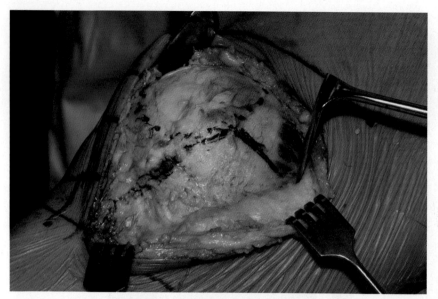

Figure 2 Intraoperative photograph demonstrates the insertion of the VMO onto the patella. Note that the VMO inserts distally at the midpole of the patella at a 50° angle relative to the long axis of the femur.

VMO that was carefully preserved during the exposure. The patella is subluxated (not everted) into the lateral gutter with relatively little tension on the VMO, and the fat pad can be excised or preserved according to surgeon preference. The knee is then flexed to 90°, providing good exposure of both femoral condyles (**Figure 1**, *D*). Before cutting the distal femur, the anterior cruciate ligament is released from the proximal tibia. If a cruciate-substituting TKA is being performed, the posterior cruciate ligament is released from the proximal tibia in full flexion, and the posterior horns of the medial and lateral menisci also are released. This will facilitate subluxation of the tibia anteriorly, which will aid visualization for proximal tibial resection.

Instruments/Equipment/Implants Required

Most manufacturers have introduced modified low-profile instruments designed specifically for MIS TKA. These instruments are more easily placed into smaller incisions and into an ideal position during surgery. We highly recommend two 90° bent Hohmann retractors for this procedure. The tapered tip effectively slides into place to protect the collateral ligaments during bone cuts, and it is also very useful for retracting the quadriceps and patella laterally. The 90° bend also aids visualization of the small surgical field by keeping the assistant's hands out of the surgeon's visual path. In addition, a large Kocher clamp placed at the time of exposure on the medial soft tissues just superior to the medial meniscus will facilitate visualization of the medial tibial side during the surgery.

Mini-Subvastus Approach

The mini-subvastus approach to the knee is a reliable, reproducible, and safe way to access the knee joint. In addition, the mini-subvastus is the only approach that maintains the integrity of the entire extensor mechanism. The VMO inserts at a 50° angle relative to the long axis of the femur, and the distal-most attachment is at the midpole of the patella on the medial side. It is important to identify the inferior aspect of this insertion, as it

tends to be more distal than expected (**Figure 2**). Therefore, any approach that extends proximally to the midpoint of the patella violates a portion of the quadriceps tendon and should not be considered "quadriceps sparing."

Procedure

The distal femur is resected with a low-profile intramedullary resection guide. Two key maneuvers can aid in visualization of the distal femur during critical steps such as placing the intramedullary guide, femoral sizing, anterior resection, and cementation. The first is bringing the knee into more extension, which decreases tension on the extensor mechanism and allows more of the distal femur to be visualized. The second is placing a small knee retractor to slightly elevate the extensor mechanism from the distal femur.

The proximal tibia is resected next. This creates more space for femoral sizing and rotation, the most difficult portion of any MIS TKA technique. Exposure of the tibia is performed by placing a bent Hohmann medially and laterally against the tibia to protect the collateral ligaments, and then placing a "pickle-fork" retractor posteriorly around the posterior cruciate ligament attachment, levering the tibia forward (**Figure 3**, *A*). The tibial resection is performed using an extramedullary guide designed for MIS. With subluxation of the patella into the lateral gutter, the patellar tendon tends to push the tibial resection block medially. As a result, it is critical to keep the distal guide toward the medial malleolus to compensate for this position and avoid a varus resection of the tibia.

Femoral rotation can be assessed accurately by referencing the transepicondylar axis, the Whiteside line, or the posterior condyles, according to the surgeon's preference. The femur is then sized precisely, and the anterior, posterior, and chamfer cuts are made

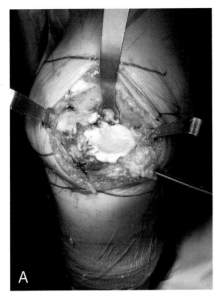
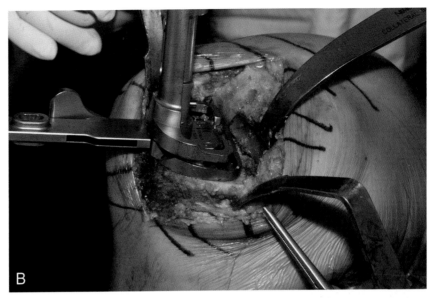

Figure 3 Tibial exposure with the mini-subvastus approach. **A,** For initial exposure, a pickle-fork retractor is placed posteriorly to provide an anterior drawer, and two bent Hohmann retractors are placed medially and laterally to both protect the collateral ligaments and define the edges of the tibial bone. **B,** Tibial exposure for final preparation is obtained by using the same three retractors as for initial exposure. This excellent visualization avoids placing the tibial component in internal rotation.

with a 4-in-one finishing guide. After the femoral cuts are made, a laminar spreader is introduced into the flexion space, and the notch osteophytes, any remaining cruciate ligament(s), medial and lateral menisci, and posterior osteophytes can be excised under direct visualization. The final ligament releases are performed, and flexion and extension gaps are checked according to the surgeon's preference. The final preparation of the tibia is performed (**Figure 3**, *B*).

The patella is then resurfaced (if desired) by turning it 90°, but not everting it. The patella can be resected free-hand from medial to lateral or by using a patellar resection guide (**Figure 4**). Resecting the patella at the end of the procedure avoids inadvertent damage to the resected surface during the remainder of the surgery. A trial reduction can then be performed and patellar tracking tested with the trials in place. The patella should track centrally with a "no-thumbs" test and should contact the medial and lateral femoral condyles equally at 90° of flexion.

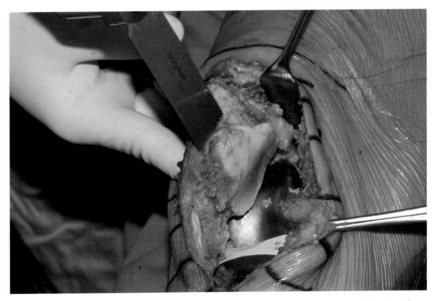

Figure 4 To resect the patella, it is turned 90° but not everted. Resection can be done freehand, cutting from medial to lateral.

The modular tibial tray is cemented first, followed by the femur and then the patella. Attention is paid to removing excess cement from the posterolateral corner of the tibia and the distal lateral surface of the femur, as these areas are obscured by a laterally subluxated patella.

Wound Closure

The tourniquet is deflated and care is taken to identify any small bleeding vessels under the VMO muscle belly. If hemostasis in that area is a concern, a drain can be placed. The arthrotomy closure begins at the midpole of the patella, reapproximating the corner of

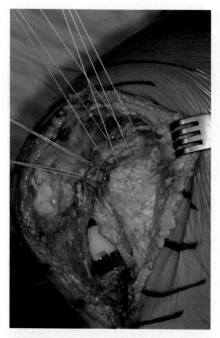

Figure 5 The mini-subvastus arthrotomy is closed by first reapproximating the corner of capsule at the midpole of the patella with two No. 0 nonabsorbable braided sutures. Three or four interrupted sutures are then placed through the synovium to close the knee joint itself and are tied in 90° of flexion to avoid creating patella baja.

the capsule to the extensor mechanism. Next, interrupted nonabsorbable braided sutures are placed deep to the VMO muscle belly (not in the muscle belly itself) in the myofascial sleeve defined at the time of exposure and reapproximated to the medial retinacular tissue (**Figure 5**). The distal vertical limb is closed by suturing the medial retinacular tissue to the medial edge of the patellar tendon with interrupted nonabsorbable braided suture. The skin and subcutaneous tissue are closed in layers.

AVOIDING PITFALLS AND COMPLICATIONS

The complication unique to the mini-subvastus approach is a subvastus hematoma. This occurs when the blood vessels that course through the adductor canal and branch through the VMO are torn with excessive retraction. This is minimized by translating

the patella and not everting it, as this decreases the tension on this area. Before the arthrotomy is closed, the tourniquet is released, the area is examined for possible bleeding, and any bleeding vessels are cauterized. If the surgeon is concerned about continued oozing after closure, a deep drain can be placed in this area.

We recommend that surgeons begin performing this procedure with a traditional skin incision and then shorten the incision as they become more comfortable with this approach. The main benefit of this exposure is that it is truly quadriceps-sparing, not that the incision is shorter. Therefore, while females with more mobile soft tissues may be operated on through a 3.5-in or shorter incision, in more muscular males, a longer incision may be required for adequate visualization.

The medial skin flap must be elevated far enough to clearly identify the inferior border of the VMO. The arthrotomy should never extend proximal to the midpole of the patella, as this will tear, split, or macerate the VMO muscle fibers during the remainder of the operation. After making the arthrotomy, the surgeon must make certain the patella is mobile by translating the patella into the lateral gutter while the knee is extended. If difficulty is encountered, the release of the medial patellofemoral ligament and any soft-tissue attachments overlying the quadriceps must be ensured to assist with patellar mobility.

Mini-Midvastus Approach

The mini-midvastus surgical approach has no absolute contraindications, but relative contraindications include the significantly obese patient (body mass index >40), men with large quadriceps muscle mass, patella baja, and substantial deformity.

PROCEDURE

A midline incision is made from the superior pole of the patella to the midpoint of the tibial tubercle distally. A

medial arthrotomy is begun distally 5 mm medial to the tibial tubercle and extended proximally just medial to the patellar border. At the superomedial corner of the patella, the arthrotomy is turned proximal-medially and a 2-cm split is made in line with the muscle fibers of the VMO. The patella is subluxated (but not everted) laterally with a bent Hohmann retractor around the margin of the lateral femoral condyle. The fat pad is then excised and the anterior horns of the medial and lateral menisci are incised. The distal femur is resected with the knee in 70° of flexion. Depending on surgeon preference, the remainder of the femoral cuts can either be made next or after the tibial resection. The anterior-posterior axis of the knee is used to assess femoral rotation. The intramedullary distal cutting guide is placed, and the cut is made. The femur is then sized, with variations in knee flexion angle needed to accommodate the guide, and the finishing cuts are made. The knee is then flexed to 90°, the tibia is exposed with bent Hohmann retractors placed medially and laterally at the tibial margins, and a posterior pickle-fork retractor is used to lever the tibia anteriorly. A modified tibial cutting guide specifically designed for small-incision surgery can be of great assistance. After removing the proximal tibial fragment, a laminar spreader can be placed in the flexion space first medially and then laterally. This facilitates removal of the osteophytes, cruciate ligaments, and posterior menisci under direct vision. The trial components are assembled and the knee reduced. The patella is prepared last. The sequence for cementation is the tibia first, followed by the femur and then the patella.

WOUND CLOSURE

The arthrotomy incision is closed with either multiple interrupted sutures or a running suture, at the discretion of the surgeon. Care should be taken not to strangulate the muscle of the VMO with the proximal sutures. Many surgeons choose to close the arthrotomy in flexion to avoid overtightening the medial side. The subcutaneous tissue and skin are closed in layers.

AVOIDING PITFALLS AND COMPLICATIONS

It is important to remember that the VMO is innervated by the terminal branches of the femoral nerve, and it can be safely dissected 4.5 cm from the patellar insertion without risk of denervation to the distal muscle. Deflating the tourniquet before polyethylene insertion allows for better visualization of bleeding vessels at the back of the knee and more thorough hemostasis.

Mini–Medial Parapatellar Approach

The mini–medial parapatellar approach is the most popular MIS TKA approach because it is simple and is familiar to most surgeons. It also has the advantage of being easily extended to a standard medial parapatellar approach at any time. The indications are similar to the other MIS TKA approaches, with the benefit being limited damage of knee structures, not necessarily a shortened incision length.

PROCEDURE

A midline or slightly medially biased incision is made from just above the superior pole of the patella to the top of the tibial tubercle. Because of the elasticity of skin, the incision can stretch, creating a mobile window that can be used throughout the procedure to gain an additional 2 to 4 cm of visualization. The medial parapatellar arthrotomy is performed like the standard medial parapatellar approach (see chapter 1), except that the proximal extent of the quadriceps tendon incision is only 2 to 4 cm. If difficulty is encountered in subluxating the patella laterally, then the success of the procedure will depend on extending the arthrotomy more proximally. Modified instruments, including alignment guides and cutting blocks that are reduced in size with contoured geometry, facilitate placement in a smaller soft-tissue window. The sequence of bone cuts can be made according to the surgeon's preference, but some favor cutting the tibia first because this increases the size of the flexion and extension space in which to perform the remainder of the operation. Placing a pickle-fork retractor posteriorly and bent Hohmann retractors medially and laterally to protect the collateral ligaments provides adequate exposure to safely cut the tibia. Next, the distal femur is cut, followed by femoral sizing and femoral finishing cuts. Adequate exposure exists to reference the anterior-posterior axis and the posterior condyles for rotational positioning of the femur. The epicondylar axis can be identified after appropriate retractor placement, moving the mobile window medially for medial visualization and moving it laterally for lateral visualization to avoid overtensioning soft tissues. Soft-tissue balancing is performed appropriately and the trial components are assembled. The patella can be prepared by either turning the patella up 90° and cutting from medial to lateral or everting the patella with the knee in full extension after the trial components have been removed. The final components are cemented with the tibia first, followed by the femur and patella. As in other MIS approaches, the surgeon should specifically assess for excess cement laterally around both the femoral and tibial components before closing because that location often is obscured when the patella is subluxated and not everted.

WOUND CLOSURE

The arthrotomy incision is closed with either multiple interrupted sutures or a running suture, at the discretion of the surgeon. Many surgeons choose to close the arthrotomy in flexion to avoid overtightening the medial side. The subcutaneous tissue and skin are closed in layers.

AVOIDING PITFALLS AND COMPLICATIONS

In male patients with large femurs, the knee is particularly difficult to expose with this approach because the wider the femur (as measured by epicondylar width), the greater the exposure needed to implant a larger femoral component. In addition, a patient with a deformity greater than 15° of varus or valgus or a flexion contracture greater than 10° will require more extensive soft-tissue dissection to release and correct the deformity, which will limit the ability to make a small incision. As in all MIS TKA approaches, a shortened patellar tendon will make it more difficult to subluxate the patella laterally and will require a longer incision.

Quadriceps-Sparing Approach

The so-called quadriceps-sparing TKA has an even more limited medial parapatellar exposure than the mini–medial parapatellar approach, with the arthrotomy stopping at the superior pole of the patella. This approach is similar to the old open medial meniscectomy approach, and it affords the poorest visualization of any of the MIS TKA approaches. Whether this approach is completely quadriceps sparing is controversial in the literature. It has been shown that the VMO tendon inserts along the medial patella from the superior pole distally to the midpole. When the arthrotomy is carried to the superior pole of the patella, however, it does involve detachment of the VMO along the upper half of the medial border of the patella.

PROCEDURE

The skin incision can be curved around the medial aspect of the patella, or a straight incision can be made just medial to the patella. The arthrotomy is from the superior pole of the patella to 2 cm below the tibial joint line, just medial to the tibial tubercle. If the patella will be resurfaced, initial resection of the patellar surface will facilitate the exposure for the remaining procedure. This has the drawback of inadvertent damage to the cut patellar surface from poorly placed retractors. The cruciate ligaments are then excised, an intramedullary femoral guide is placed, and the distal femur is cut. Because of the limited visualization, the procedure must be performed with instruments that cut from medial to lateral and demands partial cuts through resection guides followed by freehand finishing cuts. The extramedullary tibial guide is placed, and the tibia is cut from medial to lateral with great care to avoid injury to the posterior neurovascular structures. Once these cuts have been made, a spacer block is placed to check overall alignment, match flexion and extension gaps, and balance the soft tissues. The rotation of the femur is then determined using a femoral tower, and sized with a modified tower attachment. The finishing guide is then placed in extension, the knee flexed to 90°, and the finishing cuts completed. Once the trial components are placed and patellar tracking and balancing have been tested, the final components are cemented into place with the tibia first, followed by the femur and patella. The tibial component is difficult to insert because of the intramedullary stem, and special components without a stem or with shortened or modular stems are used by some surgeons.

WOUND CLOSURE

The arthrotomy incision is closed with either multiple interrupted sutures or a running suture, at the discretion of the surgeon. Many surgeons choose to close the arthrotomy in flexion to avoid overtightening the medial side. The subcutaneous tissue and skin are closed in layers.

AVOIDING PITFALLS AND COMPLICATIONS

In the more muscular male with a VMO that inserts low on the mid patella, this approach is very difficult, if not impossible, to perform without detaching a portion of the VMO. As in all MIS TKA approaches, the knee with patella baja would be better served with a traditional approach. This exposure requires custom instruments, and it is important for the operating surgeon to become thoroughly familiar with them to avoid inaccurate cuts.

———

 Postoperative Regimen

The postoperative regimen for any of the MIS TKA approaches is the same. The importance of a multimodal analgesia regimen cannot be overemphasized to allow for early mobilization and to minimize side effects of narcotic pain medications. Patients receive thromboembolism prophylaxis in accordance with the surgeon's best judgment concerning the optimal regimen. The patient is up to the edge of bed the day of surgery. The following morning, a physical therapist assists with mobilization, with weight bearing as tolerated. Almost all patients require a walker or crutches for several days and later progress to a cane. Most patients are discharged from the hospital on postoperative day 2, or when they can ambulate more than 150 feet, navigate stairs, and have pain controlled with oral pain medications. Patients may return to driving after they can ambulate with a cane and they are off all daytime narcotics. Patients are given a telephone call at 2 weeks to check on their progress and return to clinic at 2 months for formal evaluation with full-length, weight-bearing radiographs. We recommend instructing patients in the use of a compression bandage at the time of discharge from the hospital. With this surgical approach, patients are quick to regain quadriceps function and often return to more vigorous activities at 7 to 14 days after surgery. This can cause excessive swelling in the knee, which can be limited by use of the compression wrap.

———

Bibliography

Aglietti P, Baldini A, Sensi L: Quadriceps-sparing versus mini-subvastus approach in total knee arthroplasty. *Clin Orthop Relat Res* 2006;452:106-111.

Boerger TO, Aglietti P, Mondanelli N, Sensi L: Mini-subvastus versus medial parapatellar approach in total knee arthroplasty. *Clin Orthop Relat Res* 2005;440:82-87.

Dalury DF, Dennis DA: Mini-incision total knee arthroplasty can increase risk of component malalignment. *Clin Orthop Relat Res* 2005;440:77-81.

Fauré BT, Benjamin JB, Lindsey B, Volz RG, Schutte D: Comparison of the subvastus and paramedian surgical approaches in bilateral knee arthroplasty. *J Arthroplasty* 1993;8(5):511-516.

Gore DR, Sellinger DS, Gassner KJ, Glaeser ST: Subvastus approach for total knee arthroplasty. *Orthopedics* 2003;26(1): 33-35.

Hofmann AA, Plaster RL, Murdock LE: Subvastus (Southern) approach for primary total knee arthroplasty. *Clin Orthop Relat Res* 1991;269:70-77.

Horlocker TT, Kopp SL, Pagnano MW, Hebl JR: Analgesia for total hip and knee arthroplasty: A multimodal pathway featuring peripheral nerve block. *J Am Acad Orthop Surg* 2006;14(3):126-135.

Jackson G, Waldman BJ, Schaftel EA: Complications following quadriceps-sparing total knee arthroplasty. *Orthopedics* 2008;31(6):547.

King J, Stamper DL, Schaad DC, Leopold SS: Minimally invasive total knee arthroplasty compared with traditional total knee arthroplasty: Assessment of the learning curve and the postoperative recuperative period. *J Bone Joint Surg Am* 2007; 89(7):1497-1503.

Laskin RS, Beksac B, Phongjunakorn A, et al: Minimally invasive total knee replacement through a mini-midvastus incision: An outcome study. *Clin Orthop Relat Res* 2004;428:74-81.

Pagnano MW, Meneghini RM: Minimally invasive total knee arthroplasty with an optimized subvastus approach. *J Arthroplasty* 2006;21(4 suppl 1)22-26.

Pagnano MW, Meneghini RM, Trousdale RT: Anatomy of the extensor mechanism in reference to quadriceps-sparing TKA. *Clin Orthop Relat Res* 2006;452:102-105.

Roysam GS, Oakley MJ: Subvastus approach for total knee arthroplasty: A prospective, randomized, and observer-blinded trial. *J Arthroplasty* 2001;16(4):454-457.

Schroer WC, Diesfeld PJ, Reedy ME, LeMarr AR: Mini-subvastus approach for total knee arthroplasty. *J Arthroplasty* 2008; 23(1):19-25.

Scuderi GR: Minimally invasive total knee arthroplasty with a limited medial parapatellar arthrotomy. *Oper Tech Orthop* 2006;16:145-152.

Scuderi GR, Tenholder M, Capeci C: Surgical approaches in mini-incision total knee arthroplasty. *Clin Orthop Relat Res* 2004;428:61-67.

Coding

CPT Codes		Corresponding ICD-9 Codes	
Total Knee Arthroplasty			
27447	Arthroplasty, knee, condyle and plateau; medial AND lateral compartments with or without patella resurfacing (total knee arthroplasty)	715 715.80	715.16 715.89

Chapter 4

Primary Total Knee Arthroplasty: Submuscular Approaches

David F. Dalury, MD
Kimberly K. Tucker, MD

■ Indications

Originally described by von Langenbeck in 1878, the medial parapatellar (MPP) approach (**Figure 1**, *A*) is considered the standard approach for total knee arthroplasty (TKA). It is widely used as it is versatile and extensile, allowing excellent visualization of the three compartments of the knee. Some authors, however, have reported patellofemoral complications with this approach. These include patellar subluxation or dislocation, patellar osteonecrosis, patellar malalignment from disruption of the vastus medialis obliquus (VMO) insertion into the quadriceps tendon, and an increased need for lateral retinacular release (LRR). Because of these possible complications, modifications to this approach for TKA have been introduced. Insall described a midline approach (**Figure 1**, *B*), which modified the standard parapatellar approach by incising the quadriceps tendon proximally and extending the incision directly over the midline of the patella and through the patellar tendon to the tibial tubercle. The reported advantage over the MPP approach was that

this method allowed for preservation of the entire VMO insertion into the medial retinaculum.

The growing interest in less invasive surgery has led to the increased popularity of extensor mechanism–sparing approaches to the knee. The subvastus and midvastus approaches are two such examples. The subvastus approach (**Figure 2**) was first described in the English-language orthopaedic literature in 1991. With the subvastus approach, the extensor mechanism is preserved entirely. Exposure is provided by incising the medial patellar retinaculum transversely after retracting the entire VMO anteriorly and superiorly. The reported advantages of the subvastus approach include less disruption of the extensor mechanism and preservation of the patellar blood supply. This has been shown by some authors to lead to reduction in early postoperative pain, earlier recovery of quadriceps strength, decreased need for LRR, and earlier straight-leg raising.

The subvastus approach is more difficult in patients with limited range of motion, obesity, short femurs, and large deformities. The midvastus approach (**Figure 3**) was initially described in 1997 as an alternative to the subvastus approach. The midvastus approach involves incising an interval in the VMO muscle from the border of the patella, thus allowing for exposure and patellar eversion but also allowing for preservation of the fibers that insert into the quadriceps tendon. Because it mobilizes only part, rather than all, of the VMO, the midvastus approach is believed to be a compromise between the traditional MPP approach and the subvastus approach. The midvastus approach has the added benefit of allowing easier visualization of patellar tracking compared with the subvastus approach.

The potential advantages of the midvastus approach compared with the MPP approach are similar to that of the subvastus approach, including less disruption of the extensor mechanism and earlier return of function. In addition, the midvastus approach has been associated with fewer patellofemoral tracking problems and lateral releases as well as a reduced need for postoperative pain medication.

The midvastus and subvastus approaches are relatively uncomplicated and can be used as reasonable alternatives to the MPP approach in many patients undergoing primary TKA.

Dr. Dalury or an immediate family member has received royalties from DePuy; is a member of a speakers' bureau or has made paid presentations on behalf of DePuy; serves as a paid consultant to or is an employee of DePuy; and has received research or institutional support from DePuy. Neither Dr. Tucker nor any immediate family member has received anything of value from or owns stock in a commercial company or institution related directly or indirectly to the subject of this article.

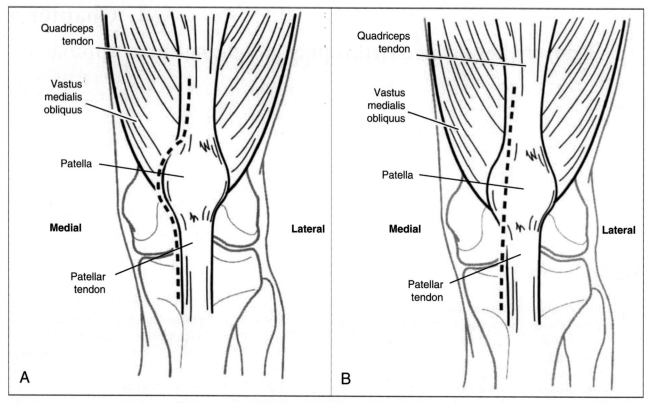

Figure 1 The medial parapatellar (MPP) approach. **A,** The classic MPP approach. **B,** Insall's modification of the MPP approach. (Adapted with permission from Engh GA, Parks NL, Ammeen DJ: Influence of surgical approach on lateral retinacular releases in total knee arthroplasty. *Clin Orthop Relat Res* 1996;331:56-63.)

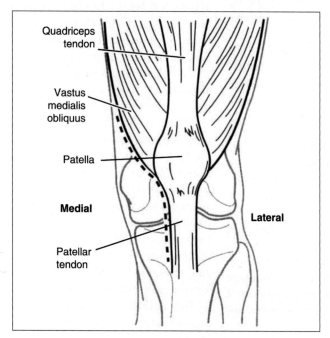

Figure 2 The subvastus approach. Note that the entire vastus medialis obliquus is elevated off the septum. (Adapted with permission from Engh GA, Parks NL, Ammeen DJ: Influence of surgical approach on lateral retinacular releases in total knee arthroplasty. *Clin Orthop Relat Res* 1996;331:56-63.)

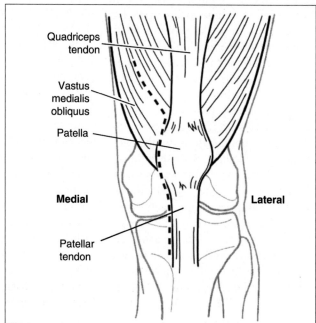

Figure 3 The midvastus approach. Note that the vastus medialis obliquus muscle fibers are split. (Adapted with permission from Engh GA, Parks NL, Ammeen DJ: Influence of surgical approach on lateral retinacular releases in total knee arthroplasty. *Clin Orthop Relat Res* 1996;331:56-63.)

Contraindications

The reported contraindications to the subvastus approach are relative rather than absolute. Contraindications to the subvastus approach include excess body weight (> 200 lb), a short femur, previous major arthrotomy (and thus revision surgery), and severe hypertrophic arthritis with secondary knee stiffness. Prior high tibial osteotomy is also a contraindication, as it is reported to cause infrapatellar scarring and patella baja, which makes visualization of the posterolateral corner of the tibia difficult and may also cause difficulty in placement of the tibial implant. This approach is also contraindicated in patients with very muscular thighs and those with a large preoperative flexion contracture.

Contraindications to the midvastus approach are similar to those for the subvastus approach. They include less than 90° of preoperative flexion, obesity, hypertrophic arthritis, and previous high tibial osteotomy.

Alternative Treatments

In patients who have the aforementioned relative contraindications, the traditional MPP approach is recommended. Additionally, in a patient with a severe valgus deformity, a lateral approach is an option. In most revision situations, submuscular approaches are not recommended because they are not extensile.

Results

Numerous articles support the use of these approaches as safe and effective (Table 1). Many authors have found that the midvastus approach yielded earlier return to function, less postoperative pain, and lower LRR rates compared with the standard MPP approach. A few authors, however, found no difference between groups.

The subvastus approach also has been compared with the MPP approach. Many authors found that the subvastus approach resulted in earlier functional return, lower LRR, less pain, and higher patient preference when compared with the MPP approach.

Technique

Subvastus Approach

A standard anterior midline incision is used. The medial aspect of the knee is dissected cleanly from the Scarpa fascia, making sure it is not tethered proximally. Blunt finger dissection is performed to identify and mobilize the entire VMO from its medial insertion. A small right-angle retractor is placed under the entire muscle belly from its insertion on the fascia, and the muscle is retracted anteriorly (Figure 4, A). An incision is made using electrocautery at the distal aspect of the muscle insertion where it blends into the capsule. This is usually at the midlevel of the patella. The synovium can either be incised at the same level (Figure 4, B), or a curvilinear arthrotomy can be used to enter the joint. The incision is then carried distally around the patella in the usual manner to the tibial tubercle. Because the entire muscle is being mobilized, sometimes the capsular dissection is extended proximally into the superior patellar pouch (Figure 4, C), although that is rarely needed.

The muscle is then slowly stretched and the patella gently everted or subluxated (Figure 4, D). The knee can be slowly flexed. The muscle can be bluntly dissected off the intermuscular septum as needed to protect the patellar tendon insertion and to avoid excess muscle tension. The key to good exposure is an adequate proximal exposure and a clean dissection of the muscle belly.

Once the TKA has been performed, the extensor mechanism is allowed to revert to its usual position. The transverse incision in the capsule is then repaired. The distal portion of the incision is handled in the usual manner (Figure 4, E).

Video 4.1 Subvastus Approach, Trivector Approach, and Midvastus Approach to the Knee. David F. Dalury, MD (8 min)

Midvastus Approach

After a standard anterior midline skin incision, the extensor mechanism is exposed. The entire VMO is identified below the Scarpa fascia (Figure 5, A). The perimuscular VMO fascia is preserved if possible. From the superomedial border of the patella, the VMO is sharply incised in the direction of its muscle fibers approximately 3 cm from the patella toward the intermuscular septum (Figure 5, B). The incision is carried deeply into the capsule in one layer (Figure 5, C). The distal peripatellar approach is identical to the standard approach. The patella can be either subluxated or everted to improve visualization. Electrocautery can be used on vessels seen in the muscle belly.

To increase exposure, the proximal patellar pouch can be incised or the VMO split can be sharply dissected toward the medial insertion. The knee is then slowly flexed, allowing the muscle to stretch. Care is taken to avoid patellar tendon avulsion or excessive stretch of the muscle.

Once the TKA has been performed, the patella is reverted to its usual place and patellar tracking can be evaluated. Closure consists of sutures placed in the capsular reticulum. The superomedial border of the VMO is then carefully repaired to its origin (Figure 6, A through C) The distal medial repair is routine (Figure 6, D).

Table 1 Results of Studies Comparing Midvastus, Subvastus, and Medial Parapatellar Approaches

Author(s) (Year)	Number of Knees	Procedure or Approach	Mean Patient Age in Years (Range)	Mean Follow-up (Range)	Results
Fauré et al (1993)	40	20 MPP 20 SV	70	3 months	SV: Greater strength (measured peak muscle torque) at 1 week and 1 month; two medial thigh hematomas (no effect on ROM) MPP: One intracapsular hematoma; increased LRR No difference in ROM between groups at any time interval No difference in strength at 3 months
Bindelglass and Vince (1996)	89	49 MPP 40 SV	66	12 months	Increased number of LRRs in MPP
Engh et al (1996)	178	90 MPP 88 MV	67 (36-92) 68 (45-93)	12 months	Increased number of LRRs in MPP (50%) versus MV (3%)
Dalury and Jiranek (1999)	48	24 MPP 24 MV	70	3 months	MV showed increased quadriceps strength at 6 weeks; no difference by 3 months MV had fewer days to SLR, lower pain scores postoperative days 1-3
Keating et al (1999)	200	100 MPP 100 MV	70 (42-86)	Unclear	No difference in ROM, SLR, terminal knee extension, extensor lag, rate of LRR 2 postoperative hematomas and 1 manipulation (all in MV group) No complications on MPP side at time of follow-up
White et al (1999)	218	109 MPP 109 MV	68 (44-87)	6 months	MV had fewer LRRs, less pain at postoperative day 8, less pain at 6 weeks, higher incidence of SLR at 8 days
Matsueda and Gustilo (2000)	336	169 MPP 167 SV	67 (30-88) 70 (32-86)	6 months	SV: required less LRR than MPP No difference in ROM, KSS, stair climbing, patellar tilt, patellar shift
Roysam and Oakley (2001)	89	43 MPP 46 SV	70	3 months	SV: Less time to SLR, greater ROM at 1 week, less blood loss, less opiate use at 1 week; Equal length of stay Equal ROM at 4 weeks
Kelly et al (2006)	51	29 MPP 22 MV	68	5.3 years (4.3-6)	No significant differences in strength, ROM, KSS, tourniquet time, proprioception, ability to SLR Increased LRR in MPP (45%) versus MV (4.5%) Increased intraoperative blood loss in MPP group EMG studied pre- and postoperatively: normal in all patients preoperatively; normal in all MPP patients postoperatively; abnormal in 43% MV (9 knees) at mean 5.8 months postoperatively (at 5 years, 7 of 9 had normal EMG and 2 had chronic EMG changes without functional limitations)
Dalury (2008)	40	20 MPP 20 MV	67 (53-86)	3 months	Intraoperative and postoperative EMGs performed Normal EMGs in all patients pre- and postoperatively No differences between MPP and MV in EMG/NCV studies

MPP = medial parapatellar, SV = subvastus, ROM = range of motion, LRR = lateral retinacular release, MV = midvastus, SLR = straight-leg raise, KSS = Knee Society score, EMG = electromyography, NCV = nerve conduction velocity.

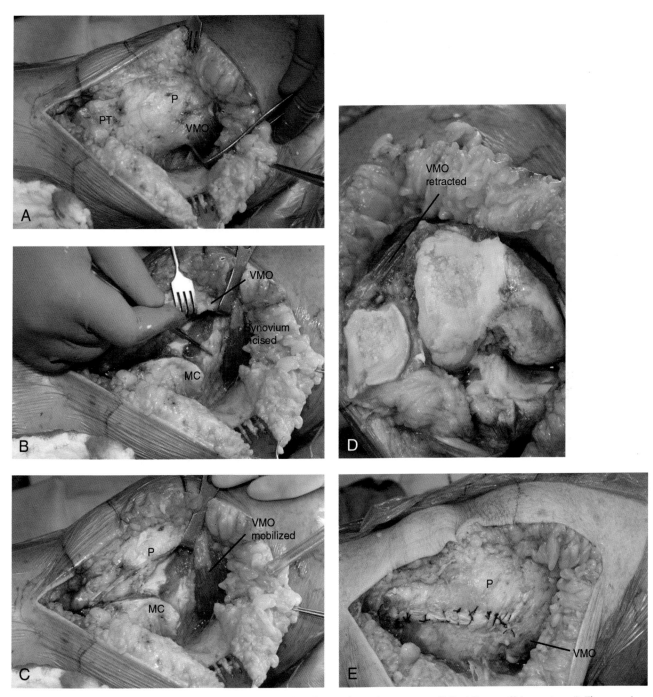

Figure 4 The subvastus approach. **A,** Blunt dissection is used to elevate the entire vastus medialis obliquus off the septum. **B,** The synovium is incised. **C,** The vastus medialis obliquus and patella are elevated to allow entry to the knee to complete the capsular incision. The capsular incision is extended proximally. **D,** The completed exposure with the subvastus approach. **E,** The completed capsular repair after the TKA has been performed. PT = patellar tendon, P = patella, VMO = vastus medialis obliquus, MC = medial capsule.

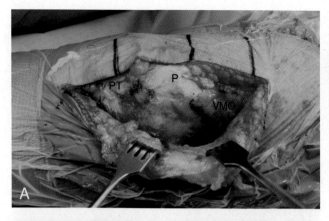

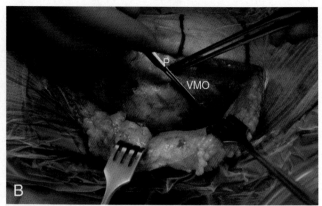

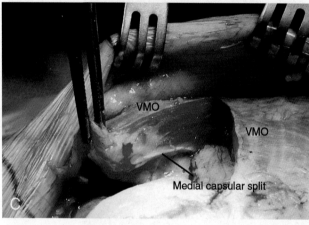

Figure 5 The midvastus approach. **A,** The vastus medialis obliquus (VMO) muscle belly and patella. **B,** The midvastus incision is made into the VMO in the direction of its fibers from the superomedial border of the patella toward the linea aspera. **C,** The incision is carried deep into the capsule in one layer. PT = patellar tendon, P = patella.

◼ Postoperative Regimen

The postoperative regimen is the same when the subvastus or midvastus approach is used as for a standard MPP arthrotomy. Patients can bear weight as tolerated, perform straight-leg raises when able, and progress their range of motion and gait as tolerated without restrictions.

———◼

◼ Avoiding Pitfalls and Complications

Some authors have reported denervation of the VMO using the midvastus approach. Other authors, however, have found no long-term denervation problems. It has been shown that 4.5

cm is the maximal distance sharp dissection can be carried into the muscle from the patellar margin before potential damage to the neurovascular supply to the muscle can occur. There have been no reports of muscle problems with the subvastus approach.

The major difficulty with these approaches is adequate exposure. Poor exposure can lead to difficulties in implant sizing and placement, ligament releases, and retained fragments of bone and cement. Extending the proximal skin incision and muscle dissection as needed is important.

Patient selection also is critical. These approaches are not proximally extensible and therefore should be avoided in revisions, in obese patients, and in patients with large muscles, large deformities, short femurs, and large patellae (factors that make mobilization more difficult). If further ex-

posure is needed, a tibial tubercle osteotomy is the solution.

Patellar tendon avulsion is a catastrophic event that can be prevented by adequate proximal dissection and mobilization. In a patient with a large patella, bony resection of the patella early in the procedure can be helpful. If there are any questions about a risk of patellar tendon avulsion, a towel clip placed into the tibial tubercle or placement of a pin to protect the tendon is advised.

Neither of these approaches is repaired tightly at the capsular layer, and there is a tendency for these patients to bruise up into the proximal thigh. Inspection of the wound before closure, especially along both sides of the split VMO, and use of electrocautery are helpful for attaining hemostasis.

———◼

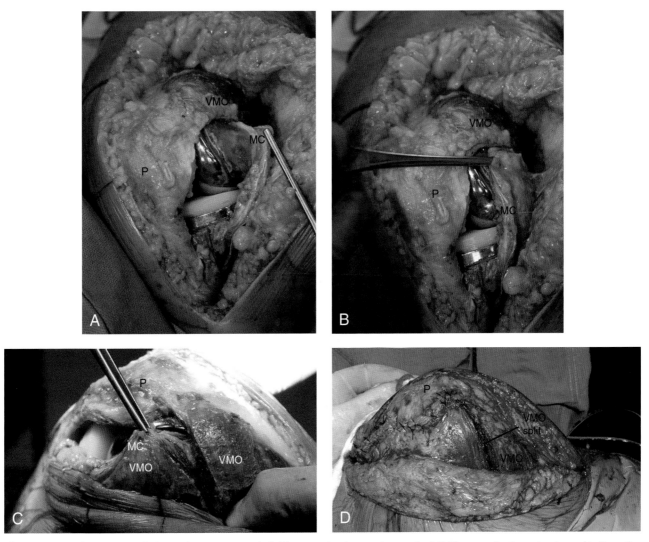

Figure 6 Capsular closure with the midvastus approach. **A,** The capsular tissue to be repaired. **B,** The capsular tissue is returned to its native position. **C,** The vastus medialis obliquus muscle split is repaired. **D,** The completed capsular closure. P = patella, VMO = vastus medialis obliquus, MC = medial capsule.

Bibliography

Berth A, Urbach D, Neumann W, Awiszus F: Strength and voluntary activation of quadriceps femoris muscle in total knee arthroplasty with midvastus and subvastus approaches. *J Arthroplasty* 2007;22:83-87.

Bindelglass DF, Vince KG: Patellar tilt and subluxation following subvastus and parapatellar approach in total knee arthroplasty: Implication for surgical technique. *J Arthroplasty* 1996;11:507-511.

Chang CH, Chen KH, Yang RS, Liu TK: Muscle torques in total knee arthroplasty with subvastus and parapatellar approaches. *Clin Orthop Relat Res* 2002;398:189-195.

Dalury DF, Jiranek WA: A comparison of the midvastus and paramedian approaches for total knee arthroplasty. *J Arthroplasty* 1999;14:33-37.

Dalury DF, Snow RG, Adams MJ: Electromyographic evaluation of the midvastus approach. *J Arthroplasty* 2008;23:136-140.

Engh GA, Ammeen DJ: The midvastus approach to the knee. *J Knee Surg* 2003;16:48-51.

Engh GA, Holt BT, Parks NL: A midvastus muscle-splitting approach for total knee arthroplasty. *J Arthroplasty* 1997;12: 322-331.

Engh GA, Parks NL: Surgical technique of the midvastus arthrotomy. *Clin Orthop Relat Res* 1998;351:270-274.

Engh GA, Parks NL, Ammeen DJ: Influence of surgical approach on lateral retinacular releases in total knee arthroplasty. *Clin Orthop Relat Res* 1996;331:56-63.

Fauré BT, Benjamen JB, Lindsey B, Volz RG, Schutte D: Comparison of the subvastus and paramedian surgical approaches in bilateral knee arthroplasty. *J Arthroplasty* 1993;8:511-516.

Hofmann AA, Plaster RL, Murdock LE: Subvastus approach for primary total knee arthroplasty. *Clin Orthop Relat Res* 1991;269:70-77.

Keating EM, Faris PM, Meding JB, Ritter MA: Comparison of the midvastus muscle-splitting approach with the median parapatellar approach in total knee arthroplasty. *J Arthroplasty* 1999;14:29-32.

Kelly MJ, Rumi MN, Kothari M, et al: Comparison of the vastus-splitting and median parapatellar approaches for primary total knee arthroplasty: A prospective, randomized study. *J Bone Joint Surg Am* 2006;88:715-720.

Matsueda M, Gustilo RB: Subvastus and medial parapatellar approaches in total knee arthroplasty. *Clin Orthop Relat Res* 2000;371:161-168.

Parentis MA, Rumi MN, Deol GS, Kothari M, Parrish WM, Pellegrini VD: A comparison of the vastus splitting and median parapatellar approaches in total knee arthroplasty. *Clin Orthop Relat Res* 1999;367:107-116.

Roysam GS, Oakley MJ: Subvastus approach for total knee arthroplasty: A prospective, randomized, and observer-blinded trial. *J Arthroplasty* 2001;16:454-457.

Scheibel MT, Schmidt W, Thomas M, von Salis-Soglio G: A detailed anatomical description of the subvastus region and its clinical relevance for the subvastus approach in total knee arthroplasty. *Surg Radiol Anat* 2002;24:6-12.

Scuderi GR, Tenholder M, Capeci C: Surgical approaches in mini-incision total knee arthroplasty. *Clin Orthop Relat Res* 2004;428:61-67.

White RE Jr, Allman JK, Trauger JA, Dales BH: Clinical comparison of the midvastus and medial parapatellar surgical approaches. *Clin Orthop Relat Res* 1999;367:117-122.

■ Video Reference

Dalury DF, Tucker KK: *Subvastus Approach, Trivector Approach, and Midvastus Approach to the Knee.* Baltimore, MD, 2009.

Coding			
CPT Codes		**Corresponding ICD-9 Codes**	
27447	Arthroplasty, knee, condyle and plateau; medial AND lateral compartments with or without patella resurfacing (total knee arthroplasty)	996.40	996.60

CPT copyright © 2010 by the American Medical Association. All rights reserved.

Chapter 5
Biomechanics of Total Knee Arthroplasty

Timothy Wright, PhD
Richard D. Komistek, PhD
Carl Imhauser, PhD
Adrija Sharma, PhD

■ Introduction

This chapter discusses kinematics and kinetics, two branches of mechanics with particular relevance to total knee arthroplasty (TKA). The study of kinematics involves the analysis of translational and rotational motion and the associated velocities and accelerations arising from that motion. Kinetics, on the other hand, deals with the forces and torques associated with a particular motion. These two groups are related, with one influencing the other. Therefore, the study of knee biomechanics and the key to successful TKA design lie in the determination and understanding of both in vivo kinematics and in vivo kinetics.

TKA designs are intended to provide adequate function and to maintain fixation to the surrounding bone. Two primary design factors are involved in reaching these biomechanical and kinematic goals: the shape of the implant components and the materials from which they are fabricated. Just as the anatomy of the natural knee

and the mechanical properties of the cartilage and bone tissue control kinematics, contact forces, and load transmission across the joint, the geometry and materials of the implant components determine kinematics, wear performance, and load transmission for the TKA. The surgeon should consider the influence of these factors in choosing the most appropriate implant for the particular indication faced in reconstructing a diseased or damaged knee joint.

TKA Function and Design

The primary motion of the natural knee joint is flexion-extension, which is controlled in TKA designs through the geometry of the femoral condyles and the tibial plateaus in the sagittal plane. Most contemporary femoral TKA components approximate the sagittal geometry of the natural femoral condyle using two radii: a large radius that contacts the tibial plateau near extension and a smaller, posterior radius that makes contact in flexion. In most designs, the two radii are

symmetric in the coronal and transverse planes, so the implant is symmetric in the sagittal plane.

Rotational laxity in a TKA is commonly provided by combining curved surfaces in the anterior-posterior direction with curvature in the medial-lateral direction, creating a toroidal shape. Many designs use a single, slightly larger radius for the tibial plateaus. Toroidal geometries consisting completely of curved contacting surfaces also have the advantage of maintaining satisfactorily large contact areas, even if the components are not ideally positioned relative to each other. This type of contact has important benefits in adequately transmitting loads across the bearing surface and to the surrounding bone (as discussed below under Load Transfer).

Posterior Cruciate Ligament Retention and Substitution

Restoring normal kinematics in TKA continues to focus on two major design aspects: posterior cruciate ligament (PCL) retention or substitution and use of a second mobile bearing. Each design has sought to provide a large range of motion in flexion by allowing posterior translation of the femur relative to the tibia. The goal of retaining the PCL is to allow it to function as a constraint against anterior

Dr. Wright or a member of his immediate family has received research or institutional support from Synthes, Zimmer, and Stryker and has stock or stock options in Exactech. Dr. Imhauser or a member of his immediate family has received research or institutional support from Stryker. Dr. Komistek or an immediate family member has received research or institutional support from Tornier, Wright Medical Technology, and Medtronic. Dr. Sharma or an immediate family member has received research or institutional support from DePuy, Medtronic, Smith & Nephew, and Zimmer.

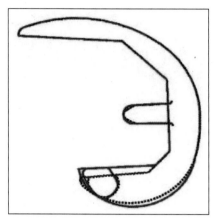

Figure 1 Schematic compares the profile of a high-flexion TKA design (red outline) with the profile of a conventional TKA design (blue dotted outline). High-flexion TKA designs, in an effort to allow greater clearance with the tibial plateau and greater range of motion, have smaller radii of curvature on the posterior condyle of the femoral component. (Reproduced with permission from Argenson JN, Scuderi GR, Komistek RD, Scott WN, Kelly MA, Aubaniac JM: In vivo kinematic evaluation and design considerations related to high flexion in total knee arthroplasty. *J Biomech* 2005;38:277-284. http://www.science direct.com/science/journal/00219290.)

femoral translation, as in the natural knee. Substituting the PCL with a cam-post mechanism provides a geometric, structural constraint to anterior translation.

PCL-retaining designs rely more heavily on soft-tissue constraints to recreate normal motion patterns of the knee. Proper balance of soft tissues during implantation is critical to ensure proper function. These devices may not restore proper function if the presence of severe arthritis has caused PCL degeneration or contracture. Furthermore, if the joint line is not restored to its preoperative level, knee kinematics will be altered as the line of action of the restraining force provided by the PCL—and hence, the constraining force provided by the ligament—is changed in both magnitude and direction.

PCL-retaining designs often use a relatively flat bearing surface on the plateau of the tibial component so that the articulating surfaces do not constrain the posterior translation created by the pull of the ligament. Flat surfaces have the advantage of providing large contact areas when the joint load is shared across both plateaus, thus providing large areas for load transmission and lower contact stresses to combat polyethylene wear. Flat surfaces have a disadvantage, however, when load transfer occurs through a single plateau, such as during large, external varus-valgus moments. These situations could pose a risk for safe load transfer to the supporting bone and for resisting wear.

In PCL-substituting (also known as posterior stabilized) designs, posterior translation is achieved by means of two aspects of implant geometry: posterior placement of the most distal point on the toroidal articulating surfaces of the tibial component, and an intercondylar cam-post mechanism between the tibial and femoral components. Limitations of posterior stabilized designs include the need to resect bone from the femoral notch to accommodate the cam-post mechanism and their susceptibility to wear damage, and, in rare instances, to fracture of the polyethylene post.

The choice of a PCL-substituting versus a PCL-retaining design is best made on a clinical basis. The PCL can be retained in the absence of significant varus or valgus malalignment without significant flexion contracture, whereas disease processes (eg, end-stage degenerative joint disease secondary to rheumatoid arthritis and posttraumatic arthritis) and conditions such as previous patellectomy and high tibial or distal femoral osteotomy are more amenable to PCL sacrifice. Clinical and functional assessments reveal little difference between PCL-retaining and PCL-substituting TKAs, although randomized clinical trials have shown that posterior stabilized designs provide slightly larger ranges of motion and in vivo fluoroscopic analyses have shown more consistent

femoral rollback during sitting and rising from a chair, stair climbing, and stepping up and down.

Greater femoral rollback is not only beneficial for achieving large amounts of flexion but also provides the biomechanical advantage of increasing the moment arm of the extensor mechanism, thus reducing the required muscle force to extend the knee under load and reducing compressive forces across the patellofemoral joint. The beneficial kinematics and biomechanics correlate with improved clinical and functional scores and quality of life indices.

High-Flexion Designs

High-flexion versions of PCL-retaining and posterior stabilized designs incorporate similar changes to accommodate higher flexion, including decreasing the femoral condyle radii at midflexion and high-flexion angles to increase contact area and reducing the anterior portion of the tibial plateau to avoid patellofemoral impingement (**Figure 1**). PCL-substituting high-flexion designs also include changes to the cam and post to avoid dislocation as the cam moves toward the top of the post in extreme flexion. High-flexion designs also require removal of additional bone from the posterior femoral condyles to accommodate the increased curvature of the posterior femoral component. Thus, less bone stock is available for subsequent revision surgery.

Postoperative range of motion in TKA depends on the preoperative range of motion. Thus, high-flexion designs that accommodate a greater range of motion will not necessarily provide an increased range of motion, but more likely will maintain range of motion compared with both the preoperative value and their conventional design counterparts. This may be why randomized clinical trials in which a high-flexion TKA was implanted in one knee and the conventional counterpart was implanted in the contralateral knee showed no differences in range of motion (or clinical and radiographic outcomes) for either PCL-retaining or PCL- substituting designs.

The necessity for smaller femoral radii in high-flexion designs is accompanied by changes in the posterior geometry of the tibial plateaus in an attempt to maintain adequate contact between the bearing surfaces in deep flexion. The changes can be beneficial as patients reach high flexion (>100°), as has been demonstrated through the combination of in vivo fluoroscopic imaging and kinematic analysis comparing high-flexion and conventional designs. Kinematics were similar in both groups, but increased conformity in the high-flexion designs suggested larger contact areas and therefore decreased polyethylene contact stresses, an important consideration given the large contact forces that can occur in high-flexion activities.

Mobile-Bearing Designs

Mobile-bearing designs attempt to facilitate normal knee kinematics through the use of a second bearing surface, allowing the articular joint surfaces to be more conforming than in fixed-bearing TKAs. The more conforming surfaces provide the benefits of a larger contact area, lower contact stresses, and, hypothetically, better wear resistance. The mobile nature of the tibial component, either as a meniscal-type bearing or as a rotating platform, is intended to allow the soft tissues (muscles, ligaments, and joint capsule) to control and constrain joint motion with the goal of creating more natural kinematics; however, this goal has proved difficult to achieve. In vivo fluoroscopic analysis of knees with meniscal-bearing TKA implants has shown little or paradoxical anterior femoral translation during flexion, resulting in lower ranges of motion (especially in extreme activities such as a deep knee bend) than either PCL-retaining or PCL-substituting fixed-bearing designs. Furthermore, the

mobile-bearing design was found to have no advantage over fixed-bearing TKA in randomized clinical trials, and it did have the added complications of bearing subluxation and dislocation. Analysis of mobile-bearing TKAs retrieved at revision surgery demonstrated considerable wear damage to the polyethylene surfaces of the rotating platform bearing, secondary to third-body polymethylmethacrylate cement particles that had become trapped between the polyethylene and metallic mobile-bearing surfaces. Thus, even when the second bearing has conforming, flat surfaces with large contact areas, mobile-bearing designs may generate more particulate debris than fixed-bearing designs.

Guided-Motion Prostheses

Most contemporary TKA designs have symmetric medial and lateral femoral and tibial geometries and thus do not simulate the natural geometry of the knee joint. The choice of symmetry is deliberate, stemming from the earliest modern designs in which condylar, toroidal geometries were used to maximize contact area (and minimize contact stress) and to provide articular constraint against anterior femoral translation and excessive rotation during daily activities. The clinical success of these designs is established by their outstanding performance and longevity. Nonetheless, as the indications for TKA have extended to young, active patients, expectations for even more normal function than is afforded by these designs has increased. Consequently, design efforts have focused on modifying implant design to more closely restore motion patterns of the native knee.

The so-called guided-motion designs move beyond the sagittal plane constraint (and, therefore, the guided anterior-posterior motion) provided by the post-cam mechanism of a PCL-substituting design. For example, medial pivot designs use asymmetric bearing surfaces with a highly con-

forming, nearly ball-and-socket articulation medially and much less conforming articulating femoral and tibial surfaces laterally. The asymmetry is intended to allow the knee to roll back laterally, simulating the internal tibial rotation that occurs as the natural knee flexes. In vivo kinematic analysis has demonstrated that a medial pivot design can indeed control rollback and provide rotation; however, similar measurements of conventional PCL-substituting designs with symmetric, toroidal geometries likewise show more rollback laterally than medially, thus providing rotation. Long-term follow-up studies are required to determine whether conventional and medial pivot designs will experience different rates of wear and osteolysis.

More complex guided-motion designs are entering the TKA marketplace. These implants include varying medial and lateral surface geometries to simulate the convexity of the native lateral tibial plateau and, with the aid of a contoured intercondylar post-cam mechanism, to control asymmetric rollback (**Figure 2**). Few clinical data exist, but early postoperative assessment of patients with such a guided-motion TKA demonstrated both functional improvement in patients with preoperative stiffness and the preservation of good flexion in patients with normal preoperative flexion.

Biomechanical concerns exist regarding guided-motion TKA designs. The first is the potential mismatch between the guiding surfaces and soft-tissue constraints, should the components be malpositioned. This mismatch could lead not only to abnormal kinematics, but also to abnormal contact mechanics at the bearing surface, increasing the possibility for excessive polyethylene wear. Naturally shaped but nonetheless nonconforming bearing surfaces increase contact stresses over those in more conforming TKA designs, even when the guided-motion components are positioned properly in the joint. Improvements in the wear

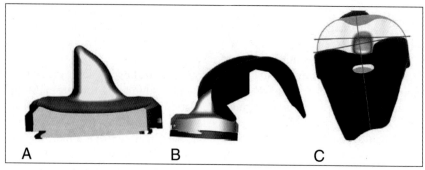

Figure 2 Photographs of a guided-motion TKA implant. Internal rotation of the tibia relative to the femur during flexion is induced by asymmetric surface geometries (**A** and **B**) and by an asymmetric PCL-substituting cam-post mechanism (**C**). The surface geometry features are intended to resemble those seen in normal knee anatomy. (Reproduced with permission from Victor J, Bellemans J: Physiologic kinematics as a concept for better flexion in TKA. *Clin Orthop Relat Res* 2006;452:53-58.)

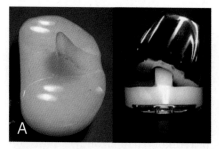 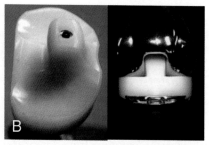

Figure 3 Photographs of posterior stabilized (**A**) and constrained condylar (**B**) knee implants. Constrained condylar designs provide added constraint in the coronal plane by incorporating a more prominent tibial post with flat, rectangular medial and lateral sides that contact the medial and lateral inner surfaces of the intercondylar femoral box when the implant experiences varus-valgus moments.

performance of polyethylene by means of modern sterilization and packaging techniques and the use of elevated cross-linking may address both concerns.

Revision TKA Implants

Revision TKA implants are designed to function in the presence of greater ligamentous laxity than are primary TKA devices. For example, constrained condylar knee (CCK) implants have been used widely in revision TKA and, more recently, in primary TKA, especially in cases with deficient collateral ligaments or joint deformity. Added constraint is provided by contact between a rectangular post between the plateaus on the superior surface of the tibial compo-

nent and an intercondylar femoral box. Unlike the cam-post mechanism in a PCL-substituting primary TKA, the larger post-box mechanism provides more constraint in rotation and, more important, to varus and valgus deforming forces (**Figure 3**).

Midterm clinical results with CCK implants show low failure rates, but complications include increased polyethylene wear and aseptic loosening, presumably caused by the added constraint. The low yield strength of polyethylene and the mechanical disadvantage of the central location of the post-box mechanism in comparison to the moments created by external functional varus-valgus moments make excessive local deformation of

the post inevitable, thus reducing the level of constraint.

In the natural knee, constraints to varus-valgus moments come from three sources. The first source is transfer of the joint contact load from both plateaus to a single plateau. As the load shifts to the plateau opposite the coronal plane angulation, it gains a mechanical advantage in generating a restoring moment. The second source is the addition of co-contraction of the hamstrings along with the quadriceps to stabilize the joint. The disadvantage of co-contraction is a further increase in the joint load; nonetheless, it is an effective mechanism that has been shown, through gait and electromyographic studies, to be used by patients for as long as 2 years after TKA. The third source for resisting external varus-valgus moments is stretching of the collateral ligaments, although this requires considerably greater angulation of the joint than the other two sources of constraint, which can be activated at much smaller angulations.

When the natural knee or failed primary TKA is replaced with a revision TKA, these three sources of constraint can still be active contributors to maintaining stability in the coronal plane. Little is known, however, about the relative constraint provided by contact between the tibial post and femoral box, by contact between the metallic and polyethylene bearing surfaces, and by stretching of the potentially compromised collateral ligaments; thus, the ability to further improve these designs is limited.

Load Transfer

Most primary TKA devices act as surface replacements, covering the surfaces of the tibia, femur, and patella and transferring load directly to the surrounding cancellous bone. The ability of an implant such as a tibial TKA component to transfer load is governed by three mechanical factors: how the joint load is distributed over the articulating surfaces, the deformations of the implant in response to that load distribution, and how the load is distributed to the bone in the presence of these deformations. The implant components must be designed so that the bone tissue does not experience load levels that are either high enough to cause local failure or, conversely, low enough to lead to stress shielding.

COMPONENT DEFORMATION

Load distribution on the bearing surfaces depends on the shape of the implant component and the elastic moduli of the surfaces that are in contact, which combine to establish the stiffness of the implant. For example, more conforming radii between the femoral and tibial components can increase the contact area between the components. This not only decreases the contact stresses in the polyethylene but also, and just as important, distributes the contact load evenly through the component to the underlying bone. Similarly, if the contacting bearing surfaces are made of materials with high-elastic moduli, little deformation will occur. The contact load will remain concentrated over a smaller area, raising contact stresses in the components themselves. Moreover, load transfer will be localized to smaller regions in the bone adjacent to the component, resulting in higher bone stress in that localized region.

The effect of a high elastic modulus is probably best understood on the basis of oxidative degradation of polyethylene. Prior to the introduction of modern sterilization and packaging, polyethylene TKA components were sterilized with gamma irradiation in air. A detrimental aspect of this process was chain scission, which reduces the molecular weight of the polymer, allowing the polymer chains to pack together more tightly, thus increasing their density. Unfortunately, the elastic modulus of polyethylene increases markedly with even small changes in density, thus increasing polyethylene contact stresses. This increased stress,

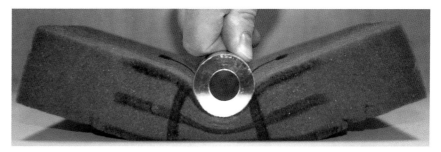

Figure 4 Photograph demonstrates that the concentrated load on the top of the structure is distributed over a larger contact area as it is transferred through the structure to the bottom. The net result is a bending moment that tips up the ends of the structure. In the tibial plateau, this deformation must be resisted by tensile fixation at the edges of the components.

together with the degradation in mechanical properties that accompanies oxidation, was responsible for much of the extreme fatigue-related wear that beleaguered TKAs over the past 30 years. Finally, the thickness of the components can affect their stiffness and hence their ability to transfer load. In general, thicker polyethylene components are beneficial, although the effect is most pronounced with extremely thin components.

The deformations of the tibial component depend on the stiffness of the implant and the loading conditions. The ideal situation is when the implant maintains its shape, allowing load to transfer evenly over as wide an area as possible. However, the contact area at the bearing surface of the tibial component is less than the contact area at the inferior portion of the component where load is transferred to the bone (**Figure 4**). If the component is not well fixed to the underlying bone, an upward bending moment develops, causing the implant to deform away from the bone. This phenomenon is lessened if the component is further stiffened by a metallic tray, but creating fixation surfaces that can withstand these tensile stresses is necessary to avoid eventual aseptic mechanical loosening.

The native knee joint transmits load through the underlying cancellous bone over a large area by means of stiff subchondral bone, which is resected to allow implantation of the

TKA component. Metal backing is particularly useful in reducing compressive stresses on the underlying cancellous bone when only a single condyle contacts the tibial plateau. In this situation, the entire implant tends to tilt, which increases tensile stresses on the opposite plateau. These tensile stresses can be carried effectively by pegs placed under the medial and lateral plateaus (such as those used in the new porous metal devices intended for uncemented fixation), provided that extensive bone growth into the porous material is achieved.

Load transfer and component stiffness are important considerations when using all-polyethylene tibial components for primary TKA. Polyethylene components are effective, provided that adequate bone underlies the all-polyethylene component and that the cement fixation to the polyethylene undersurface has the ability to transfer tensile loads (eg, through undercuts and other mechanical interlocks). Indeed, randomized clinical trials comparing TKA using all-polyethylene tibial components and TKA using metal-backed tibial components have reported equivalent clinical results at follow-up as long as 10 years, with no differences in revision rates for aseptic loosening, which is the failure mode directly affected by load transfer through the tibial component.

Similar load transfer concepts apply to the femoral and patellar TKA components, but neither of these

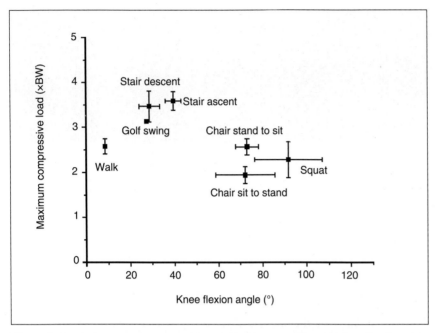

Figure 5 Graph shows maximum compressive load (measured in multiples of body weight [BW]) as a function of the knee flexion angles at which they occurred for activities of daily living in an 81-year-old man implanted with an instrumented tibial prosthesis. (Adapted with permission from Mündermann A, Dyrby CO, D'Lima DD, Colwell CW Jr, Andriacchi TP: In vivo knee loading characteristics during activities of daily living as measured by an instrumented total knee replacement. *J Orthop Res* 2008;26:1167-1172.)

components has been the subject of extensive study, primarily because aseptic loosening, an outcome of improper load transfer, is not a significant clinical problem in these components. The femur can, however, experience resorption of bone near the femoral condyles, because load is transferred proximally from the anterior and posterior flanges of the implant. The femoral condyles also have been the site of considerable osteolysis, although the contributions of implant design and load transfer on the osteolytic process remain unknown.

LOADING OF THE KNEE DURING ACTIVITIES OF DAILY LIVING

A significant limitation to understanding TKA mechanics has been the lack of reliable information regarding the loads experienced by the joint during common activities of daily living. Recently, data have become available through the direct measurement of joint loads using instrumented TKAs

implanted in consenting patients. Although data have been collected on only a small number of patients, the results are providing vital information on both the magnitude of the loads experienced across the knee and the distribution of these loads between the medial and lateral compartments of the joint. Surprisingly, golf swings generated relatively large compressive joint loads across the knee of the leading leg, approaching three to four times body weight (**Figure 5**). Other activities that produced loads of similar magnitude were jogging, tennis, and climbing stairs. Other activities—such as walking, squatting, and sitting in and rising from a chair—generated lower joint loads, in the range of 2 to 2.5 times body weight. The maximum joint load was found to be shared equally between the medial and lateral compartments for activities for which the maximum load occurred at low-flexion angles (eg, climbing stairs), but the joint load was more than seven

times higher on the medial plateau for high-flexion activities such as squatting.

The data collected from implanted TKAs show measured loads that are smaller than predicted from combining gait analysis with mathematical modeling—in some instances, by more than a factor of three. Similar discrepancies have been found in the hip joint, where mathematical models overestimated joint loads in comparison with those measured directly in total hip arthroplasty patients with instrumented femoral components. The discrepancies most likely reflect the much larger number of muscles involved in joint motion than are included in most models. The mechanical redundancy of these systems leads to an efficiency not captured by modeling.

————■

■ Knee Kinematics and Kinetics

In vivo kinematics and kinetics derived for both nonimplanted and implanted knees are discussed here. The kinematic parameters reported pertain to anterior-posterior translation and axial femorotibial rotation of the knee, analyzed using fluoroscopy and a two-dimensional (2D) or three-dimensional (3D) registration process that has been documented extensively in the literature. The kinetic parameters reported pertain to the bearing surface forces and contact stresses at the articulating surfaces and the forces in the quadriceps mechanism, derived using our mathematical modeling technique.

Kinematic Understanding of the Knee

Kinematic analyses of normal and implanted knees can be derived using either in vitro cadaveric techniques or in vivo methods. Although cadaveric techniques are useful in checking general functionality of knee implants, which is a critical step in the design process, they do not simulate actual operating conditions because the actuators used to apply joint loads do not accurately mimic muscle functionality. Therefore, in vivo methods have gained popularity. In vivo techniques can be categorized as either invasive or noninvasive techniques. Invasive techniques include the use of fracture fixation devices, bone pins, minimally invasive halo ring pin attachments, and radiographic stereophotogrammetric analysis. Because of their invasive nature, the application of these techniques has been limited.

One popular method has been the use of in vivo motion analysis techniques involving skin markers. Error analyses of gait laboratory evaluations have suggested that these systems can induce significant out-of-plane rotational and translational error owing to motion between skin markers and underlying osseous structures. Out-of-plane rotational error could be as high as 18° for internal/external knee rotation; this is quite unacceptable for analyses of TKA rotation, which is often less than 5° during certain activities. Modifications in calculations such as artifact assessment, point cluster technique, and optimization using minimization have been found to reduce errors with this technique, but errors remain high, especially when tracking out-of-plane multiple body movements. More recently, determination of in vivo kinematics of individual joints has been assessed accurately using video fluoroscopy along with a 2D or 3D registration technique; this has become the gold standard as a result of the low level of error associated with the analysis. This method has been used for the measurement of in vivo kinematics under weight-bearing, dynamic conditions.

Kinetic Understanding of the Knee

The two main techniques that have been used to determine in vivo kinetics of the knee are telemetry and mathematical modeling. Telemetry is an experimental procedure that involves sensors fitted to prosthetic components that are implanted in the human body. This method generates the most accurate results because it derives in vivo measurements directly for a specific subject. Telemetry is restricted in its use, however, because of the high costs involved in developing a telemetric implant, making it unsuitable for mass production and use. Also, being invasive in nature, this method is not feasible for nonimplanted natural joints. Recently, telemetric knee implants have been designed that have provided valuable insight about TKA contact forces during various activities.

Mathematical modeling is a theoretical approach that relies on the derivation of mathematical equations to predict the in vivo loading of the human knee. Because of the large number of muscles and soft tissues in the human body, the number of unknown factors is large and mathematically indeterminate. Therefore, mathematical modeling of the human body is a challenging task and relies on two techniques, optimization and reduction, to resolve this issue.

———————————■

■ Fluoroscopic Analyses and Kinetic Modeling Methods

Clinical Parameters of Fluoroscopy

Kinematic patterns of 1,578 knees were assessed using video fluoroscopy. The material presented is a summation analysis of more than 100 individual studies performed in our research facility during the past decade. All patients were analyzed using fluoroscopic surveillance, either during the stance phase of gait from heel strike to toe-off or during a deep knee bend from full extension through 90° of flexion. The knees analyzed included normal (nonimplanted and healthy), anterior cruciate ligament (ACL)–deficient, and those implanted with 46 different TKA designs: fixed-bearing, mobile-bearing, ACL-retaining, PCL-retaining, PCL-sacrificing, and posterior stabilized. All TKAs were considered clinically successful (Hospital for Special Surgery knee ratings >90) without any noticeable ligamentous laxity or pain. All surgical procedures were performed by experienced surgeons using a standardized technique for each implant. The postoperative follow-up for each patient was longer than 6 months.

Fluoroscopic Methods

The 3D kinematics of the knee, as well as the femorotibial contact positions, were obtained from 2D fluoroscopic images using a 2D or 3D image registration that determines the in vivo orientation of the femoral component relative to the tibia. In this process, computer-aided design models of implanted components or normal bones were overlaid on the fluoroscopic images based on their silhouettes (**Figure 6**). The implant models were obtained directly from the manufacturer, but the models of the bones were reconstructed from individual CT scan sections. This process has an in-plane error of less than 0.5 mm in translation and less than 0.5° in rotation.

Kinematic Activities

For the gait analysis, individual fluoroscopic video frames were digitized at heel strike, at 33% of stance phase, at 66% of stance phase, and at toe-off. For deep knee bend analysis, video frames were digitized at 0°, 30°, 60°, and 90° of flexion. The magnitudes of

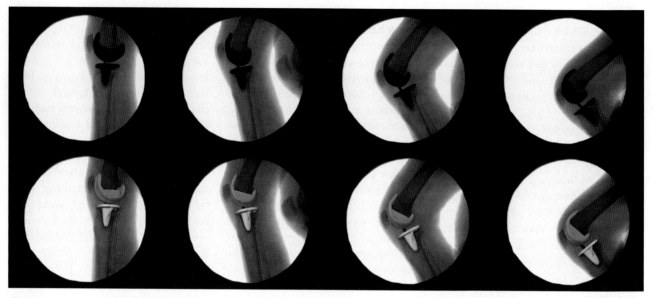

Figure 6 Computer-aided design models of TKA components are overlaid on a sequence of fluoroscopic images to determine in vivo kinematics.

anterior-posterior movement and axial rotation of the femur with respect to the tibia were then determined for six increments of gait and six flexion increments of a deep knee bend. This was done by subtracting the kinematic data obtained at the beginning of the increment from the data obtained at the end of the increment. For this analysis, anterior movement is considered positive and posterior movement is considered negative. Also, a positive (normal) axial rotation represents external rotation of the femur with respect to the tibia, whereas a negative (reverse) axial rotation value indicates internal rotation of the femur with respect to the tibia with increasing knee flexion.

Kinetic Modeling Methods

Because the knee is one of the most frequently investigated joints in the human body, a wide range of knee models are available. Newer knee models have progressed from planar 2D types to 3D anatomic models, from static to dynamic, and from rigid body to deformable body. Three-dimensional rigid-body contact analyses using multiple body simulation methods

built on subject-specific data have been the most popular method used to predict knee motion and the contact forces occurring at the joint interface. In this chapter, our findings are based on two highly accurate mathematical models that we have developed to calculate forces in normal and implanted joints. Both of these models are based on the Kane method, using the reduction technique to reduce the number of equations to keep the system determinate.

The more specific model focuses entirely on the knee joint and consists of a kinematic chain from the ankle to the hip and incorporates three rigid bodies: the femur, the tibia, and the patella. In this model, the femorotibial joint is defined by distinct medial and lateral contacts that are computed separately from the equations of motion. Also, the knee joint is modeled to roll with slip and rotate axially. The amount of slip is calculated from the difference of the theoretical distance that the femur would have traveled without slipping on the tibia to the actual distance traveled. The patellofemoral joint is modeled as a single contact point that moves within the

trochlear groove with flexion/extension of the femorotibial joint. The collateral ligaments (medial and lateral) and the cruciate ligaments (when applicable) are incorporated in the model as nonlinear elastic springs capable of carrying a load only when extended. This model is driven by the quadriceps mechanism, where the quadriceps muscle and the patellar ligament are modeled as massless and entered in the system as equal and opposite forces acting along their lengths. Wrapping of the quadriceps and the patellar ligament at higher flexion angles is taken into account. The contact force calculations of this model are validated with results obtained using a telemetric implant; these results show that the model is highly accurate at the high-flexion, high-force range.

Clinical Results

Knee Kinematics

NORMAL AND ACL-DEFICIENT KNEES
During gait, from heel strike to toe-off, 9 of 10 subjects with a normal knee

experienced posterior motion of the lateral femoral condyle and more random medial condylar motion. The average total condylar motion from heel strike to toe-off was −5.8 mm (range, 4.3 to −23.1 mm; SD, 8.1) and −0.4 mm (range, 10.6 to −19.5 mm; SD, 6.6), for the lateral and medial condyles, respectively. From heel strike to toe-off, 8 of 10 subjects with a normal knee experienced normal axial rotation. The normal knee did not experience progressively increasing axial rotation during the stance phase of gait; rather, it demonstrated an alternating internal/external rotation pattern. During a deep knee bend, all 10 subjects with a normal knee experienced posterior motion of the lateral condyle from full extension to 90° of knee flexion, whereas the medial condyle experienced less motion. On average, lateral condylar motion was −19.2 mm (range, −5.8 to −31.6 mm; SD, 8.4) and medial condylar motion was −3.4 mm (range, 3.3 to 11.8 mm; SD, 4.6). From full extension to 90° of flexion, all 10 normal knees experienced normal axial rotation. The average axial rotation from full extension to 90° of flexion was 16.5°. On average, subjects with an ACL-deficient, nonimplanted knee experienced patterns similar to the normal knee, but subject-to-subject variance was much greater, and during midflexion they experienced an anterior slide of both condyles and a decrease of axial rotation ($P < 0.05$).

TKA-IMPLANTED KNEES

During gait, patients who received an ACL-retaining TKA experienced more variable kinematic patterns than the normal knee subjects, but these patterns were more consistent than other TKAs in which one or both of the cruciate ligaments were sacrificed. Patients with a fixed-bearing or mobile-bearing PCL-retaining or a fixed-bearing or mobile-bearing posterior stabilized TKA experienced similar kinematic patterns during gait, probably

as a result of the cam-post mechanism not engaging in the traditional posterior stabilized TKA. These knees did experience posterior motion of the condyles, but of a lesser magnitude than the normal or ACL-retaining TKA and with a higher incidence of anterior sliding. On average, patients with a mobile-bearing posterior stabilized TKA experienced less femoral anterior sliding than the other TKA types. The femorotibial translation between the normal knee and any of the TKA groups during the entire stance phase of gait was found to be statistically similar ($P > 0.05$).

Among patients with an ACL-retaining TKA, 31 (91%) of 34 experienced posterior motion of the lateral condyle and less medial condylar motion during a deep knee bend. Those with a fixed-bearing or mobile-bearing PCL-retaining TKA experienced highly variable kinematic patterns. Many of these subjects experienced an anterior sliding motion with increasing knee flexion. In a single-surgeon study, 20 of 20 subjects experienced lateral condyle posterior femoral rollback (PFR) throughout deep knee bend motion. Subjects with either a fixed-bearing or mobile-bearing posterior stabilized TKA experienced a higher incidence and magnitude of posterior condylar motion than observed in the PCL-retaining TKAs, but of a lesser magnitude than the normal knee. Not all posterior stabilized TKAs produced similar results, and some experienced poor weight-bearing range of motion and more erratic kinematic patterns. Subjects with a mobile-bearing PCL-sacrificing TKA experienced a contact position that remained centralized during deep knee bend activity, often leading to posterior impingement and lessened weight-bearing range of motion. The normal and ACL-retaining TKA groups showed the highest magnitudes of PFR of both the medial and lateral femoral condyles when compared with any of the other TKA

groups ($P < 0.01$). Fixed-bearing and mobile-bearing posterior stabilized TKAs demonstrated greater PFR than did the fixed-bearing PCL-retaining, mobile-bearing PCL-retaining, or PCL-sacrificing TKAs.

During gait, patients with an ACL-retaining TKA experienced less overall rotation and greater variability than the normal knee. Patients with fixed-bearing and mobile-bearing PCL-retaining, fixed-bearing and mobile-bearing posterior stabilized, and mobile-bearing PCL-sacrificing implants experienced similar kinematic patterns, which were quite variable in nature and often opposite of the normal knee rotation pattern. Therefore, patients with a normal knee experienced the highest incidence and magnitude of axial rotation (mean, 5.7°; average maximum, 24.0°). The axial rotation patterns for the fixed-bearing and mobile-bearing posterior stabilized TKA groups were similar in pattern and magnitude, as were the axial rotation patterns for the fixed-bearing and mobile-bearing PCL-retaining TKA groups. TKA subjects experienced lesser incidence and magnitude of the normal axial rotation pattern.

During a deep knee bend, patients with an ACL-retaining TKA achieved rotational patterns similar to the normal knee. Patients with fixed-bearing and mobile-bearing PCL-retaining and fixed-bearing and mobile-bearing posterior stabilized designs experienced variable rotational patterns, and the average amount of rotation was less than in the normal knee. Often, subjects with one of these implants experienced a reverse axial rotation pattern. Patients with a mobile-bearing PCL-sacrificing TKA experienced, on average, slightly less rotation than the other subjects in this study. Again, patients with a normal knee experienced the highest incidence and magnitude of axial rotation (average, 16.5°; maximum, 27.7°).

Knee Kinetics

The magnitudes of the femorotibial contact forces, the patellofemoral forces, and the forces in the quadriceps mechanism (quadriceps and patellar ligament) were found to be highly correlated. During normal, slow walking (1.0 m/s) the maximum knee force was 2.1 times body weight for a normal knee, but it was significantly higher, up to 3.4 times body weight, for an implanted knee. The force depends on many factors, most notably the orientation of the patella and the patellar ligament, the motion of the subject being evaluated, and the individual's pattern and speed of gait. The femorotibial force variation during the stance phase of gait is characterized by an M-shaped pattern, with peaks at around 25% and 75% and a trough at 50% of the phase.

During a deep knee bend, the femorotibial contact forces were found to be affected mainly by the quadriceps, which are the principal force-producing muscles during flexion. For the same flexion angle, moving the femorotibial contact point anteriorly was found to increase the femorotibial contact force. In general, the femorotibial contact forces were characterized by three distinct regions: (1) 0° to 90° of flexion, where the forces generally increased; (2) 90° to 120° of flexion, where the forces reached a peak; and (3) beyond 120°, where the forces started to decrease. To drive the knee to a certain degree of flexion, the quadriceps muscles need to generate moment across the femorotibial interface, inducing rotation to occur. Moment is defined as the product of force and the perpendicular distance of the force from a point (moment arm) at which the moment is computed. Thus, for the same total moment, an increase in the moment arm is reflected by a decrease in the force and vice versa. The moment arm that involves the quadriceps muscle depends on the femorotibial contact points and the angle of the quadriceps with respect to the femur. As flexion increases, the femorotibial contact points move posteriorly. This action tends to increase the moment arm, but at the same time a decrease in the angle of the quadriceps with respect to the femur occurs, causing the moment arm to decrease. Thus the two effects can offset each other, causing the force to increase as the knee moves from 0° to 90° of flexion. In the flexion range of 90° to 120°, however, the quadriceps muscle wraps around the femur; therefore, its angle with respect to femur does not change. Therefore, the moment arm is always increased as a result of the posterior movement of the femorotibial contact, causing the forces in the quadriceps and the femorotibial contact forces to decrease.

The above-described pattern seen during a deep knee bend was observed routinely in the normal knees and some TKAs and is mainly a result of the PFR observed in them. Depending on the in vivo kinematics experienced by the subjects, the geometry of the knee, and speed of the activity, the maximum femorotibial contact forces varied from 1.8 to 4.5 times body weight during deep knee bend activity. Comparing normal knees with implanted knees, the variability in the femorotibial contact forces was found to be significantly higher in TKAs than in normal knees ($P < 0.05$) (**Figure 7**). In most cases, the medial condylar contact forces were found to be higher than the lateral condylar contact forces. The medial-lateral force ratio increased with the increase in flexion, varying from 65%:35% at full extension to about 75%:25% at maximum knee flexion (**Figure 8**). The patellofemoral contact force was highly correlated with the femorotibial contact force, the quadriceps force, and the patellar ligament force and varied from 2.1 to 4.6 times body weight. The ratio of the patellofemoral force to the quadriceps force varied from 0.2 to 1.2, and the ratio of the patellar ligament force to the quadriceps force varied from 1.0 to 0.5 from full extension to maximum knee flexion, respectively.

Analysis of the in vivo contact areas and contact stresses for various TKA designs using a computational model reveals that the contact behavior depends not only on the kinematics and the forces but also on the actual contours of the articulating surfaces in contact. Preliminary findings revealed that subjects with a mobile-bearing TKA experienced increased contact areas and decreased contact stresses than subjects with a comparable fixed-bearing TKA. Also, subjects with a high-flexion TKA demonstrated decreased contact stresses in deeper flexion ranges than those with a traditional TKA (**Figures 9** and **10**).

———————————————■

■ Clinical Significance

Overview of Knee Kinematics

Flexion in the normal knee is accompanied by a posterior movement of the femoral condyles on the tibia. The femoral lateral condyle moves significantly more posterior than the medial condyle, creating a medial pivot kinematic pattern. This is accompanied by an external (normal) rotation of the femur with respect to the tibia. For the normal knee, the amount of posterior movement and the magnitude of normal axial rotation depend on the degree of flexion. The magnitude of anterior-posterior translation and the amount of axial rotation are lower in lesser-flexion activities such as gait than in higher-flexion activities such as a deep knee bend. Because the gait is accompanied by cycles of increasing and decreasing flexion, a higher incidence of anterior slide and reverse axial rotation in the normal knee is observed during the activity. With a deep knee bend, on the other hand, the flexion increases monotonically; as a result, the incidence of anterior slide and reverse axial rotation in the normal knee during this activity is lower.

Posterior Femoral Rollback

Either during gait or during a deep knee bend, the magnitude of PFR in all TKA designs tested was significantly less than that of the normal knee. Among the TKA groups, the highest greatest amount of anterior-posterior translation ($P < 0.05$) was observed in the ACL-retaining TKA group. Patients with either a fixed-bearing or mobile-bearing PCL-retaining TKA experienced the highest incidence and magnitude of paradoxical anterior femoral translation of either femoral condyle. During a deep knee bend, 52% of patients with a fixed-bearing PCL-retaining TKA and 60% of patients with a mobile-bearing PCL-retaining TKA experienced more than 3.0 mm of paradoxical femoral translation at any increment of the knee flexion activity. A high incidence of anterior sliding also was observed in the PCL-sacrificing designs. These results indicate the importance of the ACL and PCL working together to maintain the anterior-posterior translational kinematic patterns as those found in the normal knee.

During gait, the fixed-bearing and mobile-bearing posterior stabilized TKA designs experienced kinematic patterns similar to those of designs that lacked a cam-post mechanism ($P > 0.1$). This is because most posterior stabilized TKAs are designed to have late engagement (at >70° of knee flexion) in the cam-post mechanism and therefore do not engage during normal gait. At higher flexion angles, however, posterior stabilized designs were found to exhibit a much lower incidence ($P < 0.01$) of anterior slide than the non–posterior stabilized designs, possibly indicating that the engagement of the cam-post mechanism prevents anterior movement.

Additionally, it was found that surgeon variability plays a significant role in eventual TKA kinematic patterns.

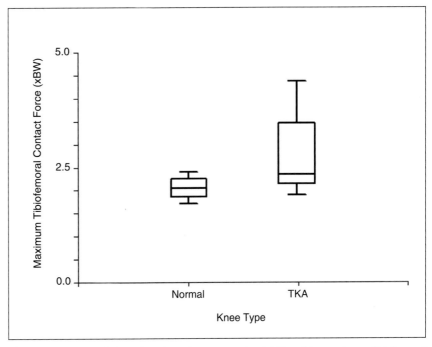

Figure 7 Box-and-whisker plots show the range and variability of the maximum tibiofemoral contact forces in normal knees and in knees with TKAs. BW = body weight.

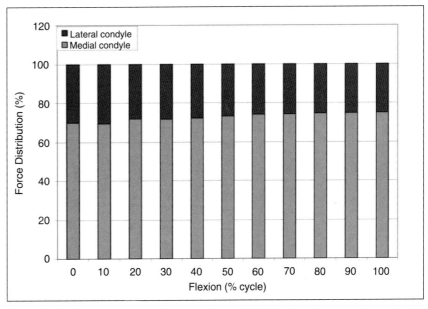

Figure 8 Graph shows mean medial-lateral force distribution found in normal knees during deep knee bend activity, from full extension to maximum flexion.

In surgeon-to-surgeon comparisons of subjects with the same fixed-bearing TKA implant, a statistically significant difference in anterior-posterior motion patterns was observed ($P < 0.05$). For example, three studies were performed by three different surgeons, all implanting the same fixed-bearing posterior stabilized TKA prosthesis. In two of these studies, 95% and 100% of patients experienced posterior rollback of the lateral femoral condyle

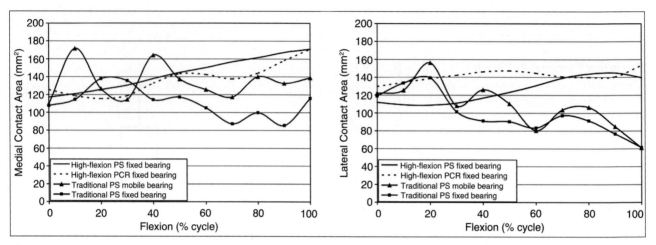

Figure 9 Graphs compare in vivo contact areas in four TKA types. PS = posterior stabilized, PCR = PCL-retaining.

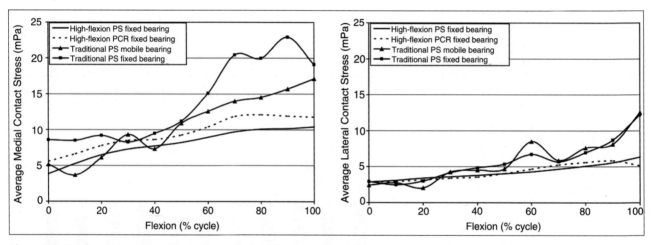

Figure 10 Graphs compare in vivo contact stress in four TKA types. PS = posterior stabilized, PCR = PCL-retaining.

during deep flexion; in the third study, only 65% of patients had posterior motion of the lateral condyle.

Implant and Patient Variability: Anterior-Posterior Translation

The actual design of the TKA significantly affects the kinematic patterns observed. Therefore, great variability was seen among TKA types within each group. For example, patients with a fixed-bearing PCL-retaining TKA with asymmetric femoral condyles experienced more posterior femoral motion and substantially less paradoxical anterior femoral translation than did patients who had a fixed-bearing PCL-retaining TKA with symmetric femoral condyles. Although it

often has been assumed that all fixed-bearing posterior stabilized TKA designs have similar kinematic patterns, the opposite is true. Different incidences and magnitudes of PFR were typically seen when comparing different fixed-bearing posterior stabilized TKA designs. For example, one showed an excessively posterior contact position throughout the flexion range, thereby never achieving cam-post engagement.

Axial Femorotibial Rotation

The percentage of subjects experiencing normal rotational patterns, as well as the magnitude of axial rotation, decreased in all TKA groups compared with normal knee subjects during

gait and deep knee bend maneuvers ($P < 0.01$). More axial rotation occurred during deep flexion than in gait in all TKA groups. Interestingly, the average axial rotational magnitudes in both gait and deep knee bend were similar in fixed-bearing and mobile-bearing designs, and in PCL-retaining and posterior stabilized designs. Thus, the mobile-bearing designs do not seem to offer any distinct advantage over fixed-bearing designs with respect to axial rotation. This might be a result of the relative slipping of the femoral component on the polyethylene insert that does not allow enough shear forces to drive the polyethylene insert. Our study may, however, underestimate the maximum magnitudes of axial rotation occurring during extreme flexion in posterior stabilized TKA designs because analysis was performed only to a maximum of 90° of flexion. Because many posterior stabilized implants are designed to have late cam-post engagement at flexion beyond 70°, additional axial rotation at flexion increments greater than 90° might be observed. Axial rotation in deep flexion was significantly higher in ACL-retaining TKA subjects than in TKA study groups in which the ACL was absent ($P < 0.01$). A more in-depth study was conducted by inserting tantalum beads in the polyethylene inserts for a mobile-bearing TKA; it was determined that all subjects achieved bearing rotation and the amount of rotation varied depending on the subject.

Reverse Axial Rotation

Reverse axial rotational patterns during individual increments of gait or a deep knee bend were common in all study groups but were observed more frequently in the TKA groups. Few subjects in most of the TKA groups demonstrated a progressive normal rotational pattern throughout all increments of deep flexion. Typically, alternating patterns of internal and external tibial rotation were observed as flexion increased. The magnitude and nature of axial rotation depend on many factors, including implant design, individual patient anatomic variances, and the surgical TKA technique. Reverse axial rotation is a concern because this kinematic pattern could lead to decreased flexion, lateralization of the patella in deep flexion, and possible soft-tissue impingement.

Bearing Surface Forces

The amount of PFR not only affects the amount of knee flexion by preventing impingement of the femoral condyles on the tibia but also has a profound influence on the contact forces experienced by these implants. As posterior movement of the condyles increases, the quadriceps moment arm increases. This is manifested by a decrease in contact forces with increasing flexion. Also, at high-flexion angles, thigh-calf contact sets in and helps to off-load contact forces at the knee. Thus, the knee does not experience drastically increased forces in deep flexion. Because a TKA knee experiences less posterior movement than the normal knee and the kinematic pattern is not as consistent as in the normal knee, the TKA bearing surface contact forces are higher than in the normal knee. Reverse axial rotation is undesirable, risking patellofemoral instability as a result of lateralization of the tibial tubercle during deep flexion. This has an adverse effect on patellofemoral and quadriceps mechanics by changing the angles at which these forces act, causing the forces to change and thereby affecting the amount of knee flexion. In general, the medial contact forces are higher in TKA knees than are the lateral contact forces. As a result of the higher forces on the medial condyle, the in vivo contact stresses at the medial condyle interface with the tibial plateau were higher than those at the lateral condyle interface, which resulted in higher posterior medial wear in TKA knees, as has been reported in retrieval studies. High-flexion TKA, designed to induce higher contact areas in deep flexion, resulted in less contact stress in deep flexion than is seen with a traditional TKA.

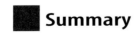

Summary

TKA surgery is a successful procedure to treat severe osteoarthritis in the knee. Because the normal soft-tissue constraints and the articulating geometry seen in the normal knee are modified with TKA, however, TKA kinematics and kinetics differ quite significantly from the normal knee, with respect to the following:

• Subjects undergoing TKA experience less PFR and a higher incidence of anterior slide. This anterior slide occurs significantly more frequently in PCL-retaining TKAs.

• Subjects with a TKA experience a lower magnitude and incidence of normal axial rotation and a higher incidence of reverse axial rotation.

• Subjects with a TKA experience significantly less weight-bearing range of motion than those with normal knees.

• Subjects with a TKA experience higher magnitudes and greater variability in the contact forces and contact stresses at the bearing surface interface. One of the most influential factors contributing to TKA wear is the bearing surface force, which directly increases the bearing surface contact stresses. Therefore, these higher forces seen in TKAs, which can be twice as high as in the normal knee, are a concern and could be a major reason why certain patients require premature revision TKA surgery.

• Because of the decreased flexion during weight-bearing motion and modified kinematic patterns, subjects with a TKA require higher magnitudes of soft-tissue forces, primarily the quadriceps muscles, to perform a deep flexion maneuver. These increased soft-tissue forces, acting at the knee joint, may be the main reason why the bearing surface forces of TKA are higher than in the normal knee.

■ Bibliography

Andriacchi TP, Alexander EJ: Studies of human locomotion: Past, present and future. *J Biomech* 2000;33(10):1217-1224.

Argenson JN, Scuderi GR, Komistek RD, Scott WN, Kelly MA, Aubaniac JM: In vivo kinematic evaluation and design considerations related to high flexion in total knee arthroplasty. *J Biomech* 2005;38(2):277-284.

Banks SA, Harman MK, Bellemans J, Hodge WA: Making sense of knee arthroplasty kinematics: News you can use. *J Bone Joint Surg Am* 2003;85-A(Suppl 4):64-72.

Bartel DL, Bicknell VL, Wright TM: The effect of conformity, thickness, and material on stresses in ultra-high molecular weight components for total joint replacement. *J Bone Joint Surg Am* 1986;68(7):1041-1051.

Bartel DL, Rawlinson JJ, Burstein AH, Ranawat CS, Flynn WF Jr: Stresses in polyethylene components of contemporary total knee replacements. *Clin Orthop Relat Res* 1995;317(317):76-82.

Catani F, Ensini A, Belvedere C, et al: In vivo kinematics and kinetics of a bi-cruciate substituting total knee arthroplasty: A combined fluoroscopic and gait analysis study. *J Orthop Res* 2009;27(12):1569-1575.

Currier JH, Bill MA, Mayor MB: Analysis of wear asymmetry in a series of 94 retrieved polyethylene tibial bearings. *J Biomech* 2005;38(2):367-375.

D'Lima DD, Patil S, Steklov N, Chien S, Colwell CW Jr: In vivo knee moments and shear after total knee arthroplasty. *J Biomech* 2007;40(Suppl 1):S11-S17.

D'Lima DD, Steklov N, Patil S, Colwell CW Jr: The Mark Coventry Award: In vivo knee forces during recreation and exercise after knee arthroplasty. *Clin Orthop Relat Res* 2008;466(11):2605-2611.

Dennis DA, Komistek RD, Mahfouz MR, Walker SA, Tucker A: A multicenter analysis of axial femorotibial rotation after total knee arthroplasty. *Clin Orthop Relat Res* 2004;428(428):180-189.

Fantozzi S, Catani F, Ensini A, Leardini A, Giannini S: Femoral rollback of cruciate-retaining and posterior-stabilized total knee replacements: In vivo fluoroscopic analysis during activities of daily living. *J Orthop Res* 2006;24(12):2222-2229.

Kane TR, Levinson D: *Dynamics: Theory and Applications.* New York, NY, McGraw-Hill Publishing, 1985.

Komistek RD, Kane TR, Mahfouz MR, Ochoa JA, Dennis DA: Knee mechanics: A review of past and present techniques to determine in vivo loads. *J Biomech* 2005;38(2):215-228.

Mahfouz MR, Hoff WA, Komistek RD, Dennis DA: A robust method for registration of three-dimensional knee implant models to two-dimensional fluoroscopy images. *IEEE Trans Med Imaging* 2003;22(12):1561-1574.

Mündermann A, Dyrby CO, D'Lima DD, Colwell CW Jr, Andriacchi TP: In vivo knee loading characteristics during activities of daily living as measured by an instrumented total knee replacement. *J Orthop Res* 2008;26(9):1167-1172.

Murphy M: *Geometry and the Kinematics of the Normal Human Knee.* [Thesis.]Cambridge, MA, Massachusetts Institute of Technology, 1990.

Sharma A, Leszko F, Komistek RD, Scuderi GR, Cates HE Jr, Liu F: In vivo patellofemoral forces in high flexion total knee arthroplasty. *J Biomech* 2008;41(3):642-648.

Victor J, Bellemans J: Physiologic kinematics as a concept for better flexion in TKA. *Clin Orthop Relat Res* 2006;452:53-58.

Wasielewski RC, Komistek RD, Zingde SM, Sheridan KC, Mahfouz MR: Lack of axial rotation in mobile-bearing knee designs. *Clin Orthop Relat Res* 2008;466(11):2662-2668.

Zelle J, Barink M, Loeffen R, De Waal Malefijt M, Verdonschot N: Thigh-calf contact force measurements in deep knee flexion. *Clin Biomech (Bristol, Avon)* 2007;22(7):821-826.

Chapter 6
Bearing Surfaces in Total Knee Arthroplasty

Joshua J. Jacobs, MD
Alexander P. Sah, MD

◼ Introduction

In general, total knee arthroplasty (TKA) is associated with excellent long-term results. Failures do occur, however, and polyethylene wear is one of the major causes. A retrospective review of 212 revision TKAs indicated that 25% of failures were due to polyethylene wear. This type of TKA failure is often the culmination of a cascade of events, beginning with polyethylene wear and followed by an adverse biologic response to debris, which subsequently initiates osteolysis. Promising results have been achieved recently with alternative bearings in total hip arthroplasty (THA), and this has generated substantial interest in attempting to achieve similar improvements in TKA bearings. For TKA materials, investigations have focused primarily on making alterations to the polyethylene insert and to the femoral prosthesis articulating surface. The potential

to improve wear characteristics must be balanced, however, with the potential to introduce other modes of implant failure. Past experience has shown that new technology can introduce unique and unforeseen complications to a procedure that is successful.

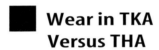

◼ Wear in TKA Versus THA

THA wear patterns have been well modeled by hip simulator studies, which have accelerated the acquisition of data relating to mid- and long-term THA longevity. It is important to realize, however, that hip and knee joint kinetics differ substantially in ways that greatly influence the performance of materials in these joints. Therefore, it cannot be assumed that material modifications

that are successful in THA will be equally successful in TKA. Furthermore, knee wear is difficult to simulate because of the increased degrees of freedom in the knee joint and the need for reduced articular conformity to maximize knee function. Therefore, no validated or reproducible methods exist of simulating in vivo wear of tibial inserts for TKA, making evaluation of the efficacy of new forms of polyethylene in TKA difficult.

In TKA, the predominant mechanism of failure is fatigue with pitting and delamination, which produces large and irregularly shaped polyethylene particles. Delamination, which is the primary cause of most polyethylene-related TKA failures, occurs after the initiation and propagation of subsurface cracks (**Figure 1**). An important difference between TKA and THA wear is that in the knee, pitting and delaminating wear can distort the geometry of the TKA bearing surface, leading to changes in joint alignment and stability, which can adversely affect the load distribution across the joint. These changes can lead to further polyethylene wear and increased bone stresses, which can result in aseptic loosening or osteolysis (**Figure 2**).

In THA, the predominant wear mechanisms are abrasion and adhesion, which produce a greater number of smaller particles than those produced in TKA. Osteolysis is less com-

Dr. Jacobs or an immediate family member serves as a board member, owner, officer, or committee member of the Bone and Joint Decade, U.S.A., the Orthopaedic Research and Education Foundation, and the NIAMS Advisory Council; serves as a paid consultant to or is an employee of Medtronic Sofamor Danek and Zimmer; has received research or institutional support from Arcus, Medtronic Sofamor Danek, National Institutes of Health (NIAMS & NICHD), Spinal Motion, Wright Medical Technology, Zimmer, and Advanced Spine Technologies; and has stock or stock options held in Implant Protection. Neither Dr. Sah nor any immediate family member has received anything of value from or owns stock in a commercial company or institution related directly or indirectly to the subject of this chapter.

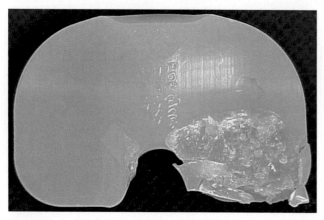

Figure 1 Photograph of a retrieved polyethylene tibial insert demonstrates failure by delamination and early wear of the bearing surface.

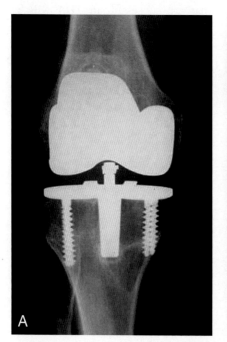
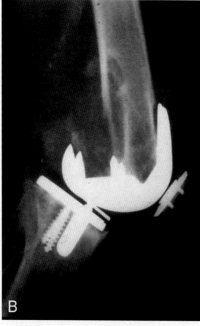

Figure 2 Wear-induced osteolysis after TKA. **A,** AP radiograph demonstrates osteolysis of the proximal tibia. **B,** Lateral radiograph reveals severe osteolysis of the distal femur.

expanding alternative bearing options in THA, the primary bearing surface in TKA remains metal on polyethylene.

Bearing Surface Materials

Ultra-High Molecular Weight Polyethylene

Ultra-high molecular weight polyethylene (UHMWPE) has been used successfully for more than 40 years and remains the gold standard for bearing surfaces for TKA. Long-term results using UHMWPE in TKA are generally excellent, and long-term failure mechanisms are predictable.

Since the mid-1990s, sterilization of polyethylene implants by gamma irradiation in air has been replaced with sterilization by ethylene oxide, gas plasma, or gamma irradiation in an inert atmosphere, and this has led to a decrease in wear-related osteolysis in THA and TKA. In UHMWPE bearing surfaces that are radiation-sterilized in air-permeable packaging, oxidative degradation occurs during shelf storage and continues in vivo after implantation. This oxidation leads to early wear and premature failure. Modern radiation sterilization techniques have addressed most concerns with shelf aging, but in vivo oxidation remains a potential problem.

Highly Cross-Linked Polyethylene

UHMWPE is a semicrystalline polymer, having both a solid crystalline phase as well as a rubbery amorphous phase. In the past, most UHMWPE components were sterilized by gamma radiation in air with a dose between 2.5 and 4.0 mrad. In contrast, highly cross-linked polyethylene (HXLPE) uses between 5 and 10 mrad of either gamma or electron beam radiation. This increase in the radiation dose is associated with increased cross-link-

mon in TKA, likely because of the size and morphologic differences in the debris. Therefore, while osteolysis does occur in TKA, the impetus to investigate improvements in bearing materials is far less urgent than for THA. In fact, a long-term study of 1,000 TKA demonstrated that mechanical failure and wear are responsible for one third of failures, but infection and periprosthetic fractures account for a substantial and increas-

ing proportion of revisions. This suggests that more attention should be directed toward these other two modes of failure.

The improvements in THA bearing technology have created enthusiasm for improving TKA bearings. These changes should be adopted in a circumspect fashion, however, until long-term data are available to show equal or improved results compared with current materials. Unlike the

ing and improved wear resistance. In addition, the sterilization is performed in an inert atmosphere to avoid the introduction of free radicals. Cross-linking of polyethylene occurs in the amorphous region but not in the crystalline region. Remelting UHMWPE by heating above the melting point effectively neutralizes free radicals, but it also decreases the amount of crystallinity, thereby reducing the mechanical properties of HXLPE, including yield stress, ultimate stress, and fatigue crack propagation resistance. In contrast, annealing, or heating below the melting point, better maintains the crystal structure and therefore has a less deleterious effect on the mechanical properties of the UHMWPE. Annealing does not reduce the number of free radicals, and thus in vivo oxidation can occur. Therefore, additional techniques such as vitamin E doping or alternating cycles of irradiation and annealing are used in an attempt to stabilize free radicals while avoiding remelting.

As described earlier, it is difficult to adequately model knee joint motion in the laboratory. Knee simulators may not demonstrate the major wear patterns of delamination or pitting. Consequently, it is extremely difficult to anticipate the consequences of new bearings in vivo because the predominant wear patterns are not predictably recreated in the laboratory. The substantial data available for HXLPE in the hip are therefore not available for the knee.

Data from the limited wear testing in the knee appear to indicate that cross-linking is effective in reducing polyethylene wear in TKA. It also appears that HXLPE is more resistant to wear when subjected to aggressive loading and accelerated aging conditions. Only one short-term retrieval study, with limited numbers of HXLPE inserts, has been published. In this study, the wear patterns for UHMWPE and HXLPE inserts were similar, with

perhaps better preservation of the original machining marks in the HXLPE inserts. These potential advantages make this material an attractive alternative for the younger, more active TKA patient.

Data have been conflicting, however, with some reports suggesting that HXLPE may be less effective for tibial inserts than for acetabular cups. Furthermore, even if HXLPE has better wear characteristics than UHMWPE, the cross-linking may have a negative effect on the mechanical properties, causing a loss in strength, ductility, fatigue crack propagation resistance, and toughness. In addition, under simulated abrasive conditions, HXLPE is substantially more sensitive to wear in the knee than in the hip, with HXLPE in the knee showing a 70-fold increase in wear under abrasive conditions versus only a 15-fold increase in the hip.

The wear-related changes in the mechanical properties of polyethylene that are most concerning in TKA are decreased resistance to cracking, insert fracture, and impaired locking mechanism integrity. These properties are more important in TKA bearings than in THA components because the lower conformity and smaller contact areas in the knee, as well as the cyclic loading with sliding and rolling, can lead to delamination. In addition, susceptibility to failure may be increased in poorly positioned knee implants. The complex motion that occurs at the tibiofemoral joint can induce increased contact and subsurface stresses on the tibial insert in the presence of differences in component sizing, tibial spine or femoral cam impingement, edge loading, or increased shear forces with unbalanced soft tissues. With the smaller contact area in the knee, contact stresses in TKA are approximately an order of magnitude higher than in a THA. Concerns exist that constrained designs with HXLPE inserts, such as posterior-stabilized or constrained condylar designs, can fail catastrophically with impingement.

Finally, wear particles from HXLPE are smaller than particles from conventional polyethylene and may be more biologically active. This could lead to increased rates of osteolysis.

Ceramics

One way to minimize wear without altering the mechanical properties of polyethylene inserts is to use a scratch-resistant ceramic counterface. Alumina ceramics have been available for THA bearings since the 1970s. Although low wear rates of ceramics in THA are reported, the brittle nature of the material, with its inability to withstand high-impact forces, is of particular concern in TKA. Several authors have reported catastrophic failure by fracture of all-ceramic bearings in THA, and it seems that knee articulations would be at similar risk.

ALL-CERAMIC

Despite concerns about the brittleness of all-ceramic components, early reports have shown durable and reliable results without catastrophic failure with all-ceramic knee components. One study followed 90 knees using a ceramic femoral and tibial component with a polyethylene insert for a mean of 56 months in patients with severe rheumatoid arthritis; no cases of osteolysis, loosening, or fracture were reported. Short-term studies show results comparable with results for cobalt-chromium components, without major complications. Nonetheless, concerns exist regarding the durability of ceramic prostheses in the knee, and long-term studies are needed to show that the performance of all-ceramic components is equivalent to or better than the performance of cobalt-chromium articulations. Previous studies have reported poor results at the ceramic-bone interface, and therefore the ceramic materials would seem to be most useful on the articulating side of knee components.

ZIRCONIUM-NIOBIUM ALLOY

As an alternative to a fully ceramic prosthesis, zirconium-niobium alloy can be used to fashion part of the prosthesis. Zirconium-niobium alloy is a metal that can be treated by oxygen diffusion hardening to provide a ceramic-like surface comprised of zirconium oxide (zirconia). Femoral components with a zirconium-niobium alloy core and a ceramic zirconia surface combine the benefits of a metal core with the wear resistance of a ceramic.

Oxidized zirconium-niobium femoral components have shown reduced wear rates in simulator studies. Oxidized zirconium-niobium is believed to reduce adhesive and abrasive wear by decreasing the coefficient of friction and lowering the potential for femoral scratching, respectively. In simulator studies, the polyethylene counterface shows less wear when the femoral components are subjected to abrasion when oxidized zirconium-niobium is used than when cobalt-chromium is used. Early clinical results are becoming available using this articulation in TKAs.

Vitamin E

Vitamin E has known antioxidant properties; it quenches free radicals by donating a hydrogen atom from its hydroxyl group. Its potential to reduce oxidation in arthroplasty bearings is attractive because it can be added to polyethylene without affecting the mechanical properties of the material. Vitamin E is believed to prevent subsurface crack or gap formation that can contribute to delamination. Vitamin E–treated polyethylene is reported to have better mechanical properties than first-generation HXLPE and better bending fatigue strength than conventional polyethylene in simulator testing, leading to the hypothesis that this material may be beneficial in TKA with post-cam impingement.

Although simulation data are promising, the improved wear characteristics of vitamin E–treated polyethylene remain to be proved. Data from early clinical studies in THA regarding wear with this material are encouraging, but fewer data are available from clinical studies of TKA. Recent knee simulator studies have suggested reduced early wear when conventional UHMWPE is mixed with vitamin E compared with UHMWPE without vitamin E. More clinical studies are needed before widespread use of this technology can be recommended.

Bibliography

Bartel DL, Bicknell VL, Wright TM: The effect of conformity, thickness, and material on stresses in ultra-high molecular weight components for total joint replacement. *J Bone Joint Surg Am* 1986;68:1041-1051.

Crowninshield RD, Muratoglu OK: Implant Wear Symposium 2007 Engineering Work Group: How have new sterilization techniques and new forms of polyethylene influenced wear in total joint replacement? *J Am Acad Orthop Surg* 2008;16(Suppl 1):S80-S85.

Fisher J, McEwen HM, Tipper JL, et al: Wear, debris, and biologic activity of cross-linked polyethylene in the knee: Benefits and potential concerns. *Clin Orthop Relat Res* 2004;428:114-119.

Koshino T, Okamoto R, Takagi T, Yamamoto K, Saito T: Cemented ceramic YMCK total knee arthroplasty in patients with severe rheumatoid arthritis. *J Arthroplasty* 2002;17:1009-1015.

Muratoglu OK, Ruberti J, Melotti S, Spiegelberg SH, Greenbaum ES, Harris WH: Optical analysis of surface changes on early retrievals of highly cross-linked and conventional polyethylene tibial inserts. *J Arthroplasty* 2003;18(7 Suppl 1):42-47.

Naudie DD, Rorabeck CH: Sources of osteolysis around total knee arthroplasty: Wear of the bearing surface. *Instr Course Lect* 2004;53:251-259.

Ries MD, Pruitt L: Effect of cross-linking on the microstructure and mechanical properties of ultra-high molecular weight polyethylene. *Clin Orthop Relat Res* 2005;440:149-156.

Ries MD, Salehi A, Widding K, Hunter G: Polyethylene wear performance of oxidized zirconium and cobalt-chromium knee components under abrasive conditions. *J Bone Joint Surg Am* 2002;84:129-135.

Schmalzried TP, Jasty M, Rosenberg A, Harris WH: Polyethylene wear debris and tissue reactions in knee as compared to hip replacement prostheses. *J Appl Biomater* 1994;5:185-190.

Shanbhag AS, Bailey HO, Hwang DS, Cha CW, Eror NG, Rubash HE: Quantitative analysis of ultrahigh molecular weight polyethylene (UHMWPE) wear debris associated with total knee replacements. *J Biomed Mater Res* 2000;53:100-110.

Sharkey PF, Hozack WJ, Rothman RH, Shastri S, Jacoby SM: Why are total knee arthroplasties failing today? *Clin Orthop Relat Res* 2002;404:7-13.

Teramura S, Sakoda H, Terao T, Endo MM, Fujiwara K, Tomita N: Reduction of wear volume from ultrahigh molecular weight polyethylene knee components by the addition of vitamin E. *J Orthop Res* 2008;26:460-464.

Vessely MB, Whaley AL, Harmsen WS, Schleck CD, Berry DJ: The Chitranjan Ranawat Award: Long-term survivorship and failure modes of 1000 cemented condylar total knee arthroplasties. *Clin Orthop Relat Res* 2006;452:28-34.

Wang A, Polineni VK, Essner A: Effect of radiation dosage on the wear of stabilized UHMWPE evaluated by the hip and knee joint simulators. *Proc Soc Biomater* 1997;23:154.

Wright TM: Polyethylene in knee arthroplasty: What is the future? *Clin Orthop Relat Res* 2005;440:141-148.

Chapter 7

Preoperative Planning and Templating for Total Knee Arthroplasty

Lawrence M. Specht, MD
Richard Iorio, MD
John F. Tilzey, MD, PhD
William L. Healy, MD

■ Introduction

Preoperative planning for primary total knee arthroplasty (TKA) begins once the patient has been evaluated and it has been determined that surgical intervention is appropriate. A detailed patient history is a critical component of the evaluation process and should include any comorbid conditions or previous surgical interventions or the specific diagnosis of arthritis of the knee. A physical examination should be conducted, with particular attention paid to the involved extremity. AP weight-bearing radiographs of both knees and lateral and axial radiographs of the operative knee should be obtained. Hip-knee-ankle (long-leg) radiographs are obtained routinely by many surgeons but are essential when hip, femoral, or tibial bone deformities exist. Any history of infection must

be investigated fully with joint aspiration, cultures, synovial fluid cell count, and serum laboratory evaluation such as erythrocyte sedimentation rate (ESR) and C-reactive protein (CRP) level. Bone quality can affect the intraoperative and perioperative management of the TKA patient. The surgeon should strive to determine if any of the following are present: osteoporosis, rheumatoid arthritis, or other metabolic disease; obesity; peripheral vascular disease or femoral popliteal bypass; anticoagulation; cardiac stenting; or systemic clotting disorders such as thrombocytopenia and hemophilia. Previous surgery, prior incision location, and retained hardware are factors that can influence approach, prosthesis selection, and intraoperative alignment guides; hence, these must be addressed before proceeding with the operation.

The physical examination must evaluate several factors that influence the degree of difficulty for the surgeon to perform TKA and for the patient to complete postoperative rehabilitation successfully. Preoperative range of motion provides a predictable indication of ultimate postoperative range of motion and joint stiffness. Relative ankylosis can affect exposure during TKA operation. Techniques such as alternative surgical approaches and alteration of steps for bony resection, quadriceps snip, or tibial tubercle osteotomy may be necessary to achieve exposure of the posterior aspect of the knee joint. Significant ligamentous laxity or subluxation is an indication that the surgeon should make sure that more highly constrained implants or grafts are available.

―――――――■

■ Previous Surgery

Scars from previous surgery on the knee may influence placement of the incision, surgical approach, and rehabilitation protocol. If multiple incisions are present and the vascularity of the proposed skin flaps is questionable, plastic surgery consultation may

Dr. Iorio or an immediate family member serves as a board member, owner, officer, or committee member of the American Association of Hip and Knee Surgeons, the New England Orthopaedic Society, and The Knee Society and has received research or institutional support from DePuy. Dr. Healy or an immediate family member serves as a board member, owner, officer, or committee member of The Knee Society and the Lahey Clinic; has received royalties from DuPuy; is a member of a speakers' bureau or has made paid presentations on behalf of DePuy; serves as a paid consultant to or is an employee of DePuy; and has received research or institutional support from DePuy. Neither of the following authors nor any immediate family member has received anything of value from or owns stock in a commercial company or institution related directly or indirectly to the subject of this chapter: Dr. Specht and Dr. Tilzey.

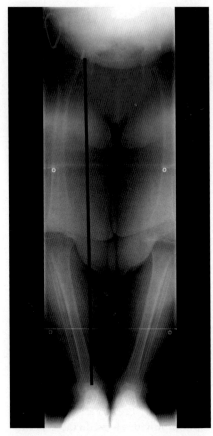

Figure 1 Standing hip-knee-ankle AP alignment radiograph of both lower extremities shows the mechanical axis (black line) drawn from the center of the femoral head to the center of the talus. This patient has a clear bilateral varus deformity, with the mechanical axis passing well medial to the center of the knee joint.

be advisable to evaluate options for surgical exposure. Preoperative tissue expansion or a trial incision with demonstrated flap healing before TKA may be helpful to judge skin flap viability. Previously operated knees and extremities must be evaluated fully for retained hardware because this can influence prosthetic choice and alignment guides.

Evaluation of ligamentous stability is critical for judging how much constraint and ligament substitution will be needed for TKA. Anterior cruciate ligament instability is relevant only if unicompartmental knee arthroplasty is considered, either alone or combined with patellofemoral arthroplasty.

Primary tricompartmental TKA generally uses posterior cruciate ligament (PCL)–retaining or PCL-substituting designs. These prostheses require functionally intact medial and lateral collateral support for balance and function. With restored alignment but relative laxity, it may be appropriate to consider a more constrained implant with greater congruity of the post and box, such as a condylar constrained knee prosthesis. With further ligamentous deficiency, still more constraint may be necessary (eg, a fully hinged rotating platform prosthesis). These components generally require intramedullary stems to distribute the increased forces, which can cause loosening.

Evaluation of gait and dynamic alignment can aid in determining forces that may detract from implant survivorship. Hip deformity and disability that affect the ipsilateral lower extremity should be addressed prior to TKA to ensure optimal alignment of the knee prosthesis. A medial thrust caused by a combination of excessive valgus alignment of the lower extremity, pes planovalgus, and/or medial collateral ligament (MCL) insufficiency must be corrected or accounted for in any knee arthroplasty. A planovalgus foot may be realigned prior to reconstruction using a brace, orthosis, or hindfoot fusion. If nonsurgical management of pes planovalgus foot deformity is chosen in a patient with a valgus knee, subsequent TKA may be compromised by MCL insufficiency because of excessive medial stress if bracing or orthotic correction is inadequate to maintain a neutral mechanical alignment of the lower extremity. Preoperative valgus deformity greater than 10° to 15°, when associated with weakened medial stabilizers, may require MCL reconstruction, MCL advancement, or use of a constrained component. More constrained implant options should be available in such cases. Similarly, significant spine pathology affecting muscle function or

balance or the weight-bearing axis must be recognized.

Mechanical Axis

Standard preoperative radiographs are used to determine static alignment and limb deformity in the coronal and sagittal planes. Hip-knee-ankle radiographs of both extremities allow evaluation of the mechanical axis of the limb and bone deformity (**Figure 1**). Care must be taken to ensure proper rotation on these images because limb rotation and flexion contracture of the knee can make normal anterior femoral bowing appear to be an increased varus deformity. Most knee surgeons attempt to position the implant to restore to neutral the mechanical axis of the lower extremity. In this position, a line drawn from the center of the femoral head through the center of the ankle joint will pass through the center of the knee joint (**Figure 2**). This axis is independent of limb position at the time of imaging. The angle of the tibiofemoral axis (or anatomic axis) drawn through the center of each shaft is then typically in the range of 5° to 7° in valgus orientation. The tibial implant typically is placed perpendicular to the anatomic and mechanical axis. This is a slight change from the anatomic 2° to 3° varus alignment of the native tibiofemoral joint. The prosthetic femoral component is placed in slight external rotation relative to the native femur (7° to 9° valgus) to create a balanced arthroplasty in flexion and extension.

Joint Line Orientation

Joint line orientation also is determined using weight-bearing hip-

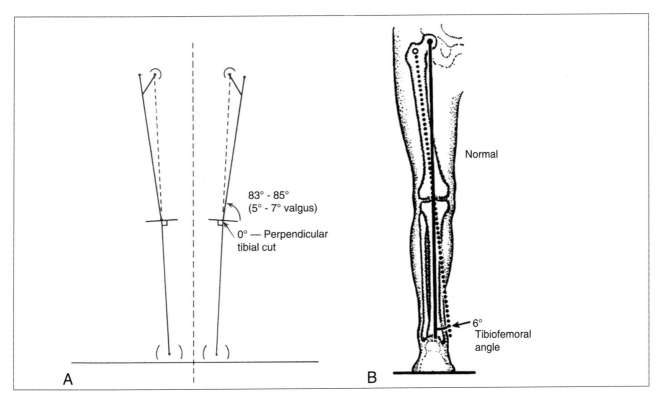

Figure 2 Anatomic and mechanical axes of the lower extremity. **A,** Drawing shows the anatomic axis (solid line) and the mechanical axis (dotted line) of the femur. Note that in the normal limb, the tibial anatomic and mechanical axes are the same, but the mechanical axis of the femur typically is in 5° to 7° of valgus relative to the anatomic axis because of the femoral neck offset and the length of the femur. **B,** The solid line indicates the mechanical axis of the limb, and the dotted line demonstrates the femoral anatomic axis, extended to show the tibiofemoral angle. (Part A reproduced with permission from Krackow KA: Preoperative assessment: Axial and rotational alignment and x-ray analysis, in Krackow KA: *The Technique of Total Knee Arthroplasty*. Philadelphia, PA, CV Mosby, 1990, p 94. Part B reproduced with permission from Healy WL, Anglen JO, Wasilewski SA, Krackow KA: Distal femoral varus osteotomy. *J Bone Joint Surg Am* 1988;70:103.)

knee-ankle alignment radiographs of both limbs. Joint line orientation can change in relation to the ground based on the position of the foot in comparison to the midline. A reasonable compromise is to place the joint line perpendicular to the mechanical axis, which would place the joint line parallel to the ground in two-legged stance when the feet are positioned shoulder width apart, consistent with normal gait patterns.

The history, physical examination, and radiographs will reveal previous trauma or operation to the femur or tibia that can lead to extra-articular deformity and/or retained hardware. Severe extra-articular deformity that cannot be corrected at the joint line in the course of routine arthroplasty can be corrected with osteotomy of the fe-

mur or tibia and fixation with either an independent device or a stemmed extension of the tibial or femoral component. Retained hardware may need to be removed or accommodated. Because intramedullary guides may be obstructed by hardware, the physician may use either extramedullary guides or computer navigation to ensure accurate alignment of the bone cuts.

Magnification

Once the surgeon has determined that alignment can be corrected at the joint line, templating for the knee implants can be performed on appropriately magnified radiographs of the knee. The magnification of the implant

templates must match the magnification of the radiographs. Lateral and weight-bearing AP radiographs are obtained with the x-ray beam located at a standard distance from the plate, usually 36 inches. In the absence of joint contracture and with average soft-tissue thickness, this results in a magnification factor of approximately 110%. This is the standard magnification assumed by most manufacturers' acetate templates.

Magnification on radiographs can be distorted by excessive soft-tissue thickness and joint contracture, as these can alter the distance of the bone from the radiographic plate. A marker of known size placed adjacent to the bone can be used to calculate the magnification factor of the radiograph. However, the marker cannot be used

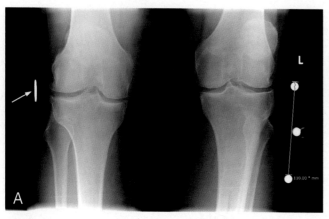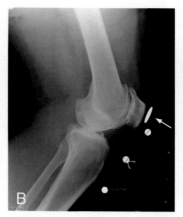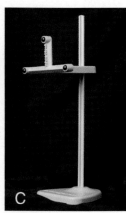

Figure 3 Calibration methods for analog and digital templating. AP (**A**) and lateral (**B**) knee radiographs with calibration markers (arrows). Alternatively, a quarter (diameter = 24.26 mm) can be used as a marker, with care taken to ensure that it is taped at the appropriate level. Note that a digital system prints the 100-mm marker at a size of 110 mm to achieve the desired printed magnification (110%) of the acetate templates. This correction should not be applied with digital templates. **C,** Photograph of a three-ball calibration unit. The balls are spaced 100 mm apart. The height of the stand is adjusted for each patient/body part to ensure accurate calibration.

for calibration if it is placed directly on the film cassette or if the distance from the marker to the plate does not match the level of the bone. Digital radiography allows the production of images equal to the magnification factors of the template by adjusting the size of the images for the magnification of the marker. Digital templating on a digital radiology format allows for seamless integration of the magnification issues of both the templating and imaging processes (**Figure 3**).

Acetate Templating Versus Digital Templating

Templating is a preoperative process that aids the physician in planning the intraoperative steps and determining the equipment required to achieve the postoperative goal of a well-aligned, stable, mobile knee joint. Templating techniques are similar whether using acetate overlays with properly magnified radiographs or a digital templating system. The advantage of digital templating is the ability to accurately record the preoperative plan and siz-

ing information, which later assists the operating room staff and implant inventory manager in having the necessary implants available. Additionally, the ability to simulate the correction of deformity digitally as part of the planning and preparation process helps prevent surprises in the operating room. Although many surgeons use a single implant system for routine cases, obtaining and maintaining a template library for several different revision systems is much easier in a digital environment.

Finally, most commercial templating programs include "wizards," or step-by-step guides, to assist with the process. These are simply guides, however; adhering to the principles outlined in this chapter is essential for obtaining the desired outcome of a stable, well-aligned primary TKA.

Acetate Templating

Acetate templating begins with good-quality, properly magnified AP and lateral radiographs of the affected knee and an axial view of the patellofemoral joint. Radiographs used for sizing im-

plants or stems or planning osteotomy cuts must have a calibration marker of known size placed at the vertical level of the affected bone at the time the radiographs are obtained (**Figure 3**). Weight-bearing hip-knee-ankle radiographs of both lower extremities are used to measure the angle between the mechanical axis and the anatomic axis on the uninvolved limb, with the goal of duplicating this anatomy on the reconstructed limb. These alignment radiographs do not need to be calibrated. Templating and radiographic evaluation also aid in the determination of bone quality, allowing the physician to identify bone defects, implant size, fit, and position.

Femoral Templating in the Coronal Plane

The mechanical axis is drawn from the center of the femoral head to the center of the talus, passing through the medial knee and the anatomic axis of the femur. If the mechanical axis is not available, most implant systems use an anatomic tibiofemoral angle of 5° to 7°. On the weight-bearing AP radiograph of both knees, a line is drawn that passes down the center of the femoral shaft and exits at the knee joint (**Figure 4**). This is the starting

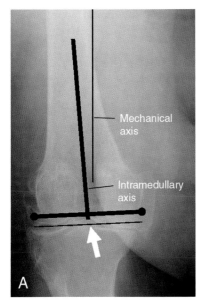

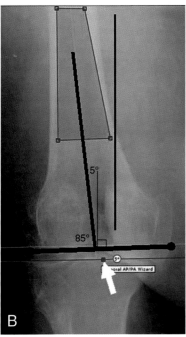

Figure 4 Femoral templating in the coronal plane. **A,** AP radiograph shows the mechanical axis (thin vertical line) and intramedullary axis (thick vertical line). Note the location of the anatomic axis at the end of the distal femur (arrow), indicating the planned entry point for the intramedullary guide. **B,** Level of the less involved condyle (blue horizontal line), planned resection level (thick horizontal line), and angle from the anatomic axis (5°). (Part A adapted with permission from Krackow KA: Preoperative assessment: Axial and rotational alignment and x-ray analysis, in Krackow KA: *The Technique of Total Knee Arthroplasty.* Philadelphia, PA, CV Mosby, 1990, p 107.)

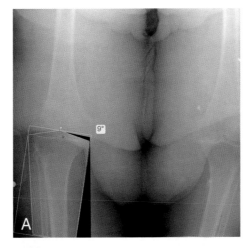

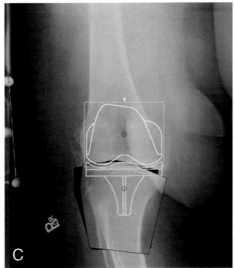

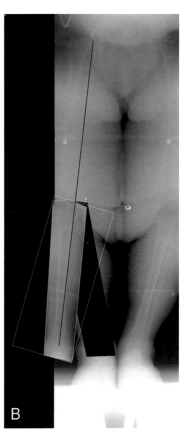

Figure 5 Simulation of the planned femoral correction in the coronal plane. **A,** Simulation of the mechanical axis preoperatively. **B,** Simulation of the proposed correction to neutral. Note that the mechanical axis point stays locked to the femoral head and talus. The femur and tibia are rotated to obtain the desired mechanical axis correction. **C,** The tibial and femoral implants in their planned correct position.

point for the intramedullary guide. Next, a second line is drawn at 5° to 7° of valgus to the anatomic femoral axis to approximate the mechanical axis. The third line is drawn perpendicular to the mechanical axis, passing through the distal femoral condyles; the distal femoral resection is parallel to this perpendicular line. Finally, the femoral template is placed along this third line. This aids in determining the width of the femoral prosthesis. The outline of the template is marked on the radiographs and the approximate size is noted (**Figure 5**).

Tibial Templating in the Coronal Plane

A line is drawn that passes along the tibial shaft and exits at the knee joint. This should represent both the anatomic and mechanical axes (**Figure 6**). A line is drawn perpendicular to this, approximately 8 to 10 mm from the higher or less involved plateau. This results in a minimal cut of the more involved compartment, usually the medial plateau in a varus knee or the lateral compartment in a valgus knee. The resected specimen should have the same amount of medial and lateral bone resected as was originally templated. If the planned resection level does not touch the more involved plateau for support, the resection level must be moved more distal to obtain bony support, or the use of bone graft, cement, or metal augments should

be considered. If bony support is not obtained, the augmented segment should be bypassed with a tibial stem. The width of the cut specimen should match the width of a tibial tray that will mate with the templated femoral size. The angle between the tibial cut

and femoral cut should approximate the planned angle correction.

Templating in the Sagittal Plane

Templating on the lateral radiographs allows the physician to check femoral and tibial sizing in the sagittal plane. The femoral size should recreate patellofemoral and tibiofemoral balance in both flexion and extension. The medial femoral condyle typically extends slightly more posteriorly on a properly rotated radiograph. The goal is to place the femoral component on the prepared distal femur without compromising the structural integrity of the anterior femur (notching) or creating a large step-off in the suprapatellar femoral flange region (**Figures 7** and **8**). The surgeon typically will not have lateral radiographs showing the entire femur (including the femoral head and talus); a full-length lateral radiograph should be obtained if needed (**Figures 9** and **10**).

The medial condyle is identified on the lateral radiograph. For a posterior referencing knee system, the template is placed so it is touching the distal femoral surface and the posterior aspect of the medial femoral condyle. Then the chosen size is adjusted until it is flush with the anterior femoral cortex without excessive notching or

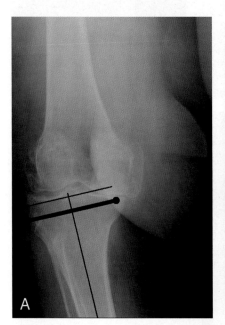
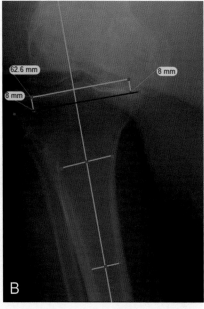

Figure 6 Tibial templating. **A,** The tibial intramedullary axis (vertical line) and the low point of the less involved lateral plateau (thin horizontal line) are shown on this AP radiograph. **B,** The planned resection level (thick horizontal line) is marked 8 mm distal to the less involved plateau in the measured resection technique. (Part A adapted with permission from Krackow KA: Preoperative assessment: Axial and rotational alignment and x-ray analysis, in Krackow KA: *The Technique of Total Knee Arthroplasty.* Philadelphia, PA, CV Mosby, 1990, p 107.)

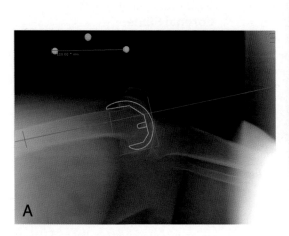
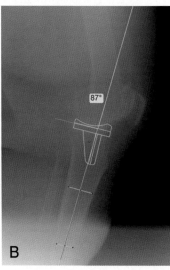

Figure 7 Templating in the sagittal plane. **A,** The femoral axis and the distal, posterior, and anterior dimensions are planned. Note the thin line extending down the center of the femoral shaft (similar to an intramedullary guide rod). A line is drawn perpendicular to this line at the most distal extent of the femur to represent the reconstructed joint line (similar to the measuring plate over the intramedullary guide rod). A second line is drawn posteriorly to represent the most posterior femoral condyle to reference flexion space. The template is fit within the two lines and the size is extended to the anterior femoral cortex. **B,** Lateral tibial templating demonstrates an appropriate-sized tibial component with proper cortical contact and a 3° posterior slope.

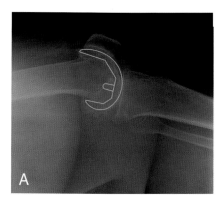 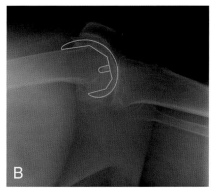 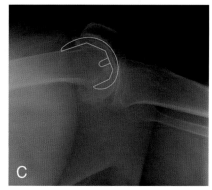

Figure 8 Lateral knee radiographs demonstrate the planned component aligned in flexion, neutral, and extension. Note how excess component flexion (**A**) leads to a step-off in the patellofemoral articulation and possible extensor mechanism irritation. It also leads to overresection of posterior supporting bone and may limit full component extension, especially with a posterior cruciate–substituting design in which the combined component flexion and the tibial post will lead to cam-post impingement before full extension. **B,** A properly aligned femoral component. **C,** Relative excess extension of the femoral component places the femoral component in this position and can lead to anterior femoral cortical violation or notching.

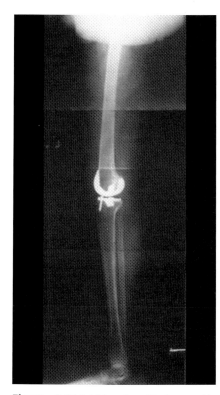

Figure 9 Weight-bearing hip-knee-ankle lateral radiograph demonstrates overall limb alignment. (Reproduced with permission from Krackow KA: Postoperative period, in Krackow KA: *The Technique of Total Knee Arthroplasty*. Philadelphia, PA, CV Mosby, 1990, p 107.)

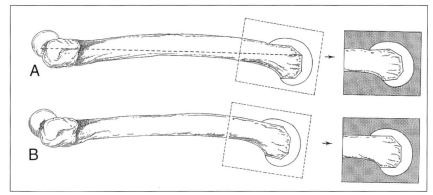

Figure 10 Drawings of a femur with physiologic anterior bowing. **A,** Lateral view. The femoral component is neutral with respect to the overall flexion-extension axis of the femur. This axis extends from the anterior distal femur to the posterior mid femur and anterior proximal femur. The inset shows that the femoral component presents the appearance of components in hyperextension. There is relative hyperextension to the distal aspect of the femur, but overall neutral flexion-extension is maintained with respect to the entire axis of the femur. **B,** The same femoral outline is shown with the component placed in neutral with respect to the distal femoral cortices. When viewed in the overall alignment scheme, this component is in relative flexion. When viewed on a small radiograph (inset), this component would appear to be in neutral with respect to distal femur. (Reproduced with permission from Krackow KA: Intraoperative alignment and instrumentation, in Krackow KA: *The Technique of Total Knee Arthroplasty*. Philadelphia, PA, CV Mosby, 1990, p 152.)

overhang (**Figure 7,** *A*). This outline should be marked on the radiograph, and it should be confirmed that the chosen implant is the correct size to properly cover the cut surface on the AP radiograph without overhang. Finally, a line is drawn along the tibial shaft in the center of the intramedullary canal and another line is drawn perpendicular to the axis of the tibial shaft. A third line with 0° to 7° of posterior slope, as indicated by implant design, is drawn at the appropriate re-section depth (**Figure 7,** *B*). Using a stemmed tibial template that has the angle incorporated within the template can be helpful even when using nonstemmed implants because it aids in aligning the implant with the shaft (**Figure 11**).

In a valgus knee, the primary deformity usually is a hypoplasia of both the distal and posterior femoral con-

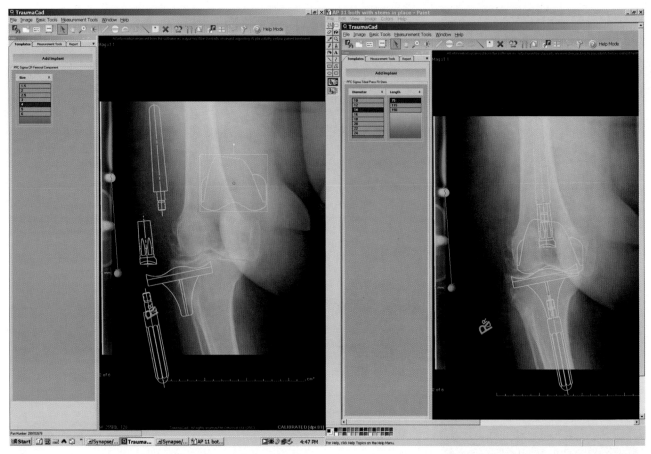

Figure 11 Templating the selected implants. **A,** Components of the available stemmed knee implants are selected. **B,** The components are assembled and placed in the planned positions. (TraumaCad, Voyant Health, Columbia, MD.)

dyles. This is often accompanied by significant lateral tibial bone loss. In such cases, templating follows the same steps, but the surgeon may need to adjust to a 3° to 5° distal femoral resection angle (or shift the intramedullary starting hole slightly to the medial side). On the tibial side, the surgeon should be cautious of lateral deformity and make sure that the resection level does not drop below the level of the fibular head.

Digital Templating

Femoral Templating in the Coronal Plane

Digital templating steps can follow a work flow similar to the intraoperative plan, addressing either the femur or the tibia first. In a femur-first work flow, the distal femoral alignment is used to place the joint line perpendicular to the mechanical axis identified on the weight-bearing hip-knee-ankle radiographs in the coronal plane. If intramedullary femoral instruments are used, the angle between the anatomic femoral axis and mechanical axis is recorded (typically 5° to 7° from the intramedullary axis). The entry point for the intramedullary guide also is templated to assist in intraoperative placement of the starting hole.

If imageless intraoperative navigation is used, the mechanical axis can be determined in the operating room by locating and registering the center of rotation of the femoral head and the distal femoral starting point. The amount of bone to be resected from the medial and lateral condyles is noted and confirmed intraoperatively. The amount of bone resected from the more prominent condyle should reproduce the thickness of the selected implant design (typically 8 to 10 mm). This measurement may be increased slightly if there is severe bone loss or flexion contracture. Note the relative thickness of the medial and lateral planned resection; the actual specimen may differ slightly based on the thickness of the cartilage.

Tibial Templating

The tibial resection is planned perpendicular to the mechanical axis on hip-knee-ankle views. Full-length views are necessary because radiographs showing only the knee are inadequate for templating. For example, on a view showing only the knee, tibial bowing and rotation will not be apparent; the knee will appear to be in slight varus (**Figure** 5). The amount of bone resected from each condyle and the depth of resection is marked again on the radiographs for intraoperative correlation between the plan and intraoperative results. The amount of bone to be resected initially is selected from the less involved condyle at a depth to match the minimum planned thickness of the tibial component, typically 6 to 10 mm. The relationship between this cut surface and the more involved condyle is then used to decide if a more extensive cut is needed to achieve adequate support without deficiency or if other supplementation techniques are required. If a significant defect is noted, then bone grafting, augments, or reinforced cement can be used with a tibial stem.

Using digital templating, the planned surgical correction of limb alignment can be simulated prior to the procedure. A lower-technology option is to use acetate and tracing paper. This simulation corresponds to intraoperative soft-tissue release or ligament advancement (**Figure** 5, *A* and *B*). The widths of the femoral and tibial cut surfaces are then recorded and used as a guide for implant sizing, with the goal of completely covering the cut cancellous surfaces without prosthetic overhang (**Figure** 5, *C*). The most important femoral sizing will be driven by the measurements obtained on the lateral view (**Figures** 7 and 8).

Digital Templating in the Sagittal Plane

Once coronal alignment is determined, the lateral view is used to address alignment in the sagittal plane. Although recreating a neutral mechanical axis and resurfacing the tibiofemoral joint are the primary goals of coronal plane templating, the situation is different in the sagittal plane. Here the focus is on creating a stable, mobile, and balanced reconstruction

throughout the arc of motion, with particular attention given to achieving full extension and maximizing flexion without impingement or instability.

The anterior-to-posterior articular surface measurement is used to determine the anterior-posterior dimension of the femoral component. A lateral radiograph that is obtained with the femur rotated will make the femur appear larger than its true anterior-to-posterior dimension (**Figure** 12). This must be accounted for in sizing or corrected by positioning the femur for a true lateral radiograph without rotation, often a cross-table lateral view. The position of the components is identified using the thickness of the planned implant both distally and posteriorly from the templates. This typically is 8 to 10 mm, but it may vary by implant family and size (**Figures** 7 and 8). In a measured resection knee arthroplasty, the distal and posterior articular surfaces are identified on properly rotated lateral radiographs (**Figure** 7). Adjustment is made at this point for a valgus knee with a hypoplastic lateral condyle or other bony deficits by templating using the less involved condyle.

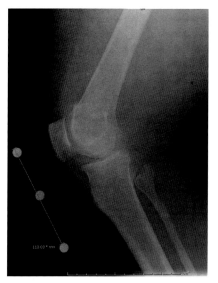

Figure 12 A malrotated lateral radiograph. Malrotation can make the sagittal dimension appear larger than it really is, leading to oversizing of the templated component. (Adapted with permission from Krackow KA: Prosthesis selection, in Krackow KA: *The Technique of Total Knee Arthroplasty.* CV Mosby, 1990, p 69.)

Balancing the Reconstruction

Selecting an implant of the proper size is critical; a too-large or too-small implant may lead to complications. An undersized femoral implant and relative extension of the anterior femoral cutting guide may result in notching of the anterior femoral cortex. Conversely, an oversized femoral implant and flexion of the anterior femoral cutting guide may lead to prominence of the femoral flange and a step-off in the patellofemoral joint, which can adversely affect the tracking and function of the patellofemoral articulation and irritation of the extensor mechan-

ism. Too much flexion of the anterior cutting guide also can lead to overresection of the posterior femur. Excess femoral flexion may prevent full extension of the knee joint, especially in a cruciate-substituting prosthesis in which the tibial post may impinge on the anterior box. Anterior translation of the femoral implant can mimic an oversized femoral component in the patellofemoral articulation, and posterior translation can tighten the flexion space, possibly inhibiting flexion. An undersized femoral component with posterior translation can violate the anterior cortex and contribute to supracondylar periprosthetic fracture. With anterior translation and an undersized femoral component, flexion instability may result.

Tibial templating is performed after sizing the femoral component. The tibial component must mate with the femoral component in an acceptable size match, which varies by manufacturer. Undersized tibial components can lead to component subsidence in

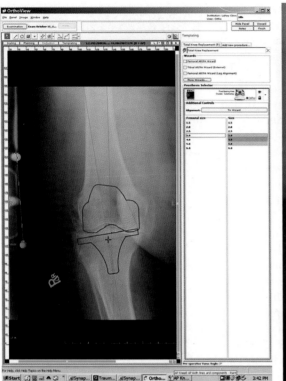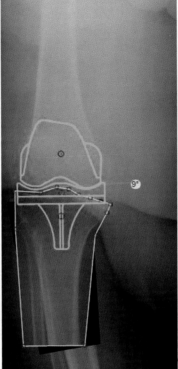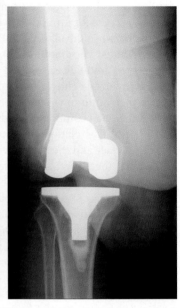

Figure 13 Final templated plan (**A**) and limb alignment correction (**B**) simulated with the selected implants in place. (**C**) AP radiograph obtained after TKA. (TraumaCad, Voyant Health, Columbia, MD.)

the central metaphyseal bone. On the other hand, oversized tibial components are associated with overhang and soft-tissue impingement. This is most common in the posterolateral corner because of the nonanatomic design of some tibial components and the need to externally rotate the component to achieve correct patellofemoral tracking. The slope of the tibial component varies from 0° to 7°, depending on the implant system and surgeon preferences. The relative merits of tibial slope are discussed in the chapters that describe surgical techniques. The effect of tibial slope on templating is twofold: first, in the case of stemmed components, the stem angle, position, and offset will dictate the component location and orientation. Second, the composite component flexion must be assessed on the lateral view. Excess combined flexion can limit full component extension or lead to excess wear of the anterior post in a posterior stabilized implant. After appropriate sizing is determined in both the sagittal and coronal planes, the final tibial and femoral templated sizes and positions are selected using AP radiographic views (**Figure 13**).

Stemmed Implants

The templating process described above works well for planning most TKAs. If stemmed implants are required, however, the surgeon's options for changing the alignment of the implants are limited. The addition of stems often dictates the position and alignment of components relative to the intramedullary canal (**Figure 11**). On the lateral femoral view, for example, the length of the stem relative to the anatomic bow often dictates the flexion-extension axis. When choosing the length of the stem, the surgeon must know whether the femoral stem can be translated relative to the component and, if so, by what degree. The anterior-posterior angle typically is 5° to 7° of valgus from the perpendicular of the distal prosthesis to the stem axis. Similarly, the tibial stem often can push a component posteriorly, requiring a smaller component to prevent posterior tibial overhang. Posterior tibial slope essentially is determined by implant design and is not adjustable.

Tibial defects on the AP view may be addressed by two methods of bypassing areas of deficiency and restoring the joint line to its predisease level. One option is to make a larger, more distal tibial resection and use a slightly larger polyethylene insert. Alternatively, bone graft, cement, or component augments can be used in conjunction with stemmed components.

Avoiding Pitfalls and Complications

Preoperative planning and templating are critical steps in the successful TKA procedure. A detailed patient history and physical examination aids implant selection and helps the surgeon to anticipate any complications that may prevent optimal reconstruction. Whether digital or analog templates are used, the principles of TKA surgical technique must not be sacrificed. The goal of templating remains to mimic and prepare for the planned surgical reconstruction. Preoperative templating can help the surgeon avoid sizing errors that may lead to suboptimal bone resection or inventory problems. With templating, when the templated sizes are outside of the range of the usual stocked inventory, special accommodation can be made to obtain appropriately sized implants prior to TKA. If preoperative templating is not completed, the surgeon may not have access to implants of the correct size for nonroutine patients, which could cause unnecessary delays.

———————■

Bibliography

Benjamin J: Component alignment in total knee arthroplasty. *Instr Course Lect* 2006;55:405-412.

Conn KS, Clarke MT, Hallett JP: A simple guide to determine the magnification of radiographs and to improve the accuracy of preoperative templating. *J Bone Joint Surg Br* 2002;84(2):269-272.

Della Valle CJ, Rosenberg AG: Indications for total knee arthroplasty, in Callaghan JJ, Rosenberg AG, Rubash HE, Simonian PT, Wickiewicz TL, eds: *The Adult Knee.* Philadelphia, PA, Lippincott Williams & Wilkins, 2003.

Healy WL, Anglen JO, Wasilewski SA, Krackow KA: Distal femoral varus osteotomy. *J Bone Joint Surg Am* 1988;70(1): 102-109.

Krackow KA: *The Technique of Total Knee Arthroplasty.* Philadelphia, PA, CV Mosby, 1990.

McAuley J, Eickman T: Choosing your implant, in Insall S, Norman SW, eds: *Surgery of the Knee,* ed 4. Philadelphia, PA, Churchill Livingstone Elsevier, 2006.

Specht LM, Levitz S, Iorio R, Healy WL, Tilzey JF: A comparison of acetate and digital templating for total knee arthroplasty. *Clin Orthop Relat Res* 2007;464:179-183.

Chapter 8

Cruciate-Retaining Total Knee Arthroplasty

Richard D. Scott, MD
C. Lowry Barnes, MD

◼ Indications

Since the advent of condylar total knee arthroplasty (TKA) in the early 1970s, controversy has existed as to whether to routinely preserve, sacrifice, or substitute for the posterior cruciate ligament (PCL). The three schools of thought are as follows: (1) almost always preserve the PCL; (2) routinely substitute for it; (3) either preserve or substitute, depending on individual patient factors such as age, weight, range of motion, and extent of deformity. Cruciate-substituting TKA is discussed in chapter 9.

Preserving the PCL has many potential advantages. Because stability is imparted by a biologic structure, the prosthesis used can be less constrained and therefore there is less force imparted to the insert-tray interface and the prosthesis-bone or bone-cement interface.

With PCL retention, it also is possible to preserve the joint line at a near-normal location. When the PCL is cut, the flexion gap increases and there is a requirement for thicker polyethylene for any given amount of bone resection. The thicker polyethylene in turn requires that more distal femoral resection be performed to allow full extension of the knee. Thus, the joint line is elevated several millimeters in both flexion and extension with cruciate-sacrificing designs, which distorts the collateral ligament kinematics. Although it is possible to equalize the 90° flexion gap with the full extension gap, midflexion laxity is likely to occur to some extent when the joint line is elevated. Finally, cruciate-retaining knees allow for preservation of intercondylar bone stock for future revision, if ever necessary.

Many surgeons have the misconception that all knees with severe angular deformity require PCL sacrifice and substitution, but in fact, in the hands of an experienced surgeon, it is likely that well over 95% of primary knees can be treated with PCL retention. This is because the PCL, to be retained, does not have to be "normal"; it merely needs to provide enough anterior-posterior stability in association with a tibial insert that is curved in the sagittal plane.

In very severe varus knees, the PCL is often encased in intercondylar osteophytes, which must be débrided to define the ligament origin. When medial structures are subsequently released to balance lax lateral structures, the PCL is often too tight relative to these structures and may have to be released to some extent to balance the knee.

In severe valgus deformity, it is not only possible to preserve the PCL, but it may in fact be preferable because of the medial stabilizing force of this ligament. Again, as in severe varus, the ligament often has to be released after the tight lateral side is released, to balance the lax medial side.

There are some potential disadvantages to preservation of the PCL. There is a possibility of late anterior-posterior instability if the PCL stretches out over time or ruptures. This is most likely the result of a combination of a flexion gap initially left too loose and a tibial topography that is flat in the sagittal plane. In addition, if the surgeon inadvertently applies an upslope to the tibial resection, posterior subluxation of the tibia on the femur is more likely.

A second possible disadvantage of PCL retention in the past was the apparent need for more frequent lat-

Dr. Scott or an immediate family member has received royalties from DePuy; serves as a paid consultant to or is an employee of DePuy; and has received nonincome support (such as equipment or services), commercially derived honoraria, or other non–research-related funding (such as paid travel) from ConforMIS and the Scientific Advisory Board. Dr. Barnes or an immediate family member serves as a board member, owner, officer, or committee member of the Southern Orthopaedic Association, the Society for Arthritic Joint Surgery, St. Vincent Infirmary (Little Rock, AR), and the Arkansas Orthopaedic Society; has received royalties from Wright Medical Technology; serves as a paid consultant to or is an employee of Wright Medical Technology; and has received research or institutional support from Johnson & Johnson, Stryker, and Wright Medical Technology.

eral release for patellar tracking. This may have been true for early experience with PCL retention, when proper attention was not given to appropriate femoral and tibial component rotational alignment. With improvements in surgical technique and prosthetic designs that promote better patellar tracking, however, there is no longer a difference in lateral release rate between cruciate-preserving and cruciate-substituting techniques.

A third disadvantage noted two decades ago was the observation of a higher incidence of late topside polyethylene wear. The earliest PCL retention designs had high contact stresses from a round-on-flat articulation, whereas cruciate-substituting designs were more conforming, with lower contact stresses. Retrievals of PCL- retaining knees that failed due to wear showed a common wear pattern. Most of these knees functioned well for several years with excellent range of motion, but patients eventually presented with late posterior wear from excessive rollback of the femur on the tibia combined with the high stresses of a round-on-flat articulation. In early experience with PCL retention, surgeons allowed the knee to adjust to the PCL. If the PCL was left too tight, the femur could have excessive rollback and possible late posterior wear. If the PCL was left too loose, the tibia could subluxate posteriorly and the wear pattern would move forward. This was in combination with the round-on-flat articulation. This experience led to the evolution of PCL-preserving designs with curved tibial topography in the sagittal plane. The knee would no longer adjust to the PCL, but the PCL would have to be adjusted to each knee. Techniques for achieving correct PCL tensioning are described below.

Contraindications and Alternative Treatments

The contraindications to PCL retention are reflected in the indications for substitution advocated by surgeons who normally preserve the PCL. One of these is severe preoperative deformity. This is because it can be easier and more forgiving to balance deformed knees when the PCL has been sacrificed, especially if the surgeon is unhappy with the PCL tensioning. It is good practice to always have a PCL-substituting device available in the operating room. Most PCL-retaining TKA systems offer methods to convert to a PCL-substituting prosthesis with relative ease.

Several other situations contraindicate retention of the PCL. They include knees with severe flexion contractures (greater than 40°), ankylosed knees, postpatellectomy knees in which the PCL lacks normal tension, and most revision TKAs.

Results

The results of TKA with PCL retention using current surgical techniques and prosthetic designs are excellent at 10 to 15 years of follow-up and competitive with results of TKA using PCL-substituting designs. Minimum 10-year results from six published series are provided in **Table 1**.

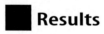

Technique

Exposure
The exposure required for the PCL retention technique is standard and can be accomplished using any of the various approaches described in chapters 1 through 4. The anterior horn of the medial meniscus is excised, and the anterior cruciate ligament, if present, is sacrificed. A 1-cm curved osteotome is passed beneath the deep medial collateral ligament along the top of the medial tibial plateau to the level of the semimembranosus bursa. The tibia can then be delivered in front of the femur by hyperflexing the knee, pulling the tibia forward, and externally rotating it.

Procedure
Following exposure of the knee joint, the bone cuts are performed (whether the femur or tibia is prepared first is according to surgeon preference). When cutting the distal femur, in the absence of a flexion contracture, it is preferable to remove 2 mm less bone than will be replaced by the femoral prosthesis, as this represents the 2 mm of articular cartilage that was present previously on the distal femur. For example, when using a 9-mm-thick femoral component, a 7-mm distal femoral bone resection is performed. This technique will not only most accurately reproduce the correct level of the joint line, but it will also minimize the chance of creating femoral-tibial gaps that are tighter in flexion than in extension, which is the more difficult imbalance to solve. A knee that is tighter in flexion requires one or a combination of maneuvers that include PCL release, downsloping the tibial resection, downsizing the femoral component, or additional tibial resection with distal advancement of the femoral component. A knee that is tighter in extension is usually corrected merely by added distal femoral resection.

At the proximal tibia, an amount of resection equal to the composite thickness of the tibial component to be implanted is removed from the less involved plateau. For example, in a varus knee, a 10-mm resection (including residual cartilage) of the lateral tibial plateau is performed to place a 10-mm composite tibial

Table 1 Results of PCL-Retaining Total Knee Arthroplasty

Author(s) (Year)	Number of Knees	Mean Patient Age in Years (Range)	Mean Follow-up in Years (Range)	Survivorship (%)
Schai et al (1999)	JRA: 14 Adult-onset RA: 67	JRA: 27 (17-37) Adult-onset RA: 61 (37-84)	11 (10-13)	97
Laskin (2001)	100 (56 PCLs retained, 44 PCLs sacrificed)	PCL retained: 69 (62-91) PCL sacrificed: 70 (55-78)	11.2 (10-12)	96
Back et al (2001)	422	69 (46-89)	5.8 (4-9.3)	97
Meding et al (2004)	220	62 (21-85)	10.2 (2-24)	97
Dixon et al (2005)	139	67 (17-89)	15.5 (15-16.9)	93
Rodricks et al (2007)	160	70.5 (34.7-94)	15.8 (14.5-17.3)	92

PCL = posterior cruciate ligament, JRA = juvenile rheumatoid arthritis, RA = rheumatoid arthritis.

component. Following completion of the bone cuts, trial components are inserted and PCL tension may be assessed.

PCL Balancing

Balancing the PCL essentially means leaving the knee with a PCL that is neither too loose nor too tight. Two intraoperative tests, the POLO (for "pull-out lift-off") and slide-back tests, have been described to help the surgeon determine proper PCL tensioning in both fixed-bearing and mobile-bearing PCL-retaining TKAs. As its name implies, the POLO test consists of two parts, pull-out and lift-off.

POLO TEST: PULL-OUT

The knee is flexed to 90° with the trial components in place. A stemless tibial trial is used with a curved or dished trial insert. If a handle is attached to the tibial tray for insertion, this is left in place. If the system being used does not have such a handle, the tray can be grasped with a clamp. An attempt is made to pull out the tibial trial component from under the prosthetic posterior femoral condyles. This essen-

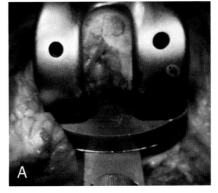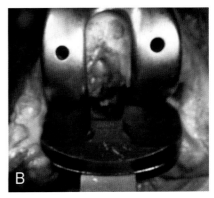

Figure 1 Intraoperative photographs demonstrate the pull-out portion of the POLO test. **A,** Pull-out of the tibial trial of a few millimeters is observed. This indicates appropriate flexion balance. **B,** In this knee, the tibial tray pulls out too easily, suggesting a loose flexion gap. (Reproduced with permission from Scott RD: Posterior cruciate ligament retention vs substitution, in Scott RD: *Total Knee Arthroplasty*. Philadelphia, PA, WB Saunders, 2006, p 12.)

tially measures how easy it is to distract the femur and tibia a certain number of millimeters in flexion depending on the amount of dishing of the insert present in the sagittal plane (**Figure 1,** *A*). If the curved tray can be easily pulled out with the knee in flexion, PCL tension and flexion stability are inadequate (**Figure 1,** *B*). In the same fashion, if the trial tibial component with a curved insert can be easily slid in place under the femoral component while the knee is in 90° of flexion, the gap and PCL are too loose.

If it is determined that the PCL is too loose, the tibial polyethylene thickness should be increased to the point where the tibial trial component cannot be pulled out from under the femur in flexion.

POLO TEST: LIFT-OFF

Following performance of the pull-out test, the handle or clamp is removed from the tibial trial component and the extensor mechanism is reduced into its anatomic position. An everted extensor mechanism may pro-

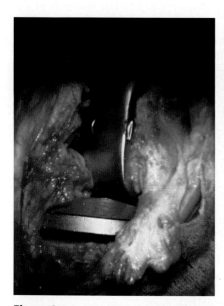

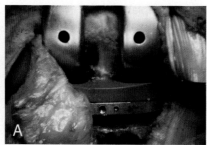

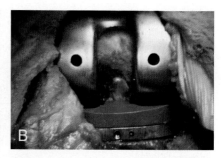

Figure 3 Intraoperative photographs demonstrate flexion gap balancing. **A,** In this knee, the PCL is too tight, pulling the femoral component posteriorly. This forces the tibial tray down posteriorly and up anteriorly (positive lift-off). **B,** After the PCL is released from the femur, the flexion gap is balanced. (Reproduced with permission from Scott RD, Chmell MJ: Balancing the posterior cruciate-retaining fixed and mobile-bearing total knee arthroplasty: Description of the pull-out lift-off and slide-back tests. *J Arthroplasty* 2008;23:605-608. http://www.sciencedirect.com/science/journal/08835403.)

Figure 2 Intraoperative photograph demonstrates positive lift-off with the POLO test. The tibial tray lifts off anteriorly with flexion, indicating the PCL is too tight. (Reproduced with permission from Scott RD: Posterior cruciate ligament retention vs substitution, in Scott RD: *Total Knee Arthroplasty*. Philadelphia, PA, WB Saunders, 2006, p 12.)

duce a falsely positive lift-off test because of the resultant eccentric pull of the patellar tendon upon the tibia; therefore, its reduction before assessing lift-off is crucial. With the knee in flexion between 90° and 100°, the anterior tibial tray–bone interface is examined. If the trial component lifts off the tibial surface anteriorly, the test is positive and the PCL is too tight (**Figure 2**). Lift-off occurs because the tight PCL pulls the femoral component posteriorly against the posterior upslope of the tibial polyethylene insert, forcing the tray down posteriorly and up anteriorly (**Figure 3, A**). When the lift-off test is positive, PCL recession is required. This may be accomplished by several techniques, either from the tibial or femoral attachments. Many surgeons prefer a selective femoral release as this can be done easily with the trials in place and the effect on lift-off can be observed as the release progresses. The tightest fibers

are usually the more lateral and anterior fibers. The release is halted when appropriate tension is achieved (**Figure 3, B**).

In some cases, the PCL will be recessed and not tight to digital palpation, and yet tibial tray lift-off still occurs. This is generally because of impingement of uncapped posterior femoral condylar bone or retained posterior femoral osteophytes on a curved or lipped tibial insert in flexion. In such a case, attention must be directed toward removal of the offending structures, rather than attempts at PCL balancing.

SLIDE-BACK TEST
In mobile-bearing TKAs, the PCL can be balanced using the slide-back test. A trial insert is placed between the femoral and tibial components (without the stabilizing post that confines its mobility in rotating platform designs). The knee is flexed 90°, and the surgeon notes the anterior-posterior position of the insert on the tray. If the PCL is too tight, the insert will slide posteriorly on the tray (**Figure 4, A**). If it is too loose, the insert will slide forward over the front of the tray (**Figure 4, B**). In a well-balanced PCL, the insert is located 1 to 3 mm posterior to the front of the tray (**Figure 4, C**).

Wound Closure
The arthrotomy/extensor mechanism is closed with 3 or 4 nonabsorbable sutures at the superior medial patellar region, and the remainder can be closed with absorbable sutures, being careful to reapproximate appropriately. Following closure, the knee is taken through a range of motion, checking for continuity of repair and also checking for any snapping, clunking, etc. Passive knee flexion against gravity is measured and recorded, as this is the best predictor of an individual patient's postoperative flexion potential. The rest of the wound is closed with absorbable suture and staples or nylon sutures.

Postoperative Regimen

Postoperative care after a PCL-retaining TKA is no different from that for a TKA with PCL substitution. Patients are mobilized quickly, getting up to a chair the evening of surgery or starting therapy on the same day if operated early in the day. Range-of-motion exercises to gain full extension and flexion are started early, and patients are encouraged to aggressively stretch the knee. In addition, patients are encour-

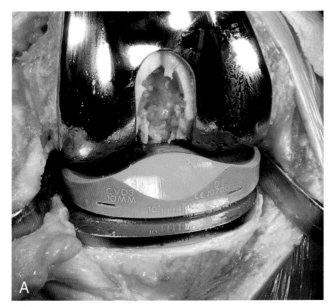

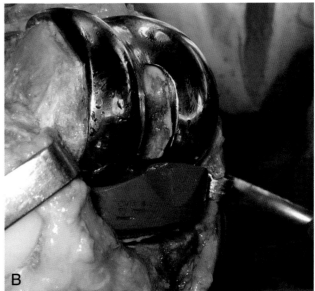

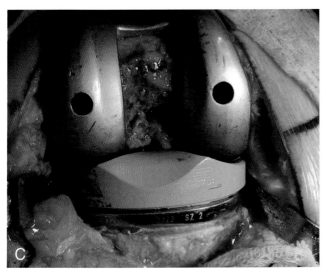

Figure 4 Intraoperative photographs demonstrate the slide-back test. **A,** Excessive posterior translation of the tibial trial indicates that the PCL is too tight. **B,** Anterior translation of the tibial trial suggests that the PCL is too loose. **C,** After appropriate PCL release, the tibial trial is properly positioned on the tibial tray. (Part A reproduced with permission from Scott RD, Chmell MJ: Balancing the posterior cruciate-retaining fixed and mobile-bearing total knee arthroplasty: Description of the pull-out lift-off and slide-back tests. *J Arthroplasty* 2008;23:605-608. http://www.sciencedirect.com/science/journal/08835403. Parts B and C reproduced with permission from Scott RD: Posterior cruciate ligament retention vs substitution, in Scott RD: *Total Knee Arthroplasty*. Philadelphia, PA, WB Saunders, 2006, p 12.)

aged to work on straight-leg raising exercises and short-arc quadriceps exercises as tolerated. Most patients are discharged home on postoperative day 2 or 3 and will use a walker or crutches until ready to progress to a cane in 1 or 2 weeks. They are usually seen daily as an outpatient in physical therapy for about 2 weeks and then 3 times per week for an additional 2 weeks. Patients are encouraged to use a stationary bicycle and to lower the seat to gain more flexion as the knee allows.

Avoiding Pitfalls and Complications

The pitfalls and complications of PCL-retaining TKA mainly occur if the PCL is left too loose or too tight. A lax PCL can lead to flexion instability that can progress over time. Symptoms might consist of a feeling of instability on stairs and inclines and the presence of a chronic effusion. The effusion can be painful.

A tight PCL can cause pain as the patient attempts to regain range of motion. The kinematics of the knee with a tight PCL are abnormal, and excessive rollback may cause the articulation to "book open" as the knee flexes beyond 90°. The problem can be diagnosed by obtaining a lateral radiograph with the knee in maximum flexion. This will show a very posterior contact point between the femur and the tibia.

A late complication that might occur as a result of a tight PCL is accelerated posterior wear of the tibial insert. This could ultimately lead to polyethylene failure.

Finally, when a PCL-retaining TKA is planned that must be converted intraoperatively to a PCL-substitutingdesign, the tibial slope applied for thepreservation technique must be reassessed. Substantial posterior slope is tolerated well with most PCL-retaining designs but can lead to post-cam impingement in most PCL-substituting articulations.

Bibliography

Back DL, Cannon SR, Hilton A, Bankes MJ, Briggs TW: The Kinemax total knee arthroplasty: Nine years experience. *J Bone Joint Surg Br* 2001;83(3):359-363.

Bourne RB, Laskin RS, Guerin JS: Ten-year results of the first 100 Genesis II total knee replacement procedures. *Orthopedics* 2007;30(8 Suppl):83-85.

Dixon MC, Brown RR, Parsch D, Scott RD: Modular fixed-bearing total knee arthroplasty with retention of the posterior cruciate ligament: A study of patients followed for a minimum of fifteen years. *J Bone Joint Surg Am* 2005;87(3):598-603.

Laskin RS: The Genesis total knee prosthesis: A 10-year followup study. *Clin Orthop Relat Res* 2001;388:95-102.

Meding JB, Keating EM, Ritter MA, Faris PM, Berend ME: Long-term followup of posterior-cruciate-retaining TKR in patients with rheumatoid arthritis. *Clin Orthop Relat Res* 2004;428:146-152.

Ritter MA, Faris PM, Keating EM: Posterior cruciate ligament balancing during total knee arthroplasty. *J Arthroplasty* 1988;3(4):323-326.

Rodricks DJ, Patil S, Pulido P, Colwell CW Jr : Press-fit condylar design total knee arthroplasty: Fourteen to seventeen-year follow-up. *J Bone Joint Surg Am* 2007;89(1):89-95.

Schai PA, Scott RD, Thornhill TS: Total knee arthroplasty with posterior cruciate retention in patients with rheumatoid arthritis. *Clin Orthop Relat Res* 1999;367:96-106.

Scott RD: *Total Knee Arthroplasty*. Philadelphia, PA, Elsevier, 2006.

Scott RD, Chmell MJ: Balancing the posterior cruciate ligament during cruciate-retaining fixed and mobile-bearing total knee arthroplasty: Description of the pull-out lift-off and slide-back tests. *J Arthroplasty* 2008;23(4):605-608.

Swany MR, Scott RD: Posterior polyethylene wear in posterior cruciate ligament-retaining total knee arthroplasty: A case study. *J Arthroplasty* 1993;8(4):439-446.

Coding

CPT Code		Corresponding ICD-9 Codes	
	Total Knee Arthroplasty		
27447	Arthroplasty, knee, condyle and plateau; medial AND lateral compartments with or without patella resurfacing (total knee arthroplasty)	715 715.80	715.16 715.89

Chapter 9

Posterior Stabilized Total Knee Arthroplasty

Giles R. Scuderi, MD

William J. Long, MD, FRCSC

■ Indications

Posterior stabilized (also called cruciate-substituting) total knee arthroplasty (TKA) provides a durable reconstruction that can be used in patients with osteoarthritis, rheumatoid arthritis, posttraumatic arthritis, and osteonecrosis. Our indications for a cemented, posterior stabilized TKA include all patients with symptomatic end-stage knee arthritis in whom nonsurgical management has failed.

A posterior stabilized design provides several advantages over cruciate-retaining designs. Soft-tissue balancing is simplified with removal of the posterior cruciate ligament (PCL), because flexion and extension balancing with respect to the retained PCL is not required. Similarly, the PCL is involved in significant angular deformities, and its removal eliminates this deforming structure. Conforming posterior stabilized designs maximize joint contact area, thus decreasing polyethylene stresses and wear of the polyethylene bearing surface.

■ Contraindications

When considering condylar TKA, there are no contraindications specific to a posterior stabilized knee prosthesis. Deep infection is a contraindication to the implantation of any reconstructive system. Deficiency of one or both collateral ligaments may require an increased degree of component stability provided by a constrained condylar or hinged prosthesis.

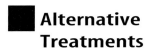

■ Alternative Treatments

Knees with primarily unicompartmental disease may be treated with a partial knee arthroplasty. Long-term studies of certain mobile-bearing prostheses and fixed-bearing unicompartmental arthroplasties for medial compartment disease have shown these procedures to be durable. With newer generations of patellofemoral replacements and better attention to soft-tissue balancing, acceptable results have been achieved for isolated patellofemoral disease. Limited follow-up data are available for new bicompartmental designs.

Cruciate-retaining TKA remains an option in most cases. Long-term studies with this design category also have demonstrated success. In some cases of significant sagittal or coronal plane deformities, it may be difficult to preserve the PCL. Patients with a plano-valgus foot deformity are not good candidates for a cruciate-retaining reconstruction. A meta-analysis of eight randomized trials comparing posterior cruciate–retaining and posterior cruciate–substituting implants failed to demonstrate a significant difference in outcomes.

■ Results

When posterior stabilized prostheses were introduced, the intent was to design implants that provided stair-climbing ability and greater range of motion and prevented tibial subluxation. A study describing 9- to 12-year follow-up with a posterior stabilized prosthesis and an all-polyethylene tibial component demonstrated 87% good to excellent results; an analysis of failures revealed a 3% rate of tibial loosening, which prompted revision to a metal-backed tibial component. In a 10- to 12-year follow-up study on this design, 96% good or excellent re-

Dr. Scuderi or an immediate family member has received royalties from Zimmer, is a member of a speakers' bureau or has made paid presentations on behalf of Zimmer, and serves as a consultant to or is an employee of Zimmer. Dr. Long or an immediate family member is a member of a speakers' bureau or has made paid presentations on behalf of Sanofi-Aventis.

Table 1 Results of Posterior Stabilized Total Knee Arthroplasty

Authors (Year)	Number of Knees	Mean Patient Age in Years (Range)	Mean Follow-up in Months (Range)	Results
Diduch et al (1997)	114	51 (22-55)	96 (36-216)	Survivorship at 18 years: 94% All excellent/good outcomes 3 revisions (2 infection, 1 wear)
Indelli et al (2002)	100	69 (57-85)	90 (64-114)	Survivorship: 92% at 10 years 97% excellent/good results Mean flexion = 116° No cases of aseptic loosening
O'Rourke et al (2002)	176	76 (69-85)	77 (60-95)	Mean flexion = 113° No revisions for osteolysis or aseptic loosening
Fuchs et al (2006)	279	66 (25-89)	48 (24-72)	Average Knee Society knee score: 96 3 late deep infections No other clinical or radiographic complications
Rasquinha et al (2006)	150	70 (29-85)	144 (120-156)	105 knees at follow-up 90% good to excellent Survivorship: 94.6% 5 revisions (2 infection, 1 dislocation, 2 osteolysis)

sults were reported. Two loose femoral components were reported, but no loose tibial components. Long-term follow-up studies of posterior stabilized designs that have been published from several centers have reported 10-year survivorship over 90% (**Table 1**). Multiple joint registries also have demonstrated survivorship over 90% at 10-year follow-up. Further modifications of patellar geometry, posterior femoral condylar offset, tibial shape, and polyethylene conformity have resulted in the modern modular, cemented, posterior stabilized prosthesis. Long-term studies do not yet exist for these designs, but at our center, at a mean follow-up of 48 months, no cases of aseptic loosening, patellar complications, or evidence of osteolysis or wear were reported, and an average Knee Society knee score of 96 was achieved in 238 TKAs.

To examine the hypothesis that the level of activity would influence the longevity of cemented TKA, the long-term results and functional outcome in 108 patients who were 55 years of age or younger at the time of the index procedure were evaluated. This was an active group of patients who regularly participated in exercises that placed high stresses on the articulating surfaces. All patients were rated good to excellent at an average follow-up of 8 years, and the 18-year cumulative survivorship was 94%. Although there was one case of polyethylene wear, there were no cases of aseptic component loosening.

━━━━━━━━━

■ Techniques

Setup/Exposure

Preoperative radiographs are obtained, including a weight-bearing AP view, a lateral view, and a patellar sunrise view. Alignment, correction, and bone cuts are anticipated using templates. A standard TKA setup is used. A sandbag is secured to the table, facilitating knee positioning at 90° of flexion. The leg is draped free, allowing the knee to be placed in a hyperflexed position during the procedure with a padded tourniquet high on the thigh (**Figure 1**).

A midline incision is made from two fingerbreadths above the patella to the tibial tubercle. Limited full-thickness flaps are elevated, followed by a short medial parapatellar approach (**Figure 2**). The distal exposure should be immediately medial to the patellar tendon. This quadriceps incision should be lengthened proximally as necessary for adequate exposure. The lateral edge of the patellar tendon insertion may be released longitudinally to reduce tension during the remainder of the procedure, similar to peeling a banana. A full-thickness subperiosteal dissection is performed along the proximal medial tibia to the semimembranosus bursa. The knee is flexed and externally rotated, and the patella is subluxated laterally. The anterior cruciate ligament is released from the tibia, allowing the tibia to be further subluxated forward.

Medial and lateral retractors are inserted, completing the exposure.

Instruments/Equipment/Implants Required

No specialized equipment is required. Smaller cutting jigs with a lower, contoured profile are helpful with more limited approaches. Bent Hohmann retractors are useful for retraction and protection of the collateral ligaments, while also keeping assistants' hands out of the surgical field. We do not routinely place a posterior retractor when subluxating the tibia forward.

Procedure

Following exposure, a conservative tibial cut is performed, opening up both the flexion and extension spaces. An extramedullary guide is lined up perpendicular to the long axis of the tibia, and a system-specific degree of posterior slope is applied. A stylus is used to measure proximal tibial resection. Approximately 10 mm is measured from the "good" (less involved) side and 2 mm from the involved side. The lesser of these two thicknesses is chosen, the guide is secured, and the cut is made. A Kocher clamp is placed on the medial tibial plateau, and a combined traction and external rotation force is applied. Cautery is used to release the meniscal roots, medial capsule, and proximal PCL insertion, allowing the fragment to be removed whole. This fragment can be used to select the appropriate-sized tibial component.

Attention is then turned to the femur. An intramedullary drill hole is made starting 1 cm anterior to the PCL, just medial to the midline. A step drill is used to "overdrill" the hole to decrease intramedullary canal pressure and fat embolization during insertion of the guide rod. The intramedullary guide is inserted atraumatically by hand. If significant resistance is encountered, the radiographs should be reexamined for excessive femoral bow, and the starting point

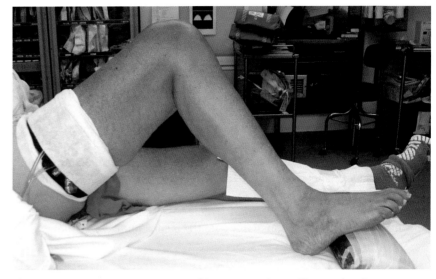

Figure 1 Preparation and positioning of the extremity for total knee arthroplasty.

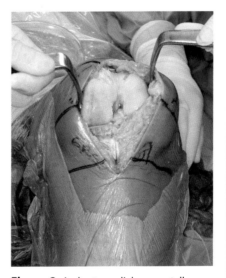

Figure 2 A short medial parapatellar approach.

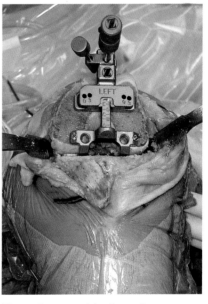

Figure 3 Sizing of the femoral component. The larger size is used when the measurement of the femur falls between sizes and notching is a concern.

and insertion angle should be reviewed. A distal femoral cut is made, usually between 4° and 6° of anatomic valgus, depending on the preexisting deformity. Some systems introduce slight flexion into the distal femoral resection to reduce the chance of notching the anterior femur.

The femoral sizer is applied with the "feet" applied to the central portions of the posterior condyles. A stylus is placed on the anterior femur to determine the appropriate femoral size. It is important to remember that

when the measurement falls between sizes, the closer size is chosen. If there is any concern regarding notching, the larger femoral component size is selected (**Figure 3**). Femoral component rotation is determined with reference to the epicondylar axis, the anterior-posterior axis of the femur, or a combination of the two. The sizer is removed and the rotational axis of the femur is confirmed. The femoral cutting guide is applied, and anterior and posterior cuts are made in a standard fashion.

The knee is then placed at 90° of flexion. A laminar spreader is placed in the lateral joint space. An osteotome is used to remove notch osteophytes and expose the cruciate ligaments (**Figure 4**). First the anterior cruciate ligament and then the PCL are resected from the femur. It is imperative to remain "on bone" and not to wander into posterior soft tissue

and fat, where the important neurovascular structures lie. A Kocher clamp is used to apply tension to the resected PCL stump, and resection proceeds along its posterior margin and the posterior margin of the ligament of Wrisberg, toward the meniscal-capsular junction of the lateral meniscus (**Figure 5**). The medial meniscus is then resected, taking care not to damage the medial collateral ligament. Posteromedial osteophytes are removed. A laminar spreader is placed in the medial joint space, allowing re-

moval of the remaining lateral meniscus while protecting the popliteal tendon, followed by any posterolateral osteophytes. Removal of thickened capsule and osteophytes is necessary to recreate the flexion space, thus allowing impingement-free flexion and extension. The flexion space symmetry from medial to lateral is then compared visually.

A spacer block is inserted and straight rods are used to assess limb alignment, followed by gap balancing (**Figure 6**). Any necessary adjustments are then made—either recutting bone to correct for alignment, or releasing contracted ligaments to correct for soft-tissue balancing.

In cases of fixed varus contractures, a medial release is performed from the tibia. A 1-in osteotome and a mallet are used to perform a subperiosteal release of the superficial medial collateral ligament and pes anserinus tendon insertions. A complete medial release may extend 15 cm or more distal to the joint line and may require further subperiosteal release around the posteromedial tibia including the semimembranosus insertion, resulting in skeletonization of the proximal medial tibia.

When addressing valgus contractures, a lateral "pie-crusting" method is used. Care is taken not to overpenetrate in the posterolateral aspect of

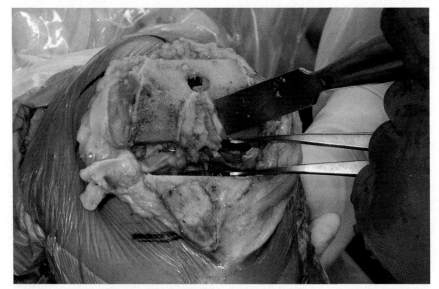

Figure 4 The knee is flexed to 90° and a laminar spreader is placed in the lateral joint space. An osteotome is used to remove notch osteophytes.

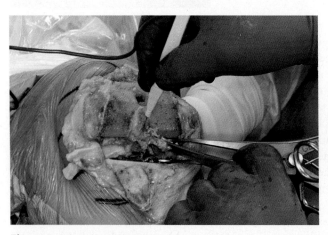
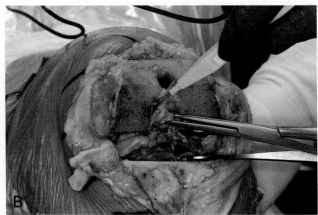

Figure 5 Subperiosteal removal of the cruciate ligaments from the femoral notch. **A,** Removal of the anterior cruciate ligament. **B,** Removal of the posterior cruciate ligament.

the joint where the peroneal nerve is at risk. In cases with a major valgus deformity (>20°), particularly when associated with a flexion contracture, a lateral epicondylar osteotomy is used instead of pie-crusting. The osteotomized fragment is not fixed down, but is allowed to "float" freely on the remaining soft-tissue attachments.

Once soft-tissue balancing is completed, the knee is flexed and the femoral finishing and box-cutting guide is applied. The femoral component should be aligned with the lateral edge of the lateral condyle, thus improving patellofemoral mechanics and avoiding medial overhang (**Figure 7**). The box cut and chamfer cuts are performed, and the lug holes are drilled. The intramedullary guide hole may be filled with a bone plug fashioned from resected bone.

The knee is then externally rotated and hyperflexed with an anterior force applied to the femur. This subluxates the tibia forward, allowing full exposure to the tibia. A tibial template is selected based on the size of the previously resected fragment. It is applied with rotation centered on the medial third of the tibial tubercle and the anterior tibial crest. The largest tibial component that does not overhang medially or in the anterior-posterior plane is selected. Most tibial baseplates are not side-specific, and overhang the posterolateral tibia slightly, which is acceptable. The template is fixed in place and an alignment rod is applied to confirm a perpendicular cut and appropriate rotation. The reamer and punch are then inserted to complete preparation of the proximal tibia. The template is removed and a tibial trial is inserted. Uncovered medial oseophytes are removed with a rongeur or saw. A trial femoral component and polyethylene insert of appropriate thickness are inserted, and the knee is reduced. Soft-tissue balance is assessed in both flexion and extension, as is patellar tracking.

The patella is then addressed. Patellar thickness is measured, and re-

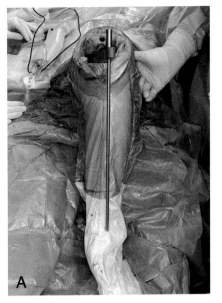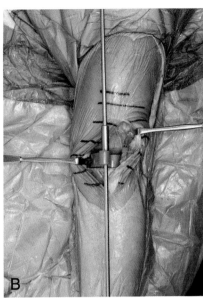

Figure 6 Alignment and gaps are assessed using a spacer block and alignment rods. **A,** With the knee in 90° of flexion, a tibial alignment rod demonstrates a perpendicular tibial surface. **B,** With the knee in extension, external alignment rods demonstrate a neutral mechanical axis and balanced soft tissues.

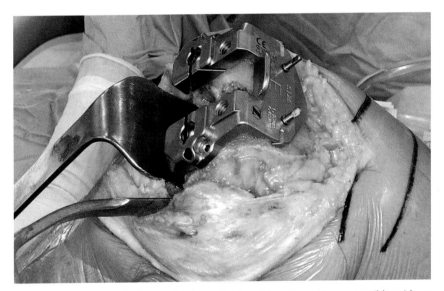

Figure 7 The femoral finishing guide is applied in as lateral a position as possible, without overhanging the cut surface of the lateral condyle.

section with a reamer or a saw is performed to recreate a patellar height within 2 mm of the existing thickness. The patellar template is applied in a relatively medial and superior position, while ensuring that the component is fully covered by bone. Uncovered lateral patellar bone is beveled

with a saw, reducing impingement on the lateral femoral condyle.

The trial patellar component is inserted and range of motion, stability, and patellar tracking are again assessed. One of two tests can be used to assess tibial-femoral flexion stability: The knee can be placed in the figure-

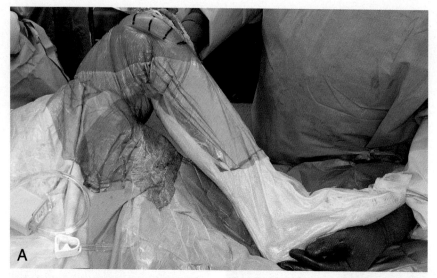

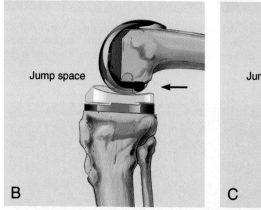
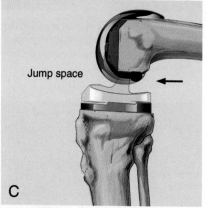

Figure 8 A, The figure-of- 4 test for flexion instability. **B,** Schematic demonstrating the jump space between the femoral cam and tibial post. **C,** The femoral cam should not rise more than halfway up the tibial post with the knee at 90° of flexion and with an upward distraction force applied to the femur.

of-4 position to look for excess lateral laxity, or the jump space can be assessed. With the knee at 90° of flexion, the femur is elevated (**Figure 8**, *A*), and if the femoral cam rises more than halfway up the tibial post, adjustments are necessary to prevent flexion instability (**Figure 8**, *B* and *C*). Care must be taken to ensure that the knee comes out into full extension without impingement of the femoral component on the tibial post (**Figure 9**). Early impingement can occur with excessive posterior tibial slope or a flexed femoral component.

Trial components are removed. Pulsatile irrigation is performed and the bony surfaces are prepared for component insertion. The cement is prepared, and the components are inserted sequentially, beginning with the tibia, then the femur, and finally the patella. Excess cement is removed. A trial insert is placed and the knee is held in full extension while the cement hardens. Appropriate soft-tissue balance, range of motion, and patellar tracking are confirmed. The trial insert is removed, along with any excess cement, and pulsatile irrigation is

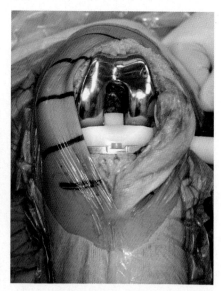

Figure 10 The completed reconstruction with the knee at 90° of flexion. Note that all components are seated securely with no soft-tissue entrapment.

Figure 9 With the final components in place, the leg is brought out into full extension to ensure that no impingement occurs.

again performed. The final polyethylene insert is placed with care to ensure complete seating without soft-tissue entrapment (**Figure 10**).

Wound Closure

The knee is flexed and the tourniquet is released. Hemostasis is obtained, ensuring that there is no significant bleeding, in particular from the inferolateral geniculate artery and the middle geniculate artery in the notch. A drain is inserted and care is taken to close the medial arthrotomy in an anatomic fashion with the sutures placed obliquely from proximal-medial to distal-lateral; this gives a mechanical advantage to the vastus medialis obliquus. A meticulous, layered interrupted closure is then performed, followed by staples and a sterile compressive dressing.

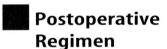

Postoperative Regimen

Radiographs are obtained in the recovery area. All patients are mobilized, allowing weight bearing as tolerated with aids, the evening of surgery or the next morning. Continuous passive motion is begun the evening of surgery and continued intermittently for 6 to 8 hours a day for the duration of the hospital stay.

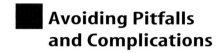

Avoiding Pitfalls and Complications

Inadequate exposure, component malalignment, and soft-tissue imbalance remain the main pitfalls of posterior stabilized TKA. Each of these concerns can be addressed with attention to surgical technique.

Coronal plane imbalances are corrected by releasing the tight side and inserting a thicker polyethylene. In some selected elderly, low-demand patients with a major valgus deformity, limited lateral soft-tissue sleeve piecrusting may be performed, with some residual imbalance left incompletely released, and a constrained condylar component inserted.

Flexion-extension imbalances may also occur. When the flexion space exceeds the extension space, a larger femoral component is necessary. Alternatively, more distal femur can be resected, thus creating symmetric laxity, which is addressed with a thicker polyethylene. When the extension space is greater than the flexion space, the distal femur can be augmented. This may also be addressed by downsizing the femoral component, again creating symmetric laxity that is addressed with a thicker polyethylene.

In obese female patients, laxity may exist in soft tissues following bony resections. To prevent this problem, in these cases a more conservative tibial resection is performed. In valgus knees, a more limited medial exposure and careful protection of the attenuated medial collateral ligament is important. In these knees we do not "spin out" the tibia during exposure.

Lateral patellar tracking, subluxation, or dislocation with range of motion is less common with appropriate attention to femoral and tibial component rotational alignment. In cases of persistent maltracking, a lateral patellar release is performed. An attempt is made to protect the superolateral geniculate arteries, but these may be a persistent tether and require transection. We have noted a greater need for lateral patellar release in valgus knees with larger femoral components. Our rate of lateral release has been reduced with attention to surgical technique.

Bibliography

Baldini A, Scuderi GR, Aglietti P, Chalnick D, Insall JN: Flexion-extension gap changes during total knee arthroplasty: Effect of posterior cruciate ligament and posterior osteophytes removal. *J Knee Surg* 2004;17(2):69-72.

Colizza WA, Insall JN, Scuderi GR: The posterior stabilized total knee prosthesis: Assessment of polyethylene damage and osteolysis after a ten-year-minimum follow-up. *J Bone Joint Surg Am* 1995;77(11):1713-1720.

Diduch DR, Insall JN, Scott WN, Scuderi GR, Font-Rodriguez D: Total knee replacement in young, active patients: Long-term follow-up and functional outcome. *J Bone Joint Surg Am* 1997;79(4):575-582.

Fuchs R, Mills EL, Clarke HD, Scuderi GR, Scott WN, Insall JN: A third-generation, posterior-stabilized knee prosthesis: Early results after follow-up of 2 to 6 years. *J Arthroplasty* 2006;21(6):821-825.

Furnes O, Espehaug B, Lie SA, Vollset SE, Engesaeter LB, Havelin LI: Failure mechanisms after unicompartmental and tricompartmental primary knee replacement with cement. *J Bone Joint Surg Am* 2007;89(3):519-525.

Indelli PF, Aglietti P, Buzzi R, Baldini A: The Insall-Burstein II prosthesis: A 5- to 9-year follow-up study in osteoarthritic knees. *J Arthroplasty* 2002;17(5):544-549.

Jacobs WC, Clement DJ, Wymenga AB: Retention versus sacrifice of the posterior cruciate ligament in total knee replacement for treatment of osteoarthritis and rheumatoid arthritis. *Cochrane Database Syst Rev* 2005;4:CD004803.

O'Rourke MR, Callaghan JJ, Goetz DD, Sullivan PM, Johnston RC: Osteolysis associated with a cemented modular posterior-cruciate-substituting total knee design: Five to eight-year follow-up. *J Bone Joint Surg Am* 2002;84-A(8):1362-1371.

Rand JA, Trousdale RT, Ilstrup DM, Harmsen WS: Factors affecting the durability of primary total knee prostheses. *J Bone Joint Surg Am* 2003;85-A(2):259-265.

Rasquinha VJ, Ranawat CS, Cervieri CL, Rodriguez JA: The press-fit condylar modular total knee system with a posterior cruciate-substituting design: A concise follow-up of a previous report. *J Bone Joint Surg Am* 2006;88(5):1006-1010.

Robertsson O, Knutson K, Lewold S, Lidgren L: The Swedish Knee Arthroplasty Register 1975-1997: An update with special emphasis on 41,223 knees operated on in 1988-1997. *Acta Orthop Scand* 2001;72(5):503-513.

Stern SH, Insall JN: Posterior stabilized prosthesis: Results after follow-up of nine to twelve years. *J Bone Joint Surg Am* 1992;74(7):980-986.

Tenholder M, Clarke HD, Scuderi GR: Minimal-incision total knee arthroplasty: The early clinical experience. *Clin Orthop Relat Res* 2005;440:67-76.

Coding

CPT Code		Corresponding ICD-9 Codes	
27447	Arthroplasty, knee, condyle and plateau; medial AND lateral compartments with or without patella resurfacing (total knee arthroplasty)	715 715.80	715.16 715.89

Chapter 10
Mobile-Bearing Total Knee Arthroplasty

John J. Callaghan, MD
Steve S. Liu, MD

Indications

Mobile-bearing total knee arthroplasty (TKA) was developed to minimize the two most common problems recognized with TKA in the early to mid-1970s, wear and loosening. At the time, there were two basic philosophies in knee prosthesis design. One concept was to use a relatively flat articulating tibial surface and preserve the posterior cruciate ligament; the other was to use a conforming articulating tibial surface and sacrifice the posterior cruciate ligament. The potential problem with the flat articulation was increased polyethylene contact stress and polyethylene wear; the potential problem with the conforming surface was increased prosthesis-bone or prosthesis–cement interface stress and component loosening. The mobile-bearing concept allowed the design of a conforming articulating surface between the femoral component and the tibial articulating surface while allowing motion between the tibial polyethylene component and the tibial metal tray (**Figure 1**). The femoral-tibial conformity could potentially decrease wear, and the mo-

tion of the tibial polyethylene component within the tibial tray could potentially decrease stress on the implant or implant–cement composite to bone. One early mobile-bearing articulation was available in two designs: as a meniscal-bearing design with independent medial and lateral polyethylene components tracking in independent tibial tray tracks, and as a rotating-platform design with a polyethylene component that had an inferior cone that articulated with a female housing unit in the tibial tray, allowing only rotational motion around the central axis of the knee. Over time, the rotating-platform designs became the most commonly used devices and remain so today.

The indications for mobile-bearing TKA are similar to the indications for a fixed-bearing design. These indications include end-stage arthritis of the knee unresponsive to exercises, injections, and anti-inflammatory medications. With the original rotating-platform knee designs, few options for increasing the constraint were available other than deepening the tibial polyethylene insert. Hence, the main indication for these early designs in

most surgeons' hands was in patients without large deformities. Today, with longer stems and the availability of posterior stabilized and constrained condylar designs, these indications can be expanded.

Contraindications

Most of the contraindications for a mobile-bearing knee prosthesis are the same as for a fixed-bearing device. These include active sepsis and some neurologic conditions; however, with constraint, we have used mobile-

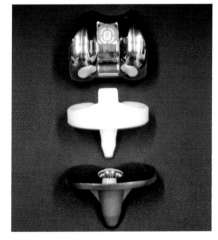

Figure 1 Contemporary posterior stabilized rotating-platform mobile-bearing knee prosthesis.

Dr. Callaghan or an immediate family member has received royalties from DePuy; serves as a paid consultant for or is an employee of DePuy; and has received research or institutional support from Biomet, DePuy, Medtronic, Synthes, Zimmer, Arthrosurface, and LifeNet Health. Neither Dr. Liu nor any immediate family member has received anything of value from or owns stock in a commercial company or institution related directly or indirectly to the subject of this chapter.

Table 1 Results for Mobile-Bearing Total Knee Arthroplasty

Authors (Year)	Number of Knees	Type of Implant	Mean Patient Age in Years (Range)	Follow-up in Years	Results
Sorrells et al (2004)	528	Uncemented LCS rotating-platform with rotating patellar component	69 (29-98)	5-12	89.5% survivorship at 12 years (revision for any reason) 1 revision for aseptic loosening 1 radiographic loosening 1 radiographic osteolysis
Callaghan et al (2005)	119	Cemented LCS rotating-platform with Townley all-polyethylene patella	70 (37-88)	≥ 15	97% survivorship at 15 years (reoperation for any reason) No revisions for aseptic loosening No radiographic loosening 3 radiographic osteolysis
Hooper et al (2009)	244	LCS mobile-bearing, both meniscal-bearing and rotating-platform	66.9 (26-87)	≥ 10	98% survivorship at 12 years (revision for aseptic loosening) 4 revisions for aseptic loosening No radiographic loosening 3 radiographic osteolysis
Callaghan et al (in press)	119	Cemented LCS rotating-platform with Townley all-polyethylene patella	70 (37-88)	≥ 20	97% survivorship at 15 years (reoperation for any reason) No revisions for aseptic loosening 1 radiographic loosening 6 radiographic osteolysis

LCS = Low Contact Stress (DePuy, Warsaw, IN).

bearing devices in some patients with polio, Charcot joints, and multiple sclerosis. The benefit we hope to achieve with these designs is decreased polyethylene wear and decreased implant loosening. Furthermore, because mobile-bearing designs are more costly than fixed-bearing designs, we tend to use them in younger patients (<65 years).

The biggest concern with mobile-bearing TKAs is the potential for bearing spinout with a loose or asymmetric flexion gap. Thus, larger deformities (varus and valgus), especially in elderly patients, are considered relative contraindications for these devices.

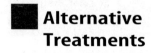

Alternative Treatments

In patients with unicompartmental end-stage arthritis, especially younger patients, osteotomy and unicompartmental replacement can be considered. The use of mobile-bearing devices may not be warranted in elderly patients (>70 years old) because of the potential risk of bearing spinout and the higher cost; fixed-bearing prostheses are indicated in this patient population.

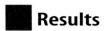

Results

Although mobile-bearing TKA has gained considerable interest among orthopaedic surgeons over the last 5 to 10 years, early mobile-bearing designs were used very selectively in the United States; for that reason, there are few studies of long-term results (Table 1). We reviewed the results of one rotating-platform design implanted in 119 knees by a single surgeon. All components were cemented,

and a cemented all-polyethylene patellar component of another design was used rather than a metal-backed mobile-bearing patellar component. In our published, minimum 15-year-results study, only three reoperations had been performed—two for periprosthetic fracture and one for hematogenous infection where bearing exchange was performed—no components had been removed over the entire follow-up interval, and there were no bearing spinouts. At further follow-up to 20 years, there have been no further reoperations; osteolysis prevalence has increased from 3 to 6 knees. In a minimum 10-year follow-up study of mobile-bearing implants in which meniscal-bearing as well as rotating-platform designs were used (192 knees followed), the survival at 10 years for wear or loosening was 97%, and for reoperation, 92%. Most, if not all, of these components were uncemented. There were three bearing spinouts. When comparing

Table 2 Results for Fixed-Bearing Knees at Long-Term Follow-up

Authors (Year)	Number of Knees	Implant	Diagnosis	Mean Patient Age in Years (Range)	Mean Follow-up in Years (Range)	Survivorship
Miyasaka et al (1997)	108 (60 at 10-year follow-up)	Cemented total condylar knee with all-polyethylene tibial components for valgus deformities	62% RA 35% OA 3% PA	61 (34-82)	14.1 (10-20)	81.9% at 17.6 years (revision for any reason) 87% at 17.1 years (revision for aseptic loosening) 3 revisions for aseptic loosening 4 radiographic loosening No radiographic osteolysis
Gill et al (1999)	159 (72 at 16-year follow-up)	Cemented total condylar knee	94% OA 4% RA 2% PA	61 (30-80)	17 (15-22)	98.6% at 20 years (revision for any reason) No revisions for aseptic loosening No radiographic loosening Radiographic osteolysis NR
Pavone et al (2001)	120 (34 at 19-year follow-up)	Cemented total condylar knee	43% OA 56% RA 1% JRA	65 (30-85)	14 (2-23)	91% at 23 years (revision for any reason) 4 revisions for aseptic loosening 4 radiographic loosening 9 radiographic osteolysis (6 tibial, 3 patellar)
Ma et al (2005)	126 (64 at 19-year follow-up)	Cemented total condylar knee	81% OA 17% RA 2% PA	59 (43-82)	19 (17-22)	83.2% at 20 years (revision for any reason) 91.9% at 20 years (revision for mechanical failure) 1 revision for aseptic loosening 1 radiographic loosening 2 radiographic osteolysis

RA = rheumatoid arthritis, OA = osteoarthritis, PA = posttraumatic arthritis, NR = not reported, JRA = juvenile rheumatoid arthritis.

our 20-year report with the long-term follow-up of fixed-bearing designs, the results are at least comparable. The one caveat in this regard is that the patients in our study group were older, with an average age at the time of surgery of 70 years compared with 59 to 65 years for the fixed-bearing designs (**Table 2**).

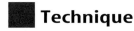

■ Technique

Setup/Exposure
A tourniquet is used if the patient has good pulses, no posterior knee vascular calcifications, and no neurologic deficits, including no peripheral neuropathy. Also, in the patient with ex-

tremely large thighs and short stature, no tourniquet is used. A midline incision with medial patellar arthrotomy is performed. In the larger patient, the proximal incision begins more laterally so that a subcutaneous lateral pouch can be made to evert the patella into the pouch rather than over the skin laterally.

Instruments/Equipment/ Implants Required
The instruments to implant a mobile-bearing knee are no different than those for a fixed-bearing knee. The important difference with mobile-bearing instrumentation is to have trialing systems that simulate the mobile-bearing motion and, most important, the ability to simulate spinout

if the gap balancing is not sufficiently tight or is too tight in flexion.

Procedure
After performing a medial parapatellar arthrotomy that extends 3 to 4 cm proximally to the patella and distally to the tibial tubercle, further exposure is obtained by removing medial femoral and tibial osteotphytes and removing half the fat pad. In a varus knee, the medial collateral ligament is incised off the proximal tibia for 4 to 5 cm distally, extending the release more distally if needed to balance the medial side of the knee to the loose lateral side. The release is extended around the posterior medial tibial plateau and can include the indirect head of semimembranosus in the tight knee. The

patella is then osteotomized, leaving the same amount of bone medially, laterally, inferiorly, and superiorly. The composite thickness of the patella and patellar component mimics the natural patellar thickness when possible. Next, the extension gap is created by cutting first the proximal tibia and then the distal femur (**Figure 2**). In the case of a varus knee, approximately 12 mm of lateral tibial bone and 8 to 10 mm of distal medial femoral bone is removed. We typically use a 7° valgus alignment jig on the femur and a neutral cutting jig on the tibia and do not set the jig to incorporate posterior tibial slope. Laminar spreaders are used to ensure medial-lateral balancing, followed by an extension block (**Figure 3**) to ensure medial and lateral balance and achievement of full extension. Anterior referencing is used to size the femoral component, placing it along the epicondylar axis for rotation. A preliminary check of the flexion gap is performed with the knee in 90° of flexion, placing the flexion block below the anteroposterior cutting block to ensure a symmetric cut to the tibia and a snug flexion gap (**Figure 4**). Anterior and posterior cuts are made on the femur, and the

flexion gap is assessed with laminar spreaders (**Figure 5**) for medial-lateral tensioning and a flexion block (**Figure 6**) to ensure appropriate tightness in flexion. After preparing chamfer cuts and cruciate-substituting femoral box cuts, trialing is performed. In addition to ensuring full extension and at least 120° of flexion with good medial-lateral stability throughout, the knee

is checked for maximum hyperflexion, with the patella located to ensure no bearing spinout. Rotation for the tibial tray is checked in extension and flexion. Tibial preparation is performed, attempting to place the tray in neutral rotation, although this does not need to be quite as precise with a rotating-platform knee because the polyethylene will self-center. After ce-

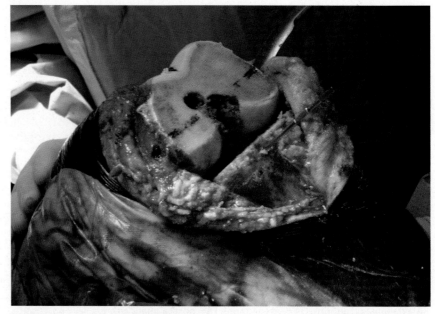

Figure 2 Left knee with medial release, proximal tibial resection, and distal femoral resection.

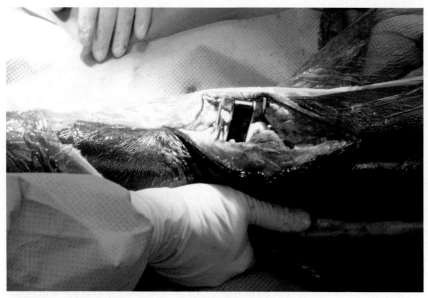

Figure 3 Evaluation of extension gap with spacer block.

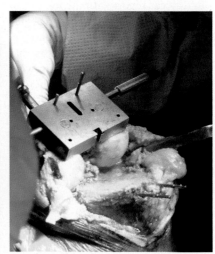

Figure 4 Anteroposterior cutting block in place using the epicondyles for rotation. Appropriate posterior femoral resection ensures tight flexion gap.

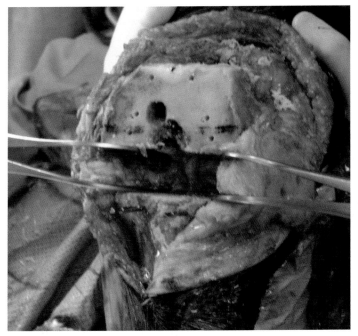

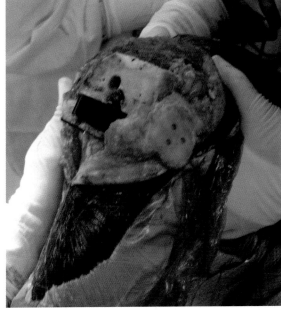

Figure 6 Femoral spacer block demonstrating snug flexion gap.

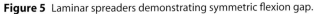

Figure 5 Laminar spreaders demonstrating symmetric flexion gap.

menting the components and trialing the tibial insert to ensure bearing stability (**Figure 7**), the polyethylene insert is placed in the tibial tray (**Figure 8**), avoiding the introduction of third-body particulates between the polyethylene insert and tray. The feel of a snapping sensation when reducing the tibia under the femur in 90° of flexion should ensure adequate tightness of the flexion gap so that bearing spinout does not occur. Before closure, the knee should be brought to hyperflexion to check for any clicking or bearing subluxation or spinout. If clicking occurs, the popliteal tendon should be evaluated (rarely, impingement occurs there). If the bearing insert subluxates or dislocates, a thicker bearing insert may be needed. Occasionally, bearing insert dislocation occurs when the knee is too tight in flexion, and this also should be evaluated. **Figure 9** illustrates a case in which a rotating-platform TKA was used in a patient with osteoarthritis.

Wound Closure

Closure is routine. We use two drains, 1-0 absorbable interrupted suture for fascia closure, 2-0 interrupted absorbable suture for subcutaneous tissue closure, running 3-0 absorbable suture for subcuticular closure, staples, fluffs, and a cotton batting dressing.

Postoperative Regimen

The postoperative regimen for mobile-bearing primary TKA is the same as for routine fixed-bearing TKA. Patients are weight-bearing with crutches until they obtain adequate quadriceps function, at which time they are switched to a cane. They receive physical therapy three times per week and stop using a cane when ambulating well without assistive devices.

Avoiding Pitfalls and Complications

The only complication that is specific to mobile-bearing TKA is bearing spinout. It is avoided by creating a symmetric flexion gap that is snug at 90°. Testing flexion stability (maximum flexion) with trials and final components is essential.

Acknowledgment

The authors would like to thank Christopher Wells, BA, for his help in preparing this chapter.

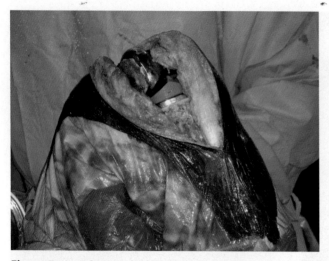

Figure 7 Hyperflexion of the knee demonstrates secure bearing liner with trial.

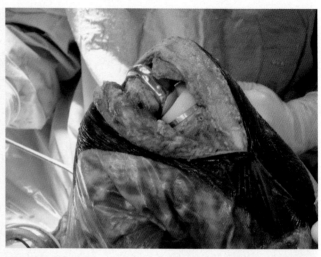

Figure 8 Hyperflexion of the knee demonstrates secure tibial insert with no bearing spinout.

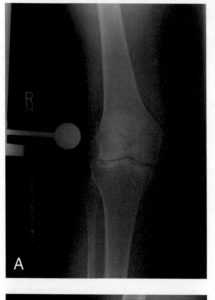

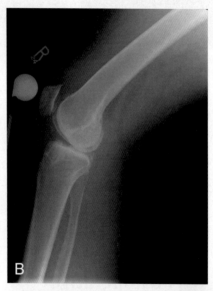

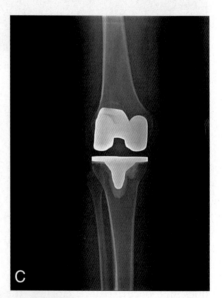

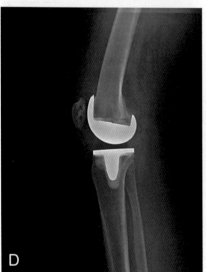

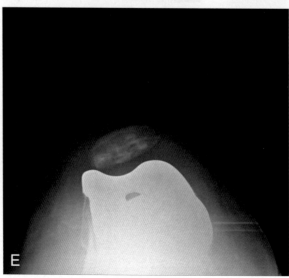

Figure 9 Preoperative AP (**A**) and lateral (**B**) and postoperative AP (**C**), lateral (**D**), and Merchant (**E**) views of a 61-year-old woman who underwent rotating-platform TKA for osteoarthritis.

■ Bibliography

Callaghan JJ, O'Rourke MR, Iossi MF, et al: Cemented rotating-platform total knee replacement: A concise follow-up, at a minimum of fifteen years, of a previous report. *J Bone Joint Surg Am* 2005;87:1995-1998.

Callaghan JJ, Wells CW, Liu SS, Goetz DD, Johnston RC. Cemented rotating platform total knee replacement: A minimum twenty year follow-up study. (Submitted to *J Bone Joint Surg Am.*)

Gill GS, Joshi AB, Mills DM: Total condylar knee arthroplasty: 16- to 21-year results. *Clin Orthop Relat Res* 1999;367: 210-215.

Hooper G, Rothwell A, Frampton C: The low contact stress mobile-bearing total knee replacement: A prospective study with a minimum follow-up of ten years. *J Bone Joint Surg Br* 2009;91:58-63.

Ma HM, Lu YC, Ho FY, Huang CH: Long-term results of total condylar knee arthroplasty. *J Arthroplasty* 2005;20:580-584.

Miyasaka KC, Ranawat CS, Mullaji A: 10- to 20-year followup of total knee arthroplasty for valgus deformities. *Clin Orthop Relat Res* 1997;345:29-37.

Pavone V, Boettner F, Fickert S, Sculco TP: Total condylar knee arthroplasty: A long-term followup. *Clin Orthop Relat Res* 2001;388:18-25.

Ritter MA: The anatomical graduated component total knee replacement: A long-term evaluation with 20-year survival analysis. *J Bone Joint Surg Br* 2009;91:745-749.

Ritter MA, Meneghini RM: Twenty-year survivorship of cementless anatomic graduated component total knee arthroplasty [published online ahead of print May 6, 2009]. *J Arthroplasty.*

Rodriguez JA, Bhende H, Ranawat CS: Total condylar knee replacement: A 20-year followup study. *Clin Orthop Relat Res* 2001;(388):10-17.

Sorrells RB, Voorhorst PE, Murphy JA, Bauschka MP, Greenwald AS: Uncemented rotating-platform total knee replacement: A five- to twelve-year follow-up study. *J Bone Joint Surg Am* 2004;86-A(10):2156-2162.

Coding				
CPT Codes			**Corresponding ICD-9 Codes**	
27447	Arthroplasty, knee, condyle and plateau; medial AND lateral compartments with or without patella resurfacing (total knee arthroplasty)		715 715.80	715.16 715.89

Chapter 11

Total Knee Arthroplasty: Tibial Component Design

Thomas S. Thornhill, MD
John P. Dunleavy, MD

Introduction

The design of total knee arthroplasty (TKA) components has evolved in response to improved understanding of failure mechanisms, in particular aseptic implant loosening secondary to implant wear and osteolysis, which was a major cause of failure in otherwise well-functioning implants in earlier reports of TKA. Component design flaws contributed to these early failures. Changes have been made to tibial component design over time with the intent to decrease aseptic loosening, thereby improving implant longevity.

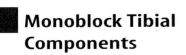

Monoblock Tibial Components

Most of the earliest metal-on-polyethylene TKA designs used separate implants for the medial and lateral compartments. In the late 1970s, after concern arose about tibial component aseptic loosening in these two-piece designs, all-polyethylene, one-piece

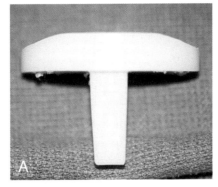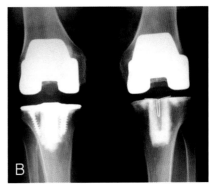

Figure 1 **A,** Photograph of an all-polyethylene tibial component. **B,** AP radiograph shows an all-polyethylene tibial component in the left knee and a metal-backed tibial component in the right knee. (Courtesy of Merrill Ritter, MD, Mooresville, IN.)

tibial components were adopted. Studies soon elucidated the biomechanical benefits of backing the plastic component with a metal tray. Soon, nonmodular metal-backed tibial components were in wide use, although relatively few sizes were available. Still, both types of nonmodular components continued to enjoy popularity for a variety of reasons.

All-Polyethylene

Polyethylene wear from the articular surface leading to implant failure was

a major concern with early TKA designs. The all-polyethylene tibial components (**Figure 1**) were designed with a high degree of conformity to the corresponding femoral component in an attempt to increase contact area and minimize surface contact stresses. The greater plastic thickness permitted by the all-polyethylene components may have been an advantage over metal-backed components, and many were implanted with good results. One review of 144 posterior cruciate–retaining condylar knees reported 94.5% good or excellent results at minimum 7-year follow-up, with only three tibial component revisions. Moreover, polyethylene wear rates from the tibiofemoral interface were relatively low. The failures of the all-polyethylene tibial components that

Dr. Thornhill or an immediate family member is a board member, owner, officer, or committee member for the Brigham and Women's PO Board; has received royalties from DePuy; is a paid consultant for or is an employee of DePuy; owns stock or stock options in SAB ConFormis; and has received nonincome support (such as equipment or services), commercially derived honoraria, or other non–research-related funding (such as paid travel) from DePuy. Dr. Dunleavy or an immediate family member has received research or institutional support from DePuy.

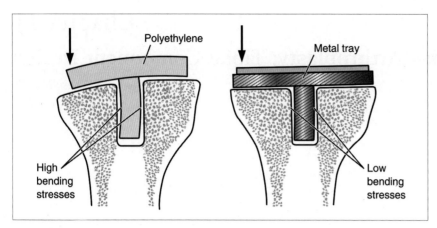

Figure 2 Schematic shows the effect of bending load (arrows) on the stresses on and around the stem for all-polyethylene and metal-backed tibial components. (Adapted with permission from Reilly D, Walker PS, Ben-Dov M, Ewald FC: Effects of tibial components on load transfer in the upper tibia. *Clin Orthop Relat Res* 1982;165:273-282.)

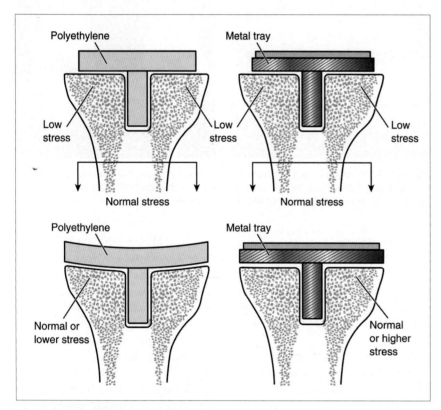

Figure 3 The effect of incomplete versus complete upper-surface coverage on load transfer with all-polyethylene and metal-backed tibial components. (Adapted with permission from Reilly D, Walker PS, Ben-Dov M, Ewald FC: Effects of tibial components on load transfer in the upper tibia. *Clin Orthop Relat Res* 1982;165:273-282.)

occurred were not attributed primarily to wear but rather to uneven loading of the underlying trabecular bone, leading to plateau subsidence and, ultimately, aseptic loosening.

High bending stresses permitted by the all-polyethylene component, poor surgical technique, and poor understanding of knee kinematics are the factors most often identified as likely causes of this uneven loading. The inherent plasticity of all-polyethylene components allows them to bend with eccentric or uneven loading, transferring high bending stresses to the cement-bone interface (**Figure 2**). The complexity of knee kinematics and alterations conferred by the arthritic soft tissues cause loading variations during normal function in even the most expertly performed TKA. Moreover, these changes are amplified in cases of malalignment or imprecise ligament balancing. Abnormally high stresses at the interface between the tibial component and the metaphyseal bone may be minimized by meticulous surgical technique. Even in the most skilled hands, however, precise ligament balancing, reproduction of anatomic extremity alignment, restoration of the proper joint-line level, and creation of symmetric flexion and extension gaps to encourage uniform loading of the articular surface may be difficult to achieve.

Even after instrumentation to promote accurate insertion and alignment became available, the all-polyethylene components remained predisposed to uneven distribution of load and subsequent loosening and failure. Early TKA designs did relatively little to reproduce the complex motion patterns of the native knee, and abnormal kinematic patterns resulted. Excessive stresses were transmitted to the tibial component–cement interface as a result of these abnormal patterns, promoting aseptic loosening. Finally, the limited range of implant sizes available also may have contributed to uneven stress distribution, because in some larger patients, the tibial surfaces remained partially uncapped (**Figure 3**).

Metal-Backed

By the early 1980s, the potential of metal-backed monoblock tibial components to solve load distribution problems on the proximal tibia led to their common use. In many of these implants, polyethylene was compression molded directly onto a metal baseplate (**Figure 4**). The baseplates were made primarily of either cast cobalt-chromium or titanium alloy. The cobalt-chromium plates required increased metal thickness for strength, were not highly polished, and had a relatively rough surface, whereas titanium alloy allowed thinner implants but were more susceptible to abrasive wear of the softer metal.

Finite-element analyses and other in vitro biomechanical studies suggested that longer-stemmed metal-backed components distributed load more evenly to the proximal tibia (**Figure 5**). Also, metal trays were manufactured with metal fins or stems to provide greater axial stability and rotational control and to help distribute stress evenly. Similarly, metal wedges, blocks, and extension stems could be attached to the undersurface of the tray, improving revision techniques and affording greater surgical options. Advantages include the ability to fill moderate-to-large bone defects of different shapes and sizes (especially noncontained), easy intraoperative assembly, and the ability to add further stability with long stems. Before the advent of metal trays, techniques for addressing large bone defects (such as in revision TKA, large angular deformity, rheumatoid arthritis, or hemophilia) were limited. For deeper proximal tibial resection, various methods were used, including shifting the tibial component away from the defect or using polymethylmethacrylate cement or cement reinforced with screws, bone autografts or allografts, or expensive custom-made devices. Many studies support the use of metal augments, including biomechanical evidence that these constructs optimize stress distribution and provide sufficient resistance to loads transmitted to the proximal tibia. As a result, augmented components are com-

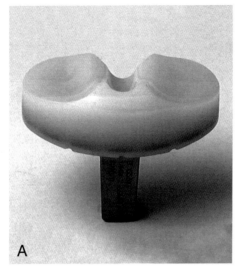
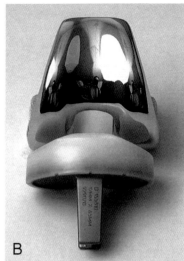
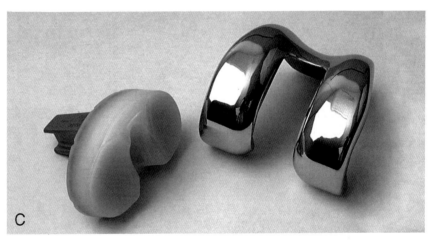

Figure 4 Metal-backed monoblock tibial component. **A,** The tibial component. The metal-backed monoblock tibial component shown articulating with a femoral component (**B**) and separate from the femoral component (**C**). (Courtesy of Merrill Ritter, MD, Mooresville, IN.)

monly used today, although mostly in revision or complex primary cases.

Adoption of metal-backed monoblock components also brought some drawbacks and new potential concerns. The metal-backed components were more costly, and a very large inventory was required to meet all possible sizing needs. Any metal augments or stems attached to the inferior surface of the tray would create a metal-on-metal articulation from which corrosion or fretting could result, leading to metal debris and accelerated polyethylene wear. Also, more of the proximal tibial bone needed to be resected to accommodate sufficient

polyethylene thickness, generally agreed to be 6 to 8 mm. Furthermore, the metal-backed implants tended to be made with less-conforming polyethylene inserts, which could lead to a reduced tibiofemoral contact area, higher point-loading stresses (especially as thin polyethylene was compressed between two metal surfaces), and, ultimately, polyethylene wear and osteolysis. For instance, some cruciate-retaining knees of this era used a flat-on-flat polyethylene design to minimize constraint and maximize conformity. These designs led to point contact and high stress, and both polyethylene damage and wear resulted.

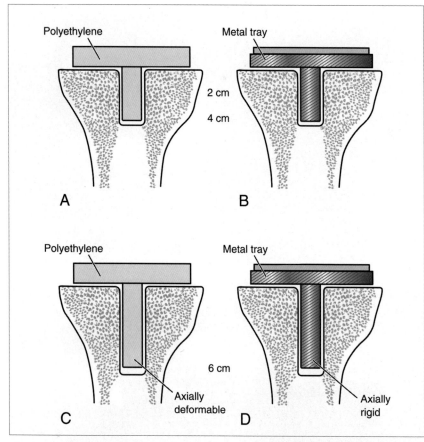

Figure 5 The effect of tibial component stem length and material on load transfer. Short polyethylene (**A**) or metal (**B**) stems transfer a small part of the load. **C,** Longer polyethylene stem transfers a small part of the load. **D,** Longer metal stem transfers about 25% of the load. (Adapted with permission from Reilly D, Walker PS, Ben-Dov M, Ewald FC: Effects of tibial components on load transfer in the upper tibia. *Clin Orthop Relat Res* 1982;165:273-282.)

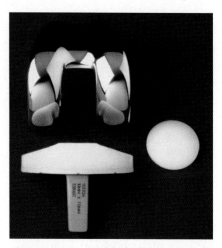

Figure 6 Anatomically graduated total knee arthroplasty components. (Courtesy of Merrill Ritter, MD, Mooresville, IN.)

Stress shielding of the proximal tibia was another concern with metal-backed components. Stress shielding refers to the process by which periprosthetic bone density is decreased over time because the neighboring implant shields the bone from the loading stress it would normally experience. If enough bone is resorbed, aseptic loosening may occur. The disparity in the Young modulus between the bone and implant has been considered the main contributing factor to stress shielding. Cast cobalt-chromium baseplates were therefore more likely to cause stress shielding than those made of titanium alloy, which has a Young modulus closer to that of bone.

Other factors, such as loading conditions varying with surface geometry and abnormal motions created by the TKA, also may impact stress shielding. Therefore, advances such as improved TKA kinematics and tibial component stems designed to reproduce normal proximal tibial bone strain have the potential to reduce proximal tibial stress shielding.

Early Results of Monoblock Components

Outcome studies seemed to contradict the many theoretical concerns associated with metal-backed components and reinforced the encouraging basic science research. Most comparative studies before 1995 found metal-backed tibial component survivorship rates to be slightly superior to those of their all-polyethylene counterparts, although both were considered "satisfactory" at mid- to long-term follow-up. For one early design, studies of posterior stabilized knees demonstrated a 94% survivorship of all-polyethylene components compared with 98% for the metal-backed version at up to 16 years of follow-up, with very low rates of aseptic loosening. Other designs also have demonstrated good results for metal-backed tibial components. A survivorship analysis of 9,200 TKAs also claimed better survival of the metal-backed components.

Other reports showed a larger disparity in the outcomes of all-polyethylene and metal-backed tibial components. One study found exceedingly poor outcomes with one all-polyethylene design with relatively flat-on-flat articulation (**Figure 6**), with 45 of 538 knees experiencing medial tibial collapse at just over 4 years of follow-up. An earlier outcome study of metal-backed knees of this design in almost 4,600 TKAs found a failure rate of 0.4% for compression-molded monoblock tibial components.

Modular Tibial Components

Metal-backed tibial components were considered efficacious by the mid 1980s. Their success soon led to the introduction of modular components, with tibial inserts of varying conformity and thickness that can be inserted into metal trays (**Figure 7**). Modularity offered many advantages, including inventory control, increased intraoperative options, and potential ease of revision. Unfortunately, modularity also created new issues, such as locking mechanism malfunction, concerns of the mechanical integrity of polyethylene, and backside wear with subsequent osteolysis.

Technical Benefits
Metal-backed modular tibial components offer several technical benefits. First, they allow the surgeon to trial different polyethylene thicknesses after fixing the tibial tray in its final position. This extra step may be more helpful in complicated cases and also may help avoid unnecessary wasting of implants. Second, a removable polyethylene trial allows easier removal of excess cement posterior to the tibial component, reducing the chance of third-body wear. Monoblock components make cement removal more difficult by blocking access to the posterior knee, especially with minimally invasive techniques. Care should be taken during the cement removal step to avoid scratching the femoral component with the empty tibial tray, as such a defect will accelerate polyethylene wear. Finally, in cases of progressive wear, it may be possible to exchange the polyethylene insert without removing other components. In one study, this liner exchange technique successfully arrested the radiographic progression of osteolytic lesions in 84% of cases at an average of 44 months. One study urged caution with this technique,

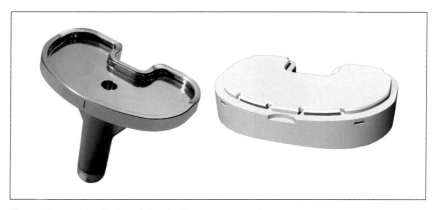

Figure 7 Metal-backed modular tibial component with separate polyethylene insert.

however, reporting some early morbidity related to instability. Moreover, others showed that liner exchange alone was inadequate in almost 89% of revisions, as metal-on-metal damage was often already present. Consistent difficulty in assessing the extent of osteolysis on routine plain radiographs has been postulated as a cause of the delay in treatment of those failed knees. Therefore, improved screening tools for osteolysis may lead to a greater frequency of successful liner exchanges.

Potential Problems
Increased polyethylene wear is a major concern with use of metal-backed fixed-bearing modular tibial trays. Decreased polyethylene thickness and backside polyethylene insert wear may contribute to this accelerated wear. As wear progresses, the tibial implant may eventually fail in either a catastrophic or insidious fashion. Catastrophic failure is relatively uncommon and occurs in one of two ways. Either the integrity of the tibial insert locking mechanism is lost, causing the polyethylene to become dissociated from the tibial tray, or the polyethylene thins to the point of fracture. Periprosthetic osteolysis, a much slower failure process, also is more common. Microscopic polyethylene debris incites a biologic response by which macrophages are upregulated. The release of cytokines, lymphokines, monokines, and other

proinflammatory peptides will stimulate osteoclasts to erode bone and amplify the response. The weaker periprosthetic bone can compromise implant fixation and accelerate aseptic loosening.

BACKSIDE WEAR
Osteolysis induced by polyethylene wear debris has emerged as a significant problem after TKA. A major source of polyethylene debris contributing to osteolysis is unintentional micromotion at the undersurface of the polyethylene, more commonly known as backside wear. The causes of backside wear have been studied extensively. This mostly abrasive wear occurs when the undersurface of the polyethylene rubs against the metal tray under loading conditions; this is known as mode-4 wear (two secondary surfaces rubbing together). Backside wear was known to occur in modular total hip arthroplasty components and was later confirmed to occur commonly in modular TKA as well. The volume of wear from the backside articulation is estimated to be from 2 to 100 times greater than wear from the tibiofemoral articulation in fixed-bearing implants. The wear particles created in backside wear also are smaller and more biologically active than those created at the tibiofemoral articulation. Clearly, backside wear presents a major concern with modular designs.

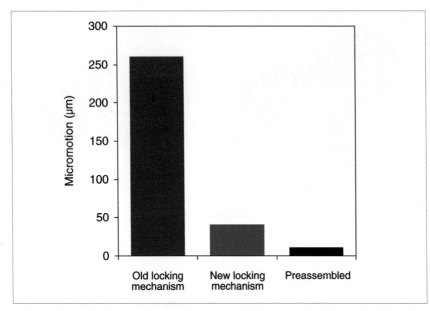

Figure 8 Graph shows micromotion generated by tibial implants with older locking mechanisms, by those with newer locking mechanisms, and by those with a preassembled, nonmodular metal-backed component.

Modular implant designs have evolved in an attempt to reduce polyethylene wear. Design improvements include use of thicker polyethylene bearings, improvements in locking mechanisms, improved manufacturing and polyethylene sterilization techniques, increased implant conformity, and the development of mobile-bearing systems.

IMPLANT THICKNESS
Contact stress studies have demonstrated rapidly increasing stresses with decreasing polyethylene thickness, leading to accelerated wear. Thickening the polyethylene insert lessens the importance of wear at the tibiofemoral articulation (mode-1 wear, which is wear between two primary surfaces inherent to function) and protects against wear-through over time. Although some authors have shown good results using tibial polyethylene components as thin as 4.4 mm, 6 to 8 mm is the accepted minimum thickness advocated by most authors. As metal trays are approximately 3 mm thick, the minimum metal-polyethylene unit thickness should be approximately 10 mm. Enough proximal tibia must be removed to accommodate such a composite implant, and concern has been raised over this amount of tibial bone resection. Proximal tibial strength has been demonstrated to be fairly constant from 4 to 10 mm below the articular surface, however, thus limiting those concerns.

LOCKING MECHANISMS
Studies have consistently found the locking mechanisms of modular tibial components insufficient to prevent undersurface fretting. Manufacturers have attempted to minimize backside wear by improving the fixation rigidity between the polyethylene and metal components. Wider-profile inserts were introduced to create a "force fit" with the metal tray that would reduce anterior-posterior, medial-lateral, and rotational motions. Also, anterior bumpers were added to reduce stress on the polyethylene snaps. Finally, the polyethylene chamfers were deepened, allowing greater ease of assembly. Despite all of these design advances, a certain amount of backside micromotion has proved unavoidable to date (**Figure 8**).

TKA Designs With Increased Conformity

Conformity refers to the degree of correspondence between the radii of curvature of two opposing articular surfaces. As conformity increases, so does contact area, reducing the subsurface polyethylene contact stress per unit area. Increasing conformity in a TKA design therefore reduces the potential for polyethylene wear. The ideal level of conformity has been widely studied. One analysis suggests that contact stresses are reduced as contact area is increased, at least until a contact area of 300 to 350 mm² is reached. Increasing contact area beyond this level reduced contact stresses further, but to a much lesser extent. Increasing coronal plane conformity is particularly critical to reducing peak polyethylene stresses in a tibial component design, as this lessens edge loading in the event of femoral condylar liftoff. Thus, the risk of prosthetic loosening and accelerated wear may be amplified in tibial designs with reduced conformity in the coronal plane (ie, flat-on-flat designs) because of increased edge loading.

The human knee is much more complex than a simple hinge joint. In reality, the knee exhibits complex motion patterns involving coronal and sagittal plane translation and axial rotation. Knee replacement designs must allow for these complex patterns (such as lateral femoral rollback during flexion) and so must limit conformity in fixed-bearing designs. Biomechanical studies have shown that highly conforming fixed-bearing TKA designs can be intolerant to higher rotational and anterior-posterior translational kinematic motion patterns that are common after TKA (and that lead to excessive polyethylene stresses). Also, subsurface polyethylene stresses can be substantially higher with malaligned, highly conforming fixed-bearing systems. To capitalize on the benefits of a highly conforming articular surface, alternative design concepts, such as mobile-bearing TKA, have been proposed.

Mobile-Bearing TKA Designs

Theoretical Advantages

Mobile-bearing TKA designs intentionally allow motion between the polyethylene and a highly polished cobalt-chromium tibial tray. This secondary articulation uncouples disparate motions, avoiding shear-generating cross-path motion. This design allows increased implant conformity and contact area without dramatically increasing torsional stresses transmitted to the polyethylene or the fixation interface.

The self-aligning behavior of highly conforming designs has been shown to maintain large, centrally located surface contact areas at the tibiofemoral articulation during both flexion-extension and axial rotation of the knee. Mobile-bearing TKA contact areas (400 to 800 mm²) are greater during gait than those typically seen in most fixed-bearing designs (200 to 250 mm²), which keeps contact stresses low, potentially improving wear and component fixation. Finite-element evaluations demonstrating reduced polyethylene contact stresses as a direct result of increased contact area further support these findings. In vitro studies have shown that these lower stresses have translated into less significant wear of the superior polyethylene articular surface.

Polyethylene mobility also reduces but does not eliminate abnormal kinematic patterns typical of fixed-bearing TKAs. Paradoxical anterior femoral translation, one of the abnormal patterns, was shown to be better controlled by the increased sagittal plane conformity of mobile-bearing designs, particularly when tested during gait. Also, the increased coronal plane conformity typical of mobile-bearing TKAs lessens the incidence and impact of femoral condylar liftoff and allows more flexion during internal and external rotation. Several studies have found low rates of aseptic loosening and revision (from 0% to 0.2%) in long-term follow-up of mobile-bearing designs, supporting these engineering concepts. Other kinematic comparisons have been more equivocal.

Mobile-bearing designs offer the additional advantage of allowing self-alignment of the polyethylene bearing with the femoral component. Malalignment of the tibial component would become less significant than in fixed-bearing devices, as the tray rotation allows some degree of self-correction. Cheng and associates reported that mobile-bearing designs reduced maximum contact pressures in malaligned TKAs better than fixed bearings, especially in regard to internal and external tibial malrotation.

This self-aligning behavior also has the potential to reduce the incidence of both patellar maltracking and post impingement, a significant source of premature polyethylene wear in posterior stabilized knees. A recent study showed a reduced rate of lateral retinacular release in mobile-bearing designs when compared with fixed bearings (5.3% versus 14.3%). The subject of patellofemoral mechanics with mobile-bearing designs remains somewhat controversial, however, and a prospective randomized trial showed no reduction of lateral release rate in mobile- versus fixed-bearing knees. Studies evaluating post impingement have been more consistent in finding less impingement-related wear in mobile-bearing component designs.

Motion Patterns in Mobile-Bearing TKA

The advantages described above are merely theoretical unless rotation of the bearing occurs in vivo. If the secondary interface did not function properly, the construct would act like a highly conforming fixed-bearing design. Many studies have been undertaken to better elucidate actual motion patterns demonstrated by mobile-bearing TKA designs, with mixed results. Two in vivo fluoroscopic kinematic studies examined motions at three articulating surfaces (femoral component–polyethylene bearing, femoral component–tibial tray, and polyethylene bearing–tibial tray) using a computer-assisted model-fitting algorithm. Most axial rotation occurred at the polyethylene bearing–tibial tray interface, with the polyethylene bearing typically following the rotation of the femoral component, as would be expected. This same finding also was observed in independent in vitro and in vivo studies of bearing mobility after TKA.

Motion at the secondary bearing can be limited. Using in vivo fluoroscopic evaluation of more than 1,000 TKAs incorporating 33 different fixed-bearing and mobile-bearing TKA designs, a large multicenter analysis demonstrated that most subjects experienced less than 10° of axial rotation with normal postoperative activities, but some knees experienced normal or reverse axial rotational magnitudes greater than 20°, which are beyond the boundaries of most fixed-bearing TKA designs. This study showed that rotating-platform TKA designs can accommodate a wide range of axial rotation without creating excessive polyethylene stresses.

Potential Problems

Potential problems are associated with mobile-bearing TKA designs when compared with fixed-bearing implants. These concerns include the need for more exacting surgical technique to prevent bearing spinout, the risk of greater polyethylene wear because of the second articulating surface (backside wear), and concern that the microparticulate wear debris created from the undersurface articulation of mobile-bearing TKA designs is smaller and has greater potential to cause osteolysis.

As previously discussed, backside polyethylene motion against a metal surface not designed to accommodate motion (ie, a relatively rough surface) results in substantial polyethylene wear and subsequent periprosthetic osteolysis if the modular locking mechanism is not rigid. In rotating-platform systems, a rotating polyethylene bearing is matched against a flat, highly polished cobalt-chromium surface with low surface roughness. The presence of a secondary articulation, however, with an increased polyethylene-metal arc of motion, or sliding distance, always predisposes to some degree of polyethylene wear.

The undersurface articulation predisposes mobile-bearing designs to third-body wear, which could accelerate wear. Even in the absence of any third bodies, polyethylene wear at the undersurface articulation is inevitable, and the debris created has been studied extensively. Recent in vitro studies found no difference in particle size or biologic activity between debris from fixed- and mobile-bearing TKAs, but they did find up to four times more debris in the fixed-bearing group. Another laboratory analysis, however, found only a slightly higher polyethylene wear rate in the fixed-bearing group (8.14 versus 6.78 mg per million cycles), a difference deemed to be insignificant. Similar retrieval analyses observed no statistical differences in particle number, shape, or size between the two groups. Also, studies examining the undersurface of retrieved rotating-platform polyethy-

lene inserts have reported minimal visual evidence of undersurface wear.

Despite theoretical concerns, backside polyethylene wear has not yet emerged as a major issue in clinical outcomes of rotating-platform designs. The lack of clinically important backside wear in mobile-bearing TKA designs can be explained in several ways, including decoupling of multidirectional motions occurring at the articular interfaces with rotating-platform designs and improved stress distribution to the proximal tibia.

———————■

■ Results

Fixed-Bearing Versus Mobile-Bearing Designs

Despite the many theoretical advantages of mobile-bearing TKAs, controversy remains as to whether they offer any clinical superiority over fixed-bearing designs. Some outcome studies suggested that the more physiologic kinematics of mobile-bearing designs do offer such a benefit, including less early postoperative anterior knee pain and improved knee flexion. Most recent studies offering longer follow-up found no significant differences between the two designs. Also, one in vivo kinematic study found no relationship between kinematics and maximal knee flexion, a result arguing against the idea that mobile-bearing designs improve maximal postoperative flexion. Patient satisfaction, functional scores, osteolysis, and revision rates were all found to be statistically similar between the two groups, as were rates of anterior knee pain.

Both fixed- and mobile-bearing designs also have been found to have a low incidence of failure. Kim and associates reported survivorship rates of 99% and 100% of fixed- and mobile-bearing TKAs, respectively, at up to 14.5 years of follow-up. Such results have led most authors to conclude that no evidence exists currently to

prove the superiority of mobile-bearing designs over fixed-bearing designs with regard to clinical and radiographic results. The theoretical benefit of increased contact area leading to lower stress and polyethylene wear rates requires longer follow-up in more active, heavier patients, who are known to experience wear and failure with fixed-bearing designs.

All-Polyethylene Versus Metal-Backed Designs

Assuming fixed-bearing designs have strong literature support, what role if any can the all-polyethylene tibial component, which is the most cost-effective tibial component, have in modern arthroplasty? Many surgeons favor metal-backed tibial components for younger, more active patients because they allow use of modularity or mobile bearings based on in vitro studies demonstrating improved knee kinematics. Early in vivo studies, however, showed at best slight clinical improvement with metal-backed designs. More recent mid- to long-term follow-up studies using more modern implants and newer surgical techniques have continued to demonstrate all-polyethylene component survival rates comparable to those of metal-backed designs. Some studies have even reported superior survival rates with the all-polyethylene components. Moreover, concerns that cemented all-polyethylene components were less stable than metal-backed components appear to be unfounded.

Despite design advances minimizing backside wear, osteolysis remains an important concern with modular components. All-polyethylene tibial components have been shown to reduce failure secondary to osteolysis when compared with modular implants, potentially an attractive option in the younger, active patient most likely to create wear. Older, less active people may not benefit greatly from metal-backed tibial implants either, as their TKAs are least likely to fail as a result of any mechanical cause. Several studies have correlated the highest long-term survival rates of all-polyethylene components with patients older than 75 years. Pagnano and associates found a 98% survival rate at follow-up of up to 14 years (patients 70 years or older), and other authors have reported survival rates greater than 99%. Blumenfeld and associates (unpublished data) stated that "the current body of literature documents the viability of the all-PE tibial component in elderly patients," a conclusion supported by numerous authors. However, Ranawat and associates recently stated that "an all-polyethylene tibial component fixed with cement can provide excellent performance and survivorship even in younger, active patients at intermediate follow up." The continued good or excellent results of all-polyethylene tibial components irrespective of patient age, combined with a relatively low cost, have led to a recent renewed interest in their use.

■ Summary

Tibial components have evolved over time in response to both real and perceived design flaws. All-polyethylene components offer relatively low cost, high conformity, and low wear rates, but they tend to fail because of uneven stress distribution to the tibial plateau. Metal-backed monoblock designs distributed stress more evenly, but they were more expensive and made surgery more technically difficult. Modular implants were developed in an attempt to improve intraoperative options, but at least in some cases they caused significant polyethylene wear from the backside, leading to osteolysis and aseptic loosening. Improvements to modular tray locking mechanisms, manufacturing and sterilization techniques, and the development of mobile-bearing designs attempt to minimize the creation of microscopic polyethylene debris and improve TKA kinematics. Despite all these changes, few significant long-term outcome differences among the various tibial component designs have been appreciated, and all are still implanted with good survival rates. Continued biomechanical, material, and outcome studies are needed to elucidate the ideal tibial component for TKA.

■ Bibliography

Blumenfeld TJ, Scott RD: The role of the cemented all-polyethylene tibial component in total knee replacement: 30-year follow-up of a single patient and review of the literature. *Knee* 2010 Jan 7. [Epub ahead of print]

Cheng CK, Huang CH, Liau JJ, Huang CH: The influence of surgical malalignment on the contact pressures of fixed and mobile bearing knee prostheses: A biomechanical study. *Clin Biomech (Bristol, Avon)* 2003;18(3):231-236.

Dennis DA, Komistek RD, Mahfouz MR, Walker SA, Tucker A: A multicenter analysis of axial femorotibial rotation after total knee arthroplasty. *Clin Orthop Relat Res* 2004;428(428):180-189.

Faris PM, Ritter MA, Keating EM, Meding JB, Harty LD: The AGC all-polyethylene tibial component: a ten-year clinical evaluation. *J Bone Joint Surg Am* 2003;85-A(3):489-493.

Griffin WL, Fehring TK, Mason JB, McCoy TH, Odum S, Terefenko CS: Early morbidity of modular exchange for polyethylene wear and osteolysis. *J Arthroplasty* 2004;19(7, Suppl 2):61-66.

Griffin WL, Scott RD, Dalury DF, Mahoney OM, Chiavetta JB, Odum SM: Modular insert exchange in knee arthroplasty for treatment of wear and osteolysis. *Clin Orthop Relat Res* 2007;464:132-137.

Haider H, Garvin K: Rotating platform versus fixed-bearing total knees: an in vitro study of wear. *Clin Orthop Relat Res* 2008;466(11):2677-2685.

Kim YH, Yoon SH, Kim JS: The long-term results of simultaneous fixed-bearing and mobile-bearing total knee replacements performed in the same patient. *J Bone Joint Surg Br* 2007;89(10):1317-1323.

Lee JG, Keating EM, Ritter MA, Faris PM: Review of the all-polyethylene tibial component in total knee arthroplasty: A minimum seven-year follow-up period. *Clin Orthop Relat Res* 1990;260(260):87-92.

Pagnano MW, Trousdale RT, Stuart MJ, Hanssen AD, Jacofsky DJ: Rotating platform knees did not improve patellar tracking: A prospective, randomized study of 240 primary total knee arthroplasties. *Clin Orthop Relat Res* 2004;428(428): 221-227.

Pereira GC, Walsh M, Wasserman B, Banks S, Jaffe WL, Di Cesare PE: Kinematics of the stiff total knee arthroplasty. *J Arthroplasty* 2008;23(6):894-901.

Ranawat AS, Mohanty SS, Goldsmith SE, Rasquinha VJ, Rodriguez JA, Ranawat CS: Experience with an all-polyethylene total knee arthroplasty in younger, active patients with follow-up from 2 to 11 years. *J Arthroplasty* 2005;20(7, Suppl 3): 7-11.

Ritter MA: Direct compression molded polyethylene for total hip and knee replacements. *Clin Orthop Relat Res* 2001; 393(393):94-100.

Rullkoetter PJ, Gabriel SM, Colleran DP, Zalenski EB: The relationship between contact stress and contact area with implications for TKR evaluation and design. *Trans Orthop Res Soc* 1999;24:974.

Windsor RE, Scuderi GR, Moran MC, Insall JN: Mechanisms of failure of the femoral and tibial components in total knee arthroplasty. *Clin Orthop Relat Res* 1989;248(248):15-19, discussion 19-20.

Yang CC, McFadden LA, Dennis DA, Kim RH, Sharma A: Lateral retinacular release rates in mobile- versus fixed-bearing TKA. *Clin Orthop Relat Res* 2008;466(11):2656-2661.

Chapter 12

Primary Total Knee Arthroplasty: Cemented Fixation

Thomas P. Sculco, MD
Roberto Rossi, MD

◼ Indications

Cemented fixation is the gold standard in total knee arthroplasty (TKA). Meticulous technique, including careful soft-tissue balancing, bone preparation, and cement handling all are fundamental to implant longevity, but obtaining rigid early fixation at the prosthesis-cement-bone interface is the most important factor in preventing mechanical loosening and achieving satisfactory long-term results in TKA. Cemented TKAs are particularly indicated in patients with poor bone quality, especially those with inflammatory conditions such as rheumatoid arthritis, but regardless of the indication, many large studies have shown overall better results with cemented fixation. Antibiotic-impregnated cement might be advisable for certain groups of patients, such as those undergoing revision arthroplasties, those with diabetes mellitus, and those on immunosuppressive medications.

◼ Contraindications

Many surgeons avoid cemented fixation in patients with a history of severe cardiopulmonary disease to minimize embolization secondary to cement pressurization, or in young patients with good bone quality, but this is a matter of surgeon preference. Good results with cement fixation can generally be demonstrated at long-term follow-up in all patients.

◼ Alternative Treatments

The alternative to cemented TKA is the use of an uncemented system. Uncemented TKA may have a role in the younger patient with robust bone, but even in this patient group ingrowth may not occur and subsidence, particularly on the tibial side, may result. Uncemented fixation of the femoral component has been successful in most patients, but the addition of porous surfaces may add cost.

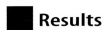

◼ Results

Long-term results of cemented fixation are excellent. Good results are seen at long-term follow-up when cement is used with various implant designs (**Table 1**).

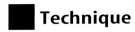

◼ Technique

Cement

Many brands of cement are commercially available. Variations exist in the elastic modulus, fatigue strength, and tensile and compressive strengths of the different preparations. The mixing and handling of bone cement must be meticulous so as to maximize the interlock of the cement with the surrounding bone. Antibiotic-containing cements available in the United States include Palacos R with gentamicin (Biomet, Warsaw, IN) and Simplex P with tobramycin (Stryker Howmedica Osteonics, Allendale, NJ).

Setup/Exposure

The patient is placed supine and the leg is prepared and draped. A tourni-

Dr. Sculco or an immediate family member serves as a board member, owner, officer, or committee member of the Arthritis Foundation and has received research or institutional support from Exactech, Smith & Nephew, and Zimmer. Neither Dr. Rossi nor any immediate family member has received anything of value from or owns stock in a commercial company or institution related directly or indirectly to the subject of this chapter.

Table 1 Results of Primary Cemented Total Knee Arthroplasty

Author(s) (Year)	Number of Knees	Implant Type	Mean Patient Age (Range)	Mean Follow-up (Range)	Results
Ranawat et al (1993)	112	Total Condylar Knee[*†]	65 years (31-79)	15 years	94% good
Gill and Joshi (2001)	268	Kinematic Condylar Knee Arthroplasty[†]	68.4 years ± 8.8	10.1 years ± 5.0	Survivorship: 98.2% at 10 years 92.6% at 17 years
Ritter (2001)	4,583	Anatomic Graduated Components (AGC) [‡]	70.4 years ± 8.9 (18-93)	11 years	98.86% at 15 years
Laskin (2001)	100	Genesis[§]	69 years	10 years	97% survivorship
Buechel et al (2002)	233	New Jersey LCS Rotating Platform Knee Replacement[‖]	NR	12.8 years	97.7% at 10 and 20 years
Callaghan et al (2005)	119	LCS rotating-platform[‖]	70 years (37-88)	(15-18 years)	94% without revision

* Johnson & Johnson, New Brunswick, New Jersey
† Howmedica, Rutherford, New Jersey
‡ Biomet Inc., Warsaw, Indiana
§ Smith & Nephew, Memphis, Tennessee
‖ DePuy, Warsaw, Indiana
LCS = low contact stress, NR = not reported

quet is applied on the proximal portion of the thigh. A midline incision 12 to 15 cm in length is made and carried down through the subcutaneous tissues. A median parapatellar arthrotomy is performed. The patellar ligament is released down to the level of the tibial tubercle and a medial release is performed, elevating the medial collateral ligament from the tibia and extending posteriorly if necessary. The quadriceps tendon is incised 2 to 3 cm proximally. The knee is maximally flexed, the anterior and posterior cruciate ligaments are detached, and the tibia is subluxated forward.

Procedure

The proximal tibial cut is performed, resecting approximately 10 mm on the better compartment to achieve a perpendicular cut. Once the intramedullary guide is in place, the femur is sized and the finishing block is applied. The cuts are performed and the notch is created. Laminar spreaders are inserted and all meniscal tissues are removed medially and laterally. The femoral component is impacted and the tibia is subluxated forward. The proximal tibia is prepared with impacted trials with the tibial block in place.

Bone Preparation

The essential bone cuts for a TKA are the proximal tibial osteotomy; resection of the distal femoral condyles angulated at 3° to the intramedullary axis of the femur (for valgus knee deformity) and 5° (for varus knee deformity); anterior and posterior condylar resections (for appropriate size); chamfers for the distal femur (anterior and posterior); resection of the intercondylar notch for the posterior cruciate ligament–substituting TKA; and retropatellar osteotomy. Once the bone cuts are performed, high-pressure and high-volume pulsatile lavage of bony surfaces is performed. Clearing of bony debris and blood from the bony surface with pulsatile lavage together with careful suction drying is important be-cause the cancellous bone surface must be kept free of debris and dry during the cementing for optimal cement interdigitation (**Figure 1**). Other drying agents, such as hydrogen peroxide, also can be used.

Prosthesis Implantation

All three components are generally cemented after one vacuum mix, beginning with the patella and followed by the femur and finally the tibia. The viscosity of the cement is an important consideration in the cementing technique. If the cement is too liquid, it can be difficult to manage, and clearing of excess cement is problematic. We prefer the cement to have a doughy consistency, and we apply it without a cement gun. The consistency of the cement is optimal when it is resistant to gravity and the surgeon can break off small pieces and roll them between the fingers without the cement adhering to the surgical gloves. This usually requires 5 to 6 minutes of setting time. Once the ce-

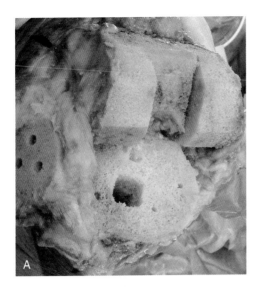
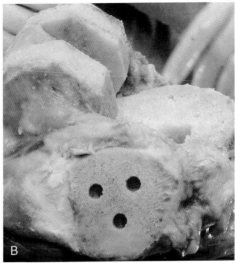

Figure 1 The bone should be pressure irrigated and dried before methylmethacrylate fixation of the components of the prosthesis. Intraoperative photographs show the appearance of the dry tibial (**A**) and patellar (**B**) cancellous surfaces.

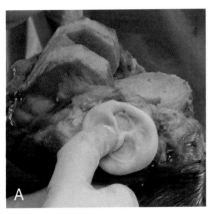
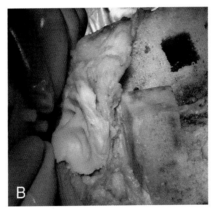
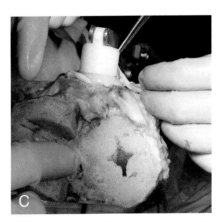

Figure 2 Implanting the patellar component. **A,** Cement is pressurized into the three holes. **B,** A three-pegged all-polyethylene patellar component is applied on the cement surface. **C,** A pressure clamp is used to hold the patellar button in place while the cement polymerizes.

ment reaches the appropriate viscosity, a three-pegged polyethylene patellar component is fixed in place with a compression clamp. All excess cement is removed from the patellar circumference. While the patellar component is held in place with the patellar clamp (**Figure 2**), cement is placed directly on the femoral component (**Figure 3,** *A*); in addition, a small amount is placed on the posterior condyles. A horseshoe-shaped segment of cement is fashioned over the anterior and distal surface of the prepared femur (**Figure 3,** *B*), and digital compression is used to force the cement into the femoral bone. Care must be taken to prevent a flexed position of the femoral

component (**Figure 3,** *C*). The implant should be seated posteriorly first, and then extended so that the anterior femoral flange is flush to the anterior femoral surface. The femoral component is impacted in place, and excess cement is carefully removed (**Figure 3,** *D*). The mantle will be about 1 mm thick when the femoral cuts are performed accurately (**Figure 3,** *E*). Once the patellar and femoral components are in place, a mushroom-shaped cement segment (**Figure 4,** *A*) is inserted into the tibial peghole (**Figure 4,** *B*). All the excess cement must be removed from around the tibial component to prevent cement

particles from breaking loose (**Figure 4,** *C*). Good exposure and attention to the exposure in the posterior lateral corner of the tibial component is important for maintaining adequate rotation and removing the remnants of cement debris. After cementing all components, the knee is brought to full extension, which places very high pressure on the cement in the femur and tibia (**Figure 5**). Once the cement has hardened, the area is irrigated copiously, eliminating most cement debris.

There are some variations in cementing the tibial component. In a hybrid system, the surface of the tibial

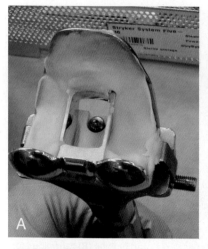

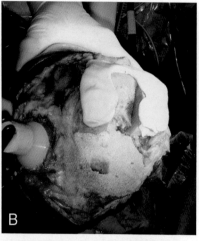

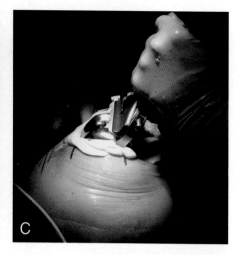

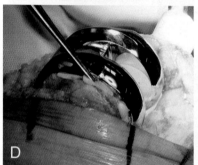

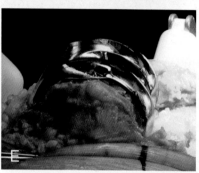

Figure 3 Implanting the femoral component. **A,** The cement is placed on the femoral component before impaction. **B,** The doughy cement is placed in a horseshoe shape around the distal femur. Avoid placing cement in the posterior cuts. **C,** A flexed position of the femoral component can be prevented by using a proper insertion device. **D,** Using a curet, all excess cement is removed from around the femoral component. **E,** With accurate femoral cuts, about 1 mm of cement mantle should be visible.

component is cemented but the stem is press-fit in the tibial physis.

 Video 12.1 Primary Total Knee Arthroplasty: Cemented Fixation. Roberto Rossi, MD; Thomas P. Sculco, MD (3 min)

Wound Closure

The knee is irrigated with pulsatile lavage to be sure that no bone or cement fragments remain, and the tourniquet is released. Bleeding points are controlled with cautery and the wound is closed over a suction drain using interrupted No. 0 absorbable sutures for the arthrotomy and 2-0 absorbable sutures for the subcutaneous closure. Staples are used for skin closure because they provide interrupted wound tension and are expeditious. The drain is used for 24 hours.

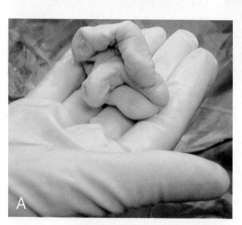

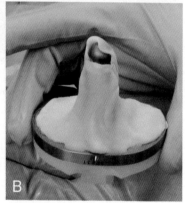

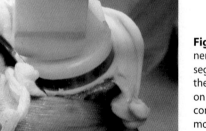

Figure 4 Implanting the tibial component. **A,** A mushroom-shaped cement segment is fashioned and inserted into the tibial peghole. **B,** Cement is placed on the surface and stem of the tibial component. **C,** Excess cement is removed from around the tibial component.

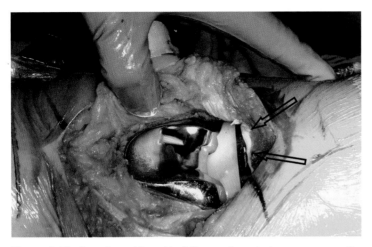

Figure 5 The knee is positioned in full extension, placing pressure on the cement (arrows).

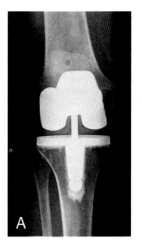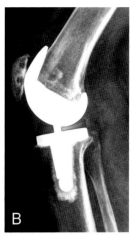

Figure 6 AP (**A**) and lateral (**B**) radiographs demonstrate a good cement mantle.

Postoperative Regimen

A continuous passive motion machine is used the first day after surgery. The patient is out of bed and usually begins walking on postoperative day 1 with a walker. The average length of hospitalization is 3 to 4 days, during which time the patient has physical therapy twice a day. Before discharge, the patient should be able to climb stairs, walk with a cane, and move in and out of bed. Patients needing inpatient rehabilitation are discharged on a walker. Patients are encouraged to be as active as they wish and are allowed to drive within 3 to 4 weeks after surgery. The skin staples are removed 10 days after the procedure.

Avoiding Pitfalls and Complications

Careful cement technique is necessary for successful cemented component fixation. The key technical factor is pressurization into carefully prepared cancellous surfaces that are dry. If sclerotic surfaces are present, they should be fenestrated with a drill to allow cement penetration to the subchondral bone. Another factor in implant longevity is obtaining a cement penetration of at least 2 to 3 mm (**Figure 6**). More than 3° of valgus or varus angulation of the tibial component on the AP view must be avoided because it can lead to asymmetric loading and early failure. Cement technique also may be compromised if there is movement of the components during polymerization of the cement.

Bibliography

Buechel FF Sr, Buechel FF Jr, Pappas MJ, Dalessio J: Twenty-year evaluation of the New Jersey LCS rotating platform knee replacement. *J Knee Surg* 2002;15:84-89.

Callaghan JJ, O'Rourke MR, Iossi MF, et al: Cemented rotating-platform total knee replacement: A concise follow-up, at a minimum of fifteen years of a previous report. *J Bone Joint Surg Am* 2005;87:1995-1998.

Callaghan JJ, Squire MW, Goetz DD, Sullivan PM, Johnston RC: Cemented rotating-platform total knee replacement: A nine to twelve-year study. *J Bone Joint Surg Am* 2000;82:705-711.

Emerson RH Jr, Higgins LL, Head WC: The AGC total knee prosthesis at average 11 years. *J Arthroplasty* 2000;15:418-421.

Gill GS, Joshi AB: Long-term results of Kinematic Condylar knee replacement: An analysis of 404 knees. *J Bone Joint Surg Br* 2001;83: 355-358.

Gill GS, Joshi AB, Mills DM: Total condylar knee arthroplasty: 16 to 21 year results. *Clin Orthop Relat Res* 1999;367:210-215.

Gioe TJ, Killeen KK, Grimm K, Mehle S, Scheltema K: Why are total knee replacements revised? Analysis of early revision in a community knee implant registry. *Clin Orthop Relat Res* 2004;428:100-106.

Laskin RS: The Genesis total knee prosthesis: A 10-year followup study. *Clin Orthop Relat Res* 2001;388388:95-102.

Ranawat CS, Flynn WF, Saddler S, Hansraj KK, Maynard MJ: Long-term results of total condylar knee arthroplasty: A 15-year survivorship study. *Clin Orthop Relat Res* 1993;286:92-102.

Ritter MA: Direct compression molded polyethylene for total hip and knee replacements. *Clin Orthop Relat Res* 2001; 393393:94-100.

Ryd L, Lindstrand A, Rosenquist R, Selvik G: Tibial component fixation in knee arthroplasty. *Clin Orthop Relat Res* 1986; 213:141-149.

 Video Reference

Rossi R, Sculco TP: Video. *Primary Total Knee Arthroplasty: Cemented Fixation.* Turin, Italy, 2009.

Coding				
CPT Codes			**Corresponding ICD-9 Codes**	
27447	Arthroplasty, knee, condyle and plateau; medial AND lateral compartments with or without patella resurfacing (total knee arthroplasty)		715 715.80	715.16 715.89

CPT copyright © 2010 by the American Medical Association. All rights reserved.

Chapter 13
Uncemented Total Knee Arthroplasty

Aaron A. Hofmann, MD
Clifford D. Clark, MD

Indications

Uncemented total knee arthroplasty (TKA) is a reliable and durable form of bone-implant fixation. For uncemented TKA to be effective, bony ingrowth into the prosthesis must occur. Bony ingrowth requires initial implant stability and a robust blood supply. Therefore, uncemented TKA is indicated only for those patients with good bone stock and uncompromised vascularity. These patients are typically younger than 70 years and do not have multiple medical problems. Uncemented TKA is indicated for both men and women; however, men tend to have greater bone density, and therefore the indications for uncemented fixation are broader in the male patient population. Uncemented TKA may be considered in all forms of arthritis but most commonly is reserved for osteoarthritis, posttraumatic arthritis, and well-controlled rheumatoid arthritis. Each patient is considered individually, however, and if sufficient bone density and blood supply are present, we proceed with uncemented fixation regardless of age or sex.

Contraindications

Uncemented TKA is contraindicated in patients with poor bone stock and poor vascularity. Diabetes, atherosclerotic vascular disease, and other diseases that impair circulation are relative contraindications. Similarly, smoking is a relative contraindication because it impairs vascularity. Osteoporosis is a contraindication to uncemented TKA, as rigid fixation is difficult to achieve in osteoporotic bone. In this setting, micromotion is likely to occur, leading to implant loosening. Advanced physiologic age and sedentary lifestyle are not absolute contraindications, but they should alert the surgeon to the possibility of poor bone stock. When soft bone is appreciated intraoperatively, converting to cement fixation is appropriate.

Alternative Treatments

For patients with poor bone stock and impaired vascular supply, cement fixation is the alternative treatment of choice. Methylmethacrylate fixation is still the most widely used form of bone-implant fixation for TKA. It has an excellent track record, with good long-term survivorship, especially when applied to older, sedentary patients or patients with rheumatoid arthritis.

Results

The long-term results of uncemented TKA can be excellent and compare very favorably with those for cemented fixation. In selected recent reports, survival rates at 7 to 15 years range from 87% to 100% (**Table 1**), with implant survivorship greater than 95% at 10 years in several series.

These long-term success rates were not always achieved. In numerous early studies of uncemented TKA, authors reported high failure rates, especially on the tibial side. Many of these reports involved the use of component designs that are no longer used in modern uncemented components. Additionally, many of these studies were published when surgical techniques for both uncemented and cemented TKA were not as refined as they are today. Some early designs included the use of tibial base plates without stems and/or screws, which

Dr. Hofmann or an immediate family member has received royalties from Zimmer, serves as a paid consultant to Zimmer, and has received research or institutional support from Zimmer. Dr. Clark or an immediate family member has received research or institutional support from Zimmer.

Table 1 Results for Uncemented Total Knee Arthroplasty

Author(s) (Year)	Number of Knees	Implant Type	Minimum Follow-up (Years)	Survival Rate (%)
Berger et al (2001)	108	MG-1 (Zimmer, Warsaw, IN)	7	88 (femur) 92 (tibia)
Hofmann et al (2001)	176	Natural Knee (Zimmer, Warsaw, IN)	10	95.1
Schroder et al (2001)	58	AGC 2000 (Biomet, Warsaw, IN)	10	97
Whiteside (2001)	184	Ortholoc Total Knee System (Wright Medical Technology, Arlington, TN)	15	98.6
Buechel (2002)	136	NJ LCS (DePuy, Warsaw, IN)	10	97.8
Goldberg and Kraay (2004)	113	MG-1 (Zimmer, Warsaw, IN)	14	87 (all) 99 (tibia)
Watanbe et al (2004)	50	Osteonics Series 3000 (Omnifit, Osteonics, Allendale, NJ)	10	100
Hardeman et al (2006)	115	Profix (Smith & Nephew, Memphis, TN)	8	97.1
Baker et al (2007)	112	PFC (Johnson & Johnson Professional, Raynham, MA)	10	93.3

MG-1 = Miller-Galante 1; AGC 2000 = Anatomically Graduated Components; NJ LCS = New Jersey Low Contact Stress; PFC = Press-Fit Condylar (Johnson & Johnson Professional, Raynham, MA).

led to fibrous attachment and component subsidence as a result of poor initial fixation. Additional problems resulted from the design of the porous coating on the tibial component. Many designs did not have circumferential porous coating on the base plate; polyethylene wear debris tracked under the smooth surfaces and then down the screw holes or stem, leading to failure due to osteolysis. Several early studies also involved the use of thin flat-on-flat tibial polyethylene, which led to early failures not only in uncemented TKA, but in cemented TKA as well. Finally, numerous authors have reported that metal-backed patellar components with thin polyethylene required early revision because of metal-on-metal abrasive wear.

With refinements in component design and improvements in surgical technique, uncemented TKA now has long-term survivorship rates equal to that of cemented TKA. Excellent results have been reported in the literature for cemented TKA (survivorship greater than 90% and excellent clinical outcomes at 15-year follow-up), and, as can be seen in **Table 1**, the rates of survivorship for uncemented TKA are equally excellent over a similar time frame. Several studies on cemented knees have shown that younger and heavier patients fare poorly relative to their lighter and older counterparts. On the contrary, studies specific to young and heavy patients found that uncemented knees in this patient group had survivorship equal to that of older and lighter patients. This suggests that uncemented TKA may be ideally suited for young and heavy patients and, in fact, may provide more durable fixation over the long term.

■ Technique

Exposure

We prefer to expose the knee via a subvastus or median parapatellar approach. The subvastus exposure should be avoided when eversion of the patella is difficult, as in patients with a history of high tibial osteotomy, obese or very muscular patients, and patients with previous medial arthrotomy. In these situations, a standard median parapatellar approach is used.

For the subvastus approach, the deep fascia of the thigh overlying the vastus medialis is incised sharply, in line with the longitudinal skin incision. The fascia is then elevated bluntly off the fibers of the vastus medialis obliquus (VMO), and the inferior edge of the VMO is identified. The VMO is bluntly separated from the intermuscular septum and lifted anteriorly. This provides tension for incision of the transverse tendinous insertion of the medial capsule, which is performed at the midpatellar level. A vertical arthrotomy is then performed adjacent to the patella and patellar tendon, leaving the fat pad mostly intact. The knee is then extended, the patella is everted or subluxated, and the knee is flexed slowly, allowing the fibers of the VMO to stretch. The distal femur will be widely exposed at this point. If the patella is difficult to evert, a partial lateral release can be performed. In addition, application of the patellar clamp can be used to serve as a counterweight to keep the patella everted.

At this point, exposure of the proximal tibia is performed. Starting medially, the anterior horn of the medial meniscus is resected, and exposure back to the posteromedial corner is obtained. In cases of marked deformity, a more generous medial release can be performed, but this is usually better titrated with trial implants in place. In similar fashion, the lateral proximal tibia is defined by resection of the anterior horn of the lateral meniscus and careful dissection back to the midtibia. Osteophytes are resected from the tibia and femur to define the true bony landmarks and relieve undue ligamentous tension. If osteophytes are present in the intercondylar notch, they must be resected to determine the true mechanical entry point of the distal femur, which lies approximately 2 mm anterior to the roof of the intercondylar notch.

Determining Alignment

Anatomic and radiographic studies have shown that the normal joint line is oriented horizontally, parallel to the floor. An average of 6° of tibiofemoral valgus results from 8° to 9° of distal femoral valgus and 2° to 3° of proximal tibia varus. Most TKA systems produce a slightly different joint line, wherein the proximal tibia is typically cut perpendicular to the long axis of the tibia, and the joint line is then ori-

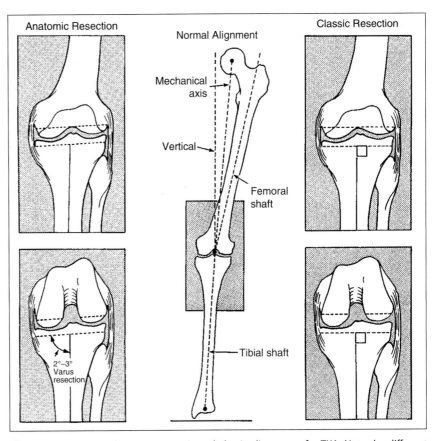

Figure 1 Schematic showing anatomic and classic alignments for TKA. Note the different orientation of the joint line in each. (Adapted with permission from Hofmann AA, Scott DF: Cementless total knee arthroplasty, in Scuderi GR, Tria AJ Jr, eds: *Knee Arthroplasty Handbook: Techniques in Total Knee and Revision Arthroplasty.* Heidelberg, Germany, Springer-Verlag, 2006, p 87.)

ented in 2° to 3° of valgus relative to the floor; this is known as classic alignment. External rotation of the femoral component is required in this situation as a result of the iatrogenic soft-tissue imbalance that this creates (**Figure 1**).

Our preference is to reproduce normal anatomy as closely as possible, and to do this we follow the principles of anatomic alignment. In doing so, the distal femur is usually cut in 5° of valgus and the proximal tibia is cut in 2° of varus. This places the mechanical axis slightly into the medial compartment and produces an even distribution of forces across an asymmetric tibia. By following anatomic alignment, there is no need for external rotation of the femoral component, and

lateral release is very rarely required. In cases of valgus, where the lateral soft tissues are contracted, we cut the tibia perpendicular to the long axis of the tibia.

Equally as important as this alignment in the coronal plane is reproduction of the patient's normal joint line in the sagittal plane. Normal posterior tibial tilt ranges from 4° to 12°, and this slope must be matched to reproduce the patient's anatomy and kinematics. To aid in matching the slope, a long, smooth pin is placed in the top hole of the tibial cutting block, and the slope is adjusted so that the pin is parallel to the patient's proximal tibia (**Figure 2**). Failure to reproduce the tibial slope leads to abnormal kinematics, and if the posterior cruciate

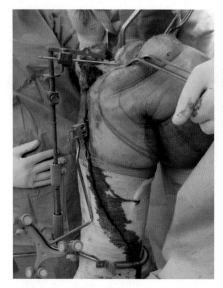

Figure 2 Measurement and reproduction of tibial slope. Note the long, smooth pin parallel to tibial joint surface.

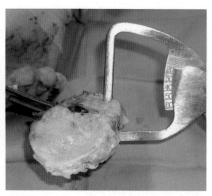

Figure 3 Method of measured resection. The tibial wafer is measured to determine the tibial polyethylene thickness required for replacement.

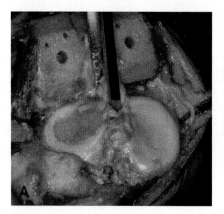 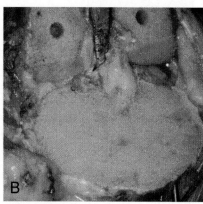

Figure 4 PCL retention. **A,** A 0.25-in osteotome is placed anterior to the PCL for protection during the tibial cut. **B,** The tibia after the tibial cut has been made. Note the complete preservation of the PCL.

ligament (PCL) is retained, tension is either too tight or too loose. An additional benefit to matching the patient's posterior slope is an increase in the load-carrying capacity of the proximal tibia. An improvement of 40% in the maximum compressive strength has been shown when the tibia is resected parallel to the joint line versus perpendicular to the tibial shaft. This is important to prevent anterior subsidence of the tibial component in uncemented TKA.

Measured Resection

A measured resection technique is used for resurfacing the knee by referencing the least-diseased portion of the distal femoral condyle and tibial plateau. For the patella, the thickest portion of the medial facet of the patella is referenced. All bony cuts are measured after resection (**Figure 3**), taking into account the 1 mm lost from the thickness of the saw blade. Replacement of resected bone by an equal amount of prosthesis ensures

restoration of the anatomic joint line with near-normal varus-valgus balance. Soft-tissue releases are rarely required after initial exposure; when they are needed, they are much less extensive.

PCL Retention or Substitution

Our preference is to retain the PCL during TKA if it appears healthy. We argue that this preserves the normal kinematics of the knee as closely as possible. Retention of the PCL maintains femoral rollback, allowing femoral clearance and an increased range of motion. Additional benefits include decreased patellar/femoral complications and decreased anteroposterior shear stress across the bone-implant interface. The procedure we choose to balance the flexion-extension gaps is dependent on the preoperative state of the PCL. If the PCL is to be retained, we recommend protecting it by placement of a 0.25-in osteotome anterior to the PCL during the tibial cut (**Figure 4**). In cases of marked valgus or fixed flexion deformity greater than 10°, the PCL is contracted, and achieving proper balance is more difficult. In these cases, we sacrifice the PCL. When the PCL is inadequate, such as in inflammatory arthritis or severe degenerative arthritis, we also sacrifice the PCL. When the PCL is sacrificed, a substitute must be provided. Traditionally, this is achieved with a central polyethylene post that articulates with a cam on the femoral component. This design has proved to be effective, but it is not without complications, including post failure and dislocation. We prefer to substitute for the PCL by implanting a deep-dished (ultracongruent) tibial polyethylene component (**Figure 5**). The femur is stabilized anterior to posterior by an ultracongruent articular surface with an anterior buildup of the tibial polyethylene. This has proved to be clinically reliable since the early 1990s, and several implant manufacturers now have this technology available.

Bone Preparation

Bone resorption and connective tissue formation can occur when bone is excessively traumatized or heated above 55°C. To prevent this, the saw blade should be cooled by constant irrigation and all bone cuts should be made with a new, sharp saw blade (**Figure 6**). Flat saw cuts are of paramount importance to maximize the amount of bone-implant contact. To ensure this, a precisely toleranced saw capture should be used, and all bone cuts should be sighted in two planes against cutting blocks once cuts have been made. A central "high spot" near the intercondylar notch may persist after the distal femoral cut and must be eliminated. This can be easily eliminated by additional planing with a slight upward spring of the blade against the bone. Flatness also can be checked with the use of an auxiliary cutting block.

In the average tibia, cortical and cancellous bone account for only 6% and 18% of the total surface area, respectively. The remaining space is composed of bone marrow. The surface area available for attachment can be markedly increased with the use of autologous cancellous bone graft, which acts as a form of biologic cement (**Figure 7**). The autologous bone chips are obtained from the cut surface of the resected fragment of tibia by use of a patellar reamer. Several studies performed on paired porous-coated devices have shown improved bony ingrowth with the use of autologous bone graft, and postmortem analyses of retrieved tibial base plates have corroborated this as well.

Trial Reduction

Before trial reduction, the femur is lifted anteriorly to allow the removal of osteophytes with the use of a curved 0.75-in osteotome. Osteophyte resection is essential to obtain maximal knee extension. Stability is checked in full extension, 20° of flexion, and maximum flexion. When the PCL is

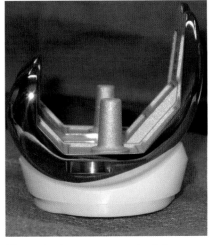

Figure 5 Ultracongruent polyethylene component used when the PCL must be sacrificed. Note the substantial anterior buildup for resistance to posterior displacement.

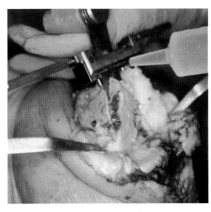

Figure 6 Bone preparation. Note that the saw blade is cooled with irrigation to prevent bone necrosis, which can occur as a result of thermal injury.

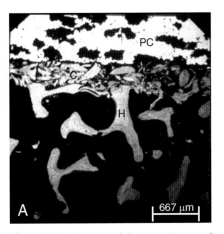

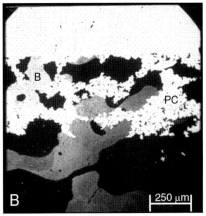

Figure 7 Backscattered electron micrographs show incorporation of autologous bone chips. **A,** Autologous bone chips (C) are interposed between the porous coating (PC) and the host cancellous bone (H). Note that the bone chips significantly increase the porous-coating surface area exposed for bony ingrowth. **B,** Living, mature autologous bone chips (B) incorporated into the porous coating.

preserved, slight medial-to-lateral laxity should be allowed and full extension must be obtained. If the PCL has been sacrificed, the next size thicker tibial polyethylene component should be selected. A slight flexion deformity that is manually correctable to neutral should exist. This flexion deformity will stretch out over the next 6 months. If varus or valgus imbalance persists, soft-tissue releases can be titrated at this point.

Component Implantation

After removal of the trial components, cancellous bone slurry is obtained from the cut undersurface of the tibial wafer by use of a patellar reamer (**Figure 8**, *A* and *B*). Large amounts of bone graft can be obtained easily using this technique. The bone slurry is applied to all cut bony surfaces, ensuring that a flat surface is obtained (**Figure 8**, *C*). In a standard varus knee, it is important to apply plenty of slurry to the more porotic lateral tibial surface in order to obtain maximum interface between porous coating and bone. This additionally reinforces the weaker bone and helps rebuild the subchondral plate. At this point, the tibial component is solidly driven into place. Placement of screws that provide extra tibial component fixation is highly recommended to ensure a tight press-fit and provide for rigid initial fixation. We use 6.5-mm × 50-mm cancellous screws placed medially and laterally. To prevent perforation of the tibia by screws, the lateral screw is angled approximately 20° medially, and the medial screw is placed straight, aligned with the tibial axis. Because of the porosity of the proximal tibia, no predrilling deeper than 1 cm is performed. With the tibial component in place, the polyethylene component is implanted and the femoral component is driven into place. After final implantation of all components (**Figure 8,** *D*) we take fluoroscopic spot images in the operating room to ensure proper implant position and to document the true bone-implant interface, as this can be more difficult to obtain in the outpatient setting (**Figure 9**).

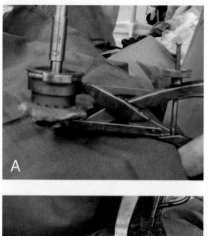
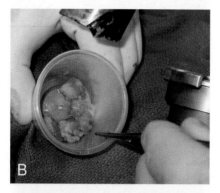
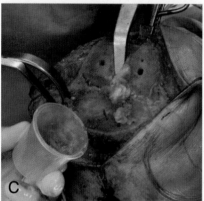
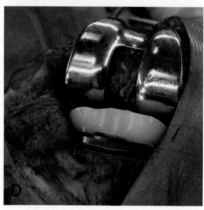

Figure 8 Component implantation. **A,** A patellar reamer is used on the backside of the tibial wafer to obtain autologous bone slurry (**B**). **C,** Bone slurry is applied to all cut bony surfaces, but especially on the lateral tibia. **D,** The implants are placed after the bone slurry has been applied.

Wound Closure

Prior to closure, the posterior capsule may be injected with 30 mL of 0.25% bupivacaine. The wound is then irrigated thoroughly, and a closed suction drain is placed in the lateral gutter. The knee capsule is closed with No. 2 nonabsorbable sutures. The subcutaneous layer is apposed with 2-0 absorbable sutures, and the skin is closed with staples. A sterile, occlusive dressing is applied, along with a continuous cooling device. Finally, the lower extremity is wrapped in a bulky Jones dressing.

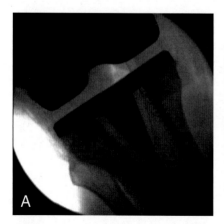
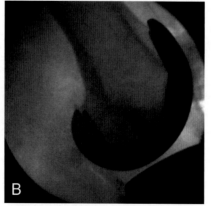
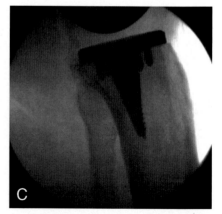

Figure 9 Fluoroscopic spot views in the AP and lateral planes document bone-implant interfaces immediately after implantation. **A,** AP view of tibial component. **B,** Lateral view of femoral component. **C,** Lateral view of tibial component.

Postoperative Regimen

Our postoperative TKA protocol involves the use of a multimodal pain-control regimen. It first involves the use of an indwelling femoral nerve catheter that is managed by the anesthesia pain service. This is typically discontinued on postoperative day 1 or 2. The patient uses a knee immobilizer during ambulation until the femoral nerve block has fully worn off, to prevent falls. We also use low-dose, sustained-release oxycodone twice a day for patients younger than 70 years of age, celecoxib (200 mg) once per day, and immediate-release oxycodone as needed for breakthrough pain control. With this protocol, we very rarely need to administer intravenous narcotics.

Continuous passive motion is begun the day of surgery and continued until the patient is discharged from the hospital, usually 72 hours postoperatively. Patients are mobilized with immediate weight bearing as tolerated; however, some form of assistive device is required until postoperative week 6, to prevent falls. Deep vein thrombosis prophylaxis consists of rapid mobilization, sequential compressive devices, thigh-high compression stockings, and warfarin administered for a 2-week period.

Avoiding Pitfalls and Complications

Sound surgical technique and proper patient selection are critical to avoid pitfalls and complications associated with uncemented TKA. One key surgical consideration is attaining correct alignment of components, which will prevent edge-loading and shear stresses across the bone-implant interface. These shear stresses can result in micromotion and the development of fibrous rather than bony ingrowth; this is especially true on the tibial side. Precise bone cuts are also critical for producing a flat, level surface. Remaining high spots can result in toggling of the components and limits the surface area available for bony ingrowth. We also believe that the use of autologous bone slurry is an extremely important factor. Not only does it markedly improve surface area available for ingrowth, but it also can make up for residual high and low spots left behind by imperfect cuts.

Of equal importance is proper patient selection. As stated earlier, uncemented TKA should be avoided in patients with soft bone and impaired vascularity.

Bibliography

Baker PN, Khaw FM, Kirk LM, Esler CN, Gregg PJ: A randomised controlled trial of cemented versus cementless press-fit condylar total knee replacement: 15-year survival analysis. *J Bone Joint Surg Br* 2007;89(12):1608-1614.

Berger RA, Lyon JH, Jacobs JJ, et al: Problems with cementless total knee arthroplasty at 11 years followup. *Clin Orthop Relat Res* 2001;392(392):196-207.

Bloebaum RD, Bachus KN, Mitchell W, Hoffman G, Hofmann AA: Analysis of the bone surface area in resected tibia. Implications in tibial component subsidence and fixation. *Clin Orthop Relat Res* 1994;309(309):2-10.

Bloebaum RD, Rubman MH, Hofmann AA: Bone ingrowth into porous-coated tibial components implanted with autograft bone chips: Analysis of ten consecutively retrieved implants. *J Arthroplasty* 1992;7(4):483-493.

Buechel FF Sr: Long-term followup after mobile-bearing total knee replacement. *Clin Orthop Relat Res* 2002;404(404):40-50.

Goldberg VM, Kraay M: The outcome of the cementless tibial component: A minimum 14-year clinical evaluation. *Clin Orthop Relat Res* 2004;428(428):214-220.

Hardeman F, Vandenneucker H, Van Lauwe J, Bellemans J: Cementless total knee arthroplasty with Profix: A 8- to 10-year follow-up study. *Knee* 2006;13(6):419-421.

Hofmann AA, Bachus KN, Wyatt RW: Effect of the tibial cut on subsidence following total knee arthroplasty. *Clin Orthop Relat Res* 1991;269(269):63-69.

Hofmann AA, Evanich JD, Ferguson RP, Camargo MP: Ten- to 14-year clinical followup of the cementless Natural Knee system. *Clin Orthop Relat Res* 2001;388(388):85-94.

Hofmann AA, Heithoff SM, Camargo M: Cementless total knee arthroplasty in patients 50 years or younger. *Clin Orthop Relat Res* 2002;404(404):102-107.

Moran CG, Pinder IM, Lees TA, Midwinter MJ: Survivorship analysis of the uncemented porous-coated anatomic knee replacement. *J Bone Joint Surg Am* 1991;73(6):848-857.

Peters PC Jr , Engh GA, Dwyer KA, Vinh TN: Osteolysis after total knee arthroplasty without cement. *J Bone Joint Surg Am* 1992;74(6):864-876.

Schrøder HM, Berthelsen A, Hassani G, Hansen EB, Solgaard S: Cementless porous-coated total knee arthroplasty: 10-year results in a consecutive series. *J Arthroplasty* 2001;16(5):559-567.

Watanabe H, Akizuki S, Takizawa T: Survival analysis of a cementless, cruciate-retaining total knee arthroplasty: Clinical and radiographic assessment 10 to 13 years after surgery. *J Bone Joint Surg Br* 2004;86(6):824-829.

Whiteside LA: Long-term followup of the bone-ingrowth Ortholoc knee system without a metal-backed patella. *Clin Orthop Relat Res* 2001;388(388):77-84.

Whiteside LA, Viganò R: Young and heavy patients with a cementless TKA do as well as older and lightweight patients. *Clin Orthop Relat Res* 2007;464:93-98.

Coding

CPT Code		Corresponding ICD-9 Codes	
27447	Arthroplasty, knee, condyle and plateau; medial AND lateral compartments with or without patella resurfacing (total knee arthroplasty)	715 715.80	715.16 715.89

Chapter 14

Primary Total Knee Arthroplasty: Patellar Resurfacing

Jess H. Lonner, MD

Indications

Although many surgeons consider patellar resurfacing a prerequisite for the ultimate success of total knee arthroplasty (TKA) and therefore routinely resurface the patella except in highly unusual circumstances, others resurface selectively. For those who opt to resurface selectively, the relative indications for patellar resurfacing include the presence of anterior knee pain, notably damaged articular cartilage, inflammatory arthritis, patellar subluxation and maltracking on the femoral prosthesis, and a nonanatomic trochlear groove of the femoral prosthesis.

Contraindications

Even surgeons who choose to resurface the patella routinely may consider leaving the patella unresurfaced in young patients who have noninflammatory arthritis and no patellar cartilage wear, especially if the femoral component has an anatomic trochlear groove. Perhaps the strongest contraindication to resurfacing the patella

is the presence of a very thin and severely eroded patella, which can occur in patients with inflammatory arthritis and chronic patellar subluxation, when thickness of the patella even after conservative resection would be less than 10 to 12 mm.

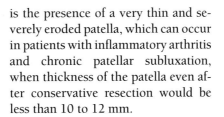

Alternative Treatments

No alternative treatment options exist except to not resurface the patella.

Results

Historically, complication rates and the need for secondary surgeries referrable to the patellofemoral articulation after patellar resurfacing in TKA were high, but these numbers have improved substantially over the last decade owing to improved trochlear designs and better understanding of femoral, tibial, and patellar prosthesis positioning, rotational alignment, and improved techniques of patellar resur-

facing. Complications include patellar fracture, patellar subluxation, patellofemoral pain, aseptic loosening, patellar clunk, extensor mechanism disruption, osteonecrosis, and patellar component wear. Data are available to support both resurfacing and nonresurfacing of the patella in TKA, but the trend over the last decade, especially in North America, appears to favor patellar resurfacing on a routine basis. An analysis of a large number of patients in the Swedish Knee Arthroplasty Register demonstrated that 19% of the nonresurfaced knees in patients with osteoarthritis were considered unsatisfactory, compared with 15% of the knees in which the patella was resurfaced. In patients with rheumatoid arthritis, 15% of the nonresurfaced knees were considered unsatisfactory compared with 12% of resurfaced knees. Other prospective randomized studies provided conflicting data: some showed superior results when the patella was resurfaced, some showed better results when the patella was left unresurfaced, and others showed no benefit of one approach over the other.

Technique

The patella can be resurfaced at any time during TKA. Although some surgeons prefer to prepare the patella

Dr. Lonner or an immediate family member has received royalties from Zimmer; serves as a member of a speakers' bureau or has made paid presentations on behalf of Zimmer and MAKO Surgical; serves as a paid consultant to or is an employee of Zimmer and MAKO Surgical; has received research or institutional support from Zimmer; and owns stock or stock options in MAKO Surgical.

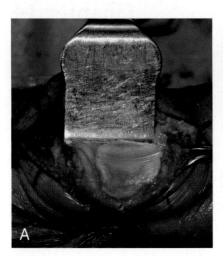 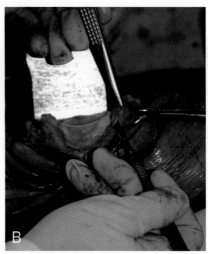 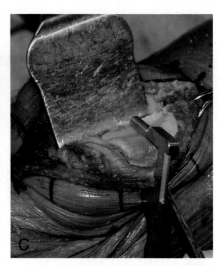

Figure 1 Assessing the patella. **A,** Advanced patellar arthritis is seen. **B,** The synovium from the undersurface of the quadriceps tendon is excised. **C,** The patellar thickness is measured with calipers.

early in the procedure, drilling lug holes in a resected articular surface of the patella may create a stress riser that could, in theory, predispose to inadvertent patellar fracture during retraction. It is advisable, therefore, to consider delaying drilling of the lug holes until after completion of the femoral and tibial preparation.

First, the extent of patellar arthritis and erosion is assessed (**Figure 1,** *A*). The synovial tissue surrounding the patella should be excised so that the margins of the articular surface of the patella are adequately exposed, focusing primarily on the synovial tissue on the undersurface of the quadriceps tendon at the proximal edge of the patella, to reduce the risk of patellar clunk or soft-tissue crepitus (**Figure 1,** *B*).

The thickness of the patella at the prominent point of the median ridge of the patella is measured using calipers (**Figure 1,** *C*). The amount of patellar bone resection depends in part on the thickness of the native patella and the patellar prosthesis, which typically is between 8 and 10 mm, depending on the manufacturer. In general, "overstuffing" the patella should be avoided because this may predis-

pose to anterior knee pain, loss of flexion, or fracture. Ideally, the prosthesis should be the same thickness or 1 mm thinner than the thickness of the removed bone. The composite thickness of the remaining patella and the patellar button should typically be the same as, or 1 mm less than, the native patellar thickness. At times, however, the patella is thin and underresection is necessary, which results in a patella-component composite that is thicker than the native patella. Some newer femoral prosthesis designs accommodate this with a thinner anterior flange, which reduces the risk of overstuffing the patellofemoral space when the patella is underresected.

My preference for patellar resection is an onlay-style preparation. The alternative preparation is an inlay technique. Resection is made from the medial patellar facet to the lateral patellar facet, keeping the saw blade parallel to the anterior surface of the patella (**Figure 2,** *A*). The saw blade is positioned at the edge of the articular cartilage on the medial patellar facet and directed to the junction of the patella and the quadriceps tendon proximally, the patella and patellar tendon distally (exposing the "patellar nose"), and the lateral facet at the junction of the ar-

ticular cartilage and the underlying subchondral bone. In cases of chronic patellar subluxation, the lateral facet can be extremely sclerotic; patience should be used in resecting this bone (**Figure 2,** *B*). After resecting the bone, calipers are used to ensure adequate thickness and symmetry of patellar resection. The patellar thickness should be equal in all quadrants of the bone after resection. The patellar sizing template is selected so that the button will be medialized as far as possible on the patella without hanging over the edges (**Figure 3,** *A*). It is also applied toward the proximal edge to reduce the risks of patellar clunk and catching within the intercondylar region of the femoral prosthesis in flexion. Typically, the patella is smaller when medialized than when it is placed centrally on the patella because of the oval shape of most patellae and because proximal-distal overhang must be avoided. Once the position is confirmed, the three lug holes are drilled (**Figure 3,** *B*). The trial patellar prosthesis is applied to the prepared surface. The uncovered bone of the lateral patellar facet (lateral to the lateral-most edge of the patella trial) is marked with a methylene blue pen and then removed with either a rongeur or saw blade to avoid a potential source of bony impingement and enhance patellar tracking (**Figure 4**). Patellar tracking is then assessed. Tilt or subluxation is addressed by first ensuring appropriate position of all three components of the TKA both coronally and rotationally. Additionally, appropriate bony preparation of the patella should be confirmed. If all components are appropriately positioned and the composite thickness of the patella is accurate, then a lateral retinacular recession can be performed, releasing the lateral retinaculum directly off the resected patellar surface. Downsizing the patellar prosthesis as described earlier and removing the uncovered lateral patellar facet in essence creates a bony decompression, substantially reducing the need for formal retinacular release with this technique.

The bony surfaces are then copiously irrigated and dried and the prosthesis is cemented into place (**Figure 5, A**). Extruded cement is removed (**Figure 5, B**). The uncovered portion of the patella is beveled to eliminate a potential source of pain from bone impingement. Additionally, removing this bone very likely removes tension on the lateral retinaculum, improving patellar tracking and reducing the need for lateral release. Once again, patellar tracking is assessed before closure and the wound is closed in the standard fashion (**Figure 5, C**). Figure 6 shows a knee before and after patellar resurfacing.

———————————————■

Video 14.1 Technique to Resurface the Patella. Robert Bourne, MD (4 min)

■ Postoperative Regimen

The postoperative regimen for primary TKA is the same for resurfaced and nonresurfaced patellae. Range-of-motion and isometric exercises begin immediately. Full weight bearing is al-

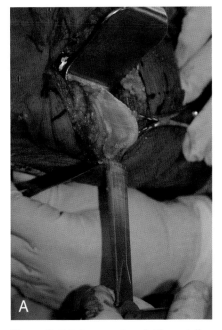
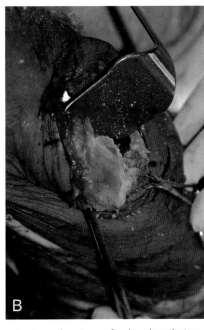

Figure 2 Patellar resection. **A,** The patellar resection is made using a "freehand" technique, starting from the medial facet and aiming toward the lateral facet. **B,** The patellar resection is completed. Note that sclerotic bone remains on the lateral facet. Measuring with calipers confirms equal depth of resection in all areas of the patella.

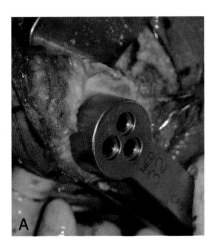
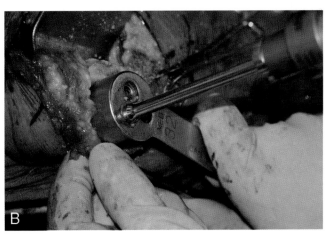

Figure 3 Preparing the patella for resurfacing. **A,** The patella sizing guide is medialized. **B,** Lug holes are drilled.

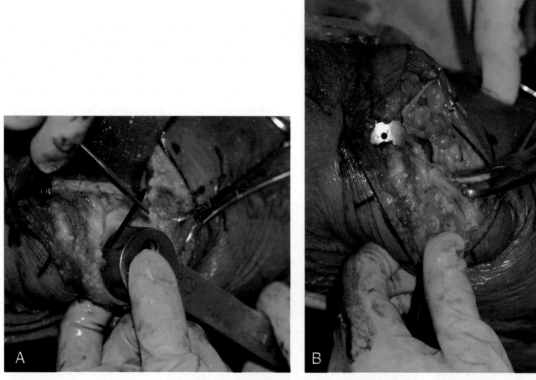

Figure 4 Removing excess patellar bone. **A,** The bone lateral to the lateral border of the patella sizing guide is marked with a methylene blue marker. **B,** The lateral bone that will not be covered by the patellar prosthesis is excised.

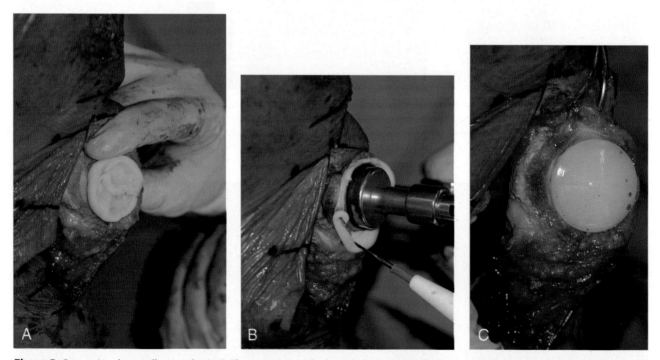

Figure 5 Cementing the patellar prosthesis. **A,** The cement is applied to the prepared patella. **B,** The patella and prosthesis are clamped until the cement hardens. Extruded cement is removed. **C,** The patellar prosthesis is in place, medialized to the edge of the patella, and the uncovered portion of the lateral patella has been beveled.

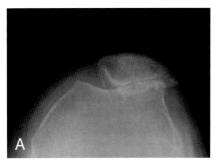 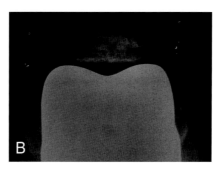

Figure 6 Radiographs of a knee with advanced patellar arthritis. **A,** Preoperative sunrise view showing advanced patellofemoral arthritis with patellar tilt and subluxation. **B,** Postoperative sunrise view demonstrating symmetric patellar preparation with centralization of the patellar prosthesis within the trochlear groove and elimination of patellar tilt or subluxation. The patellar prosthesis is medialized on the resected patella and the exposed lateral facet was excised.

lowed, initially with support; discontinuation of ambulation aids is allowed once reasonable quadriceps strength returns.

Avoiding Pitfalls and Complications

Historical data attributed nearly 50% of secondary surgeries after TKA to problems related to the patellofemoral articulation or extensor mechanism, but contemporary studies show that far fewer TKAs are failing due to patellofemoral complications. Nonetheless, while the incidence of problems attributable to the patellofemoral compartment has decreased, the challenges inherent in managing these complications and their ultimate implications are no less significant. These problems include patellar instability, fracture, patellar clunk/crepitus, osteonecrosis, extensor mechanism disruption, and patellar component loosening or wear. When the patella is resurfaced in TKA, patellar preparation and component positioning are important variables that may impact the clinical and functional outcomes. Even in the perfectly resurfaced patella, some degree of postoperative anterior knee or peripatellar pain and

compromised function after TKA may occur. The surgeon must be careful to avoid overresection, underresection, asymmetric bone preparation, and improper positioning of the patellar component or the presence of exposed bone, which may increase the risk of problems even further.

Patellar Instability
Symptomatic patellar instability occurs in less than 1% of TKAs thanks to improvement in prosthesis design and technical proficiency with proper implant alignment, positioning, and sizing. Internally rotated components, an overstuffed patellofemoral compartment, asymmetric patellar resection, medialized tibial or femoral components, lateralized patellar components, and improper soft-tissue balancing may predispose to patellar instability, which may compromise the outcome after TKA. Intraoperative performance of lateral retinacular release can correct patellar tilt and subluxation, but the need for lateral release has been reduced substantially by improved component design and by avoiding the errors noted earlier.

Patellar Fracture
The incidence of periprosthetic patellar fractures after TKA is less than 1%. Several factors may increase the risk for periprosthetic patellar fractures

during or after TKA. Predisposing intraoperative factors include overzealous clamping of the patella during implantation, aggressive bone resection leaving less than 10 to 15 mm of patellar bone stock, thermal injury and bone necrosis due to polymethylmethacrylate cement, and revision of the patellar component, particularly with poor bone stock. Periprosthetic patellar fractures can result from direct trauma or an indirect mechanism from an eccentric quadriceps muscle contraction. They can occur as a result of fatigue failure, particularly when there is osteonecrosis or very thin residual patellar bone. Sacrifice of a branch of the superior lateral geniculate artery during lateral release has been reported to be a risk factor for patellar osteonecrosis and subsequent patellar fracture following TKA, but this is not universally supported in all studies. Osteolysis and patellar component loosening put the patella at risk for fracture due to poor bone quality. Inadequate bony resection, overstuffing the anterior compartment (from an underresected patella or an anteriorized femoral component), and patellar maltracking also can increase the risk for postoperative patellar fractures due to transfer of higher contact stresses to the patella. Femoral and tibial component malalignment, either rotational or angular, can promote abnormal loading of the patellofemoral compartment, resulting in subluxation, dislocation, or fracture of the patella. Several patient factors have been suggested as increasing the risk of patellar fracture after primary TKA, including osteoporosis, bone cysts, poor bone stock, rheumatoid arthritis, male sex, increased activity, and excessive range of motion. Certain implant design features have been implicated as risk factors for patellar fracture after patellar resurfacing, such as a central peg design or uncemented or press-fit implants, especially metal-backed prostheses, which have higher contact stresses across the patellofemoral joint than cemented patellar implants. Periprosthetic patellar fractures are more likely in revision surgery.

Extensor Mechanism Rupture

Extensor mechanism disruption is one of the most devastating complications after TKA. Many features are required for an optimally functioning TKA, but loss of active extension profoundly compromises the basic functions of gait, stair-climbing, standing at rest, and knee stability. In the setting of TKA, surgical strategies aimed at reconstructing a disrupted extensor mechanism are fraught with complications and poor results. Quadriceps and patellar tendon ruptures have been reported to occur after 0.1% to 1.4% of primary TKAs. In addition to technical factors such as overresection of the patella, comorbidities such as rheumatoid arthritis, systemic and local corticosteroid use, obesity, and diabetes can put these tendons at risk. The patellar tendon is at particularly high risk for avulsion in stiff, tight, multiply operated, and revised knees, and therefore it must be protected during exposure and manipulation of the knee.

Patellar Component Loosening/Wear

Patellar component loosening and/or wear is unusual in cemented all-polyethylene patellar components that are well positioned, but loosening or wear can occur when there is chronic patellar subluxation, overstuffing, asymmetric bone preparation, component malposition, patellar osteonecrosis, obesity, elevated joint line, osteolysis, failure of ingrowth of porous prostheses, or component oxidation.

Patellar Clunk Syndrome and Synovial Impingement

Patellar clunk and synovial impingement represent a spectrum of patellar impingement complications following TKA, including painful crepitus, synovial entrapment, peripatellar fibrous hyperplasia, and full-blown patellar clunk. The incidence of patellar clunk has been reported to range from 0% to 7.5%, depending on femoral prosthesis design features.

In the classic sense, patellar clunk syndrome is the development of painful anterior knee catching or clunk, which results from the engagement of a hyperplastic prepatellar fibrous nodule in the intercondylar notch of the femoral component in knee flexion that displaces (clunks) as the knee is extended from approximately 45° to 30° of flexion. The nodule appears to be the result of fibrous hyperplasia and irritation at the level of the quadriceps insertion, but it also can arise from retained synovial tissue. Patellar clunk rarely occurs in patients with poor range of motion, because reasonably good flexion (90°) is required before the superior pole of the patella comes into contact with the intercondylar box and allows soft-tissue impingement. The etiology is multifactorial and has been attributed to femoral component design, alteration in the joint line, patellar height, patellar thickness, and patellar tracking. Patellar clunk has largely been described in first-generation posterior stabilized knee designs. Its incidence has declined with the use of contemporary posterior stabilized femoral designs that include modifications such as a raised lateral flange, deepened trochlear groove, and a more posterior intercondylar box, which allow the patella to be engaged in the component for a greater arc of motion.

———■

■ Bibliography

Barrack RL, Bertot AJ, Wolfe MW, Waldman DA, Milicic M, Myers L: Patellar resurfacing in total knee arthroplasty: A prospective, randomized, double-blind study with five to seven years of follow-up. *J Bone Joint Surg Am* 2001;83(9):1376-1381.

Burnett RS, Haydon CM, Rorabeck CH, Bourne RB: Patella resurfacing versus nonresurfacing in total knee arthroplasty: Results of a randomized controlled clinical trial at a minimum of 10 years' followup. *Clin Orthop Relat Res* 2004;428:12-25.

Clarke HD, Fuchs R, Scuderi GR, Mills EL, Scott WN, Insall JN: The influence of femoral component design in the elimination of patellar clunk in posterior-stabilized total knee arthroplasty. *J Arthroplasty* 2006;21(2):167-171.

Dobbs RE, Hanssen AD, Lewallen DG, Pagnano MW: Quadriceps tendon rupture after total knee arthroplasty: Prevalence, complications, and outcomes. *J Bone Joint Surg Am* 2005;87(1):37-45.

Hsu HC, Luo ZP, Rand JA, An KN: Influence of patellar thickness on patellar tracking and patellofemoral contact characteristics after total knee arthroplasty. *J Arthroplasty* 1996;11(1):69-80.

Hsu HC, Luo ZP, Rand JA, An KN: Influence of lateral release on patellar tracking and patellofemoral contact characteristics after total knee arthroplasty. *J Arthroplasty* 1997;12(1):74-83.

Kim BS, Reitman RD, Schai PA, Scott RD: Selective patellar nonresurfacing in total knee arthroplasty: 10 year results. *Clin Orthop Relat Res* 1999;367:81-88.

Lonner JH: Lateral patellar chamfer in total knee arthroplasty. *Am J Orthop* 2001;30(9):713-714.

Lynch AF, Rorabeck CH, Bourne RB: Extensor mechanism complications following total knee arthroplasty. *J Arthroplasty* 1987;2(2):135-140.

Mihalko W, Fishkin Z, Krackow K: Patellofemoral overstuff and its relationship to flexion after total knee arthroplasty. *Clin Orthop Relat Res* 2006;449:283-287.

Pollock DC, Ammeen DJ, Engh GA: Synovial entrapment: a complication of posterior stabilized total knee arthroplasty. *J Bone Joint Surg Am* 2002;84(12):2174-2178.

Reuben JD, McDonald CL, Woodard PL, Hennington LJ: Effect of patella thickness on patella strain following total knee arthroplasty. *J Arthroplasty* 1991;6(3):251-258.

Sheth NP, Pedowitz DI, Lonner JH: Periprosthetic patellar fractures. *J Bone Joint Surg Am* 2007;89(10):2285-2296.

Waters TS, Bentley G: Patellar resurfacing in total knee arthroplasty: A prospective, randomized study. *J Bone Joint Surg Am* 2003;85(2):212-217.

Yoshii I, Whiteside LA, Anouchi YS: The effect of patellar button placement and femoral component design on patellar tracking in total knee arthroplasty. *Clin Orthop Relat Res* 1992;275:211-219.

Video Reference

Bourne R: Video. *Technique to Resurface the Patella*, in DVD-video supplement to Helfet DL, Greene WB: *Instructional Course Lectures 53*. Rosemont, IL, American Academy of Orthopaedic Surgeons, 2004.

Coding				
CPT Codes			**Corresponding ICD-9 Codes**	
Total Knee Arthroplasty				
27447	Arthroplasty, knee, condyle and plateau; medial AND lateral compartments with or without patella resurfacing (total knee arthroplasty)		715 715.80	715.16 715.89

CPT copyright © 2010 by the American Medical Association. All rights reserved.

Chapter 15

Pain Management and Rehabilitation After Primary Total Knee Arthroplasty

Michael A. Mont, MD

Michael G. Zywiel, MD

Mike S. McGrath, MD

Anil Bhave, PT

Introduction

As the number of total knee arthroplasties (TKAs) performed each year increases, patient expectations also have grown, and an increasing number of patients desire higher activity levels, including a return to recreational sports activities. This desire to perform at a higher functional level requires effective pain management, in addition to a carefully planned and aggressive rehabilitation regimen.

Pain control and rehabilitation are two crucial aspects of postoperative care after TKA. They are important for patients to maximize range of motion, improve muscle strength, ambulate, and resume activities of daily living.

Some patients who undergo TKA may experience poor function as a result of soft-tissue limitations, such as flexion contractures or deficits, even if the prosthesis is well aligned and well fixed. Specialized intensive rehabilitation and pain management techniques may successfully treat patients who have arthrofibrosis or other soft-tissue dysfunctions.

This chapter describes a multimodal pain management and rehabilitation protocol that has been used to treat patients who have undergone TKA. Results of several randomized controlled studies that followed patients managed with multimodal pain and rehabilitation protocols are listed in **Table 1**. Standard rehabilitation methods are described for the immediate postoperative period. In addition, specialized therapeutic techniques for patients who have specific postoperative functional problems are described.

Pain Management

Patients who have undergone TKA may experience severe postoperative pain, which may slow their functional progression. A multimodal approach to pain management uses multiple strategies synergistically. This may be more effective than a single pain control technique, because the multimodal approach uses smaller doses of each treatment, lowering the risk of side effects from any single modality. In addition, various treatments are used preoperatively, intraoperatively, and postoperatively to improve pain control at all stages of recovery. We will describe these approaches for pain management, illustrating them with our own pain protocol (**Table 2**) and comparing it with other protocols.

Preemptive Analgesia

Preemptive analgesia refers to any pain management medication or other treatment that is given before the surgical procedure. This may reduce sensitization of the central nervous system to the pain stimulus and decrease immediate postoperative pain. A cyclooxygenase-2 (COX-2) inhibitor or other nonsteroidal anti-inflammatory

Dr. Mont or an immediate family member has received royalties from Stryker; serves as a paid consultant to or is an employee of Stryker and Wright Medical Technology; and has received research or institutional support from Stryker, Wright Medical Technology, Biomet, Brainlab, DePuy, Finsbury, Smith & Nephew, and Salient Surgical Technologies. Dr. Zywiel or an immediate family member has received research or institutional support from Stryker, Wright Medical Technology, Biomet, Brainlab, DePuy, Finsbury, Smith & Nephew, and Salient Surgical Technologies. Neither of the following authors nor any immediate family member has received anything of value from or owns stock in a commercial company or institution related directly or indirectly to the subject of this chapter: Dr. McGrath and Mr. Bhave.

Table 1 Results of Multimodal Pain and Rehabilitation Protocols After Total Knee Arthroplasty

Authors (Year)	Number of Knees or Patients	Procedure or Approach	Mean Patient Age in Years (Range)	Mean Follow-up	Results
MacDonald et al (2000)	120 knees randomized to one of three groups	Group I: no CPM* Group II: CPM* from 0° to 50°, increased as tolerated Group III: CPM* from 70° to 110°	NR	52 weeks	No differences in cumulative postoperative analgesic requirements, range of motion and final or interval follow-up, length of stay, or Knee Society scores at final follow-up
Avramidis et al (2003)	30 patients randomized to one of two groups	Group I: standard physical therapy only Group II: electromuscular stimulation of vastus medialis 4 hours/day from postoperative day 2 for 6 weeks + standard physical therapy	Group I: 71 ± 7.8 Group II: 68 ± 10.6	Final follow-up: 12 weeks Interval follow-up: 6 weeks	Significantly faster walking speed at all follow-up periods with stimulation; similar physiologic cost index and Hospital for Special Surgery knee scores
Vendittoli et al (2006)	42 patients randomized to one of two groups	All patients operated under spinal anesthesia Group I: intraoperative periarticular injection of analgesic cocktail + postoperative PCA Group II: postoperative PCA only	NR	5 days	Significantly lower narcotic consumption over first 40 hours postoperatively in group I (47 vs 69 mg; $P = 0.044$) Group I had significantly lower pain scores on postoperative day 1 during exercise (4.7 vs 6.6; $P = 0.008$) and on postoperative day 2 at rest ($P = 0.01$) Both groups achieved similar active knee flexion on postoperative day 5 (85° vs 86°; $P = 0.815$)
Busch et al (2006)	64 knees randomized to one of two groups	All patients received the same postoperative analgesia consisting of 24 hours of PCA followed by standard analgesia Group I: intraoperative periarticular injection of analgesic cocktail Group II: no injection	Group I: 66 (51-78) Group II: 70 (51-80)	6 weeks	Significantly lower use of PCA in group I over first 24 hours postoperatively (mean, 25 vs 45 mg; $P < 0.001$) Group I had significantly higher patient satisfaction scores ($P = 0.016$) and significantly lower pain scores ($P = 0.007$) 4 hours postoperatively No significant difference in range of motion at 6-week follow-up
Parvateneni et al (2007)	60 knees randomized to one of two groups	All patients operated on under spinal anesthesia Group I: intraoperative periarticular injection of analgesic cocktail Group II: postoperative femoral nerve block and PCA	Group I: 69 Group II: 71	All patients followed for 3 months	Significantly higher number of patients in group I able to achieve straight-leg raise on postoperative day 1 (63% vs 21%; $P < 0.05$) Group I mean pain scores were lower and satisfaction levels were higher on postoperative day 1, but difference was not significant (P value NR) Mean range of motion was higher in group I at 3 months postoperatively (118 vs 114), but not significant (P value NR)

* CPM was initiated in the recovery room for 18 to 24 hours.
PCA = patient-controlled analgesia, NR = not reported, CPM = continuous passive motion.

Table 2 Authors' Protocol for Total Knee Arthroplasty Pain Management

Preemptive	Intraoperative	Postoperative	Discharge
Anti-inflammatory: ketorolac 15-30 mg intravenous (continue every 8 h postoperatively) Oxycodone 10 mg in preoperative holding area	Lumbar spinal anesthesia (10 mg 0.5% tetracaine) Femoral nerve block (40 mL 0.125% bupivacaine) Injections: 20 mL 0.25% bupivacaine HCl with epinephrine (skin and subcutaneous tissues preincision) 10 mL morphine sulfate injected at end (capsule and other tissues)	Femoral nerve block (10 mL/h 0.125% bupivacaine), left in until postoperative day 2 Oxycodone 5-19 mg every 3-4 h Hydromorphone 0.2 mg every 6 min PCA, discontinued on postoperative day 1 Toradol 15-30 mg every 8 h postoperatively Acetaminophen 650 mg every 6 h as needed If pain not controlled, add oxycodone (10 mg every 12 h orally)	Oxycodone/acetaminophen 5-10 mg orally every 4 h as needed Acetaminophen 650 mg every 8 h as needed

PCA = patient-controlled analgesia.

drug (NSAID) is given before the surgery. This may reduce the inflammation associated with the tissue damage as well as lower the response of the central nervous system to the painful stimuli. In addition, a sustained-release narcotic medication may be given to further reduce the transmission of the nociceptive (pain) signals. We use a combination of ketorolac and oxycodone for preemptive analgesia (**Table 2**).

We use lumbar spinal anesthesia that is induced in the operating room by the anesthesiologist with a continuous infusion of a long-acting local anesthetic for the duration of the surgery. Next, the anesthesiologist performs a femoral nerve block. A nerve stimulator is used to find the femoral nerve in the surgical limb, and a 40-mL bolus of a long-acting local anesthetic is injected through a nerve catheter. The catheter is left in place for 48 hours following the surgery and is attached to a peripheral nerve pump for a continuous infusion of the local anesthetic at 10 mL per hour. Other anesthesia methods include epidural anesthesia (for longer surgeries than those for which spinal anesthesia is appropriate) or general anesthesia (in patients who prefer this modality to regional anesthesia, who are anticoagulated, or who have indications such as an intervertebral disk prolapse or a history of previous back surgery.

Intraoperative Analgesia

Before making the incision, the skin and subcutaneous tissues in the region of the incision are infiltrated with 20 mL of a short-acting local anesthetic to block pain transmission in this region. At the end of the procedure, after closure of the capsule, the capsule and all other soft tissues within the surgical wound are infiltrated with a solution that contains 10 mL of a long-acting opioid medication. This is applied directly to the soft tissues in an attempt to reduce transmission of pain signals. Various authors have described different anesthetic agents and techniques for instillation of local anesthetics at the surgical site.

Postoperative Analgesia

As described previously, the femoral nerve catheter is left in place for 48 hours with a continuous infusion of a long-acting local anesthetic at 10 mL per hour after the surgery. The patient is given a patient-controlled analgesia (PCA) device with an opioid medication. The dose and lockout times of the PCA device are titrated to give the patient adequate analgesia, and the device is discontinued the following day.

When the patient can tolerate oral intake, a sustained-release opioid, a COX-2 inhibitor or other NSAID, and a centrally acting analgesic such as acetaminophen (650 mg, every 8 hours) are prescribed. Breakthrough narcotic medications are also given orally or intravenously every 3 hours as needed. At discharge, prescriptions are given for an opioid/acetaminophen combination (5 to 10 mg orally every 4 hours as needed) and for acetaminophen (650 mg every 8 hours, with instructions to not exceed 4,000 mg of acetaminophen from all sources in 24 hours). In addition to these medications, other pain control methods are occasionally used. Various authors have described other anti-inflammatory, analgesic, and narcotic regimens.

Epidural infusions of a long-acting local anesthetic medication in addition to an opioid medication are used for patients who have severe preoperative pain or who exhibit a low tolerance for pain. The benefits of this technique must be weighed against the potential risks, which include spinal hematoma, hypotension, urinary retention, or motor inhibition. Iontophoresis has been used to apply anti-inflammatory or local anesthetic medications transdermally into the knee joint, although little scientific data exist on the use of this technique. Cryotherapy has been found by some to be a useful method of pain control. It has occasionally been shown to reduce length of stay after TKA, and it may improve walking velocity. Although cryotherapy may not reduce the need for narcotic analgesics in the early postoperative phase, it may be a useful adjunct, which is best used before and after therapy sessions.

————————■

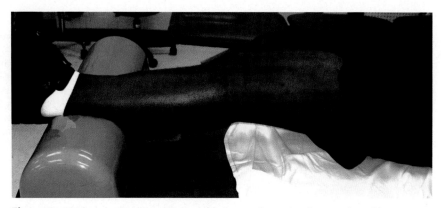

Figure 1 A bolster is placed under the ankle for gravity-assisted promotion of knee extension.

■ Rehabilitation

Rehabilitation protocols can be divided broadly into an acute phase of postoperative recovery, which takes place during the hospital stay, and an outpatient phase, in which the patient returns home and may require outpatient rehabilitation. Patients who have undergone TKA most commonly report increased pain during flexion exercises. Despite the pain, early flexion range of motion is one of the critical factors to achieve good function postoperatively. Patients are not restricted by weight-bearing protocols, only by their own abilities, tolerance to pain, and improvement of strength as well as range of motion.

Acute Phase
The acute phase of rehabilitation may last up to 3 to 4 days after surgery. Physical therapy sessions are performed at least once per day, with twice-daily sessions useful for most patients. It is best to provide therapy coverage through the weekend for all patients.

Patients often have better results during the acute phase if they have been assessed for risk factors that might increase the length of stay. Patients with risk factors such as obesity, diabetes, preoperative knee stiffness, or other comorbidities may respond well to a more targeted and intensive regimen during this early phase. Patients who are identified as high risk receive a targeted therapy approach,

with two sessions per day of therapy in the acute rehabilitation phase. Patients are encouraged to begin therapy once a day, five times a week, immediately on discharge from the hospital. When contractures are exhibited before discharge, the patient is fitted with a customized knee device (CKD) brace to improve extension. Patients typically use the brace for up to three sessions daily, each lasting up to 45 minutes. Patients with flexion deficits (<70° of knee flexion) may receive continuous passive motion (CPM) machines to use at home and intensive hands-on knee joint mobilization therapy daily. Once the staples are removed, these patients can be fitted for a CKD brace or begin treatment with an off-the-shelf stretch orthosis to improve flexion as well. Patients are requested to follow up every 2 weeks instead of at 6 weeks after surgery as otherwise practiced.

Postoperative rehabilitation starts on the day of surgery and is focused on helping the patient get out of bed and teaching transfers from the bed to a chair. Moderate-intensity isometric contractions of the gluteal, quadriceps, and calf muscles are started at the same time. Patients are encouraged to perform deep breathing exercises. A gentle regimen is started that consists of active assisted flexion and passive extension exercises, followed by the slide and flex, tighten, extend

(SAFTE) protocol, as described by Kolisek and associates. Active exercises of the hamstring muscles relax the quadriceps mechanism by reciprocal inhibition and reduce pain associated with knee flexion. Aggressive passive flexion exercises should be avoided in the early postoperative phase; however, passive knee extension exercises of moderate intensity are recommended to avoid development of flexion contractures. Patients are positioned with a towel roll or bolster under the ankle for several hours each day to promote gravity-assisted knee extension (**Figure 1**).

Routine use of CPM machines for all patients after TKA may be unwarranted. Several published reports have found no additional benefit from routine use of CPM in patients after TKA when compared with a standardized physical therapy regimen. A CPM protocol might be reserved for patients who have preoperative stiffness, poor tolerance to pain, and inadequate participation in therapy. In our practice, we use this modality if patients have less than a 90° total arc of motion preoperatively or have heavy preoperative narcotic usage per day (>20 mg morphine or equivalent usage per day), or after knee manipulations or revision surgery with known range-of-motion problems. Patients who have preoperative stiffness with reduced flexion range of motion may benefit from an early flexion protocol with CPM (70° to 110° of flexion followed by increased extension daily as tolerated). Patients who have preoperative flexion contractures are better suited for periods of extension bracing followed by the use of a CPM protocol that ranges from full extension to flexion. Care should be taken to avoid development of flexion contractures, as most CPM machines allow the knee to stay flexed. It is important to use additional padding under the heel to avoid development of knee flexion contractures while using CPM.

Neuromuscular electrical stimulation (NMES) of the quadriceps muscle is a very useful modality for promoting knee extension and improving strength in selected patients. Specifically, it is used in patients with excessive postoperative pain or pain at rest that interferes with rehabilitative efforts (**Figure 2**). It involves applying electrodes over the vastus medialis obliquus muscle and over the proximal aspect of the vastus lateralis muscle. NMES is recommended for 20 to 30 minutes, with a 5-second on time and a 15-second off time, and a waveform at 70 to 90 pps with a pulse duration of 400 μsec. During the early postoperative phase, the intensity of the stimulator can be set to produce submaximal contractions.

Several precautions should be followed for ambulation during rehabilitation. Patients are typically allowed to bear weight as tolerated after a TKA and to gradually increase the loading of the joint. They also are allowed unlimited ambulation on a level surface. Early use of a unilateral assistive device such as a cane may cause increased torsional stress and pain in the knee joint, however, so bilateral support, such as crutches or a walker, is sometimes encouraged. A knee immobilizer is recommended for ambulation during rehabilitation for patients who have quadriceps muscle weakness and who demonstrate knee extension lag. This ensures axial weight

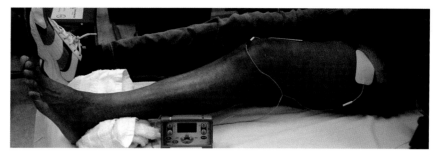

Figure 2 Neuromuscular electrical stimulation (NMES) can help to improve knee extension strength after total knee arthroplasty. Clinical photograph shows electrodes applied over the vastus medialis obliquus and vastus lateralis muscles; a stimulus is used to promote quadriceps contractions.

bearing and reduces the risk of torsional or angular forces on the prosthesis. Patients are instructed to ascend stairs one at a time and to use the nonoperated side as the leading leg for each step during the early postoperative phase. When going down stairs, patients are encouraged to descend one step at a time, leading with the operated leg.

Outpatient Phase

After the acute phase, the patient may be discharged to home or to an inpatient rehabilitation unit. Many patients are sent home on postoperative day 2 or 3 without negative consequences. The decision to send a patient to an inpatient rehabilitation unit should be made in a team setting after evaluating the physical, social, and psychologic needs of the patient. There is an increasing trend in many hospitals to refer patients to an inpatient rehabilitation unit to reduce the length of stay in the acute setting. This can lead to inadequate therapy services for the patient, which may result in the premature onset of knee stiffness. A reduced length of stay in the acute setting has been correlated with an increased incidence of manipulations under anesthesia.

After discharge, most patients who have undergone a TKA are not restricted in any specific way. They are allowed unlimited ambulation on a

level surface and are encouraged to exercise at least 1 hour daily, focusing on increasing range of motion to attain full extension, increasing lower extremity strength, and improving balance and gait. However, for patients with considerable knee instability associated with an extensor lag of 30° or more, the use of a knee immobilizer, supportive devices such as crutches or a cane, and a gradual increase in the loading of the joint are recommended.

In the outpatient setting, NMES therapy is modified to provide maximal contractions for short durations. Simple biofeedback measures, such as inflated cuffs, also are useful to promote knee extension with isometric quadriceps muscle exercises.

Most patients can return to driving a motor vehicle 4 to 6 weeks after TKA. The decision to return to driving should be based on improvement in reaction time, ability to sit for prolonged periods of time, and strength of the operated side. A gradual return to activities of daily living, followed by increased joint loading in ambulation as tolerated, may lead to the best results. At this point, patients are eager to return to some form of recreational sports. Patients who have undergone TKA should be encouraged to engage in light recreational activities such as swimming, golf, bowling, bicycling, and doubles tennis. Patients can resume sexual activity shortly after

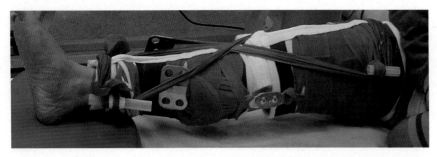

Figure 3 A customized knee device is used to provide a low-load progressive stretch to the knee joint in extension.

TKA. Patients who have undergone TKA rarely ask questions about safe sexual positions during a clinic visit, but they do welcome information when it is supplied.

Treatment of Soft-Tissue Impairments

Some patients may have soft-tissue impairments that require special attention, such as quadriceps muscle weakness, knee flexion contracture, knee flexion deficit, peroneal neuropathy, or limb-length discrepancy. Quadriceps muscle weakness is defined as an active extension lag exceeding 15° in the early postoperative phase, or muscle strength that is less than 50% compared with the contralateral limb as measured by a dynamometer in the later stages of recovery. A knee flexion contracture is defined as a lack of extension of 10° or more, and a knee flexion deficit is defined as knee flexion range of motion less than 90°. Peroneal nerve entrapment produces burning pain down to the dorsum of the foot, paresthesias of the foot, increased foot pain, mild extensor hallucis longus muscle weakness, and a positive Tinel sign. In addition to these symptoms, patients who have a previous history of sciatica can develop increased peroneal nerve tension and symptoms postoperatively. Patients who have undergone a TKA occasionally demonstrate a limb-length discrepancy, with the TKA side being longer than the contralateral side; this might result in a compensa-

tory flexed knee posture and a subsequent knee flexion contracture. Patients who have a bilateral genu varum deformity may develop a limb-length discrepancy after a unilateral TKA, as a result of increased length on the operated side due to the correction of the varus deformity.

The causes of knee flexion contractures include preoperative loss of motion with muscle shortening; previous surgery with excessive scar-tissue formation; knee effusion, which may result in pain as well as quadriceps muscle inhibition with associated hamstring overactivity; unrecognized gastrocnemius muscle tightness; a limb-length discrepancy, with a resultant flexed-knee posture, as described previously; periarticular remodeling; joint subluxation; and peroneal nerve entrapment.

All patients who develop knee flexion contractures should receive a fitted splint to wear at home. A splint can hold the knee in a position of maximally tolerated extension for a period of time, which may lead to plastic remodeling of the soft tissues and subsequent improvement of the contracture. Two types of off-the-shelf devices are commercially available. The Dynasplit brace (Dynasplint Devices, Severna Park, MD) uses the principles of low-load prolonged stretch and might need to be used up to 8 hours per day. The JAS device (Joint Active Systems, Effingham, IL) uses the principles of stress relaxation and static progressive stretch, in which the pa-

tients apply incrementally greater degrees of stretch across the joint for 30-minute sessions, three times per day. An alternative is the use of a low-cost CKD. This device is custom-fitted for each patient and uses a graded elastic band attached in a figure-of-8 fashion to produce an extension moment at the knee (**Figure 3**). Patients typically use the CKD at the maximally tolerated tension for three 30- to 45-minute sessions per day. The device is helpful for maintaining prolonged knee extension positioning at home, and it is sometimes used at night.

In addition to splinting, an adjunctive therapy consisting of moist heat, aggressive soft-tissue mobilization of the posterior knee, manual maximal knee extension, NMES, and weight-bearing exercise at least 4 to 5 days per week is recommended. Knee joint mobilization is performed to position the knee at the end range of extension, with the patient in a supine position and the proximal tibia supported by a bolster (**Figure 4**). The gastrocnemius muscle is stretched with the patient supine, the heel propped, and the knee joint positioned in maximum extension. It is important to mobilize the patella superiorly during knee extension mobilization, as this promotes easier knee extension. NMES also is used, initially at submaximal intensity until this is well tolerated by the patient, followed by a short-duration protocol of burst superimposition technique with maximal isometric contraction, which may rapidly increase quadriceps muscle strength. Weight-bearing exercises, including leg-press movements for closed-chain end-range knee extension, also are used. This aggressive treatment regimen for flexion contractures is successful in most patients. Gait training is used to improve active heel strike at initial contact once the flexion contracture has resolved, and any limb-length discrepancy is managed with an appropriate shoe lift. Special attention is given to terminal knee extension strength. Patients who have weakness in this range will flex the knee during walking to put the quadriceps muscle under tension for stance-phase stability, which can result in recurrence of the knee flexion contracture.

Knee flexion deficits (<90° of flexion) result in functional impairments in stair ascent or descent, sitting in or rising from a chair, prolonged sitting, and sexual activities. These problems may be caused by joint effusion, quadriceps muscle tightness, rectus femorus muscle tightness, or patellar tendon tightness or inflammation. In a subset of patients who fail to achieve adequate knee flexion with physical therapy alone, additional mechanical therapy is recommended. A simple adaptation of the overhead pulley system could be used to do self-stretching exercises. Another method of self-stretching can be performed with the CKD, which can be fitted to stretch the knee in flexion (**Figure 5**). Patients are asked to use it for 30 to 45 minutes per session, three times per day, to improve knee flexion. In addition to splinting, careful knee joint mobilization with posterior glides of the tibia, inferior patellar mobilization, and mobilization of the quadriceps muscle and patellar tendon may be used to increase knee flexion. Physical therapy and customized bracing alone are successful in most cases.

Significant quadriceps muscle weakness is considered to be present when there is either an active extension lag of greater than 15°, or quadriceps muscle strength that is less than 50% of the contralateral side, as measured with a dynamometer. A high incidence of quadriceps muscle weakness is seen in patients who have undergone TKA, and this may continue up to 2 years postoperatively if not specifically addressed. Patients should be counseled that regular daily activities in addition to walking may not improve quadriceps strength, and that a targeted strengthening exercise

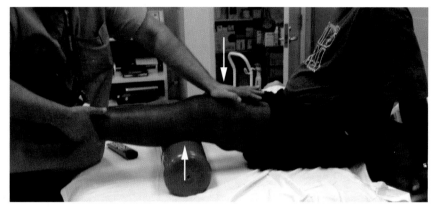

Figure 4 Anterior-posterior mobilization of the femur is used to position the knee at the end range of extension. The patient is placed in the supine position with a bolster under the proximal tibia. The applied forces are indicated by the white arrows.

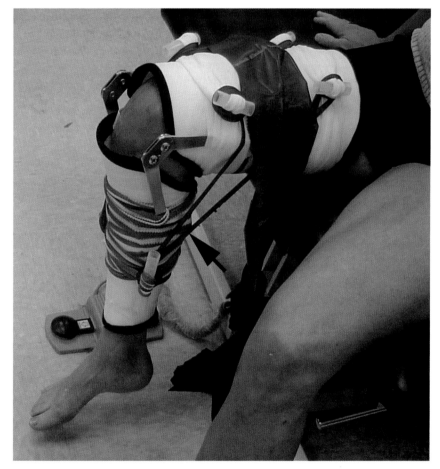

Figure 5 A customized knee device is positioned to apply low-load progressive stretch in flexion. A graded elastic band provides the stretching force (arrow). A second elastic band (not seen) is similarly placed on the lateral aspect of the device.

may be needed. Several techniques can be used to increase motor unit recruitment. Our protocol is to begin with closed-chain exercises such as leg presses. These are followed by open-chain exercises such as active knee extension exercises with ankle weights, and finally isokinetic exercises. NMES can be used to augment the muscle contraction during strengthening. This regimen may be more effective than voluntary contractions alone because of the neural overflow produced by the electrical stimulation. In addition to this targeted regimen, functional activities such as step-ups and mini-squats may be beneficial.

Peroneal nerve entrapment can result in a lack of knee extension, because knee extension can place tension on the entrapped peroneal nerve, which can result in foot pain; accordingly, patients who have this condition will keep the knee flexed to avoid this symptom. These patients may show no frank motor involvement except for mild weakness of the extensor hallucis longus muscle. In the presence of peroneal nerve symptoms, rehabilitation is difficult and may not improve the results. Surgical release of the peroneal nerve typically results in quick resolution of symptoms, and aggressive rehabilitation can immediately begin to address contractures as well as muscle weakness.

Manipulation Under Anesthesia

Patients who fail these methods may require manipulation under anesthesia to improve flexion range of motion. The best results of manipulation are obtained around 6 weeks postoperatively. Patients who have not attained 90° of motion by 6 weeks postoperatively are candidates for manipulation. In addition, some patients who are making less progress at earlier time points can be considered for manipulation. We do not like to perform manipulations after 8 weeks postoperatively. We typically use general anesthesia (ie, propofol 4 mg/kg) for outpatient manipulations, which occasionally are combined with femoral nerve blocks. If patients are being admitted for prolonged pain control, an epidural with or without a continuous femoral nerve block is an option. Once analgesia is achieved, the manipulation is performed by applying gentle downward pressure on the tibia with one hand, with the knee being flexed against the femur, which is stabilized by the other hand. We often put an ear to the knee to auscultate the "snap, crackle, pop" of the breaking up of adhesions. When sounds cease, the manipulation should be discontinued to avoid complications such as skin tears or fracture. Postoperatively, patients resume physical therapy immediately (the same day if possible), either as an inpatient or an outpatient. Patients should be followed up often after manipulation to ensure the best results.

Bibliography

Ashburn MA, Stephen RL, Ackerman E, et al: Iontophoretic delivery of morphine for postoperative analgesia. *J Pain Symptom Manage* 1992;7(1):27-33.

Avramidis K, Strike PW, Taylor PN, Swain ID: Effectiveness of electric stimulation of the vastus medialis muscle in the rehabilitation of patients after total knee arthroplasty. *Arch Phys Med Rehabil* 2003;84(12):1850-1853.

Bonutti PM, McGrath MS, Ulrich SD, McKenzie SA, Seyler TM, Mont MA: Static progressive stretch for the treatment of knee stiffness. *Knee* 2008;15(4):272-276.

Busch CA, Shore BJ, Bhandari R, et al: Efficacy of periarticular multimodal drug injection in total knee arthroplasty: A randomized trial. *J Bone Joint Surg Am* 2006;88(5):959-963.

Kolisek FR, Gilmore KJ, Peterson EK: Slide and flex, tighten, extend (SAFTE): A safe, convenient, effective, and no-cost approach to rehabilitation after total knee arthroplasty. *J Arthroplasty* 2000;15(8):1013-1016.

Lavernia C, Cardona D, Rossi MD, Lee D: Multimodal pain management and arthrofibrosis. *J Arthroplasty* 2008;23(6, Suppl 1)74-79.

MacDonald SJ, Bourne RB, Rorabeck CH, McCalden RW, Kramer J, Vaz M: Prospective randomized clinical trial of continuous passive motion after total knee arthroplasty. *Clin Orthop Relat Res* 2000;380:30-35.

Mahomed NN, Koo Seen Lin MJ, Levesque J, Lan S, Bogoch ER: Determinants and outcomes of inpatient versus home based rehabilitation following elective hip and knee replacement. *J Rheumatol* 2000;27(7):1753-1758.

Mauerhan DR, Mokris JG, Ly A, Kiebzak GM: Relationship between length of stay and manipulation rate after total knee arthroplasty. *J Arthroplasty* 1998;13(8):896-900.

Oldmeadow LB, McBurney H, Robertson VJ, Kimmel L, Elliott B: Targeted postoperative care improves discharge outcome after hip or knee arthroplasty. *Arch Phys Med Rehabil* 2004;85(9):1424-1427.

Seyler TM, Marker DR, Bhave A, et al: Functional problems and arthrofibrosis following total knee arthroplasty. *J Bone Joint Surg Am* 2007;89(Suppl 3):59-69.

Silva M, Shepherd EF, Jackson WO, Pratt JA, McClung CD, Schmalzried TP: Knee strength after total knee arthroplasty. *J Arthroplasty* 2003;18(5):605-611.

Parvataneni HK, Shah VP, Howard H, Cole N, Ranawat AS, Ranawat CS: Controlling pain after total hip and knee arthroplasty using a multimodal protocol with local periarticular injections: A prospective randomized study. *J Arthroplasty* 2007;22(6, Suppl 2):33-38.

Vendittoli PA, Makinen P, Drolet P, et al: A multimodal analgesia protocol for total knee arthroplasty: A randomized, controlled study. *J Bone Joint Surg Am* 2006;88(2):282-289.

Youm T, Maurer SG, Stuchin SA: Postoperative management after total hip and knee arthroplasty. *J Arthroplasty* 2005; 20(3):322-324.

	Coding		
CPT Codes		**Corresponding ICD-9 Codes**	
20974	Electrical stimulation to aid bone healing; noninvasive (nonoperative)	733.82	
27447	Arthroplasty, knee, condyle and plateau; medial AND lateral compartments with or without patella resurfacing (total knee arthroplasty)	715 715.80	715.16 715.89
27570	Manipulation of knee joint under general anesthesia (includes application of traction or other fixation devices)	718.46	

Chapter 16
Unicondylar Knee Arthroplasty

Gerard A. Engh, MD
William G. Hamilton, MD

▮ Indications

Unicompartmental knee arthroplasty (UKA) has been performed worldwide since the 1970s. The popularity of UKA compared with total knee arthroplasty (TKA) has oscillated over time. Early enthusiasm for UKA was tempered in the orthopaedic community by reports of short-term and midterm failures. Researchers continue to improve UKA implant designs, however, and surgical techniques have been refined. Accordingly, the indications for UKA are evolving as well.

Currently in North America, several classic indications for UKA are reasonably well accepted. An anteromedial wear pattern in the medial compartment is desirable because this pattern of wear correlates with a functional anterior cruciate ligament (ACL), which most consider important to the success of UKA. If cartilage loss is evident either radiographically or intraoperatively in the posterior region of the medial tibial plateau or

femoral condyle, it is likely that the ACL has lost its functional integrity. Because early degeneration of the ligament may result in functional deficiency in the knee, many authors emphasize the wear pattern as more important than the appearance of the ACL. In younger (<60 years of age) patients with a nonfunctional ACL, performing ACL reconstruction concomitantly with a medial UKA has shown promising short-term results.

The other classic indications for UKA include preoperative range of motion and ligament laxity of the knee within acceptable parameters. An arc of flexion greater than 90° with a flexion contracture of less than 15° is considered acceptable. A varus deformity of up to 10° can be accepted; however, physical examination should reveal this deformity to be passively correctable to neutral when a valgus stress is placed on the knee at 20° of flexion. Stress radiographs can be used preoperatively to confirm the ability to passively correct alignment of the knee.

Other indications for UKA that are more controversial relate to patient age, weight, and degenerative changes in the unresurfaced compartments. Early in the evolution of UKA, authors considered the ideal patient for UKA to be thin, elderly, and sedentary. Currently, there is no well-accepted age criterion for UKA. Most publications report a wide age range in the study population, as UKA has become a more widely accepted option for patients with unicompartmental disease. In the younger (<50 years of age), more active patient, UKA can be used as a pre-TKA procedure in an effort to postpone TKA to a time when the prosthesis would be expected to have better longevity. Some of these patients may avoid TKA altogether, but for those in whom TKA does become necessary, several recent studies have shown that conversion of a failed UKA to TKA can be done with relative ease. In the elderly population (>75 years of age), UKA is an attractive alternative to TKA because of lessened surgical trauma, reduced blood loss, and accelerated recovery time. In this population, UKA may reduce the risk of perioperative complications. At the present time, age is a less important selection criterion than pattern of wear, degree of deformity, or the functional status of the ligaments.

UKA for obese patients remains controversial. The obesity epidemic in

Dr. Engh or an immediate family member has received royalties from DePuy and Innomed; is a member of a speakers' bureau or has made paid presentations on behalf of Smith & Nephew; serves as a paid consultant to or is an employee of Smith & Nephew and DePuy; has received research or institutional support from DePuy, Smith & Nephew, US Army Medical Research & Material Command & the Telemedicine & Advanced Technology Research Center, Medtronic, and Inova Health Systems; owns stock or stock options in Alexandria Research Technologies; and has received nonincome support (such as equipment or services), commercially derived honoraria, or other non-research-related funding (such as paid travel) from DePuy and Smith & Nephew. Neither Dr. Hamilton nor any immediate family member has received anything of value from or owns stock in a commercial company or institution related directly or indirectly to the subject of this chapter.

North America has increased the prevalence of this consideration. Neither UKA nor TKA is ideal in the morbidly obese patient (body mass index ≥ 40). In addition, the increased stresses that are placed on the implant in patients with a body mass index greater than 30 may increase the risk of aseptic loosening. Because of the larger surface area of a TKA implant, it has been theorized that loosening rates will be lower with TKA than with UKA. Resolution of this debate cannot be settled with the available published data. A frank discussion with the patient of the pros and cons of arthroplasty surgery is of paramount importance in the management of obese patients.

The ideal candidate for a UKA has a knee with disease that is isolated to one compartment. The amount of cartilage degeneration that is acceptable in the unresurfaced compartments of the knee is debatable. In medial UKA, up to grade 3 cartilage loss in the patellofemoral compartment appears to be acceptable; little difference in outcomes is seen in these patients. Some authors suggest ignoring nearly all patellofemoral lesions, treating only the worst grade 4 lesions on both the patellar and trochlear surfaces with a TKA. However, concern remains for knees with persistent patellofemoral pain after UKA. Some studies report a need for conversion to a TKA because of degeneration in the patellofemoral compartment. In lesions involving the contralateral compartment, full-thickness cartilage loss of the weight-bearing surface should be considered a contraindication to UKA.

Contraindications

In addition to the relative contraindications mentioned earlier, absolute contraindications for UKA include rheumatoid arthritis, recent infection, and arthritis that is clearly evident in all three compartments of the knee. Osteonecrosis can be successfully treated by UKA as long as the underlying bone is adequate to support the component. For an extensive lesion that might jeopardize the structural support beneath a unicondylar implant, TKA is preferable to UKA.

Patients with a previous high tibial osteotomy (HTO) can be treated with UKA, although some reports indicate less predicable results in this population. Overcorrected mechanical alignment, altered flexion-extension balance, the presence of previously placed hardware, and patella infera are contraindications that commonly present after an HTO; TKA is preferred in most of these patients.

Alternative Treatments

The debate between UKA and HTO in the young, active patient has waned with the decreasing popularity of HTO in North America. Although early results with HTO have been acceptable, deteriorating results into the second decade have been observed. The potential advantages of UKA versus HTO include faster pain relief, early weight bearing, no compromise to the extensor mechanism, fewer complications, better range of motion, and an easier conversion to a TKA. Current indications for HTO include younger patients whose activity demands exceed the acceptable limits of an arthroplasty. A full discussion of the pros and cons of each surgical option is especially important in these patients.

Results

When reviewing UKA results in the literature, readers must carefully evaluate the data to avoid misinterpreting the information and reaching incorrect conclusions. The natural tendency is to compare survivorship directly to the published results of TKA; in reality, however, significant differences often exist between these cohorts. To our knowledge, only one prospective, randomized study comparing UKA with TKA has been published, with results showing UKA to yield better results than TKA in terms of fewer perioperative complications, more rapid knee motion in the immediate postoperative interval, and shorter hospitalization. In addition, better range of motion in the knee was achieved and maintained through 5-year follow-up. No survivorship data were included in this study.

Studies of UKA often include a patient cohort that is younger and more active, a known risk factor for earlier revision. Another factor that is not usually considered is polyethylene shelf age, which is known to negatively influence survivorship. Storage time is likely to be longer with UKA components than with TKA components because fewer UKAs are performed. Also, given that a smaller fraction of patients qualify for UKA compared with TKA, it is common for surgeons to perform only a small number of UKA surgeries annually. Results with one mobile-bearing UKA design have been directly linked to annual surgeon volume, with low-volume surgeons producing inferior results.

Direct comparison of revision rates of UKA and TKA is inappropriate because of the current treatment algorithm used by many surgeons. In the face of a painful TKA with no known cause for the pain, conventional wisdom is to avoid surgical intervention. In the case of a painful UKA with no obvious cause, revision surgery is more likely to be performed simply because conversion to a TKA is an available and less-complex option.

Table 1 displays several of the available longer-term follow-up stud-

Table 1 Results of Unicondylar Knee Arthroplasty

Authors (Year)	Number of Knees	Implant Type	Mean Patient Age in Years (Range)	Results Survivorship (Interval)	Comments
Scott et al (1991)	100	Custom UKA design	71 (41-85)	85% (10 years)	Includes medial and lateral UKAs
Murray et al (1998)	143	Oxford (Biomet, Warsaw, IN)	71 (35-91)	98% (10 years) (with intact ACL)	Surgeon experienced with UKA technique
Squire et al (1999)	140	Marmor (Richards Manufacturing Company, Memphis, TN)	71 (51-94)	90% (10 years) 84% (20 years)	Disease progression a major long-term problem
Collier et al (2004)	100	SCR Uni (Osteonics, Allendale, NJ)	68 (46-88)	96% (6 years) (non–shelf-aged) 71% (6 years) (shelf-aged)	Greater shelf age had higher failure rate
Berger et al (2005)	62	Miller-Galante (Zimmer, Warsaw, IN)	68 (51-84)	98% (10 years)	Slow rate of disease progression in other compartments
Furnes et al (2007)	2,288	Multiple UKA implants	66 (25-91)	80.1% (10 years)	UKA inferior to TKA; volume of surgeries important
Koskinen et al (2007)	1,819	Multiple UKA implants	65 (38-91)	73% (10 years)	Survivorship for all UKA implants
Emerson and Higgins (2008)	55	Oxford (Biomet, Warsaw, IN)	64 (38-85)	85% (10 years)	Failure from progression of arthritis

UKA = unicondylar knee arthroplasty, TKA = total knee arthroplasty.

ies reporting UKA. Registry studies show 10-year survivorship ranging from 73% to 89%, but it should be recognized that several different implants were used in these studies, surgeon volume is typically low, and factors such as shelf age are not reported.

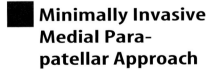

Minimally Invasive Medial Parapatellar Approach

The surgical techniques used to perform UKA have changed with the introduction of minimally invasive surgery. For more than two decades, a standard medial parapatellar incision with patellar dislocation was used for both medial and lateral UKAs. Because of its small size, a unicondylar implant is particularly suitable for implantation through a small incision. Currently, most surgeons use a minimally invasive surgical approach for medial UKA, because the option to extend a minimally invasive medial parapatellar incision is available should it become necessary in difficult cases.

Most surgeons use a standard medial parapatellar approach for lateral UKA because the patella must be fully displaced for adequate exposure of the lateral compartment. A lateral approach is less invasive, but it compromises the surgical exposure if the UKA procedure must be abandoned intraoperatively in favor of TKA. TKA performed through a lateral approach is more difficult, particularly for surgeons not experienced with a lateral approach.

Setup/Exposure

The patient is positioned supine. A footrest, sandbag, or leg positioner is placed so that the knee is relatively stable at a 90° angle. A tourniquet is placed, and the standard surgical skin preparation is completed. Surgical drapes should be positioned with maximum visualization of the upper thigh for orientation of extramedullary alignment guides. The planned skin incision is marked on the leg and a betadine-impregnated adhesive draping is applied.

The skin incision begins at or just above the superior pole of the patella and ends along the medial border of the patella 1 to 2 cm distal to the joint line. The joint capsule is opened along the medial border of the patella, leaving a cuff of soft tissue along the edge of the patella and patellar tendon for suture repair of the capsule at closure. The capsular incision extends proximally to the edge of the quadriceps tendon. If the surgeon needs to translate the patella laterally in the trochlear groove, the proximal end of the incision can be extended into the medial border of the quadriceps tendon. Alternatives for opening the upper end of the capsular incision include following the inferior border of the vastus medialis muscle with a subvastus capsular opening, or extending the incision from the superior pole of the patella in the direction of the vastus medialis muscle with a so-called "mini-midvastus" approach.

The inferior end of the capsular in-

cision should stop just medial of the proximal insertion of the patellar tendon into the tibia. The capsule is released along the medial side of the incision from the upper end of the tibial metaphysis to allow exposure of the anterior aspect of the medial tibial plateau (**Figure 1**). The anterior portion of the medial meniscus is removed to complete the surgical exposure.

Video 16.1 Incision and Exposure; Medial Unicompartmental Knee Arthroscopy. Craig J. Della Valle, MD (5 min)

Procedure

INSPECTION OF THE JOINT

The lateral and patellofemoral compartments of the knee are inspected to rule out pathology that would contraindicate a UKA and to correct any meniscal pathology that might be present. The patellofemoral joint is inspected visually and by palpating the articular surfaces with the knee fully extended. The lateral compartment is inspected by placing the knee in a figure-of-4 position and retracting the fat pad with a right-angle retractor. To identify cartilage defects, a nerve hook is useful for probing the border of the meniscus and the articular surfaces.

TIBIAL RESECTION

A gap-balancing technique begins with resection of the proximal surface of the medial tibial plateau. In a knee with varus degenerative arthritis and an intact ACL, the wear typically is located on the distal portion of the femur and on the anteromedial portion of the medial tibial plateau. This wear pattern creates laxity of the knee in extension but not in flexion. A gap-balancing technique is designed to balance the gaps in both flexion and extension.

The goal of the tibial resection is to retain strong subchondral bone at the

upper end of the tibia for optimal bone quality to support the tibial component. An extramedullary alignment guide is used to set the coronal and sagittal alignment for the tibial resection and the depth of the tibial cut. Most authors recommend a 90° coronal cut, although some surgeons prefer a more anatomic varus slope to the tibia of 2° or 3°. A stylus can be used to set the depth of the resection on the medial tibial plateau to the highest point or to the lowest point (the point of deepest wear). If the highest point is used as the reference for the resection, the depth of the resection should be set so that no more than 7 mm of cartilage and bone is removed from the highest point on the medial tibial plateau. If the lowest point is referenced, the depth of the resection should be no more than 2 to 4 mm below the point of deepest wear. The coronal slope of the tibial cut should correspond to the anatomic slope of the patient's tibial plateau. The slope usually is between 3° and 7°. The extramedullary tibial alignment guide is adjusted to achieve the correct amount of posterior slope.

It is important to pin the tibial cutting block in a position that avoids weakening the metaphyseal bone beneath the tibial resection. One pin (or two at most) is placed toward the midline of the tibia. The first tibial bone cut is usually the vertical cut and is made with a saber-type saw. If osteophytes inhibit positioning the saber blade through the intercondylar notch along the lateral border of the medial femoral condyle, the osteophytes need to be removed with a 0.25-in osteotome (**Figure 2, A**). The saber blade should hug the lateral border of the medial femoral condyle and not damage the insertion of the cruciate ligaments to the tibia. The saber blade should be placed through the intercondylar notch to the posterior edge of the tibial plateau (**Figure 2, B**).

The depth of the vertical cut with the saber saw should be equal to the

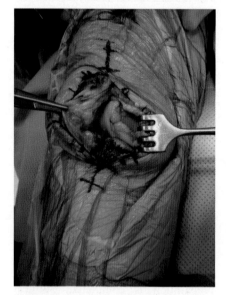

Figure 1 A medial incision is made, extending from the superior pole of the patella to 1 or 2 cm inferior to the tibial plateau. A capsular sleeve is raised from the medial tibial plateau.

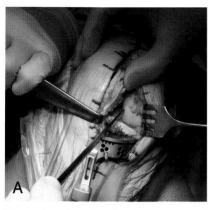 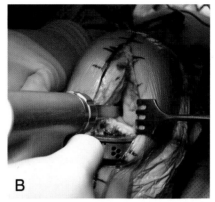 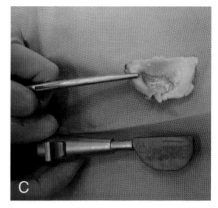

Figure 2 Making the tibial bone cut. **A,** To facilitate proper positioning of the saber blade, osteophytes are removed from the lateral side of the medial femoral condyle. **B,** A saber blade is placed through the intercondylar notch for a vertical tibial bone cut. **C,** The resected bone from the medial tibial plateau is sized against a tibial spacer block.

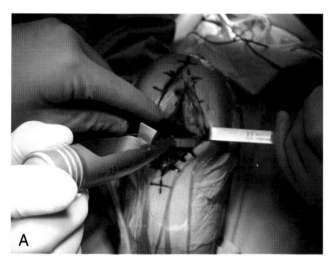 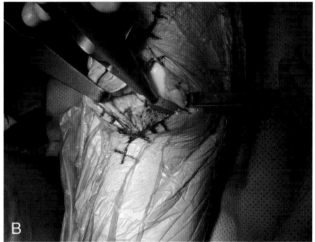

Figure 3 Gap balancing. **A,** This flexion gap is too tight for a 7-mm spacer block. A pen is used to mark cartilage that will be removed from the posterior femoral condyle. **B,** A 7-mm spacer block fills the extension gap.

anticipated depth of the resection from the tibial plateau. Because the intercondylar eminence is the highest point on the tibial plateau, the depth is typically about 7 mm from the flat part of the intercondylar eminence. After the vertical cut, the saber blade can be left in place as a barrier to avert undercutting the tibial eminence during the horizontal resection of the medial tibial plateau. The horizontal cut of the medial tibial plateau is made with an oscillating saw.

Removal of the resected tibial bone is facilitated by extending the knee to approximately 20° from full extension and applying valgus stress to the knee.

Laxity in extension from wear on the distal end of the femur creates a larger gap in extension and makes bone removal easier. The resected tibial bone wafer is held against a trial tibial component to confirm the appropriate size for the tibial implant (**Figure 2,** *C*).

GAP BALANCING

As noted above, with varus degenerative arthritis, wear occurs on the distal but not the posterior aspect of the femur. Therefore, the flexion gap is almost always tighter than the extension gap. A 6- to 7-mm spacer block is trialed in both the flexion and extension gaps. In many knees, the block

will fit in the extension gap but will not fit in the flexion gap. A spacer block can be firmly pushed into the flexion gap until it is blocked by the posterior femoral condyle. The condyle is then marked at the top of the spacer block to identify the amount of cartilage that will need to be removed to enlarge the flexion gap (**Figure 3,** *A*). The flexion gap is enlarged by removing a small amount of cartilage from the posterior femoral condyle with a curved 0.5-in osteotome. Trial spacer blocks are again inserted until the spacer block fills the flexion gap and provides appropriate ligament tension (**Figure 3,** *B*).

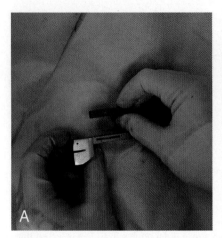 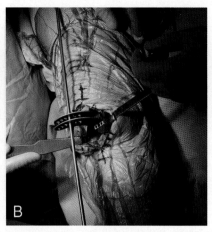 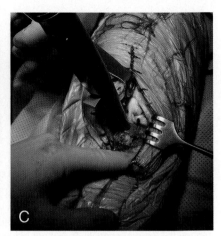

Figure 4 Distal femoral resection. **A,** The distal femoral cutting block is the same thickness as the spacer block that provides stability after the tibial bone resection. **B,** Sagittal alignment is checked with an outrigger and alignment rod. **C,** A spacer block that is the combined thickness of the distal femoral and tibial resections is placed to check stability and mark the correct rotation for the femoral component.

In some instances, the spacer block fits the flexion gap but is loose with the knee in extension. Gap balancing is achieved by adding a shim to the distal femoral resection block and resecting less distal femoral bone. The distal femoral resection will then be thinner than the distal thickness of the femoral component. Taking less bone from the end of the femur thereby equalizes the size of the gaps. For example, if a 7-mm-thick spacer block is stable in flexion and loose in extension, and a 9-mm spacer block is stable in extension, a 2-mm shim added to the distal femoral cutting block will result in 2 mm less bone removal from the distal femur, effectively tightening the extension gap and restoring flexion/extension balance.

DISTAL FEMORAL RESECTION

Although it is possible to use an intramedullary guide to align the distal femoral cutting block, the preferred method for achieving optimal implant alignment and knee stability is to align the femoral component to the tibial resection with the knee in extension, with appropriate tension on the medial collateral ligament. Ligament releases are not advocated for patients undergoing UKA. The basic concept is to align the components to each other

optimally and restore the patient's natural knee alignment by filling the flexion/extension gap with an implant of the thickness that properly tensions the patient's ligaments.

The distal femoral cutting block is designed to fill the gap created by the tibial resection. Usually, the distal femoral cutting block is 7 mm thick. This block is appropriate if the correct spacer block for gap balancing after the tibial resection was 7 mm (**Figure 4,** *A*). If the gap created by the tibial resection is greater than 7 mm, a shim is added to the underside of the distal femoral cutting block to create the appropriate block thickness to achieve knee stability.

The distal femoral cutting block has a slot for performing a resection that is the thickness of the distal portion of the femoral component. When completed, the distal femoral resection will create a space that, in conjunction with the tibial resection, is the combined thickness of the tibial and femoral components with the knee in extension. If the extension gap was larger than the flexion gap, a shim is added to the resection side of the distal femoral cutting block to reduce the thickness of the distal femoral resection. In this situation, the distal thickness of the femoral component is

greater than the distal femoral resection, and stability in extension is restored to the knee.

The orientation of the distal femoral cutting block in the sagittal plane is dictated by the slope of the tibial bone cut in the sagittal plane. For example, if the distal femoral cutting block is positioned and pinned with the knee in full extension, a tibial cut made with a 5° posterior slope will hyperextend the distal femoral cutting block by 5°. The alignment of the distal femoral cutting block in the sagittal plane can be evaluated with an alignment rod added to an outrigger that is attached to the distal femoral cutting block (**Figure 4,** *B*). If the alignment rod is not parallel to the long axis of the femur in the sagittal plane, the knee can be flexed to position the cutting block to the correct orientation with the long axis of the femur. The distal femoral cutting block is then pinned to the end of the femur in a neutral position of flexion/extension relative to the shaft of the femur.

The distal femoral resection can be performed with the knee either in extension or in flexion. The thickness of the distal femoral resection is equal to the distal thickness of the femoral component unless a shim has been added to reduce the thickness of the resection for gap balancing. The final extension gap created should be equal to the combined thickness of the distal portion of the femoral component plus the thickness of the tibial component. After both the tibial and distal femoral resections are completed, a spacer block (the combined thickness of the distal femoral component plus the thickness of the tibial component) is used to confirm that the extension gap is correct and that the distal femoral resection is parallel to the tibial resection.

The correct rotation of the femoral component is determined by placing the knee in full extension with a spacer block in place that fills the extension gap. A line or groove present on the spacer block is used to position and mark the distal femur for the correct rotation for the femoral component relative to the rotation and position of the tibial component (**Figure 4, C**). This block is also used to mark the most anterior point of the tibial component relative to the end of the femur when the knee is in full extension. The correctly sized femoral component should not extend farther forward on the distal femur than this mark.

FEMORAL SIZING GUIDE
With the knee in 90° of flexion, a Z-retractor or intercondylar notch retractor is placed into the intercondylar notch to slightly subluxate the patella. This retractor works best if positioned over the ACL. Next, a femoral sizing guide is placed flush against the posterior femoral condyle (**Figure 5**). A spacer that is thinner than the flexion gap can be used to hold the femoral sizing block against the posterior femoral condyle. In most cases, a smaller femoral guide is used initially to evaluate component size for average-size female patients and a medium- or large-sized guide used for male patients. The appropriately sized femoral component should not extend beyond the line or mark on the distal femur that was made to correspond to

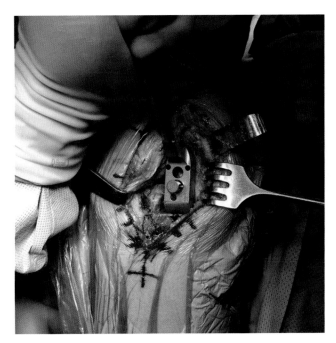

Figure 5 The femoral sizing guide is placed flush against the posterior femoral condyle and rotated to the mark on the anterior surface of the medial femoral condyle.

the anterior tip of the tibial component with the knee in full extension. Rotation is set by referencing the mark on the anterior femur that identifies correct femoral component rotation with the knee in extension. Drill holes are made through this sizing guide to set the correct position and rotation for the cutting block for the posterior condylar and chamfer femoral bone cuts.

Selecting the appropriately sized femoral component involves several considerations. Patient size is the first consideration, as women usually require an implant one size smaller than men. Using a template on a lateral radiograph, determine the implant size that best matches the size of the posterior femoral condyle but does not extend beyond the anterior tip of the intercondylar notch. The final decision regarding the size of the femoral component is made intraoperatively, after the tibial plateau has been resected. A spacer block is placed and the knee extended so that the position in which the spacer block contacts the anterior edge of the femoral condyle can be marked with methylene blue. This mark should not be anterior to

the femoral tidemark. When the sizing block is placed against the femoral condyle, the anterior lip of the implant should not extend anterior to this mark.

POSTERIOR CONDYLAR AND CHAMFER CUTS
The remaining femoral bone cuts are made through slots or flat surfaces on the femoral cutting block designed to guide the posterior femoral resection and chamfer cuts. Usually, the anterior chamfer and posterior condylar cuts are made first. The posterior chamfer cut is the last cut because removing the bone from this area reduces the stability of the femoral cutting block. The resection from the posterior femoral condyle should be the same thickness as the posterior condyle of the implant. The thickness of the resection is confirmed with a caliper (**Figure 6**). The posterior chamfer cut is made, being careful not to tilt the cutting block. The remaining posterior horn of the meniscus is removed along with any posterior condylar osteophytes that might interfere with knee flexion.

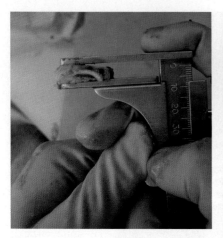

Figure 6 Calipers are used to confirm the correct thickness of the posterior condylar resection.

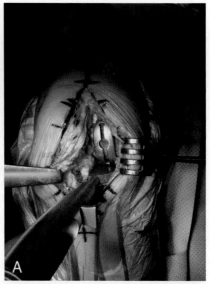

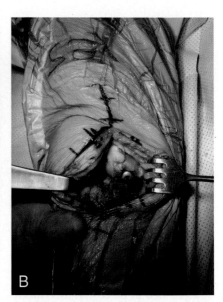

Figure 7 Trialing the components. **A,** A trial femoral component is centered on the trial tibial component with the knee in flexion. **B,** The femoral component is correctly aligned relative to the tibial component with the knee in full extension.

TRIAL COMPONENTS

A trial femoral component is placed, orienting the component in a medial/lateral position to the previous mark on the anterior femur made for femoral rotation. For the femoral component to be centered over the tibial implant, it is best to place the femoral component relatively laterally on the medial femoral condyle (**Figure 7, A**). The implant must fit flat against the resected posterior femoral condyle. It may help to place a tibial spacer first, and then insert a trial femoral component with the knee in flexion. Stability of the knee is evaluated in flexion and in extension. As the knee is taken to extension, the components should remain parallel to each other and the femur should remain centered over the tibia (**Figure 7, B**). When a valgus stress is applied, a gap of 1 to 2 mm should be present between the components in both flexion and extension. The tibial component should not lift off anteriorly as the knee is flexed. The ACL can be palpated to confirm normal tension in the ligament.

Trial components or templates are used to position the implants for proper orientation of drill guides for pegs and posts and slots for fins that are integral on the anchorage side of the components. Slots are created with a saber-type saw, a high-speed burr, or a chisel osteotome. It is important to carefully avoid fracturing the bone at the front or rear of any groove or slot. If a tibial template is used, the plate can be held in place by placing the knee in 90° of flexion and using a lamina spreader placed on the tibial plate and against the posterior femoral condyle. The lamina spreader stabilizes the template by tensioning the medial collateral ligament.

COMPONENT IMPLANTATION

Bone of the distal femur or the tibial plateau that is not porous in nature should be prepared for component implantation by using a small drill (1/8 inch or smaller) to allow adequate cement penetration for secure component fixation. The drill holes should be shallow (2 or 3 mm).

After cleaning the bone with pulsatile lavage, the tibial component is implanted. A thin layer of acrylic bone cement is applied to the tibial plateau and the undersurface of the tibial component. The tibial baseplate or the component itself (an all-polyethylene tibial component) is positioned and impacted until fully seated on the bone. Excess bone cement is removed from the margins of the tibial component with a Freer elevator or a nerve hook. On the femoral side, bone cement is injected into post or peg holes and finger-packed into cancellous bone. Acrylic cement is applied to the underside of the femoral component, the component is impacted, and excess bone cement is removed with a Freer elevator. Retained cement is not a problem with modular tibial components. The margins of both the femoral and tibial baseplates can be inspected and cleared of cement before placing the modular polyethylene insert. With an all-polyethylene tibial component, several methods can be used to avoid leaving retained fragments of cement in the knee. One method of removing extruded cement is to place a 4 × 4-in sponge around the margins of the tibia before placing the component. After the tibial implant is impacted but before the cement cures, the sponge is removed, bringing any extruded cement with it. Another method is to use a right-angled nerve hook and a Freer elevator to reach over and around the margins of the components to free any extruded cement. Once the cement has cured, the

Freer elevator also can be used to break free any extruded fragments of cement that remain. The knee is placed in 45° of knee flexion and varus alignment so that a central load across the fixation interface is applied while the cement cures. During final inspection of the components, any extruded cement is removed from around the margins of both components.

Wound Closure

The knee is irrigated with pulsatile lavage and inspected for any loose fragments of bone or cement. The tourniquet does not need to be deflated before closure. The deep capsular layers are injected with a mixture of 0.25 bupivacaine with epinephrine 1:200,000 plus 10 mg morphine sulfate. The knee is placed in 45° of flexion so that the capsule and soft tissues are in tension. The deep capsular layer is closed with 2-0 resorbable sutures in a figure-of-8 fashion. The subcutaneous tissue is closed with 3-0 resorbable sutures. A subcuticular suture that gives a watertight seal to the skin and does not require suture removal is used for the final skin closure. A transparent mesh dressing is applied to cover the incisional area. A sterile gauze pack is applied to the wound area underneath a surgical stocking.

Alternative Surgical Techniques

Intramedullary Technique

An intramedullary alignment guide can be used for alignment and placement of cutting guides for preparation of the medial femoral condyle. A 9-mm drill is used to make a pilot hole in the intercondylar notch just above the insertion of the posterior cruciate ligament. After the intramedullary alignment guide is inserted into the femoral canal, cutting blocks for per-

forming the distal femoral resection are oriented and pinned to the guide. The same pilot hole anchors a retractor connected to the intramedullary rod that holds the patella laterally in the patellofemoral groove. This retractor is particularly helpful in providing adequate exposure for the posterior condylar and chamfer cuts from the medial femoral condyle.

Bone Preparation With a High-Speed Burr

Although bone cuts traditionally have been made with an oscillating saw, the use of a high-speed burr offers some advantages with less invasive surgical techniques. A high-speed burr is essential if an inlay rather than an onlay surgical technique is preferred. A smaller surgical exposure is needed with a dental-type burr. Bone preparation for an inlay procedure is more of a bone-sculpting technique, as cutting guides are not of benefit. High-speed burrs and inlay surgical techniques are particularly beneficial when used in conjunction with computer-aided navigation integrated with surgical robotics. Precise bone preparation can be performed in a safe and precise manner through a very small incision. Additional time and preparation are required for these surgical procedures, as the robotic instrument must be programmed preoperatively from patient-specific digital information and further programmed intraoperatively for surgical navigation.

Mobile-Bearing UKA

Although many of the technical aspects of performing a mobile-bearing UKA are similar to a fixed-bearing UKA, there are a few distinct differences. Currently, the mobile-bearing device is recommended for use only in the medial compartment. With the possibility of bearing spinout as a unique complication for this surgery, soft-tissue balancing is of paramount importance. To balance a mobile-bearing knee, the knee is positioned over a

leg holder so that the leg hangs freely. This permits gravity to distract the knee in flexion, a position that aids in accurate gap balancing.

The approach can be performed in the same fashion as a fixed-bearing UKA, with special emphasis to preserve the deep medial collateral ligament and to avoid overcorrecting knee alignment. Using an extramedullary guide, the tibial cut is made with 7° of posterior slope and the flexion gap is tested with a feeler gauge (spacer) to determine the flexion gap size. Both the feeler gauges and polyethylene inserts are available in 1-mm increments.

Once the flexion gap thickness is determined, a thin intramedullary rod is placed in the femur. A femoral positioning guide is used in conjunction with the intramedullary rod, and a cutting guide is used to make a posterior femoral bone cut the same thickness as the posterior aspect of the femoral component. A spigot is inserted into the drill hole in the distal femur and a reamer is placed over the distal end of the spigot to shape the femoral bone. The flexion and extension gaps can be evaluated with a trial component in place and an appropriate amount of distal femoral bone removed to equalize the gaps. Once the gaps are equal, the bony surfaces are prepared for the implants, and the final components are cemented into place.

Lateral UKA

Positioning the leg in the figure-of-4 position is critical to performing a lateral UKA. In this position, the lateral compartment of the knee opens fully, allowing cutting blocks and implants to be moved into and out of the joint space. With lateral UKA, the amount of knee flexion is altered. Knee flexion increases tension in the extensor mechanism, making it more difficult to displace the patella.

A medial or lateral approach can be used to perform a lateral UKA. If a medial incision is used, the incision should follow the medial border of the patellar tendon and extend proximally along the medial border of the quadriceps tendon so that the patella can be fully dislocated laterally. The attachments of the anterior horn of the medial meniscus are not disturbed. The lateral tibial plateau is accessed by removing a substantial portion of the fat pad. The leg is placed in the figure-of-4 position to open the lateral compartment and remove the lateral meniscus. The knee is returned to a neutral varus/valgus position and placed in 90° of knee flexion to resect bone from the lateral tibial plateau. A standard extramedullary tibial alignment guide is positioned and pinned to resect a thin wafer of cartilage and bone (3 to 4 mm thick) from the lateral tibial plateau.

Alternatively, a lateral UKA can be performed through a lateral parapatellar incision following the lateral border of the patellar tendon. The incision is extended proximally and can include a partial lateral retinacular release to improve exposure. The capsule is opened along the lateral tibial plateau just above the Gerdy tubercle. When using this approach, the vertical tibial cut just lateral to the intercondylar eminence can be made either along the lateral border of the patellar tendon or by making a vertical split in the patellar tendon and passing a saber saw through the tendon.

As a general rule with lateral UKA, it is most appropriate to use a smaller femoral component than anticipated preoperatively. The lateral condyle is somewhat hypoplastic, and using a small component minimizes the potential for impingement with the patella. Unlike a medial UKA, where the femoral component is usually positioned toward the intercondylar notch, in lateral UKA, the femoral component is best positioned to the lateral side of the lateral condyle. Because of the shape of the lateral tibial plateau, the tibial component is in the best position if it is slightly internally rotated on the lateral tibial plateau.

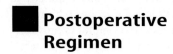

Postoperative Regimen

When the surgical procedure is complete, spinal or epidural anesthesia is discontinued so that the patient will be able to get out of bed, stand, and ambulate the day of surgery. While the patient is in the postoperative anesthesia recovery unit, the leg is placed in a continuous passive motion machine and foot pumps are used for deep vein thrombosis prophylaxis. This is our preferred regimen; however, some surgeons use chemoprophylaxis in addition to compression devices.

The postoperative hospital regimen is designed with the goal of next-day discharge from the hospital. Full weight bearing is permitted, and the patient is encouraged to ambulate with a walker or crutches. Physical therapy is initiated the day of surgery and progresses to more advanced exercises the morning after surgery. The patient is discharged with instructions for home exercises and a plan for initiating outpatient therapy within 4 days from discharge.

Avoiding Pitfalls and Complications

Inadequate Surgical Exposure: Malpositioned Components/Ligament Damage. Adequate surgical exposure is a prerequisite of any operation. The incision should extend proximally into the border of the quadriceps tendon to allow the patella to be easily subluxated laterally. Failing to move the patella laterally makes it difficult to position the femoral cutting guide to make the posterior condylar and chamfer bone cuts. The patella is held tightly in the patellofemoral groove as the knee is flexed. This reduces exposure to the medial side of the knee. Releasing the distal end of the quadriceps tendon enhances exposure as the knee is flexed. Inadequate exposure can result in an internally rotated femoral component.

Inadequate surgical exposure also can result in damage to the medial collateral ligament. The anterior portion of the medial joint capsule can be released from the upper end of the tibia to expose the anterior third of the medial tibial plateau. The medial collateral ligament is less likely to be damaged if it is freed and retracted when performing tibial and femoral bone cuts. A properly placed retractor holds the ligaments and capsule away from the cutting end of a saw blade. An incorrect placement of a retractor tenses the ligaments and makes the ligament vulnerable to damage from a saw cut.

Aggressive Bone Resection: Implant Loosening/Bone Collapse/Instability. The tibial resection should remove bone at or just below the subchondral bone plate. As the wear pattern with varus osteoarthritis is anteromedial on the tibial plateau, a bone resection 6 or 7 mm deep in this area will likely be 10 or 11 mm in depth from the posterior aspect of the tibial plateau. This posterior depth may be greater than the thickest tibial component available, as they usually are no more than 10 mm thick. A resection too deep in the tibia can result in residual knee instability. In addition, the tibial metaphyseal bone is weaker with a thicker cut, and the plateau becomes narrower. A thinner component placed on weakened bone may not provide adequate support for the implant and can result in tibial bone collapse or early component loosening.

Gap imbalance is often the result of inadequate experience with gap-balancing techniques or improper place-

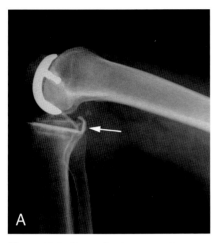 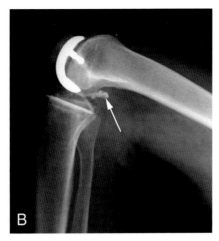

Figure 8 Radiographs demonstrating cement debris. **A,** Extruded bone cement (arrow) is seen on a lateral radiograph taken at 6-week follow-up. **B,** A lateral radiograph taken 1 month later demonstrates that the large fragment of cement had broken away (arrow). The knee had become acutely painful. The loose body was removed arthroscopically.

ment of cutting guides. The surgeon must first understand that the tibial cut influences both the flexion and extension gap relatively equally. The distal femoral cut influences only the extension gap, and the posterior condylar cut influences only the flexion gap. A helpful step to achieving proper gap balance is to measure the thicknesses of the bone cuts and compare them to the thickness of the implant. As an example, if the posterior condylar cut is 4 mm thick and the posterior condyle of the implant is 7 mm thick, the knee will most definitely be too tight in flexion. The surgeon also should take into consideration cartilage that has been worn from the condyles when measuring bone resec-

tions. As an example, if it appears that 3 mm of cartilage has been worn from the end of the medial femoral condyle, then it would be appropriate to remove approximately 3 mm less bone and cartilage.

Gap imbalance is evaluated by testing the stability of the trial implants before final component implantation. The trial components are placed and the knee is articulated through a full range of motion while the stability of the components is carefully observed. The tibia should not lift off in front (or "yawn," so to speak) and the femur should not rock or shift forward. Failure to correct gap imbalance is likely to result in early component loosening.

Inadequate Bone Cement Penetration: Implant Loosening. Adequate cancellous bone exposure is essential for rigid component fixation. Cement provides excellent component fixation when loaded in compression, but acrylic bone cement has relatively poor adhesive properties. If cement does not adequately penetrate cancellous bone, the implant is at risk for aseptic loosening. Aseptic loosening is largely prevented by placing multiple small drill holes (3 to 5 mm deep) in all areas of dense bone with a drill bit (9/64 inch or smaller).

Extruded Cement: Painful Cement Debris. Cement debris is usually the consequence of inadequate surgical exposure. Cement often extrudes from the back of the components as the cement is compressed after the components are placed and the knee is extended. With a small incision, it is hard to visualize the space behind the components and even harder to access this area. Cement fragments can become loose bodies either during the process of implantation or when the surgeon attempts to clear cement from the back of the components after the cement has cured. A free cement fragment can cause acute episodes of sharp, recurrent pain, and another surgical procedure generally is necessary to remove the fragment (**Figure 8**).

——————————■

■ Bibliography

Annual Report of the Swedish Knee Arthroplasty Register (SKAR), 2007. http://www.knee.nko.se/english/online/thePages/contact.php (Accessed April 5, 2010.)

Australian Orthopaedic Association—National Joint Replacement Registry 2007. http://www.dmac.adelaide.edu.au/aoanjrr/publications.jsp (Accessed April 5, 2010.)

Beard DJ, Pandit H, Gill HS, et al: The influence of the presence and severity of pre-existing patellofemoral degenerative changes on the outcome of the Oxford medial unicompartmental knee replacement. *J Bone Joint Surg Br* 2007;89:1597-1601.

Beard DJ, Panditt H, Ostlere S, et al: Pre-operative clinical and radiological assessment of the patellofemoral joint in unicompartmental knee replacement and its influence on outcome. *J Bone Joint Surg Br* 2007;89:1602-1607.

Berger RA, Meneghini RM, Jacobs JJ, et al: Results of unicompartmental knee arthroplasty at a minimum of ten years of follow-up. *J Bone Joint Surg Am* 2005;87:999-1006.

Collier MB, Engh CA Jr, Engh GA: Shelf age of the polyethylene tibial component and outcome of unicondylar knee arthroplasty. *J Bone Joint Surg Am* 2004;86:763-769.

Emerson RH Jr, Higgins LL: Unicompartmental knee arthroplasty with the Oxford prosthesis in patients with medial compartment arthritis. *J Bone Joint Surg Am* 2008;90:118-122.

Furnes O, Espehaug B, Lie SA, et al: Failure mechanisms after unicompartmental and tricompartmental primary knee replacement with cement. *J Bone Joint Surg Am* 2007;89:519-525.

Hernigou P, Deschamps G: Patellar impingement following unicompartmental arthroplasty. *J Bone Joint Surg Am* 2002; 84:1132-1137.

Koskinen E, Paavolainen P, Eskelinen A, et al: Unicondylar knee replacement for primary osteoarthritis: A prospective follow-up study of 1,819 patients from the Finnish Arthroplasty Register. *Acta Orthopaedica* 2007;78:128-135.

Murray DW, Goodfellow JW, O'Connor JJ: The Oxford medial unicompartmental arthroplasty: A ten year survival study. *J Bone Joint Surg Br* 1998;80:983-989.

Newman JH, Ackroyd CE, Shah NA: Unicompartmental or total knee replacement: Five-year results of a prospective, randomized trial of 102 osteoarthritic knees with unicompartmental arthritis. *J Bone Joint Surg Br* 1998;80:862-865.

Scott RD, Cobb AG, McQuery FG, Thornhill TS: Unicompartmental knee arthroplasty: Eight- to 12-year follow-up evaluation with survivorship analysis. *Clin Orthop Relat Res* 1991;271:96-100.

Squire MW, Callaghan JJ, Goetz DD, Sullivan PM, Johnston RC: Unicompartmental knee replacement: A minimum 15 year followup study. *Clin Orthop Relat Res* 1999;367:61-72.

Video Reference

Della Valle CJ: Video. *Incision and Exposure: Medial Unicompartmental Knee Arthroplasty.* Video clip from *Medial Unicompartmental Arthroplasty Using an Intramedullary Guide,* in Della Valle CJ, Stuchin SA, eds: *Surgical Techniques in Orthopaedics: Arthroplasty for Unicompartmental Arthritis.* DVD. Rosemont, IL, American Academy of Orthopaedic Surgeons, 2007.

Coding			
CPT Codes			**Corresponding ICD-9 Codes**
Unicompartmental Knee Arthroplasty			
27446	Arthroplasty, knee, condyle and plateau; medial OR lateral compartment	715 715.80	715.16 715.89
High Tibial Osteotomy			
27705	Osteotomy; tibia	755.64 905.4	736.9 905.5

CPT copyright © 2010 by the American Medical Association. All rights reserved.

Chapter 17

Primary Total Knee Arthroplasty: Patient Factors Affecting Outcomes

Douglas K. Ayres, MD, MBA
Ayesha Abdeen, MD, FRCSC

More than 35 years have passed since the earliest form of the contemporary tricompartmental total knee arthroplasty (TKA), the Total Condylar Knee prosthesis, was designed and implanted by Dr. John Insall at the Hospital for Special Surgery in 1974. Long-term studies have revealed an exceptionally low failure rate for this design, with implant survival of 95% at 15 years and 91% at 21 years. Long-term studies involving a variety of subsequent designs have produced similar results. These studies have demonstrated that results after TKA are predictable with respect to implant survival and pain control when conventional indications for the procedure (eg, severe osteoarthritis of the knee in an elderly, low-demand patient) are observed. Thus, TKA has been established as a durable operation with favorable clinical outcomes.

As the population has aged, the incidence and prevalence of osteoarthritis has increased, and the number of TKAs performed has increased accordingly. In 2003, a total of 402,100 primary TKAs were performed in the United States; by 2030, the demand is projected to increase dramatically (by 673%), to 3.48 million procedures annually. Although 90% of patients who undergo TKA experience significant pain relief, success with respect to functional improvement has not been as widespread; as many as 30% of patients report only minimal gains in function following TKA. Long-term outcome studies of primary TKA measure implant success in terms of Kaplan-Meier survival curves, with revision of the implant as the end point. As described above, studies have shown that at 15 to 20 years, less than 10% of TKAs have failed and required revision due to complications such as infection or aseptic loosening. This indicates that something other than technical failure must account for the remainder of patients who report dissatisfaction and poor physical function.

Outcomes following TKA depend on several factors. Despite consistency in implants used, surgical technique, postoperative analgesic protocols, and rehabilitation programs, postoperative functional gain varies greatly in patients who undergo TKA. Several clinical rating systems have been validated for the purpose of measuring postoperative function after TKA. These instruments have demonstrated that the wide variance in outcome can be accounted for by a variety of patient-specific factors, including demographic and medical variables. This knowledge is valuable because it allows identification of the "problem patient" before surgery. Being able to clearly identify the attributes that are associated with lower functional gains following TKA facilitates appropriate decision making, patient selection, and patient education before surgery.

■ Outcome Evaluation Systems

More than 34 clinical rating systems have been used to assess outcomes after TKA; however, only a few of them have been shown to be reliable and valid in published studies (**Table 1**). Two self-reported patient scores, the Western Ontario and McMaster University Osteoarthritis Index (WOMAC) and the Short Form–36 (SF-36), have undergone rigorous psychometric evaluation in the context of assessing patients before and after TKA.

Neither of the following authors nor any member of their immediate families has received anything of value from or owns stock in a commercial company or institution related directly or indirectly to the subject of this chapter: Douglas K. Ayres, MD, and Ayesha Abdeen, MD, FRCSC.

Table 1 Factors Measured by Evaluation Systems for Total Knee Arthroplasty

Western Ontario and McMaster University Osteoarthritis Index (WOMAC)
 Joint pain
 Physical joint function
 Joint stiffness

Short Form-36 (SF-36)
 Physical function
 Role limitation
 Bodily pain
 Mental health
 Emotional role function
 Social function
 Vitality
 General health perception

Knee Society Clinical Rating System (KSS)
 Knee rating
 Pain
 Stability
 Range of motion
 Functional assessment
 Walking distance
 Stair climbing
 Walking aids

The WOMAC questionnaire is a self-administered instrument designed to evaluate disability specifically related to knee and hip arthritis. The WOMAC score is an aggregate of three subscales: joint pain, physical joint function, and joint stiffness. The SF-36 is a generic measure of health status that evaluates eight dimensions of health: physical function, role limitation, bodily pain, mental health, emotional role function, social function, vitality, and general health perception. These eight dimensions are then categorized into two larger subdivisions—the Physical Component Summary (PCS) and Mental Component Summary (MCS). Both tests have been accepted as reliable and valid for the evaluation of this specific patient population.

Another measurement tool, the Knee Society Clinical Rating System (KSS), has been used widely to assess outcome in this population since its

introduction in 1989. The KSS has an objective scoring component based on clinical features (pain, range of motion, joint stability, and alignment) and a functional scoring component (distance tolerated on a flat surface, ability to walk stairs, and the use of an assistive walking device). The KSS was modified by Insall in 1993 to incorporate the objective clinical score and functional outcome with the patient's subjective perception of how well the knee functions during specific activities. The KSS was validated as an outcome measure for TKA in 2001; however, it was found to be a less responsive measure than the WOMAC and the SF-36. The KSS, WOMAC, and SF-36 have been applied to large populations of patients undergoing TKA to evaluate the effect of patient-specific factors on postoperative function.

Patient Factors

Patient factors that have been shown by reliable evaluation systems to be associated with less satisfactory patient outcomes after TKA are summarized in **Table 2**.

Age

Many studies have identified age as a predictor of outcome following TKA, although whether increasing age is a negative or positive predictor of outcome depends greatly upon the outcome that is measured. A national (United States) registry of 8,050 patients who underwent TKA from 2000 to 2005 revealed progressively less postoperative functional gain for each 5-year increase in patient age. Furthermore, increased age is an independent predictor of systemic complications. A study performed at the University of California, Los Angeles, measured outcome in more than 222,000 patients registered in a state database.

Probability analysis with respect to a base patient age of 65 years revealed that in patients younger than the base age, the probability of mortality was reduced by 73%, and the probability of pulmonary embolism was decreased by 34%. Young patients report greater preoperative pain than older patients as measured by the WOMAC pain score. Although younger patients have an increased probability of achieving better function overall, young patient age is associated with reduced postoperative range of motion as well as reduced patient satisfaction. Other authors have suggested that age does not have a linear relationship with outcome after TKA; rather, the effect of age on function occurs at the extremes of age, with patients 50 years of age or younger and patients older than 80 years demonstrating lower physical function after TKA as measured by the SF-36 functional score.

Sex

Women also have lower preoperative and postoperative function scores than men, as measured by the SF-12 physical function subset of the SF-36 in the national United States registry from 2000 to 2005. In patients with varus alignment, female sex has been associated with less improvement in range of motion after TKA than is seen in men. However, a combined United Kingdom, Australia, and United States study showed that although women tend to have worse function than men before and in the first 2 years after surgery, these differences do not persist beyond 2 years postoperatively, at which time functional gains are equal in men and women.

Obesity

Morbid obesity (body mass index [BMI] ≥ 40) is predictive of lower functional outcome after TKA. The PCS component of the SF-36 was applied to the 8,050 patients in the national registry to measure functional gain at 12 months after TKA. Lower

Table 2 Risk Factors for Primary Total Knee Arthroplasty

Factor	Effect on Outcome
Age	Extremes of age are associated with reduced ROM, lower satisfaction
Sex	Women have less-improved function than men up to 2 years postoperatively After 2 years, outcomes similar
Obesity	BMI ≥ 40 is associated with decreased functional gain
Arthritis type	Osteoarthritis is associated with better outcomes than "nonosteoarthritis" diagnoses
Emotional health	MCS < 50 predicts little to no improvement postoperatively
Preoperative physical function	Worse preoperative knee flexion correlates with worse postoperative function and overall function
Quadriceps strength	Worse preoperative quadriceps strength correlates with worse outcomes
Comorbidities	CCI > 2 is associated with a significant increase in mortality and infection

ROM = range of motion, BMI = body mass index, MCS = Mental Component Summary (of the Short Form-36), CCI = Charlson comorbidity index.

gains were found in patients with a BMI greater than or equal to 40 compared with patients with a BMI of 30 to 40 or a BMI less than 30.

Arthritis Type

A diagnosis of osteoarthritis is predictive of better outcome after TKA than is rheumatoid arthritis or another "nonosteoarthritis" diagnosis, as demonstrated in many studies of functional outcome as measured by the SF-36 and WOMAC.

Emotional Health

Preoperative emotional health (as assessed by the MCS component of the SF-36) is one of the most important factors in predicting function at 12 months following surgery as measured by the PCS of the SF-36 and the WOMAC physical function score.

TKA patients with MCS scores higher than 50 report significant improvement in physical function postoperatively. Conversely, those with poor preoperative emotional health (MCS scores lower than 50) demonstrate very little to no improvement in physical function following TKA. In addition, the MCS score before TKA correlates directly with postoperative pain, with patients with higher MCS scores preoperatively reporting less postoperative pain. Mental health, as assessed by the SF-36, was found to be one of the strongest correlations with postoperative WOMAC pain scores in patients in the United States, United Kingdom, and Australia assessed at 1 and 2 years following surgery.

Preoperative Physical Function

Preoperative physical function—specifically, knee flexion—is one of

the strongest predictors of postoperative range of motion of the knee. A rigorous analysis of more than 4,000 knees after TKA examined the effect of preoperative and intraoperative flexion and extension, preoperative alignment, age, sex, and soft-tissue release on postoperative range of motion. The single most important predictor of postoperative range of motion was found to be knee flexion before surgery. Preoperative joint function is one of the most important predictors of both postoperative joint function (as measured by the WOMAC score) and overall function (as demonstrated by the SF-36). General preoperative physical function is another strong predictor of postoperative physical function. The most dramatic improvements in postoperative function in terms of stiffness, pain, and physical function measured by the WOMAC have been observed to occur in patients who rate their preoperative status as "excellent," "very good," or "good." Conversely, the smallest gains in function are demonstrated in those who rate their preoperative status as "fair" or worse.

Quadriceps Strength

Weakness of the quadriceps femoris is implicated in the progression of degenerative osteoarthritis of the knee. Quadriceps muscle weakness also contributes to functional decline in patients with osteoarthritis. After TKA, quadriceps function declines in the acute postoperative phase, and although function is regained with time, most patients do not regain normal strength at long-term follow-up. Preoperative quadriceps strength is another independent predictor of improved overall physical function as measured by the PCS score of the SF-36 at 1-year follow-up. In addition to self-reported tests such as the SF-36, functional performance tests such as the "timed up and go" test (the time it takes a patient to rise from an armchair, walk 3 m, turn, and return to sitting in the same chair) and the stair-climbing test (the time it takes a subject to ascend and descend a flight of 12 steps) show that preoperative quadriceps function is also predictive of outcome. Unlike many of the other inherent patient attributes that correlate with postoperative function such as sex, age, pain, and medical comorbidities, quadriceps function is modifiable. Therefore, preoperative quadriceps strengthening may positively affect functional outcome following TKA.

Comorbidities

The Charlson comorbidity index (CCI) is a validated tool used in administrative databases that predicts 1-year mortality based on a range of medical conditions including cardiovascular disease, renal disease, liver disease, malignancy, acquired immunodeficiency syndrome, and diabetes. A CCI score greater than 2 is associated with a significant increase in both mortality and infection following TKA. Multiple comorbidities are associated with decreased overall postoperative physical function as measured by the SF-36.

Summary

In summary, preoperative predictors of low functional outcome at 1 year include extremes of age, BMI ≥ 40, poor mental health, poor physical function, and multiple comorbidities. Factors specific to the knee that predict postoperative function include a diagnosis other than osteoarthritis, preoperative knee range of motion (particularly flexion), and quadriceps strength. Although no given attribute is independently a surgical contraindication, it is critical that the surgeon be aware of the patient-specific features that are associated with poor functional outcome following TKA. Such knowledge can guide patient selection and enable the surgeon to appropriately counsel patients with regard to postoperative expectations. Although many of the factors deemed to be predictive of postoperative function are inherent and fixed (such as age, sex, and comorbidities), others (such as emotional well-being, obesity, and quadriceps strength) are to some degree modifiable. It has yet to be determined whether intervention to improve these modifiable patient factors preoperatively will result in superior function after TKA.

Bibliography

Bellamy N, Buchanan WW, Goldsmith CH, Campbell J, Stitt LW: Validation study of WOMAC: A health status instrument for measuring clinically important patient relevant outcomes to antirheumatic drug therapy in patients with osteoarthritis of the hip or knee. *J Rheumatol* 1988;15:1833-1840.

Bombardier C, Melfi CA, Paul J, et al: Comparison of a generic and a disease-specific measure of pain and physical function after knee replacement surgery. *Med Care* 1995;33:AS131-AS144.

Drake BG, Callahan CM, Dittus RS, Wright JG: Global rating systems used in assessing knee arthroplasty outcomes. *J Arthroplasty* 1994;9:409-417.

Font-Rodriguez DE, Scuderi GR, Insall JN: Survivorship of cemented total knee arthroplasty. *Clin Orthop Relat Res* 1997; 345:79-86.

Franklin PD, Li W, Ayers DC: The Chitranjan Ranawat Award: Functional outcome after total knee replacement varies with patient attributes. *Clin Orthop Relat Res* 2008; 466:2597-2604.

Husted H, Holm G, Jacobsen S: Predictors of length of stay and patient satisfaction after hip and knee replacement surgery: Fast-track experience in 712 patients. *Acta Orthop* 2008;79:168-173.

Insall JN, Dorr LD, Scott RD, Scott WN: Rationale of the Knee Society clinical rating system. *Clin Orthop Relat Res* 1989; 248:13-14.

Jones CA, Voaklander DC, Suarez-Alma ME: Determinants of function after total knee arthroplasty. *Phys Ther* 2003;83: 696-706.

Kurtz S, Ong K, Lau E, Mowat F, Halpern M: Projections of primary and revision hip and knee arthroplasty in the United States from 2005 to 2030. *J Bone Joint Surg Am* 2007;89:780-785.

Lingard EA, Katz JN, Wright EA, Sledge CB, Kinemax Outcomes Group: Predicting the outcome of total knee arthroplasty. *J Bone Joint Surg Am* 2004;86:2179-2186.

Lingard EA, Katz JN, Wright RJ, Wright EA, Sledge CB, Kinemax Outcomes Group: Validity and responsiveness of the Knee Society Clinical Rating System in comparison with the SF-36 and WOMAC. *J Bone Joint Surg Am* 2001;83:1856-1864.

Long MJ, McQueen DA, Bangalore VG, Schurman JR II: Using self-assessed health to predict patient outcomes after total knee replacement. *Clin Orthop Relat Res* 2005;434:189-192.

Mizner RL, Petterson SC, Stevens JE, Axe MJ, Snyder-Mackler L: Preoperative quadriceps strength predicts functional ability one year after total knee arthroplasty. *J Rheumatol* 2005;32:1533-1539.

Ranawat CS, Flynn WF Jr , Saddler S, Hansraj KK, Maynard MJ: Long-term results of the total condylar knee arthroplasty: A 15-year survivorship study. *Clin Orthop Relat Res* 1993;286:94-102.

Ritter MA, Harty LD, Davis KE, Meding JB, Berend ME: Predicting range of motion after total knee arthroplasty: Clustering, log-linear regression, and regression tree analysis. *J Bone Joint Surg Am* 2003;85-A:1278-1285.

SooHoo NF, Lieberman JR, Ko CY, Zingmond DS: Factors predicting complication rates following total knee replacement. *J Bone Joint Surg Am* 2006;88:480-485.

Coding

CPT Codes		Corresponding ICD-9 Codes	
27447	Arthroplasty, knee, condyle and plateau; medial AND lateral compartments with or without patella resurfacing (total knee arthroplasty)	715 715.80	715.16 715.89

SECTION 2
Complex Total Knee Arthroplasty

Section Editors
Daniel J. Berry, MD
Jay R. Lieberman, MD

Chapter 18

Overview and Strategies for Complex Total Knee Arthroplasty

Jay R. Lieberman, MD

Indications

In this section of the book there are 7 chapters that review the management of patients with deformities of the knee that require a so-called complex total knee arthroplasty (TKA). There are a wide variety of issues that may add to the complexity of a TKA including: (1) significant soft-tissue deformities with or without flexion contractures (ie, severe valgus or varus deformities); (2) extensor mechanism problems; (3) bony deformities (intra-articular or extra-articular deformities) related to prior trauma or prior surgery including osteotomy; (4) poor skin quality; (5) neuropathic joints, osteoporotic fractures, obesity, and bilateral TKA. Despite the variety of these clinical problems, there are certain critical principles that can be followed to enhance outcomes after a complex TKA.

The indications are the same for an uncomplicated and a complex TKA. However, because the complex TKA carries a greater level of risk, the threshold to perform surgery may be higher than for routine primary TKA. Prior to proceeding with any TKA, it is important that patients receive appropriate nonoperative management. Because some knee deformities may develop secondary to trauma or as a result of congenital deformities, the patients may have had these problems for many years and multiple surgeries may have been performed on the knee over time. A trial of conservative management is important because many of the complex TKA population is often younger than the typical TKA population.

Contraindications

Infection is a definite contraindication for TKA. Therefore, it may be appropriate in patients who have had prior surgical procedures or sustained a significant trauma such as an open fracture to obtain a C-reactive protein and erythrocyte sedimentation rate. A knee aspiration for culture and cell count is indicated if these blood tests are elevated or there are continued concerns about infection even if these lab tests are normal. In some circumstances there may be medical contraindications to surgery as a result of cardiac or pulmonary dysfunction, and medical consultation should be obtained prior to surgery if appropriate. This medical evaluation is particularly important in patients undergoing bilateral TKA because of the duration of the procedure.

Relative contraindications for TKA include extensor mechanism disruption and poor quality of the skin. In patients with extensor mechanism problems, reconstruction can be performed at the time of the procedure including use of an extensor mechanism allograft, but this will add to the complexity of the procedure. Patients with multiple surgical scars or atrophic skin need to be carefully evaluated. Plastic surgery consultation may be useful (**Table 1**).

Alternative Treatments

These patients should receive a complete nonoperative treatment regimen prior to proceeding with TKA. This regimen may include anti-inflammatory medication, physical therapy, corticosteroid, hyaluronic acid injections, and weight loss. In some patients an unloader brace may be useful. Even though these patients may have significant deformities if they are minimally symptomatic, in many cases it is best to wait to perform the total knee arthroplasty. Knee arthrodesis may be necessary for pa-

Dr. Lieberman or an immediate family member serves as a paid consultant to DePuy; has received research or institutional support from Amgen and Arthrex; and serves as a board member, owner, officer, or committee member of the American Academy of Orthopaedic Surgeons and the American Association of Hip and Knee Surgeons.

Table 1 Checklist for Complex Total Knee Arthroplasty

1. Surgical approach: Placement of incision and type of surgical approach

2. Template: Location of bony cuts, use of stems, necessity of hardware removal, and whether an osteotomy is needed

3. Component and instrument selection: Level of constraint, osteotomy fixation devices, hardware removal tools

4. Pain management: Multimodal pain regimen, peripheral nerve block, and/or epidural catheter

5. Rehabilitation protocol: Variations from standard total knee arthroplasty regimen with respect to weight-bearing status and osteotomy protection

tients with significant soft tissue problems, extensor mechanism failure, neuropathic conditions, and chronic infection.

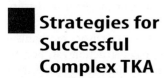

Strategies for Successful Complex TKA

Patient Evaluation

A critical element for successful management of a complex problem is thorough preoperative planning, including a thorough history and physical examination. The patient's disability and quality of life should be evaluated. Any history of prior infection must be determined. In addition, all prior surgical procedures need to be delineated. It is useful to obtain prior operative reports to discern the extent of the intra-articular pathology and identify the types of hardware used.

A thorough physical examination must be performed. An evaluation of the skin, soft tissues, and neurovascular status of the limb is essential. All soft tissue, ligamentous, and bony deformities must be thoroughly assessed. Plastic surgery consultation should be considered for patients who have very poor skin (which may require some type of flap) or to determine the best incision to use. Rarely, patients with significant scarring may require the placement of soft-tissue expanders in advance of TKA. Physi-

cal examination includes assessment of the range of motion and the stability of the knee to varus and valgus stress testing. The patient's gait should be closely examined to determine if there is varus or valgus thrust. The quality of the extensor mechanism should be established by having the patient straight-leg raise in order to look for the presence of an extensor lag and by manual strength testing. A thorough examination of the hip should be performed to determine if there is any hip pathology that will have an impact on the function or the deformity of the knee.

Plain radiographs of the knee that include full-length hip-to-ankle films are recommended for complex cases. (See templating section.)

Finally, these patients require a thorough preoperative medical assessment. This is especially true for patients that are candidates for bilateral TKA or patients that are going to have a more extensive procedure such as an osteotomy with a TKA or distal femoral replacement. In elderly patients or patients with significant cardiac or pulmonary disease, it may be wise to stage the osteotomy or hardware removal. It may also be preferable to remove the hardware in a separate procedure if there are concerns about appropriate healing of the soft tissues and the skin incision.

Templating

Standard TKA has three major goals, including: restoration of the mechan-

ical axis, balancing the soft tissues, and attaining equal flexion and extension gaps. These goals are usually accomplished by appropriate soft-tissue releases and by bony resections using standard cutting jigs. In the complex TKA it is critical to evaluate the overall limb alignment. For example, if there is a significant extra-articular deformity, it will be more difficult to adequately restore the mechanical axis and this must be identified preoperatively. Therefore, when dealing with a patient with a more complex knee deformity it is usually advisable to obtain long-leg films from the hip to the ankle joint and a lateral view of the knee on a long film cassette (**Figure 1**). It is essential to assess the height of the joint line and any coronal and/or sagittal plane deformity. The degree of the deformity and its location (distance from the joint) must be determined especially if an extra-articular deformity is present. The general rule is the closer the deformity is to the joint, the greater the impact the deformity has on the bony resection. A significant deformity near the knee joint may require a corrective osteotomy. It is essential to determine if an intra-articular correction without an osteotomy will jeopardize the collateral ligaments. Although a corrective osteotomy has the potential advantage of maintaining the normal relationship of the collateral ligaments, it requires the use of internal fixation and it prolongs the surgical procedure. Osteotomy may be performed at the time of TKA or as a separate staged procedure. An alternative to corrective osteotomy in some cases is to use a more constrained implant, which makes balancing the ligaments less of a problem. However, this may not be optimal in a younger patient. Templates can be used to determine if hardware, particularly screws in the proximal tibia or distal femur, will interfere with placement of a tibial or femoral stem in the intramedullary canal and prevent

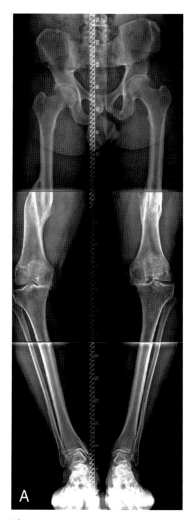
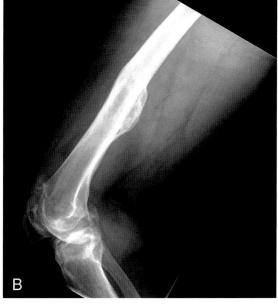
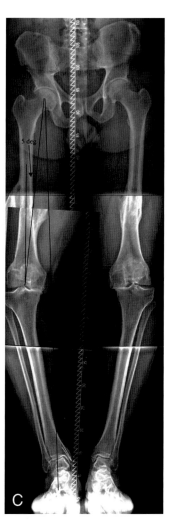

Figure 1 Images of a 60-year-old man who presented approximately 25 years after bilateral femur fractures treated in traction. **A,** Full-length radiograph demonstrates complete displacement of the distal femoral fragment in the right knee. **B,** Lateral radiograph demonstrates acceptable alignment in the sagittal plane. **C,** Preoperative templating demonstrates that alignment can be restored with a femoral osteotomy. A retrograde nail can be used to obtain fixation in this patient.

seating of the femoral or tibial component.

Preoperative evaluation should also include the size of the components and stems if they are needed. A decision should be made whether to use cemented or cementless stems. Finally, there should be an assessment of whether bone grafts, metal augments, or prosthetic sleeves may be necessary. Thorough preoperative planning is important to ensure that the various implant and fixation devices are available at the time of the surgical procedure. Finally, in some cases of severe deformity the use of an intramedullary guide may not be feasible, and computer-assisted surgery can be advantageous in these cases.

Surgical Approach

The surgeon needs to determine the appropriate surgical approach. In a complex TKA there may be patients who have had multiple incisions in the past or have significant atrophy of the skin or soft-tissue defects. As stated previously, consultation with a plastic surgeon may be very helpful. In general, the most laterally based skin incision should be used for exposure but this may have to be adjusted according to the type of deformity and the location of hardware that needs to be removed. Patients with significant scarring that prevents mobilization of the patella may require a quadriceps snip or tibial tubercle osteotomy. When performing a complex TKA, more extensile exposures may be necessary. Therefore, midvastus or subvastus approaches that are routinely

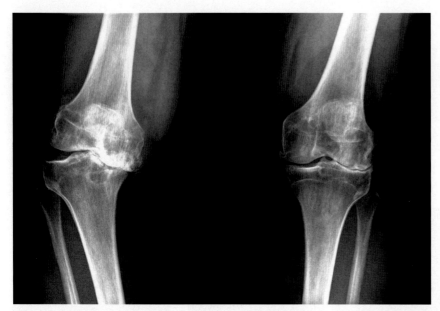

Figure 2 Weight-bearing AP radiograph of the knees of a 55-year-old man. Note the severe varus deformity, flexion contracture, and bone loss in the proximal tibia of the right knee. Preoperative planning should include selection of the type of implant and the level of constraint and a decision whether to use a cemented or uncemented stem for the tibia. The medial bone loss can be managed with either metal augments or local bone graft.

used in a primary TKA may not provide satisfactory exposure. In a patient with a severe valgus knee, a lateral approach may facilitate exposure.

Instruments/ Equipment/ Implants

The surgeon must make sure that the appropriate implant systems and fixation devices are available to perform the TKA. A number of critical decisions will need to be made during the surgical procedure. In many cases a variety of total knee systems that can provide different types of constraint should be available in case there is significant ligamentous instability present. It may not be possible in some patients to balance the knee using either a cruciate-retaining prosthesis or

posterior stabilized knee. Therefore, a total knee system with more constraint should be available. Bone obtained from the bony resections or metal augments can be used to treat bone defects. Another decision is to determine the necessity for the use of a stem to provide further implant stability (**Figure 2**). The type (cemented or press fit), length, and size of the stem will be determined during the course of the procedure. Stems will be needed if using semiconstrained systems or if bone grafts or augments are used to manage the bone defects. Different types of patellar implants may be needed if the patient has had prior surgery on the patella. When dealing with patients with osteoporotic fractures of the distal femur a distal femoral replacement may be appropriate. A careful evaluation of the plain radiographs and a CT scan to evaluate the quality of the bone and the extent of the comminution present is helpful.

The appropriate tools and systems must be available to remove hardware. During the preoperative templating it should be determined if screws and plates need to be removed.

Intraoperative images can often be helpful, so the surgeon should decide preoperatively if fluoroscopy or plain radiographs will be needed. Finally, in some cases with severe deformity, the use of an intramedullary guide may not be possible, and computer-assisted surgery may be advantageous in these situations.

Anesthesia and Pain Management

The complex total knee often involves more extensive dissection and patients may have more postoperative pain. A multimodal pain regimen that is used in an uncomplicated TKA may be very effective. Some surgeons prefer to use indwelling epidural or peripheral nerve catheters because of the large soft-tissue dissections that can be associated with increased pain. Protection of the quadriceps mechanism with a knee immobilizer during ambulation should be considered in patients with a femoral nerve block.

Rehabilitation

Specific consultation with physical therapy may be appropriate if the knee requires a different type of postoperative rehabilitation regimen than an uncomplicated TKA. Special considerations for these patients include weight-bearing status, especially if an osteotomy has been performed.

Bibliography

Berend KR, Lombardi AV Jr: Distal femoral replacement in nontumor cases with severe bone loss and instability. *Clin Orthop Relat Res* 2009;467(2):485-492.

Clarke HD, Fuchs R, Scuderi GR, Scott WN, Insall JN: Clinical results in valgus total knee arthroplasty with the "pie crust" technique of lateral soft tissue releases. *J Arthroplasty* 2005;20(8):1010-1014.

Haslam P, Armstrong M, Geutjens G, Wilton TJ: Total knee arthroplasty after failed high tibial osteotomy: Long-term follow-up of matched groups. *J Arthroplasty* 2007;22(2):245-250.

Lonner JH, Siliski JM, Lotke PA: Simultaneous femoral osteotomy and total knee arthroplasty for treatment of osteoarthritis associated with severe extra-articular deformity. *J Bone Joint Surg Am* 2000;82(3):342-348.

Mullaji A, Shetty GM: Computer-assisted total knee arthroplasty for arthritis with extra-articular deformity. *J Arthroplasty* 2009;24(8):1164-1169, e1.

Parvizi J, Marrs J, Morrey BF: Total knee arthroplasty for neuropathic (Charcot) joints. *Clin Orthop Relat Res* 2003;416: 145-150.

Ranawat AS, Ranawat CS, Elkus M, Rasquinha VJ, Rossi R, Babhulkar S: Total knee arthroplasty for severe valgus deformity. *J Bone Joint Surg Am* 2005;87(2, Suppl 1):271-284.

Weiss NG, Parvizi J, Hanssen AD, Trousdale RT, Lewallen DG: Total knee arthroplasty in post-traumatic arthrosis of the knee. *J Arthroplasty* 2003;18(3, Suppl 1):23-26.

Wolff AM, Hungerford DS, Pepe CL: The effect of extra-articular varus and valgus deformity on total knee arthroplasty. *Clin Orthop Relat Res* 1991;271:35-51.

Chapter 19

Total Knee Arthroplasty: Extra-Articular Deformity

Thomas K. Fehring, MD

Indications

Total knee arthroplasty (TKA) is an extremely successful operation. Surgical techniques are standardized and outcomes are consistently good. The long-term success of TKA depends on re-creating the mechanical axis, balancing the soft tissues appropriately, and equalizing the flexion and extension gaps. Most arthritic knees have some degree of bony and soft-tissue deformity preoperatively. These deformities can usually be handled by asymmetric intra-articular bony resection and soft-tissue release. Occasionally, however, bony deformity above or below the joint makes restoration of the mechanical axis difficult. Despite such deformities, it is still important to obtain proper mechanical alignment to ensure a successful result. Malalignment can cause off-axis loading and increased polyethylene wear, as well as early or late coronal instability. Additionally, malalignment can lead to altered gait mechanics and subsequent implant loosening.

Proper axial alignment is traditionally obtained through the use of intramedullary instruments on the femoral side and either intramedullary or extramedullary guides on the tibial

side. These techniques have remained relatively unchanged over the past 25 years, demonstrating the utility and consistency of this method. Extra-articular deformity can prevent the use of intramedullary guides, however. Although this problem can be circumvented easily on the tibial side with extramedullary jigs, extramedullary techniques are difficult on the femoral side, requiring radiographic identification of the femoral head and free-hand pinning of the distal femur. An alternative to extramedullary alignment in these situations is the use of computer-assisted surgery. This technology has been used successfully when extra-articular deformity prevents the use of traditional intramedullary instrumentation.

A variety of femoral and/or tibial deformities can affect proper alignment in TKA. Coronal plane deformity, sagittal plane deformity, and rotational deformities can occur in isolation or in combination to make surgical planning and surgical execution much more difficult (**Figures 1 and 2**).

The etiology of extra-articular bony deformities can be diverse. Malunion of femoral or tibial fractures is the most common cause of extra-articular deformity affecting subsequent TKA. Con-

genital malformations or metabolic problems such as rickets or Paget disease are less common but can be equally troubling to the patient and surgeon. Finally, previous corrective osteotomies in the distal femur or proximal tibia also can lead to problems in reestablishing alignment or obtaining proper ligamentous balance.

The degree of deformity and location of the deformity are important parameters to consider in dealing with extra-articular deformity. The closer the deformity is to the joint, the greater impact the deformity has on the orientation of resection. For example, Wolff and associates noted that a 20° deformity in the proximal femur has a negligible effect on the distal femoral joint line because the hip is able to abduct or adduct to bring the foot back to the midline. A 20° deformity in the supracondylar area, however, requires an intra-articular compensatory wedge resection of nearly 20° to restore neutral alignment. Therefore, not only the extent of the deformity is important, but also the location of the deformity relative to the knee joint. Deformities farther from the knee joint may be less in need of corrective osteotomy than those that are closer to the knee joint.

Beyond alignment issues, the effect of intra-articular correction of extra-articular deformities on ligamentous stability remains a concern. In the presence of large extra-articular defor-

Dr. Fehring or an immediate family member has received royalties from DePuy; is a member of a speakers' bureau or has made paid presentations on behalf of DePuy; serves as a paid consultant for or is an employee of DePuy; and has received research or institutional support from DePuy.

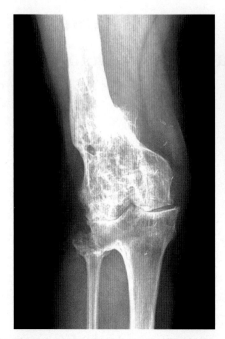

Figure 1 AP radiograph of a right knee demonstrates a severe coronal plane extra-articular deformity.

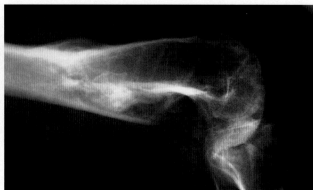

Figure 2 Lateral radiograph demonstrates a severe sagittal plane extra-articular deformity of the knee. (Reproduced with permission from Fehring TK, Mason J, Bohannon J, et al: When computer-assisted knee replacement is the best alternative. *Clin Orthop Relat Res* 2006;452:132-136.)

mities, significant imbalance of the collateral ligaments may result if intra-articular correction is used. In the presence of extra-articular deformity of 10° or more in the coronal plane or 20° or more in the sagittal plane, one author recommends simultaneous or staged osteotomy to reduce the need for constrained implants. Although extra-articular osteotomy has the advantage of maintaining the normal relationship of the collateral and posterior cruciate ligaments to the joint, it involves an additional procedure requiring the use of adjunct internal fixation. The concerns about ligamentous problems with intra-articular correction are more important to surgeons who use a measured resection surgical technique and retain the posterior cruciate ligament. Such ligamentous imbalance can more easily be dealt with in a balanced-gap surgical technique with posterior cruciate ligament substitution.

Contraindications

Contraindications in these cases do not differ from those for TKA without deformity. Proper patient selection is critical to the success of any arthroplasty. The surgeon should be sure that the degree of pain and functional disability correlates with the radiographic findings. The severity of the extra-articular deformity itself, although sometimes dramatic, should not take priority over the condition of the articular surface in assessing the timing of intervention.

Results

The literature concerning TKA and extra-articular deformities is limited. Most series have small numbers of patients and results that reflect the complexity of these problems (**Table 1**).

Technique

Preoperative Planning
A variety of techniques can be used to deal with extra-articular deformity at the time of TKA. Options include two-stage osteotomy, one-stage osteotomy, and one-stage intra-articular correction. The optimal technique for a given patient depends on patient age,

bone quality, and the location and extent of the deformity. The most important tool in making a proper decision is the 36-inch weight-bearing radiograph, on which a line is drawn from the center of the femoral head to the center of the knee. Another line is drawn from the middle of the talus to the center of the knee. Perpendiculars from these lines at the level of the joint line will help determine the relative difference between the medial and lateral resection of the distal femur. A similar differential calculation is made for the proximal tibia (**Figure 3**). Any planned resection that would compromise the integrity of the collateral ligament must be dealt with either by an osteotomy or by using metallic augmentation on the deficient side and limiting the resection on the prominent side to preserve the collateral ligament.

TWO-STAGE OSTEOTOMY
A two-stage osteotomy can be performed for extra-articular deformities that are thought to be too severe for intra-articular correction. The osteotomy is usually done at the apex of the deformity and fixed with either intramedullary or, in most cases, extramedullary hardware following wedge resection. A TKA is then performed once the osteotomy has healed. The advantage of this technique is that ligamentous balancing at the time of knee replacement is less challenging. Bone resection is more

Table 1 Results of Total Knee Arthroplasty for Extra-Articular Deformity

Authors (Year)	Number of Knees	Procedure	Mean Patient Age in Years (Range)	Mean Follow-up in Months (Range)	Results
Lonner et al (2000)	11	Osteotomy	63 (40-70)	46 (26-88)	Mean postoperative ROM = 89° 1 nonunion
Wang and Wang (2002)	15	Intra-articular correction	65 (57-78)	38 (24-60)	Mean postoperative ROM = 104° No complications No ligamentous imbalance
Klein et al (2006)	5	Intra-articular computer-assisted correction	60 (50-75)	NA	All within 2° of neutral mechanical axis
Fehring et al (2006)	17	Intra-articular computer-assisted correction	NA	NA	16 of 17 within 3° of neutral mechanical axis
Bottros et al (2008)	9	Intra-articular computer-assisted correction	NA	NA	Mean postoperative ROM = 98° Mean mechanical axis deviation = 1.3°

ROM = range of motion, NA = not available.

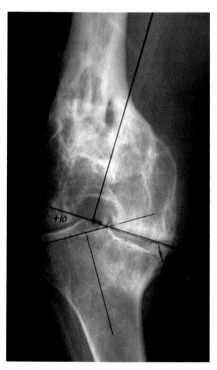

Figure 3 Lines are drawn on a 36-inch radiograph to indicate the femoral and tibial mechanical axes. Perpendiculars to those lines are drawn at the joint line to calculate the amount of resection anticipated. In this case, 10 mm more bone is resected from the lateral femoral condyle compared to the medial femoral condyle.

conservative and the surgeon has the freedom to use a posterior cruciate–retaining or substituting implant. The major disadvantage of this protocol is the need for a second procedure, with an unpredictable time period between stages to allow for bony healing. Additionally, retained hardware that may preclude the use of intramedullary alignment guides may have to be removed before or during the second stage. Risks of this protocol include nonunion at the osteotomy site and/or arthrofibrosis.

ONE-STAGE OSTEOTOMY

As an alternative to two different operations for the arthritic patient presenting with a degenerative knee and a significant extra-articular deformity, some authors have recommended a one-stage osteotomy. In these cases, an extensile incision is made, through which either a wedge osteotomy with plating or a wedge osteotomy fixed with a long-stemmed, uncemented fluted implant is performed (**Figure 4**). Lonner and associates described 11 knees in which this one-stage extra-articular osteotomy combined with a TKA was performed. The average range of motion preoperatively was 56°, and the average range of motion postoperatively was only 84°. Seven tibial tubercle osteotomies were required in 11 knees to perform the procedures. The authors reported one nonunion and one pulmonary embolus that was nonfatal. Radke and Radke described ten cases of tibial osteotomies for proximal tibial deformities along with a TKA. They had one delayed union in the ten cases. The average hospital stay was 25 days, and full weight bearing was delayed 9.5 weeks. Booth (Instructional Course Lecture presented at the American Academy of Orthopaedic Surgeons annual meeting, 2001) described an elegant oblique osteotomy technique that allows for correction primarily by rotation through an oblique osteotomy (**Figure 5**).

INTRA-ARTICULAR CORRECTION

The decision as to whether an intra-articular correction can be made depends primarily on the amount of resection anticipated based on the 36-inch radiograph. On this radiograph, a line from the middle of the femoral head to the middle of the knee is

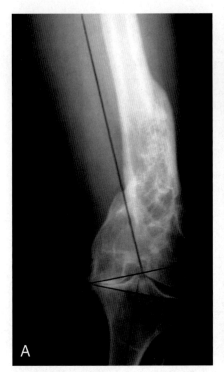
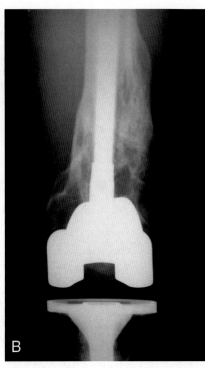

Figure 4 Radiographs of a severe extra-articular deformity of the left knee. **A,** Preoperative templating on a 36-inch radiograph indicates that an extra-articular deformity requiring osteotomy will be necessary. **B,** Postoperative AP view after one-stage extra-articular osteotomy with press-fit, fluted rod fixation.

drawn to re-create the femoral mechanical axis. A line drawn perpendicular at the level of the joint line indicates the anticipated bone resection. Frequently, despite significant deformity, an intra-articular correction can be made without jeopardizing the collateral ligaments (**Figure 6**). If it appears intraoperatively that so much bone would be resected off one of the femoral condyles that the insertion of a collateral ligament might be jeopardized, the surgeon has two options. The first option is to perform an extra-articular osteotomy at that time. The second option is to make a cut of ≤10 mm on the prominent side, avoiding the collateral ligament, and then build up the opposite side with metallic augmentation. Similarly, to plan the tibial resection, a line is drawn on the 36-inch radiograph from the middle of the talus to the middle of the knee, and another line is drawn perpendicular to this line at the joint line. Once

again, if it appears that more than 10 mm of bone would be taken from one of the tibial condyles, a smaller resection can be made on the prominent condyle and metallic augmentation can be used on the other side.

Most cases of severe deformity can be managed intra-articularly. Wang and Wang described 15 patients with fracture malunions, all corrected intra-articularly. There were no complications, and the range of motion improved from 77° to 104° following surgery. They concluded that if the femoral deformity was less than 20° and the tibial deformity was less than 30°, an intra-articular correction could be made.

Procedure: Intra-articular Correction

With intra-articular correction of severe extra-articular femoral deformities, the use of intramedullary alignment jigs often is not feasible because

of bony deformity. In these situations, preoperative cuts are drawn out carefully on a 36-inch radiograph. The femoral head must be identified intraoperatively. Preoperatively, the surgeon needs to know how much more bone must be taken off one distal femoral condyle than the other (**Figure 3**). These resected pieces of distal femur can then be measured with calipers to ensure a proper distal femoral resection perpendicular to the mechanical axis. For the tibial side, similar measurements are made on the 36-inch radiograph. The surgeon should calculate preoperatively the difference between the amount of bone to be resected from the lateral plateau and that resected from the medial plateau. In doing this, proper mechanical axis can be obtained. The resected plateau is then measured with calipers to ensure a proper proximal tibial resection perpendicular to the mechanical axis.

With computer-assisted surgery, proper alignment can be more predictably ensured when treating extra-articular deformities. My colleagues and I described the use of computer-assisted surgery to manage these difficult deformities in 17 cases of significant femoral deformity and were able to successfully use the computer to help reestablish the mechanical axis. In subsequent case series, Klein and associates and Bottros and associates also demonstrated the efficacy of using computer-assisted surgery to obtain proper mechanical alignment with significant extra-articular deformities.

■

Postoperative Regimen

The postoperative regimen is not dissimilar from that used after routine TKA if an intra-articular correction technique is used. Because many of

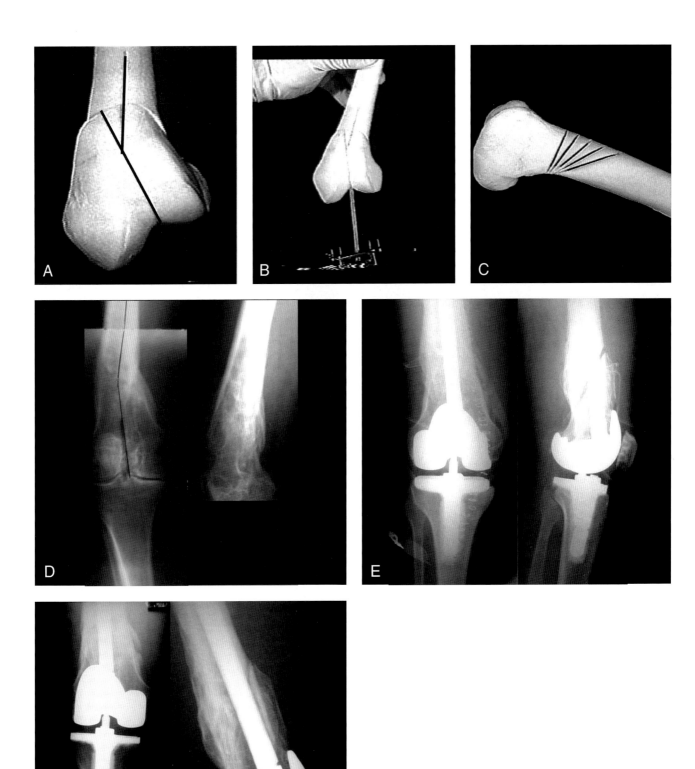

Figure 5 Oblique femoral osteotomy described by Booth. **A** and **B,** Bone model showing femoral deformity and oblique distal femoral osteotomy. **C,** Potential oblique osteotomy angles. The more oblique osteotomy allows greater angular correction without removal of a bone wedge. **D,** AP and lateral radiographs of a patient with knee arthritis and extra-articular supracondylar bone deformity. **E,** AP and lateral radiographs after TKA with oblique distal femoral osteotomy fixed with a long-stemmed femoral component. **F,** AP and lateral radiographs of patient shown in **D** and **E** after osteotomy healing.

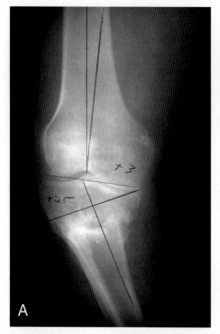
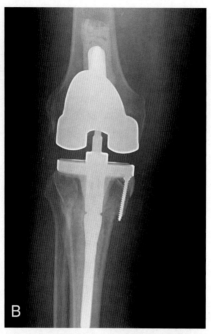

Figure 6 Radiographs of severe extra-articular deformity of the right knee. **A,** Templating shows that significantly more bone will need to be resected from the lateral tibial condyle (25 mm) than from the medial tibial condyle (3 mm). **B,** Postoperative AP view after intra-articular correction with limited resection laterally and cement and screw augmentation medially.

these patients have had previous incisions about the knee, it is important to incorporate the most lateral skin incision in the surgical approach. Range-of-motion exercise may be delayed to ensure adequate wound healing in cases where large flaps are required for exposure.

If an osteotomy has been performed, weight bearing should be restricted. The amount of weight bearing allowed and the timing of these restrictions depend on the type of osteotomy, the stability of fixation, and bone quality.

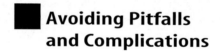

Avoiding Pitfalls and Complications

The key to dealing with extra-articular deformity and arthritis of the knee is preoperative planning. Bowing of the femur or tibia as well as previous fractures that may have gone unnoticed since childhood can be identified on the 36-inch radiograph. The surgeon must then draw out the mechanical axis to determine the difference between resection on the medial and lateral sides of the femoral and tibial condyles, respectively (**Figure 3**). Once this is done, the surgeon can make a decision as to whether an intra-articular or extra-articular approach is called for. The vast majority of these deformities can be managed by intra-articular resection and careful ligamentous balancing. Even in severe deformities, the surgeon has the option of using metal augmentation on the deficient side and limiting the amount of resection on the prominent side to 10 mm. Resection much greater than 10 mm may jeopardize the origin of the collateral ligaments on the femoral side or affect the strength of the tibial bone stock on the tibial side. In the rare case of a severe extra-articular deformity that cannot be handled intra-articularly, stable fixation with locking plates after a wedge resection probably is the most predictable form of fixation. Whether to do this in one stage or two stages is at the discretion of the surgeon.

Bibliography

Bottros J, Klika AK, Lee HH, Polousky J, Barsoum WK: The use of navigation in total knee arthroplasty for patients with extra-articular deformity. *J Arthroplasty* 2008;23(1):74-78.

Fehring TK, Mason JB, Moskal J, Pollock DC, Mann J, Williams VJ: When computer-assisted knee replacement is the best alternative. *Clin Orthop Relat Res* 2006;452:132-136.

Klein GR, Austin MS, Smith EB, Hozack WJ: Total knee arthroplasty using computer-assisted navigation in patients with deformities of the femur and tibia. *J Arthroplasty* 2006;21(2):284-288.

Lonner JH, Booth RE: Total knee arthroplasty in outliers, in Barrack RL, Booth RE, Lonner JH, McCarthy JC, Mont MA, Rubash HE, eds: *Orthopaedic Knowledge Update: Hip and Knee Reconstruction 3.* Rosemont, IL, American Academy of Orthopaedic Surgeons, 2006, pp 111-121.

Lonner JH, Siliski JM, Lotke PA: Simultaneous femoral osteotomy and total knee arthroplasty for treatment of osteoarthritis associated with severe extra-articular deformity. *J Bone Joint Surg Am* 2000;82(3):342-348.

Mason JB, Fehring TK, Estok R, Banel D, Fahrbach K: Meta-analysis of alignment outcomes in computer-assisted total knee arthroplasty surgery. *J Arthroplasty* 2007;22(8):1097-1106.

Radke S, Radke J: Total knee arthroplasty in combination with a one-stage tibial osteotomy: A technique for correction of a gonarthrosis with a severe (>15 degrees) tibial extra-articular deformity. *J Arthroplasty* 2002;17(5):533-537.

Wang JW, Wang CJ: Total knee arthroplasty for arthritis of the knee with extra-articular deformity. *J Bone Joint Surg Am* 2002;84-A(10):1769-1774.

Wolff AM, Hungerford DS, Pepe CL: The effect of extraarticular varus and valgus deformity on total knee arthroplasty. *Clin Orthop Relat Res* 1991;271:35-51.

Coding

CPT Codes		Corresponding ICD-9 Codes	
Intramedullary Rod			
27712	Osteotomy; multiple, with realignment on intramedullary rod (eg, Sofield type procedure)	715 756.11	715.16
Bony and Soft Tissue Resection/Release			
27422	Reconstruction of dislocating patella; with extensor realignment and/or muscle advancement or release (eg, Campbell, Goldwaite type procedure)	715 718.26	715.16 718.36
27425	Lateral retinacular release, open	715	715.16
27435	Capsulotomy, posterior capsular release, knee	718.26 715	718.36 715.16
29873	Arthroscopy, knee, surgical; with lateral release	718.4 715.16 715.36	715.26 716.6
Computer Assisted Surgical Navigation			
20985	Computer-assisted surgical navigational procedure for musculoskeletal procedures, image-less (List separately in addition to code for primary procedure)	715 715.80	715.16 715.89
Total Knee Arthroplasty			
27447	Arthroplasty, knee, condyle and plateau; medial AND lateral compartments with or without patella resurfacing (total knee arthroplasty)	715 715.80	715.16 715.89
Tibial Osteotomy			
27705	Osteotomy; tibia	715 733.81	715.16 736.9

CPT copyright © 2010 by the American Medical Association. All rights reserved.

Chapter 20

Total Knee Arthroplasty: Posttraumatic Osteoarthritis

Michael D. Ries, MD

Indications

Total knee arthroplasty (TKA) is indicated for the treatment of posttraumatic osteoarthritis and limb malalignment when nonsurgical measures fail to provide symptomatic relief of pain and functional impairment. Posttraumatic arthritis develops from intra-articular proximal tibial or distal femoral fractures, metaphyseal or diaphyseal fractures that result in limb malalignment and eccentric joint loading, patellar fractures, or a combination of fracture mechanisms. Prior trauma may have resulted in soft-tissue injury or open fractures with subsequent infection, loss of soft-tissue coverage, and limited knee motion. Prior trauma can result in a wide spectrum of limb and joint problems that affect the complexity of reconstructive surgery. The expected outcome of TKA for posttraumatic arthritis therefore depends on many factors, including the integrity of soft-tissue coverage, the severity of extra-articular and intra-articular deformities, preoperative knee motion, history of prior infection, and other associated limb injuries.

Contraindications

TKA is contraindicated when active infection is present, although staged treatment of septic arthritis with use of an antibiotic-impregnated cement spacer followed by delayed TKA after infection is controlled can permit restoration of joint function. Extensor mechanism disruption is a relative contraindication to TKA. Extensor mechanism reconstruction can be performed before or during TKA with allograft or autologous tissue, although the functional results are quite variable. Multiple scars, atrophic skin, and/or inadequate soft-tissue coverage after knee arthrotomy may be relative contraindications to TKA. However, improved soft-tissue coverage can be achieved with soft-tissue transposition as a staged procedure or during TKA to minimize the risk of skin necrosis after surgery.

Alternative Treatments

Nonsurgical alternative treatments to TKA include activity restrictions, nonsteroidal anti-inflammatory drugs or analgesic medications, cortisone or viscosupplementation injections, physical therapy, and bracing. If these measures fail to provide adequate relief, reconstructive surgery may be a more appropriate option. Surgical alternatives to TKA include arthroscopic débridement, osteotomy, and arthrodesis. However, arthroscopic débridement for the treatment of osteoarthritis has not been associated with favorable results, although it may be beneficial for treatment of mechanical symptoms. Osteotomy is indicated for correction of extra-articular angular deformity associated with asymmetric joint loading and unicompartmental arthritis. This may be performed as an alternative to TKA, as a staged procedure before TKA, or simultaneously with TKA. Arthrodesis is most appropriate when TKA is contraindicated, particularly with active infection and extensor mechanism disruption.

Results

TKA for posttraumatic arthritis can be expected to result in improvement in pain and function. A review of the published reports of TKAs for posttraumatic arthritis indicates that the Knee Society pain and function scores improved from a preoperative average of 41 and 50, respectively, to an average of 82 and 75, respectively, after

Dr. Ries or an immediate family member is a board member, owner, officer, or committee member of the Foundation for the Advancement of Research in Medicine; has received royalties from Smith & Nephew; and serves as a paid consultant for or is an employee of Smith & Nephew.

Table 1 Results of Total Knee Arthroplasty for Posttraumatic Arthritis

Authors (Year)	Number of Knees	Mean Patient Age (Range)	Prior Trauma	Mean Follow-up (Range)	Results	Complications
Lonner et al (1999)	31	60 (36-78)	Distal femur fracture (*n* = 11) Proximal tibia fracture (*n* = 20)	46 months (28-114)	KSS score improved from 36 to 78 (pain) and from 44 to 72 (function)	8 aseptic loosening 3 deep infection 1 patellar tendon rupture 1 patellar subluxation 2 skin necrosis
Saleh et al (2001)	15	56 (37-68)	Proximal tibia fracture	6.2 years (5.4-11.1)	HSS score improved from 51 to 80	3 manipulation 3 deep infection 2 patellar tendon rupture
Papadopoulos et al (2002)	48	65 (19-84)	Distal femur fracture	74.4 months (24-192)	KSS score improved from 40 to 84 (pain) and from 48 to 66 (function)	4 manipulation 2 aseptic loosening 3 deep infection
Weiss et al (2003)	62	63 (19-89)	Proximal tibia fracture	56.4 months (24-144)	KSS score improved from 44 to 83 (pain) and from 52 to 84 (function)	5 manipulation 2 aseptic loosening 2 deep infection 5 patellar tendon rupture 1 medial collateral ligament avulsion 2 instability 2 skin necrosis 1 reflex sympathetic dystrophy

KSS = Knee Society score, HSS = Hospital for Special Surgery score.

surgery (**Table 1**). However, bony deformity, prior infection, stiffness, and poor soft-tissue coverage can increase the technical complexity of the procedure and risk of complications. The overall reported rates of loosening (8%), deep infection (7%), patellar tendon rupture (5%), and skin necrosis (3%) at 3- to 6-year follow-up are considerably higher than the expected complication rates after TKA for nonposttraumatic arthritis.

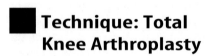

Technique: Total Knee Arthroplasty

Setup/Exposure

Prior trauma that has resulted in extra-articular deformity can cause asymmetric joint loading and lead to posttraumatic arthritis. Correction of malalignment can be achieved with TKA and soft-tissue release or osteotomy. The decision between the two methods depends primarily on the severity of deformity and proximity to the knee. Deformities that are more severe and closer to the knee generally require corrective osteotomy, whereas those that are farther from the knee and less severe can be corrected with TKA.

Full-length weight-bearing alignment radiographs and full-length lateral views of the femur and tibia should be obtained to determine the degree and location of extra-articular deformity and retained hardware (**Figure 1**, *A*).

Instruments/Equipment/ Implants Required

Prior trauma with intra-articular fracture is often associated with stiffness requiring soft-tissue release. A posterior stabilized implant is needed if complete release of the posterior cruciate ligament is necessary. The orientation of the distal femoral and proximal tibial bone cuts should be templated to assess any asymmetry in the extension space and the relative soft-tissue correction that will be needed during TKA (**Figure 1**, *B* and *C*). If correction of extra-articular deformity with intra-articular bone resections results in significant asymmetry of the extension or flexion spaces that cannot be corrected with soft-tissue release, then a constrained implant will be required.

Retained hardware should be removed if it is causing pain. The type of hardware should be identified preoperatively if possible so that appropriate screwdrivers and extraction equipment can be available. A universal

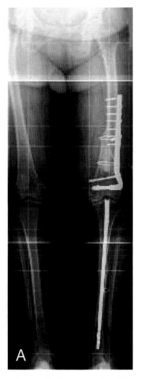 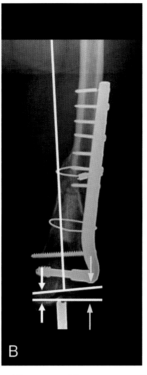 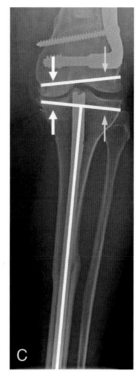

Figure 1 Images of a 62-year-old woman with posttraumatic arthritis. **A,** Full-length alignment AP radiograph demonstrates retained hardware in the femur and tibia. **B,** The line drawn on the AP view from the femoral head to the intercondylar notch of the distal femur demonstrates the mechanical axis of the femur. The line perpendicular to the mechanical axis represents the planned distal femoral bone resection for TKA. This will result in more lateral than medial bone resection because the femur is aligned in varus. The joint line is also drawn. The distance between the lateral (yellow) arrows represents the amount of lateral distal condylar resection, and the distance between the medial (white) arrows represents the amount of medial distal femoral resection. **C,** The line drawn on the AP view demonstrates the mechanical axis of the tibia. The line perpendicular to the tibial mechanical axis represents the planned tibial resection for TKA, which will remove more lateral than medial bone. The planned distal femoral resection is also illustrated. The greater distance between the lateral (yellow) arrows compared to the medial (white) arrows indicates that relative lateral laxity can be expected after bone resections are made, which will require medial collateral soft-tissue release or use of a constrained implant. If the asymmetry in the space between the distal femoral and proximal tibial bone resections can be balanced into a rectangular space by soft-tissue releases, then a constrained implant or corrective osteotomy is not needed.

placement of the TKA components. However, hardware removal also leaves defects from screw holes or other areas of bone loss that can leave the bone at risk of refracture during or after TKA. If plates and screws are removed, the surgeon may consider bypassing the screw holes with an intramedullary stem or rod to minimize the risk of refracture.

If patella infera is present, then tibial tubercle osteotomy can also permit slight proximal recession of the tibial tubercle to minimize postoperative patella infera.

The distal femoral and proximal tibial bone cuts are made perpendicular to the mechanical axis of each bone to restore axial limb alignment and orientation of the joint line perpendicular to the mechanical axis. However, if angular bony deformity is present, this will create soft-tissue imbalance between the collateral ligaments, which can be treated with release of contacted collateral soft-tissue constraints, advancement of the attenuated collateral ligament, or use of a constrained implant.

Technique: Simultaneous Supracondylar Osteotomy and TKA

Setup/Exposure
If prior trauma has resulted in significant extra-articular femoral or tibial deformity, correction of limb alignment and treatment of posttraumatic arthritis may require both osteotomy and TKA. Osteotomy can be performed as a separate staged procedure or simultaneously with TKA. Simultaneous osteotomy and TKA rather than a staged procedure offers the advantage of a single surgical procedure, and the resected cancellous bone obtained during the TKA can be used to graft the os-

screw removal set that can accommodate a variety of screw head sizes and geometries may be helpful. Because broken screws may not be apparent on preoperative radiographs, screw removal tools should include a cannulated bore to extract broken screws. Retained hardware or bony deformity can preclude use of intramedullary instrumentation. If intramedullary alignment is not feasible, then extramedullary alignment or computer navigation should be used to orient the bone cuts for TKA.

Procedure
Prior scars are used or incorporated into the knee incision when possible to minimize devascularization of soft tissues. A medial parapatellar arthrotomy provides exposure for most knees. However, particularly for knees with limited range of motion and contracture of the extensor mechanism, more extensile exposures using rectus snip or tibial tubercle osteotomy may be necessary.

Hardware should be removed if it is painful or interferes with proper

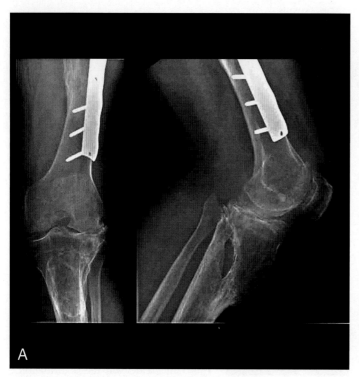
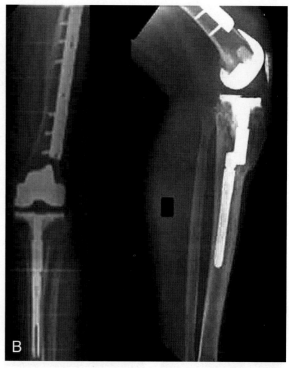

Figure 2 Radiographs of a 55-year-old man with posttraumatic osteoarthritis that developed as a result of prior femoral and proximal tibial fractures. **A,** Preoperative AP (left) and lateral (right) views. Overall limb alignment was relatively well maintained, but the proximal tibia had healed in an anteriorly displaced position relative to the diaphysis and a large defect was present in the tibial metaphysis. **B,** Postoperative AP (left) and lateral (right) views demonstrate treatment with a custom offset tibial stem to bypass the metaphyseal defect.

teotomy site. Osteotomy at the time of TKA can be stabilized using plate or intramedullary rod fixation, or with the intramedullary stem of the TKA.

The desired correction of an extraarticular tibial or femoral deformity should be determined preoperatively based on radiographs and an appropriate wedge of bone removed at the site of bony deformity. A biplanar osteotomy is required to correct combined axial (varus/valgus) and flexion or recurvatum deformity. A TKA and supracondylar osteotomy site can be exposed through a single incision and medial parapatellar approach, or with an anterior approach for the TKA and a separate lateral approach to the femur, particularly if plate fixation of the osteotomy is required.

Instruments/Equipment/ Implants Required

The osteotomy can be fixed using an intramedullary rod inserted proximal to the TKA bone cuts or with plate fixation. The osteotomy also can be stabilized using the stem portion of a stemmed TKA. However, this may require additional fixation at the osteotomy because the TKA stem typically does not provide adequate rotational stability in the proximal bone fragment. This method appears best suited for treatment of supracondylar nonunion, where there is fibrous tissue or irregularity of the bone surfaces at the nonunion site that provides rotational stability.

Extra-articular deformity resulting in medial or lateral displacement of the articular surface relative to the diaphysis may not require corrective osteotomy. However, bony deformity may require use of custom or modular offset stems to bypass areas of bony deformity and minimize risk of postoperative periprosthetic fracture (Figure 2).

Procedure

Preoperative AP and lateral radiographs are obtained to determine the amount of angular correction needed (**Figure 3**). The knee is exposed through a medial parapatellar approach, and the site of maximal extra-articular deformity is dissected subperiosteally. A transverse saw cut is made partially through the bone perpendicular to the long axis of the femur, and then a saw blade is inserted to orient the second angular osteotomy cut. A second saw cut is made at the desired angle of correction, and the angle between the two saw cuts is measured with a protractor to ensure accurate correction of deformity before completing the osteotomy (**Figure 4, *A***).

After completion of the osteotomy, the bone surfaces are opposed to correct the extra-articular deformity and an intramedullary alignment rod is in-

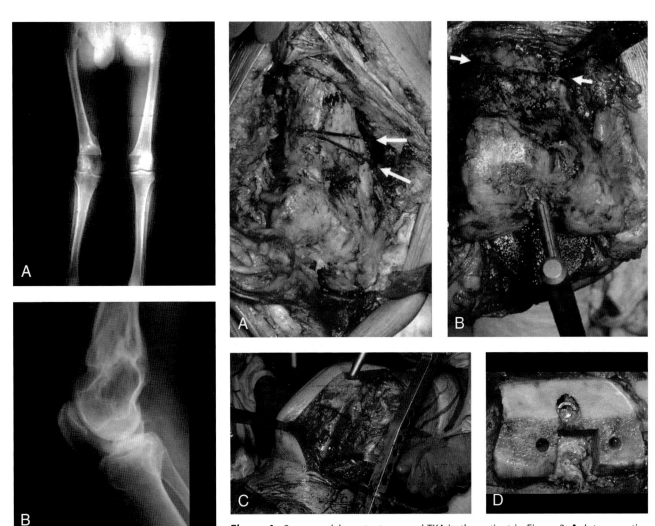

Figure 3 A 72-year-old man presented with valgus and extension deformity associated with lateral compartment osteoarthritis. Supracondylar osteotomy and TKA were performed simultaneously. Full-length weight-bearing alignment AP (**A**) and lateral (**B**) preoperative radiographs illustrate supracondylar malunion.

Figure 4 Supracondylar osteotomy and TKA in the patient in Figure 3. **A,** Intraoperative photograph illustrates saw cuts through the supracondylar region of the femur to remove a medial-based wedge (arrows) to correct valgus and extension deformity. **B,** The osteotomy was reduced (arrows) and an intramedullary rod was inserted to orient the distal femoral cutting block and remaining femoral bone cuts. **C,** The osteotomy was fixed with a supracondylar nail. **D,** The distal end of the nail was positioned proximal to the level of the bone cuts used for the TKA.

serted to hold the osteotomy reduced and orient the distal femoral TKA bone cuts (**Figure 4**, *B*). Once the distal femoral TKA bone cut is made, the osteotomy can be reduced and fixed because the remaining femoral bone cuts are based on the position of the resected distal femoral bone surface. The osteotomy can be fixed with a supracondylar nail, using the same technique required for fixation and stabili-

zation of a supracondylar femur fracture (**Figure 4**, *C*). The remainder of the TKA can then be performed in a routine fashion (**Figure 4**, *D* and **Figure 5**). Alternatively, the osteotomy can be performed to correct extra-articular deformity and stabilized using intramedullary rod or plate fixation, following which extramedullary alignment methods or computer-assisted navigation may be used to perform the TKA.

Technique: Treatment of Nonunion

Setup/Exposure

Nonunion following prior open reduction and internal fixation can be associated with infection. Preoperative evaluation should include an erythrocyte sedimentation rate and C-reactive protein level. Further evaluation with aspiration or nuclear medicine scans may help to establish or rule out the presence of infection. Nonunion can be treated either by stabilization of the nonunion with a stemmed TKA or excision of the non- united bone segment and replacement with a distal femoral replacement (tumor prosthesis).

Instruments/Equipment/Implants Required

For young patients who may require future revision surgery, the nonunited bone should be retained if possible. The nonunion can be treated with a stemmed revision TKA, using the stem to stabilize the nonunion. Cancellous bone from the resected articular surfaces that is removed during TKA can be used as bone graft at the nonunion site (**Figure 6**).

If the bone is osteoporotic or the nonunited segment of metaphyseal bone is relatively small, then salvage of the bone fragment may not be feasible. For elderly, low-demand patients with osteoporosis, excision of the fragment and implantation of a distal femoral hinged replacement is a good option. This permits early weight-bearing activity and restoration of knee function.

Procedure

The knee should be exposed through a medial parapatellar arthrotomy. If a lateral plate is present, the proximal lateral hardware can be removed through

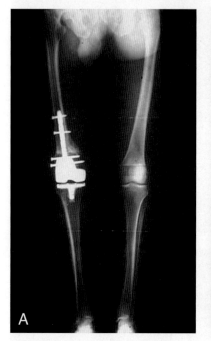
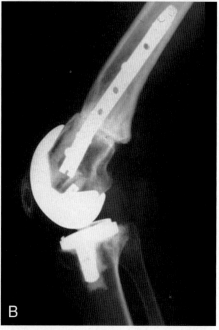

Figure 5 Full-length weight-bearing alignment AP radiograph (**A**) and lateral radiograph (**B**) of the patient in Figure 3 obtained 2 years after surgery demonstrate healing of the osteotomy and correction of malalignment.

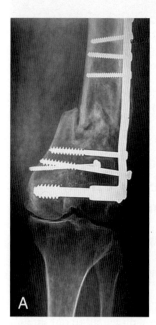
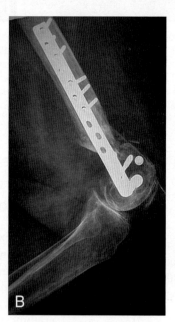
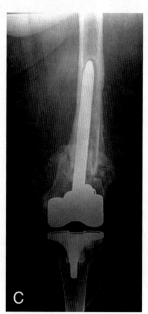
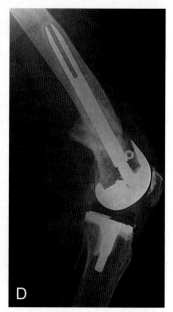

Figure 6 A 58-year-old woman who had sustained a supracondylar femur fracture presented with nonunion and degenerative arthritis. Preoperative AP (**A**) and lateral (**B**) radiographs demonstrate irregularity at the fracture site and fibrous union, which provided adequate rotational stability so that a press-fit long intramedullary stem could be used for fixation of the nonunion. Postoperative AP (**C**) and lateral (**D**) radiographs after TKA with a long stem was used to stabilize the osteotomy.

a separate lateral approach to the femur. However, the distal extent of the lateral incision and proximal extent of the anterior knee incision should not overlap excessively. If both lateral and anterior incisions are needed, the anterior incision should be made more medial to increase the distance between the two incisions and the vascularity to the lateral soft-tissue flap.

For revision TKA after supracondylar nonunion, revision instrumentation should be used to prepare the femur. The femoral canal is reamed to a diameter that engages the isthmus, and a stem length is selected that will provide adequate stability of the nonunion. The distal femoral bone cuts are then based on the position of the revision stem. If the collateral ligaments are preserved and a nonconstrained prosthesis is used, the tibial cuts can be prepared as for a standard TKA. If additional constraint is required, then a stemmed tibial component should be considered to provide additional fixation.

For replacement of a supracondylar nonunion with a distal femoral replacement prosthesis, removal of the distal bone segment is associated with a risk of neurovascular injury due to the proximity of the neurovascular structures to the posterior bone fragment. The segment of bone should be removed by subperiosteal dissection of all surrounding soft tissues with the knee in a flexed position. Cemented stemmed femoral and tibial components should be used to provide adequate fixation for the hinge mechanism, particularly in osteoporotic bone.

Technique: Management of Soft-Tissue Defects

Preoperative Planning

Prior scars, skin that is adherent to underlying bone, previous skin grafts, and other soft-tissue flaps may be present. The vascularity of the remaining soft tissues should be assessed preoperatively. If necessary, a plastic surgeon should be consulted to evaluate the risk of postoperative soft-tissue necrosis and determine if additional soft-tissue transposition procedures are likely to be required during TKA.

Additional Materials Required

If wound closure cannot be achieved after TKA, soft-tissue coverage can be obtained with local muscle or fasiocutaneous transposition, or a free flap. Most defects can be effectively treated with medial gastrocnemius muscle–flap transposition. The decision regarding which flap to use depends on the size and location of the soft-tissue defect and the donor material available. This requires an assessment during surgery after the prosthesis is implanted. Intraoperative consultation with a plastic surgeon can be helpful for assessing the condition of the soft tissues, relative need for soft-tissue coverage, risk of postoperative soft-tissue necrosis, and selection of soft-tissue coverage procedure.

Procedure

The lateral skin edge of a vertical incision over the knee is more hypoxic than the medial skin edge (**Figure 7**, *A* and *B*). In general, when multiple scars are present, the more lateral scar should be used. However, the decision to incorporate prior scars into the TKA incision also depends on several other factors, including the proximity of the scar to the medial parapatellar arthrotomy, the length of the scar, and the relative vascularity of the underlying subcutaneous layer.

If medial gastrocnemius muscle–flap transposition is required, the entire lower leg should be prepared and draped to the ankle to provide access to the distal extent of the medial gastrocnemius tendon. An area for skin grafting should also be selected and prepared, such as the contralateral thigh.

For medial gastrocnemius muscle–flap transposition, a vertical incision is made along the muscle in the lower leg, extending distally toward the Achilles tendon. The medial gastrocnemius tendon is transected distally, leaving the remaining Achilles tendon intact, and the muscle is rotated proximally to direct the distal portion of the muscle and tendon over the anterior knee defect. The muscle can be passed underneath a skin and subcutaneous bridge to the knee, and the lower leg incision from the medial gastrocnemius exposure can be closed primarily (**Figure 7**, *C*). A skin graft is then used to cover the transposed muscle over the knee (**Figure 7**, *D*).

Postoperative Regimen

Restrictions to postoperative range of motion and weight bearing should be determined based on the stability of bony fixation and vascularity of soft tissues. If an osteotomy is performed or a nonunion is fixed and stable fixation is achieved, knee range of motion can be started immediately after surgery, using the same protocol as for postoperative primary TKA patients. Use of a hinged knee brace is appropriate to protect the osteotomy or nonunion site if necessary until healing occurs. Weight bearing should be restricted until callus has formed at the osteotomy or nonunion site, usually 6 to 12 weeks after surgery.

Avoiding Pitfalls and Complications

Previous trauma may have resulted in diminished vascularity to the soft tis-

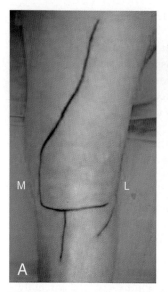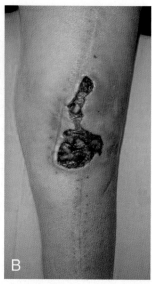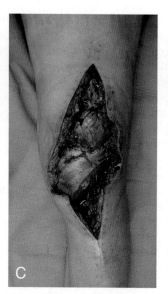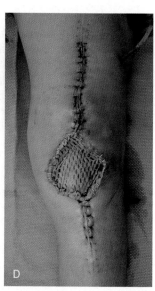

Figure 7 Clinical photographs of a 49-year-old woman with a history of cigarette smoking who had posttraumatic arthritis and multiple prior scars over the knee. **A,** The longest, most vertical scar was oriented relatively medially (M) and required elevation of a lateral (L) skin flap. **B,** Necrosis of the lateral skin flap developed 10 days after TKA. **C,** The wound was débrided and covered with a medial gastrocnemius flap. The muscle fibers are oriented relatively vertically to cover the patellar tendon. **D,** A skin graft was used to cover the exposed medial gastrocnemius muscle. (Reproduced with permission from Ries MD, Bozic K: Medial gastrocnemius flap coverage for treatment of skin necrosis after total knee arthroplasty. *Clin Orthop Relat Res* 2006;446:186-192.)

sues over the knee. Early knee flexion can further decrease circulation to the soft tissues. For knees with compromised soft-tissue coverage, delaying early knee range of motion for 2 to 3 days after surgery can reduce the risk of wound complications.

Exposure of knees with limited motion and quadriceps contracture can be associated with risk of patellar ligament disruption. More extensile approaches with tibial tubercle os-teotomy, rectus snip, or V-Y quadriceps turndown may be needed to minimize risk of extensor mechanism disruption.

If infection had occurred previously, intraoperative tissue cultures should be obtained. Use of antibiotic-impregnated cement is appropriate in patients considered to be at increased risk of developing infection.

Previous hardware may be present and require removal if the hardware is painful or interferes with positioning the TKA. Prior trauma or hardware may also result in bone defects that are associated with risk of postoperative periprosthetic fracture. Stress risers from removed hardware and bone defects should be bypassed with use of stemmed components or prophylactic internal fixation.

Bibliography

Bottros J, Klika AK, Lee HH, Polousky J, Barsoum WK: The use of navigation in total knee arthroplasty for patients with extra-articular deformity. *J Arthroplasty* 2008;23(1):74-78.

Lonner JH, Pedlow FX, Siliski JM: Total knee arthroplasty for post-traumatic arthrosis. *J Arthroplasty* 1999;14(8):969-975.

Lonner JH, Siliski JM, Lotke PA: Simultaneous femoral osteotomy and total knee arthroplasty for treatment of osteoarthritis associated with severe extra-articular deformity. *J Bone Joint Surg Am* 2000;82(3):342-348.

Mullaji AB, Padmanabhan V, Jindal G: Total knee arthroplasty for profound varus deformity: technique and radiological results in 173 knees with varus of more than 20 degrees. *J Arthroplasty* 2005;20(5):550-561.

Mullaji A, Shetty GM: Computer-assisted total knee arthroplasty for arthritis with extra-articular deformity. *J Arthroplasty* 2009;24(8):1164-1169, e1.

Papadopoulos EC, Parvizi J, Lai CH, Lewallen DG: Total knee arthroplasty following prior distal femoral fracture. *Knee* 2002;9(4):267-274.

Ries MD, Bozic KJ: Medial gastrocnemius flap coverage for treatment of skin necrosis after total knee arthroplasty. *Clin Orthop Relat Res* 2006;446:186-192.

Saleh KJ, Sherman P, Katkin P, et al: Total knee arthroplasty after open reduction and internal fixation of fractures of the tibial plateau: A minimum five-year follow-up study. *J Bone Joint Surg Am* 2001;83-A(8):1144-1148.

Wang JW, Wang CJ: Total knee arthroplasty for arthritis of the knee with extra-articular deformity. *J Bone Joint Surg Am* 2002;84-A(10):1769-1774.

Weiss NG, Parvizi J, Hanssen AD, Trousdale RT, Lewallen DG: Total knee arthroplasty in post-traumatic arthrosis of the knee. *J Arthroplasty* 2003;18(3, Suppl 1):23-26.

Coding

CPT Code		Corresponding ICD-9 Codes	
27447	Arthroplasty, knee, condyle and plateau; medial AND lateral compartments with or without patella resurfacing (total knee arthroplasty)	715 715.80	715.16 715.89

Chapter 21
Total Knee Arthroplasty Following Prior Osteotomy

John F. Tilzey, MD, PhD
William L. Healy, MD

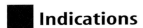 **Indications**

Total knee arthroplasty (TKA) following prior osteotomy of the proximal tibia or distal femur can be technically more difficult than a routine primary TKA. Despite several published clinical evaluations, no consensus exists in the orthopaedic literature regarding the outcome of TKA following prior osteotomy and internal fixation. Our indications for TKA following osteotomy are pain secondary to arthrosis, joint stiffness, recurrence of deformity, progression to tricompartmental arthrosis, and nonunion of the osteotomy or fracture.

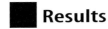 **Contraindications**

Active infection is an absolute contraindication to TKA. Relative contraindications include prior infection, a nonfunctional extensor mechanism, neuromuscular disease leading to loss of function of the lower extremity, severe peripheral vascular disease, severe osteoporosis, or metabolic bone disease.

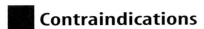 **Results**

High Tibial Osteotomy

Clinical results of TKA following prior high tibial osteotomy (HTO) have demonstrated variable patient outcomes (**Table 1**). Most of these studies report on outcome at short-term or intermediate-term follow-up. Parvizi and associates and Haslam and associates reported longer follow-up, at 15.1 years and 12.6 years, respectively. Parvizi and associates found that the overall functional outcome and radiographic outcome were slightly inferior for knees that have undergone a prior tibial osteotomy, including higher rates of limb malalignment, patella infera (patella baja), and instability. Despite an increased prevalence of radiolucent lines and higher rate of revision, prosthetic survival rate following TKA in patients who have had a previous HTO was still high, at 92.3% at 10 years. Haslam and associates reported no difference in knee scores between TKA performed on patients with prior HTO compared with a matched group undergoing primary TKA. However, the authors did note more patients from the osteotomy group with a poor result or failure, reduced flexion, and higher reoperation rate.

Distal Varus Femoral Osteotomy

Few studies exist that report the outcome of TKA following varus-producing distal femoral osteotomy performed for isolated lateral compartment gonarthrosis with valgus alignment. Nelson and associates reported the results of 11 consecutive knees that had undergone TKA following prior distal femoral varus osteotomy with average follow-up of 5.1 years. Three patients also had previous ipsilateral proximal tibial osteotomy. Seven knees had a good or excellent result, and four had a fair result. Five knees received a constrained implant, and one knee required a rotating-hinge prosthesis. The authors commented that TKA following distal femoral varus osteotomy is technically demanding and is associated with results inferior to those with primary TKA.

Table 1 Clinical Outcomes of Total Knee Arthroplasty Following Prior High Tibial Osteotomy

Authors (Year)	Number of Knees	Mean Patient Age in Years (Range)	Mean Follow-up (Range)	Mean Outcome Score (% good or excellent)	Average Range of Motion	Outcome
Katz et al (1987)	21 HTO 21 control	62 (31-76)	35 months (24-69)	HTO: 86* (81%) Control: 93*	HTO: 95° Control: 103°	Inferior
Staeheli et al (1987)	35	67 (48-87)	44 months (24-70)	84† (89%)	HTO: 92°	No difference
Windsor et al (1988)	45 (26 women, 15 men)	Women: 66 (37-81) Men: 62 (36-83)	4.6 years (minimum, 2 years)	83† (80%)	HTO: 98°	Inferior
Amendola et al (1989)	42 HTO 41 control	64 (52-82)	37 months (24-50)	HTO: 86† (88%) Control: 89† (90%)	HTO: 101° Control: 115°	No difference
Mont et al (1994)	73 HTO 73 control	62 (29-79)	73 months (24-132)	(64%)	HTO: 102° (40°-135°)	Inferior
Nizard et al (1998)	63 HTO 63 control	71.8	4.6 years (1.1-10.1)	HTO: 74.4‡ (56%) Control: 80.9‡ (87.7%)	HTO: 100.6° Control: 105.4°	Inferior
Haddad and Bentley (2000)	50 HTO 50 control	HTO: 65 (54-74) Control: 66 (59-76)	6.2 years (5-10.6)	HTO: 87† (84%) Control: 89† (82%)	HTO: 95° Control: 103°	No difference
Meding et al (2000)	39 HTO 39 control (bilateral TKAs)	HTO: 66.9 (50-80) Control: 67.4 (52-80)	HTO: 7.5 years (3-16) Control: 6.8 years (2-10)	HTO: 89‡ Control: 89.6‡	HTO: 113° Control: 117.8°	No difference
Haslam et al (2007)	51 HTO 51 control	78	12.6 years (8-18)	HTO: 79† (55%) Control: 80† (67%)	HTO: 91° Control: 106°	No difference

HTO = high tibial osteotomy, TKA = total knee arthroplasty.
* Baltimore Knee Score
† Hospital for Special Surgery score
‡ Knee Society Score

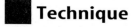

Technique

Preoperative Radiographic Evaluation

Routinely, preoperative radiographs include hip-knee-ankle alignment views, weight-bearing AP views, and lateral and tangential views (**Figure 1**). A 10° posterior-tilt AP radiograph to visualize the proximal tibia may be helpful in assessing proximal tibial bone stock, and a PA weight-bearing radiograph in 40° of flexion may better define the tibiofemoral articular cartilage.

Exposure

Prior skin incisions around the knee should be evaluated carefully to plan an appropriate surgical approach that will minimize the potential for wound complications. All previous skin incisions are marked with a skin marker once the limb is prepared and draped (**Figure 2**). A straight midline incision is optimal for exposure, closure without tension, and healing, but previous skin incisions may compromise this approach. We recommend trying to use the most recent or most lateral incision if possible. Narrow skin

bridges between incisions should be avoided. Transverse incisions can be safely crossed at a 90° angle; angles less than 60° should be avoided. When we encounter prior anterior and medial incisions, we often use a full-thickness, laterally based fasciocutaneous flap incorporating the superficial fascia. The blood supply to the skin is from deep to the superficial fascia (**Figure 3**, *A*). The lateral-based wound flap also can be raised over the lateral proximal tibia to remove retained hardware that may interfere with the tibial reconstruction (**Figure**

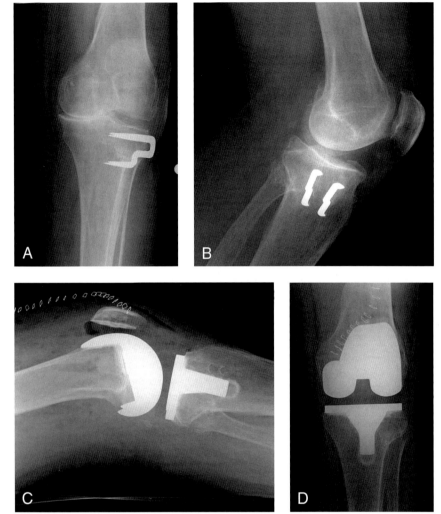

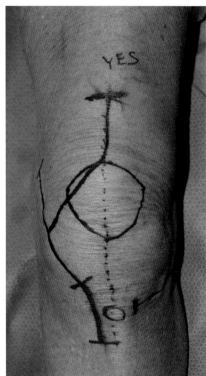

Figure 2 Photograph of a left knee with previous incisional scars marked. A previous oblique medial joint line incision and a transverse lateral joint line incision are marked as solid lines. The planned incision is medially based, incorporating the distal half of the previous incision. The planned incision is at an angle greater than 60° to the previous incisional scar.

Figure 1 Radiographs of a left knee that had undergone prior high tibial osteotomy. Preoperative weight-bearing AP (**A**) and lateral (**B**) views show presence of a lateral staple requiring removal, as this would affect tibial tray placement. Postoperative AP (**C**) and lateral (**D**) views.

3, *B*). Alternatively, a second lateral incision may be used for hardware removal, or the hardware can be removed in a separate staged operation.

Procedure

Once the skin incision exposes the joint capsule, the quadriceps tendon, and the patellar tendon, we prefer a standard medial parapatellar arthrotomy. Proximal medial tibial exposure is performed with subperiosteal dissection of the medial retinaculum and deep medial collateral ligament that is continued posteromedially to the semimembranosus

tendon insertions. If additional medial release is required, the subperiosteal dissection is carried more distally on the medial tibia to release the superficial medial collateral ligament. The lateral gutters are débrided of synovium and fibrous tissue. The patellofemoral ligament can be released. The patella can be everted or retracted posterolaterally with a bent Hohmann retractor. If this is difficult, a quadriceps snip, V-Y turndown, or tibial tubercle osteotomy may be required.

With the knee in flexion, the distal femoral osteotomy is performed to achieve a 5° valgus alignment. In a

knee with prior HTO, this can be performed with intramedullary femoral instrumentation. Following distal femoral varus osteotomy, this may require extramedullary instrumentation or computer navigation because of distal femoral deformity.

Following the distal femoral osteotomy, the remaining distal femoral bone cuts can be performed in accordance with a measured resection technique. Alternatively, attention may be turned to the proximal tibia using a gap-balancing technique.

Closing wedge osteotomy of the proximal tibia may create bony deficiency of the lateral column of the proximal tibia. The tibial osteotomy is performed perpendicular to the anatomic axis of the tibia. A minimum

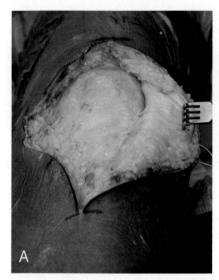
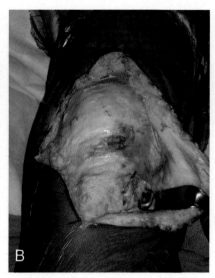

Figure 3 Intraoperative photographs show exposure. **A,** A fasciocutaneous wound flap is raised from medial to lateral. Note that the superficial fascia is incorporated in the lateral flap. **B,** The fasciocutaneous wound flap is elevated over the proximal lateral tibia. Retained hardware is removed without requiring an additional skin incision.

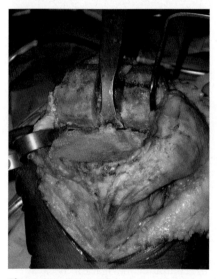

Figure 4 Intraoperative photograph shows excellent exposure. A proximal tibial osteotomy required only a "skim" cut of the lateral tibial plateau.

"skim" cut of bone from the lateral tibial plateau may be all that is required (**Figure 4**); rarely, tibial wedges may be required.

The flexion and extension gaps are balanced with soft-tissue releases and removal of osteophytes. The appropriate trials are placed; stemmed implants are not required if there is suf-

ficient host bone stock to obtain varus-valgus, anterior-posterior, and rotational stability. The components are cemented following irrigation of the bony surfaces.

Wound Closure

The arthrotomy is closed, and the skin is closed without tension. When a fasciocutaneous flap is used, the flap is closed in two layers. When the anterolateral extensor muscles are elevated to remove proximal tibial hardware, use of a drain to reduce the risk of compartment syndrome may be considered.

Postoperative Regimen

Our TKA protocol consists of a clinical pathway and pain management program with a multimodal approach, including femoral nerve blocks. Deep vein thrombosis prophylaxis is with mechanical compression, warfarin, and early ambulation. The average hospital stay is 3 to 4 days. The path-

way includes continuous passive motion beginning in the recovery room, or 24 or 48 hours postoperatively if there are concerns about wound healing. When a fasciocutaneous flap is used, we hold the knee in extension for 24 to 48 hours to maintain optimal blood supply and oxygenation of the flap without tension created by knee flexion.

Avoiding Pitfalls and Complications

TKA following osteotomy can be technically demanding. Meticulous preoperative planning of surgical approach and anticipated implants is mandatory. Adequate exposure is necessary; therefore, TKA following HTO is not a setting for minimal incision techniques.

TKA Following HTO
Potential technical challenges associated with TKA following HTO performed with a closing wedge osteotomy of the proximal tibia include surgical exposure, prior incisions about the knee, retained hardware, lateral proximal tibial insufficiency, patella infera, sclerotic proximal tibial bone that is prone to fracture, and achieving range of motion (0° to 120°).

Surgical Exposure and Prior Surgical Incisions
In the multiply operated knee, careful planning of the intended incision is mandatory to minimize risk of wound complications secondary to dermal vascular insufficiency. The vascular supply to the skin of the anterior knee is derived primarily from the medial side; accordingly, when multiple incisions are present, the most laterally based incision is preferable if adequate exposure can be obtained. Plastic surgery consultation and balloon tissue

expanders can be helpful in some circumstances, although there is an increased risk of complications with this technique around the knee. When a knee has multiple prior incisions or when fasciocutaneous flaps are used, we do not flex the knee for 24 to 48 hours following TKA.

Retained Hardware

Retained hardware in the proximal tibia may need to be removed if it is painful or if it is in the way of proposed tibial cuts as determined on preoperative radiographs. Removal may require increased exposure or a separate incision. If a separate incision is anticipated, staging of the TKA may be considered to avoid wound healing problems, especially in the multiply operated knee. The first stage is removal of hardware, followed 6 to 12 weeks later by TKA. In some cases hardware or portions of hardware can be left in place (**Figure 5**). For example, in the case of a lateral tibial plate, the proximal screws may be removed so as not to interfere with the tibial tray, and the plate and distal screws may be retained intact to minimize tissue dissection and reduce the risk of distal fracture through stress risers from empty screw holes.

Patella Infera

Closing wedge osteotomies performed proximal to the tibial tubercle can lower the joint line and cause scarring in and around the patellar tendon, leading to patella infera. This can be determined using the Insall-Salvati ratio of patellar height to tibial patellar tendon length from the preoperative radiograph. If this ratio is less than 0.6, eversion of the patella and exposure of the lateral compartment may be difficult. In such cases, lateral subluxation of the patella without eversion may be used. Occasionally, a more extensile exposure may be needed.

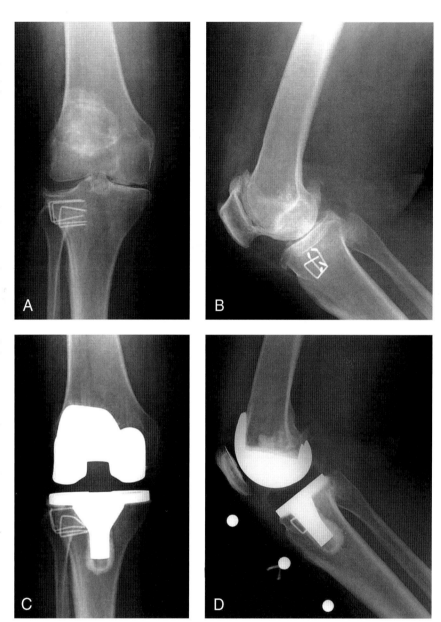

Figure 5 Radiographs of a left knee that had undergone prior high tibial osteotomy. Weight-bearing AP (**A**) and lateral (**B**) views. The staple may be retained, as it will not impede placement of the tibial component. Postoperative AP (**C**) and lateral (**D**) views.

Range of Motion

Some patients may develop flexion contractures following HTO, thus adding to the complexity of TKA. Preoperative range of motion is an important predictor of postoperative range of motion, and patients should be informed preoperatively that they may be at risk for less than the ideal 0° to 120° arc of motion.

Nonunion

Nonunion of the HTO or proximal tibial fracture may have to be bone grafted as a staged procedure (**Figure 6**). Alternatively, in a single-stage TKA, bone grafting and a stemmed tibial component may provide stable proximal tibial reconstruction.

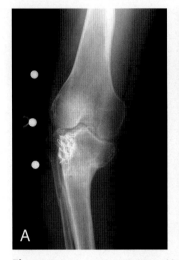
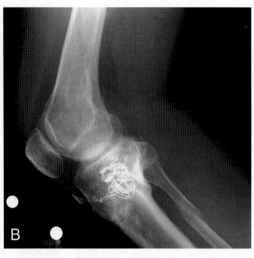

Figure 6 Preoperative AP (**A**) and lateral (**B**) radiographs of a right knee demonstrate proximal tibial malunion with varus malalignment. An infected nonunion healed with antibiotic-impregnated cement beads still in situ.

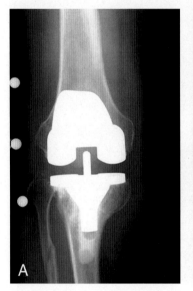
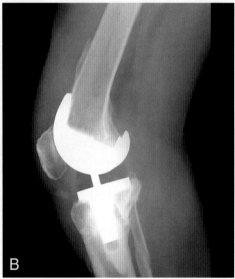

Figure 7 Postoperative AP (**A**) and lateral (**B**) radiographs of the same knee shown in Figure 6 following total knee arthroplasty. Note adequate lateral tibial bone stock. The cemented tibial component did not require a tibial stem for stability.

Osteonecrosis

Osteonecrosis of the proximal tibia following HTO is unusual but has been described. When osteonecrosis is encountered, tibial augments placed on viable bone, structural allograft, or metaphyseal cones may be required with a stemmed tibial component.

Tibial Implant Alignment

Closing wedge HTO may affect lateral positioning of the tibial component secondary to alteration of the normal proximal tibial metaphyseal anatomy. The major concerns are lateral tibial bone deficiency and/or offset of the plateau relative to the tibial shaft. The usual proximal tibial resection perpendicular to the tibial anatomic axis may resect the tibial tubercle and excessive medial bone, thereby compromising the medial collateral ligament insertion. In these cases, wedges, bone grafting, offset tibial stems, or even extra-articular proximal tibial osteotomy may be necessary. Preoperative templating will determine if the tibial stem, fins, pegs, or screws will be difficult to place secondary to this deformity (**Figure 7**).

TKA Following Distal Femoral Osteotomy

TKA following osteotomy of the distal femur also has been described as being a technically difficult operation, and it has been associated with patient outcomes inferior to those with routine primary TKA. Achieving a 5° to 7° valgus alignment of the distal femoral cut can be a problem because of altered distal femoral anatomy and inability to use intramedullary femoral guides. Extramedullary femoral alignment guides and computer-assisted navigation may be helpful. The deformity following distal femoral varus osteotomy is extra-articular, and it may create difficulties with intra-articular ligament balancing and instability; therefore, it is useful to have a constrained condylar prosthesis available in the operating room. Preoperative joint aspiration as well as intraoperative Gram staining and frozen section analysis may be considered, given the higher infection rates encountered for TKA following distal femoral varus osteotomies.

■ Bibliography

Amendola A, Rorabeck CH, Bourne RB, Apyan PM: Total knee arthroplasty following high tibial osteotomy for osteoarthritis. *J Arthroplasty* 1989;4(Suppl):S11-S17.

Coonse K, Adams JD: A new operative approach to the knee joint. *Surg Gynecol Obstet* 1943;77:344-347.

Haddad FS, Bentley G: Total knee arthroplasty after high tibial osteotomy: A medium-term review. *J Arthroplasty* 2000;15(5):597-603.

Haslam P, Armstrong M, Geutjens G, Wilton TJ: Total knee arthroplasty after failed high tibial osteotomy: Long-term follow-up of matched groups. *J Arthroplasty* 2007;22(2):245-250.

Katz MM, Hungerford DS, Krackow KA, Lennox DW: Results of total knee arthroplasty after failed proximal tibial osteotomy for osteoarthritis. *J Bone Joint Surg Am* 1987;69(2):225-233.

Meding JB, Keating EM, Ritter MA, Faris PM: Total knee arthroplasty after high tibial osteotomy: A comparison study in patients who had bilateral total knee replacement. *J Bone Joint Surg Am* 2000;82(9):1252-1259.

Mont MA, Antonaides S, Krackow KA, Hungerford DS: Total knee arthroplasty after failed high tibial osteotomy: A comparison with a matched group. *Clin Orthop Relat Res* 1994;299:125-130.

Nelson CL, Saleh KJ, Kassim RA, et al: Total knee arthroplasty after varus osteotomy of the distal part of the femur. *J Bone Joint Surg Am* 2003;85(6):1062-1065.

Nizard RS, Cardinne L, Bizot P, Witvoet J: Total knee replacement after failed tibial osteotomy: Results of a matched-pair study. *J Arthroplasty* 1998;13:847-853.

Parvizi J, Hanssen AD, Spangehl MJ: Total knee arthroplasty following proximal tibial osteotomy: Risk factors for failure. *J Bone Joint Surg Am* 2004;86(3):474-479.

Scott RD, Siliski JM: The use of a modified V-Y quadricepsplasty during total knee replacement to gain exposure and improve flexion in the ankylosed knee. *Orthopedics* 1985;8(1):45-48.

Staeheli JW, Cass JR, Morrey BF: Condylar total knee arthroplasty after failed proximal tibial osteotomy. *J Bone Joint Surg Am* 1987;69(1):28-31.

Whiteside LA, Ohl MD: Tibial tubercle osteotomy for exposure of the difficult total knee arthroplasty. *Clin Orthop Relat Res* 1990;260:6-9.

Windsor RE, Insall JN, Vince KG: Technical considerations of total knee arthroplasty after proximal tibial osteotomy. *J Bone Joint Surg Am* 1988;70(4):547-555.

Yoshino N, Takai S, Watanabe Y, Nakamura S, Kubo T: Total knee arthroplasty with long stem for treatment of nonunion after high tibial osteotomy. *J Arthroplasty* 2004;19(4):528-531.

Coding				
CPT Codes			**Corresponding ICD-9 Codes**	
Total Knee Arthroplasty				
27447	Arthroplasty, knee, condyle and plateau; medial AND lateral compartments with or without patella resurfacing (total knee arthroplasty)		996.67	996.78

Chapter 22

Recurvatum/Flexion Contracture in Total Knee Arthroplasty

Adolph V. Lombardi, Jr, MD, FACS
Keith R. Berend, MD

 Indications

Most patients undergo total knee arthroplasty (TKA) because of primary osteoarthritis; however, some have inflammatory arthropathy, posttraumatic arthritis, or osteonecrosis. Whatever the diagnosis, patients present with severe pain, limited function, loss of motion, and increasing deformity. Many TKA candidates present with either fixed varus or valgus deformities, which are deformities in the coronal plane. Most sagittal plane deformities are flexion contractures; a few are recurvatum deformities. The etiology of flexion contractures is related to the recurrent effusions present in a knee with end-stage degenerative joint disease secondary to the associated inflammatory process. These recurrent effusions cause increased pressure within the knee, which results in pain and discomfort. Patients will always seek a position of comfort, which in

this situation is with the knee in slight flexion. Flexion decreases the painful stimulus by decreasing the pressure within the knee and relaxing the posterior capsule. This is a self-perpetuating process that leads to a greater degree of contracture as the disease progresses. Furthermore, patients rarely maintain the knee in full extension. Even during the gait cycle, the knee is slightly flexed. As the disease progresses, patients limit ambulation and spend more time in a seated position. Patients often report that they sleep in the fetal position or with a pillow under the knee. All of these actions increase the flexion contracture deformity.

Recurvatum is less common; it is subdivided into deformities with neurogenic etiologies and those with non-neurogenic etiologies. The status of the extensor mechanism is extremely critical in patients with recurvatum. Significant weakness of the extensor mechanism secondary to neurogenic

conditions such as multiple sclerosis or postpolio syndrome presents significant challenges that are beyond the scope of this particular chapter. On the other hand, generalized laxity and associated recurvatum can be addressed similar to flexion contractures, with bone resection and soft-tissue balance.

 Contraindications

Patients with severe deformity (ie, flexion contracture greater than 40° or recurvatum greater than 20°) should be counseled regarding the complexities of the surgical procedure that will be required. These patients should be advised that implants with increasing constraint may be required and, specifically in patients with excessive recurvatum, a rotating hinge design may be indicated.

Dr. Lombardi or an immediate family member serves as a board member, owner, officer, or committee member of the American Board of Orthopaedic Surgery, The Hip Society, and the New Albany Surgical Hospital Foundation; has received royalties from Biomet; serves as a paid consultant to or is an employee of Biomet; has received research or institutional support from Biomet; and has received nonincome support (such as equipment or services), commercially derived honoraria, or other non–research-related funding (such as paid travel) from Biomet, Medtronic, GlaxoSmith-Kline, Merck, Tornier, Allergan, New Albany Surgical Hospital, Pivotal Research Solutions, and Pozen. Dr. Berend or an immediate family member serves as a board member, owner, officer, or committee member of Mount Carmel New Albany Surgical Hospital and the American Association of Hip and Knee Surgeons Education Committee; has received royalties from Biomet; serves as a paid consultant to or is an employee of Biomet, Salient Surgical, and Synvasive; and owns stock or stock options in Angiotech.

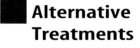 **Alternative Treatments**

The algorithm for the treatment of end-stage degenerative joint disease of the knee starts with use of over-the-counter analgesics and nonsteroidal

Table 1 Results of Total Knee Arthroplasty in Patients With Flexion Contracture or Recurvatum

Authors (Year)	Number of Knees	Mean Preoperative Degrees of Deformity* (Range)	Mean Patient Age in Years (Range)	Mean Follow-up in Years (Range)	Results
Lu et al (1999)	37	78 (60-100)	42 (20-57)	4.3 (2-8)	12° average residual contracture (range, 0°-15°) 1 revised for deep infection 3 transient peroneal nerve palsies
Whiteside and Mihalko (2002)	552 (542 flexion contracture, 10 recurvatum)	Flexion contracture: 14.5 (11-40) Recurvatum: 11.1 (6-25)	73.0 ± 18.9	Minimum, 2	Flexion contracture: 95% had <3° residual contracture Recurvatum: No residual
Bellemans et al (2006)	130 (95 moderate, 35 severe)	Moderate: 23 (15-30) Severe: 54.3 (minimum, 30)	Moderate: 64.4 ± 11.8 Severe: 61.5 ± 11.7	Minimum, 2	Moderate: 99% had <5° residual contracture at follow-up 94% had <5° residual contracture at follow-up 2 peroneal nerve palsies (1 permanent)
Berend et al (2006)	52	28 (minimum, 20)	63 (42-95)	3.2 (0.1-6.4)	94% had <10° residual contracture at follow-up 1 revised for instability 1 revised for deep infection No nerve injuries

*Flexion contracture unless otherwise specified.

anti-inflammatory drugs (NSAIDs). Many patients are initially able to control symptoms with medications such as acetaminophen, aspirin, and ibuprofen. Nutraceuticals such as glucosamine and chondroitin sulfate have demonstrated some limited value over placebo in several studies. Patients should be counseled on an appropriate exercise regimen that focuses on quadriceps rehabilitation and range of motion and avoids impact loading of the knee. Corticosteroid injections can be extremely helpful in alleviating acute inflammatory reactions, and viscosupplementation has demonstrated more sustained relief of symptoms in several studies. Varus or valgus deformities in the early stages can be treated with appropriate osteotomies. Arthroscopic intervention has a limited role in patients with end-stage degenerative joint disease unless they have associated mechanical symptoms. The duration of pain relief will be directly proportional to the amount of disease

present. There is an increasing use of partial knee arthroplasty (patellofemoral arthroplasty and isolated medial or lateral unicompartmental knee arthroplasty). The success of these procedures is directly related to careful patient selection. TKA, therefore, represents the ultimate treatment of patients with end-stage degenerative joint disease of the knee. Upon electing to undergo TKA, patients should be instructed in preoperative physical therapy. The major focus of therapy both for patients with flexion contracture and for those with recurvatum should be quadriceps rehabilitation. Patients with preoperative flexion contractures also should be instructed in stretching techniques. Preoperative casting and bracing with dynamic-type braces play a limited role. Additionally, patients who present with spasticity of the hamstrings should be sent for neurologic evaluation and for consideration of botulism toxin injection.

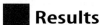

Results

We have used the techniques described in this chapter to treat flexion contractures as detailed by Berend and associates in a cohort of 52 patients. Of 52 knees with flexion contractures of 20° or greater, 49 (94%) had less than 10° residual contracture at an average follow-up of 37 months. A cruciate-retaining prosthesis was used in 31 (60%) of the knees, a posterior stabilized design in 14 (27%), a posterior stabilized constrained type in 5 (10%), and a rotating-hinge prosthesis in 2 (4%). No peroneal nerve injuries occurred despite large flexion contractures and preoperative fixed valgus deformity greater than 10° in 7 (14%) of the knees.

Other studies have reported excellent results using various techniques, including the use of both posterior and anterior referencing systems (Table 1). Bellemans and associates used posterior referencing techniques combined with an algorithm that included four steps: (1) mediolateral ligament balancing with resection of all osteophytes and overresection of 2 mm of distal femur, (2) progressive posterior capsular release, (3) additional resection of up to 4 mm of distal femur, and (4) hamstring tenotomy. They reported excellent results in 95 patients with preoperative flexion contractures between 15° and 30°, with all patients having less than 10° residual contracture at 2-year follow-up. Two patients who underwent biceps tenotomy for contractures greater than 30° sustained a peroneal nerve injury.

Whiteside and Mihalko treated 542 knees with preoperative flexion contracture greater than 10° with the use of an anterior referencing technique, with emphasis on collateral ligament contracture as a cause of the flexion contracture. Ninety-five percent of the cases resolved with medial-lateral ligament balancing and osteophyte resection. Only 3% required release of the posterior capsule, 2% required overresection of the distal femur, and no cases required the use of constrained or hinged components. Overall, a 1° mean residual contracture was present at 2-year follow-up. Consistent in all reports is the concept that overresection of the distal femur by more than 2 mm should be avoided in the treatment of flexion contracture until all osteophytes have been removed and the knee has been balanced medially and laterally. Finally, complete correction of deformity must be attained intraoperatively at the time of surgery. Whiteside and Mihalko also reported on 10 knees with significant preoperative recurvatum. They were able to successfully treat the recurvatum in all cases. The technique involved underresection of the distal femur by 4 to 6 mm, downsizing the femoral component, overresecting the posterior femoral condyles, and resecting the tibia with added posterior slope. The overresection of the posterior femoral condyles and the additional posterior tibial slope in-

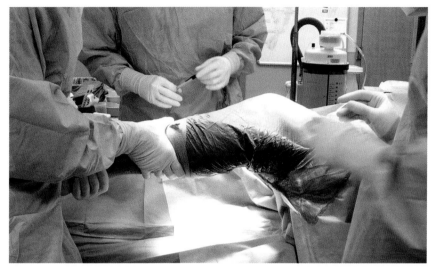

Figure 1 Final preoperative evaluation. The surgeon holds the extremity by the heel and raises the leg to evaluate the degree of deformity present, the potential for correcting the deformity to neutral, the status of the medial and lateral collateral ligaments, the presence of flexion contracture or excessive recurvatum, and the potential for obtaining full extension. (Photograph © Joint Implant Surgeons.)

creased the flexion gap, which balanced the flexion and extension gaps.

Technique

Preoperative Preparation and Surgical Setup

Patients are seen preoperatively by a physical therapist and given a prearthroplasty conditioning program. Patients with excessive flexion contracture are specifically instructed in stretching techniques, and patients with excessive recurvatum are instructed to avoid full extension. Both types of patients are also instructed to focus on quadriceps rehabilitation exercises. Patients are offered an instruction manual, which guides them through all phases of this surgical intervention. When patients are admitted to the hospital, they are seen and evaluated by an anesthesiologist, who commences the preemptive analgesia protocols, which include NSAIDs and oral analgesics. Single-shot spinal anesthetic with appropriate dosing of bupivacaine and morphine sulfate is

recommended. This provides the analgesia for the surgical intervention and sustained analgesia in the early postoperative period. Femoral nerve blocks are discouraged because their use requires ambulation with an immobilizer, which is contrary to the needs of patients with flexion contractures or recurvatum to have well-functioning extensor mechanisms.

At the completion of suitable and adequate induction of anesthesia, the patient is positioned supine, a tourniquet is placed on the upper thigh, and the extremity is prepared and draped in a standard fashion. At this point the surgeon should evaluate the degree of deformity present and the ability to correct the deformity (**Figure 1**). Can the varus or valgus malalignment be corrected to neutral? What is the status of the medial and lateral collateral ligaments? When holding the extremity by the heel and raising the leg, is there a flexion contracture? Does the knee come to full extension, or is there excessive recurvatum? This information is extremely critical at the time of exposure. For example, a fixed varus deformity and associated flexion contracture can be addressed immediately with an extensive soft-tissue release from the proximal medial tibia to include the deep medial collateral ligament, meniscal capsular ligament, semimembranosus, and perhaps some of the superficial medial collateral ligament, whereas in the patient with a fixed valgus deformity, medial exposure should not go beyond the midcoronal plane. We recommend selecting an implant system that offers a continuum of constraint so that the appropriate implant is available for the specific indications presented by the patient.

Procedure

The goals of the surgical procedure are to achieve balanced flexion/extension gaps with reconstruction of the mechanical axis. This is accomplished with a combination of appropriate bony resections and soft-tissue releases. In knees with notable flexion contractures, this involves not only release of contracted medial or lateral structures but also release of the posterior capsule. Surgeons typically choose one of two methods to obtain alignment and balance, the measured resection technique or the gap-balancing technique, while recognizing the importance of maintaining the joint line for kinematic function of the knee. Regardless of the technique used, correction of flexion contractures and recurvatum depends on basic fundamental principles that apply to all techniques.

A standard surgical approach is performed. In the varus knee, the deep medial collateral ligament, the meniscal capsular ligament, and the semi-membranosus are released from the proximal medial tibia. If the knee has a valgus malalignment, this exposure is taken only to the midcoronal plane. Osteophytes on the distal femur and proximal tibia are removed (**Figure 2**). The distal femoral resection is one of the keys to successful correction of both flexion contracture and recurva-

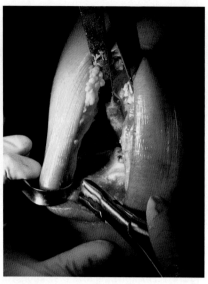

Figure 2 Intraoperative photograph of a rongeur being used to clear osteophytes from the proximal tibia. (Photograph © Joint Implant Surgeons.)

tum. In knees with a flexion contracture, we prefer to remove the amount of bone that is being replaced with metal, thereby maintaining the joint line. Additional bony resection will be performed later only if all other techniques have failed to obtain full extension (**Figure 3**).

With recurvatum, the extension gap is greater than the flexion gap. To balance this generalized laxity, distal femoral resection should be set to remove at least 2 mm less bone than will be replaced with the prosthesis. This will in essence tighten the extension gap by moving the joint line distally by 2 mm or more if necessary. Upon completion of the distal femoral resection, we prefer to resect the proximal tibia next. The goals of tibial resection are similar to femoral resection—ie, to re-establish the tibial joint line. In most systems, the minimal tibial thickness is 10 mm, so tibial resection is planned to remove 10 mm from the intact tibial plateau. The exact amount of resection required, however, depends on the degree of deformity (and, therefore, relative ligamentous laxity) that is present. For example, in a varus

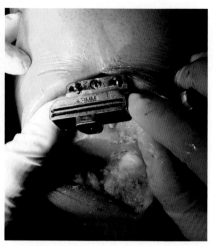

Figure 3 Femoral resection. The distal femoral resection guide shown in this intraoperative photograph is available with three pin locations for the purpose of adapting the resection to the deformity. In this case, the cutting guide was positioned to remove an additional 2 mm of distal femur. However, in a case of recurvatum, the guide would be positioned to remove 2 mm less of distal femur than will be replaced by the prosthesis. (Photograph © Joint Implant Surgeons.)

knee with significant lateral laxity, tibial resection from the more intact lateral tibial plateau may be only 6 mm (**Figure 4**). This is also true with recurvatum, which requires minimizing the amount of tibial resection, again in an effort to balance the ligamentous structures. The resection is planned to be perpendicular to the tibial shaft axis in the coronal plane. The amount of posterior slope depends on the deformity and the implant chosen. In posterior cruciate–retaining TKA, the slope should be set at 5° to 10°, whereas in posterior cruciate–substituting designs, the slope should be set at neutral because sacrificing the cruciate ligament will generally increase the flexion gap by 2 mm more than the extension gap. The surgeon also should be cognizant of the fact that in flexion contractures, the flexion gap is generally greater than the extension gap and, therefore, a resection without posterior slope will facilitate balance of the flexion/extension gap; however, in recurvatum, a resection with posterior slope that will increase the flexion gap will better facilitate balance of the flexion/extension gap.

Upon completion of the tibial resection, attention should be turned to completion of the distal femoral preparation. The AP axis of the femur should be outlined, as well as the transepicondylar axis. These axes are generally perpendicular to each other (**Figure 5**). The posterior condylar axis often is internally rotated 3° to the transepicondylar axis, and the tibial shaft axis is generally perpendicular to the transepicondylar axis. After identifying these axes, an appropriate sizing guide is placed. In posterior referencing systems, posterior condylar resection follows the concept of measured resection—ie, the amount of bone removed is equal to the amount of metal that will replace it. Appropriate sizing is accomplished by varying the amount of bone resected from the anterior femur. In anterior referencing systems, resection is set flush with the anterior cortex, and the amount of posterior condylar resection varies depending on the size chosen. To facilitate balance of the knee with flexion contracture, the largest size possible is chosen; in recurvatum, a smaller size is selected to resect more posterior condyle.

Upon completion of the femoral resections, the most important part of the surgical intervention ensues, especially in cases of flexion contracture. This involves removal of posterior osteophytes and reestablishment of the posterior recess of the knee by release of the posterior capsule, which is accomplished by subperiosteal stripping of the capsule with a curved osteotome (**Figure 6**). Our technique involves placing a custom femorotibial spreader with parallel arms in the side opposite the one the surgeon is working on. A curved osteotome is used to remove the posterior osteophytes, and a curet is used to remove all of the bony fragments. The posterior capsule is then stripped subperiosteally from

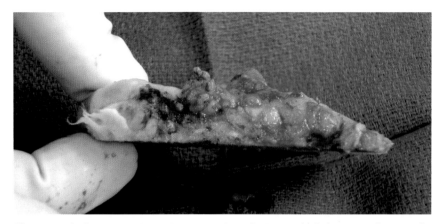

Figure 4 Tibial resection. Removing 10 mm from the intact tibial plateau conforms to the minimal tibial component thickness in most systems, but the actual amount removed depends on the degree of deformity and relative ligamentous laxity that is present. In this case of a varus knee with significant lateral laxity, tibial resection from the more intact lateral tibial plateau was less than 10 mm. (Photograph © Joint Implant Surgeons.)

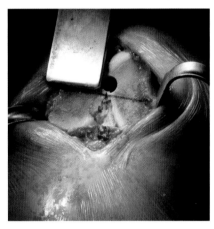

Figure 5 Femoral preparation. In this intraoperative photograph, the AP and transepicondylar axes of the femur are outlined; these are generally perpendicular to each other. The posterior condylar axis is frequently 3° internally rotated to the transepicondylar axis, and the tibial shaft axis is generally perpendicular to the transepicondylar axis. After identifying these axes, an appropriate femoral sizing guide is placed. (Photograph © Joint Implant Surgeons.)

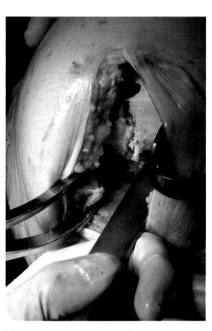

Figure 6 Preparation of the posterior capsule. In this intraoperative photograph, a custom femorotibial laminar spreader is placed on one side with arms open to parallel at a 20-mm gap while the surgeon débrides the opposite side, using a curved osteotome and then a curet to remove posterior osteophytes and all fragments of bone. (Photograph ©Joint Implant Surgeons.)

the posterior aspect of the femur. Care is taken to avoid damage to the popliteal vessels and nerve. The femorotibial spreader is then removed and placed in the opposite compartment and the procedure is repeated. In cases of recurvatum, the capsule does not need to be released, but the posterior osteophytes should be removed. At

this point in the surgical procedure, all peripheral osteophytes from the proximal tibia and distal femur have been removed and all bony resections have been accomplished (**Figure 7**). Bal-

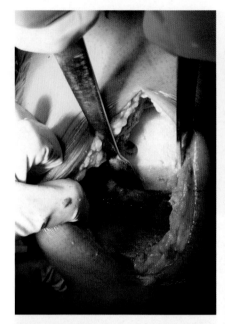

Figure 7 In this intraoperative photograph, all bony resections have been accomplished, all peripheral osteophytes have been removed from the proximal tibia and distal femur, and the posterior capsule has been débrided. (Photograph ©Joint Implant Surgeons.)

ance of the flexion/extension gap and of the medial and lateral collateral ligaments can now be determined with either spacer blocks or trial components; we prefer the latter. The trial tibial and femoral components are placed and the appropriate trial tibial bearing insert is inserted to balance the flexion/extension gaps and the medial and lateral collateral ligaments. Fine adjustment of the varus and valgus structures is accomplished and then balance of the flexion/extension gaps is assessed. If continued flexion contracture remains after all releases have been accomplished, then further distal femoral resection will be required to balance the flexion/extension gap and obtain full extension. We prefer to remove an additional 2 mm of bone, especially if the posterior cruciate ligament is to be retained (**Figure** 8). In posterior cruciate–sacrificing designs, the joint line elevation can be extended by 4 or even 6 mm. Therefore, if an additional 2 mm of distal

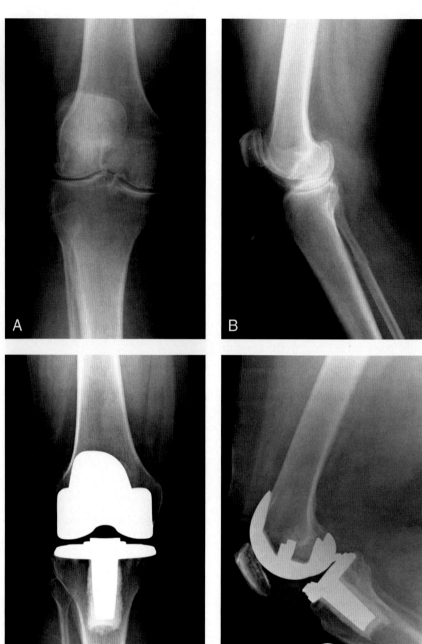

Figure 8 Radiographs of the right knee of a 69-year-old woman who presented with severe pain, instability, and stiffness secondary to osteoarthritis and severe flexion contracture. Preoperative AP (**A**) and lateral (**B**) views demonstrate joint space narrowing and varus deformity. AP (**C**) and lateral (**D**) radiographs taken 6 years after TKA with a cruciate-retaining device show well-fixed components in satisfactory position and alignment. The patient has 125° range of motion with no flexion contracture. (Radiographs ©Joint Implant Surgeons.)

femoral resection does not accomplish full extension, we would advise converting to a posterior stabilized prosthesis and removing additional distal

femoral bone (**Figure 9**). With severe flexion contracture, where greater amounts of distal femoral resection are required to obtain full extension, all structures anterior to the posterior capsule are somewhat lax in full extension. Therefore, a posterior stabilized constrained device may be required for varus/valgus stabilization through the entire arc of motion. For cases of recurvatum, distal femoral augmentation may be required to balance the flexion/extension gaps. However, if there is gross laxity of the posterior capsule, the surgeon may need to resort to a rotating-hinge device that has a built-in stop to hyperextension. We believe that full correction of flexion contractures at the time of surgical intervention is required for full postoperative extension.

Wound Closure

Wound closure follows the standard techniques for TKA, with the exception that patients who have a severe flexion contracture (greater than 30°) or recurvatum may require a proximal realignment of the extensor mechanism (ie, a lateral and distal advancement of the vastus medialis obliquus) in an effort to strengthen the extensor mechanism and place the quadriceps at a mechanical advantage.

▪ Postoperative Regimen

The postoperative protocols for patients who present with flexion contracture are distinctively different from those for patients who present with recurvatum. For patients with a flexion contracture, the goal at the time of surgical intervention is to obtain full extension. Therefore, these patients are immobilized for the first 24 hours in full extension with plaster splints. We prefer a modified Robert Jones dressing—a heavy cotton dressing with anterior and posterior plaster splints to maintain the extremity in full extension. This dressing is removed on postoperative day 1. The

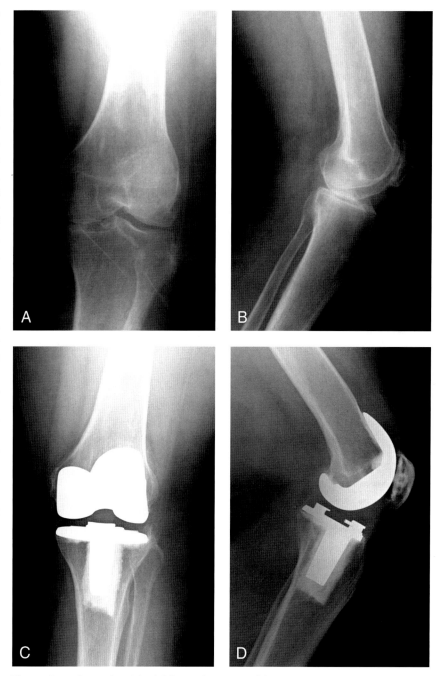

Figure 9 Radiographs of the left knee of a 39-year-old woman who presented with severe pain, spasticity, and stiffness secondary to osteoarthritis and severe flexion contracture. Preoperative AP (**A**) and lateral (**B**) views demonstrate narrowing of the joint space and varus deformity. AP (**C**) and lateral (**D**) views obtained 3.5 years after a TKA with a posterior stabilized device show well-fixed components in satisfactory position and alignment. The patient has 110° range of motion with no flexion contracture. (Radiographs ©Joint Implant Surgeons.)

patient is then placed in a knee immobilizer and instructed to wear the knee immobilizer during bed rest, during ambulation, and in the evening.

The immobilizer is removed only for range-of-motion exercises. In cases of severe flexion deformity (>30°), patients are maintained in full extension for 3 to 4 weeks, until initiation of flexion. It should have been stressed to the patient preoperatively that the goal of the surgical procedure is to obtain full extension. Therefore, the focus will be on obtaining full extension not only at the time of surgical intervention but also in the postoperative physical therapy rehabilitation program via appropriate stretching regimes. Patients are encouraged to use a knee immobilizer for at least the first 6 weeks postoperatively.

In patients who present with recurvatum, the goal at the time of surgical intervention is to decrease the laxity that enables the recurvatum deformity. This is accomplished by attention to bony resection and soft-tissue balance. These patients are actually encouraged to maintain the knee in slight flexion postoperatively to promote scarring of the posterior capsule

and further assist in preventing recurrent hyperextension. These patients also must be involved in a very aggressive quadriceps rehabilitation program.

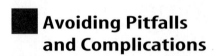

Avoiding Pitfalls and Complications

When treating patients with flexion contracture or recurvatum, it is imperative to understand that the treatment involves a combination of bone resection and soft-tissue balance. Furthermore, every effort must be made to preserve both the femoral and tibial joint lines. In flexion contracture, a common error is to begin by resecting too much distal femur. This may result in an elevation of the joint line

and midflexion instability. The distal femoral resection should remove the same amount of bone that is being replaced with metal. Attention should be directed at careful and meticulous balance of the soft tissues and release of the contracted posterior capsule with reestablishment of the posterior recess of the knee. This will correct most flexion contractures. With recurvatum, on the other hand, one should pay specific attention to the amount of distal femur being resected. Depending on the degree of laxity and recurvatum, 2 to 5 mm less bone resection should be performed. Furthermore, a minimal tibial resection should be performed. This will allow for balance of the flexion/extension gap and for correction of the recurvatum.

Bibliography

Bellemans J, Vandenneucker H, Victor J, Vanlauwe J: Flexion contracture in total knee arthroplasty. *Clin Orthop Relat Res* 2006;452:78-82.

Berend KR, Lombardi AV Jr, Adams JB: Total knee arthroplasty in patients with greater than 20 degrees flexion contracture. *Clin Orthop Relat Res* 2006;452:83-87.

Firestone TP, Krackow KA, Davis JD IV, Teeny SM, Hungerford DS: The management of fixed flexion contractures during total knee arthroplasty. *Clin Orthop Relat Res* 1992;284(284):221-227.

Lombardi AV Jr: Soft tissue balancing of the knee—flexion, in Callaghan JJ, Rosenberg AG, Rubash HE, Simonian PT, Wickiewicz TL, eds: *The Adult Knee.* Philadelphia, PA, Lippincott Williams & Wilkins, 2003, Volume II, pp 1223-1232.

Lombardi AV Jr, Berend KR: Posterior cruciate ligament-retaining, posterior stabilized, and varus/valgus posterior stabilized constrained articulations in total knee arthroplasty. *Instr Course Lect* 2006;55:419-427.

Lombardi AV, Berend KR: Soft tissue balancing of the knee—flexion contractures. *Tech Knee Surg* 2005;4(3):193-206.

Lombardi AV Jr, Berend KR, Ellison BA: Correction of flexion contractures in total knee arthroplasty, in Lotke PA, Lonner JH, eds: *Master Techniques in Orthopaedic Surgery: Knee Arthroplasty,* ed 3. Philadelphia, PA, Lippincott Williams & Wilkins, 2009, pp 127-138.

Lombardi AV Jr, Mallory TH: Dealing with flexion contractures in total knee arthroplasty: Bone resection versus soft tissue releases, in Insall JN, Scott WN, Scuderi GR, eds: *Current Concepts in Primary and Revision Total Knee Arthroplasty.* Philadelphia, PA, Lippincott-Raven Publishers, 1996, pp 191-202.

Lombardi AV Jr, Mallory TH, Adams JB, Herrington SM: A stepwise algorithmic approach to flexion contractures in total knee arthroplasty. *Arch Am Acad Orthop Surg* 1997;1:1-8.

Lu H, Mow CS, Lin J: Total knee arthroplasty in the presence of severe flexion contracture: A report of 37 cases. *J Arthroplasty* 1999;14(7):775-780.

Massin P, Petit A, Odri G, et al: Total knee arthroplasty in patients with greater than 20 degrees flexion contracture. *Orthop Traumatol Surg Res* 2009;95(4 Suppl):7-12.

McPherson EJ, Cushner FD, Schiff CF, Friedman RJ: Natural history of uncorrected flexion contractures following total knee arthroplasty. *J Arthroplasty* 1994;9(5):499-502.

Mihalko WM, Whiteside LA: Bone resection and ligament treatment for flexion contracture in knee arthroplasty. *Clin Orthop Relat Res* 2003;406(406):141-147.

Scuderi GR, Kochhar T: Management of flexion contracture in total knee arthroplasty. *J Arthroplasty* 2007;22(4 Suppl 1) 20-24.

Whiteside LA, Mihalko WM: Surgical procedure for flexion contracture and recurvatum in total knee arthroplasty. *Clin Orthop Relat Res* 2002;404:189-195.

Coding

CPT Code		Corresponding ICD-9 Codes	
Total Knee Arthroplasty			
27447	Arthroplasty, knee, condyle and plateau; medial AND lateral compartments with or without patella resurfacing (total knee arthroplasty)	715 715.80	715.16 715.89

Chapter 23

Total Knee Arthroplasty: Neuropathic Joint

Terence J. Gioe, MD
Patrick Morgan, MD

 ## Indications

Neuropathic arthropathy of the knee typically is a chronic destructive process associated with neurosensory loss that may result in significant deformity of a joint that the patient perceives as being painless. Charcot originally described the disorder in association with tabes dorsalis, but the term "Charcot joint" is often used to describe neuropathic arthropathy of any etiology, and Charcot-like neuropathic arthropathy may be seen in several conditions, including leprosy, congenital insensitivity to pain, syringomyelia, and, perhaps most commonly, diabetes mellitus. The pathophysiology of neuropathic arthropathy remains poorly defined.

Because neuropathic arthropathy is characterized by bone destruction, ligamentous instability, and a wide spectrum of clinical presentations, total knee arthroplasty (TKA) cannot be universally recommended. The underlying diagnosis (eg, neurosyphilis or diabetes), the stage of the arthropathy (fragmentation, coalescence, or reconstitution), and the overall status of the patient (eg, ataxia or normal gait) all are prognostic factors that the astute clinician should consider.

TKA remains controversial as a treatment for neuropathic arthropathy. We use TKA in the nonsyphilitic patient without ataxia in whom nonsurgical management has failed and in whom radiographs demonstrate late coalescence or reconstitution of the joint; however, reconstitution is sometimes difficult to discern. Patients should be counseled that the operation is fraught with potential complications. We proceed cautiously after advising patients that they should be prepared for arthrodesis or amputation as a salvage procedure should the arthroplasty fail.

Contraindications

Neuropathic arthropathy of the knee was long considered to be an absolute contraindication to TKA. As surgical techniques and modern revision TKA instrumentation have improved, however, and as the condition has become better understood, satisfactory outcomes can be expected in properly selected patients.

Active joint sepsis is an absolute contraindication, as is a knee in the early inflammatory fragmentation phase of the neuropathic process. Because both joint sepsis and neuropathic arthropathy can present with swelling, erythema, warmth, and variable pain responses, serologic studies (C-reactive protein, erythrocyte sedimentation rate) and knee aspiration may help confirm the diagnosis.

Diagnosing a neuropathic knee may be difficult because the disorder has varied presentations and because no single specific diagnostic test exists for a neuropathic joint. In addition, fragmentation, coalescence, and reconstitution may be seen simultaneously. Delaying surgery until clear evidence of bone reconstitution and bone formation exists is prudent.

Relative contraindications include those associated with the underlying disease process itself, such as diabetic skin ulcerations or concerns regarding vascular status. Neurosyphilis is uncommon now as a result of improved antibiotic management and detection techniques, but patients who do have this disease may have both multiple involved joints and a deteriorating neurologic status that renders the anticipated outcome less favorable.

Dr. Gioe or an immediate family member serves as a board member, owner, officer, or committee member of the American Association of Hip and Knee Surgeons, the American Board of Orthopaedic Surgery, and The Knee Society; has received research or institutional support from DePuy, Stryker, and Zimmer; and owns stock or stock options in Johnson & Johnson. Dr. Morgan or an immediate family member has received research or institutional support from Arthrex, Biomet, DePuy, Medtronic, Smith & Nephew, Stryker, Synthes, Wright Medical Technology, and Zimmer.

In addition, development of ataxia in this or other conditions associated with neuropathy may place unusual stresses on the prosthetic construct during gait.

Alternative Treatments

Preventing destruction of the knee joint remains the mainstay of management of this difficult problem. Patients with known neuropathy should be warned of this potential complication and advised to avoid repetitive trauma, maintain muscle strength, and report any unusual swelling or warmth about the knee. Early recognition of a neuropathic knee condition is paramount. Both the patient and the surgeon should be alert for the common presentation of a swollen, painless, warm knee joint with increased ligamentous laxity in the absence of a history of significant trauma. Evidence of peripheral neuropathy (symmetric sensory loss of all modalities in a stocking distribution) and reduced or absent knee and ankle reflexes are common. Motor weakness is uncommon, and pronounced asymmetric motor findings are suspicious for nondiabetic neuropathy.

The knee joint should be adequately protected during the acute destructive phase. This may involve prolonged bracing and non–weight-bearing ambulation to prevent further destruction. Anti-inflammatory agents can help to control the surrounding inflammation, and aspiration can help to relieve ligamentous and capsular pressure when large effusions are present. Bisphosphonates, through their inhibition of osteoclastic activity, may play a role as well. Physical therapy to maintain muscle tone and promote appropriate gait with assistive devices may prevent exacerbations.

If nonsurgical measures fail and the neuropathic process is believed to be in the late coalescence-reconstitution phase, surgery may be considered. The surgeon should keep in mind that these patients are often relatively mobile and have no pain despite significant radiographic and clinical deformity and ligamentous laxity. Arthrodesis of the knee is the most widely recommended alternative to TKA for the neuropathic knee, despite a relatively high incidence of failure, and can still be considered the procedure of choice when TKA is contraindicated. Arthrodesis is contraindicated in patients with bilateral neuropathy of the knee and in patients who are predominantly wheelchair ambulators.

Results

In the last 20 years, only six studies in the English language literature have documented the results of TKA in the neuropathic knee (**Table 1**). The studies are relatively small, level-IV-evidence retrospective case series that represent experience with 75 TKAs in total. Despite these limitations, some pertinent conclusions can be drawn. TKA in patients with neuropathic arthropathy of the knee has the potential for significant complications, and patients must be well aware of the possibility of failure, because subsequent salvage options often are limited to arthrodesis or above-knee amputation. Neuropathy secondary to diabetes mellitus carries a more favorable prognosis than neuropathy associated with neurosyphilis or other diagnoses associated with ataxia. Radiographic evidence of late coalescence or reconstitution of the joint fragmentation should be present before surgical intervention. A complete synovectomy should be performed at the time of surgery; the histologic finding of cartilage and bone fragments embedded

in the synovium is typical of neuropathic processes. Revision TKA surgical techniques are often necessary, including supplemental bone grafting, metal augmentation, use of stems, and appropriate prosthetic constraint. Stems for both femoral and tibial components should be used liberally to distribute stress more efficiently, and constrained condylar designs should be considered to compensate for significant ligamentous laxity. Hinged designs play a larger role than in most primary TKA situations, but their use must be balanced against the increased stresses transmitted to the bone-cement and cement-implant interface. Postoperative bracing is advisable, and continued long-term follow-up is necessary to monitor possible complications. When these principles are implemented, durable results can be expected in the intermediate term (5 to 10 years) in appropriately selected candidates.

Technique

Because of the bone loss and ligamentous instability typically associated with the neuropathic knee, the technical considerations of TKA reconstruction in these knees resemble those of revision TKA surgery. Thorough preoperative planning is essential. Bone loss may be substantial, and the quality of the remaining bone may be poor or questionable. Knee instability may be global in nature, and postoperative instability can occur as soft tissues "stretch out." If the diagnosis is in doubt, neurologic consultation and electromyography should precede any surgical consideration. A careful history and exhaustive physical examination focusing on knee stability, presence of other neuropathic joints, and signs of ataxia, are essential. In the setting of a warm, swollen, erythematous knee, infectious processes should first be ruled out, and if the symptoms are

Table 1 Results of Total Knee Arthroplasty for Neuropathic Arthropathy

Authors (Year)	Number of Knees	Patient Condition	Patient Age in Years (Range)	Type of Implant	Mean Follow-up in Years (Range)	Results
Soudry et al (1986)	9 (7 patients)	Syphilis, DM Charcot-like	72 (56-80)	2 posterior-stabilized condylar type 7 custom posterior-stabilized (for tibial or femoral bone defects)	3 (2-4.25)	AKS score improved from 50 (range, 25-70) preoperatively to 92 (range, 83-98) Complications: 4 asymptomatic VTEs
Yoshino et al (1993)	5 (3 patients)	Tabes dorsalis	58 (56-60)	Yoshino total knee 1 tibial stem	(~ 8-10)	1 revision for periprosthetic fracture
Chong et al (1995)	1	Cerebral and cerebellar atrophy with peripheral neuropathy	56	Uncemented, posterior stabilized	2.5	ROM 0°-60° HSS knee score improved from 35 to 75
Kim et al (2002)	19 (10 patients)	Tabes dorsalis	52 (48-64)	1 uncemented hinged knee 1 cemented semiconstrained 17 cemented constrained 11 with autogenous structural bone graft to tibial plateau	5.2 (5-6)	HSS knee score improved from 36.5 (range, 30-42) preoperatively to 76 (range, 58-90) Major complications in 47%: 3 knee dislocations 2 supracondylar femur fractures 1 patellar dislocation 1 periprosthetic fracture at stem of hinged prosthesis with aseptic loosening after ORIF 1 quadriceps tendon rupture "Satisfactory" result in 53% at final follow-up
Lambert and Close (2002)	1	Type I DM	27	Cemented, constrained revision component with femoral/tibial stems	4	"Good knee function"
Parvizi et al (2003)	40 (29 patients)	16 familial sensorimotor deficit 11 idiopathic 7 DM 4 neurosyphilis 1 lacunar infarct 1 syringomyelia	67.5 (37-91)	27 stemmed components 8 cruciate condylar prostheses 5 rotating hinge	Clinical: 7.9 (2-15) Radiographic: 6.4 (2-15)	AKS pain score improved from 44 preoperatively (range, 0-65) to 78 AKS function improved from 51 (range, –10-70) to 78 82.5% free of mechanical failure at final follow-up 42.5% complication rate: 4 intraoperative complications including MCL avulsion, tibial tubercle avulsion, patellar tendon avulsion 3 postoperative complications including hematoma, wound infection, DVT 6 revisions for aseptic loosening, periprosthetic fracture, instability, infection

DM = diabetes mellitus, AKS = American Knee Society, HSS = Hospital for Special Surgery, VTE = venous thromboembolism, ROM = range of motion, ORIF = open reduction and internal fixation, MCL = medial collateral ligament, DVT = deep vein thrombosis.

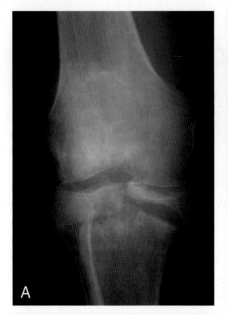 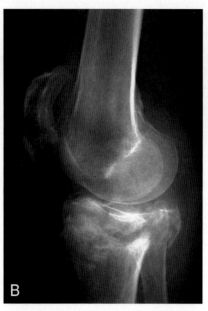

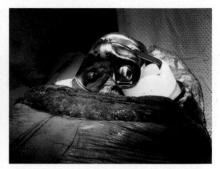

Figure 2 Intraoperative photograph demonstrating a rotating hinge design that shares load transmission through the articular surface and that may be appropriate in patients with significant bone loss or ligamentous instability.

Figure 1 AP (**A**) and lateral (**B**) radiographs show a neuropathic tibial plateau fracture in the early coalescence phase in a patient with diabetes. Note the uncoalesced fragments. Further coalescence and reconstitution should occur before attempting surgical reconstruction

determined to indicate the acute destructive phase of neuropathic arthropathy, protective care should be offered while surgery is deferred. Before surgery can be performed on a knee with a destructive neuropathic process, radiographs must be obtained (**Figure 1**) to confirm that the knee is in the late coalescence-reconstitution phase, and long weight-bearing radiographs are used to assess overall limb alignment and for templating purposes.

Setup/Exposure

The exposure of the neuropathic knee is the same as that for routine primary TKA, because it is uncommon to encounter notable preoperative stiffness. Extensile exposures, including a quadriceps snip, V-Y quadriceps turndown, or tibial tubercle osteotomy, are rarely needed. A "femoral peel" with release of both collateral ligaments and skeletonization of the distal femur may be used in settings in which bone loss or ligamentous instability requires use of a hinged prosthesis. Typically, a medial parapatellar approach

is used, with subluxation rather than eversion of the patella. Minimally invasive approaches are contraindicated in these demanding cases.

Equipment/ Implants Required

The issues of bone loss and ligamentous instability routinely encountered in the neuropathic knee require preoperative planning for proper implant and graft choices. Structural allograft may be necessary in certain circumstances and should be available. Modular revision TKA systems, which allow for different levels of constraint, modular augments, and diaphyseal stem fixation, typically are used because of their intraoperative flexibility. In rare circumstances of significant bone loss or ligamentous instability that compromises the collateral ligaments, a rotating hinged prosthesis design that shares load through the articular interface may be appropriate (**Figure 2**).

Procedure

Loss of metaphyseal bone and the generally poor quality of the remaining

bone often compromise the support of the components. All viable host bone should be preserved, and bone loss should be addressed with metal augments or allograft bone to maintain a relatively anatomic joint line. Radiographs of the contralateral knee, if normal, may be helpful in determining the position of the native joint line in relation to the fibular head. Options for addressing the bone loss encountered include structural allograft (**Figure 3**, *A*), impaction grafting of cortical-cancellous bone chips, metal augments, and trabecular metal cones/augments (**Figure 3**, *B*). Where possible, we prefer to use metal augments on modular devices or bone-replacing implants rather than allografts in patients with ongoing neuropathic processes and higher infection risks (**Figure 3**, *C*).

Stems should routinely be considered part of the reconstruction. They help to extend the component fixation to diaphyseal bone, relieving stress on the deficient bone or allograft and providing axial alignment. Most important, they provide overall stability to the reconstruction in patients with an increased risk of aseptic loosening and given the common use of increased prosthetic constraint. Short cemented stems have the advantage of allowing more latitude in implant placement

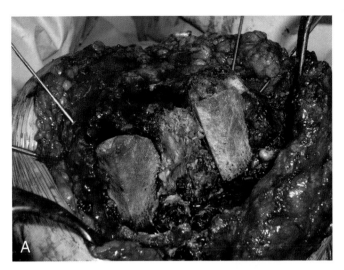
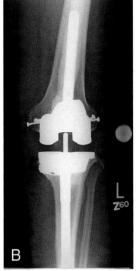
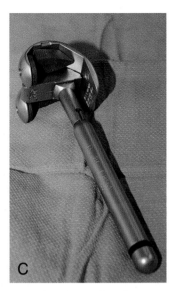

Figure 3 Options for addressing bone loss. **A,** Intraoperative photograph showing structural allografts shaped from femoral heads temporarily transfixed for management of femoral bone loss. This technique is used only rarely in the neuropathic joint. **B,** AP radiograph shows a tantalum cone, which was used to accommodate the significant tibial bone loss present in this neuropathic joint. **C,** Photograph of a trial modular augmentation component with a long press-fit stem, which is an excellent option when poor-quality bone is present.

and are helpful in capacious canals and osteoporotic bone. Longer uncemented stems (with metaphyseal cementing of the condylar component) can assist with axial alignment and can typically be removed with minimal bone loss if necessary (**Figure 4**). Ideally, uncemented stems should extend beyond the metaphyseal-diaphyseal junction to engage the diaphysis, and cemented stems should be as short as is consistent with achieving the surgical goal. When used in conjunction with cement restrictors, these short stems minimize the cement column and extraction difficulties.

Ligamentous laxity is a common component of the neuropathic knee process, and may be associated with the destructive process at the knee or present as subluxation or dislocation of the joint (**Figure 5**). Although it is generally advisable to use the least constrained device consistent with a stable TKA, as in revision TKA surgery, the surgeon must be aware of the tendency for the soft tissues of the neuropathic knee to "stretch out" over

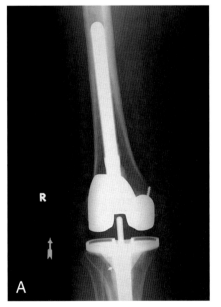
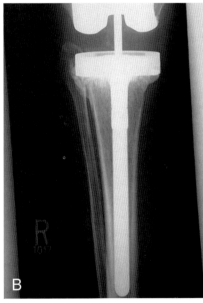

Figure 4 AP radiographs of TKAs with uncemented stems. Press-fit stems should engage the diaphysis on both the femur (**A**) and the tibia (**B**).

time, resulting in late instability. Posterior cruciate–substituting implants provide some measure of improved anterior/posterior stability but do little to improve varus/valgus constraint. Constrained condylar designs, which have taller posts and more congruent surfaces, are used most commonly because they offer improved stability in both the anterior/posterior and varus/valgus planes. Hinged implants play a role only when less constrained implants cannot address instability. The primary indication for a hinged TKA

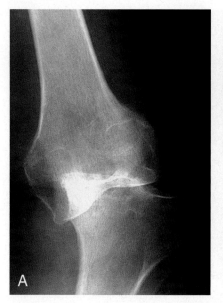 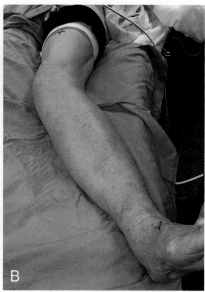

Figure 5 Ligamentous laxity in the neuropathic knee. **A,** AP radiograph of a neuropathic knee that presented as a painless dislocation. **B,** Clinical photograph of a neuropathic knee with significant preoperative laxity to valgus stress.

would be significant distal femoral bone loss with concomitant loss of ligamentous attachment associated with neuropathic fracture.

Wound Closure

Wound closure is routine, but the surgeon should keep in mind the often impaired sensibility of the neuropathic patient, the high incidence of diabetes in this population, and the increased risk of infection. The deep tissues are closed with interrupted sutures. A nonabsorbable suture material is used for the repair of the extensor mechanism in a quadriceps snip or V-Y turndown. The wound is closed in layers, including both a subcutaneous interrupted layer and a running suture layer to ensure tight repair. Skin closure may be performed with staples or with a subcuticular absorbable stitch. We routinely use a deep drain that is pulled within 24 hours.

Postoperative Regimen

Postoperative management is tailored to the individual patient and to the disease process that resulted in the neuropathic joint. Patients with diabetes require vigilant hyperglycemia management. Other neuropathic joints require ongoing monitoring, and, in the patient with painful neuropathy, neurologic consultation and the use of gabapentin or pregabalin may be considered. Vigilant nursing care is critical to prevent skin breakdown in insensate distal extremities.

The rehabilitation regimen follows the revision TKA pathway, because the procedure typically uses revision techniques and implants. Routine mobilization, continuous passive motion, and physical therapy are used unless extensor mechanism issues preclude such an approach. Protected weight bearing may be advocated for up to 3 months if extensive bone grafting was required. Long-leg hinged knee braces

are used routinely during ambulation in the postoperative period for 8 to 12 weeks to protect the reconstruction, preserve the soft-tissue envelope, encourage ligamentous healing, and remind patients of the need to protect the joint. Patients and caregivers are instructed to monitor the skin under the brace at each removal and reapplication.

Antibiotic prophylaxis is typically achieved using a first-generation cephalosporin for 24 hours (barring allergy) or until intraoperative culture results are known. Bladder catheters and wound drains are routinely removed within 24 hours. Pain management parallels that of our TKA patients in general, with pre- and postoperative celecoxib, regional anesthesia, femoral nerve blocks, and oral oxycodone.

Unless unusual risk factors exist (eg, a prior venous thromboembolic event or hypercoagulability), a combination of mechanical pressure devices (foot pumps) and warfarin is used as prophylaxis against thromboembolic disease. Target international normalized ratios are in the 1.8 to 2.2 range to minimize the risk of bleeding, and patients are rapidly mobilized.

Physical therapy often is continued in an outpatient facility or in the home. Patients are followed routinely with radiographs for the first year and annually thereafter. The importance of continued follow-up is repeatedly stressed to patients.

Avoiding Pitfalls and Complications

Managing patient expectations is critical. Complications are more common than in routine primary TKA, and salvage is more difficult and less predictable. Cemented or diaphyseally engaging press-fit stems are encouraged, and the prudent surgeon should err on the side of more prosthetic constraint rather than less. As with all cases, meticulous wound closure and soft-tissue handling is emphasized, as is strict management of diabetes. Postoperative bracing allows the soft-tissue envelope to heal in a protected fashion and acts as a reminder to patients that the joint must be preserved. Routine follow-up is encouraged to detect aseptic loosening or recurrent ligamentous laxity.

Bibliography

Chong A, Bruce W, Goldberg J: Treatment of the neuropathic knee by arthroplasty. *Aust N Z J Surg* 1995;65(5):370-371.

Drennan DB, Fahey JJ, Maylahn DJ: Important factors in achieving arthrodesis of the Charcot knee. *J Bone Joint Surg Am* 1971;53(6):1180-1193.

Fullerton BD, Browngoehl LA: Total knee arthroplasty in a patient with bilateral Charcot knees. *Arch Phys Med Rehabil* 1997;78(7):780-782.

Johnson JT: Neuropathic fractures and joint injuries: Pathogenesis and rationale of prevention and treatment. *J Bone Joint Surg Am* 1967;49(1):1-30.

Kim YH, Kim JS, Oh SW: Total knee arthroplasty in neuropathic arthropathy. *J Bone Joint Surg Br* 2002;84(2):216-219.

Lambert AP, Close CF: Charcot neuroarthropathy of the knee in Type 1 diabetes: Treatment with total knee arthroplasty. *Diabet Med* 2002;19(44):338-341.

Parvizi J, Marrs J, Morrey BF: Total knee arthroplasty for neuropathic (Charcot) joints. *Clin Orthop Relat Res* 2003;(416): 1416 145-150.

Rathur HM, Boulton AJ: Recent advances in the diagnosis and management of diabetic neuropathy. *J Bone Joint Surg Br* 2005;87(12):1605-1610.

Soudry M, Binazzi R, Johanson NA, Bullough PG, Insall JN: Total knee arthroplasty in Charcot and Charcot-like joints. *Clin Orthop Relat Res* 1986;(208):199-204.

Yoshino S, Fujimori J, Kajino A, Kiowa M, Uchida S: Total knee arthroplasty in Charcot's joint. *J Arthroplasty* 1993;8(3): 335-340.

Coding				
CPT Codes			**Corresponding ICD-9 Codes**	
27447	Arthroplasty, knee, condyle and plateau; medial AND lateral compartments with or without patella resurfacing (total knee arthroplasty)		715 715.80	715.16 715.89
27580	Arthrodesis, knee, any technique		711.16 714.0 717.9	711.46 716.16

Total Knee Arthroplasty Following Patellectomy or Other Extensor Mechanism Problems

E. Michael Keating, MD
John B. Meding, MD
Trevor R. Pickering, MD

■ Indications

Extensor mechanism problems that exist before a primary total knee arthroplasty (TKA) is performed can be obstacles to a satisfactory outcome. Therefore, careful consideration of such problems by both the surgeon and patient is required if an optimal result is to be obtained. Although the results of TKA following patellectomy and other extensor mechanism issues are generally inferior to those in patients without such problems, significant improvements in pain and function can be achieved.

In the past, patellectomy was indicated for rheumatoid arthritis, trauma, and many other conditions, but it is performed less frequently today. Nevertheless, the arthroplasty surgeon undoubtedly will see some patellectomized knees that warrant consideration for TKA. In this population, only patients with severe osteoarthritis should be considered, as mild tibiofemoral arthritis is associated with a poor outcome. Other factors associated with a good outcome are excellent quadriceps function, fewer prior knee surgeries, and a longer time since patellectomy.

Patients with patellofemoral dysplasia and/or a history of chronic patellar dislocation or subluxation may be considered for TKA provided they meet the standard criteria. An additional proximal soft-tissue procedure to properly align patellar tracking (eg, medial reefing) can be performed at the time of TKA. Distal bony procedures (tibial tubercle osteotomy and transposition) sometimes are performed in primary TKAs by some surgeons to achieve exposure and can be done for realignment purposes in this scenario as well.

TKA after high tibial osteotomy is well described. Care must be taken to address exposure difficulties due to patella infera (patella baja) or joint line elevation, which also may cause impingement of the native patellar bone or the prosthetic replacement on the tibial polyethylene.

Patients with a previous patellar fracture can undergo TKA successfully provided the fracture is well healed and the extensor mechanism is intact.

Previous quadriceps or patellar tendon rupture should not exclude a patient from consideration for a TKA. However, the disruption must be fully healed and good active quadriceps function must be present. An extensor mechanism reconstruction or allograft should not be performed at the time of primary TKA.

Recurvatum and flexion contracture do not preclude a successful TKA, provided quadriceps function is good. On the other hand, conversion of a knee arthrodesis to TKA is associated with a high complication rate, including the need for a repeat arthrodesis, and should be undertaken only by surgeons experienced with the procedure. The details of TKA in these populations are described in other chapters.

Dr. Keating or an immediate family member has received royalties from Biomet; serves as a paid consultant for or is an employee of Biomet; has received research or institutional support from Biomet; and has received nonincome support (such as equipment or services), commercially derived honoraria, or other non–research-related funding (such as paid travel) from Biomet. Dr. Meding or an immediate family member has received royalties from Biomet; serves as an unpaid consultant for Biomet; and has received research or institutional support from Biomet. Neither Dr. Pickering nor any immediate family member has received anything of value from or owns stock in a commercial company or institution related directly or indirectly to the subject of this chapter.

Contraindications

Acute injuries to the extensor mechanism are contraindications to TKA. Before TKA is undertaken, quadriceps and patellar tendon ruptures as well as patellar fractures must be repaired and fully healed, and active knee extension must be restored. The soft-tissue envelope, which can change significantly in the months following repair or reconstruction of the extensor mechanism, can be properly balanced and the degree of constraint correctly determined in a TKA only after the patient has completed rehabilitation and the tissues have attained their permanent resting tension and range of motion.

Patients without active quadriceps function are poor candidates for TKA. The inability to extend the knee or use the quadriceps for ambulation necessitates the use of a locking knee brace and other assistive devices after TKA and can significantly increase energy consumption while walking. In addition, the lack of quadriceps tension can lead to instability in the TKA, necessitating a higher degree of constraint that, in turn, can lead to higher rates of failure. Our institution has had good results with TKA in patients with recurvatum and active quadriceps function. With neuropathic loss of quadriceps function, however, such as in poliomyelitis, recurvatum provides a biologic locking mechanism for the knee, allowing ambulation. TKA provides poorer results in this population and is relatively contraindicated.

TKA is contraindicated in patients who have extensor mechanism problems and mild to moderate osteoarthritis. These patients do more poorly in terms of pain after knee replacement than do patients with severe arthritis.

The existence of an extensor lag is not a contraindication to TKA. Patients should be made aware, however, that knee extension may not improve significantly following TKA. Despite techniques such as patellar tendon bone grafting in patients with previous patellectomy, the mechanical advantage provided by the patella is not easily restored once lost, and soft-tissue reconstructive techniques cannot predictably restore biologic extensor tension. Therefore, patient expectations must be weighed carefully when deciding whether to proceed with TKA. In addition, patients must understand that a history of previous knee surgeries puts them at greater risk for infection, reoperation, and implant failure.

Alternative Treatments

For patients who are not candidates for TKA, nonsurgical treatment, consisting of physical therapy, bracing, and walking aids, should be considered. For patients with severe and painful arthritis, arthrodesis should be considered.

Results

Results of TKA following prior patellectomy are mixed in the literature, largely because of differences in implant designs, primary versus revision setting, and outcome classification schemes (**Table 1**). Clearly, residual postoperative pain is more likely and results are less predictable in these patients than in patients who have patellae and undergo TKA. Overall knee scores are also comparably lower. Extensor lag and difficulty climbing stairs are more common in the patellectomized patient. Despite these problems, most authors report significant improvement in knee scores after TKA in these patients. Anterior-posterior instability in knees that have undergone TKA after patellectomy has been noted in several studies and is theorized to be a source of postoperative pain. There is no consensus regarding the degree of constraint that is optimal in patients with prior patellectomy, but most authors recommend use of a cruciate-substituting TKA.

Technique

Setup/Exposure

No changes to the standard setup and positioning for a TKA are needed for the patellectomized patient. Draping must allow maximum exposure of the femur for access to the myotendinous junction of the quadriceps if proximal realignment is needed. In obese or short patients, a sterile tourniquet should be used so that it can be removed easily if more exposure is necessary. Distally, draping should allow exposure to several centimeters below the tibial tubercle to permit an osteotomy.

Prior incisions should be used if at all possible. We use a standard medial parapatellar arthrotomy for these TKAs. The incision can be extended on both ends as needed for soft-tissue balancing and proximal or distal realignment. In addition, in a knee with a significant lack of flexion preoperatively, such as in an ankylosed or arthrodesed knee, the extensor mechanism can be lengthened by converting the arthrotomy to a simple V-Y quadricepsplasty. There is no role for minimally invasive techniques in these patients.

In the patient with a contracted patellar tendon, we prefer a quadriceps snip to facilitate exposure to the knee joint. A tibial tubercle osteotomy is another option.

Instruments/Equipment/ Implants Required

In addition to the surgeon's standard TKA equipment, wires or cables should be available for an osteotomy,

Table 1 Results of Total Knee Arthroplasty Following Prior Patellectomy

Authors (Year)	Number of Knees	Implant Design Type	Mean Patient Age in Years (Range)	Mean Follow-up (Years)	Outcome
Bayne and Cameron (1984)	14	6 hinged 2 unlinked hinge 6 semiconstrained	68.5 (51-83)	2.5	Hinged: 6/6 good/excellent Unlinked hinge: 1/2 good/excellent Semiconstrained: 2/6 good/excellent Anterior-posterior shift may cause pain.
Lennox et al (1987)	11	CR	51 (29-80)	3.75	5/11 good/excellent 18% required fusion for continued pain. Good outcome associated with ≤3 knee surgeries, severe arthritis, good quadriceps function.
Railton et al (1990)	7	Unconstrained, cruciate-sacrificing	65.3 (58-75)	4	6/7 pain free 4/7 required help getting out of chair.
Larson et al (1991)	26 (14 primary, 12 revision)	Multiple types	53.6 (24-77)	8.5 (primary) 7.6 (revision)	Primary: 7/14 good/excellent Revision: 7/12 good/excellent Study noted that patellectomized patients are at higher risk for TKA failure.
Szalapski et al (1994)	22	CR	69 (53-83)	5	18/22 good/excellent Difficulty stair climbing after TKA
Martin et al (1995)	22	CR and PS	67 (36-89)	7	13/22 good/excellent Longer interval between patellectomy and TKA correlated with better results.
Paletta and Laskin (1995)	22	CR and PS	69 (59-74)	5	CR: mean Knee Society score of 67 PS: mean knee score of 89 More predictable results when patellectomy was for fracture rather than for patellofemoral arthritis
Cameron et al (1996)	16	PS	NA	5.5	11/16 good/excellent 81% could use operated leg as lead in stair-climbing.

CR = cruciate-retaining, PS = posterior stabilized, TKA = total knee arthroplasty, NA = not available.

as well as heavy-gauge permanent suture if needed for deep soft-tissue repair. In most cases, the primary TKA implant preferred by the surgeon can be used, but posterior stabilized and constrained trials and implants must be available at the time of surgery in the event that significant soft-tissue laxity and instability are found during trialing with the initial implant design.

Procedure

TKA IN THE PATELLECTOMIZED KNEE

The procedure for a TKA in the patellectomized knee does not differ signif-icantly from one for a knee with a pa-tella. When possible, we prefer retention of the posterior cruciate lig-ament (PCL), which assumes a greater role in anterior-posterior stabilization in patients who have undergone a pre-vious patellectomy (**Figure 1**). Al-lograft and autograft bone reconstruc-tion of the patella has been described with mixed results. At our institution, we have found it to be unreliable and unnecessary.

Despite the fact that these knees lack a patella, it is important to re-establish the alignment of the exten-sor mechanism, which is often lat-erally displaced. Realignment is achieved by external rotation of the femoral component in line with the transepicondylar axis, as in a standard TKA, to balance the extensor mechan-ism forces across the knee (**Figure 2**). If necessary, we perform a proximal re-alignment as described by Insall and associates, by advancing the medial quadriceps muscle over the lateral portion of the arthrotomy in a pants-over-vest manner. A lateral release also may be needed to centralize the extensor tendon in the trochlear

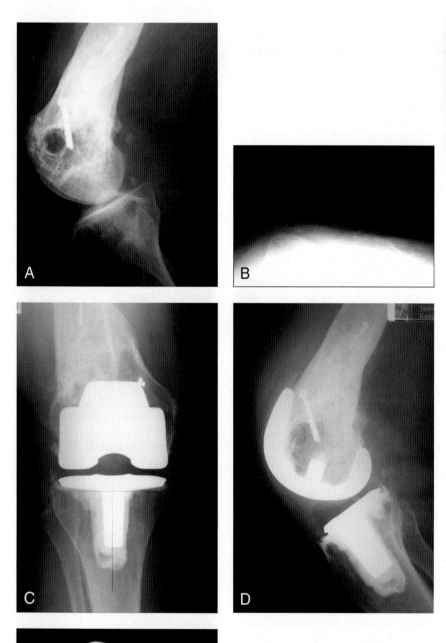

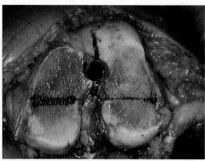

Figure 2 The transepicondylar axis and the Whiteside line are used to establish the appropriate external rotation of the femoral component and realign patellar tracking.

Figure 1 Radiographs of a patient with a patellectomized knee with significant post-traumatic arthritis. Preoperative lateral (**A**) and sunrise (**B**) views. AP (**C**), lateral (**D**), and sunrise (**E**) views obtained after TKA with a PCL-retaining implant. If intraoperative stability is good with the trial components, greater constraint is unnecessary.

at this time. The implant with the least constraint needed to stabilize the knee should be used.

TKA IN THE KNEE WITH PATELLAR SUBLUXATION

In the knee with subluxation or dislocation of the patella due to hypoplasia of the lateral femoral condyle or patella, the patella is resurfaced in the standard manner, as long as native patellar thickness after resection is adequate (12 to 14 mm) (**Figure 3**). Appropriate external rotation of the femur according to the transepicondylar axis, as described above in TKA in the Patellectomized Knee, is especially important to correct patellar tracking. Residual medial capsular laxity, if present, is generally corrected with closure. **Figure 4** shows a completed TKA.

For the chronically dislocated patella undergoing TKA, advancement of the medial quadriceps muscle (proximal realignment) is indicated. Tibial tubercle transfer to a more medial position is considered, although rarely needed, in cases of severe malalignment. Lateral release also may be required, but it may be associated with osteonecrosis of the patella and failure of the patellar implant.

PATELLA INFERA

Patella infera can be congenital or secondary to prior surgeries on the knee. Patella infera can cause anterior knee

groove. With trial components in place, the soft tissue is balanced in the medial-lateral and anterior-posterior planes, with special care to assess the anterior-posterior laxity of the femur on the tibia at 30° and 90° of flexion. The need for a posterior stabilized or constrained prosthesis is determined

pain, decreased range of motion, and impingement of the patellar implant on the tibial polyethylene after TKA. Care should be taken to prevent over-resection of the distal femur, which can elevate the joint line and exacerbate the effect of patella infera. When the patella is being resurfaced, placement of the patellar polyethylene in a cephalad position can help symptoms of a contracted patellar tendon, but a tibial tubercle osteotomy that moves the tubercle more proximal may be needed in severe cases. In the most severe cases, the patella can be left unresurfaced.

Wound Closure

Special care is taken to ensure that the arthrotomy is closed securely, because closure of the capsule contributes to proper extensor mechanism alignment. If the quadriceps tendon is released for exposure, lengthening, or realignment, strong nonabsorbable suture is used. We recommend that the same suture be used in an interrupted fashion on the medial capsule if tension is needed to ensure good patella or extensor mechanism position throughout the range of motion. In knees with limited preoperative flexion, closure is undertaken with the

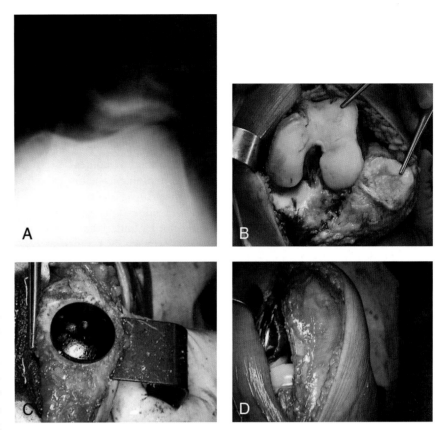

Figure 3 TKA in a knee with hypoplasia of the patella and lateral femoral condyle. **A,** Preoperative Merchant view demonstrating subluxation of the patella. **B,** Intraoperative photograph demonstrating hypoplasia of the patella and lateral femoral condyle with significant degenerative changes. The patella was assessed intraoperatively and found to be sufficiently thick to allow resurfacing. **C,** The patellar polyethylene is placed medially in the standard manner. **D,** Patellar tracking is assessed intraoperatively with all components in place. With good tracking and no medial tension, there is no need for additional proximal or distal realignment procedures.

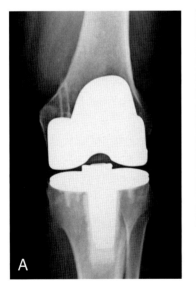
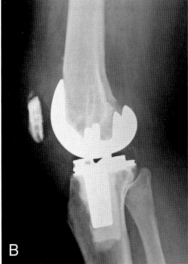
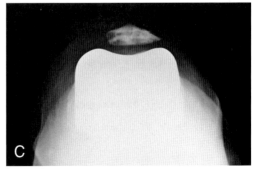

Figure 4 Postoperative radiographs of the patient in Figure 3. A PCL-retaining implant was used. AP **(A)**, lateral **(B)**, and sunrise **(C)** views.

knee in 30° of flexion. If the patella tracks well with no tension on the medial capsule, the surgeon's preferred closure can be used. The remaining layers are closed in a standard manner.

Postoperative Regimen

If an osteotomy is performed, patients are kept non–weight bearing for 6 to 8 weeks, until evidence of healing at the osteotomy site appears on radiographs. Passive range of motion is begun immediately postoperatively. Patients who did not undergo an osteotomy begin weight bearing as tolerated, with passive and active range of motion immediately postoperatively.

Avoiding Pitfalls and Complications

It is important to address extensor mechanism problems before TKA. Extensor mechanism reconstruction and repair of tendon ruptures or fractures should not be undertaken in the setting of a primary TKA. Once such issues are addressed and the reconstruction or repair has healed, TKA can proceed using the same principles as any primary TKA to ensure correct extensor alignment. Exposure difficulties in knees that have undergone pre- vious surgeries are addressed with revision techniques proximally (quadriceps snip) and distally (tibial tubercle osteotomy) as needed.

Another important issue to address before surgery is patient expectations. TKA will likely not correct an extensor lag, and patients must understand this before surgery. A patient who has had prior surgery on the knee also must understand the additional risks after TKA, including infection, failure, and the need for reoperation. Nonetheless, with proper preoperative planning, patients with a prior patellectomy or other extensor mechanism problem can expect significant pain relief and improved function following TKA.

Bibliography

Bayne O, Cameron HU: Total knee arthroplasty following patellectomy. *Clin Orthop Relat Res* 1984;186:112-114.

Cameron HU, Hu C, Vyamont D: Posterior stabilized knee prosthesis for total knee replacement in patients with prior patellectomy. *Can J Surg* 1996;39(6):469-473.

Insall JN, Aglietti P, Tria AJ Jr: Patellar pain and incongruence. II: Clinical application. *Clin Orthop Relat Res* 1983;176: 225-232.

Larson KR, Cracchiolo A III, Dorey FJ, Finerman GA: Total knee arthroplasty in patients after patellectomy. *Clin Orthop Relat Res* 1991;(264):243-254.

Lennox DW, Hungerford DS, Krackow KA: Total knee arthroplasty following patellectomy. *Clin Orthop Relat Res* 1987; 223:220-224.

Martin SD, Haas SB, Insall JN: Primary total knee arthroplasty after patellectomy. *J Bone Joint Surg Am* 1995;77(9):1323-1330.

Nazarian DG, Booth RE Jr : Extensor mechanism allografts in total knee arthroplasty. *Clin Orthop Relat Res* 1999;367: 123-129.

Paletta GA Jr, Laskin RS: Total knee arthroplasty after a previous patellectomy. *J Bone Joint Surg Am* 1995;77(11):1708-1712.

Railton GT, Levack B, Freeman MA: Unconstrained knee arthroplasty after patellectomy. *J Arthroplasty* 1990;5(3):255-257.

Rand JA: The patellofemoral joint in total knee arthroplasty. *J Bone Joint Surg Am* 1994;76(4):612-620.

Sledge CB, Ewald FC: Total knee arthroplasty experience at the Robert Breck Brigham Hospital. *Clin Orthop Relat Res* 1979;145:78-84.

Szalapski EW, Siliski J, King TV, Ritter MA: Total knee replacement in the patellectomized knee. *Am J Knee Surg* 1994; 7(2):73-76.

	Coding		
CPT Code		**Corresponding ICD-9 Codes**	
27447	Arthroplasty, knee, condyle and plateau; medial AND lateral compartments with or without patella resurfacing (total knee arthroplasty)	715 715.80	715.16 715.89

Chapter 25

Total Knee Arthroplasty in the Obese Patient

Ray C. Wasielewski, MS, MD

Sharat K. Kusuma, MD, MBA

Indications

Although significant advances in both nutrition and exercise science have been made over the last century, there has been a concomitant and nearly geometric increase in obesity rates. By the year 2006, more than one third of adults in the United States were obese (body mass index [BMI] ≥ 30). Obese patients experience increased joint reactive forces, which can accelerate the degenerative process in the knee and thereby lower the age at which total knee arthroplasty (TKA) is required. Recent literature has demonstrated that severely obese patients (BMI = 35 to 39.9) undergo TKA 8 years earlier than patients who are not obese, and morbidly obese patients (BMI ≥ 40) undergo TKA a mean 13 years earlier than normal-weight patients.

Obesity increases the risks associated with TKA. Obese patients have an increased risk of perioperative complications, including wound infections and dehiscence, deep vein thrombosis (DVT), and medial collateral ligament avulsion. They are also at a higher risk for early failure and early revision surgery. Accordingly, obese patients should undergo extensive preoperative counseling regarding the potential for complications and inferior results to ensure appropriate expectations regarding the outcome of their TKA. Because of inferior outcomes, significant controversy exists as to whether TKA is contraindicated in morbidly obese patients. To determine TKA candidacy, the patient's BMI, knee girth, and medical and musculoskeletal comorbidities must be considered. The decision to operate also should take into account the willingness of the surgeon and patient to accept the increased risk of postoperative complications.

Despite unfavorable statistics, TKA in morbidly obese patients with knee arthritis frequently provides pain relief and functional improvements. As in any cohort of patients, however, TKA should be performed only when the risks of surgery are outweighed by the benefits.

Contraindications

The presence of major comorbidities may be a contraindication to TKA in the morbidly obese patient. Patients with multiple medical comorbidities are already at an increased risk of complications after TKA. It has been shown that patients with greater medical and musculoskeletal comorbidity (Knee Society class C) experience longer hospital stays, incur higher hospital charges, and are more often discharged to a rehabilitation facility than are TKA patients without significant comorbidity (Knee Society class A). Greater anesthesia severity assessment (ASA) scores (ASA ≥3) also have been found to correlate with increased hospital charges and discharge to a rehabilitation facility instead of home. The addition of morbid obesity may render a patient unfit for TKA. Unfortunately, because morbid obesity contributes to both the onset and exacerbation of a myriad of medical morbidities, including diabetes mellitus, hypertension, pulmonary hypertension, and sleep apnea, medical comorbidities are more common in patients with morbid obesity. Because of the numerous potential complications to which they are exposed, the successful and complication-free navigation of these patients through elective TKA can be extremely challenging.

Dr. Wasielewski or an immediate family member has received royalties from DePuy and Zimmer; is a member of a speakers' bureau or has made paid presentations on behalf of Zimmer; and has received research or institutional support from King Pharmaceuticals. Dr. Kusuma or an immediate family member is a member of a speakers' bureau or has made paid presentations on behalf of Genzyme and serves as a paid consultant to or is an employee of Graftys.

Diabetes often is seen concurrently with obesity and worsens the prognosis for obese patients who undergo TKA. To minimize infection risk, TKA should be avoided in patients with a hemoglobin A1C level greater than 7%. Selected patients may benefit from rigorous perioperative insulin administration to reduce wide variations in their blood glucose levels. Fibromyalgia commonly accompanies diabetes and obesity and also should be maximally treated before TKA. Patients with fibromyalgia and diabetes typically have higher hemoglobin A1C levels compared with patients with diabetes only.

Even obese patients who are otherwise reasonable candidates for TKA should be encouraged to lose weight preoperatively. However, many obese TKA candidates are unable to tolerate exercise other than very low impact activities; in these cases, the primary modality of weight loss must be modification of eating behaviors. In our practice, we have found that exercises such as water walking and aqua jogging, in which the patient simulates a jogging motion while suspended by a flotation device in the deep section of the swimming pool, are usually very well tolerated by these patients. These types of exercise have demonstrated reasonable success in helping patients to lose weight. We have found that patients who lose at least 10% of their body weight preoperatively tend to continue their weight loss after TKA, at which time more exercise can be added to their weight loss regimen. Bariatric surgery also may be an option for some morbidly obese patients who are not TKA candidates at their present weight and in whom multiple nonsurgical weight loss measures have failed. Results of TKA after bariatric surgery are excellent, with acceptable complication rates. For some very young patients with morbid obesity and severe knee arthritis, preoperative gastric bypass surgery may be advisable to both reduce the risk of complications and improve the odds of increased implant longevity.

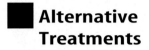

Alternative Treatments

Nonsurgical treatments can be used in obese patients who are not candidates for TKA. Nonsurgical treatments offer variable amounts of pain relief, but they neither restore lost articular cartilage nor correct joint deformity, and therefore they must be performed on a repeated basis for sustained pain relief. Common pharmacologic treatment options include nonsteroidal anti-inflammatory drugs and nonnarcotic (eg, tramadol) medications. Neuroleptic agents and muscle relaxants are occasionally helpful, particularly for patients with fibromyalgia. Unfortunately, valgus knee bracing, a commonly used nonsurgical treatment, is rarely a viable option for obese patients because of knee girth and soft-tissue impingement. When knee girth precludes bracing, alternative limb realignment measures such as heel wedges (varus knee) or arch supports (valgus knee) remain an option. Although heel wedges may no longer be considered a mainstream or first-line treatment for knee arthritis, they may be indicated in obese patients who are suboptimal surgical candidates, to avoid TKA. Other nonsurgical treatments include viscosupplementation injections, corticosteroid injections, physical therapy, and assistive walking devices.

Arthroscopic knee procedures may be considered as a way of delaying TKA in young, obese, high-risk patients. Arthroscopy may provide some benefit to patients with mechanical symptoms, such as locking and catching, resulting from meniscal tears or loose bodies. Arthroscopy also may allow the débridement of osteophytes in the proximity of the collateral ligaments, thereby providing some pain relief and perhaps minor deformity correction. Unfortunately, obese patients often have severe and advanced degenerative disease, in which setting arthroscopy is almost uniformly ineffective in relieving pain and improving symptoms. Moreover, several recent prospective studies have failed to demonstrate major benefit from knee arthroscopy for most patients with advanced arthritis.

Once significant bone loss or ligament laxity is present, TKA may be seriously considered despite the potential drawbacks. If surgery is delayed further, allowing laxities to worsen, a highly constrained prosthesis may become necessary. Highly constrained prostheses are likely to have higher rates of failure and early loosening in obese patients.

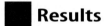

Results

Obese and normal-BMI patients typically achieve similar magnitudes of improvement in knee scores from the preoperative to the postarthroplasty period, indicating similar amounts of functional improvement. Obese patients nonetheless usually have lower postoperative knee scores and more complications, including DVT, wound complications, and infection. Namba and associates reported a significantly higher postoperative infection rate in morbidly obese (BMI ≥ 35) TKA patients than in obese (BMI = 30 to 35) TKA patients (1.1% versus 0.3%). Odds ratio calculations indicate that the risk of infection was 6.7 times higher for morbidly obese patients.

Because obesity increases the risk of DVT, patients who are obese and who also have other DVT risk factors require extra perioperative vigilance. A preoperative duplex Doppler ultrasonogram and temporary or permanent inferior vena cava filter placement may be considered for obese patients with a history of lower extremity blood clots. Discretion should be exercised before operating on obese patients who are unable to stop anticoagulation agents preoperatively or who must resume this medication immediately after surgery.

Diabetic patients undergoing TKA are already at increased risk of postoperative complications, including infection, wound complications, blood transfusion, urinary tract infection, pneumonia, ileus, and stroke. Diabetes is often coupled with obesity, further increasing the risk of complication. A recent study demonstrated that diabetic TKA patients had a deep periprosthetic infection rate 6.87 times that of nondiabetic TKA patients, yet no periprosthetic infections occurred in patients with diabetes who were not obese.

Although obesity is a negative risk factor for osteoporosis, the unfortunate patient with both conditions is occasionally seen. Because of the additional weight demands obesity puts on osteoporotic bones, the tibial baseplate may need extra support, and strong consideration should be given to the use of stemmed implants.

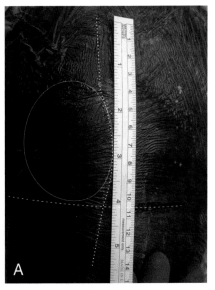
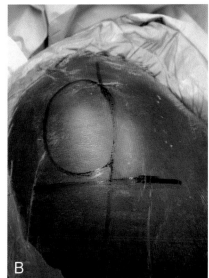
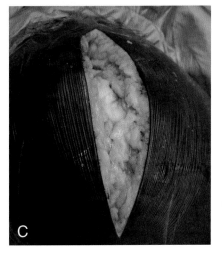
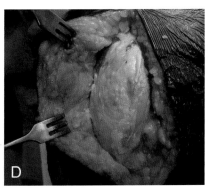

Figure 1 Surgical approach for TKA in an obese patient. **A,** The planned medial incision (dotted line), patellar outline (circle), and joint line (dashed line) are indicated on this extended knee. **B,** The planned medial incision, patellar outline, and joint line are marked on this flexed knee. **C,** The incision reveals a thick subcutaneous layer. **D,** The thick subcutaneous layer is separated from the superficial patellar fascia.

Technique

Setup/Exposure

In general, obese patients should not be considered candidates for muscle-sparing or minimally invasive surgical approaches for TKA. To gain adequate exposure, the skin and quadriceps incisions often have to be extended proximally. The patella may either be subluxated or fully everted, depending on the surgeon's preference. Both techniques are safe in the obese patient.

The successful execution of a stable and well-balanced TKA in the obese patient requires meticulous attention to detail with a focus on adequate exposure and a systematic, stepwise approach to careful ligament balancing and bone cuts. Because exposure is often challenging in these patients, the surgeon must be especially careful to avoid errors related to inadequate exposure, such as incorrect bone cut alignment or overresection of bone, because these errors can lead to significant instability. Additionally, the surgeon must vigilantly avoid overreleasing critical ligamentous structures, as these structures are more prone to intraoperative rupture in obese patients.

Consistent with other gap-balancing techniques, bone cuts should be made after adequate exposure but before aggressive ligament releases. The sequential and safe removal of adequate bone can optimize and sequentially increase the exposure. A consistent sequence of bone cuts that commences with the patellar resection, followed by the distal femoral cut and then the tibial cut, provides for the creation of an extension gap that can be used to assess ligament integrity and exten-

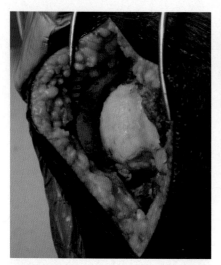

Figure 2 The cut patella is protected with a metal button.

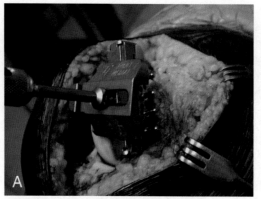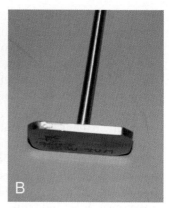

Figure 3 Femoral resection. **A,** An intramedullary alignment guide and a four-pin fixation cutting jig are positioned on the medial distal femur to verify correct distal femoral cut angulation. **B,** An intramedullary guide used to check bone cut alignment.

sion gap balance. The surgeon must choose a femoral component, degree of rotation, and anterior-posterior position that creates an equivalent flexion gap. We describe this technique for TKA in obese patients in more detail below.

With the knee flexed, the skin incision is made along the medial border of the patella. The incision begins 2 to 3 cm proximal to the superior pole of the patella and ends 2 to 3 cm distal to the joint line (**Figure 1**, *A* through *C*), but it may need to be lengthened. To optimize mobility of the patella, the thick subcutaneous layer is separated from the superficial patellar fascia (**Figure 1**, *D*). Using the medial parapatellar approach, the extent of division into the quadriceps tendon is determined by extensor mechanism tightness. Careful dissection of any scar tissue between the infrapatellar fat pad and the patellar tendon will significantly improve patellar mobility for the remainder of the procedure. The entire perimeter of the patella is carefully exposed to facilitate a very accurate patellar resection. The patella is then cut and a protective metal button is used for the remainder of the procedure to prevent fracture (**Figure 2**).

A partial and conservative medial release is performed to improve medial exposure. The distal femur is cut from medial to lateral using a cutting guide anchored to the medial femur. The medial incision location facilitates placement of this cutting guide (**Figure 3**, *A*), but a more standard anterior-to-posterior distal cutting guide can be used. Regardless of the cutting guide used, the critical factor is that the distal femoral cut is in the appropriate coronal and sagittal plane alignment. After the cut is complete, an intramedullary distal femoral cut check guide can then be used to verify correct distal femoral angulation (**Figure 3**, *B*).

Once the patellar and distal femoral bone has been removed, exposure is significantly improved. Because we use a posterior stabilized component in nearly every case, the next step of the exposure involves the removal of osteophytes from the femoral notch. Upon removal of these osteophytes, exposure is nearly complete and the anterior and posterior cruciate ligaments are safely removed. Partial anterior subluxation of the tibia is now possible; it is accomplished by the careful placement of a Hohmann-type retractor in the femoral notch, just behind the tibial plateau. During placement of this retractor, great care must be taken to avoid damage to the pos-

terior neurovascular structures. The tibial subluxation allows close inspection of the medial tibial plateau, the medial collateral ligament, and the posterior medial capsular structures. This medial exposure is important because it allows the surgeon to obtain an early indication of the extent of medial contracture and to anticipate the amount of medial soft-tissue release that will be required later in the procedure. It also allows the preliminary removal of medial tibial osteophytes that may be tenting the medial collateral ligament and medial and lateral meniscal tissue.

Procedure

The tibia is relocated, and an extramedullary tibial cutting guide is placed. Our preferred cutting guide anchors to the medial tibial plateau and permits the cut to be made from a medial to lateral direction (**Figure 4**). In obese patients, the surgeon must diligently confirm that the tibial cut is aligned perpendicular to the mechanical axis. Because obese patients generally have significant soft-tissue girth in the ankle region, the surgeon may easily become confused about alignment of the cut and inadvertently cut the tibia in excessive varus or valgus, or with an inappropriate amount of anterior-posterior slope. The surgeon should carefully check the position of

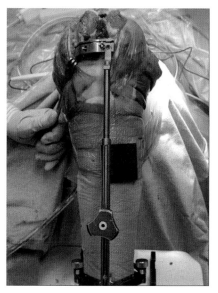

Figure 4 An extramedullary tibial cutting jig in place. Note that it allows access to the medial tibia.

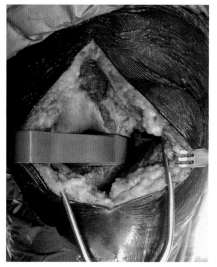

Figure 5 Rectangular extension gap.

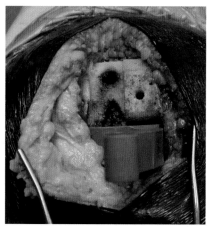

Figure 6 A spacer block is used to assess flexion gap symmetry.

the tibial cutting jig and use any type of additional alignment device, such as an external alignment rod, to further confirm the cut alignment. After the tibia is cut medial to lateral perpendicular to the mechanical axis, spacer blocks of varying thickness are used to accurately gauge the size of the extension gap and assess overall limb alignment. The size of the spacer block chosen is one that allows the knee to achieve both full extension and equal medial and lateral ligament tension (**Figure 5**). Accurate measurement of the size of the extension gap allows the surgeon to estimate the anticipated size of the flexion gap that will be required to achieve matched gaps; this measurement will allow the surgeon to anticipate the size of femoral component that will achieve this balance.

Once a rectangular extension gap is created with appropriate ligament releases (**Figure 6**), the knee is flexed to 90° and the femoral component rotation is determined by referencing the Whiteside line. We have found that rotating the femoral component such that the cut anterior surface is either perpendicular to the Whiteside line or

externally rotated 1° to 2° from this line reliably achieves congruent femoral component positioning with excellent patellar tracking and rectangular flexion and extension gaps through the entire range of motion in most cases. We have also found that positioning the femoral cutting guide such that it is parallel to the cut tibial surface provides an additional check and confirmation of appropriate femoral component rotation. Once the appropriate rotation is set, the next step is to choose the correct size of the femoral cutting block to produce a flexion space that matches the extension space. Because of the extreme weight of the leg, however, and the tightness of the extensor mechanism in obese patients, the strict use of the gap-balancing technique is often very difficult. The extreme weight of the leg can mislead the surgeon into overestimating the tightness of the flexion gap. Therefore, we recommend the placement of a laminar spreader centrally under the posterior edge of the femoral cutting block to assess the flexion gap (**Figure 7**). With the laminar spreader tensioned, a spacer block can be inserted into the flexion space to help determine whether an appropriate flexion space has been created. This laminar spreader technique can

help offset the effect of the heavy leg and extensor mechanism tightness, particularly when the patella has not been everted.

The anterior and posterior femoral condylar and chamfer cuts are made using a 4-in-1 cutting block. After the cuts have been made, a laminar spreader is placed with the knee in 90° of flexion, and any remaining posterior femoral osteophytes are removed. The removal of these osteophytes is critically important, as they can tent the posterior capsule in both flexion and extension and result in loss of some motion.

After the femoral preparation is complete, attention is turned to final preparation of the cut tibial surface. Anterior subluxation of the tibia facilitates accurate tibial baseplate positioning and external rotation. Subluxation and exposure of the tibia are aided when the flexion gap is at least 12 to 14 mm (**Figure 8**). During preparation of the tibial surface, the surgeon should seriously consider using a stemmed tibial baseplate, which can increase the accuracy of tibial component alignment and improve component fixation. If revision becomes necessary in the future, a stemmed baseplate may ease the conversion to a revision constrained prosthesis by potentially eliminating the requirement

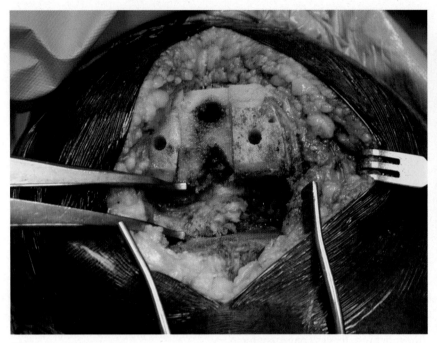

Figure 7 A laminar spreader is used to distract the lateral compartment.

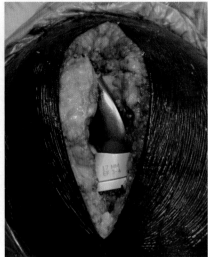

Figure 8 Implant trials in place, showing a well-located patella and a 17-mm spacer.

that the tibial component be removed and revised; most current knee systems require the use of a stemmed tibial baseplate before conversion to a constrained knee.

Wound Closure and Management

The literature is replete with evidence that obese patients have a higher wound complication rate than do patients with a normal body habitus. We advocate the use of several layers of interrupted sutures to decrease wound tension and wound dehiscence. Additionally, meticulous hemostasis can reduce hematoma formation and the risk of wound complications. We advocate the complete release of tourniquet pressure prior to closure of the arthrotomy layer, to allow the surgeon to carefully inspect the knee for visual evidence of profuse bleeding. Control of excessive bleeding at this stage of the closure can prevent later hematoma formation.

To achieve a completely watertight closure of the deep arthrotomy layer, the use of interrupted 1-0 absorbable sutures with close spacing is advocated. We routinely use a second layer of 1-0 absorbable suture in the deep adipose layer to reduce wound tension in the more superficial skin layers. The structural integrity of this layer is not significant; however, the use of several interrupted sutures spaced approximately 2 to 3 cm apart can reduce wound tension at the level of the dermis. For closure of the dermis, which is another critical layer of structural integrity, we favor the use of an absorbable 2-0 suture in an interrupted pattern. It is extremely important that these sutures are placed so that accurate skin eversion is achieved. Finally, for the superficial skin layer, the use of skin staples or interrupted nylon sutures is favored over an absorbable subcuticular running suture. Interrupted sutures or staples provide a stronger barrier to wound dehiscence and also allow for early range-of-motion physical therapy and ambulation without the fear of wound dehiscence.

Postoperative Regimen

In the immediate postoperative period, daily and careful wound inspection should be performed. Any persistent wound drainage should be addressed with serious consideration of a return to the operating room for irrigation and débridement. With regard to postoperative rehabilitation, as with other TKA patients, obese patients should be aggressively encouraged to mobilize, as they are at increased risk of atelectasis, pulmonary embolus, decubitus ulcers, heel sores, and other medical complications. Such complications can be minimized by early mobilization.

Avoiding Pitfalls and Complications

Several potential pitfalls are associated with TKA in morbidly obese patients. Because the patella has to withstand higher forces during the exposure and subsequent procedure in these patients, the patella must not be cut too thin, to avoid the risk of intraoperative fracture. Additionally, great care must be taken during flexion and/or hyperflexion of the knee for exposure, as obese patients have a higher risk of intraoperative medial collateral ligament avulsion.

During the distal femoral and the tibial resections, the surgeon should recognize that valgus alignment is poorly tolerated by obese patients. Valgus alignment in heavy patients can result in tension on the medial collateral ligament and persistent pain. Therefore, when placing the distal femoral and tibial cutting guides, the surgeon must be absolutely certain that a valgus cut is not being made. Slight varus alignment is much preferred over a valgus cut.

Another potential pitfall occurs during the setting of the depth of the distal femoral resection. In obese patients with flexion contractures, the surgeon may be tempted to resect additional distal femoral bone to achieve full extension. However, such overresection elevates the joint line and can adversely affect the amount of postoperative flexion achieved. Moreover, an overly aggressive distal femoral resection combined with an extensive tibial resection may result in a large extension gap, causing recurvatum deformity.

The identification of pathologic medial or lateral ligament laxities in extension after the distal femur and tibia cuts allows the surgeon to make an early decision regarding whether ligament releases can sufficiently balance the knee or whether a constrained prosthesis is necessary. During these steps, the surgeon must be careful not to overrelease the medial or lateral collateral ligament to accommodate pathologic laxities in the opposite ligament. Medial or lateral overrelease can result in large gap sizes, which can adversely affect knee stability and patellar tracking.

Acknowledgment

The authors would like to acknowledge the help of Kate C. Sheridan, BS, in preparing this manuscript.

———————■

Bibliography

Amin AK, Clayton RA, Patton JT, Gaston M, Cook RE, Brenkel IJ: Total knee replacement in morbidly obese patients: Results of a prospective, matched study. *J Bone Joint Surg Br* 2006;88(10):1321-1326.

Bolognesi MP, Marchant MH Jr , Viens NA, Cook C, Pietrobon R, Vail TP: The impact of diabetes on perioperative patient outcomes after total hip and total knee arthroplasty in the United States. *J Arthroplasty* 2008;23(6 Suppl 1):92-98.

Changulani M, Kalairajah Y, Peel T, Field RE: The relationship between obesity and the age at which hip and knee replacement is undertaken. *J Bone Joint Surg Br* 2008;90(3):360-363.

Clark CR: Perioperative medical management, in Barrack R, Booth RE Jr, Lonner JH, McCarthy JC, Mont MA, Rubash HE, eds: *Orthopaedic Knowledge Update: Hip and Knee Reconstruction 3*. Rosemont, IL, American Academy of Orthopaedic Surgeons, 2006, pp 205-216.

Dowsey MM, Choong PF: Obese diabetic patients are at substantial risk for deep infection after primary TKA. *Clin Orthop Relat Res* 2009;467(6):1577-1581.

Eknoyan G: A history of obesity, or how what was good became ugly and then bad. *Adv Chronic Kidney Dis* 2006;13(4): 421-427.

Messier SP, Gutekunst DJ, Davis C, DeVita P: Weight loss reduces knee-joint loads in overweight and obese older adults with knee osteoarthritis. *Arthritis Rheum* 2005;52(7):2026-2032.

Moseley JB, O'Malley K, Petersen NJ, et al: A controlled trial of arthroscopic surgery for osteoarthritis of the knee. *N Engl J Med* 2002;347(2):81-88.

Namba RS, Paxton L, Fithian DC, Stone ML: Obesity and perioperative morbidity in total hip and total knee arthroplasty patients. *J Arthroplasty* 2005;20(7 Suppl 3):46-50.

Parvizi J, Trousdale RT, Sarr MG: Total joint arthroplasty in patients surgically treated for morbid obesity. *J Arthroplasty* 2000;15(8):1003-1008.

Rajgopal V, Bourne RB, Chesworth BM, MacDonald SJ, McCalden RW, Rorabeck CH: The impact of morbid obesity on patient outcomes after total knee arthroplasty. *J Arthroplasty* 2008;23(6):795-800.

Tishler M, Smorodin T, Vazina-Amit M, Ramot Y, Koffler M, Fishel B: Fibromyalgia in diabetes mellitus. *Rheumatol Int* 2003;23(4):171-173.

Wasielewski RC, Weed H, Prezioso C, Nicholson C, Puri RD: Patient comorbidity: Relationship to outcomes of total knee arthroplasty. *Clin Orthop Relat Res* 1998;356:85-92.

Winiarsky R, Barth P, Lotke P: Total knee arthroplasty in morbidly obese patients. *J Bone Joint Surg Am* 1998;80(12):1770-1774.

York DA, Rössner S, Caterson I, et al: Prevention Conference VII: Obesity, a worldwide epidemic related to heart disease and stroke. Group I: Worldwide demographics of obesity. *Circulation* 2004;110(18):e463-e470.

Coding			
CPT Codes		**Corresponding ICD-9 Codes**	
Total Knee Arthroplasty			
27447	Arthroplasty, knee, condyle and plateau; medial AND lateral compartments with or without patella resurfacing (total knee arthroplasty)	715 715.80	715.16 715.89

CPT copyright © 2010 by the American Medical Association. All rights reserved.

Chapter 26
Total Knee Arthroplasty in the Valgus Knee

Amar S. Ranawat, MD
Chitranjan S. Ranawat, MD
Yossef C. Blum, MD

■ Indications

A valgus deformity may present a significant challenge when performing a total knee arthroplasty (TKA). The deformity, as defined by an anatomic valgus greater than 10°, is encountered in approximately 10% of knees undergoing a TKA. A valgus deformity is often found in patients with rheumatoid arthritis, osteoarthritis, posttraumatic arthritis, and metabolic bone disease. The overall results, as well as the correction of the deformity and instability, are variable because of the technical challenges of the surgery.

Typically, two anatomic components make up the valgus deformity. One component is lateral bone loss with metaphyseal remodeling, usually from the lateral femoral condyle. The other component is a lateral soft-tissue contracture; the tight lateral structures include the lateral collateral ligament, iliotibial band (ITB),

popliteus tendon, posterolateral capsule, and hamstring muscles.

Valgus deformities have been classified by Krackow and associates into three subtypes. A type I deformity is characterized by minimal valgus angulation and minimal soft-tissue stretching. A type II deformity (**Figure 1**) is characterized by a more notable deformity (>10°) with medial soft-tissue stretching. A type III deformity is characterized by a severe osseous deformity that occurs after a prior osteotomy; an incompetent medial soft-tissue sleeve is present. Type III deformities are best treated with a constrained or hinged TKA. The "inside-out" technique described in this chapter applies to correction of type I and type II deformities.

Valgus deformities may be managed by one of three general methods. In the first method, the contracted lateral structures are released until the lateral compartment is balanced with the more lax medial compartment. This re-

quires placing a larger polyethylene insert. In the second method, the lax medial soft-tissue structures are tightened until the medial compartment is balanced with the more contracted lateral compartment. In the third method, a component that is constrained in the coronal plane is placed.

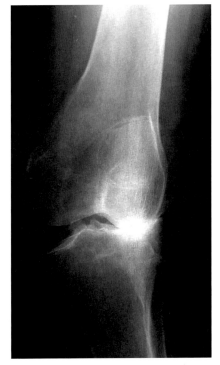

Figure 1 AP radiograph of the knee shows a type II valgus deformity.

Dr. Amar Ranawat or an immediate family member has received royalties from DePuy and Stryker; is a member of a speakers' bureau or has made paid presentations on behalf of DePuy and Stryker; is a paid consultant for or is an employee of DePuy, Stryker, MAKO, and ConforMIS; and has received research or institutional support from DePuy and Stryker. Dr. Chitranjan Ranawat or an immediate family member is a board member, owner, officer, or committee member of The Hip Society; has received royalties from DePuy and Stryker; serves as a paid consultant for or is an employee of DePuy; and has received research or institutional support from DePuy and the Hospital for Special Surgery. Neither Dr. Blum nor any immediate family member has received anything of value from or owns stock in a commercial company or institution related directly or indirectly to the subject of this chapter.

Table 1 Results of Total Knee Arthroplasty for Valgus Knees

Author(s) (Year)	Number of Knees	Deformity	Technique	Implant Type
Miyasaka et al (1997)	60	> 10° valgus	Released lateral retinaculum and ITB; LCL and popliteus released if needed	PS, cemented
Whiteside (1999)	231	12°-45° of valgus	Tight laterally in both flexion and extension: LCL and popliteus released Tight in extension only: ITB released Tight in flexion only: LCL ± popliteus released	CR
Easley et al (2000)	28	11°-25° of valgus	CCK with uncemented stem extension	CCK
Politi and Scott (2004)	35	>15° of valgus	Lateral cruciform retinacular release Partial PCL release in 5 knees LCL and popliteus released in 3 knees	CR
Elkus et al (2004)	35	>10° of valgus	Inside-out soft-tissue balancing technique	PS, cemented
Clarke et al (2005)	24	9°-30° of valgus	Selective pie-crusting of tight lateral structures	PS, cemented
Aglietti et al (2007)	53	> 5° valgus	Selective pie-crusting of tight lateral structures	16 knees: PS 37 knees: CR, mobile-bearing
Kubiak et al (2008)	31	20°-32° of valgus 10°-21° of varus	ITB release (6 knees) LCL release (7 knees) PCL recession (9 knees), constrained polyethylene liner used in these cases	CR

ITB = iliotibial band, LCL = lateral collateral ligament, PS = posterior stabilized, CR = cruciate-retaining, CCK = constrained condylar knee, PCL = posterior cruciate ligament, MCL = medial collateral ligament.

Table 1 *(Continued)*

Mean Age in Years (Range)	Mean Follow-up (Range)	Results	Comments
61 (34-82)	14.1 years (10-20)	Mean postoperative Knee Society score 88.7 75% of knees corrected to 2°-7° of valgus 3 revisions for aseptic loosening 91% of prostheses retained at 13 years 24% incidence of postoperative instability	The senior author (C.S.R.) developed inside-out soft-tissue balancing technique based on high incidence of instability seen in this study.
NR	6 years	Average final alignment 6.0° of valgus (SD = 1.1) No knees required CCK implants for additional stability 13 knees with preoperative deformity >15° required PCL sacrifice/PS implant for persistent lateral tightness No cases of postoperative instability	
72.7 (60-88)	7.8 years (5-11)	Average Knee Society score improved from 27.4 to 95.2 Average clinical score improved from 32.4 to 67.2 Postoperative alignment 3°-7° of valgus No flexion instability No clinical failures or radiographic loosening	Elderly, low-demand patients with MCL incompetence
63.6 (18-81)	41.6 months (24-67)	Average postoperative valgus 4.8° (range, 4°-6°) No cases of postoperative instability No revisions for loosening	
67	>5 years	Average Knee Society score improved from 30 to 93 Mean functional score improved from 34 to 81 Mean coronal alignment improved from 15° of valgus to 5° of varus postoperatively Mean range of motion was 110° both before and after surgery Three knees revised: one for delayed infection, one for premature polyethylene wear, one for patellar loosening No incidence of late-onset instability Average 5° of valgus postoperatively No cases of postoperative instability No revisions for tibia or femur loosening	
68 (40-82)	54 months (24-69)	Average Knee Society score 97 (range, 87-100) No postoperative instability No clinical failures No radiographic evidence of loosening/wear	
68 (44-78)	8 years (5-12)	1 transient peroneal nerve palsy (spontaneously resolved) 96% achieved alignment within 5° from neutral 1 case of varus instability in extension No cases of revision	
71 (36-89)	12 years (10-17)	93% revision-free survivorship for valgus knees No revisions for instability or loosening	

Contraindications

In a type III valgus deformity, the excessive medial laxity and degree of deformity are not amenable to correction by the inside-out technique. In these circumstances, a constrained or hinged prosthesis is advised.

Alternative Treatments

Over the years, various techniques for addressing valgus deformity have been advocated in response to the poor results that were initially obtained. These have not been universally successful, however, and some have been fraught with complications.

One of the proposed methods of addressing the valgus knee is with a lateral approach and capsulotomy. This approach does have several potential advantages. It is more direct, because it offers better exposure of the contracted lateral and posterolateral structures. With a medial approach, a more extensive lateral release, which compromises vascularity, was once thought to be necessary; lateral exposure can potentially preserve more of the blood supply to the patella. Good early results have been reported using a modified lateral capsular release with repositioning of the vastus lateralis; authors have reported that this avoided the need for tibial tubercle osteotomy and more consistently restored patellofemoral tracking. A disadvantage of the lateral approach is that it is technically demanding.

Another proposed method for obtaining stability and soft-tissue balance in valgus knees is medial reconstruction. The femoral origin of the medial collateral ligament is advanced into the medial femoral condyle to obtain appropriate medial soft-tissue tension. This method relies on osse-ous healing and requires postoperative bracing for 6 weeks.

As correction of the valgus knee can be technically demanding, some surgeons approach valgus deformities by placing constrained components. It is our opinion, however, that constrained implants often are not required if attention is paid to appropriate soft-tissue and osseous balancing. In many cases, use of the inside-out technique may obviate the need for constrained implants; this will likely result in improved longevity of the TKA. If there is concern that appropriate coronal balance has not been achieved, however, a more constrained prosthesis should be used.

Results

Results of TKA for severe valgus deformity have generally been poorer than for the more common varus deformity. The results are summarized in **Table 1**.

Recurrent instability associated with the use of the total condylar knee replacement was originally described in 1979. Based on this experience, one of us (C.S.R.) developed the inside-out technique in 1985 to prevent late-onset instability after deformity correction and to avoid the primary use of constrained implants.

Elkus and associates previously reported our results of 35 patients with a preoperative valgus deformity greater than 10° using the surgical technique that is described in detail in the next section. We have had no instances of neurovascular compromise, despite the fact that we often perform "pie-crusting" of the ITB and release of the posterolateral capsule. To determine the risk to the peroneal nerve when this technique is performed, Clarke and associates evaluated 60 MRI studies of adult knees. They found that at the level of the standard proximal tibial resection, the mean distance of the peroneal nerve to the bone is 1.49 cm (range, 0.91 to 2.18 cm). In addition, the lateral head of the gastrocnemius muscle was found to be interposed between the nerve and the capsule at this level. They concluded that the peroneal nerve was adequately protected at this level. In our own unpublished cadaveric study, we found that the nerve is at risk during release of the posterolateral capsule but not during pie-crusting of the ITB. For this reason, we recommend the use of electrocautery during capsular release because the current often will indicate when the nerve is nearby. For pie-crusting of the ITB, we recommend using a fresh No. 11 blade, as this provides more control.

Techniques

Radiographic Evaluation

After weight-bearing AP, lateral, and sunrise views have been obtained, the knee should be assessed for overall coronal alignment both radiographically and clinically. Full-length weight-bearing radiographs of the lower extremity can be used to determine overall limb alignment and may reveal anatomic abnormalities not visualized on standard knee radiographs.

The surgeon should focus on both osseous and soft-tissue deformities. Osseous deformities include distal femoral hypoplasia, posterior femoral condylar erosion, and unusual proximal femoral neck-shaft angles. In addition, one should look for metaphyseal remodeling of the femur and the tibia, which can lead to malalignment or malrotation of the femoral component. Soft-tissue deformities include the lateral soft-tissue contracture described above.

The amount of bone to be resected can be planned preoperatively using measurements made on the preoperative radiographs. The amount of medial joint space opening, as well as any fixed flexion contractures, may deter-

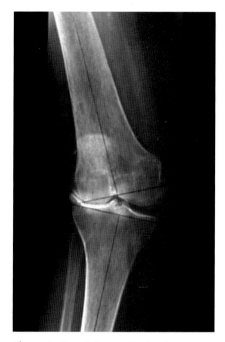

Figure 2 Templating on the AP view.

mine the amount of osseous resection needed for deformity correction. In most cases of type II valgus deformities in which the medial joint space is greater than 1 cm on a weight-bearing AP radiograph, less bone than usual should be resected from the distal femur and proximal tibia. The purpose of decreasing the amount of osseous resection is to allow for appropriate soft-tissue balancing while maintaining the position of the joint line. A "normal" osseous resection in a type II valgus deformity can result in elevation of the joint line or can create an extension gap that is too large.

Templating

Templating on the AP radiograph (**Figure 2**) begins with drawing a vertical line down the center of the tibial diaphysis. A perpendicular line is then drawn at the level of the lateral plateau, which is more involved in a valgus deformity. This allows the surgeon to plan the level of the proximal tibial resection, as well as to judge the medial:lateral ratio of bone resection. Valgus correction using the inside-out

technique is based on a tibial cut that is perpendicular to the shaft.

To template the femoral side, a line should be drawn down the center of the femoral diaphysis. A second line is then drawn at the level of the lateral distal femoral condyle that is in 3° of valgus in relation to the first line; based on this, the quantity of osseous resection can be planned, as well as the ratio of resection of the medial and lateral femoral condyles. A 3° valgus resection, as opposed to the usual 5° to 7° cut, is made to prevent undercorrection of the valgus deformity.

The lateral radiograph is then evaluated. Any posterior osteophytes should be noted and circled. These osteophytes should be removed during the surgery because they may impede soft-tissue balancing and postoperative range of motion. The size of the femoral component is determined on the lateral view, as the magnification of the femoral condyles is greater on the AP view by 5% to 7%. The sunrise radiograph is assessed for patellar tilt and subluxation.

Implant Selection

We prefer a posterior stabilized design when correcting a valgus deformity. This design is better suited for correcting deformities than is the cruciate-retaining design because of the post-cam mechanism and the more conforming articulation. In addition, the inside-out technique mandates resection of the posterior cruciate ligament. Resection of the posterior cruciate ligament also allows for lateralization of the femoral component, which can optimize patellar tracking and decrease the need for lateral retinacular release.

Setup/Exposure

The patient is positioned supine, and a tourniquet is placed. A sandbag is then placed under the foot to allow the knee to be positioned in 90° of flexion. A lateral thigh post can be helpful in stabilizing the knee in this position of flexion.

The leg is then prepared and draped. A straight midline incision is marked with the knee in extension. The knee is then flexed to 90°, and a midline incision is made from 5 to 10 cm proximal to the patella down to an equal distance distal to the inferior pole, just medial to the tibial tubercle. The incision is carried down to the level of the extensor mechanism without creating substantial flaps. The quadriceps tendon, vastus medialis obliquus, patella, and patellar tendon are exposed. A standard medial parapatellar arthrotomy is then performed.

After subperiosteal release of the medial soft tissues from the proximal tibia, the knee is extended, and the patella is everted. The knee is then flexed again, and the lateral patellofemoral ligament is released. The menisci are excised, and both cruciate ligaments (in a posterior stabilized TKA) are released. The knee is then hyperflexed in preparation for the tibial osseous resection.

Procedure

TIBIAL RESECTION

The tibial resection should be made perpendicular to the anatomic axis of the tibia; the quantity of resection depends on the degree of deformity. In a type II valgus deformity, less bone than usual should be resected. Approximately 6 to 8 mm of bone should be resected from the more intact side (in this case, the medial side), as opposed to the usual 10 mm for many TKA designs. Tibial alignment also should be confirmed with the use of an external jig; coronal alignment is assessed by centering the distal aspect of the jig on the center of the talus, and sagittal alignment should be evaluated by aligning the rod parallel to the tibial crest.

The tibial resection is then performed. A varus or valgus cut will affect femoral component rotation if this is referenced off the tibial "platform" using this technique. After the tibial resection is performed, the tibial tray should be sized based on the anterior-posterior dimension of the lateral condyle. Proper rotation of the tray usually is obtained by placing the anterior aspect of the tray flush with the anterior aspect of the medial tibial condyle.

FEMORAL RESECTION

The entry site for the femoral medullary canal is at the intersection of the patellofemoral and tibiofemoral articular surfaces; this point is entered with a gauge to assist in drill placement. A drill is used to gain entrance to the canal, enlarging the entry site with circular motions (to decrease canal pressure) before progressing up the canal. The drill should not come into contact with the femoral cortices.

The intermedullary jig is then placed and advanced until it is flush with the medial femoral condyle. It should be grossly parallel to the cut tibial surface. An anterior rough cut is made. A 3° valgus cut should then be made to prevent undercorrection of the valgus deformity and to compensate for any coronal metaphyseal-diaphyseal remodeling that has taken place (**Figure 3**). No more than 10 mm of bone should be resected from the medial side; in a valgus deformity, this often corresponds to only a minimal resection of the lateral femoral condyle (eg, 1 to 2 mm).

The knee is then extended, and a spacer block is placed. Patellar resurfacing may now be performed.

EXTENSION GAP BALANCING

The extension gap is now evaluated. The goal should be a rectangular extension gap; this is assessed by placing an appropriate-size spacer block with the knee in full extension. Medial-lateral stability is judged by applying varus and valgus stresses. In a valgus deformity, lateral tightness often is present (**Figure 4**). The spacer block is then removed, and a lamina spreader is placed centrally in the knee. If there is lateral-sided tightness, a trapezoidal

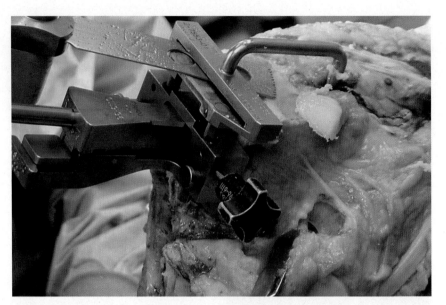

Figure 3 The distal femoral valgus cut is performed at a 3° angle to the intramedullary guide (anatomic axis). (Reproduced with permission from Ranawat AS, Chitranjan CS, Elkus M, Rasquinha VJ, Rossi R, Babhulkar S: Total knee arthroplasty for severe valgus deformity. *J Bone Joint Surg Am* 2005;87(Suppl 1):271-284.)

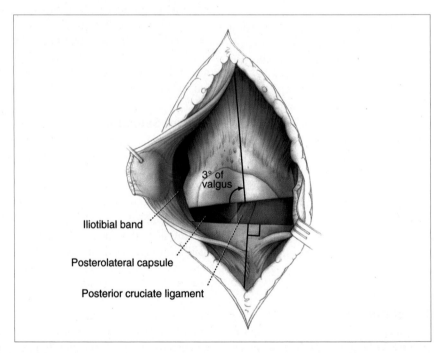

Figure 4 Schematic shows an asymmetrically tight lateral compartment, resulting in a trapezoidal extension gap. (Reproduced with permission from Ranawat AS, Chitranjan CS, Elkus M, Rasquinha VJ, Rossi R, Babhulkar S: Total knee arthroplasty for severe valgus deformity. *J Bone Joint Surg Am* 2005;87(Suppl 1):271-284.)

extension gap will be apparent. This trapezoidal extension gap may be converted to a rectangular gap by using the inside-out technique (**Figure 5**).

There are nine steps to the inside-out technique (**Table 2**); these should be performed in sequence until the knee is balanced in extension. At this

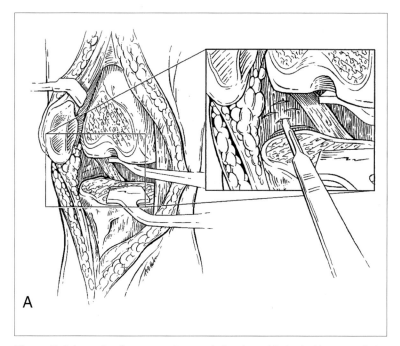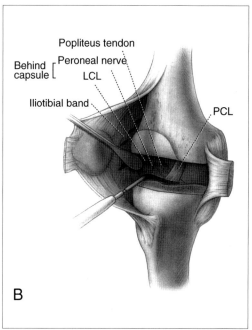

Figure 5 Schematics show extension gap balancing with the inside-out technique. **A,** The iliotibial band is lengthened by making multiple stab incisions (the "pie-crusting" technique) several centimeters proximal to the cut tibial surface (Reproduced with permission from Clarke HD, Schwarz JB, Math KR, Scuderi GR: Anatomic risk of peroneal nerve injury with the "pie crust" technique for valgus release in total knee arthroplasty. *J Arthroplasty* 2004;19:40-44). **B,** The balanced extension gap. The trapezoidal extension gap has been converted to a rectangular (symmetric) extension gap (Reproduced with permission from Ranawat AS, Chitranjan CS, Elkus M, Rasquinha VJ, Rossi R, Babhulkar S: Total knee arthroplasty for severe valgus deformity. *J Bone Joint Surg Am* 2005;87(Suppl 1):271-284.). LCL = lateral collateral ligament, PCL = posterior cruciate ligament.

Table 2 Steps of the Inside-Out Technique for Correction of Valgus Deformities

1. Remove any peripheral osteophytes.

2. Extend the knee and distract the tibiofemoral joint with a lamina spreader.

3. Irrigate and dry the joint.

4. Palpate the posterior cruciate ligament, posterolateral corner, and iliotibial band with a finger or with a Cobb elevator to determine which structures are tight.

5. Release the posterior cruciate ligament completely.

6. Release the posterolateral capsule intra-articularly using electrocautery at the level of the cut tibial surface from the posterior cruciate ligamant to the posterior border of the iliotibial band. Electrocautery is used to avoid injuring the peroneal nerve, which is less than 1 cm from the articular side.

7. Make an effort to preserve the popliteus, unless it is too tight.

8. Lengthen the iliotibial band as necessary from the inside with multiple transverse stab incisions a few centimeters proximal to the joint line (the pie-crusting technique).

9. Manually apply valgus and varus stresses in extension to determine medial and lateral compartment balance; repeat these steps as necessary if the lateral compartment remains tight.

point, applying a valgus or varus force to the knee will result in a "springy" and symmetric opening of 2 to 3 mm on both the medial and lateral sides (**Figure 6**). At least one of the lateral structures should be maintained for stability. Should instability be detected after the releases are performed, a constrained implant may be indicated.

FLEXION GAP BALANCING

The flexion gap can be evaluated only after the extension gap has been balanced. Whereas the extension gap is balanced by addressing the soft-tissue structures, the flexion gap is balanced primarily by adjusting the anterior-posterior femoral osseous resection. Excessive release of the medial soft-tissue structures may result in internal rotation of the femoral component.

After the knee is flexed to 90°, the anterior-posterior cutting block of the same size as the tibial tray size is placed on the distal femur, with its posterior surface roughly parallel to the tibial cut (**Figure 7**). In this position, it usually is perpendicular to the Whiteside line. In a valgus knee, referencing off the posterior femoral con-

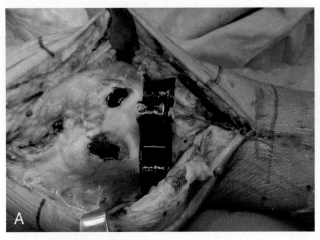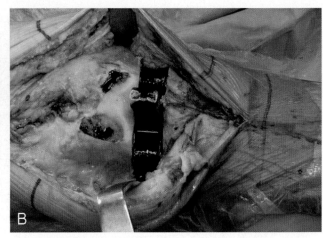

Figure 6 Evaluating the extension gap. **A,** A spacer block has been placed to evaluate the extension gap, and a varus stress has been applied. Note the appropriate (2- to 3-mm) opening on the lateral side. **B,** A valgus stress has been applied, resulting in the same amount (2 to 3 mm) of medial opening. This represents a balanced extension gap. (Reproduced with permission from Ranawat AS, Chitranjan CS, Elkus M, Rasquinha VJ, Rossi R, Babhulkar S: Total knee arthroplasty for severe valgus deformity. *J Bone Joint Surg Am* 2005;87(Suppl 1):271-284.)

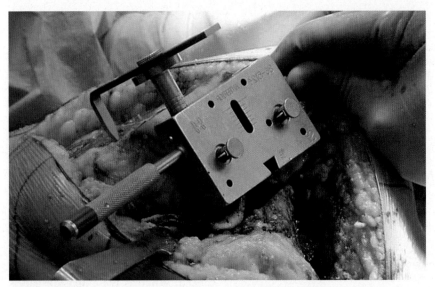

Figure 7 The femoral anterior-posterior cutting block is applied in a position that is roughly parallel to the tibial cut. (Reproduced with permission from Ranawat AS, Chitranjan CS, Elkus M, Rasquinha VJ, Rossi R, Babhulkar S: Total knee arthroplasty for severe valgus deformity. *J Bone Joint Surg Am* 2005;87(Suppl 1):271-284.)

dyles should be avoided because associated lateral condylar hypoplasia and posterior condylar wear often are present, so resection based on referencing the posterior femoral condyles may result in excessive internal rotation of the femoral component.

Medial-lateral flexion gap balancing is then performed. A lamina spreader is placed laterally between the anterior-posterior cutting block and the proxi-mal tibia. The femur is lifted medially and a ruler is used to ensure that the medial compartment flexion space is symmetric to the lateral compartment flexion space (**Figure 8,** *A*). If the medial and lateral spaces are unequal, the cutting block should be rotated until symmetry is obtained.

The size of the flexion gap should then be compared with that of the extension gap. This is done by using the same spacer block that was used to evaluate the extension gap and placing it between the femoral cutting block and the proximal tibia (**Figure 8,** *B*). The flexion gap should be the same as or 2 mm smaller than the extension gap. If the spacer block is too big or too small, the anterior-posterior femoral cutting block should be raised or lowered until the spacer block fits properly. Medial-lateral stability can again be verified by internally and externally rotating the leg in flexion and ensuring a snug fit with no medial or lateral opening. If there is any doubt as to whether the appropriate femoral rotation will be obtained, the rotation should be compared with the White-side line and the epicondylar axis.

After ensuring that the anterior femoral cortex will not be notched, the final anterior and posterior femoral cuts should be performed (**Figure 9**). This should be followed by the box and chamfer resections, being careful to place the box laterally to optimize patellofemoral tracking. Trial components should then be placed to evaluate stability throughout range of motion. Patellofemoral tracking should be assessed by the "no-thumbs" test.

Patellar tracking should be reassessed with the tourniquet deflated. If

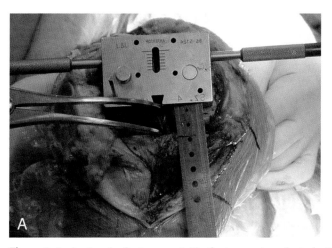 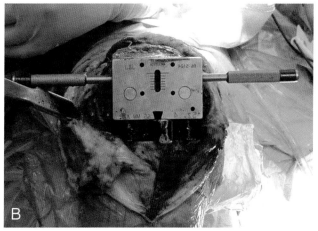

Figure 8 Evaluating the flexion gap. **A,** The flexion gap is evaluated with a lamina spreader. The block should be rotated to create a symmetric flexion gap. **B,** Further evaluation of the flexion gap using a spacer block. (Reproduced with permission from Ranawat AS, Chitranjan CS, Elkus M, Rasquinha VJ, Rossi R, Babhulkar S: Total knee arthroplasty for severe valgus deformity. *J Bone Joint Surg Am* 2005;87(Suppl 1):271-284.)

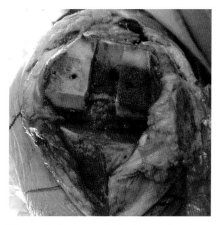

Figure 9 A symmetric flexion gap has been created by bone cuts, not by soft-tissue balancing. (Reproduced with permission from Ranawat AS, Chitranjan CS, Elkus M, Rasquinha VJ, Rossi R, Babhulkar S: Total knee arthroplasty for severe valgus deformity. *J Bone Joint Surg Am* 2005;87(Suppl 1): 271-284.)

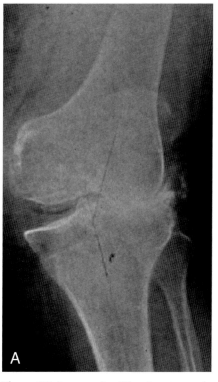 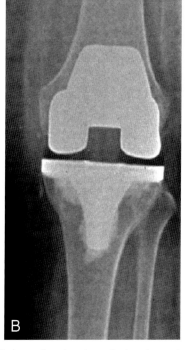

Figure 10 Preoperative (**A**) and postoperative (**B**) AP views of a valgus knee that underwent TKA using the inside-out technique.

maltracking is still evident, the surgeon should reevaluate the position of the trial components. If the trial implants are well aligned and well positioned, we prefer to pie-crust the lateral retinaculum as opposed to performing a formal lateral release.

After irrigating the knee, the osseous surfaces are dried to allow for cement interdigitation. The implants are then cemented into place. Excess ce-

ment is removed, and the cement is allowed to polymerize. A drain is placed, and the capsule is closed with the knee in flexion (**Figure 10**).

Postoperative Regimen

Postoperative management of the valgus knee generally is identical to the regimen used following TKA in a varus knee. One must be vigilant for a peroneal nerve palsy in the early postoperative setting, especially in the setting of correction of a flexion contracture. If any sign of peroneal nerve dysfunction becomes evident, the knee should be flexed and the bandage loosened. Patients begin physical therapy and continuous passive motion on the first postoperative day, and weight bearing is allowed as tolerated.

Bibliography

Aglietti P, Lup D, Cuomo P, Baldini A, De Luca L: Total knee arthroplasty using a pie-crusting technique for valgus deformity. *Clin Orthop Relat Res* 2007;464:73-77.

Anderson JA, Baldini A, MacDonald JH, Pellicci PM, Sculco TP: Primary constrained condylar knee arthroplasty without stem extensions for the valgus knee. *Clin Orthop Relat Res* 2006;442:199-203.

Clarke HD, Fuchs R, Scuderi GR, Scott WN, Insall GN: Clinical results in valgus total knee arthroplasty with the "pie crust" technique of lateral soft tissue releases. *J Arthroplasty* 2005;20:1010-1014.

Clarke HD, Schwartz JB, Math KR, Scuderi GR: Anatomic risk of peroneal nerve injury with the "pie crust" technique for valgus release in total knee arthroplasty. *J Arthroplasty* 2004;19:40-44.

Easley ME, Insall JN, Scuderi GR, Bullek DD: Primary constrained condylar knee arthroplasty for the arthritic valgus knee. *Clin Orthop Relat Res* 2000;380:58-64.

Elkus M, Ranawat CS, Rasquinha VJ, Babhulkar S, Rossi R, Ranawat AS: Total knee arthroplasty for severe valgus deformity: Five to fourteen year follow-up. *J Bone Joint Surg Am* 2004;86-A:2671-2676.

Fiddian NJ, Blakeway C, Kumar A: Replacement arthroplasty of the valgus knee: A modified lateral capsular approach with repositioning of vastus lateralis. *J Bone Joint Surg Br* 1998;80:859-861.

Healy WL, Iorio R, Lemos DW: Medial reconstruction during total knee arthroplasty for severe valgus deformity. *Clin Orthop Relat Res* 1998;356:161-169.

Keblish PA: The lateral approach to the valgus knee: Surgical technique and analysis of 53 cases with over two-year follow-up evaluation..*Clin Orthop Relat Res* 1991;271:52-62.

Krackow KA, Jones MM, Teeny SM, Hungerford DS: Primary total knee arthroplasty in patients with fixed valgus deformity. *Clin Orthop Relat Res* 1991;273:9-18.

Kubiak P, Archibeck MJ, White RE Jr: Cruciate-retaining total knee arthroplasty in patients with at least fifteen degrees of coronal plane deformity. *J Arthroplasty* 2008;23:366-370.

McAuley JP, Collier MB, Hamilton WG, Tabaraee E, Engh GA: Posterior cruciate-retaining total knee arthroplasty for valgus osteoarthritis. *Clin Orthop Relat Res* 2008;466:2644-2649.

Mihalko WM, Krackow KA: Anatomic and biomechanical aspects of pie crusting posterolateral structures for valgus deformity correction in total knee arthroplasty. *J Arthroplasty* 2000;15:347-353.

Miyasaka KC, Ranawat CS, Mullaji A: 10- to 20-year followup of total knee arthroplasty for valgus deformities. *Clin Orthop Relat Res* 1997;345:29-37.

Politi J, Scott R: Balancing severe valgus deformity in total knee arthroplasty using a lateral cruciform retinacular release. *J Arthroplasty* 2004;19:553-557.

Ranawat AS, Ranawat CS, Elkus M, Rasquinha VJ, Rossi R, Babhulkar S: Total knee arthroplasty for severe valgus deformity. *J Bone Joint Surg Am* 2005;87(Suppl 1):271-284.

Whiteside LA: Selective ligament release in total knee arthroplasty of the knee in valgus. *Clin Orthop Relat Res* 1999;367:130-140.

Coding

CPT Codes		Corresponding ICD-9 Codes	
27447	Arthroplasty, knee, condyle and plateau; medial AND lateral compartments with or without patella resurfacing (total knee arthroplasty)	715 715.80	715.16 715.89

CPT copyright © 2010 by the American Medical Association. All rights reserved.

Chapter 27

Total Knee Arthroplasty: Varus Knee

Russell E. Windsor, MD
Yoowang Choi, MD

◼ Indications

Deformity is common in total knee arthroplasty (TKA) patients with osteoarthritis. The deformity can be valgus or varus (coronal plane) or a flexion contracture (sagittal plane). Varus is the type of deformity most commonly encountered. Standard TKA can be performed without release in most knees with correctable varus alignment, but soft-tissue release of the medial collateral ligament (MCL) and medial soft-tissue sleeve is indicated in knees with rigid varus deformity that shows minimal passive correction on valgus stress. Correctable varus alignment may allow the operation to proceed without the need for soft-tissue release. A medial release also is indicated if asymmetry of the flexion and extension spaces with a tight medial space is observed upon tensioning with a laminar spreader or spacer block.

The mechanical axis of the knee is defined by a line drawn from the center of the femoral head to the middle of the mortise of the ankle. A knee is considered to have a neutral mechanical axis when this line passes through the center of the knee at the intercondylar notch. If the line passes to the medial side, the knee is in varus; if the line passes to the lateral side, the knee is in valgus. The mechanical axis can be difficult to determine precisely intraoperatively, so many surgeons instead use the anatomic axis, a line drawn along the long axis of the femur and tibia, to align the knee joint. Using this anatomic axis, the goal in most patients is to preserve or attain final alignment of 4° to 7° of anatomic valgus between the medullary canal axis of the femur and tibia.

Varus knee deformity develops from medial compartment overload, which in turn accelerates articular surface wear. The increased stress on the underlying bone frequently leads to sclerosis of the tibial plateau and a marked decrease in the medial joint space. Usually, in the early stages of the degenerative process, the knee is somewhat symmetric or in slight varus. In knees with this early form of substantial arthritis, the deformity is ordinarily flexible and reducible, and minimal soft-tissue procedures are required to properly balance the knee during replacement.

As the degenerative arthritis progresses, this varus moment in the knee causes the medial soft tissues (MCL, posteromedial capsule, pes anserinus, and semimembranosus muscle) to contract over time, and a fixed, asymmetric deformity of the knee develops. Often, a flexion contracture will accompany a severe varus deformity. Osteophytes frequently develop on the posteromedial aspect of the tibial plateau and can impinge on the MCL, worsening the contracture. The semimembranosus tendon in particular limits exposure of the tibia in its contracted state. Adaptive changes occur in the lateral soft-tissue sleeve as well. Attenuation of the lateral collateral ligament (LCL) and lateral joint capsule appears in severe stages of the arthritic varus deformity, resulting in a lateral thrust during gait. Even though the medial femoral condyle may become eroded in the late stage of arthritis, femoral bone loss on the medial side is less profound than lateral condylar loss in the valgus knee (**Figure 1**). A fixed varus deformity (**Figure 2**), seen in long-standing, advanced arthritis, requires additional soft-tissue procedures to correctly balance the knee when performing a TKA.

Dr. Windsor or a member of his immediate family has received royalties from Zimmer and has received research or institutional support from Ortho Biotech. Neither Dr. Choi nor any immediate family member has received anything of value from or owns stock in a commercial company or institution related directly or indirectly to the subject of this chapter.

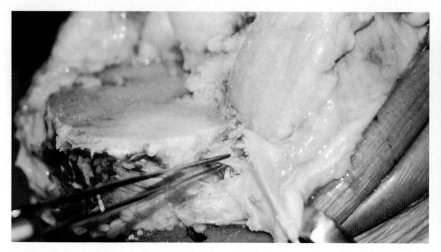

Figure 1 Medial anatomy of the knee, after resection of the proximal tibia. Note the semi-membranosus tendon (held by forceps) and eburnated medial femoral condyle. Residual medial tibial plateau sclerosis is present after resection.

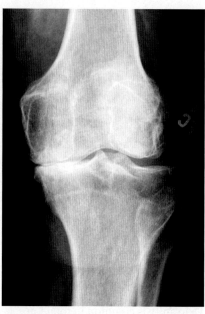

Figure 2 AP radiograph demonstrates advanced medial joint osteoarthritis and a fixed varus deformity of the knee.

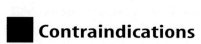

Contraindications

Medial collateral release is contraindicated in knees with correctable varus deformity because of the danger of rendering the medial side unstable by overcorrection of the deformity. The surgeon must assess the medial side carefully by performing a valgus stress test. With a rapidly progressive arthritic deformity, medial opening of the joint is commonly demonstrated when a valgus stress is applied to the knee. With long-standing arthritis and long-term progressive varus deformity, frequently no medial side opening is seen on valgus stress, and a medial release is required.

Alternative Treatments

There are no alternative treatments. To address varus knees with a significant lateral thrust, imbrication of the LCL has been described by Krackow. This technique involves a transection of the LCL and "pants-over-vest" repair to shorten the ligament. This technique or imbrications of the LCL in a similar manner may not provide sufficient stability in flexion and extension and will not address tightness on the medial side of the knee.

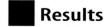

Results

The importance of alignment and soft-tissue balance after TKA cannot be overemphasized because they play an important role in the long-term results of TKA. Asymmetry of the medial and lateral flexion spaces may cause excessive tightness on the medial side. This asymmetric stress due to an excessive tensioning of an unreleased MCL has been implicated in premature polyethylene wear and stiffness. This clinical situation also may contribute to continuous, unexplained pain because of excessive tightness on the medial side leading to pain at the proximal and distal insertions of the ligament.

Clinical studies have shown that malalignment greater than 3° in varus or valgus may be associated with earlier failure of the tibial component. Similarly, alignment of the components in neutral position is an important predictor of favorable long-term results. This can be explained by the increased contact pressure created by varus tibial alignment with edge loading.

Biomechanical studies conducted by Green and associates found varus tibial malalignment increases posteromedial and anteromedial tibial surface strains. This can cause medial tibial cancellous bone overload with failure through medial tibial collapse. Keating and associates described how this overload can lead to an osteolytic lesion that may heal or progress to implant failure.

Techniques

Setup/Exposure

The patient is placed in the supine position. A standard medial parapatellar approach is preferred because it allows full exposure of the distal femur and proximal tibia and can be extended proximally or distally to give greater exposure (**Figure 3**). This approach permits excellent exposure to the medial and lateral soft-tissue sleeves and allows soft-tissue procedures to be performed on either the medial or lat-

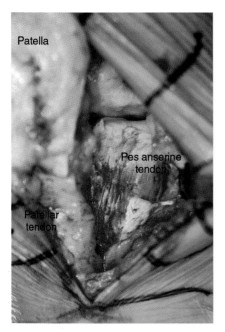

Figure 3 Midline longitudinal incision with medial arthrotomy. The patella is to the left of the joint line. A bent Hohmann retractor is placed beneath the MCL around the posterior aspect of the tibia, and the pes anserine tendons are seen inserting on the tibia to the left of the retractor.

eral side of the knee. Alternatively, the subvastus or midvastus approach may be used, but the exposure will be more limited.

Instruments/Equipment/ Implants Required

No special instruments are required other than straight and curved osteotomes. Laminar spreaders are useful for assessing the flexion space and extension space by opening up the flexion space and placing tension on the collateral ligaments before, during, and after medial release. In cases of severe, fixed varus deformity greater than 25°, a constrained condylar implant system should be readily available on standby, if significant instability remains after full release of the medial soft-tissue structures.

Procedure

The technique chosen depends on the severity of varus deformity. **Table 1**

Table 1 Surgical Techniques Indicated for Varus Deformities

Technique	Indication
Standard medial exposure	Least severe rigid deformity
Distal release of superficial MCL	Moderately severe rigid deformity
Medial femoral epicondylar osteotomy (controversial)	Very severe rigid deformity
Tibial downsizing and vertical resection of medial proximal tibia and osteophytes (used as adjunct to medial soft-tissue release)	Very severe rigid deformity with medial tibial erosion
Lateral ligament advance (controversial)	The most severe deformities, with significant lateral collateral laxity and lateral thrust during gait

MCL = medial collateral ligament.

presents an outline of how to proceed when correcting this deformity.

Varus deformity can be corrected with either a posterior cruciate ligament (PCL)–retaining design or a PCL-substituting design. Sacrificing the PCL will change the tension of the ligaments in both flexion and extension. The relative merits of these two main design categories remain somewhat controversial, but both can yield equally good results in knees with mild varus deformities. Some data show, however, that a cruciate-substituting design may provide advantages in knees with severe varus deformity.

Fixed varus deformity can be corrected by a single, progressive release of the superficial MCL. Intermittent checks on stability should be performed either manually or by laminar spreaders to avoid overzealous release and overcorrection of the deformity.

TECHNIQUE 1

A standard medial exposure of the knee, which involves a sequential release of medial soft tissues, is performed most frequently for standard fixed varus deformities. Using subperiosteal dissection with a scalpel or electrocautery, the anteromedial tibial soft-tissue sleeve is released 2 cm below the medial joint line (**Figure 4, A**)

and osteophytes are removed (**Figure 4, B**). Next, the posteromedial capsule and tibial attachment of the semi-membranosus are released (**Figure 4, C**). Progressive release of the semimembranosus tendon does not affect MCL balancing, but it can contribute to the balancing of an accompanying flexion contracture. These steps are performed sequentially, and medial soft-tissue release and osteophyte removal may be sufficient to attain balanced tension and an equal flexion/extension space (**Figure 4, D**).

A subperiosteal dissection of the medial tibia is performed. The tibial bone resection should be perpendicular to the long axis of the tibia. Less than 10 mm of bone should be removed from the lateral (intact) side. A small sclerotic surface of the medial tibial plateau may remain, or a bone defect may still be present. "Chasing" a medial bone defect (ie, making the tibial resection at the lowest point of the medial tibial defect) by performing a more aggressive proximal tibial resection is not recommended in most cases, especially when severe medial tibial bone loss is present. By chasing the defect, softer cancellous bone is encountered and the proximal coverage of the resected tibia may become smaller. On occasion, the tibial component can be shifted slightly laterally,

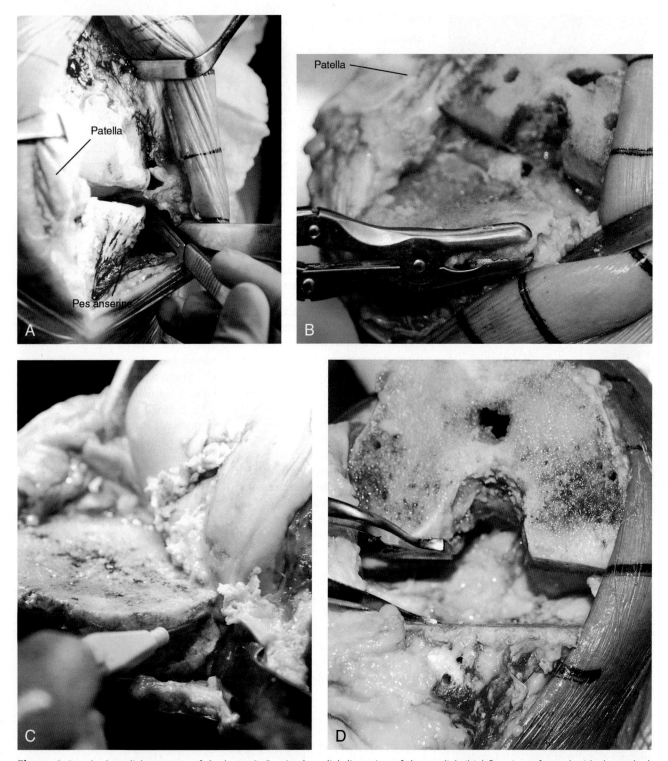

Figure 4 Standard medial exposure of the knee. **A,** Proximal medial dissection of the medial tibial flare is performed with the scalpel. Electrocautery also may be used. The deep portion of the MCL is released from its proximal tibial insertion. The pes anserine tendons remain attached distally to the right of the scalpel. The patella is everted. **B,** Complete removal of residual medial osteophytes is mandatory to eliminate their tethering effect on the MCL. **C,** The distal insertion of the semimembranosus tendon is frequently released in contracted varus deformities. The release also facilitates exposure of the proximal tibial plateau during tibial stem preparation and implantation. **D,** A laminar spreader is placed to apply maximum tension on the MCL. A symmetric space is seen here; no MCL release is necessary.

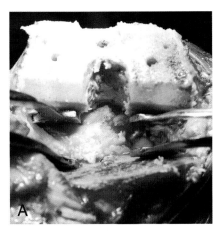
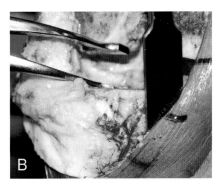
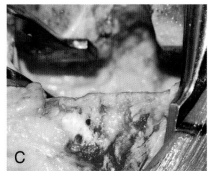

Figure 5 Balancing the flexion/extension space. **A,** Tensioning of the flexion space with laminar spreaders gives a good indication of the need for MCL release. Notice the asymmetric, trapezoidal space that is seen in this patient. **B,** An osteotome is used to strip the distal insertion of the MCL. **C,** The osteotome is passed subperiosteally until it is fully stripped from its insertion. With minimally invasive approaches, the osteotome face frequently disappears down the medial side of the tibia.

away from a medial bone defect, so that it rests on healthier, intact bone. Residual medial osteophytes are removed after tibial resection (**Figure 5**). For the sclerotic surface, fixation holes are created for fixation of polymethylmethacrylate (PMMA). Defects of the medial tibial plateau can be addressed with cement, a metal augment, or bone grafts.

TECHNIQUE 2

Release of the superficial MCL at the point of maximum tension enables balancing of the flexion and extension spaces in cases of severe, rigid varus deformities. The deep insertion of the MCL at the joint line is released during normal exposure. When further release of the superficial insertion of the MCL is required, however, it is performed at its distal tibial insertion. The release of the superficial MCL is particularly useful in treating moderate to severe varus deformity. Bone resections are done first to allow tensioning of the MCL as the flexion and extension gaps are assessed. A trapezoidal space that is narrower medially indicates the need for MCL release (**Figure 5,** *A*). The release is done by using a straight or curved osteotome to strip the distal insertion of the MCL (**Figure 5,** *B*). The knee is placed in

either flexion or extension and a laminar spreader is inserted to tension the MCL. The tightest portion of the superficial MCL can be felt to release as the osteotome is passed distally and subperiosteally. The release is continued until tension on the laminar spreader is reduced and the deformity is corrected. Essentially, the superficial MCL is "stripped and stretched" and the trapezoidal gap becomes rectangular and symmetric. Sometimes, it is necessary to tension a laminar spreader placed in the medial compartment of the knee with the knee in flexion to release the ligament (**Figure 6**). After release, particular attention should be given to using a spacer block to assess proper sizing of the tibial insert required to maintain this symmetry with stability. After release, an increase of one size of tibial insert may be necessary to account for the released dimension, especially if the patient demonstrated a lateral thrust with attenuation of the LCL. This technique is widely considered the standard MCL release for varus deformity.

TECHNIQUE 3

Medial femoral epicondylar osteotomy is indicated for the most severe rigid varus deformities. This

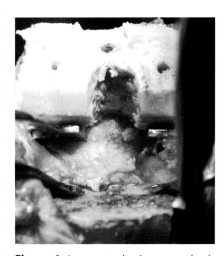

Figure 6 A separate laminar spreader is placed in the medial and lateral parts of the flexion gap. After the osteotome is passed distally to release the distal MCL insertion, the laminar spreader on the medial side is tensioned to further fine-tune the release and stretch the MCL insertion from the site of its distal release.

technique, developed by Engh and Ammeen, is performed infrequently. A medial epicondylar osteotomy can be used in severe varus deformity with a fixed flexion contracture of the knee and can be performed either before or after the bone resections. The reported advantage of the epicondylar osteotomy is that the integrity of the MCL is maintained and it facilitates the approach to the posterior femoral condyle for additional capsular release.

The procedure is performed by excising the synovial tissue from the medial femoral condyle to expose the epicondyle. The osteotomy is performed with a 1.25-in osteotome directed in the long axis of the femur with the knee placed in 90° of flexion. A wafer of bone approximately 1 cm thick and 4 cm in diameter is separated from the condyle. The insertion of the adductor magnus tendon provides proximal stability to the osteotomized segment of bone while the knee is in extension. The knee is temporarily unstable in flexion on the medial side. The deep and superficial MCL segments are not damaged. Stability in extension is maintained by the proximal to distal continuity of the collateral ligaments and the adductor magnus tendon. Electrocautery release of the posteromedial joint capsule can be performed, if necessary, to correct a flexion contracture. After implantation of total knee components, the epicondylar osteotomy is repaired by reattaching the epicondyle to the medial femoral condyle with No. 2 or heavier nonabsorbable suture. The repair is done with the knee in 90° of flexion to ensure proper placement of the osteotomized wafer of bone, usually placed somewhat distal and posterior to the original location. Sutures are placed through the epicondyle and then beneath a bridge of metaphyseal cortical bone that represents the junction between the anterior femoral resection and the adjacent epicondylar osteotomy. A minimum of two to three sutures is recommended to restore the knee stability in flexion.

TECHNIQUE 4

As an alternative for the very severe, rigid varus deformity, tibial downsizing and vertical resection of the medial proximal tibia and resection of osteophytes can be performed. The procedure, first described by Dixon and associates, is recommended as an adjunct to the medial soft-tissue release described earlier for moderate to severe varus deformity. The bone resections are made in the usual manner, and trial components are used to assess mediolateral balancing. If a trapezoidal extension gap with tightness on the medial side is observed, the tibial tray that demonstrates good coverage of the cut tibial surface is downsized by one size. The downsized tibial component is lateralized to the lateral tibial cortical margin and the remaining medial tibial overhang is removed flush with the medial edge of the tibial tray by a vertical saw cut.

By downsizing and lateralizing the tibial component and removing the exposed medial proximal tibial bone around the component, the MCL is indirectly lengthened. This technique shortens the distance between the origin and insertion of the medial ligamentous structures without the need for an extensive medial soft-tissue release.

The disadvantage of this technique is that the forces across the joint through the polyethylene and fixation interface are increased slightly as a result of downsizing the tibial component. However, an even distribution is always preferred over uneven stress. This procedure is best reserved for cases when the tibial component is found to be between sizes.

TECHNIQUE 5

Ligament advancement on the attenuated lateral side as described by Krackow is indicated for severe varus deformities with significant lateral collateral laxity and large lateral thrust during gait. It is done to prevent overlengthening of the leg after release of the MCL. In a severely deformed varus knee, the LCL and lateral joint capsule can be attenuated or, on rare occasions, even ruptured, causing instability and overlengthening of the leg to compensate for the instability. On these infrequent occasions, ligament advancement procedures or reconstruction of lateral ligaments can be done. Lateral ligament advancement is done by resecting the attachment of the LCL from a segment of proximal fibula and then reattaching the fibular head by an intramedullary screw distally, tightening the ligament. Also, the LCL can be advanced proximally at the femoral attachment and fixed with a washer and screw.

Wound Closure

Wound closure after TKA with medial release is the same regardless of the technique used to correct the varus deformity. The medial arthrotomy is closed with interrupted No. 0 Vicryl suture. The distal aspect of the medial arthrotomy not infrequently becomes somewhat difficult to approximate because of the relative stripping of the soft tissues and lengthening of the leg on the medial side. Usually the medial and lateral portions of the arthrotomy in this area can be brought together using figure-of-8 sutures with absorbable No. 0 Vicryl suture. The subcutaneous layer is closed with a combination of No. 0 and No. 2-0 Vicryl suture. Staples are used to close the skin.

———————————————■

■ Avoiding Pitfalls and Complications

Several key principles must be adhered to when performing a TKA for varus knee. Orientation of the tibial bone resection should be perpendicular to the long axis of the tibial intramedullary canal. Distal femoral resection aims to attain 4° to 7° of valgus relative to the femoral medullary canal. A rectangular flexion and extension gap should be produced after soft-tissue balancing, with less than 2 to 3 mm of movement during varus and valgus stress. Proper femoral rotational alignment should be achieved for proper symmetry with the proximal tibial resection and to ensure that the patellar mechanism is not tilting or subluxating in flexion.

Overrelease of the MCL usually can be avoided by intermittently checking the balance while doing the soft-tissue release. When adequate flexion and extension balance cannot be achieved, conversion to a constrained implant is appropriate. This is required less often for varus deformities than for valgus deformities, but some severe medial varus deformities may require added constraint.

Rotational alignment of the femoral component will affect balancing of the varus knee, especially if the component is placed in an internally rotated orientation. Care should be taken to reference femoral resections from the epicondylar axis and the Whiteside line. The flexion gap on the medial side will be tight in flexion if the femoral component is medially rotated with a balanced extension gap.

Thus, internal rotation of the femoral component in varus knee deformities should be avoided.

If the surgeon prefers to use a cruciate-retaining design, the PCL may have to be balanced. If this cannot be achieved, conversion to a PCL-substituting design may be considered.

Bibliography

Dixon MC, Brown RR, Parsch D, Scott RD: Modular fixed-bearing total knee arthroplasty with retention of the posterior cruciate ligament: A study of patients followed for a minimum of fifteen years. *J Bone Joint Surg Am* 2005;87(3):598-603.

Engh GA, Ammeen D: Results of total knee arthroplasty with medial epicondylar osteotomy to correct varus deformity. *Clin Orthop Relat Res* 1999;367(367):141-148.

Green DL, Bahniuk E, Liebelt RA, Fender E, Mirkov P: Biplane radiographic measurements of reversible displacement (including clinical loosening) and migration of total joint replacements. *J Bone Joint Surg Am* 1983;65(8):1134-1143.

Keating EM, Meding JB, Faris PM, Ritter MA: Long-term followup of nonmodular total knee replacements. *Clin Orthop Relat Res* 2002;404(404):34-39.

Krackow KA: Deformity, in Krackow KA, ed: *The Technique of Total Knee Arthroplasty*. St. Louis, MO, CV Mosby, 1990, pp 329-332.

Laskin RS, Rieger M, Schob C, Turen C: The posterior-stabilized total knee prosthesis in the knee with a severe fixed deformity. *Am J Knee Surg* 1989;1:199-203.

Rand JA, Ilstrup DM: Survivorship analysis of total knee arthroplasty: Cumulative rates of survival of 9200 total knee arthroplasties. *J Bone Joint Surg Am* 1991;73(3):397-409.

Coding

CPT Code		Corresponding ICD-9 Codes	
27447	Arthroplasty, knee, condyle and plateau; medial AND lateral compartments with or without patella resurfacing (total knee arthroplasty)	711.15 711.35 736.6	711.25 711.45 755.64

Chapter 28

Total Knee Arthroplasty for Distal Femoral Fracture in the Elderly Patient

Michael E. Berend, MD
Keith R. Berend, MD

Indications

Primary total knee arthroplasty (TKA) is indicated in an elderly patient following distal femoral fracture in the presence of severe fracture comminution and concurrent bone loss and for some fractures that disrupt the collateral and cruciate ligamentous insertions on the femur (**Figure 1**). The term *elderly* is used here to describe patients with lower functional goals and potential for rehabilitation; it therefore is related to both physiologic and chronologic age. The patient with significant joint destruction, arthrosis prior to the fracture, or hardware retained from prior surgery about the knee also may be a candidate for primary TKA. Other candidates for primary TKA include the patient with multiple medical problems who would benefit from early rehabilitation and the patient with severe osteo-porosis for whom it would be difficult to perform open reduction and internal fixation (ORIF) with or without bone grafting.

TKA provides immediate knee stability and the ability to bear weight, allowing rapid mobilization of elderly (and low-demand) patients. The primary TKA implant most likely to avoid nonunion, malunion, and the morbidity associated with fracture treatment in these patients is a rotating-hinge prosthesis. The patient with extensor mechanism dysfunction or injury may be a candidate for a rigid or linked-hinge–type prosthesis. Diaphyseal implant fixation in the femur is most often necessary, and therefore the proximal femur and hip should be evaluated for the presence of any implants that might interfere (**Figure 2**).

Contraindications

Active infection, severe soft-tissue fracture blisters, and limited blood supply to the extremity are contraindications to primary TKA in this population.

Alternative Treatments

Younger patients with adequate bone stock and without severe comminution may be appropriate candidates for ORIF with bone grafting. Locking plates and intramedullary rods are the most common treatment options in these patients. Concerns about adequate protected weight bearing, range of motion, and facilitating a stable fracture union must be balanced when deciding between ORIF and primary TKA in patients with a distal femoral fracture.

Results

Results of primary TKA after distal femoral fracture are inferior to those

Michael E. Berend or an immediate family member serves as a board member, owner, officer, or committee member of the Piedmont Orthopaedic Society, the American Association of Hip and Knee Surgeons, The Knee Society, and the Mooresville Ambulatory Surgery Center; has received royalties from Biomet; is a member of a speakers' bureau or has made paid presentations on behalf of Biomet; serves as a paid consultant to or is an employee of Biomet; and has received research or institutional support from Biomet, MCS, St. Francis Hospital, and ERMI. Keith R. Berend or an immediate family member serves as a board member, owner, officer, or committee member of Mount Carmel New Albany Surgical Hospital and the American Association of Hip and Knee Surgeons Education Committee; has received royalties from Biomet; serves as a paid consultant to or is an employee of Biomet, Salient Surgical, and Synvasive; has received research or institutional support from Biomet; and owns stock or stock options in Angiotech.

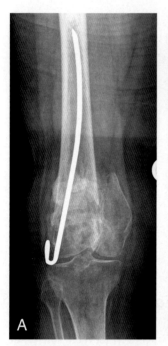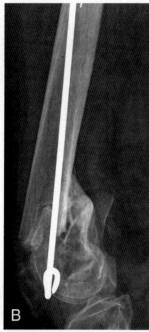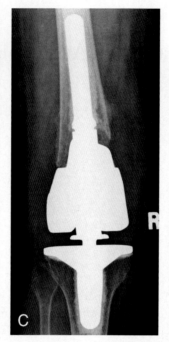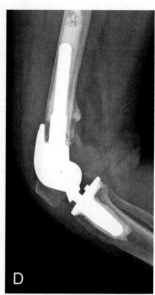

Figure 1 Radiographs of a comminuted distal femoral fracture in an elderly patient. Because the patient had cardiac instability, rod fixation was used to achieve temporary fixation until the patient could be cleared for TKA. Preoperative AP (**A**) and lateral (**B**) views. The patient was treated with TKA using a rotating-platform prosthesis with cemented stems. A temporary rod that had been placed to achieve stability was removed during the TKA. Postoperative AP (**C**) and lateral (**D**) views.

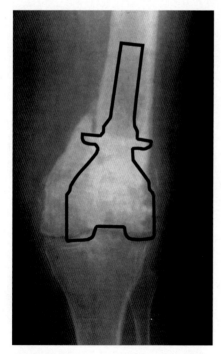

Figure 2 Preoperative planning for a TKA in a patient with a distal femoral fracture is demonstrated on an AP radiograph. The distance from the proximal extent of the fracture to the joint line is measured with a template. This serves as a starting point for creating the implant trial.

of primary TKA for other diagnoses such as osteoarthritis or inflammatory arthritis in this unique subset of elderly patients. Postoperative Knee Society scores, when grouped with other patients receiving similar implants, ranged from 100 to 131 points. Postoperative range of motion averaged 93° to 97°, which is more limited than the range of motion seen in patients who undergo primary TKA with standard implants without fracture, who average a 114° arc of motion, or those who undergo revision TKA with similar prostheses without fracture, who average 112°.

Reported survivorship at midterm, considering revision as an end point, ranges from 67% to 94%. Reliable data on long-term survivorship are limited; the mean follow-up in most studies is less than 7 years (**Table 1**). Failures have been reported in similar patients treated with ORIF, but it may not be appropriate to compare these different cohorts. Patient selection bias likely plays a strong role in these outcomes

and should be considered when weighing the multiple medical risks, differences in mobilization, and restoration of function of ORIF versus TKA.

Technique

Setup/Exposure

The patient is positioned supine on the operating table. Additional assistance is required to maintain longitudinal traction on the limb during skin preparation. After administration of prophylactic antibiotics, a thigh tourniquet is placed well proximal to the knee and inflated to 250 mg Hg. Exposure is achieved through an extensile medial parapatellar arthrotomy. A quadriceps snip obliquely across the superior portion of the quadriceps tendon proximal to the patella can provide additional proximal exposure. Soft-tissue dissection is continued about the fracture site subperiosteally;

Table 1 Results for Rotating-Hinge Devices

Authors (Year)	Number of Knees	Implant Type	Mean Patient Age (Range)	Mean Follow-up in Months	Survivorship
Barrack et al (2000)	16	S-ROM (DePuy Orthopaedics, Warsaw, IN)	69	51	94%
Westrich et al (2000)	24	Finn (Biomet, Warsaw, IN)	63	33	92%
Springer et al (2001)	69	Kinematic (Stryker Orthopaedics, Mahwah, NJ)	72	75	67%
Springer et al (2004)	26	Kinematic (Stryker Orthopaedics)	72	59	73%
Berend and Lombardi (2009)	39	Orthopaedic Salvage System (OSS) (Biomet)	76	46	87%

comminuted distal femoral fragments are removed. When dissecting in the posterior aspect of the knee, it is critical to protect the neurovascular bundle as it emerges from the adductor hiatus; this often is adjacent to the proximal extent of the fracture. Elevating the limb and using electrocautery to subperiosteally skeletonize the distal femur may be helpful. Dissection is carried proximally to the level of the diaphyseal portion of the fracture, at which point a transverse osteotomy is made to freshen the end of the femoral diaphysis.

Procedure

BONE PREPARATION AND IMPLANT CONSIDERATIONS

The femoral canal is prepared with tapered reamers to a depth of 100 to 150 mm. This allows the positioning of either a straight or bowed femoral stem to obtain proximal implant fixation. More distal fractures may require a bowed femoral stem to bypass the diaphyseal bow of the femur, whereas more proximal fractures may be better matched with a straight stem. The tibia and patella are prepared in routine fashion for knee arthroplasty and insertion of a rotating-hinge–type prosthesis. Most often, a short-

stemmed tibial component can be used in the patient with minimal tibial deformity. Patellar resurfacing may be indicated in the patient who has severe osteoporosis. If extensor mechanism dysfunction, subluxation, a prior patellar problem, or acute trauma is present, a linked-hinge–type device should be available, because the extensor mechanism is critical for appropriate balance and control of the flexion gap. The absence of the extensor mechanism in flexion creates a soft-tissue imbalance in which the flexion gap is much larger than the extension gap, so in these situations, a linked-hinge–type device, which prevents implant subluxation in flexion, should be considered.

TRIAL REDUCTION AND IMPLANT ROTATION

Trial reduction is performed with distal femoral replacement segments of various lengths to determine which length reestablishes the joint line at the appropriate level. The joint line also can be referenced relative to the inferior pole of the patella, which is approximately 1 cm proximal to the joint line. In addition, radiographs of the contralateral knee are helpful for showing the position of the joint line

relative to the patella in the patient's unoperated knee (**Figure 3**).

Because the epicondylar landmarks are no longer present in these patients, assessing the rotational position of the femoral prosthesis is challenging. The femoral rotation is most easily determined in reference to the tibia at 90° of flexion with the trial tibial component and rotating-platform polyethylene in place. Medial-lateral flexion gap balance, symmetry with respect to the extension gap, and femoral length should be assessed simultaneously during trial reduction. Evaluating the extensor mechanism tension, including patellar tracking, with the trial implants in place also helps assess femoral rotation (**Figure 4**). Despite the fact that the collateral ligament soft-tissue envelope has no femoral attachments following fracture removal, the tension in this soft-tissue envelope about the knee may help guide extension gap balance and femoral length.

The rotation of the trial femoral prosthesis is marked on the remaining proximal femoral bone and recreated at the time of final implant insertion. Various thicknesses of rotating-hinge bearings may be trialed to re-create soft-tissue tension, full extension, and a stable flexion gap with the extensor

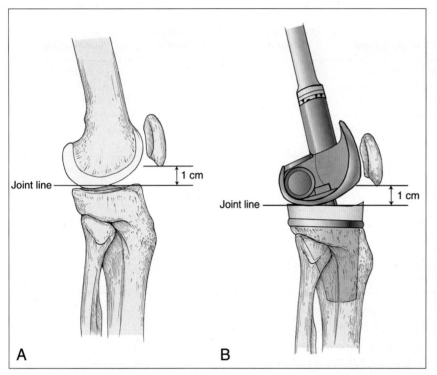

Figure 3 Drawings demonstrate the use of the patella as a reference point for joint line restoration when the distal femur is fractured or absent. **A,** Using the contralateral knee as a reference, the joint line is placed approximately 1 cm from the inferior pole of the patella. **B,** The implant is shown in place.

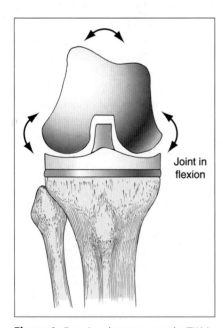

Figure 4 Drawing demonstrates the TKA in flexion. Determining the correct rotational position of the femoral implant is challenging when the epicondyles are absent. The medial and lateral soft-tissue balance is assessed using the tibia as a reference.

mechanism repositioned. The surgeon should take care not to insert the implant too proximal, as this results in insufficient implant polyethylene thickness to balance the final gaps after cementation.

PROSTHESIS IMPLANTATION

Trial implants often are complex and use many modular parts; therefore, prior to implantation, the implant should be assembled on the back table according to the manufacturer's specifications for tapers and stem attachments. Following this, a proximal cement restrictor is inserted in the femur to the appropriate depth. The bony surfaces are prepared with pulsatile lavage and dried. Femoral preparation parallels the technique used for cemented hip replacement stem insertion. Antibiotic-impregnated polymethylmethacrylate (PMMA) is mixed and pressurized into the femo-

ral canal and applied to the metaphyseal tibial bone; then the components are cemented in place. The tibia is cemented first, followed by the femoral implant. A trial rotating-platform bearing is inserted, and the knee is held in extension while the cement hardens. The routine use of antibiotic in cement in the elderly patient with medical comorbidities remains controversial; however, this practice is standard at both authors' centers.

Following cementation, the final polyethylene insert selection is made, and the rotating platform yoke assembly is inserted. When selecting a polyethylene bearing, the surgeon should keep in mind the goal of re-creating remaining soft-tissue tension and joint line balance. Care should be taken to avoid hyperextension caused by leaving the extensor gap too loose because this may increase the likelihood of early implant failure, especially in the patient with a high body mass index or high activity level.

Wound Closure

Wound closure begins with thorough irrigation and closure of the medial arthrotomy with figure-of-8 absorbable sutures. If a quadriceps snip was performed, this is reinforced with nonabsorbable sutures in a figure-of-8 fashion. We do not modify the postoperative physical therapy prescription if a quadriceps snip was performed. Subcutaneous closure is performed with absorbable sutures over a drain, and the skin is reapproximated with staples. A bulky, soft dressing is applied, and the tourniquet is let down at the completion of the surgery. Many surgeons' anesthesia programs include a periarticular injection in the knee prior to closure, with the goal of reducing postoperative pain and bleeding.

Postoperative Regimen

The postoperative course begins with appropriate risk stratification for deep vein thrombosis. This patient population often is considered to be at a higher risk because of age, reduced activity level, and multiple medical comorbidities. A multimodal prophylaxis treatment program should be used, including mechanical and pharmacologic modalities such as pneumatic compression devices, compression stockings, and warfarin. Bridge therapy with low-molecular-weight heparin also may be considered.

Physical therapy involves ambulation on postoperative day one, with immediate full weight bearing with supervised walker assistance and progressive ambulation. Continuous passive motion is not routinely used. Care should be taken to protect the heels, buttocks, and other bony prominence to avoid skin breakdown in the perioperative period. A primary advantage of prosthetic reconstruction in contrast to ORIF is that weight bearing and range-of-motion exercises can start immediately and do not have to be delayed during fracture healing. Radiographs are obtained either intraoperatively or in the recovery room, with follow-up at 2 months, 6 months, 1 year, and then biannually.

Avoiding Pitfalls and Complications

We strongly believe in a multidisciplinary approach to caring for the arthroplasty patient, and even more so with elderly patients with fractures treated with immediate TKA. The multidisciplinary approach includes an internal medicine evaluation; treatment of any underlying cardiopulmonary or renal diseases, hypertension, or diabetes; and coordination of care, particularly in patients taking multiple medications. Common complications in this patient population include pneumonia, deep vein thrombosis, skin ulceration, and urinary tract infection. Some complications can be avoided with discontinuation of Foley catheters early in the postoperative course (postoperative day 1 or 2), rapid mobilization, incentive spirometry, and a team approach. Because of the extent of the surgery, there is an increased likelihood of superficial and deep wound infection. Appropriate prophylactic intravenous antibiotics should be administered preoperatively, as well as three to four doses within the 24 hours following the surgery operation. We also use antibiotic-impregnated bone cement in these patients to further reduce the risk of infection. The risks and possible complications of the surgery should be discussed preoperatively with the patient and family. Periprosthetic fracture around the tip of a long-stemmed prosthesis may be an inherent risk in this population because of osteoporosis and increased risk of falls postoperatively. In the patient with a peripheral nerve block, the use of a knee immobilizer may prevent falls during the early hospitalization period. Internal rotation of the femoral prosthesis may result in patellofemoral dysfunction, lateral subluxation, and uncontrolled flexion or rotational instability in this complex patient population.

Bibliography

Appleton P, Moran M, Houshian S, Robinson CM: Distal femoral fractures treated by hinged total knee replacement in elderly patients. *J Bone Joint Surg Br* 2006;88(8):1065-1070.

Barrack RL: Evolution of the rotating hinge for complex total knee arthroplasty. *Clin Orthop Relat Res* 2001;392:292-299.

Barrack RL, Lyons TR, Ingraham RQ, Johnson JC: The use of a modular rotating hinge component in salvage revision total knee arthroplasty. *J Arthroplasty* 2000;15(7):858-866.

Berend KR, Lombardi AV Jr: Distal femoral replacement in nontumor cases with severe bone loss and instability. *Clin Orthop Relat Res* 2009;467(2):485-492.

Harrison RJ Jr, Thacker MM, Pitcher JD, Temple HT, Scully SP: Distal femur replacement is useful in complex total knee arthroplasty revisions. *Clin Orthop Relat Res* 2006;446:113-120.

Hossain F, Patel S, Haddad FS: Midterm assessment of causes and results of revision total knee arthroplasty. *Clin Orthop Relat Res* 2010;468(5):1221-1228.

Jones RE, Barrack RL, Skedros J: Modular, mobile-bearing hinge total knee arthroplasty. *Clin Orthop Relat Res* 2001;392:306-314.

Jones RE, Skedros JG, Chan AJ, Beauchamp DH, Harkins PC: Total knee arthroplasty using the S-ROM mobile-bearing hinge prosthesis. *J Arthroplasty* 2001;16(3):279-287.

Petrou G, Petrou H, Tilkeridis C, et al: Medium-term results with a primary cemented rotating-hinge total knee replacement: A 7- to 15-year follow-up. *J Bone Joint Surg Br* 2004;86(6):813-817.

Ritter MA, Berend ME, Meding JB, Keating EM, Faris PM, Crites BM: Long-term followup of anatomic graduated components posterior cruciate-retaining total knee replacement. *Clin Orthop Relat Res* 2001;388:51-57.

Springer BD, Hanssen AD, Sim FH, Lewallen DG: The kinematic rotating hinge prosthesis for complex knee arthroplasty. *Clin Orthop Relat Res* 2001;392:283-291.

Springer BD, Sim FH, Hanssen AD, Lewallen DG: The modular segmental kinematic rotating hinge for nonneoplastic limb salvage. *Clin Orthop Relat Res* 2004;421:181-187.

Westrich GH, Mollano AV, Sculco TP, Buly RL, Laskin RS, Windsor R: Rotating hinge total knee arthroplasty in severely affected knees. *Clin Orthop Relat Res* 2000;379:195-208.

Coding

CPT Code		Corresponding ICD-9 Codes	
27447	Arthroplasty, knee, condyle and plateau; medial AND lateral compartments with or without patella resurfacing (total knee arthroplasty)	711.15 711.35 711.55	711.25 711.45 711.65

CPT copyright © 2010 by the American Medical Association. All rights reserved.

Chapter 29

Bilateral Total Knee Arthroplasty

Robert E. Booth, Jr, MD

Indications

Several strategies are currently used for the surgical treatment of severe arthritis of both knees. Total knee arthroplasty (TKA) procedures can be staged, staggered, or simultaneous. Staged bilateral TKA, which requires a second hospital stay, a second anesthetic, and a surgical interval of weeks or months, is the most common. Staggered procedures, which involve a single hospital stay but a second anesthetic exposure, are the least popular. Simultaneous bilateral total knee arthroplasty (SBTKA), which involves either concurrent (two-team) or sequential (one-team) surgeries, are the most controversial strategy. Evaluating these strategies is complicated by the fact that various anesthesia choices, surgical volumes and skill levels, instrumentation options, patient selection criteria, and postoperative regimens are involved. No one strategy can be clearly substantiated and endorsed; however, the following discussion is intended to guide those who choose to perform SBTKAs.

Strong indications for SBTKA include nonambulators, patients with insurance that does not allow two hospitalizations, and most particularly those with such severe deformity—in

addition to pain and dysfunction—that the rehabilitation of the operated knee would be severely compromised by the contralateral knee (**Figure 1**). Several centers performing SBTKA have demonstrated improved outcomes as a result of this approach. A difficult situation that sometimes occurs is when a patient presents with one severely radiographically arthritic knee and one knee that is less deformed yet clinically more painful (**Figure 2**). Ideally, the patient can be persuaded to allow surgery on the less painful side or SBTKA, but if not, the surgeon is in the uncomfortable position of operating on less severe pathology, with a less salubrious outcome and with a second procedure required expeditiously.

Softer indications for SBTKA include a patient who insists on a single surgery, a patient who fears losing a job by being out of work twice, and a high-demand patient in whom a solitary arthroplasty would diminish pain but not restore the function the patient requires. Some elderly patients who live alone and have no family support opt for SBTKA to ensure their admission to an acute care rehabilitation center rather than a subacute nursing home. The cost-effectiveness of SBTKA is unquestionable; however, most of the

benefits accrue to the hospitals and insurance companies, because since 1992, surgeons in the United States have been paid only 50% for the "second side" in SBTKA. This dispensation may modify the enthusiasm of some surgeons for SBTKA.

Contraindications

The primary contraindications to SBTKA are age and fragility, which are often hard to quantify. Even a single TKA is a biologic insult, and SBTKA creates at least twice the physiologic stress. The impact of comorbidities, particularly cardiopulmonary disease, is important in assessing a patient's risk for SBTKA. Many institutions that perform a high percentage of SBTKAs require extensive medical clearance—including a cardiac stress test—to filter out the frail patients. This effort is facilitated by using a small but select team of cardiologists and internists who become familiar with the preoperative assessment and postoperative management issues associated with SBTKA. My practice is to perform not only primary SBTKA but also simultaneous revision TKA on one knee and primary TKA on the other (**Figure 3**) as well as bilateral revisions, all of which elevate even further the need for preoperative scrutiny.

Dr. Booth or an immediate family member serves as a paid consultant to or is an employee of Zimmer.

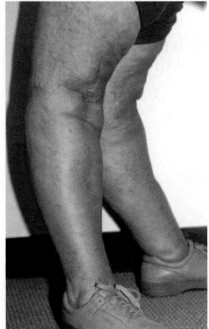
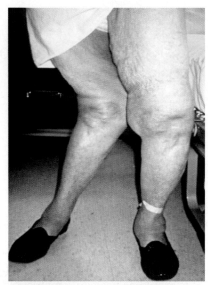
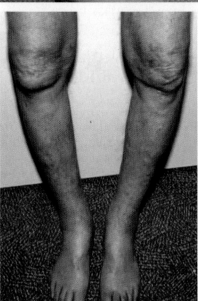
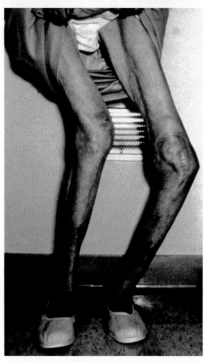

Figure 1 Bilateral knee deformities of a severity that would encourage simultaneous bilateral total knee arthroplasty (SBTKA).

Alternative Treatments

If staged TKA is elected rather than SBTKA, the patient may require closer postoperative scrutiny—as well as a contralateral shoe lift—to avoid a flexion contracture in the operated knee.

Especially in cases of severe deformity, surgery on the second knee should be scheduled as soon as possible, with a critical assessment of hemoglobin, serum proteins, and patient energy levels guiding the decision. Aggressive treatment of the unoperated knee with corticosteroids or viscosupplementa-

tion may reduce complications and increase the functional result, as long as they are terminated well before the anticipated second procedure.

Results

The wide variability in approaches, patient selection criteria, anesthesia techniques, surgical instrumentation, anticoagulation prophylaxis, postoperative rehabilitation, and surgeon skill and volume make interstudy comparisons difficult. The salient issue is postoperative mortality and significant complications, with high volume and efficient surgeons (and their patients) predictably enjoying the best results (**Table 1**).

From January 2000 through December 2008, I performed 10,961 TKAs, of which 3,646 were SBTKAs. These included 230 primary TKAs with contralateral revision and 117 simultaneous bilateral revisions or TKAs. Only six deaths occurred in that entire population, including three from Ogilvie syndrome, one liver failure 3 months after surgery, one myocardial infarction, and one multiorgan systemic failure. This is an overall mortality rate of 0.02%. Interestingly, none of the fatalities was in the most challenging populations, those who underwent revision/contralateral primary or bilateral revision.

Pain Management

Although SBTKA is not the appropriate venue for time-consuming minimally invasive techniques, analgesic regimens developed for minimally invasive surgery are very helpful in this population. Preoperative oral narcotics and nonsteroidal anti-inflammatory drugs are followed by intraoperative local anesthetic (bupivacaine hydrochloride) injections. Our anesthetic of choice is a combination spinal/epidural placed through a sin-

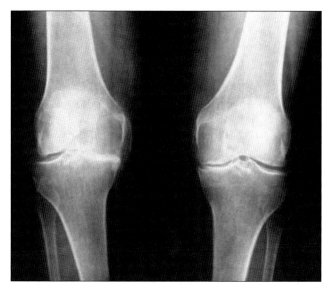

Figure 2 AP view of the knees of a patient who presented with pain in the left knee despite far worse arthrosis in the right.

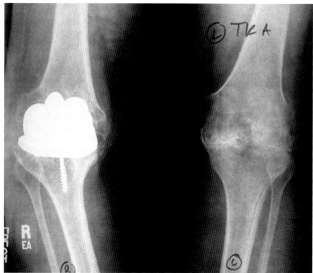

Figure 3 AP view demonstrates a failed right TKA and advanced arthritis and deformity in the left knee. This patient is a good candidate for simultaneous right revision TKA and left primary TKA.

Table 1 Results of Bilateral Total Knee Arthroplasty

Authors (Year)	Number of Bilateral TKAs	Mean Patient Age in Years (Range)	Mean Follow-up in Years (Range)	Results
Alemparte et al (2002)	604 SBTKAs	70 (30-92)	NR	Morbidity/mortality: 5.1%/0.7%
Ritter et al (2003)	2,050 SBTKAs 152 staged bilateral TKAs	69.9	4.3 (4 months to 17.8 years)	Morbidity/mortality: 0.5%/0.6%
Pavone et al (2004)	501 SBTKAs	66 (18-88)	NR	Morbidity/mortality: 21.8%/0%
Sliva et al (2005)	241 staggered bilateral TKAs 26 SBTKAs 65 staged bilateral TKAs	65 (35-90)	NR	Morbidity/mortality for SBTKAs: 0%

SBTKA = simultaneous bilateral total knee arthroplasty, NR = not reported.

gle small-needle puncture. The spinal is short-acting and provides not only analgesia but also motor blockade for the procedure, whereas the epidural is activated in the recovery room once the patient has demonstrated full neurovascular function in the distal extremities. Although the deep vein thrombosis prophylaxis of choice is low-dose warfarin initiated the night of surgery, the epidural catheter can be safely removed without a normal International Normalized Ratio (INR)

48 hours later. In my experience, it seems to provide the best pain relief for SBTKA patients. At the discretion of the anesthesiologist, some patients receive a Swann-Ganz catheter to monitor pulmonary hypertension. Despite the pharmacologic phlebotomy of regional anesthesia, the anesthesiologist should avoid large fluid administration to support hypertension because this may create postoperative cardiopulmonary overload. The use of a tourniquet is appropriate to

expedite the surgery, except in patients with vascular grafts, severe peripheral vascular disease, significant radiographic vascular calcification, or morbid obesity.

Setup/Patient Positioning

Both knees are prepared and draped simultaneously, using a double-fenestrated impervious sheet. A split sheet is put down to cover the second limb and then removed while sterile dressings are applied to the operated knee.

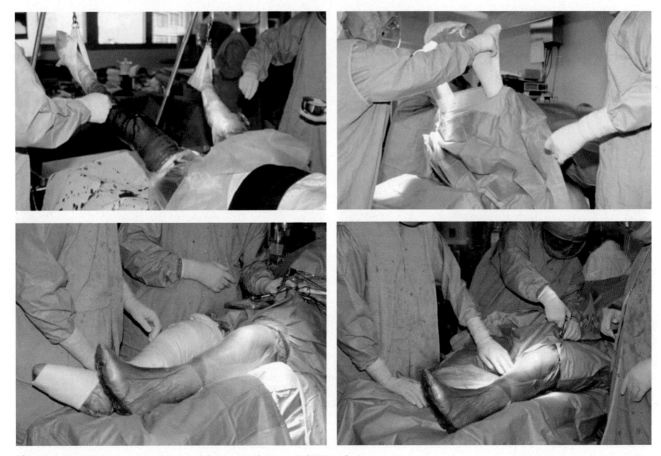

Figure 4 Simultaneous preparation and draping and sequential TKA techniques.

A second split sheet is then used for the second side (**Figure 4**). Many SBTKA surgeons prefer to do the "worst first" to ensure that the more severely affected knee is completed before any medical issues arise, although it is extremely rare to abort the second side.

Procedure

The approach is a median parapatellar arthrotomy with as little intrusion into the quadriceps tendon as possible. Patellar eversion is optional. I believe that intramedullary instrumentation should be avoided on the tibia and used only sparingly on the femur, to reduce the risk of marrow embolism. If intramedullary guidance is necessary, overdrilling of access holes and suctioning of the intramedullary canal are important. The primacy of soft-tissue balancing for successful ar-

throplasties is accommodated by the routine use of a tensor or distractor.

Despite the caution to avoid intramedullary instrumentation, it should be noted that my series of bilateral revisions with contralateral TKA and bilateral revisions—both using routine intramedullary reaming with frequent and substantial stems—have yet to generate any embolic complications.

Perhaps most important of all, SBTKA needs to be performed by experienced surgeons who perform TKA regularly and with a familiar and dedicated team of assistants. The absolute elimination of instrumentation or prosthetic deficiencies, the use of a planned and organized standard approach, and the elimination of delays between surgical steps are essential for an expeditious operation. Capsular closures are performed over double

drains with either No. 1 figure-of-8 interrupted sutures or (currently) running barbed continuous suture. The latter is also used for subcutaneous tissue and secured with staples. The drains are connected to a washed cell saver, which is used in the recovery room to restore lost blood. Patients capable of autotransfusion provide one or two units preoperatively, of which at least one is used postoperatively in the recovery room. Sterile compressive dressings with toe-to-groin elastic bandages are applied, and a continuous passive motion device is applied to one leg at a time, alternating every 4 hours, during hospitalization. With all this in place, the average surgical and tourniquet time for some surgeons can be less than 30 minutes for a straightforward primary TKA and well under an hour for a full three-component revision. If this level of efficiency cannot be approximated, it may be appropriate to consider sequential surgeries.

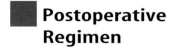

Postoperative Regimen

All patients are up and standing with minimal ambulation the morning after surgery. The continuous passive motion devices begin at 30° of flexion and are moved to 70° to 90° by the second day. Almost all SBTKA patients go to a rehabilitation center for approximately 1 week before being discharged with in-home therapy. Antibiotics are given intravenously for 24 hours, except in revisions, where they are maintained until the surgical culture results are known. Warfarin is used for 6 weeks with a target INR of 1.5 to 2 and is monitored by the internist who cleared and covered the patient for surgery. Patients are forbidden to use weights or do resistive exercises of any nature postoperatively until a range of motion of 0° to 100° is achieved, with particular focus on extension. Patients are seen in the office at 6 weeks and 12 weeks unless other issues mandate closer attention.

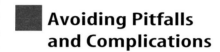

Avoiding Pitfalls and Complications

Patient selection is clearly crucial, and the surgeon must never discount or second-guess the advice of the clearing cardiologist. Careful administration of regional anesthetics with minimal fluid shifts, careful pre- and postoperative analgesic regimens, and early postoperative mobilization of the patient are essential. Surgically, SBTKAs demand the surgeon's most skillful effort, with minimal surgical times and with techniques that avoid known problems such as embolization. SBTKA patients do well under epidural anesthesia, but this places an increased demand on nursing and physical therapy personnel to avoid pressure sores, bowel obstructions, and delayed motion exercises. Indeed, when all these variables can be controlled and sufficient resources are marshaled, the recuperation and outcome of SBTKA should be almost identical to a single or staged procedure.

Bibliography

Alemparte J, Johnson GV, Worland RL, Jessup DE, Keenan J: Results of simultaneous bilateral total knee replacement: A study of 1208 knees in 604 patients. *J South Orthop Assoc* 2002;11(3):153-156.

Bezwada HP, Nazarian DG, Booth RE Jr: Simultaneous revision and contralateral primary total knee arthroplasty. *J Bone Joint Surg Am* 2003;85(10):1993-1998.

Bullock DP, Sporer SM, Shirreffs TG Jr: Comparison of simultaneous bilateral with unilateral total knee arthroplasty in terms of perioperative complications. *J Bone Joint Surg Am* 2003;85(10):1981-1986.

Della Valle CJ, Idjadi J, Hiebert RN, Jaffe WL: The impact of Medicare reimbursement policies on simultaneous bilateral total hip and knee arthroplasty. *J Arthroplasty* 2003;18(1):29-34.

Dennis DA: Debate: Bilateral simultaneous total knee arthroplasty. *Clin Orthop Relat Res* 2004;428:82-83.

Gill GS, Mills D, Joshi AB: Mortality following primary total knee arthroplasty. *J Bone Joint Surg Am* 2003;85(3):432-435.

Kim YH, Choi YW, Kim JS: Simultaneous bilateral sequential total knee replacement is as safe as unilateral total knee replacement. *J Bone Joint Surg Br* 2009;91(1):64-68.

Kim YH, Kim JS: Incidence and natural history of deep-vein thrombosis after total knee arthroplasty: A prospective, randomised study. *J Bone Joint Surg Br* 2002;84(4):566-570.

Leonard L, Williamson DM, Ivory JP, Jennison C: An evaluation of the safety and efficacy of simultaneous bilateral total knee arthroplasty. *J Arthroplasty* 2003;18(8):972-978.

Lombardi AV, Mallory TH, Fada RA, et al: Simultaneous bilateral total knee arthroplasties: Who decides? *Clin Orthop Relat Res* 2001;392:319-329.

Oakes DA, Hanssen AD: Bilateral total knee replacement using the same anesthetic is not justified by assessment of the risks. *Clin Orthop Relat Res* 2004;428:87-91.

Parvizi J, Sullivan TA, Trousdale RT, Lewallen DG: Thirty-day mortality after total knee arthroplasty. *J Bone Joint Surg Am* 2001;83(8):1157-1161.

Pavone V, Johnson T, Saulog PS, Sculco TP, Bottner F: Perioperative morbidity in bilateral one-stage total knee replacements. *Clin Orthop Relat Res* 2004;421:155-161.

Restrepo C, Parvizi J, Dietrich T, Einhorn TA: Safety of simultaneous bilateral total knee arthroplasty: A meta-analysis. *J Bone Joint Surg Am* 2007;89(6):1220-1226.

Ries MD, Rauscher LA, Hoskins S, Lott D, Richman JA, Lynch F Jr: Intramedullary pressure and pulmonary function during total knee arthroplasty. *Clin Orthop Relat Res* 1998;356:154-160.

Ritter MA, Harty LD, Davis KE, Meding JB, Berend M: Simultaneous bilateral, staged bilateral, and unilateral total knee arthroplasty: A survival analysis. *J Bone Joint Surg Am* 2003;85(8):1532-1537.

Sliva CD, Callaghan JJ, Goetz DD, Taylor SG: Staggered bilateral total knee arthroplasty performed four to seven days apart during a single hospitalization. *J Bone Joint Surg Am* 2005;87(3):508-513.

Stefansdottir A, Lidgren L, Robertsson O: Higher early mortality with simultaneous rather than staged bilateral TKAs: Results from the Swedish Knee Arthroplasty Register. *Clin Orthop Relat Res* 2008;466(12):3066-3070.

Coding

CPT Codes		Corresponding ICD-9 Codes	
27447	Arthroplasty, knee, condyle and plateau; medial AND lateral compartments with or without patella resurfacing (total knee arthroplasty)	715 715.80	715.16 715.89

CPT copyright © 2010 by the American Medical Association. All rights reserved.

SECTION 3
Complications Following Total Knee Arthroplasty

Section Editors
Jay R. Lieberman, MD
Daniel J. Berry, MD

Chapter 30

Management of the Infected Total Knee Arthroplasty

Tad M. Mabry, MD
Arlen D. Hanssen, MD

■ Indications

Infection is one of the most feared complications of total knee arthroplasty (TKA). It has been shown to be one of the dominant causes of failure requiring revision or removal of the prosthesis. Deep prosthetic infection has been shown to affect 1% to 2% of primary TKAs, with even higher rates reported after revision surgery. Despite its relatively low incidence, infection will become an increasingly important issue as the number of TKAs performed annually continues to rise. Every patient who presents with a painful TKA should be evaluated for the possibility of an infectious etiology. Other common causes of pain following TKA include polyethylene wear/osteolysis, aseptic loosening, instability, extensor mechanism complications, arthrofibrosis, and periprosthetic fracture; it should be noted that prosthetic joint infection can occur concomitantly with each of these aseptic diagnoses. Effective management of the infected TKA begins with a rapid and accurate diagnosis of the underlying problem.

■ Contraindications

Surgical treatment is indicated for all but a few patients with an infected TKA. Patients with multiple medical comorbidities that preclude surgery can be offered antibiotic suppression if the implant is well fixed and the infecting organism is characterized by low virulence and is responsive to oral agents with low toxicity. Antibiotics in isolation cannot eradicate the infection and should be avoided if the above-mentioned criteria are not met or if there is a risk of seeding other implants.

In most cases, implant revision via a delayed exchange protocol will provide the best functional result. The potential functional advantage of a new prosthesis must be weighed against the potential infection risk. Contraindications to the implantation of a new prosthesis at the site of an infected TKA include persistent or recalcitrant infection, medical conditions that preclude multiple reconstructive attempts, severe disruption of the local soft-tissue envelope (eg, extensor mechanism disruption, failed muscle flaps), or systemic conditions that predispose to reinfection.

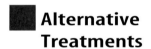

■ Alternative Treatments

The primary goals of treatment in this setting include pain relief, maintenance of function, and eradication of infection. Five surgical options are available for treatment of the infected TKA: (1) débridement with retention of components, (2) resection arthroplasty, (3) arthrodesis, (4) amputation, and (5) exchange arthroplasty. Consideration of host factors, the local environment of the knee, the nature of the infecting organism, and the timing of the infection diagnosis with respect to the arthroplasty allow the treating surgeon to develop the most effective management strategy.

Surgical débridement with component retention is indicated for patients with acute infection in the early postoperative period and for patients with acute hematogenous infection at the

Dr. Mabry or an immediate family member is a member of a speakers' bureau or has made paid presentations on behalf of DePuy; has received research or institutional support from DePuy, Stryker, and Zimmer; and owns stock or stock options in Pfizer. Dr. Hanssen or an immediate family member serves as a board member, owner, officer, or committee member of the American Association of Hip and Knee Surgeons, the Hip Society, and the Knee Society; has received royalties from Stryker Orthopaedic Development Corp.; serves as a paid consultant to or is an employee of Stryker; and has received research or institutional support from Biomet, DePuy, Implex, Stryker, Tornier, and Zimmer.

site of a functional, well-fixed implant. Attempts to salvage a chronically infected TKA (symptom duration longer than 2 to 4 weeks) with this technique almost always fail. Most surgeons recommend the exchange of modular components at the time of débridement to gain better access to the posterior knee joint and to allow irrigation of the nonarticular surface of the polyethylene insert. Improved results are reported when the symptoms of infection have been short-lived and no draining sinus is present. Antibiotic regimens containing rifampin have been shown to improve the chances of success when treating infections caused by biofilm-producing organisms such as *Staphylococcus aureus*.

Definitive resection arthroplasty involves removal of the infected knee prosthesis with no subsequent attempts at reimplantation. This procedure has a very high cure rate, but the functional result is often poor. The resulting flail knee can be considered an alternative to arthrodesis that allows motion during flexion for sitting, but at the expense of instability during ambulation. Most patients now treated with this technique are low-demand individuals, often in the setting of polyarticular rheumatoid arthritis.

Knee arthrodesis, or fusion, remains a viable method of limb salvage at the site of an infected TKA. The ultimate goal of a knee arthrodesis is to achieve a painless, stable joint, but motion is sacrificed. Relative indications for arthrodesis include high functional demand, single-joint disease, young age, extensor mechanism deficiency, poor soft-tissue coverage, host immunocompromise, and highly virulent infecting organisms. Individuals with ipsilateral hip or ankle disease, bilateral knee disease, or contralateral amputations are not considered suitable candidates for this type of reconstruction.

External fixation and intramedul-

lary fixation are the two most commonly described methods used to obtain fusion at the site of an infected TKA. Each has its advantages and disadvantages. In addition to producing excellent femorotibial compression, an external fixator may be adjusted in the postoperative period to maintain proper limb alignment. The fixator may be applied at the time of TKA resection, which may reduce the overall number of invasive surgical procedures. Finally, the knee is left free of indwelling hardware once the arthrodesis site has united. Two potential disadvantages of external fixation are that it does not allow early weight bearing and it is associated with a relatively high frequency of pin-site complications (eg, infection and/or fracture). Several authors also have noted a substantial risk of nonunion with the use of external fixation in this setting. Intramedullary fixation allows early weight bearing and has been associated with a very low risk of nonunion. This procedure is best performed in a staged manner, however, to avoid the potential spread of the articular infection up and down the femoral and tibial canals. The risk of persistent deep infection following intramedullary fixation may be higher than the risk following external fixation. The surgical time and estimated surgical blood loss are also typically higher when intramedullary rods are used. Overall, the use of intramedullary rods may be considered a trade-off between fusion rate and infection cure rate. The surgeon must weigh the potential risks and benefits for each patient on a case-by-case basis.

Transfemoral amputation is performed only very rarely after TKA, and is usually the result of issues unrelated to the prosthesis itself, such as tumor recurrence or peripheral vascular disease with critical ischemia. Less than 5% of patients with an infection diagnosis will ever require a transfemoral amputation. Indications for amputation in this setting include life-threat-

ening sepsis, multiple failed attempts at the eradication of infection, nonreconstructible bone loss, and intractable pain. Given the large burden of medical issues carried by most transfemoral amputees, very few will ever regain ambulatory capacity with a prosthetic limb.

———————————■

Results

The success rate for eradication of infection at the site of an infected TKA when a modern, two-stage protocol is used ranges from 85% to 95%, depending on the time of follow-up (**Table 1**). The beneficial effects of delayed exchange and the use of antibiotic-loaded bone cement (ALBC) have been demonstrated (**Table 2**).

———————————■

Technique

Classification of Infection
The critical first step in the treatment of patients with an infected TKA is to establish the diagnosis. This process requires a high index of suspicion in conjunction with a comprehensive history and physical examination, radiographic evaluation, blood tests, and arthrocentesis. Once the diagnosis has been established, management principles are generally guided by a simple classification scheme based on the onset and duration of infection symptoms (**Table 3**).

Pain is the most common presenting symptom in the setting of an infected TKA. Patients with acute postoperative infections also may present with wound drainage and cellulitis. Occasionally, these patients are systemically ill, with high fevers and chills. Patients with acute hematogenous infections typically report the sudden onset of pain and swelling in a previously well-functioning joint with

Table 1 Results of Two-Stage Exchange Total Knee Arthroplasty

Authors (Year)	Number of Knees	Spacer Type	Mean Patient Age in Years (Range)	Mean Follow-up (Range)	Results
Haleem et al (2004)	96	Static ALBC	69 (37-89)	7.2 years (2.5-13.2)	Survivorship free of implant removal for reinfection: 93.5% at 5 years; 85% at 10 years
Hofmann et al (2005)	50	Articulating ALBC	67 (38-92)	73 months (24-150)	Eradication rate 88% at last follow-up. Reinfection seen at a mean of 35 months (range, 7-60) following reimplantation
Freeman et al (2007)	76	Static ALBC (*n* = 28) Articulating ALBC (*n* = 48)	67 (41-87)	71.2 months (24-196)	Eradication rate at last follow-up: 94.7% in articulating group, 92.1% in static group

ALBC = antibiotic-loaded bone cement.

or without constitutional symptoms related to the underlying bacteremia. Identification of the source of bacteremia and screening of other potentially infected joints should be completed expeditiously.

Unlike patients with acute infections, patients with chronic knee infections describe a much more insidious clinical course. Persistent pain and night pain are two typical symptoms. Many of these patients have an effusion or significant stiffness that has failed to resolve over time despite appropriate therapies. Patients reporting a history of prolonged postoperative wound drainage or intermittent treatment with antibiotics for knee symptoms should be considered infected until proven otherwise.

High-quality plain radiographs should be scrutinized as part of the evaluation of the patient with a suspected infection. Areas of periosteal new bone formation or progressive radiolucency could indicate an infection. The knee should also be assessed for overall alignment, fixation status, and bone stock remaining to most effectively plan subsequent reconstructive efforts.

Analysis of the erythrocyte sedimentation rate (ESR) and C-reactive protein (CRP) is useful in all cases of

Table 2 Results of Treatment of Infected Total Knee Arthroplasty

Type of Procedure	Prosthesis Fixation	Success Rate (%)
Direct exchange	Plain cement	58
Direct exchange	ALBC	74
Delayed exchange	Plain cement	88
Delayed exchange	ALBC	92

ALBC = antibiotic-loaded bone cement.
Data from Leone JM, Hanssen AD: Management of infection at the site of a total knee arthroplasty. *J Bone Joint Surg Am* 2005;87:2335-2348.

Table 3 Classification of Infected Total Knee Arthroplasty

Type	Timing	Definition	Treatment
1	Positive intraoperative culture	≥2 deep cultures positive for the same organism(s) obtained intraoperatively	Antibiotics
2	Acute postoperative infection	Infection ≤4 weeks postoperatively	Débridement with component retention and antibiotics
3	Acute hematogenous infection	Infection in a previously well-functioning total knee arthroplasty subsequent to bacteremia	Débridement with component retention and antibiotics versus component removal
4	Chronic infection	Infection >4 weeks postoperatively with a more insidious clinical course	Component removal

Data from Segawa H, Tsukayama DT, Kyle RF, Becker DA, Gustilo RB: Infection after total knee arthroplasty: A retrospective study of the treatment of eighty-one infections. *J Bone Surg Am* 1999;81:1434-1445.

Table 4 Synovial Fluid Analysis in the Evaluation of the Painful Total Knee Arthroplasty

Authors (Year)	Indicator	Sensitivity (%)	Specificity (%)	Positive Predictive Value (%)	Negative Predictive Value (%)
Trampuz et al (2004)	Leukocyte count >1,700/μL	94	88	73	98
	Neutrophils >65%	97	98	94	99
Parvizi et al (2006)	Leukocyte count >1,760/μL	90	99	99	88
	Neutrophils >73%	93	95	96	91
Ghanem et al (2008)	Leukocyte count >1,100/μL	91	88	87	92
	Neutrophils >64%	95	95	92	97

suspected infection. These two tests are useful both for infection screening and for monitoring the effects of treatment over time. Although both tests demonstrate a rise postoperatively, the CRP tends to peak more quickly and then return to baseline. A rising CRP more than 1 week after surgery strongly indicates the presence of infection. In general, an ESR greater than 30 mm/h and a CRP level greater than 10 mg/L warrants further investigation.

We recommend analysis of the synovial fluid as part of the routine evaluation of the painful TKA. The fluid should be sent for both aerobic and anaerobic bacterial culture. In some instances, expanding the cultures to include fungi and mycobacteria may be indicated. Many recent studies have noted the value of the synovial-fluid cell count and differential. These values may resemble a native joint infection in the setting of acute postoperative or acute hematogenous infection, with a neutrophil differential exceeding 90% and total nucleated cell counts greater than 50,000/μL. However, it must be noted that much lower values can indicate chronic TKA infection (**Table 4**). A leukocyte count greater than 1,100/μL with a neutrophil differential greater than 60% is suggestive of infection.

In large part because of the ease and utility of synovial fluid analysis, nuclear medicine imaging is rarely needed to evaluate for infection at the site of a TKA. Combination indium In 111 leukocyte and technetium Tc 99m scanning has been shown to be a very accurate test, but it is limited in its usefulness by its lack of specificity.

The use of sonication to dislodge adherent bacteria from removed total joint prostheses has been described recently as a novel diagnostic tool. This method may be more sensitive than standard sampling of periprosthetic tissue, most notably when the patient has been recently exposed to antibiotics that have sterilized this tissue while not penetrating the biofilm layer. The utility of this method will be analyzed further once its use becomes more widespread.

Setup/Exposure

When a patient with an infected TKA is brought to the operating room for surgical treatment, antibiotics are typically withheld until all of the deep-tissue cultures have been obtained, so that the infecting organism can be identified and the most effective antibiotic agent is used. In most cases, the knee should be accessed through the previous anterior incision after excision of the previous scar. When multiple incisions are present, the more lateral longitudinal incision that will allow appropriate access to the knee is typically used, to avoid devascularizing the skin flaps. Transverse incisions should be transected at right angles where possible. Plastic surgery consultation is occasionally necessary in the preoperative period to plan skin incisions or to evaluate the need for flap coverage.

The medial parapatellar arthrotomy is the typical capsular approach to the knee at the time of prosthesis removal. The surgeon must be able to expose the knee in such a way as to facilitate component removal and débridement while protecting the soft tissues, with great care given to maintaining the integrity of the extensor mechanism. In most cases, the patella can be subluxated rather than everted to minimize tension on the patellar tendon insertion. The quadriceps snip and the tibial tubercle osteotomy are two of the most commonly used extensile approaches when enhanced exposure is required.

Instruments/Equipment/ Implants Required

Removal of infected prostheses may be facilitated with the use of a variety of instruments. The use of flexible osteotomes and oscillating saw blades is standard. Many implant-specific extraction devices also are available. Ultrasonic cement extraction tools may be needed when removing cemented stems from the femoral or tibial canal.

Procedure

BONE PREPARATION

The goal of the débridement is to remove all foreign material and necrotic tissue while maintaining the vascular supply to the bone. Once the components have been removed, the bone must be evaluated carefully for any retained cement on the condylar or intramedullary surfaces. Intraoperative plain radiographs are occasionally useful to assess the knee after débridement. Several areas where cement is commonly left behind include the posterior femoral condyles, the femoral and patellar lug holes, and the anterior intramedullary surface of the tibia behind the tibial tubercle. It is helpful to reassess the final soft-tissue débridement after complete bony débridement has been ensured, as the capsular recesses will now be fully exposed. The surgeon should then assess and document any areas of bone or soft-tissue deficiency that will need to be addressed at the time of any future knee reconstruction.

PROSTHESIS IMPLANTATION

The vast majority of patients treated with a two-stage exchange protocol will have a high-dose ALBC spacer implanted at the time of prosthesis removal. The antibiotic dosages used for the treatment of deep prosthetic infection are much higher than the doses used at the time of definitive joint reconstruction. The use of premixed, low-dose antibiotic formulations should be avoided in this setting. We typically use 3 to 4 g of vancomycin and 3.6 to 4.8 g of an aminoglycoside antibiotic (gentamicin or tobramycin) per 40-g batch of cement. An additional 100 to 150 mg of amphotericin B will be added to each 40-g batch of cement in the setting of a fungal infection. Methylene blue dye can be added to the ALBC to aid in its identification and removal at the time of the next operation. When using high doses of antibiotics in the cement, it is helpful to mix the cement into its liquid phase before the addition of the antibiotic.

There is no consensus with respect to the use of articulating (mobile) versus nonarticulating (static) ALBC spacers after removal of the infected TKA. Each type of spacer allows for

the delivery of antibiotics to the site of infection, stabilization of the soft-tissue envelope, facilitation of the subsequent reconstruction, and improvement in the ultimate clinical outcome. The unique goal of a mobile spacer is to preserve joint motion during the treatment period, which may further facilitate the surgical exposure at the time of reimplantation when compared to a static spacer. A wide variety of articulating designs are available, including both cement-on-cement and metal-on-polyethylene bearing surfaces. Each design requires its own specific technique of implantation and rehabilitation. The rates of infection cure with the use of these spacers have been very good despite the presence of prosthetic materials within the joint. Although some studies have demonstrated a trend toward better long-term function with the use of articulating spacers, there have been no randomized, prospective studies to date. We typically reserve the use of mobile spacers for patients presenting with simultaneous, bilateral infected TKAs.

The original static spacers were simple, preformed blocks of ALBC. These incongruous shapes were placed into the remaining femorotibial space after the infected knee prosthesis had been resected. A host of problems directly related to spacer migration were noted, including bone loss, instability, and erosion of periarticular soft tissues. To address the issue of migration, the "molded arthrodesis block" was developed. This nonarticulating spacer is easily made and is applicable across the entire range of bone loss patterns commonly

Video 30.1 Preparation of Molded Articulating Cement Spacers for Treatment of Infected Total Knee Arthroplasty. Adolph V. Lombardi, Jr, MD, FACS; Keith R. Berend, MD; Joanne B. Adams, BFA (3 min)

encountered at the site of an infected TKA.

Once the knee débridement has been completed, local hemostasis is attained. Before the arthrodesis block spacer is placed, ALBC dowels are placed in the intramedullary canals of the femur and tibia. These dowels are easily created with standard operating room equipment (**Figure 1**, *A*). As noted previously, the cement is mixed into its liquid state before the addition of the high-dose antibiotics (**Figure 1**, *B*). This mixture is injected into the nozzle of a standard cement gun until the desired length is achieved (**Figure 1**, *C*). Care must be taken to shape the proximal end of the dowel to avoid overstuffing the joint. It is critically important to pull the cement out from underneath the threads of the nozzle. The dowels are then set aside until the cement has completely hardened, at which time they are easily removed with retrograde impaction. One 40-g batch of cement can easily make the two dowels typically used in these cases (**Figure 1**, *D*).

Once the dowels have been placed, the knee is then held in a slightly flexed position over a small bolster. The knee joint is distracted to maintain appropriate tension of the soft-tissue envelope. Typically, two 40-g batches of cement are mixed with the chosen concentration of antibiotics to fabricate the spacer. Once the mixture has settled into a doughy phase, it is introduced into the joint space and allowed to macrointerdigitate with the unique contours of the patellofemoral and tibiofemoral surfaces (**Figure 2**). Due to the mechanical properties of high-dose ALBC, microinterdigitation of the cement within the interstices of the exposed cancellous bone is not an issue. With the knee held in position during cement curing, the extensor mechanism should be reduced manually and the spacer adjusted as needed to avoid overstuffing of the joint. This simple, yet effective static construct will result in a very stable knee joint and will min-

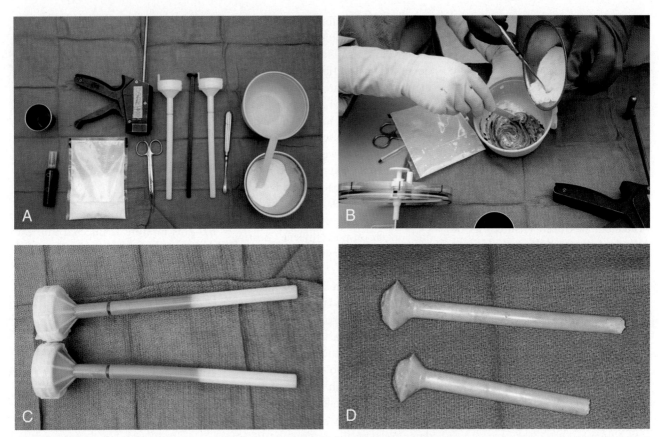

Figure 1 Producing a molded arthrodesis block spacer with two intramedullary dowels. **A,** The basic equipment needed includes a cement gun with two nozzles, cement, antibiotics, and a mixing bowl. **B,** High-dose antibiotics are mixed with liquid cement dyed with methylene blue. **C,** The antibiotic-loaded bone cement mixture has been injected to the desired length with the cement-gun nozzles. These will be allowed to completely harden before removal with retrograde impaction. **D,** The final antibiotic-loaded cement dowels.

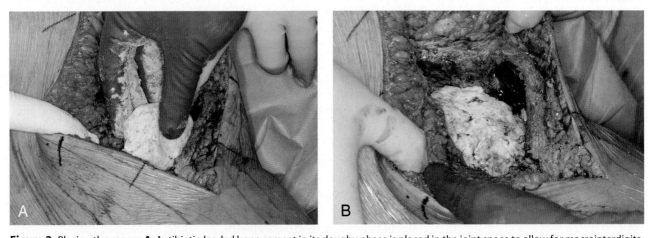

Figure 2 Placing the spacer. **A,** Antibiotic-loaded bone cement in its doughy phase is placed in the joint space to allow for macrointerdigitation with the osseous surfaces, which enhances the stability of the spacer. **B,** The spacer is folded into the patellofemoral space to avoid a fusion between the resected surfaces of the patella and the anterior femur.

imize the risks associated with spacer migration (**Figure 3**).

Wound Closure

The extensor mechanism is closed over suction drains with interrupted, absorbable, monofilament suture. The skin is closed with a combination of heavy (No. 2) retention-type and standard (2-0) monofilament sutures. The use of braided suture is typically avoided in the setting of infection.

Postoperative Regimen

Wound healing is of paramount importance after the removal of infected TKA components. Appropriate nutrition should be ensured for all patients. Retention sutures are removed before hospital discharge, and the remaining sutures are removed 2 to 3 weeks postoperatively. We use the molded arthrodesis block in the vast majority of cases. These patients are maintained in toe-touch weight bearing in a long-leg cast until the time of reimplantation. Adjusted-dose warfarin is typically used for deep vein thrombosis prophylaxis during this same period. The prothrombin time must be monitored very carefully to avoid postoperative hematoma formation.

Rehabilitation instructions following the implantation of an antibiotic spacer vary according to technique. In the setting of a nonarticulating spacer, the focus of physical therapy is maintenance of general conditioning rather than maintenance of joint motion. As noted above, we typically use a long-leg cast during this phase of treatment. When a mobile spacer is chosen, the patient is generally encouraged to initiate range-of-motion exercises once the wound has healed. The intensity of these exercises and the amount of weight bearing allowed is influenced by the type of mobile spacer and the quality of the host bone and ligamentous structures.

Patients are typically given organism-specific intravenous antimicrobial therapy for 4 to 6 weeks after removal of the components. Serum inflammatory markers (CRP, ESR) are obtained at the antibiotic stop date and again immediately before the next

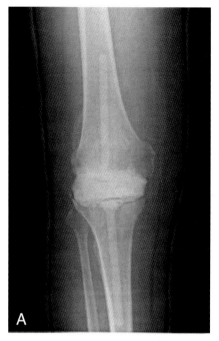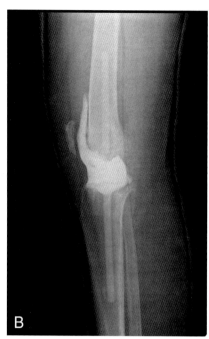

Figure 3 AP (**A**) and lateral (**B**) radiographs obtained 8 weeks after resection of a right knee with a molded arthrodesis block spacer. Note the presence of the intramedullary dowels and the customized fit of the spacer within the patellofemoral and tibiofemoral spaces. The leg is immobilized in a full-length fiberglass cast pending reimplantation.

stage of knee reconstruction. These values can be compared with the preoperative values to assess the effectiveness of treatment. An antibiotic holiday lasting at least 2 to 4 weeks is recommended to assess for any relapse of infection.

If the clinical and serologic parameters appear satisfactory and the patient is an acceptable host, reimplantation of a new prosthesis is undertaken. This usually occurs 8 to 10 weeks after component removal when a static spacer is used. The preservation of joint motion afforded by a mobile spacer may allow for a longer interval between surgeries without excessive soft-tissue contracture. The final decision to implant a new prosthesis is made at the time of surgery, based on the intraoperative judgment of the surgeon as to the resolution of the infection, which is based on an evaluation of the gross appearance and the microscopic appearance of the tissues. At least three tissue cultures should be obtained at the time of the

reimplantation in all cases. Unlike the resection of an infected prosthesis, when reinsertion of a new prosthesis is intended, intravenous antibiotics are recommended before the skin incision.

We typically use antibiotics in the cement at the time of reimplantation at a concentration of 1 g vancomycin and 1.2 g tobramycin per 40-g batch of cement. We occasionally substitute daptomycin for vancomycin, if the patient is allergic to vancomycin. Amphotericin B is typically added in the event of prior fungal infection. We generally use fully cemented constructs at the time of reimplantation (**Figure 4**), but the use of so-called hybrid fixation techniques with metaphyseal cement and cementless stems is favored by some to facilitate extraction in the event of recurrence of infection. Most bone deficiencies can be managed with modular metal augments on the femur and/or the tibia. At our institution, larger defects are typically managed with porous metal

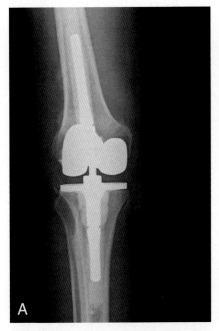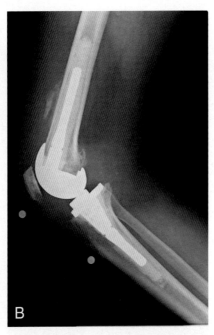

Figure 4 AP (**A**) and lateral (**B**) radiographs of a right knee following reimplantation TKA with fully cemented stems.

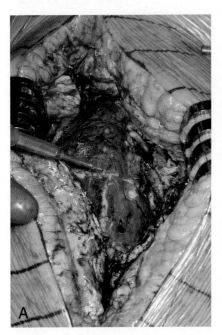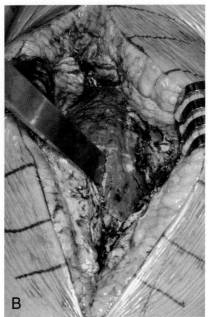

Figure 5 Removal of the spacer. **A,** Piecemeal extraction of the static spacer is facilitated through the creation of "fault lines" with a small-diameter burr. **B,** These fault lines are then opened with a medium osteotome, allowing the cement to be removed from the knee.

metaphyseal cones. Allograft bone is used less frequently in this situation, given persistent concerns over the infection risk.

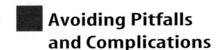

Avoiding Pitfalls and Complications

Given the value of synovial fluid analysis for cell count, differential, and culture, it is critical to obtain this fluid before any revision surgery. Low-grade infection can mimic, or be superimposed upon, many of the aseptic causes of failure. It is the responsibility of the surgeon to thoroughly investigate the knee before revision to avoid missing a septic complication. Synovial fluid analysis is best performed when the patient has been free of all antibiotics for 2 to 3 weeks.

Once the infection diagnosis has been made, the patient should be evaluated and treated for any reversible contributing factors (eg, poor dentition, lymphedema, diabetes mellitus). Consultation with an infectious disease specialist can be very valuable in all phases of treatment of the patient with an infected TKA. The surgeon must not overlook any condition that may jeopardize the outcome of future reconstructive procedures.

To avoid unnecessary delays in treatment, and perhaps to avoid emerging antibiotic resistance, it is very important to avoid the use of protracted oral antibiotic suppression of infected joints.

Several pitfalls associated with ALBC are easily avoided. First, it is best to add the antibiotics after the cement has been mixed into its liquid phase. Next, it is best to avoid the use of premixed, low-dose formulations at the time of treatment. These formulations are usually intended for definitive joint reconstruction and often are mixed at a concentration of around 2 g of antibiotic per 40 g of cement. As noted previously, the recommended treatment dose is typically around 8 g of antibiotic per 40 g of cement. Finally, the shaping of the cement dowels is very important to facilitate their use. This is very easily performed, and requires reducing the size of the proximal flare to a low profile. The most common mistake is to leave this segment too large, and then overstuff the joint.

Removal of the static spacer at the time of reimplantation is straightforward. This is best done piecemeal.

"Fault lines" through the cement can be made quickly with a small-diameter burr and then finished with a wide osteotome (**Figure 5**). This will reduce the force required to disrupt the spacer and minimize the risk of iatrogenic fracture during spacer removal.

As previously noted, the final decision to implant a new prosthesis is made at the time of surgery based on the intraoperative judgment of the surgeon, which is based on an evaluation of the gross and microscopic appearance of the tissues. At our institution, pathologists describe acute inflammation consistent with ongoing infection when there are 5 or more neutrophils per high-power field in multiple separate fields. When a cutoff value of 10 or more neutrophils per high-power field is used, there will be a greater specificity but a lower sensitivity for the diagnosis of ongoing infection. If the knee appears to remain infected at the time of intended reimplantation, we obtain deep cultures, perform a thorough débridement, and insert a new antibiotic cement spacer. Although infection remains the primary contraindication to placement of a new prosthesis, other issues may arise at the time of intended reimplantation that could alter the plan. At the time of reimplantation, the surgeon should be prepared to manage any issues related to bone loss, extensor mechanism disruption, or collateral ligament injury, as in all other types of complex knee reconstruction.

Bibliography

Burnett RS, Kelly MA, Hanssen AD, Barrack RL: Technique and timing of two-stage exchange for infection in TKA. *Clin Orthop Relat Res* 2007;464:164-178.

Freeman MG, Fehring TK, Odum SM, Fehring K, Griffin WL, Mason JB: Functional advantage of articulating versus static spacers in 2-stage revision for total knee arthroplasty infection. *J Arthroplasty* 2007;22(8):1116-1121.

Ghanem E, Parvizi J, Burnett RS, et al: Cell count and differential of aspirated fluid in the diagnosis of infection at the site of total knee arthroplasty. *J Bone Joint Surg Am* 2008;90(8):1637-1643.

Haleem AA, Berry DJ, Hanssen AD: Mid-term to long-term followup of two-stage reimplantation for infected total knee arthroplasty. *Clin Orthop Relat Res* 2004;428:35-39.

Hofmann AA, Goldberg T, Tanner AM, Kurtin SM: Treatment of infected total knee arthroplasty using an articulating spacer: 2- to 12-year experience. *Clin Orthop Relat Res* 2005;430:125-131.

Leone JM, Hanssen AD: Management of infection at the site of a total knee arthroplasty. *J Bone Joint Surg Am* 2005;87(10):2335-2348.

Mabry TM, Jacofsky DJ, Haidukewych GJ, Hanssen AD: Comparison of intramedullary nailing and external fixation knee arthrodesis for the infected knee replacement. *Clin Orthop Relat Res* 2007;464:11-15.

Parvizi J, Ghanem E, Menashe S, Barrack RL, Bauer TW: Periprosthetic infection: What are the diagnostic challenges? *J Bone Joint Surg Am* 2006;88(Suppl 4):138-147.

Segawa H, Tsukayama DT, Kyle RF, Becker DA, Gustilo RB: Infection after total knee arthroplasty: A retrospective study of the treatment of eighty-one infections. *J Bone Joint Surg Am* 1999;81(10):1434-1445.

Trampuz A, Hanssen AD, Osmon DR, Mandrekar J, Steckelberg JM, Patel R: Synovial fluid leukocyte count and differential for the diagnosis of prosthetic knee infection. *Am J Med* 2004;117(8):556-562.

Trampuz A, Piper KE, Jacobson MJ, et al: Sonication of removed hip and knee prostheses for diagnosis of infection. *N Engl J Med* 2007;357(7):654-663.

Video Reference

Lombardi AV Jr, Berend KR, Adams JB: Video. *Preparation of Molded Articulating Cement Spacers for Treatment of Infected Total Knee Arthroplasty*, from *Molded Articulating Cement Spacers for Treatment of Infected Total Knee Arthroplasty*. Columbus, OH, 2008.

Coding

CPT Codes		Corresponding ICD-9 Codes	
27486	Revision of total knee arthroplasty, with or without allograft; one component	996.4	996.6
27487	Revision of total knee arthroplasty, with or without allograft; femoral and entire tibial component	996.4	996.6
27488	Removal of prosthesis, including total knee prosthesis, methylmethacrylate with or without insertion of spacer, knee	996.4	996.6
27580	Arthrodesis, knee, any technique	711.16 714.0 717.9	711.46 716.16
29877	Arthroscopy, knee, surgical; debridement/shaving of articular cartilage (chondroplasty)	717.7	
27559	Treatment of tibial shaft fracture (with or without fibular fracture) by intramedullary implant, with or without interlocking screws and/or cerclage	733.16	
27880	Amputation, leg, through tibia and fibula	172.7	
27881	Amputation, leg, through tibia and fibula; with immediate fitting technique including application of first cast	172.7	
20690	Application of a uniplane (pins or wires in one plane), unilateral, external fixation system	733.16	
20692	Application of a multiplane (pins or wires in more than one plane), unilateral, external fixation system (eg, Ilizarov, Monticelli type)	733.16	

CPT copyright © 2010 by the American Medical Association. All rights reserved.

Chapter 31

Management of the Unstable Total Knee Arthroplasty

Steven J. MacDonald, MD, FRCSC
Keegan P. Au, MD, FRCSC

Introduction

Instability is one of the most common causes of failure in total knee arthroplasty (TKA). When it occurs early following the index procedure, it is often attributable to improper surgical technique, such as component malposition, failure to restore an appropriate mechanical axis, suboptimal soft-tissue balancing, or compromise of ligamentous structures. Late instability typically relates to polyethylene wear, component loosening, dysfunction of the extensor mechanism, or ligamentous instability, such as delayed posterior cruciate ligament (PCL) rupture. Instability can be classified by mode or direction of failure: (1) recurvatum, (2) anterior-posterior instability, (3) varus-valgus instability, or (4) global instability.

Recurvatum may represent a weakness in the extensor mechanism causing secondary compensations in gait, such as that which occurs in the quadriceps musculature in poliomyelitis. Additionally, an extension space that is larger than the flexion space, either one that occurs at the time of the in-dex procedure due to improper gap balancing or one that develops over time secondary to component loosening and subsidence, will create a recurvatum deformity.

Anterior-posterior flexion space instability usually represents an improperly balanced index arthroplasty with a relatively large flexion gap. It also can be observed in cruciate-retaining implants where the PCL has been injured intraoperatively or becomes incompetent postoperatively.

Varus-valgus instability, also known as extension space instability, is secondary to medial or lateral laxity. This can be seen secondary to mechanical malalignment, collateral laceration or rupture, or failure to deal appropriately with pathologic tightness or laxity related to preoperative deformity.

Global instability refers to laxity that can be elicited in multiple planes. It can, in its most severe form, result from polyethylene wear debris that contributes to destruction of periarticular soft-tissue supports and osteolysis, causing implant subsidence. Causes of anterior-posterior and varus-valgus instability, discussed earlier, also may contribute to global instability.

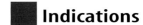

Indications

The indication for revision surgery in the unstable TKA is symptomatic instability in clinical situations in which the pattern and cause for the instability can be identified and addressed.

Contraindications

Although most TKAs that fail because of instability issues require revision procedures, caution is necessary. The underlying cause of the instability must be identified and addressed with the revision. Failure to do so may result in persistent instability and recurrent failure. For example, a valgus instability secondary to component malalignment that is managed with a medial collateral ligament (MCL) reconstructive procedure is destined to recur. Similarly, pain following TKA is a very nonspecific symptom, and in the absence of other findings or convincing evidence for the presence of coexisting instability, pain should not

Dr. MacDonald or an immediate family member has received royalties from DePuy; serves as a paid consultant for or is an employee of DePuy; has received research or institutional support from DePuy, Stryker, and Smith & Nephew; and is a board member, owner, officer, or committee member for The Knee Society. Neither Dr. Au nor an immediate family member has received anything of value from or owns stock in a commercial company or institution related directly or indirectly to the subject of this chapter.

Table 1 Results of Revision Total Knee Arthroplasty for Instability

Authors (Year)	Number of TKAs	Instability Pattern	Management	Outcomes
Peters et al (1997)	57	Extension space	Revision to VVC	80% good results at minimum 5 years Complications related to extensor mechanism
Pagnano et al (1998)	25	Flexion space	Revision from CR to PS	Reliable success No further instability KSS significantly improved
Hofmann et al (2000)	100	Flexion space	Ultracongruent polyethylene insert in primary TKA	No revisions for instability
Easley et al (2000)	44	Extension space	VVC in primary TKA for elderly patients with valgus knees	No failures or instability Improvement in HSS knee scores
Giori and Lewallen (2002)	16	Recurvatum	TKA primary and revision, mixed components	High complication rate, especially if no antigravity quadriceps strength

TKA = total knee arthroplasty, VVC = varus-valgus constrained; CR = cruciate-retaining; PS = posterior stabilized; KSS = Knee Society score; HSS = Hospital for Special Surgery.

be interpreted as an indication to offer a revision TKA with increased constraint.

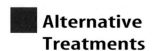

Alternative Treatments

The management of instability following TKA is primarily surgical. In the setting of recurvatum following primary TKA secondary to extensor weakness from neuromuscular disease, however, bracing may be the most practical lifelong option. In addition, because revision TKA to address instability issues is often lengthy and complicated, it may be worthwhile to consider bracing as an alternative in patients who are considered very high medical risk for such procedures. In the rare circumstance in which bracing is determined to be appropriate, the orthosis prescribed should offer the specific support necessary to assist in the pattern of instability. We have found that in most circumstances, the most appropriate device is a custom hinged brace with

derotational properties and options for static blocks to restrict range of motion, such as that prescribed for ligamentous insufficiency in native knees.

Results

Table 1 lists results of selected studies reporting on various options in revision TKA for different instability patterns. These studies indicate that revision can be successful when performed for TKA instability when appropriate soft-tissue balancing and, most critically, flexion/extension gap balancing are performed. Increased constraint is commonly needed. The preoperative plan must include the ability to increase constraint, and posterior stabilized, constrained, and hinged implants may be required. An absent or poorly functioning extensor mechanism is a predictor of a potentially poorer outcome, and extensor mechanism reconstructive options must be considered in these cases.

Technique

Clinical Evaluation

Evaluation of an unstable TKA begins with a careful history and physical examination. Patients with TKA instability have variable clinical presentations. In some patients, symptoms are very specific and obviously related to knee instability with accounts of positional laxity. Other patients report vague symptoms, including pain, stiffness, and strange sensations. Many patients present after a period of using a series of nonprescription braces and walking aids, particularly in the setting of varus-valgus instability, which tends to cause more symptoms of laxity and involuntary buckling. Some patterns can be suspected based on subtle clues in the history that may not be uncovered unless asked about specifically. For instance, a patient with cruciate-retaining components who had impressive early flexion after primary TKA but later reports pain over the pes anserine insertion and difficulty descending stairs may have anterior-posterior instability from PCL insufficiency. Recurrent effusions

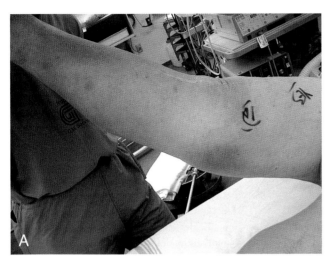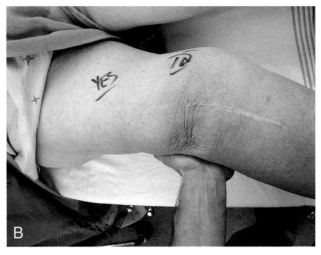

Figure 1 Clinical photographs of an 80-year-old woman who presented with global instability with both recurvatum and varus-valgus instability 5 years after TKA and 3 years after patellar tendon rupture and primary repair with semitendinosus autograft. **A,** Passive straight-leg raise demonstrates recurvatum. **B,** Valgus stress demonstrates moderate instability.

are a relatively common symptom in patients with varus-valgus instability.

The components of the physical examination assessing knee joint stability, and the documentation of the findings, should be a routine part of regular follow-up assessments in the orthopaedic clinic in an attempt to more accurately measure both abnormalities and their progression. Standing position and gait should be observed carefully for hyperextension, malalignment, or thrusts. Measurement of range of motion may reveal relative deficits of flexion or extension that indicate gap inequality. Assessment of medial and lateral structures should be performed in flexion, in extension, and in the midflexion position, whereas anterior-posterior motion is evaluated most effectively at a right angle, with a drawer maneuver. Care also should be taken to evaluate competency of the extensor mechanism, including the presence or absence of an extensor lag.

A focused clinical examination should be performed, looking for findings that can indicate specific patterns of instability (**Figure 1**). Anterior-posterior laxity may be indicated by anterior structure tenderness, relative laxity in the anterior-posterior plane

with the knee in flexion, sag of the tibia relative to the femur, and a positive quadriceps active test. Varus-valgus instability is best detected by stressing the knee in extension.

Radiographic Assessment

The routine preoperative set of knee radiographs at our institution consists of an AP weight-bearing view, a weight-bearing notch view, a weight-bearing long-leg (hip-to-ankle) view, individual lateral views of both knees, and skyline patellofemoral views. Osteolysis and component wear patterns may suggest global patterns of laxity. Obvious malalignment on weight-bearing radiographs strongly suggests both the presence and cause of varus-valgus instability (**Figure 2**). The relative position of the components as seen on the lateral view should be especially noted, such as the posterior sag seen in flexion-space instability. If angular deformity is not apparent on weight-bearing views, further assessment can be accomplished with stress radiographs, although this would be indicated only rarely.

Surgical Options

Surgical options for the treatment of the unstable TKA include focused sys-

tematic soft-tissue balancing/reconstruction with or without polyethylene liner exchange, polyethylene liner exchange with an increased constraint option, revision TKA with various constraint options, or revision to a hinged TKA. In all patterns of instability, the axis of the limb must be taken into account, and correction of any component malposition should be included in the surgical plan. The surgeon also must recognize that the foundation of instability correction is the appropriate balancing of flexion and extension spaces. The resection level at the proximal tibia affects both the flexion and extension space, the resection level at the distal femur selectively affects the extension space, and the resection level at the posterior femur affects the flexion space.

RECURVATUM

In the setting of neuromuscular disease, a nonsurgical solution such as bracing should be considered. Although hinged components with hyperextension blocks may appear attractive, significant implant-bone interface forces occur in these constructs, and implant fixation can be a long-term challenge. A common challenge in revision TKA is that distal

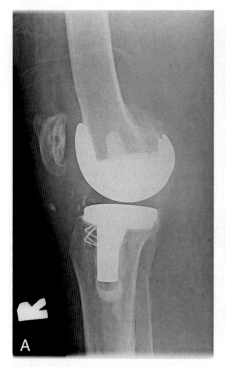

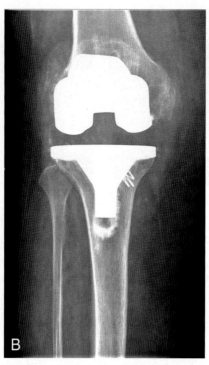

Figure 2 Preoperative radiographs of the patient shown in Figure 1. **A,** Lateral radiograph confirms recurvatum deformity. **B,** A weight-bearing AP radiograph demonstrates no malalignment.

femoral bone loss creates the tendency to raise the joint line by placing the femoral component more proximal than in the primary setting, which can create the potential for a recurvatum deformity. The solution is to restore the joint line by distalizing the femoral component, restoring the bone loss via cement, augments, or bone grafts. These techniques are discussed in detail in chapters 47, 48, and 49.

ANTERIOR-POSTERIOR INSTABILITY
If the index operation used PCL-retaining components, the first option for addressing flexion space instability is conversion to posterior stabilized implants. With the advent of high-conformity polyethylene inserts, another option is a simple conversion to a deep-dished polyethylene component, although our experience with these is limited. A common approach is to simply exchange to a larger polyethylene insert, but recognizing the

concomitant effects on the extension gap with this approach, we advocate using this technique only if there is a degree of coexisting extension instability such that with a larger polyethylene trial in place there is no significant loss of terminal extension. This approach is best reserved for the older, lower demand patient who has had a well-functioning TKA for many years and is only now experiencing a new onset of instability due to PCL incompetence. In all primary and revision TKAs, care should be taken to balance the flexion and extension gaps effectively. The most commonly encountered scenario in revision TKA gap balancing is when the flexion gap is larger than the extension gap. This is best managed by upsizing the femoral component (which has a larger anterior-posterior diameter), thereby effectively independently tightening the flexion gap and using posterior augments as necessary to maximize

contact between the femoral component and host bone.

VARUS-VALGUS INSTABILITY
Options for correcting extension space instability include soft-tissue reconstruction or revision TKA, often to implants with increased constraint. Once again, this decision depends on the exact pattern of instability. Joints that demonstrate symmetric laxity of both medial and lateral structures in both flexion and extension may be addressed by revision to a thicker polyethylene insert (**Figure 3**). Symmetric laxity in extension alone indicates a femoral component with appropriate anterior-posterior diameter that has been placed in a more proximal position than desired. Once again, this requires revision to lower the joint line and selectively tighten the extension space.

Treatment of the more common asymmetric extension space instability can be challenging both intellectually and technically. In elderly, lower demand patients, the best option is often conversion to components with increased constraint. In younger patients, however, the larger forces associated with hinged components may lead to early failure. The preferred management in this setting is correction of any malalignment and selective soft-tissue balancing, using a varus-valgus constrained prosthesis only if necessary to support any soft-tissue procedures. For varus instability, we recommend subperiosteal release of the superficial MCL, which is best completed with a Cobb or similar elevator, while leaving the tendons of the pes anserinus intact. For valgus instability, we prefer a sequential lateral release as described by Insall, which includes releasing the tightest structures in the position of greatest imbalance.

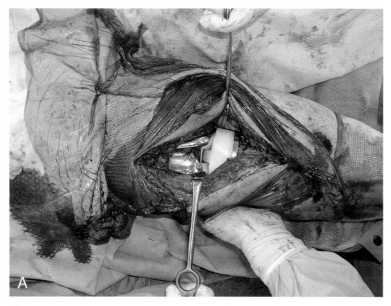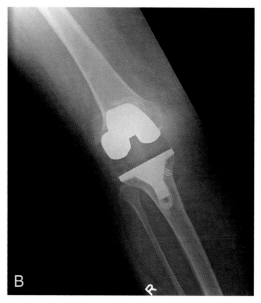

Figure 3 Images of the patient shown in Figure 1. **A,** Intraoperatively, the extensor mechanism was found to be intact, and the instability pattern was thought to be a symmetrically loose flexion and extension gap, which was managed with a thicker polyethylene insert and component retention. **B,** Postoperative weight-bearing AP radiograph demonstrates the thicker polyethylene insert.

Postoperative Regimen

There is nothing particularly unique about the postoperative regimen in a revision TKA that has been performed for instability. Postoperative bracing has no significant role unless an extensor mechanism allograft also has been performed, in which case the TKA is kept locked in extension for at least 6 weeks. Bracing should not be used to try to achieve postoperative varus-valgus stability. Instead, the intraoperative techniques discussed in this chapter should be used to achieve stability.

Avoiding Pitfalls and Complications

Obviously, the best way to avoid problems with an unstable TKA is to avoid instability at the time of initial component implantation. If a PCL-retaining implant is used, careful preservation of the PCL and verification of its func-

tion intraoperatively should be a part of the surgical procedure. Careful attention to soft-tissue balancing as well as appropriate component sizing intraoperatively is critical. This is particularly true when it is noted at the time of revision surgery that the anterior-posterior dimension has been underestimated and the femoral component is undersized, which has led to a relatively wide flexion space that clinically manifests as flexion space instability. The correct approach in such a scenario has already been discussed: a larger femoral component should be used to correct this flexion-extension gap imbalance, supplemented with augments beneath the posterior flanges of the component as necessary.

In centers where revision surgery for instability is undertaken, the importance of the availability of options for varying degrees of constraint, as well as surgeon familiarity with the use of such systems, cannot be overemphasized. The surgeon must be certain that the correct indication is present before using constrained components. Increased constraint in

the cam-post mechanism leads to increased stresses at the implant-bone interface and theoretically may lead to earlier failure. We believe that the primary indications for the use of highly constrained prostheses are either flexion instability that persists despite placement of the largest posterior stabilized femoral component that the coronal dimension will accommodate or extension instability resulting from collateral ligament rupture or incompetence.

Careful attention to the basic principles of TKA will avoid many of the causes of instability, particularly those occurring in the early postoperative period, as most of these issues relate to surgical technique. Late instability is more often related to issues of polyethylene wear and component failure. An understanding of the various instability patterns, their clinical presentations, and appropriate management techniques will allow the reconstructive surgeon to have an approach to address these challenging cases.

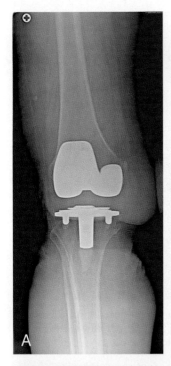
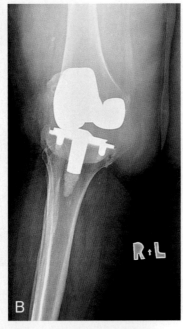
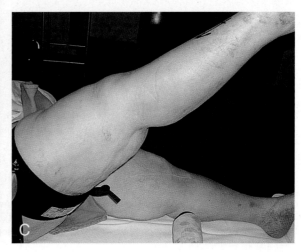
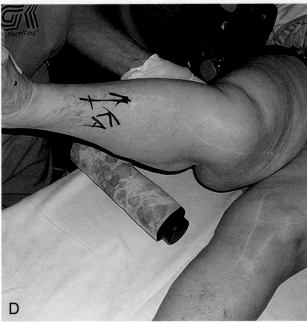

Figure 4 Images of a 76-year-old woman who underwent a primary TKA 18 years previously. She presented with recent-onset varus-valgus instability and a subjective sense of the knee dislocating. **A,** Non-weight-bearing AP radiograph shows no obvious abnormality. **B,** Weight-bearing AP radiograph demonstrates the instability pattern. **C,** Clinical photograph demonstrates no clinical recurvatum evident with passive straight-leg raise. **D,** Valgus stress demonstrates significant instability.

▮ Case Discussion

A 76-year-old woman presented 18 years after a primary TKA (**Figure 4**). She had done well until approximately 12 months before presentation, when generalized instability symptoms with activities of daily living began to develop. She had no symptoms when at rest. Additionally, she was experiencing increasing generalized knee pain and recurrent effusions. She had no constitutional symptoms and no history of infection or wound problems. All screening laboratory test results were within normal limits. Although a supine AP radiograph (**Figure 4**, *A*) did not show any significant findings, a weight-bearing image (**Figure 4**, *B*) demonstrated a significant valgus deformity. No significant recurvatum deformity was seen clinically (**Figure 4**, *C*). Both varus and valgus instability were present (**Figure 4**, *D*), but with firm end points, demonstrating probable collateral ligament competence. A routine medial parapatellar ar-

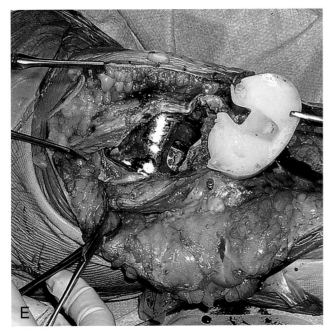 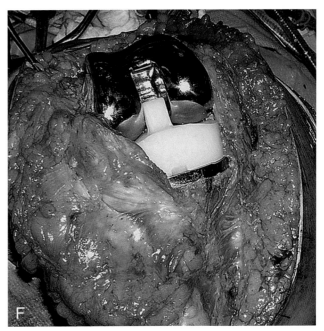

Figure 4 continued E, Intraoperative photograph demonstrates significant polyethylene wear. **F,** Intraoperative photograph shows the revision TKA with a constrained polyethylene insert.

throtomy was performed. As is typical in cases of ligamentous instability, no additional extensile exposure techniques were required because the soft tissues were already very lax. The polyethylene component demonstrated very significant damage both posteromedially and posterolaterally (**Figure 4,** *E*). The polyethylene component removed was a 10-mm insert. To achieve proper flexion-extension balancing, the joint was distalized 8 mm with distal augments, and a 22.5-mm polyethylene insert was required (**Figure 4,** *F*). Our routine in all revisions is to use a femoral component that has a cam design that can accept both posterior stabilized and constrained polyethylene inserts. An intraoperative trial is performed and a final polyethylene insert is selected that provides acceptable stability. Although the classic teaching is to avoid the use of increased constraint unless absolutely necessary, we prefer to use a constrained polyethylene insert in older, lower demand patients at the time of the revision TKA if this provides a more stable construct.

Bibliography

Callaghan JJ, O'Rourke MR, Liu SS: The role of implant constraint in revision total knee arthroplasty: Not too little, not too much. *J Arthroplasty* 2005;20(4, Suppl 2):41-43.

Dennis DA, Berry DJ, Engh G, et al: Revision total knee arthroplasty. *J Am Acad Orthop Surg* 2008;16(8):442-454.

Easley ME, Insall JN, Scuderi GR, Bullek DD: Primary constrained condylar knee arthroplasty for the arthritic valgus knee. *Clin Orthop Relat Res* 2000;380(380):58-64.

Giori NJ, Lewallen DG: Total knee arthroplasty in limbs affected by poliomyelitis. *J Bone Joint Surg Am* 2002;84-A(7): 1157-1161.

Hofmann AA, Tkach TK, Evanich CJ, Camargo MP: Posterior stabilization in total knee arthroplasty with use of an ultracongruent polyethylene insert. *J Arthroplasty* 2000;15(5):576-583.

McAuley JP, Engh GA: Constraint in total knee arthroplasty: When and what? *J Arthroplasty* 2003;18(3, Suppl 1):51-54.

McAuley JP, Engh GA, Ammeen DJ: Treatment of the unstable total knee arthroplasty. *Instr Course Lect* 2004;53:237-241.

Mihalko WM, Krackow KA: Flexion and extension gap balancing in revision total knee arthroplasty. *Clin Orthop Relat Res* 2006;446:121-126.

Naudie DD, Rorabeck CH: Managing instability in total knee arthroplasty with constrained and linked implants. *Instr Course Lect* 2004;53:207-215.

Pagnano MW, Hanssen AD, Lewallen DG, Stuart MJ: Flexion instability after primary posterior cruciate retaining total knee arthroplasty. *Clin Orthop Relat Res* 1998;356(356):39-46.

Parratte S, Pagnano MW: Instability after total knee arthroplasty. *Instr Course Lect* 2008;57:295-304.

Peters CL, Hennessey R, Barden RM, Galante JO, Rosenberg AG: Revision total knee arthroplasty with a cemented posterior-stabilized or constrained condylar prosthesis: A minimum 3-year and average 5-year follow-up study. *J Arthroplasty* 1997;12(8):896-903.

Pour AE, Parvizi J, Slenker N, Purtill JJ, Sharkey PF: Rotating hinged total knee replacement: use with caution. *J Bone Joint Surg Am* 2007;89(8):1735-1741.

Sculco TP: The role of constraint in total knee arthoplasty. *J Arthroplasty* 2006;21(4, Suppl 1):54-56.

Vince KG, Abdeen A, Sugimori T: The unstable total knee arthroplasty: Causes and cures. *J Arthroplasty* 2006;21(4, Suppl 1):44-49.

Whiteside LA: Ligament balancing in revision total knee arthroplasty. *Clin Orthop Relat Res* 2004;423(423):178-185.

Coding

CPT Codes		Corresponding ICD-9 Codes	
Revision Total Knee Arthroplasty			
27486	Revision of total knee arthroplasty, with or without allograft; one component	996.40 996.42	996.41
27487	Revision of total knee arthroplasty, with or without allograft; femoral and entire tibial component	996.40 996.42	996.41
Lateral Retinacular Release			
27425	Lateral retinacular release, open	996.40 996.42	996.41
Removal of Prosthesis			
27488	Removal of prosthesis, including total knee prosthesis, methylmethacrylate with or without insertion of spacer, knee	996.40 996.42	996.41
Arthroscopic Posterior Cruciate Ligament Repair			
29889	Arthroscopically aided posterior cruciate ligament repair/augmentation or reconstruction	996.40 996.42	996.41

HCPCS Codes*			
Dynamic Extension Braces			
L1843	Knee orthosis, single upright, thigh and calf, with adjustable flexion and extension joint (Unicentric or polycentric), medial-lateral and rotation control, with or without varus/valgus adjustment, prefabricated, includes fitting and adjustment		
L1844	Knee orthosis, single upright, thigh and calf, with adjustable flexion and extension joint (Unicentric or polycentric), medial-lateral and rotation control, with or without varus/valgus adjustment, custom fabricated		
L1845	Knee orthosis, double upright, thigh and calf, with adjustable flexion and extension joint (Unicentric or polycentric), medial-lateral and rotation control, with or without varus/valgus adjustment, prefabricated, includes fitting and adjustment		
L1846	Knee orthosis, double upright, thigh and calf, with adjustable flexion and extension joint (Unicentric or polycentric), medial-lateral and rotation control, with or without varus/valgus adjustment, custom fabricated		

*HCPCS codes (supply codes) are separately reportable by the physician when provided in the office setting. If ordered in the hospital or outpatient facility, supply codes are not separately reportable.
CPT copyright © 2010 by the American Medical Association. All rights reserved.
HCPCS copyright © 2010 by the Centers for Medicare and Medicaid Services. All rights reserved.

Chapter 32

Management of Periprosthetic Fractures Around a Total Knee Arthroplasty

George J. Haidukewych, MD

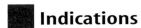 Indications

The incidence of periprosthetic fracture after total knee arthroplasty (TKA) ranges from 0.3% to 2.5%. These fractures most commonly involve the distal femoral metaphysis above the flange of the femoral component. Patellar and tibial fractures are rare compared with supracondylar distal femur fractures. This chapter focuses on the most common clinical situation, which is a distal femoral fracture above a well-fixed, well-functioning TKA. Fractures around loose prostheses generally are treated with revision arthroplasty, not internal fixation. These revision techniques are covered elsewhere in this text.

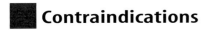 Contraindications

Potential contraindications to internal fixation include a loose TKA or a situation where distal bone stock is inadequate for internal fixation, such as with massive osteolysis (**Figure 1**).

Active infection also is a contraindication to internal fixation and should be managed by other strategies.

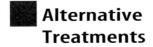 Alternative Treatments

In general, two types of fixation implants are useful for supracondylar periprosthetic fractures: retrograde nails and plates. Each has advantages and disadvantages, which should be considered when deciding which type of implant to use. The type of arthroplasty and surgeon preference will also influence implant choice. For example, if the distal fragment is of sufficient length to allow purchase with multiple locking screws and the arthroplasty allows intracondylar notch access (as with a cruciate-retaining femoral component design), then a retrograde nail can be quite effective (**Figure 2**). Careful control of alignment and the use of multiplanar distal locking screws to ensure excellent distal fragment fixation is recommended.

Newer-generation retrograde nails offer "angle stable" locking screw fixation that may be advantageous in this setting. Nails offer limited fixation in short distal fragments, however, and I rarely find them useful in these situations.

Because of the challenges posed by short distal fragments and intercondylar notch access, locked plates are used more commonly than retrograde nails. Modern locked plating designs allow the use of multiple large-diameter, fixed-angle locking screws to secure short distal fragments. With modern percutaneous targeting equipment and clamps, such procedures can be performed in a tissue-friendly fashion, without requiring an arthrotomy through a scarred tissue bed. Additionally, there are no concerns with intracondylar notch access or incorrect nail starting points that may be necessitated by a particular trochlear design. For example, some cruciate-retaining femoral components have "long" trochlear designs that may interfere with proper nail trajectory, even though notch access exists. Studies of modern methods of fixation of periprosthetic fractures using retrograde nailing or locked plating techniques have documented clear superiority over older methods of fixing these fractures with nonlocked plates with or without allograft strut aug-

Dr. Haidukewych or an immediate family member serves as a board member, owner, officer, or committee member of the Orthopaedic Trauma Association and the American Academy of Orthopaedic Surgeons; has received royalties from DePuy; is a member of a speakers' bureau or has made paid presentations on behalf of DePuy; serves as a paid consultant to or is an employee of DePuy; and holds stock or stock options in Surmodics and Orthopediatrics.

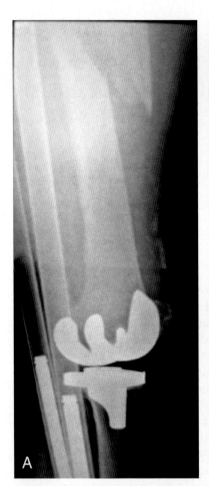
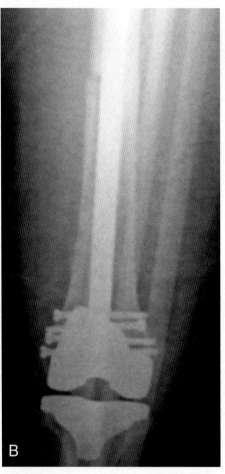

Figure 1 Radiographs of the knee of an elderly patient with a periprosthetic fracture above a loose femoral component. **A,** Preoperative lateral view shows massive distal osteolysis. **B,** Postoperative lateral view after revision using a distal femoral replacement. (Courtesy of George J. Haidukewych, MD, Orlando, FL.)

mentation. The surgical technique section below describes my preferred locked plating technique for periprosthetic fractures of the distal femur.

Results

The results of internal fixation of distal femur fractures above a TKA have been documented in several studies (**Table 1**). Excellent outcomes have been documented for both retrograde nailing and locked plating techniques. Studies also have shown that modern plating and nailing techniques are associated with a dramatic decrease in the requirement for allograft strut augmentation and delayed bone grafting to achieve union. Concerning rates of malalignment remain with both techniques, however, and therefore careful alignment technique using fluoroscopic guidance is required to avoid distal fragment malalignment.

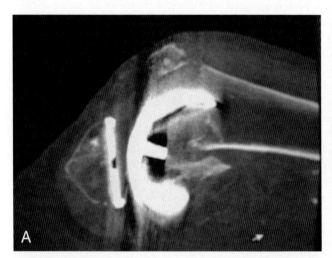
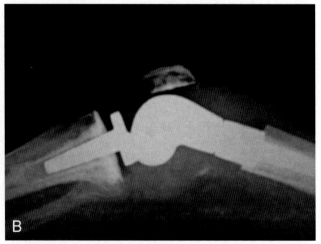

Figure 2 Radiographs of a knee with a periprosthetic fracture with a long distal fragment above a cruciate-retaining femoral component. **A,** Preoperative lateral view. **B,** Lateral view after treatment with a retrograde nail with multiple locking screws in the distal fragment. (Courtesy of George J. Haidukewych, MD, Orlando, FL.)

Table 1 Results of Internal Fixation of Periprosthetic Fractures of the Distal Femur

Authors (Year)	Number of Fractures	Procedure or Approach	Mean Patient Age (Range)	Mean Follow-up (Range)	Results
Gliatis et al (2005)	10	Retrograde nailing	NR	35 months (25-52)	100% union 1 with malalignment
Ricci et al (2006)	22	Minimally invasive locked plating	74 years	15 months	19 of 22 healed
Fulkerson et al (2007)	24	LISS locked plating	69.4 years	6 months	21 of 24 united
Large et al (2008)	50	29 locked plating 21 nonlocked plating or intramedullary nail	NR	1.7 years	Locking plating outperformed retrograde nailing and nonlocked plating
Han et al (2009)	8	Retrograde nailing	NR	39 months	100% union
Chettiar et al (2009)	14	Retrograde nailing	NR	To union	100% union

NR = not reported, LISS = less invasive stabilization system.

■ Technique (Locked Plating)

Setup/Exposure

I prefer to position the patient supine on a flat fluoroscopic table. The C-arm is brought in from the side opposite that of the fractured extremity. Both limbs are prepared and draped into the field. This is done for several reasons. First and foremost, this position facilitates imaging of the entire fractured femur because the unaffected leg can simply be lifted out of the way to allow the fluoroscope to obtain an unobstructed lateral view of the fractured extremity. Preparing both limbs into the field also provides the surgeon immediate access to the contralateral limb to verify appropriate limb length, rotation, and alignment. Intravenous antibiotics are administered (typically a first-generation cephalosporin), and careful attention is paid to making sure good muscle relaxation has been achieved. The limbs are prepared and draped in the usual fashion; typically, a small towel "bump" is placed under the limb to be operated on. The bump should be positioned somewhat proximal to the fracture site to avoid the

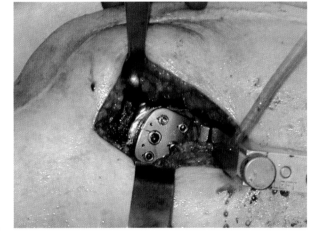

Figure 3 Intraoperative photograph demonstrates minimally invasive plate insertion through a small anterolateral incision. (Courtesy of George J. Haidukewych, MD, Orlando, FL.)

typical hyperextension deformity of the distal fragment that is noted if the bump is placed directly under the knee. An anterolateral incision is made, typically just lateral to the flange of the femoral component. The fascia is incised, and a small lateral subvastus exposure is performed (**Figure 3**).

Procedure

A plate of appropriate length is slid along the lateral aspect of the femoral cortex in a submuscular, extraperiosteal fashion. Gentle traction is applied to the limb, and gross fracture alignment is obtained. Plate position is then verified in two planes fluoroscopically. A guide pin is placed in the distal fragment, typically parallel to the articular condylar surfaces of the femoral component distally. If the surgeon is satisfied with this alignment, then the plate can be secured to the shaft proximally either with a percutaneous pin or with a percutaneous clamp. At this critical point, the reduction is carefully scrutinized in the AP and lateral planes, and limb length, alignment, and rotation can be finely

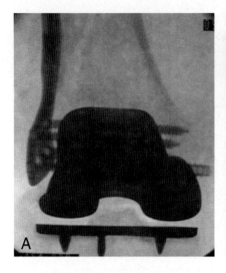
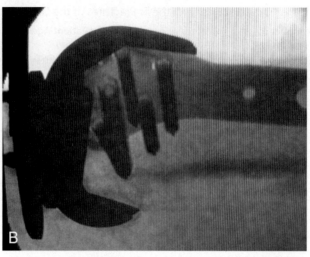

Figure 4 AP (**A**) and lateral (**B**) fluoroscopic views of a locked plate used for a distal femoral periprosthetic fracture. Note the multiple distal locking screws. (Courtesy of George J. Haidukewych, MD, Orlando, FL.)

adjusted (**Figure 4**). If necessary, comparison with the contralateral nonfractured limb can be performed at this point.

When the surgeon is completely satisfied with the alignment of the limb, screws can be inserted in the usual fashion using the standard drilling, measurement, and insertion techniques recommended by the plate manufacturer. Typically, nonlocking screws are placed first, to either lag fragments or "pull" the plate down to bone if necessary. Locking screws are then placed in the usual fashion to "lock" the construct in place. I prefer to use all distal locking screws, as many as allowed by plate design, targeting areas around the lugs of the femoral component. Plates that allow screw angulation (so-called "polyaxial" plates) have a unique advantage in this situation because long locking screw fixation can be obtained, even if obstacles to distal fixation are encountered during drilling. In general, femoral proximal shaft fixation should include at least four bicortical screws. In excellent bone, such as that found in younger patients, locking screws are typically unnecessary in the shaft; traditional screws are sufficient. In osteopenic patients, I prefer to use bicortical locking screw fixation. All clamps and wires are then removed. The entire construct is again carefully checked fluoroscopically in both the AP and lateral planes. It should be noted that the most common errors include valgus alignment of the distal fragment, hyperextension of the distal fragment, and fracture distraction. Rotation is also compared with the arc of the contralateral hip.

Wound Closure

The wounds are irrigated and closed in layers with absorbable sutures for the deep layers and standard sutures or stainless steel clips for the skin. The neurovascular status of the limb is evaluated and the limb is placed in a bulky plaster splint.

Postoperative Regimen

The splint is removed on the first postoperative day and the patient is typically placed in a hinged knee brace. If the fixation is deemed excellent and the patient is compliant, then gentle range of motion is begun on the first postoperative day. Weight bearing is typically delayed for 6 to 12 weeks, depending on the bone quality and the fracture pattern. For example, I typically progress weight bearing at 6 weeks for simple fractures with good bony contact and good bone quality, and I delay weight bearing for 12 weeks for severely osteopenic or comminuted fractures. Radiographs are typically obtained 6 weeks, 12 weeks, and 6 months after surgery.

Avoiding Pitfalls and Complications

Avoiding malalignment is perhaps the most challenging part of internal fixation of periprosthetic fractures above a TKA. Common pitfalls to avoid include valgus alignment of the distal fragment, hyperextension of the distal fragment, fracture distraction, and plate malposition. To avoid excessive valgus alignment of the distal fragment, careful radiographic scrutiny is important as well as careful attention to the initial alignment guide pin placement into the distal fragment. If this placement is parallel to the distal articular surface of the femoral component and the plate is affixed to the shaft, in most plating systems a 5° valgus angle will be obtained. To avoid hyperextension, careful lateral radiographic fluoroscopic scrutiny is recommended. Placing the bump slightly proximal to the fracture site will allow the distal fragment to tip "over the bump" into a position of relative flexion. Also, avoiding excessive traction on the limb will avoid a pull on the gastrocnemius origin and therefore will minimize the tendency for the fragment to hyperextend. Fracture distraction should be avoided by not applying too much traction when affixing the plate to the shaft. I generally recommend maintaining bony contact, even if slight limb shortening of a few millimeters is necessary. This is most useful in very elderly and severely osteopenic patients. Plate malposition can be avoided by using percutaneous clamps and fluoroscopic scrutiny, especially in the lateral plane. The proximal aspect of the plate tends to slide anteriorly on the femoral shaft. Palpating the plate with a finger inserted through a small incision proximally can also help avoid this common complication.

Premature weight bearing can cause construct failure, especially in patients with osteopenia and comminuted fractures. Aggressive range of motion also can "cycle" the construct, causing loss of fixation. In severely osteopenic, elderly patients or those with comorbidities including mental status changes, dementia, or other noncompliance issues, a period of immobilization with bed-to-chair restrictions may be wise to avoid early construct failure.

■ Bibliography

Anakwe RE, Aitken SA, Khan LA: Osteoporotic periprosthetic fractures of the femur in elderly patients: Outcome after fixation with the LISS plate. *Injury* 2008;39(10):1191-1197.

Chettiar K, Jackson MP, Brewin J, Dass D, Butler-Manuel PA: Supracondylar periprosthetic femoral fractures following total knee arthroplasty: Treatment with a retrograde intramedullary nail. *Int Orthop* 2009;33(4):981-985.

Fulkerson E, Tejwani N, Stuchin S, Egol K: Management of periprosthetic femur fractures with a first generation locking plate. *Injury* 2007;38(8):965-972.

Gliatis J, Megas P, Panagiotopoulos E, Lambiris E: Midterm results of treatment with a retrograde nail for supracondylar periprosthetic fractures of the femur following total knee arthroplasty. *J Orthop Trauma* 2005;19(3):164-170.

Haidukewych GJ: Innovations in locking plate technology. *J Am Acad Orthop Surg* 2004;12(4):205-212.

Haidukewych GJ, Sems SA, Huebner D, Horwitz D, Levy B: Results of polyaxial locked-plate fixation of periarticular fractures of the knee: Surgical technique. *J Bone Joint Surg Am* 2008;90(suppl 2 pt 1):117-134.

Han HS, Oh KW, Kang SB: Retrograde intramedullary nailing for periprosthetic supracondylar fractures of the femur after total knee arthroplasty. *Clin Orthop Surg* 2009;1(4):201-206.

Herrera DA, Kregor PJ, Cole PA, Levy BA, Jönsson A, Zlowodzki M: Treatment of acute distal femur fractures above a total knee arthroplasty: Systematic review of 415 cases (1981-2006). *Acta Orthop* 2008;79(1):22-27.

Large TM, Kellam JF, Bosse MJ, Sims SH, Althausen P, Masonis JL: Locked plating of supracondylar periprosthetic femur fractures. *J Arthroplasty* 2008;23(6, suppl 1):115-120.

Norrish AR, Jibri ZA, Hopgood P: The LISS plate treatment of supracondylar fractures above a total knee replacement: a case-control study. *Acta Orthop Belg* 2009;75(5):642-648.

Parvizi J, Jain N, Schmidt AH: Periprosthetic knee fractures. *J Orthop Trauma* 2008;22(9):663-671.

Parvizi J, Kim KI, Oliashirazi A, Ong A, Sharkey PF: Periprosthetic patellar fractures. *Clin Orthop Relat Res* 2006;446: 161-166.

Ricci WM, Borrelli J Jr: Operative management of periprosthetic femur fractures in the elderly using biological fracture reduction and fixation techniques. *Injury* 2007;38(suppl 3):S53-S58.

Ricci WM, Loftus T, Cox C, Borrelli J: Locked plates combined with minimally invasive insertion technique for the treatment of periprosthetic supracondylar femur fractures above a total knee arthroplasty. *J Orthop Trauma* 2006;20(3): 190-196.

Coding

CPT Codes		Corresponding ICD-9 Codes	
Femoral Fixation, Plate/Screws			
27507	Open treatment of femoral shaft fracture with plate/screws, with or without cerclage	821.10	821.20
Femoral Fixation, Intramedullary Implant			
27506	Open treatment of femoral shaft fracture, with or without external fixation, with insertion of intramedullary implant, with or without cerclage and/or locking screws	821.10	821.20

CPT copyright © 2010 by the American Medical Association. All rights reserved.

Chapter 33

Management of Nerve and Vascular Injuries Associated With Total Knee Arthroplasty

James A. Rand, MD

Introduction

Neurovascular complications are some of the most feared problems associated with total knee arthroplasty (TKA). Avoidance of these complications, which is preferable to treatment, is facilitated by an understanding of the neurovascular anatomy of the knee, recognition of patient risk factors, use of appropriate postoperative management, and careful surgical technique. Prompt recognition of a vascular injury is essential for minimizing sequelae. High-risk patients must be counseled about the potential of a neurovascular complication before they undergo TKA.

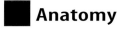

Anatomy

Vascular Anatomy

Although many aspects of anatomy are relevant to TKA, a brief review of the nerves and vascular supply around the knee are important for avoiding complications. Five main channels provide arterial supply to the knee: (1) the descending (supreme) genicular, (2) the medial and lateral superior genicular, (3) the medial and lateral

inferior genicular, (4) the middle genicular, and (5) the anterior tibial recurrent arteries. The descending genicular artery arises from the femoral artery just above the opening of the adductor canal and divides into three branches: the saphenous branch, which accompanies the saphenous vein and nerve; the articular branch, which runs between the tendon of the adductor magnus and the lower margin of the vastus medialis and supplies the vastus medialis; and the deep oblique branch, which descends along the medial aspect of the femoral shaft. The descending genicular artery lies at a mean distance of 13.5 mm (range, 6.9 to 22.4 mm) from the superomedial border of the patella and enters the vastus medialis at an angle of 33°. A midvastus exposure of the knee should extend no farther than 15 mm from the superior border of the patella, to avoid injury to the descending genicular artery. The popliteal artery, vein, and tibial nerve enter the popliteal space at the junction of the middle and lower thirds of the femur. The popliteal vessels initially lie medial, then anterior, and finally lateral to the nerve. In the proximal popliteal space, the vessels are separated from the femur by fat. As the vessels prog-

ress distally, they lie close to the posterior capsule proximal to the popliteus muscle. The popliteal vessels lie posterior to the popliteus muscle. At the lower border of the popliteus muscle, the popliteal artery divides into the anterior and posterior tibial arteries. There is considerable variability in the popliteal vein.

The genicular arteries arise from the popliteal artery. The superior medial genicular artery passes anteriorly above the medial femoral condyle deep to the tendon of the adductor magnus to supply the vastus medialis. The lateral superior genicular artery travels anterior to the biceps femoris above the femoral condyle to supply the vastus lateralis. The lateral superior genicular artery is at risk of injury when a lateral retinacular release is performed to correct patellar maltracking. The middle genicular artery arises behind the popliteal surface of the femur, penetrates the posterior capsule, and supplies the cruciate ligaments and posterior portions of the menisci. The medial inferior genicular artery arises below the level of the joint line, travels deep to the medial collateral ligament, and supplies the infrapatellar fat pad and periphery of the medial meniscus. The medial inferior genicular artery may be injured with the distal portion of a medial parapatellar incision, excision of the

Dr. Rand or an immediate family member is a member of a speakers' bureau or has made paid presentations on behalf of Zimmer and serves as a paid consultant for or is an employee of Zimmer.

medial meniscus, or a medial soft-tissue release from the tibia. The lateral inferior genicular artery arises deep to the lateral head of the gastrocnemius, passes around the lateral tibial plateau above the fibular head, and courses deep to the lateral collateral ligament. The lateral inferior genicular artery is frequently injured during excision of the lateral meniscus. The anterior tibial recurrent artery arises from the anterior tibial artery and supplies the anterior aspect of the knee. The genicular and recurrent tibial arteries form a complex anastomosis around the knee (**Figure 1**).

Tibial and femoral bone cuts in TKA are usually performed with the knee in at least 90° of flexion. In some techniques that are called minimally invasive, however, bone resections are performed with the knee in less than 90° of flexion. With the knee in extension, the popliteal vessels are a mean of 5.9 to 6.8 mm (range, 3 to 12 mm) from the tibia at the level of resection for a TKA; with the knee in 90° of flexion, this distance increases to a mean of 9.1 to 10.2 mm (range, 4.6 to 17 mm). In one study, however, the popliteal artery was found to move toward the tibia upon knee flexion in 2 of 9 patients. A high-branching (proximal to the popliteus muscle) anterior tibial artery was identified in 6 of 100 knees, and in all 6 of these knees, the artery passed anterior to the popliteus, placing it directly against the posterior tibial cortex. Therefore, it is essential to keep the saw blade from progressing farther posterior than the posterior tibial cortex.

Neuroanatomy

The tibial nerve arises from the sciatic nerve at the midfemoral level and passes into the popliteal fossa (**Figure 2**). In the popliteal space, the tibial nerve proximally lies lateral to the popliteal vessels, and then passes behind the vessels to a medial location. The tibial nerve passes with the popliteal vessels between the two

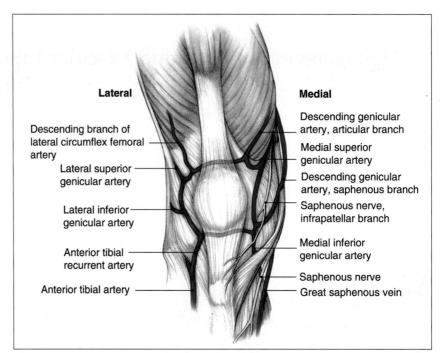

Figure 1 Vascular anatomy of the anterior aspect of the knee. (Modified with permission from Clarke HD, Scott WN, Insall JN, et al: Anatomy, in Insall JN, Scott WN, eds: *Surgery of the Knee*, ed 3. New York, NY, Churchill Livingstone, 2001, pp 13-76.)

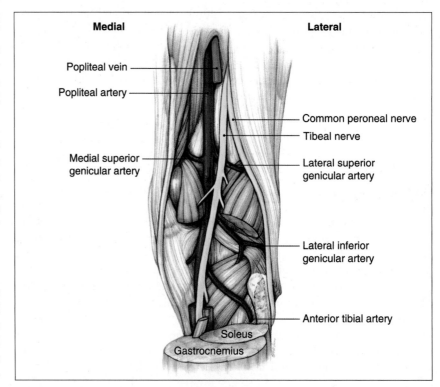

Figure 2 Vascular and nerve anatomy of the posterior aspect of the knee. (Modified with permission from Clarke HD, Scott WN, Insall JN, et al: Anatomy, in Insall JN, Scott WN, eds: *Surgery of the Knee*, ed 3. New York, NY, Churchill Livingstone, 2001, pp 13-76.)

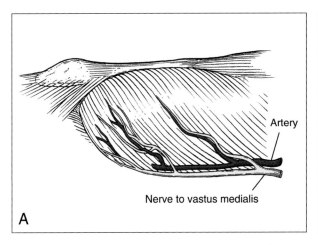

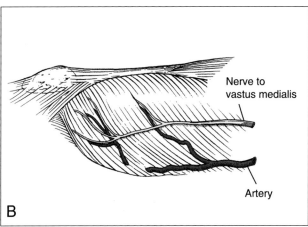

Figure 3 Diagram of posterior (**A**) and central (**B**) patterns of innervation of the vastus medialis muscle. (Reprinted with permission from Jojima H, Whiteside LA, Ogata K: Anatomic considerations of nerve supply to the vastus medialis in knee surgery. *Clin Orthop Relat Res* 2004;423:157-160.)

heads of the gastrocnemius muscle, then anterior to the soleus and posterior to the tibialis posterior muscle. The peroneal nerve arises from the sciatic nerve, enters the popliteal fossa on the lateral side of the tibial nerve, and runs along the medial side of the biceps femoris. The peroneal nerve passes between the tendon of the biceps femoris and the lateral head of the gastrocnemius. The peroneal nerve wraps around the lateral neck of the fibula and pierces the peroneus longus; it divides into superficial and deep branches at the level of the fibular neck. The superficial location and relatively fixed position of the peroneal nerve at the fibular neck places the nerve at risk of injury by direct pressure from dressings or external force such as a continuous passive motion (CPM) machine. The saphenous nerve arises from the femoral nerve. At the lower end of the Hunter canal, the saphenous nerve pierces the fascia between the sartorius and gracilis. The infrapatellar branch of the saphenous nerve passes through the sartorius to supply the skin on the medial side of the knee medial to the patellar ligament. The infrapatellar branch is subject to injury by an anteromedial arthrotomy and medial soft-tissue releases from the tibia. The nerve supply to the vastus medialis is poten-

tially at risk with a midvastus approach to the knee. The vastus medialis is innervated by two nerves arising from the posterior division of the femoral nerve. A short lateral branch enters the proximal portion of the muscle, and a larger medial branch, which has a variable presentation, runs along the anteromedial border of the muscle distally and supplies the middle and distal thirds of the vastus medialis. Two patterns of distribution of the medial branch have been observed (**Figure 3**). In the posterior pattern, the medial branch courses along the posterior edge of the muscle and terminates in three to four branches sent into the vastus medialis obliquus fibers posteriorly. In the central pattern of innervation, the medial branch enters the main body of the muscle, sending branches through the substance of the muscle into the distal vastus medialis obliquus. In addition, a branch of the saphenous nerve that leaves the adductor canal just proximal to the infrapatellar branch supplies the vastus medialis obliquus in 10% of knees. In a midvastus approach to the knee, the potential for muscle denervation is greater with the central pattern of innervation.

Arterial Injury

Prevalence

Vascular injuries associated with TKA are infrequent. I have reported the prevalence of arterial injury to be 0.03% (3 of 9,022 TKAs), and Calligaro and associates reported a prevalence of 0.17% (24 of 23,199 TKAs). The prevalence of injury is greater following revision TKA (0.36% [6 of 1,665]) than following primary TKA (0.15% [18 of 11,953]).

Types of Injury

Arterial injury may be acute bleeding from a vessel laceration, arterial occlusion from thrombosis or embolization of plaque, compartment syndrome, pseudoaneurysm, or mycotic aneurysm. The popliteal artery is the most frequent site of injury, but any of the vessels around the knee may be affected. The most frequent injury is thrombosis, followed by direct vessel laceration; the least frequent problem is an arteriovenous fistula. Multiple problems may coexist, such as compartment syndrome and thrombosis. False aneurysms of the popliteal, lateral superior genicular, medial inferior genicular, and lateral inferior genicular arteries have been observed.

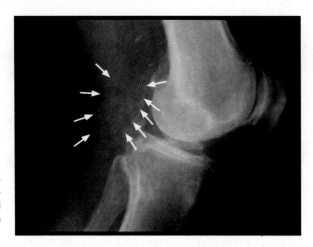

Figure 4 Lateral radiograph of the knee demonstrating a calcified popliteal artery aneurysm (arrows).

There are two case reports of a mycotic aneurysm associated with an infected TKA.

Risk Factors

A major risk factor for a vascular complication is preexisting peripheral vascular disease. Vascular disease should be suspected in the patient with absent pedal pulses, dystrophic skin or hair loss on the lower limb, or a history of other vascular surgery (carotids, cardiac, abdominal aortic aneurysm) or of intermittent claudication, rest pain, diabetes mellitus, popliteal aneurysm, smoking, or malignancy. A local anesthetic injection into the knee followed by ambulation can help to distinguish between local arthritic knee pain and pain from ischemia. In a prospective study, 15 of 207 patients undergoing TKA (7%) had evidence of chronic lower extremity ischemia. Ischemic complications occurred in three of these patients following TKA. The preoperative ankle-brachial pressure index (ABPI) ranged from 0.55 to 0.89. DeLaurentis and associates advised that a TKA be performed in a patient with an ABPI greater than 0.5. If the ABPI is less than 0.5, however, vascular surgery should be considered before TKA. In a study of 54 knees with either an absent dorsalis pedis or posterior tibial pulse, all but four had a pulse identified by a Doppler probe. Thirty-five of

the 54 knees had an ABPI less than 0.9 (the lowest was 0.73), but no vascular compromise occurred following TKA. In another study of 7 patients with chronic lower extremity ischemia with an ABPI of 0.65 to 0.9 before TKA, there were no vascular complications.

Vascular calcification visible on plain radiographs (**Figure 4**) should raise a suspicion of peripheral vascular disease. However, Calligaro and associates believe that calcification of the superficial femoral artery is not associated with a higher prevalence of vascular complications after TKA.

Patients with a preexisting vascular bypass graft in the lower limb are at high risk for vascular complications. In a study of nine patients with an ipsilateral peripheral arterial reconstruction, two of ten knees developed an arterial complication following TKA. A tourniquet was used during TKA in six knees. Of the two thromboses, one occurred with and one without the use of a tourniquet. A preoperative ultrasound study of the graft before TKA should be obtained, and intravenous heparin should be used before tourniquet inflation. Another risk factor is a preoperative large fixed flexion contracture.

Mechanisms of Injury

The popliteal vessels may be injured directly by surgical cutting instru-

ments such as scalpels or saws. In one study, 12 of 19 popliteal vessel injuries were the result of direct trauma. Dissection of the popliteal area during revision surgery for scar removal from the posterior capsule places the vessels at risk of injury. The knee that requires distal femoral or proximal tibial segmental bone replacement with either a prosthesis or allograft bone is at high risk. "Past-pointing" (an instrument progressing deeper into tissue than intended) with a saw can injure the popliteal vessels. The tendency to past-point with a saw may be greater when TKA is performed through a small incision with limited visibility and retraction. A high-branching anterior tibial artery passing anterior to the popliteus places it directly against the posterior tibial cortex, where it can easily be injured by a saw blade. Caution should be used during retractor placement. A posterior retractor placed lateral and deep to the posterior cruciate ligament will directly displace the popliteal vessels. Screw fixation of the tibial component can result in direct vessel injury. Screws placed between the 11 o'clock and 3 o'clock positions (with the 6 o'clock position defined as directly anterior and the 3 o'clock position defined as lateral) places neurovascular structures at risk.

Indirect trauma is a more common mechanism of injury than direct trauma. Thrombosis, intimal tears in a diseased artery, or embolization of plaque can result in acute ischemia. Pressure from a tourniquet on a diseased artery that has decreased elasticity is a potential etiology. Manipulation of the limb into hyperextension can result in popliteal vessel compression. Hyperextension of the knee after the femoral and tibial osteotomies can result in tenting of the popliteal vessels over the sharp bone edge of the tibial plateau. Correction of a large fixed flexion contracture can result in soft-tissue compression of the popliteal vessels. Unusual causes of vascular compromise include impingement resulting from a tibial component or a large fragment of extruded bone cement overhanging the posterior tibial plateau. Instability with recurrent dislocation of the knee is a rare etiology of popliteal vessel injury.

Diagnosis

Prompt diagnosis of an arterial injury is essential for a satisfactory outcome. Acute bleeding is readily identifiable at the time of surgery if the tourniquet is released before wound closure. The lateral inferior genicular artery is a frequent source of substantial hemorrhage and is easily treated. Popliteal vascular injury is unmistakable in the magnitude of bleeding. Diagnosis of acute hemorrhage is more difficult if the wound is closed and a compressive dressing is applied before release of the tourniquet. The classic findings of ischemia—a cool, pale foot with absent pulses—are indicative of vascular compromise. False aneurysms present with pain, local tenderness, palpable mass, and a bruit. Arteriovenous fistulae present with pain, swelling, and a palpable thrill, or they may present as a hemarthrosis. Isolated compartment syndromes in the thigh or leg following TKA have been reported following anticoagulation therapy or knee dislocation. A tightly swollen muscle compartment with extreme pain and decreased distal sensation is indicative of a compartment syndrome. Diagnosis of a compartment syndrome is accomplished by measuring the pressure with a slit catheter. Loss of sensation from the use of postoperative epidural analgesia may cause a delay in diagnosis of a compartment syndrome.

The time of diagnosis of an acute vascular injury or thrombosis has been reported to range from during the operation to 10 days after TKA. The prognosis for arterial injury is determined largely by the rapidity of diagnosis and treatment. A delay of more than 6 hours from injury to treatment will result in permanent

muscle and/or nerve dysfunction. Calligaro and associates studied 32 cases and found that the arterial injury was diagnosed on the day of the surgery in only 18 patients (56%) and was not diagnosed until the first to fifth day postoperatively in 14 (44%). Patients with acute arterial insufficiency who are treated after the day of surgery are more likely to require fasciotomy, sustain muscle necrosis, and have foot drop than patients who receive immediate treatment. Vascular surgery consultation should be obtained as soon as possible. Angiography is useful in identifying the location and type of injury before treatment (**Figure 5**). Calligaro and associates performed lower extremity angiography in 17 of 32 patients with acute arterial injuries. In 15 of the 32 cases, emergent vascular intervention was necessary and angiography was not obtained, as angiography should not be performed if it would result in a prolonged delay in treatment.

Management

Management of vascular complications depends on the time to diagnosis, type of injury, and associated complications such as a compartment syndrome. A thrombosis may occasionally be successfully managed by percutaneous thrombus aspiration or thrombolytic therapy with intra-arterial urokinase. Calligaro and associates found that surgical thrombectomy was successful in only 5 of 18 patients (28%); revascularization with arterial bypass surgery was necessary in the other 13 patients. They recommended arterial bypass surgery in most instances because of underlying chronic occlusive arterial disease. Angiography is recommended after either bypass or thrombectomy to rule out an intimal flap and to ensure that a thrombosis does not occur. Arterial transections are preferentially treated by end-to-end anastomosis. If a direct repair is under tension, either a polyfluoroethylene graft or below-

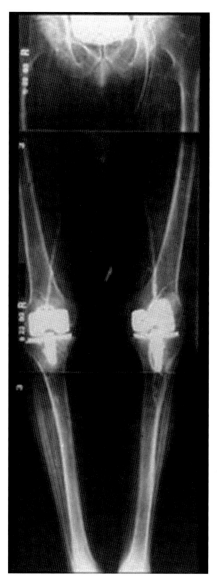

Figure 5 Angiogram performed for right popliteal arterial occlusion after TKA. (Reproduced with permission from Rand JA: Vascular complications of total knee arthroplasty. *J Arthroplasty* 1987;2:89-93).

knee bypass graft is recommended. Pseudoaneurysms can be treated by percutaneous thrombin injection or open interposition vein grafts. Ancillary techniques such as sympathectomy and fasciotomy for compartment syndrome may be required.

Outcomes

Of 131 reports of arterial complications after TKA in the literature, the outcomes were: retained TKA in 103, amputation in 24 (**Figure 6**), death in 3, and unknown in 1. Data from larger studies are listed in **Table 1**. In patients with a salvaged limb, muscle loss and residual dysfunction are not uncommon. Recommendations for management of an arterial complication are outlined in **Figure 7**.

Prevention

Prevention of arterial injuries is preferable to treatment. Careful preoperative assessment of the patient for risk factors combined with a physical examination of popliteal and pedal pulses will identify the patient at risk. Arterial vascular laboratory studies are useful in the patient with absent pedal pulses. DeLaurentis stated that a patient with an ABPI less than 0.5 usually can be treated by TKA. If evidence of a popliteal aneurysm, extensive vascular calcification, or ischemia is present, a vascular surgeon should be consulted about possible vascular bypass surgery before TKA. In the high-risk patient, use of a tourniquet should be avoided. Acute traumatic arterial injury can best be recognized at the time of operation by release of the tourniquet before wound closure. If a large fixed deformity is corrected at the time of TKA, the limb initially should be splinted in flexion in the immediate postoperative period to avoid soft-tissue compression of the popliteal vessels. Dissection of posterior capsular scar during revision TKA can be performed with the tourniquet deflated. An intraoperative Doppler can be used to identify the location of the popliteal artery. The neurovascular status of the extremity must be assessed in the recovery room. In the presence of postoperative epidural analgesia, frequent physical examination of the patient is essential for assessing the vascular status of the limb, as the patient may be unable to detect pain associated with vascular compromise. In the event of ischemic changes in the foot, care must be taken to avoid pressure on areas of compromised skin from foot pumps, compressive stockings, dressings, or bed linen.

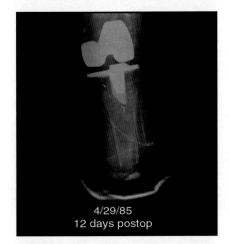

4/29/85
12 days postop

Figure 6 Radiograph of below-knee amputation in a patient with acute vascular compromise after TKA. (Reproduced with permission from Rand JA: Vascular complications of total knee arthroplasty. *J Arthroplasty* 1987; 2:89-93).

Table 1 Arterial Injury Associated With Total Knee Arthroplasty

Author(s) (Year)	Number of Knees at Risk	Number of Arterial Injuries	Prevalence (%)	Complications	Outcomes
Rand (1987)	9,022	3	0.03	3 thromboses	1 retained TKA 2 amputations
Rush (1987)	NR	12	NR	4 popliteal lacerations 1 arteriovenous fistula 7 thromboses	5 retained TKAs 5 amputations 1 death 1 unknown
Calligaro et al (1994)	4,097	7	0.17	7 thromboses	7 retained TKAs
Kumar (1998)	NR	14	NR	3 popliteal lacerations 10 thromboses	6 retained TKAs 6 amputations 1 death
DaSilva and Sobel (2003)	NR	19	NR	12 popliteal lacerations 7 thromboses 2 compartment syndrome	17 retained TKAs 2 amputations
Calligaro et al (2003)	23,199	24*	0.17	9 popliteal lacerations 5 false aneurysms 18 thromboses	24 retained TKAs

*Includes 8 total hip arthroplasties for a total of 32 total joints.
TKA = total knee arthroplasty, NR = not reported.

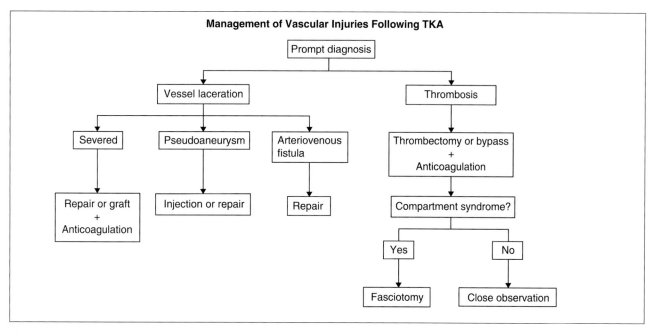

Figure 7 Algorithm for management of arterial compromise following TKA.

Nerve Palsy

Prevalence

Nerve palsy following TKA is an infrequent complication, but it is more common than arterial injury. The prevalence of peroneal nerve palsy in large series has been reported to be from 0.3% to 2.2% (**Table 2**). The highest reported prevalence was in a small series, in which 4 of 42 patients with rheumatoid arthritis had peroneal nerve palsy after TKA. The peroneal is the most frequently injured nerve, but the tibial nerve may be affected as well.

Risk Factors and Mechanisms of Injury

A variety of risk factors for peroneal palsy have been identified. A diagnosis of rheumatoid arthritis has been associated with a high risk of peroneal palsy. In a study of 42 TKAs in patients with rheumatoid arthritis, electromyograms (EMGs) were performed before and 34 days after TKA in 16 of the knees. Four knees developed clinical symptoms, and three additional knees had EMG signs of peroneal nerve dysfunction. The high prevalence of pero-

neal palsy was attributed to stretching of the nerve from the correction of the combined sagittal and coronal deformity. Bilateral peroneal palsy following bilateral TKA in four patients has been reported. The prevalence of peroneal palsy is higher following revision TKA than following primary TKA. Preoperative valgus and flexion contracture are risk factors. Asp and Rand found valgus >15° was present in 13 of 26 patients and flexion contracture >10° in 12 of 26 patients. Idusuyi and Morrey identified risk factors for nerve palsy after TKA and found the relative risk of palsy to be 12 times greater for a knee with preoperative valgus deformity, 6.5 times greater for patients with a prior laminectomy, and 2 times greater for knees with a prior proximal tibial osteotomy. The role of epidural anesthesia has been controversial, with Idusuyi and Morrey reporting the risk of palsy to be 2.8 times greater with epidural anesthesia than with general anesthesia. Another review from the same institution, however, stated that postoperative epidural analgesia was not a risk factor.

Surgical technique may affect the

risk of peroneal nerve palsy. One study found a significantly longer mean tourniquet time of 141 minutes in the group with nerve palsy, compared with 103 minutes in the patients without nerve palsy. Placement of long, pointed Hohmann-type retractors over the cut edge of the lateral tibial condyle can injure the peroneal nerve. Rose and associates stated that prophylactic dissection and release of the peroneal nerve at the time of correction of large, fixed valgus deformities does not prevent peroneal palsy and potentially may injure the nerve. Excessive postoperative bleeding also has been identified as a risk factor for nerve palsy. Idusuyi and Morrey reported on peroneal palsy caused by lateral hematoma in two knees. Poorly padded or tight dressings over the peroneal nerve also have been suggested as a cause of peroneal nerve palsy.

The time to diagnosis of a peroneal nerve palsy has ranged from the day of surgery to 10 days later. Unusual causes should be sought for peroneal nerve palsies that present late, such as years following a successful TKA. Such reported late causes include sy-

Table 2 Peroneal Nerve Palsy Following Total Knee Arthroplasty

Authors (Year)	Number of TKAs	Number of Cases of Peroneal Nerve Palsy	Prevalence (%)	Complications/Outcomes
Rose et al (1982)	2,626	23	0.9	Extent of palsy: NR Neurologic deficit: 3 motor, 20 combined Recovery: 2 full, 19 partial, 2 unknown
Asp and Rand (1990)	8,998	26	0.3	Extent of palsy: 18 complete, 8 partial Neurologic deficit: 3 motor, 23 combined Recovery: 13 full, 12 partial, 1 unknown
Horlocker et al (1994)	361	8	2.2	Extent of palsy: NR Neurologic deficit: 4 sensory, 4 combined Recovery: 4 full, 4 partial
Idusuyi and Morrey (1996)	10,361	32	0.3	Extent of palsy: 15 complete, 17 partial Neurologic deficit: 4 motor, 3 sensory, 25 combined Recovery: 16 full, 16 partial
Schinsky et al (2001)	1,476	19	1.3	Extent of palsy: NR Neurologic deficit: 19 combined Recovery: 13 full, 6 partial

TKA = total knee arthroplasty, NR = not reported.

novial cyst of the proximal tibiofibular joint, polyethylene granuloma in a popliteal cyst from wear, and an extruded tibial component of a lateral unicompartmental TKA.

Prognosis

Of 108 patients with nerve palsies studied in large series, only 48 had complete recovery (**Table 2**). Asp and Rand noted in their study that the prognosis following nerve injury is related to the extent of injury: 6 of 7 patients whose palsies were incomplete neurologic deficits had complete recovery, whereas only 6 of 18 patients whose palsies were complete neurologic deficits had complete recovery. Hospital for Special Surgery knee scores at follow-up evaluation were higher for knees with an initial partial palsy than in those with a complete palsy. Idusuyi and Morrey found that 13 of 17 patients with partial palsies had complete recovery, compared with only 3 of 15 patients with complete palsies.

Management

Management of the patient with nerve palsy should consist of removing any compressive dressings and flexing the knee to decrease tension on the nerves. Pressure on the peroneal nerve can occur with external rotation of the limb; placing a rolled towel under the greater trochanter can prevent limb external rotation. If a CPM machine is being used, care must be taken to avoid pressure from the device over the region of the fibular head. The patient with an indwelling epidural catheter for postoperative analgesia may be at increased risk for local nerve compression because of lack of protective sensation. The use of a foot drop brace (ankle-foot orthosis) will help prevent equinus contracture and improve gait while awaiting nerve recovery.

Mont and Krackow and their colleagues have recommended surgical decompression of the peroneal nerve for a nerve palsy that is not demonstrating signs of recovery. Confirmation by EMG of peroneal palsy with conduction delays at the level of the fibular neck should be obtained to document the location of the nerve injury. Dissection of the peroneal nerve extending from the biceps femoris tendon to the passage of the nerve deep to the peroneus longus is performed. The fibrous tunnel over the fibular neck is released. Krackow and associates performed surgical decompression at 5 to 45 months after onset in a series of five peroneal nerve palsies, resulting in four with complete resolution of symptoms and one with mild improvement in sensation. Mont and associates reported on a series of 31 patients treated by surgical decompression of the peroneal nerve for peroneal nerve palsy (6 of which were after TKA); 30 had subjective and functional improvement. The time between the onset of palsy and surgical decompression of the peroneal nerve affected the outcome. Full recovery of motor function occurred in all 8 patients treated within 6 months, 4 of 5 treated between 7 and 12 months, 7 of 11 treated between 13 and 24 months, and 6 of 7 treated after 24 months. Of the six palsies after TKA, five had complete recovery; the sixth recovered motor function but had residual sensory impairment. Therefore, if the patient with peroneal palsy after TKA is not showing clinical and EMG evidence of recovery after 5 to 6 months from onset, surgical decompression of

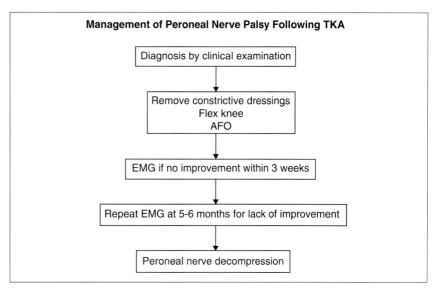

Figure 8 Algorithm for management of peroneal nerve palsy following TKA. AFO = ankle-foot orthosis, EMG = electromyography.

the peroneal nerve should be considered.

In summary, the patient at risk for nerve palsy has combined fixed valgus and flexion deformity, prior laminectomy, or rheumatoid arthritis. Prompt diagnosis combined with removal of constrictive dressings, flexion of the knee, and avoidance of pressure on the peroneal nerve are appropriate treatment. Surgical decompression of the peroneal nerve is indicated for a nerve palsy that does not demonstrate any improvement over a 5- to 6-month period. An algorithm for management of peroneal nerve palsy is outlined in **Figure 8.**

Bibliography

Asp JP, Rand JA: Peroneal nerve palsy after total knee arthroplasty. *Clin Orthop Relat Res* 1990;(261):233-237.

Calligaro KD, DeLaurentis DA, Booth RE, Rothman RH, Savarese RP, Dougherty MJ: Acute arterial thrombosis associated with total knee arthroplasty. *J Vasc Surg* 1994;20(66):927-930, discussion 930-932.

Calligaro KD, Dougherty MJ, Ryan S, Booth RE: Acute arterial complications associated with total hip and knee arthroplasty. *J Vasc Surg* 2003;38(66):1170-1177.

Clarke HD, Scott WN, Insall JN, et al: Anatomy, in Insall JN, Scott WN, eds: *Surgery of the Knee*, ed 3. New York, NY, Churchill Livingstone, 2001, pp 13-76.

Da Silva MS, Sobel M, Surgeons of the Southern Association of Vascular Surgery: Popliteal vascular injury during total knee arthroplasty. *J Surg Res* 2003;109(22):170-174.

DeLaurentis DA, Levitsky KA, Booth RE, et al: Arterial and ischemic aspects of total knee arthroplasty. *Am J Surg* 1992; 164(33):237-240.

Farrington WJ, Charnley GJ, Harries SR, Fox BM, Sharp R, Hughes PM: The position of the popliteal artery in the arthritic knee. *J Arthroplasty* 1999;14(77):800-802.

Horlocker TT, Cabanela ME, Wedel DJ: Does postoperative epidural analgesia increase the risk of peroneal nerve palsy after total knee arthroplasty? *Anesth Analg* 1994;79(33):495-500.

Idusuyi OB, Morrey BF: Peroneal nerve palsy after total knee arthroplasty: Assessment of predisposing and prognostic factors. *J Bone Joint Surg Am* 1996;78(22):177-184.

Jojima H, Whiteside LA, Ogata K: Anatomic consideration of nerve supply to the vastus medialis in knee surgery. *Clin Orthop Relat Res* 2004;423(423423):157-160.

Krackow KA, Maar DC, Mont MA, Carroll C IV: Surgical decompression for peroneal nerve palsy after total knee arthroplasty. *Clin Orthop Relat Res* 1993;292(292292):223-228.

Kumar SN, Chapman JA, Rawlins I: Vascular injuries in total knee arthroplasty: A review of the problem with special reference to the possible effects of the tourniquet. *J Arthroplasty* 1998;13(22):211-216.

Mont MA, Dellon AL, Chen F, Hungerford MW, Krackow KA, Hungerford DS: The operative treatment of peroneal nerve palsy. *J Bone and Joint Surg Am* 1996;78:863-869.

Rand JA: Vascular complications of total knee arthroplasty: Report of three cases. *J Arthroplasty* 1987;2(22):89-93.

Rose HA, Hood RW, Otis JC, Ranawat CS, Insall JN: Peroneal-nerve palsy following total knee arthroplasty: A review of The Hospital for Special Surgery experience. *J Bone Joint Surg Am* 1982;64(33):347-351.

Rush JH, Vidovich JD, Johnson MA: Arterial complications of total knee replacement: The Australian experience. *J Bone Joint Surg Br* 1987;69(33):400-402.

Schinsky MF, Macaulay W, Parks ML, Kiernan H, Nercessian OA: Nerve injury after primary total knee arthroplasty. *J Arthroplasty* 2001;16(88):1048-1054.

Coding

CPT Codes		Corresponding ICD-9 Codes	
Total Knee Arthroplasty and Revision Total Knee Arthroplasty			
27447	Arthroplasty, knee, condyle and plateau; medial AND lateral compartments with or without patella resurfacing (total knee arthroplasty)	715 715.80	715.16 715.89
27487	Revision of total knee arthroplasty, with or without allograft; femoral and entire tibial component	996.4 996.77 715	996.6 996.78
Decompression of the Peroneal Nerve			
64708	Neuroplasty, major peripheral nerve, arm or leg; other than specified	355	354

Chapter 34

Prevention and Management of Stiffness Following Total Knee Arthroplasty

Michael H. Bourne, MD
E. Marc Mariani, MD

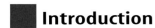

Introduction

Patients and physicians expect excellent results following total knee arthroplasty (TKA). Most patients experience dramatic pain relief and obtain good motion and stability; however, a host of studies following TKAs have found problematic postoperative limitation of motion in 1% to 7% of patients. The definition of satisfactory knee motion depends on several factors, including patient expectations, the degree of improvement following surgery, and overall pain relief. Daily activities require varying degrees of knee motion. Normal gait, for example, requires less than 90° of flexion; rising from a chair without assistance requires from 90° to 120°; and getting out of a bath requires approximately 135°. In general, 110° of knee motion is a suitable postoperative goal for most patients. Walking patterns require less than 5° of flexion contracture for proper heel strike and at heel off.

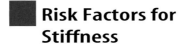

Risk Factors for Stiffness

Many factors in the preoperative, operative, and postoperative phases of TKA will affect the overall motion and stability of the knee. The best way to treat stiffness is to avoid it. The surgical procedure is in some ways a balance between the extremes of instability and stiffness.

Preoperative Risk Factors
Some patients may be predisposed to stiffness following TKA. When patient-related risk factors are known to be present, greater vigilance in patient care and extra effort in attempting to gain and preserve motion are required. Many inflammatory arthropathies, such as rheumatoid arthritis, may predispose to postoperative stiffness. Patients with previous knee surgery or those with posttraumatic arthritis also are at risk for stiffness.

This risk of postoperative stiffness is especially great when significant motion limits from any cause exist preoperatively. Indeed, the greatest predictor of postoperative knee motion is preoperative range of motion. Previous corrective osteotomy has been shown to have an effect on subsequent TKA results and may predispose to limitation of motion. Some obese patients may have flexion limits due to posterior soft-tissue impingement. A preexisting patella baja (patella infera) may cause early flexion impingement on the tibia or tibial component, thus limiting flexion, and can be difficult to deal with at the time of surgery. Finally, in patients with chronic pain, an exaggerated pain response may limit motion.

Intraoperative Risk Factors
SURGICAL TECHNIQUE
The low incidence of stiffness in TKA indicates that most knee surgeons are well versed in proper surgical techniques. Surgical factors that might

Dr. Bourne or an immediate family member has received royalties from Ortho Development Corp; is a member of a speakers' bureau or has made paid presentations on behalf of DePuy; has received research of institutional support from Ortho Development Corp; and owns stock or stock options in Ortho Development Corp. Dr. Mariani or an immediate family member serves as a board member, owner, officer, or committee member of the Board of Directors at St. Mark's Hospital; has received royalties from Ortho Development Corp; is a member of a speakers' bureau or has made paid presentations on behalf of DePuy; serves as a paid consultant for or is an employee of DePuy; and owns stock or stock options in Ortho Development Corp.

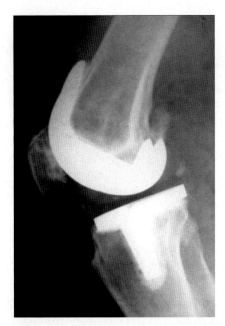

Figure 1 Lateral radiograph of a TKA with a retained posterior femoral osteophyte.

contribute to knee stiffness in the postoperative period are those most directly under the control of the surgeon, including equalization of the flexion/extension gaps and proper balancing of soft tissues. Many authors have described specific techniques of soft-tissue release unique to either the medial or the lateral side of the joint (chapters 26 and 27). Motion not established at the time of surgery will not be gained secondarily with physical therapy.

Frequent testing of the extension and flexion limits at the time of surgery with both trial components and real components in place before final wound closure is recommended.

Modern cutting jigs and instrumentation aid surgeons in performing accurate bone resection, alignment, and preservation of the tibial joint line. Pitfalls include excessively elevating the joint line, which may cause an unintended patella baja, and overstuffing the patellofemoral joint, which might limit knee flexion.

Synovial tissues at the superior patellar pole and quadriceps junction

should be removed at the time of surgery to prevent the formation of a possible nodule of scar. The nodule of scar may become entrapped in the box portion of a posterior stabilized design with flexion, and a "clunk" occurs as it suddenly releases when the knee moves into extension. This painful clunk may inhibit motion and require subsequent resection.

APPROACH

Minimal incision surgery may affect postoperative knee motion. Supporters of the technique claim that smaller incisions and variations that are less disruptive of soft tissues, such as the mini-midvastus or mini-subvastus, may cause less pain and permit more rapid return of motion. Stretching of the soft tissues occurs with smaller incisions, however, and may increase inflammation as well as increase postoperative pain, and both of these factors may hinder motion. Furthermore, and perhaps more important, exact placement of components may be compromised with limited incisions, especially during the early learning curve. Despite this controversy, longer-term follow-up shows similar motion after TKAs done with the smaller, less invasive incisions and TKAs done with the more traditional approaches.

PROSTHESIS SELECTION

Several types of prostheses are available for TKA. Acceptable motion may be achieved with either cruciate-retaining or posterior stabilized prostheses. Attention to detail in balancing is important. With cruciate-retaining designs, care must be taken to ensure that the posterior cruciate ligament (PCL) is not too tight and does not limit flexion. Recession and balancing of the PCL may be important to ensure adequate flexion. In either knee component design, removal of posterior femoral osteophytes and balancing to include posterior capsule release are important. Retained posterior femoral osteophytes may impinge in flexion

and cause excessive tightening of the posterior capsule, limiting full extension (**Figure 1**).

Some studies have shown differences in motion between the so-called high-flexion knee arthroplasty designs and standard implants, whereas others have shown no differences. Both designs can provide adequate motion. Satisfactory knee scores and results are reported for both ingrowth and cemented TKAs, without any significant differences in motion results.

SURGICAL CHECKS PRIOR TO CLOSURE

A trial reduction is performed to assess stability and range of motion. The extensor mechanism can be approximated with sharp towel clips to reproduce the appropriate tightness in flexion (**Figure 2**).

Full range of motion should be obtained. The tibial component should not "lift off" during flexion, nor should the knee hyperextend (**Figure 3**). Varus-valgus stress testing should demonstrate a very firm feel with the knee in full extension but slight medial lateral opening at 20° of flexion (Sato test). The appropriate trial polyethylene spacer is then placed.

WOUND CLOSURE

It is postulated that closure of the wound in flexion may ensure adequate soft-tissue tension by preventing overtightening of the extensor mechanism. Intraoperative checks of motion during the wound closure, by ranging the knee into full flexion, may accomplish the same thing, ensuring that the extensor mechanism is not overly snug (**Figure 4**).

Perioperative Risk Factors/Adjunctive Measures

During the early phases of rehabilitation, several measures may assist in gaining adequate motion. None is mandatory; good results can be obtained if any one is lacking. However, these measures may be helpful in com-

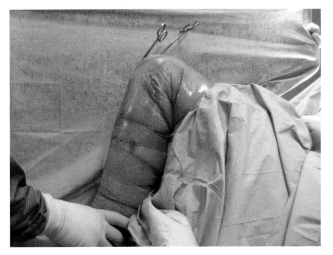

Figure 2 Interoperative motion is assessed with the extensor mechanism approximated by use of penetrating towel clamps.

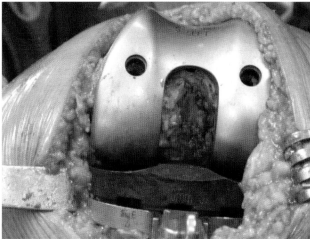

Figure 3 Intraoperative photograph demonstrating tibial trial polyethylene lift off due to excessive tightness in flexion.

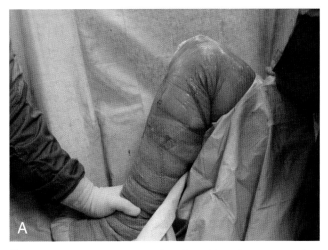
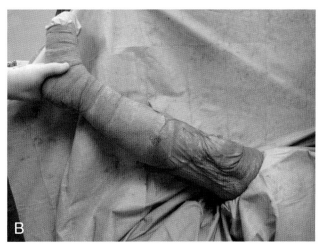

Figure 4 Intraoperative range of motion with real components in position and the wound closed. **A,** Flexion. **B,** Extension.

bination, especially with patients at risk for stiffness.

NERVE BLOCKS

Pain is a significant inhibitor of motion, and all patients appreciate minimization of pain whenever possible. Administration of femoral and sciatic nerve blocks, as well as knee injections and epidural or spinal anesthetics, can be useful. This may be particularly important in patients with a low pain threshold, although these patients may be difficult to identify. Adjunctive pain blocks help mitigate pain in two ways:

First, preemptive analgesia blocks nerve transmission before surgery, thus diminishing the overall pain experience significantly. Second, adjunctive analgesia improves patient comfort, diminishes the use of narcotics, and permits early motion.

POSTOPERATIVE ROUTINE

Anything that quells inflammation and swelling and thus reduces patient discomfort will help to reestablish knee motion and generally assist in overall recovery and patient satisfaction. Cryotherapy, such as a cooling

pad for the first 48 hours at 50° F, may be helpful. Compressive dressings and compression stockings may help limit swelling.

ANTICOAGULATION

Some evidence suggests that the type of anticoagulation used may influence knee motion and stiffness after TKA. For example, excessive bleeding with hematoma formation may decrease motion in the short term. The impact of this swelling on the ultimate motion of the joint has not been studied in a systematic fashion.

DRAINS

Drains are used for two reasons. First, drains facilitate the use of a cell-saver device, which can limit the need for postoperative transfusion. Second, drains minimize the accumulation of blood within the joint, thus decreasing irritation, swelling, and pain—all of which may inhibit early motion. However, there are no evidence-based data available indicating that using drains enhances range of motion after TKA.

CONTINUOUS PASSIVE MOTION DEVICES

There is no definitive evidence demonstrating that the use of a continuous passive motion (CPM) machine leads to an increase in range of motion.

PHYSICAL THERAPY

Formal physical therapy usually begins the day after surgery. The motion goals are 80° to 90° of flexion by postoperative day 3 and 100° to 110° by day 14. Patient education about the proposed goals and use of the CPM device is important. Similarly, separate extension stretches must be taught to avoid a flexion contracture.

MEDICAL COMPLICATIONS

A severe reactive depression or major medical complication may significantly retard motion obtained at the time of surgery. At times, a patient may be willing to accept inadequate motion, accepting instead the newfound pain relief as sufficient gain. When issues such as these arise, including regional pain syndromes, adjunctive appropriate help is sought. Use of antidepressant agents and/or nerve blocks may prove helpful.

Postoperative Risk Factors

INFECTION

One cause of painful limited motion and swelling about a recent TKA is infection. When a joint arthroplasty that has initially performed well develops swelling and tenderness, infection

must be considered. This is especially true if the patient has undergone a recent procedure such as bladder or colon manipulation or invasive dental work. When infection is suspected, an appropriate evaluation would include blood work (C-reactive protein level, erythrocyte sedimentation rate, complete blood cell count), radiographs, possibly a bone scan, and knee joint aspiration with synovial studies and cultures.

SYNOVITIS

A reactive synovitis may create swelling and tenderness, mimicking a low-grade infection. Once infection has been ruled out, the synovitis should be treated appropriately with nonsteroidal anti-inflammatory drugs (NSAIDs) or a prednisone taper. Synovial entrapment has been reported as a cause of painful extension in some posterior stabilized knees with active extension from 90° of flexion. In rare cases, an arthroscopic débridement or an open synovectomy may be required.

TENDINITIS

Inflammation of any of the soft-tissue structures, including tendons, may adversely influence knee motion through pain inhibition. In extreme cases, shortening or soft-tissue contractures, as of the patellar tendon, may result in a patella infera. Tendinitis may be treated with pharmacologic agents (NSAIDs and corticosteroids), local modalities such as heat and ice, and physical therapy.

HETEROTOPIC OSSIFICATION

Heterotopic ossification (HO) is the formation of abnormal true bone in the soft tissues; it has been reported in up to 9% of TKAs. Although this can be painful and may reduce the mobility of the soft tissues and contribute to stiffness about a knee prosthesis, it is rarely a significant problem. Factors that predispose to this condition include Paget disease, a history of HO,

osteonecrosis, ankylosing spondylitis, rheumatoid arthritis, posttraumatic arthritis, and diffuse idiopathic skeletal hyperostosis. Preventive measures include meticulous surgical technique and wound lavage to remove all residual bone debris. In high-risk patients, NSAIDs or radiation may be used. If HO is established, maturation is permitted for approximately 6 to 12 months, followed by surgical resection and adjunctive irradiation.

COMPONENT LOOSENING

Loosening of the components or lack of bone ingrowth with resultant micromotion may cause pain and thereby limit motion of the knee.

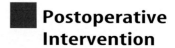

Postoperative Intervention

If a patient has not achieved the expected motion goals, several factors should be considered. If adequate motion was achieved at the time of initial surgery, this motion can potentially be restored. The component size and position must be assessed. If these are appropriate, then treatment consideration is given in a stepwise approach: (1) nonsurgical measures such as an intensified physical therapy program in conjunction with bracing and pharmacologic agents to deal with inflammation and pain; (2) manipulation under anesthesia; and (3) possibly surgery, including arthroscopy or revision TKA.

Nonsurgical Treatment

PHYSICAL THERAPY

Patients must assert themselves to maintain the motion obtained at surgery. Most patients welcome the help of a physical therapist to guide them through this process. Emphasis is on teaching and self-directed therapy to the extent the patient is capable. Rea-

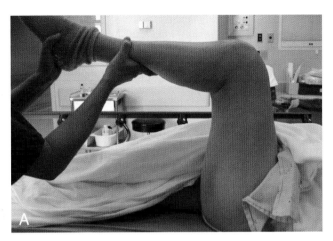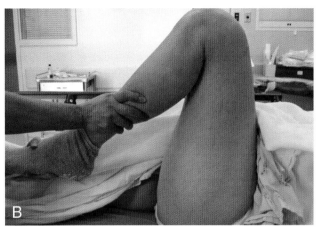

Figure 5 Clinical photographs demonstrating results of manipulation under anesthesia for a stiff knee following TKA. **A,** Premanipulation flexion limit (patient anesthetized). **B,** Flexion after manipulation under anesthesia.

sonable range-of-motion goals are 5° to 90° by day 3, 0° to 110° by day 14, and 0° to ≥120° by week 4. When a patient lags behind these goals, re-education and supervised physical therapy are valuable.

MEDICATIONS

Some patients are inhibited by pain and improve when pain is alleviated through medication. Adjunctive use of NSAIDs may be helpful in diminishing inflammation and pain. On occasion, a brief prednisone taper also can be used. Although every attempt to avoid long-term use of narcotics is advised, short-term use of pain medications is usually necessary.

Complex regional pain syndromes may be responsible for painful and limited knee motion. Because these can be difficult to diagnose, consultation with a pain management specialist and adjunctive nerve blocks may prove invaluable.

BRACING

A static flexion or extension brace to provide a constant force across the knee joint may occasionally be helpful, especially if a patient has difficulty gaining full terminal extension. If the knee has a flexion contracture of 10° or 15° and is not progressing, a dynamic extension brace can be worn in-

termittently during the day. Note, however, that this approach presumes that there is bona fide hamstring tightness and that full extension was gained at the time of surgery.

Manipulation Under Anesthesia

About 1% of primary TKA patients ultimately undergo manipulation. If stiffness occurs and the nonsurgical measures described earlier do not advance motion sufficiently, a formal knee manipulation under anesthesia should be considered. For the patient to be a candidate for manipulation, the knee components must be properly positioned, sized, and aligned. Manipulation under anesthesia may be indicated when a patient feels the motion of the knee is blocked and the knee has not progressed past 90° of flexion or has a 10° flexion contracture by week 4.

Manipulation is most successful when provided as an adjunct to physical therapy no later than 6 to 8 weeks after surgery. If an adequate range of motion was obtained after wound closure at the time of surgery, manipulation will likely provide significant benefit in restoring that degree of motion (**Figure 5**). Manipulation is not without risks, however, as sudden, forceful pressure has been known to cause femoral fractures or quadriceps or patellar tendon disruptions, and therefore the

procedure should be undertaken with care. Intraoperative notching of the anterior femoral cortex may predispose the femur to fracture.

The manipulation is performed with either a general anesthetic or an indwelling epidural or spinal anesthetic. True flexion angles are best appreciated radiographically; however, safe manipulation does not require the use of a C-arm. During the procedure, we move slowly and palpate carefully to feel the tearing of adhesions within the knee. The patient needs to be relaxed because co-contraction of muscles will make the manipulation more difficult and impair an accurate feel of adhesions breaking. Some knees exhibit an initial tight end point at 70° to 90°. Gentle, constant pressure, with one hand pushing on the ankle and the other hand on the knee, creates a palpable and audible release of adhesions with a subsequent large gain in the end point of flexion.

Some knees exhibit a softer end point, requiring a slow and steady but forceful exertion throughout the full range of motion. These knees may not have a palpable or audible tearing of adhesions but rather a more uniform release of stiffness while gaining motion. Often we lower the surgical table and use the surgeon's body weight on the leg to apply gentle, constant flex-

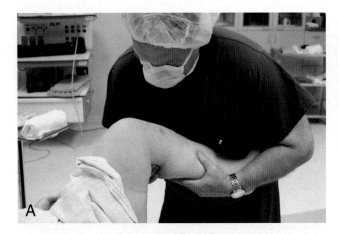

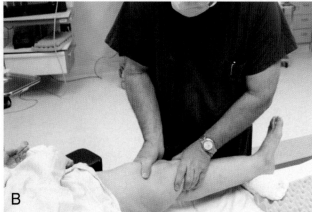

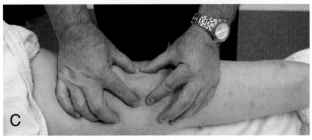

Figure 6 Manipulation under anesthesia. **A,** Flexion manipulation. **B,** Extension manipulation. **C,** Patellar manipulation.

ion pressure (**Figure 6**, *A*). Regardless of technique, the goal is to gain the maximum possible flexion at the time of manipulation, usually to allow 130° of flexion.

Manipulation of the knee in extension is also important and is accomplished by placing a bolster under the ankle and then applying a gentle force in extension (**Figure 6**, *B*). Often, the posterior capsule stretches and an audible pop may occur. Gaining 5° to 10° of extension is reasonable. Finally, patellar mobility is gained through gentle manipulation of the patella using a medial and lateral displacement force (**Figure 6**, *C*).

The manipulation can be performed as an outpatient procedure or, in cases where an indwelling epidural catheter is used, overnight observation. The patient uses compressive wraps, ice, and other local modalities, including a CPM machine. Outpatient physical therapy begins on the first postoperative day. Although an early rebound stiffness may occur, with some loss of the motion gained at the

time of manipulation, the patient will note that the "block" experienced preoperatively that prevented progress has been relieved. The patient can now steadily progress in flexion over the weeks to come.

Surgical Treatment

Once 8 to 12 weeks have passed since the initial surgery, the window for a safe manipulation under anesthesia likely has closed. At this point, arthroscopic débridement or open lysis of adhesions and débridement could be considered. A revision surgery is much less likely to be successful when the primary cause of failure has not been identified.

Arthroscopic Procedures

Arthroscopy has a limited role in the stiff knee after TKA, but has been used for débridement in cases of persistent synovitis and removal of scar, as in patellar clunk syndrome. When a symptomatic patellar clunk is present, it is fairly easily treated with arthroscopic resection (**Figure 7**).

When isolated flexion tightness is present in cruciate-retaining TKAs, an arthroscopic PCL release may be considered. This can be very technically demanding and may, in some cases, result in a secondary synovitis due to PCL instability. An open revision to a posterior stabilized TKA or exchange of the spacer to a lipped stabilized polyethylene design would then be required.

When specific causes of stiffness are not identified, arthroscopic evaluation is not considered to be productive.

Open Procedures

Precise diagnosis of the cause of stiffness will direct optimal open surgical treatment. Open treatments range from soft-tissue débridement to full component revision.

OPEN DÉBRIDEMENT

Arthrofibrosis is a condition produced by inflammation and the presence of abundant, extensive, dense scar tissue within the knee. It is more commonly associated with immobilization, infection, and previous hematoma. When arthrofibrosis exists, an open resection of the scar and synovial tissues provides a more complete excision than an arthroscopic technique.

The knee is approached through the previous incision. Cultures and tissue specimens are sent following the arthrotomy. The patella is mobilized through débridement and possible lateral release. When initial patellar mobilization is extremely difficult and risk of extensor disruption is high, a quadriceps snip should be used to expose the joint. This approach permits a normal postoperative rehabilitation protocol. Synovial tissues and periprosthetic scar are resected. Clearing both the lateral and medial gutters aids in visualization as well as mobilization of the joint. Removal of the polyethylene spacer helps gain early motion without overstressing the extensor mechanism. Release of the capsule off the posterior aspect of the tibia is made possible by removal of the polyethylene spacer. This aids in mobilization and helps with release of a flexion contracture. The polyethylene should be inspected to see if there is posterior wear, which is often seen in cruciate-retaining knees with a tight PCL. A medial or lateral posterior capsular release with a curved osteotome will also help restore the flexion and extension gaps. Throughout the procedure, care is taken to avoid forceful flexion, which risks tendon disruption.

Careful assessment of components is essential. Inspection should confirm appropriate component sizing, position, and stability, indicating that scarring is responsible for the stiffness. If component malposition, loosening, or overstuffing of the patella exist, then component revision is undertaken. In addition, component revision may be necessary if there is significant overhang at either the femoral or tibial components.

Soft tissues should be balanced. Appropriate polyethylene spacer trials

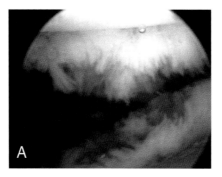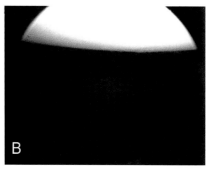

Figure 7 Arthroscopic views of a knee with patellar clunk syndrome. **A,** Preresection view showing retropatellar synovial hypertrophy. **B,** Postresection view showing polyethylene patellar component.

should confirm flexion and extension balance with knee stability throughout a full range of motion. If the knee is still too stiff, then removal of components may be necessary to further adjust the flexion and extension gaps.

POSTERIOR CAPSULAR RELEASE

An isolated flexion contracture (inability to gain passive full extension of the knee) may be more difficult to treat than lack of flexion. If complete extension was once obtained and the original distal femoral cut was adequate, isolated capsular release to lengthen the posterior femoral capsule might be attempted. We perform this through polyethylene removal and capsular stripping from the posterior femur with a curved osteotome. Any residual posterior osteophytes should be removed. Further extension can be obtained by releasing the capsule off the posterior aspect of the tibia.

POLYETHYLENE EXCHANGE

Isolated polyethylene exchange for knee stiffness has met with disfavor. Decreasing the thickness of the polyethylene spacer affects both the flexion and the extension gaps of the knee. Therefore, it may have a limited role in TKAs that are equally tight in flexion and extension.

COMPONENT REVISION

Complete revision of the femoral and tibial components may be required if

the knee alignment is inaccurate, the size of the components is incorrect, component loosening or rotational deformity exists, or a flexion-extension gap mismatch has occurred.

An isolated tibial revision with further proximal tibial resection is indicated if the knee is stiff in extension and flexion and the thinnest polyethylene component is already in place, eliminating the possibility of polyethylene downsizing.

If the knee is tight only in extension, an isolated femoral component revision that includes further distal resection of the femur will improve extension. If the knee is tight only in flexion, downsizing the size of the femoral component by resecting only the posterior femoral bone will widen and open the flexion gap.

In some instances, only a full revision of both the femoral and the tibial component will give acceptable balancing and the potential to reestablish full motion. In cases of long-standing significant stiffness, even when the components are adequately aligned and sized, a full revision may be required. Release of the appropriate soft tissues is also necessary, as outlined earlier.

QUADRICEPSPLASTY

In rare circumstances, both postoperative adhesions in the knee and the entire quadriceps mechanism will limit knee motion. Surgical correction is a large undertaking that can be fraught with difficulties, including blood loss and recurrent stiffness. Recently, arthroscopically assisted quadricepsplasty has been described. Whether performed open or arthroscopically, a complete quadricepsplasty should perhaps be reserved for those familiar with the technique.

——————■

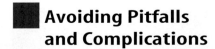

Avoiding Pitfalls and Complications

Stiffness following TKA is a concern. There are preoperative, intraoperative, and postoperative factors that contribute to stiffness. Identifying potentially at-risk patients preoperatively will permit a more concerted effort to avoid this complication. Diligent efforts to balance the knee intraoperatively,

combined with careful postoperative management, may minimize but not eliminate this complication. Several treatment options exist postoperatively to help preserve or reestablish adequate knee motion. Following the recommendations of this chapter will help ensure that TKA patients have a satisfactory range of motion.

——————■

Bibliography

Bae DK, Yoon KH, Kim HS, Song SJ: Total knee arthroplasty in stiff knees after previous infection. *J Bone Joint Surg Br* 2005;87(3):333-336.

Bong MR, Di Cesare PE: Stiffness after total knee arthroplasty. *J Am Acad Orthop Surg* 2004;12(3):164-171.

Brinkmann JR, Perry J: Rate and range of knee motion during ambulation in healthy and arthritic subjects. *Phys Ther* 1985;65(7):1055-1060.

Christensen CP, Crawford JJ, Olin MD, Vail TP: Revision of the stiff total knee arthroplsty. *J Arthroplasty* 2007;17(4): 409-415.

Gonzalez MH, Mekhail AO: The failed total knee arthroplasty: Evaluation and etiology. *J Am Acad Orthop Surg* 2004;12(6): 436-446.

Hunt KJ, Bourne MH, Mariani EM: Single-injection femoral and sciatic nerve blocks for pain control after total knee arthroplasty. *J Arthroplasty* 2009;24(4):533-538.

Kim J, Nelson CL, Lotke PA: Stiffness after total knee arthroplasty: Prevalence of the complication and outcomes of revision. *J Bone Joint Surg Am* 2004;86(7):1479-1484.

Laskin RS, Beksac B: Stiffness after total knee arthroplasty. *J Arthroplasty* 2004;19(4, suppl 1):41-46.

Mont MA, Seyler TM, Marulanda GA, Delanois RE, Bhave A: Surgical treatment and customized rehabilitation for stiff knee arthroplasties. *Clin Orthop Relat Res* 2006;446:193-200.

Nicholls DW, Dorr LD: Revision surgery for stiff total knee arthroplasty. *J Arthroplasty* 1990;5(suppl):S73-S77.

Ritter MA, Lutgring JD, Davis KE, Berend ME, Pierson JL, Meneghini RM: The role of flexion contracture on outcomes in primary total knee arthroplasty. *J Arthroplasty* 2007;22(8):1092-1096.

Ritter MA, Stringer EA: Predictive range of motion after total knee replacement. *Clin Orthop Relat Res* 1979;143(143): 115-119.

Rowe PJ, Myles CM, Walker C, Nutton R: Knee joint kinematics in gait and other functional activities measured using flexible electrogoniometry: How much knee motion is sufficient for normal daily life? *Gait Posture* 2000;12(2):143-155.

Scuderi GR: The stiff total knee arthroplasty: Causality and solution. *J Arthroplasty* 2005;20(4 suppl 2):S23-S26.

Wang JH, Zhao JZ, He YH: A new treatment strategy for severe arthrofibrosis of the knee: Surgical technique. *J Bone Joint Surg Am* 2007;89(suppl 2, pt 1):93-102.

Yercan HS, Sugun TS, Bussiere C, Ait Si Selmi T, Davies A, Neyret P: Stiffness after total knee arthroplasty: Prevalence, management and outcomes. *Knee* 2006;13(2):111-117.

Coding

CPT Codes		Corresponding ICD-9 Codes	
Open Knee Débridement			
27310	Arthrotomy, knee, with exploration, drainage, or removal of foreign body (eg, infection)	711.96 998.5	958.3 996.4
Capsular Release			
27435	Arthroplasty, knee, condyle and plateau; medial AND lateral compartments with or without patella resurfacing (total knee arthroplasty)	715 715.80 996.4	715.16 715.89
Total Knee Arthroplasty Revision			
27447	Arthroplasty, knee, condyle and plateau; medial AND lateral compartments with or without patella resurfacing (total knee arthroplasty)	715 715.80 996.4	715.16 715.89
27486	Revision of total knee arthroplasty, with or without allograft; one component	996.4 996.77	996.6 996.78
27487	Revision of total knee arthroplasty, with or without allograft; femoral and entire tibial component	996.4 996.77	996.6 996.78
Knee Manipulation			
27570	Manipulation of knee joint under general anesthesia (includes application of traction or other fixation devices)	718.46 715.56	715.36 996.4
Arthroscopic PCL Release			
29873	Arthroscopy, knee, surgical; with lateral release	715.16 717.7	718.36 996.4
Arthroscopic Knee Débridement			
29877	Arthroscopy, knee, surgical; debridement/shaving of articular cartilage (chondroplasty)	717 718.36	715.16 996.4

HCPCS Codes*

L1843	Knee orthosis, single upright, thigh and calf, with adjustable flexion and extension joint (unicentric or polycentric), medial-lateral and rotation control, with or without varus/valgus adjustment, prefabricated, includes fitting and adjustment
L1844	Knee orthosis, single upright, thigh and calf, with adjustable flexion and extension joint (unicentric or polycentric), medial-lateral and rotation control, with or without varus/valgus adjustment, custom fabricated
L1845	Knee orthosis, double upright, thigh and calf, with adjustable flexion and extension joint (unicentric or polycentric), medial-lateral and rotation control, with or without varus/valgus adjustment, prefabricated, includes fitting and adjustment
L1846	Knee orthosis, double upright, thigh and calf, with adjustable flexion and extension joint (unicentric or polycentric), medial-lateral and rotation control, with or without varus/valgus adjustment, custom fabricated

*HCPCS codes (supply codes) are separately reportable by the physician when provided in the office setting. If ordered in the hospital or outpatient facility, supply codes are not separately reportable.
CPT copyright ©2010 by the American Medical Association. All rights reserved.
HCPCS copyright © 2010 by the Centers for Medicare and Medicaid Services. All rights reserved.

Chapter 35

Management of Skin Problems Associated With Total Knee Arthroplasty

Fred Cushner, MD
William J. Long, MD, FRCSC
Michael Nett, MD

■ Introduction

Nothing ruins the good results following total knee arthroplasty (TKA) more than wound failure. Soft-tissue considerations must always be at the forefront when planning surgical intervention. This is especially true in high-risk patients, including those with prior incisions. Although several plastic surgery techniques are available to treat wound complications, much of the damage is already done once the complication occurs. Even the best outcome of salvage techniques involves functional loss and cosmetic deficit. Therefore, the surgeon's primary goal should be to avoid postoperative wound complications. Despite appropriate planning and meticulous technique, however, wound complications will still occur. The orthopaedic surgeon must work in conjunction with the plastic surgeon and be aware of the nonsurgical and surgical techniques available to minimize

functional loss. Inappropriate management of postoperative skin problems can result in failure of the reconstruction, deep infection, a nonfunctioning extremity, amputation, and/or a potentially life-threatening situation.

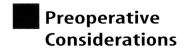

■ Preoperative Considerations

General Considerations

The knee has a thin overlying soft-tissue envelope that must be protective, well vascularized, and supple enough to allow for the large degrees of stretch and shear required for a functional range of motion. Although most TKAs can be performed with standard protocols, an understanding of when to apply specific soft-tissue management principles is required. Preoperative evaluation for TKA should include not only a complete history and physical examination, including radiographic

and clinical assessment of degree of deformity and joint space narrowing, but also a thorough history and evaluation of the skin. Systemic concerns include vascular compromise, obesity, malnutrition, prolonged corticosteroid or nonsteroidal anti-inflammatory drug use, diabetes mellitus, an immunocompromised state, and a history of smoking. Local factors that affect wound healing include the inability to incorporate a previous incision into the planned incision, a small skin bridge between the previous incision and the planned incision, local radiation or burns, and dense, adherent scar tissue. Other local factors may play a role as well. The correction of severe deformity may make subsequent closure difficult. Special caution should be used in patients with severe varus and rotational deformity because as the deformity is corrected, there may not be enough skin to close the inferior aspect of the wound over the subcutaneous surface of tibia. Prior trauma may play a role because of previously placed skin incisions, significant scarring, and loss of skin mobility.

Preoperative consultation regarding medical optimization and early plastic surgery consultation for soft-tissue management should be consid-

Dr. Cushner or an immediate family member is a member of a speakers' bureau or has made paid presentations on behalf of Sanofi-Aventis, Bayer, and Angiotech Pharmaceuticals; serves as a paid consultant for or is an employee of Limvatec, Sanifo-Aventis, Smith & Nephew, Clearant, and Angiotech Pharmaceuticals; and owns stock or stock options in Angiotech Pharmaceuticals. Dr. Nett or an immediate family member is a member of a speakers' bureau or has made paid presentations on behalf of Angiotech Pharmaceuticals. Neither Dr. Long nor any immediate family member has received anything of value from or owns stock in a commercial company or institution related directly or indirectly to the subject of this chapter.

ered in any complex case. Not only will this help minimize complications, but it will help ensure comprehensive involvement should complications be encountered.

Planning the Skin Incision

Previous anterior incisions present a concern regarding both the planned approach and the healing potential of the skin and underlying tissue. A balance must be achieved between the ability to expose the knee through a prior incision and avoiding extensive undermining of the subcutaneous flaps. A clear history of the previous incision should be obtained, including the age of the wound, the subcutaneous dissection and procedure performed, and any wound complications encountered. The previous surgical reports often provide critical information.

An understanding of the local anatomy and blood supply is also necessary. Terminal branches of the peripatellar anastomotic ring of arteries are responsible for most of the blood supply to the anterior skin and subcutaneous tissues. This occurs through a subdermal plexus supplied by arterioles in the subcutaneous fascia. Thus, flap formation over the anterior aspect of the knee must be limited and performed deep to the subcutaneous fascia. A midline skin incision is optimal and should be used whenever possible. This approach reduces the dimensions of the lateral skin flap where lower skin oxygen tension is noted. Previous longitudinal incisions can be used safely. Some degree of modification is often required to incorporate previous paramedian incisions. If multiple parallel longitudinal incisions exist, the most lateral incision is chosen, as the predominant blood supply enters medially.

Transverse skin incisions, such as those from previous patellar surgery or osteotomy, can be safely approached at a 90° angle. Short oblique incisions, such as from previous meniscectomies,

can often be ignored. Caution should be exercised when crossing longer oblique incisions or oblique incisions that cross the midline, as crossing these incisions may result in a narrow point where the incisions intersect. When the planned surgical incision and prior incision create an angle of less than 60°, alternative techniques should be considered.

Alternative Techniques

If the previous skin incision cannot be incorporated and other concerns exist, several techniques can be considered. One option is the sham incision. This technique has limited applications today; we mention it here mainly for historic reasons. A sham incision involves making the planned skin incision, performing the necessary subcutaneous dissection, developing flaps, then closing the wound and waiting a period of time to observe how the wound heals. This provides information regarding the ability of the tissues to heal and creates a "delay phenomenon" with increased local perfusion. If the sham incision heals, then the TKA can proceed as planned 1 to 3 weeks later. Disadvantages to this approach include the need for two procedures and, in cases where the sham incision does not heal, the need for further prearthroplasty management but with more limited options.

Another option is prophylactic flap coverage. The best candidates for prophylactic flap coverage are patients with prior skin graft, local irradiation, or densely adherent scar tissue. The choice of flap depends on the location of the lesion, the extent of coverage required, and the status of the limb. Most lesions can be covered adequately with a medial or lateral gastrocnemius muscle flap or myocutaneous flap. Lesions proximal to the

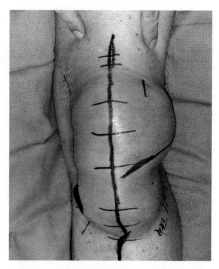

Figure 1 Clinical photograph shows a soft-tissue expander in place, with skin expansion achieved. The planned incision and previous incisions are marked.

superior pole of the patella may require a free flap. The principles involve excision of the area of concern followed by soft-tissue coverage. A minimum of 12 weeks should be allowed between coverage and subsequent arthroplasty. Available data demonstrate successful outcomes in most patients. However, as the indications for this procedure are few, results are extremely limited.

Indications for Soft-Tissue Expansion

Our preferred technique is soft-tissue expansion. Soft-tissue expanders are indicated when insufficient or inadequate soft tissue is present for wound healing (**Figure 1**). This may occur with multiple crossing and combined incisions, previous skin grafts or flaps, or severe preoperative deformity, or when expanded soft-tissue coverage is required. For example, when extensor mechanism allograft as well as a TKA is to be performed, the added bulk of

Table 1 Results of Techniques to Manage Soft-Tissue Problems Associated With Total Knee Arthroplasty

Author(s) (Year)	Number of Procedures	Mean Age in Years (Range)	Mean Follow-up (Range)	Limb Salvage %	Prosthesis Salvage %	Results/Comments
Markovich et al (1995)	4 prophylactic flap coverage	56 (30-80)	4.1 years (1-8)	100	NA	Prophylactic flap: 1 deep infection, 3 good to excellent results
	7 free flaps (3 prophylactic, 4 treating)			100	72	Free flap: 2 infections in treating group
Nahabedian et al (1999)	27 medial gastrocnemius-soleus complex flaps	65 (36-87)	NA	97	83	Secondary procedures: 5 plastic surgery, 4 orthopaedic
	5 anterolateral thigh flaps			100	100	1 major reoperation requiring gastrocnemius-soleus complex flap
Ries (2002)	2 STSGs	NA	NA	100	100	Treatment was successful.
Wei et al (2002)	121 anterolateral thigh flaps	NA	NA	NA	NA	12 total flap failures 17 partial flap failures
Ries and Bozic (2006)	12 medial gastrocnemius-soleus complex flaps	61 (39-72)	28 months (18-48)	92	92	1 above-knee amputation 3 major reoperations
Scott and Reiffel (2006)	64 soft-tissue expansions	57 (33-89)	35 months (24-64)	100	NA	14 minor complications 6 major complications requiring reoperation
Galat et al (2009)	59 I & D and closure	66	5.1 years	98	98	4 patients developed deep infection. 3 patients required major reoperation.

NA = not available; STSG = split-thickness skin graft; I & D = irrigation and débridement.

the extensor mechanism reconstruction may necessitate soft-tissue expansion. Eight to 10 weeks must be allocated for this procedure. Good long-term results have been reported from our institution.

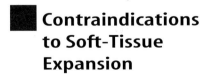

Contraindications to Soft-Tissue Expansion

Contraindications to soft-tissue expansion include previous local irradiation or skin graft that is directly adherent to underlying bone or fascia. This limits the mobility of the sur-

rounding tissue and eliminates the plane necessary for safe soft-tissue expansion. Other contraindications include open wounds, active infection, local drainage, and active anticoagulation or a significant bleeding disorder. Relative contraindications include a history of local infection with drainage or of significant deep vein thrombosis (DVT) in the involved extremity.

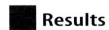

Results

Little conclusive clinical evidence is available regarding the outcomes of soft-tissue expansion in the setting of TKA (**Table 1**). Our institution em-

braced the use of soft-tissue expansion over the last decade. Refinement in technique has led to minimal complications, successful functional and cosmetic results, and the avoidance of wound failure. Our most recent review included 64 knees. One major wound complication occurred in a patient with previously irradiated skin, which required abandoning the planned arthroplasty. Fourteen minor complications (22%) were noted during the expansion phase. These all responded to local treatment. Six major complications (9%) occurred that required reoperation.

Techniques for Soft-Tissue Expansion

Setup/Patient Positioning

The patient is placed in the supine position. The limb is prepared and draped in the usual fashion for a TKA. The tourniquet is in place but is not inflated. All previous incisions are marked. The planned incision is marked on the anterior aspect of the knee.

Procedure

A mixture of diluted local anesthetic is infiltrated into the subcutaneous tissue in the area of the planned incision until the overlying skin blanches (Figure 2, A). This usually requires 250 to 300 mL, which is injected through a Tuohy needle with a blunt tip and an opening at 90°. The injectate dissects the soft-tissue plane ahead of the advancing needle.

A small access incision (2 to 4 cm) is made at the proximal aspect of the planned TKA incision. The expanders are inserted through this small incision. This incision must not be in the area of planned soft-tissue expansion. A pocket is developed with blunt dissection between the subcutaneous fat and the underlying musculotendinous layer (Figure 2, B). The pocket is irrigated with antibiotic solution, and hemostasis is obtained with direct pressure.

Rectangular expanders are inserted (Figure 3, A), which can be up to 350 mL in volume. Typically, two expanders are placed at right angles to each other. Up to four expanders can be used, depending on the size of the limb, the pliability of the soft tissue, and the extent of expansion required. The expansion ports are secured at ei-

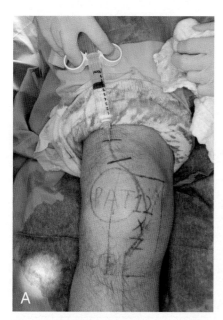
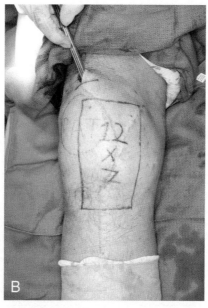

Figure 2 Soft-tissue expansion. **A,** Pocket expansion is performed before expander placement. **B,** Local dissection for placement of expander port.

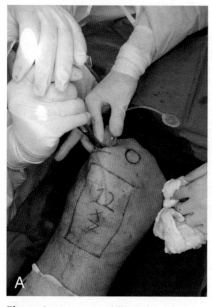
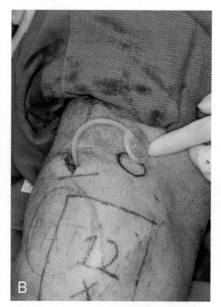
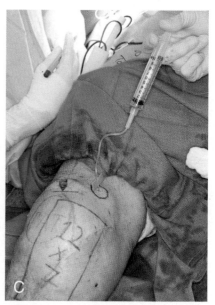

Figure 3 Inserting and filling the soft-tissue expander. **A,** Placement of the expander into pocket. **B,** Mobile port is placed in a location where it can be palpated. **C,** Primary inflation and testing of the expander.

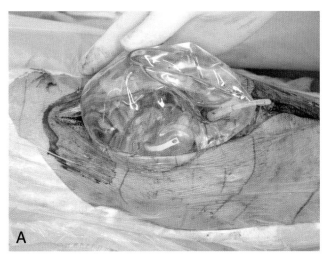
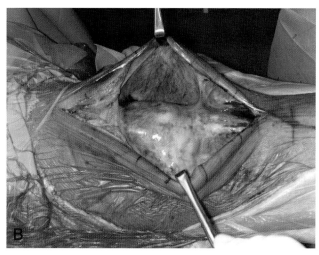

Figure 4 The knee at the time of the indicated TKA, after soft-tissue expansion has been accomplished. **A,** The expander at time of removal. **B,** Pocket of expanded skin with new vascularized flap.

ther side of the access incision, superior to the expanders (**Figure 3,** *B*). The expanders are then inflated until the remaining dead space is filled (**Figure 3,** *C*). The access incision is closed and a bulky sterile dressing is applied. The knee is placed in a knee immobilizer and elevated.

Expansion is postponed and the knee immobilizer is continued during postoperative week 1. The following week, gradual soft-tissue expansion is initiated, at a rate of 10% of the expander volume per week. Expansion should be limited if the capillary refill of the overlying skin is longer than 5 seconds or if the patient experiences significant discomfort. During this phase, range of motion and weight bearing are not limited.

At the time of final reconstruction, the soft-tissue expanders are easily removed from the subcutaneous pocket (**Figure 4,** *A*). Care is taken to not violate the reflected margins or pseudocapsule of the pocket, which provides the blood supply to the full-thickness flaps (**Figure 4,** *B*).

Wound Closure

Following reconstruction, primary closure is usually performed easily (**Figure 5**). Often, excess skin is present, which presents a "nice problem."

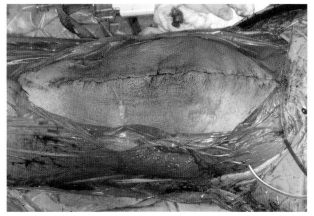

Figure 5 Appearance of skin at closure.

This allows the excision of previous broad incisions or small intervening skin planes.

Hemostasis is then obtained and subcutaneous drains are placed in the medial and lateral aspect of the pocket. The pseudocapsule is closed as a separate layer. Skin closure is performed in the usual fashion. Again, a compressive dressing is applied and the leg is elevated. The patient is allowed to bear weight as tolerated, but elevation is encouraged at all times when at rest. The drains are removed when daily output is less than 40 mL/d (usually 48 hours postoperatively). Continuous passive motion (CPM) and chemical DVT prophylaxis is held until drain removal. In our experi-

ence, subcutaneous drain placement has reduced the incidence of hematoma formation and persistent drainage.

Postoperative Considerations

Appropriate postoperative wound management depends on the severity and timing of the complication. These are discussed below in order of severity. The failure of the soft tissues to heal following TKA has serious complications. Careful examination at the time of the first dressing change can often alert the clinician to a potentially problematic wound. Early indications may include ecchymosis, blistering, and persistent or large amounts of wound drainage. The goal is early intervention when possible to prevent further wound breakdown and complication.

Local Care

Local care measures begin with frequent dressing changes, elevation of the extremity, and limiting mobilization, including range-of-motion activities. When a wound is identified to be at risk in the early postoperative period, we routinely discontinue CPM, apply a compressive dressing, place the knee in an immobilizer, and hold physical therapy. When superficial epidermal loss occurs in an area of less than 2 to 3 cm^2, several modified dressing protocols can be instituted to protect the underlying tissues and allow secondary healing. These include antibacterial ointments or gels and enzymatic débriding agents. During this phase, we may consider temporary discontinuation of the anticoagulant agent, as a hematoma related to overaggressive anticoagulation can be devastating at this stage of healing. The use of mechanical devices for DVT prophylaxis should be considered until the wound stabilizes.

Irrigation and Débridement

Early surgical intervention may be helpful and is indicated in certain situations. In cases of imminent wound compromise due to a large or expanding hematoma or prolonged wound drainage beyond 1 week postoperatively, early surgical interventions should be considered. The goal of irrigation and débridement (I & D) is to prevent further wound breakdown and deep infection. Studies have shown that each day of persistent drainage greatly increases the risk of wound infection. In addition, other studies have shown a lower incidence of deep infection when postoperative

hematoma or persistent drainage is treated with I & D versus nonsurgical management.

Once the decision is made to proceed with surgery, the patient is taken to the operating room expediently. The setup is the same as with the index arthroplasty. Thorough I & D is performed. Deep cultures should be obtained to direct antibiotic therapy if indicated. If an opening in the arthrotomy exists, or if the hematoma is deep to the arthrotomy, then the entire prosthesis should be exposed and irrigated, and a tibial polyethylene component exchange is performed. It is best to assume that deep infection is present and perform a thorough I & D with antibiotic irrigation. After hemostasis is attained, the wound is closed in a layered fashion over a drain. A compression dressing is applied. Occasionally, when a tension-free closure cannot be obtained, a gastrocnemius muscle flap may be necessary. This should be anticipated before surgery. Appropriate accommodations should be made preoperatively, including the involvement of a plastic surgeon.

Postoperatively, the limb is elevated, while range of motion and chemical DVT prophylaxis is initially held. Broad-spectrum antibiotics are given until pending cultures are final. An infectious disease consultation is obtained in cases where infection is suspected or cultures return positive. Decisions regarding range of motion, DVT prophylaxis, and continued antibiotic therapy are made on an individual basis.

Split-Thickness Skin Graft

If large areas of superficial skin loss have occurred, split-thickness skin graft (STSG) is an option. A healthy dermal-epidermal layer is taken from a harvest site and is used to cover the area over the knee. The graft relies on serum inhibition for the initial 48 hours. Therefore, a healthy bed with an intact dermal layer is required at the time of the application. Re-

cently, wound vacuum-assisted closures (VACs) have been used to prepare the knee before the tissue graft procedure. A bed of healthy granulation tissue provides the best environment for skin graft healing.

The patient is placed supine. The limb is prepared in the usual fashion, and the thigh from which the graft will be taken is included. Initial focus is on the recipient site. Débridement of all necrotic tissue must be performed. Deep extension of soft-tissue compromise or evidence of local infection must be ruled out before performing the STSG. The STSG is harvested and meshed. It is then applied to the recipient site and secured with staples. A VAC dressing is applied over the skin graft. The harvest site is dressed with petroleum gauze.

Postoperatively, the leg is elevated and bed rest is encouraged for 5 days. No motion of the knee is allowed during this time. The VAC dressing is removed on day 5. If the STSG shows signs of incorporation, mobilization and range of motion is initiated at this point.

Very few results have been reported for isolated STSG after TKA (**Table 1**). The soft-tissue envelope surrounding the knee is limited and extremely tenuous; thus, few scenarios call for isolated STSG without additional soft-tissue coverage.

Local Fasciocutaneous Flaps

Both the condition of surrounding tissue and the size of the defect determine whether a local fasciocutaneous flap may be used. Preoperative planning must include designing a flap appropriate for coverage based on arterial fasciocutaneous patterns. Ideally, the flap should be oriented in an axial direction and the ratio of length to width should not exceed 2.5:1. Anterolateral thigh fasciocutaneous flaps are frequently available for coverage in the area of the knee.

The surgical setup is similar to that for an STSG. The limb and ipsilateral thigh are prepared and draped in the usual fashion. Often an STSG will be necessary to cover the flap after it is applied. A donor site for the STSG must be identified and prepared into the surgical field. The recipient site is débrided and all necrotic tissue is removed. The region is irrigated copiously with antibiotic solution. Signs of local infection must not be present. If local infection is present, surgery is delayed until the infection has been treated and has resolved. Doppler outlining of the specific planned fasciocutaneous flap is performed, as vascular supply can vary significantly. The flap is raised with the deep areolar tissue left attached. The flap is mobilized to cover the recipient site. An STSG is then applied over the deep areolar tissue to cover the flap. Hemostasis is obtained and a layered closure is performed. A compression or VAC dressing is applied. If STSG is not required, mobilization can proceed early, with care to avoid excessive knee flexion that may cause ischemia to the tissues over the anterior aspect of the knee. If STSG is required, then the protocol outlined above for STSGs should be followed.

The use of the fasciocutaneous flap to cover wounds on the lower extremity was originally described in 1981. Several authors have reported success with modifications of this technique around TKAs. However, a more recent study demonstrated a 43% failure rate with fasciocutaneous grafts. We suggest limiting their use to small, superficial defects without evidence of infection.

Muscle and Myocutaneous Flaps

Large areas of soft-tissue breakdown or wounds with exposed tendon or bone require greater coverage than the local fasciocutaneous flap. The workhorse for local coverage about the knee is the gastrocnemius muscle. The two heads are divided by a median raphe and are usually supplied by individual arteries, which provide the pedicle about which they are rotated. The medial head is larger and longer and thus can be used in most cases. In far lateral wounds, the lateral head may be used, but care must be taken to avoid the peroneal nerve as it passes around the proximal fibula.

The involved extremity is prepared and draped freely. The recipient site is débrided of all necrotic or devitalized tissue. If the prosthesis is exposed, a thorough I & D is performed along with a tibial polyethylene component exchange. A longitudinal incision is made along the anterior border of the medial head of the gastrocnemius. The overlying deep fascia is split in line with the incision. The long saphenous vein is protected as the plane anterior to the gastrocnemius is developed bluntly between the gastrocnemius-soleus complex and the soleus muscle. If a myocutaneous flap is needed, the perforators off the posterior aspect of the muscle belly are preserved. These provide the blood supply to the skin. Otherwise, these perforators can be divided. Dissection is then carried proximally. The short saphenous vein and sural nerve traveling along the midline raphe are preserved. Small crossing fibers and vessels are divided. Distally, the insertion into the Achilles tendon is divided with a small cuff of tendon attached to later aid in securing the flap. A subcutaneous tunnel is then created to allow passage of the flap into the area of tissue deficiency. If additional length is needed, the deep fascia can be incised or striped. This allows further lengthening or widening. An alternative or supplemental technique is to release the proximal origin of the muscle without disrupting the pedicle. The flap is secured at the recipient site by suture to the deep tissue layers and insetting it under the skin edges. Finally, hemostasis is obtained and the wound is closed in layers over a deep drain. STSG is often required to cover the flap. A compressive dressing or VAC is applied and the knee is immobilized.

Postoperatively, the extremity is elevated. Mobilization and motion are restricted for 5 to 7 days. The dressing is changed on day 5. Weight bearing and motion are gradually begun after day 7. Mobilization progresses as tolerated and as dictated by the status of the flap.

Specific complications involve injury to the nearby neurovascular structures, including the sural nerve and short and long saphenous veins. Other complications include hematoma formation in the calf due to failure to achieve hemostasis, graft strangulation secondary to an insufficiently wide subcutaneous tunnel, and damage to the vascular pedicle from excessive stretch. Cosmetic concerns include a decrease in calf girth and the excessive soft-tissue mass on the anterior aspect of the knee.

Results with gastrocnemius flap coverage following TKA have been good, with series reporting up to a 96% success rate (**Table 1**). Poor results have been demonstrated in the face of chronic infection and delayed soft-tissue coverage. Complication rates increase with attempted coverage of more-proximal lesions over the patella or quadriceps tendon.

Free Flaps

Free flaps around the knee are indicated when local flaps are insufficient due to the location or size of defect or the compromised status of the traditional (and our preferred) gastrocnemius flap. Certainly, the technique of a free flap is beyond the scope of most orthopaedic surgeons, and plastic surgery consultation is needed. Any of several harvest sites may be used to obtain the graft. Common sites include the latissimus dorsi, the rectus abdominus, or the serratus anterior muscles. Relative contraindications to the free flap include severe peripheral vascular disease, smoking, diabetes mellitus, and chronic renal failure.

Common complications include the development of a hematoma or seroma at the harvest site due to the large dead space created. The use of a surgical drain and an alternative to low-molecular-weight heparin for DVT prophylaxis can reduce these risks, as does obtaining intraoperative hemostasis. The rare complication of microvascular occlusion or graft failure requires a second free flap or an above-knee amputation.

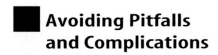

Avoiding Pitfalls and Complications

The best way to deal with wound problems associated with TKA is to avoid them. This begins with obtaining a thorough history to recognize at-risk patients and maximizing their preoperative status. In most cases, this involves optimizing nutritional status, maintaining tight control of blood glucose, quitting smoking, and perhaps controlling lower extremity edema when significant venous stasis exists. More complex cases may require more aggressive intervention, however, occasionally including soft-tissue expansion. Despite meticulous attention to detail and preoperative planning, wound complications will still occur. The key, then, becomes early identification and intervention. If persistent drainage occurs or a large postoperative hemarthrosis is noted, aggressive management is indicated.

Several authors have shown that prolonged wound drainage increases the incidence of infection. Therefore, aggressive management is warranted. The appropriate intervention will decrease infection and prevent potential soft-tissue loss. Although most wound complications can be handled with routine early intervention, an established relationship with a plastic surgeon is advantageous for all total joint arthroplasty surgeons. Not only can preoperative consultation minimize complication, but the more complex complications tend to occur on a semiemergent basis. Having a skilled and established team to assist in these cases will save critical time and improve outcomes.

Bibliography

Craig SM: Soft tissue considerations in the failed total knee arthroplasty, in Scott WN, ed: *The Knee*, vol 2. St. Louis, MO, Mosby Yearbook, 1994, pp 1279-1295.

Galat DD, McGovern SC, Larson DR, Harrington JR, Hanssen AD, Clarke HD: Surgical treatment of early wound complications following primary total knee arthroplasty. *J Bone Joint Surg Am* 2009;91(1):48-54.

Gold DA, Scott SC, Scott WN: Soft tissue expansion prior to arthroplasty in the multiply-operated knee: A new method of preventing catastrophic skin problems. *J Arthroplasty* 1996;11(5):512-521.

Manifold SG, Cushner FD, Craig-Scott S, Scott WN: Long-term results of total knee arthroplasty after the use of soft tissue expanders. *Clin Orthop Relat Res* 2000;(380):133-139.

Markovich GD, Dorr LD, Klein NE, McPherson EJ, Vince KG: Muscle flaps in total knee arthroplasty. *Clin Orthop Relat Res* 1995;(321):122-130.

Møller AM, Pedersen T, Villebro N, Munksgaard A: Effect of smoking on early complications after elective orthopaedic surgery. *J Bone Joint Surg Br* 2003;85(2):178-181.

Nahabedian MY, Mont MA, Orlando JC, Delanois RE, Hungerford DS: Operative management and outcome of complex wounds following total knee arthroplasty. *Plast Reconstr Surg* 1999;104(6):1688-1697.

Pontén B: The fasciocutaneous flap: Its use in soft tissue defects of the lower leg. *Br J Plast Surg* 1981;34(2):215-220.

Rehman HU, Mohammed K: Perioperative management of diabetic patients. *Curr Surg* 2003;60(6):607-611.

Ries MD: Skin necrosis after total knee arthroplasty. *J Arthroplasty* 2002;17(4, Suppl 1)74-77.

Ries MD, Bozic KJ: Medial gastrocnemius flap coverage for treatment of skin necrosis after total knee arthroplasty. *Clin Orthop Relat Res* 2006;446:186-192.

Ruberg RL: Role of nutrition in wound healing. *Surg Clin North Am* 1984;64(4):705-714.

Scott SC, Reiffel RS: Soft-tissue healing, in Scott WN, ed: *Surgery of the Knee*, ed 4. Philadelphia, PA, Churchill Livingstone, 2006, vol 2, pp 1105-1108.

Wei FC, Jain V, Celik N, Chen HC, Chuang DC, Lin CH: Have we found an ideal soft-tissue flap? An experience with 672 anterolateral thigh flaps. *Plast Reconstr Surg* 2002;109(7):2219-2226, discussion 2227-2230.

Weiss AP, Krackow KA: Persistent wound drainage after primary total knee arthroplasty. *J Arthroplasty* 1993;8(3):285-289.

Coding

CPT Codes		Corresponding ICD-9 Codes	
Total Knee Arthroplasty			
27447	Arthroplasty, knee, condyle and plateau; medial AND lateral compartments with or without patella resurfacing (total knee arthroplasty)	715 715.80	715.16 715.89
Incision and Drainage			
27301	Incision and drainage, deep abscess, bursa, or hematoma, thigh or knee region	958.3	998.1
Split-Thickness Skin Graft			
15220	Full thickness graft, free, including direct closure of donor site, scalp, arms, and/or legs; 20 sq cm or less	958.3	998.1
15221	Full thickness graft, free, including direct closure of donor site, scalp, arms, and/or legs; each additional 20 sq cm, or part thereof (List separately in addition to code for primary procedure)	958.3	998.1
Local Fasciocutaneous Flaps			
14020	Adjacent tissue transfer or rearrangement, scalp, arms and/or legs; defect 10 sq cm or less	958.3	998.1
14021	Adjacent tissue transfer or rearrangement, scalp, arms and/or legs; defect 10.1 sq cm to 30.0 sq cm	958.3	998.1
Muscle or Myocutaneous Flaps			
15756	Free muscle or myocutaneous flap with microvascular anastomosis	958.3	998.1
Free Flaps			
15757	Free skin flap with microvascular anastomosis	958.3	998.1

Chapter 36

Management of Extensor Mechanism Rupture

Craig J. Della Valle, MD
Aaron Rosenberg, MD
Alexander P. Sah, MD
Bryan D. Springer, MD

◼ Indications

Extensor mechanism disruption is one of the most feared, disabling, and difficult complications to treat following total knee arthroplasty (TKA). We use an extensor mechanism allograft (EMA) for the treatment of patients with a chronic rupture of the quadriceps or patellar tendon or a nonunion of a patellar fracture (**Figure 1**). Patients often describe difficulty ambulating (secondary to a loss of active extension required for the swing phase of gait) as well as instability of the knee. Instability is typically severe enough that patients often report a history of frequent falls, which can be associated with significant morbidity given the risk of fragility fractures in this typically elderly patient population. On physical examination, patients have an extensor lag (usually 50° or more) that prevents active extension of the knee,

but full passive extension (and sometimes hyperextension) is possible. Physical examination characteristically also reveals a palpable defect of the extensor mechanism and substantial anteroposterior and, in some cases, global knee instability.

———————◼

◼ Contraindications

The primary contraindication for an EMA is the patient who can actively extend the knee. Given the morbidity and complexity of the procedure, as well as the lack of long-term results, only patients with severe disability should be considered for this treatment. The presence of active periprosthetic infection is another contraindication, and all patients in whom this procedure is considered should have an erythrocyte sedimentation rate and C-reactive protein level obtained pre-

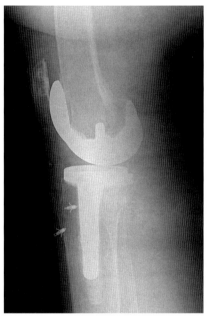

Figure 1 Lateral preoperative radiograph showing patella alta associated with a chronic rupture of the patellar tendon.

operatively to screen for infection. If either or both of these laboratory values are elevated, strong consideration should be given to a preoperative knee aspiration. The synovial fluid should be sent for a white blood cell count and differential, along with cultures, to more thoroughly assess the patient for the presence of infection. The presence of more than 1,100 to 3,000 white blood cells per mm³, or a differ-

Dr. Della Valle or an immediate family member serves as a paid consultant to or an employee of Biomet, Kinamed, Smith & Nephew, and Zimmer; has received research or institutional support from Zimmer; and has received nonincome support (such as equipment or services), commercially derived honoraria, or other non–research-related funding (such as paid travel) from Stryker. Dr. Rosenberg or an immediate family member has received royalties from Zimmer, has received research or institutional support from Zimmer, and has stock or stock options held in Zimmer. Dr. Springer or an immediate family member is a member of a speakers' bureau or has made paid presentations on behalf of DePuy and has received research or institutional support from DePuy and Zimmer. Neither Dr. Sah nor any immediate family member has received anything of value from or owns stock in a commercial company related directly or indirectly to the subject of this chapter.

ential showing more than 60% to 80% neutrophils, is highly suggestive of infection, even if the aspirated fluid does not show growth on culture.

The surgeon must also evaluate the prosthetic knee components to decide if revision is required at the time of EMA reconstruction. Components that are loose, malaligned, sized improperly, or malrotated require concomitant revision. Although loosening, axial malalignment, and inappropriate sizing are often apparent on the preoperative plain radiographs, rotational alignment can be more difficult to judge preoperatively (using the plain radiographs) and intraoperatively. Preoperative CT scans of the extremity, as described by Berger and associates, should be strongly considered if retention of the implanted tibial and femoral components is being considered. Preoperative consultation with the radiologist performing the test is critical to ensure that the correct images are obtained, along with the use of metal-suppression sequences to allow for an accurate assessment of the rotation of the tibial and femoral components. Components that are internally rotated can contribute to extensor mechanism failure, and the retention of such malrotated components can predispose to recurrent failure of the reconstruction.

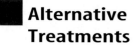

Alternative Treatments

Nonsurgical treatment in the form of physical therapy is typically not successful in these cases of extensor mechanism disruption. Although bracing can alleviate some symptoms of instability, patients normally will not accept this as a long-term solution to their lack of active knee extension and instability. Attempts at primary repair in the setting of a postoperative extensor mechanism disruption have been

met with an unacceptable rate of failure and are not recommended. The use of local autograft tissue (such as harvesting the hamstring tendons) to augment a primary repair have similarly had disappointing results when applied to a chronic postoperative extensor mechanism disruption.

An alternative to the use of a full EMA is the use of an Achilles tendon allograft. The primary principles for this procedure are similar to those for a full EMA; the graft is secured distally in the proximal tibia using a calcaneal bone block, and the allograft tissue is used to augment the extensor mechanism. The primary advantage of this technique is retention of the native patella. Proximal fixation of the allograft, however, can be more difficult than with an EMA, and, similarly, full coverage of allograft tissue with native extensor mechanism can be more difficult.

A final reconstructive option is the use of a medial gastrocnemius muscle flap to reconstruct the extensor mechanism. Published results on this technique are available on only a small number of patients, however, and the reported risk of recurrent extensor lag appears to be higher than for EMA. This technique may be attractive, however, in the patient who is being treated for a concomitant deep infection, or where wound healing problems are experienced or anticipated in the area of the tibial tubercle and/or the proximal-medial portion of the tibia.

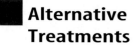

Results

The results of extensor mechanism allograft reconstruction are highly dependent on the surgical techniques used (**Table 1**). Specifically, it is imperative to fully tighten the graft in full extension at the time of surgery; failure to do so has resulted in a higher percentage of failures second-

ary to recurrent extensor lag and instability.

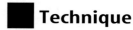

Technique

Setup/Exposure
The leg must be prepared and draped widely to allow for full access to the knee from approximately the midtibia distally to the apex of the quadriceps tendon proximally. The tourniquet should be placed as high on the ipsilateral thigh as possible; if the patient's body habitus precludes high placement of the tourniquet underneath the drapes, a sterile tourniquet can be used.

Instruments/Equipment/ Implants Required
Beyond the instruments and implants required to perform either a modular polyethylene liner exchange or a complete revision, a fresh-frozen graft for the appropriate side (right or left) is required. It is preferable to obtain the allograft with the proximal tibia, to ensure adequate bone is available for fashioning the bone block that will be secured to the proximal tibia (**Figure 2**). Heavy nonabsorbable suture and 16-gauge wire also are required.

Procedure
The prior skin incision can typically be used; however, if multiple prior incisions are present, the most lateral one that will allow adequate exposure is selected. Exposure from the apex of the quadriceps tendon to a point approximately 10 cm from the cut surface of the tibial plateau will be required. Once full-thickness skin flaps are developed on either side of the extensor mechanism, a midline arthrotomy is performed that runs down the center of the extensor mechanism from the center of the quadriceps tendon, down the midline of the patella to the middle of the tibial tubercle; a

Table 1 Results of Extensor Mechanism Allograft Reconstruction

Authors (Year)	Number of Knees	Mean Patient Age in Years (Range)	Mean Follow-up in Months (Range)	Results/Comments
Emerson et al (1994)	9	69 (36-81)	49 (28-84)	3 graft failures/complications 3 knees with extensor lag >30° Durability of reconstruction a concern
Nazarian and Booth (1999)	36	71	43 (24-120)	8 graft failures/complications Average extensor lag of 13° in 15 of 36 patients
Barrack et al (2003)	14	61	42 (26-40)	1 graft failure/complication 2 knees with extensor lag >30° Mixture of 8 Achilles-calcaneal and 6 quadriceps-patella-tubercle allografts
Prada et al (2003)	3	65 (59-70)	57 (48-72)	No complications Average range of motion 3° to 110°
Burnett et al (2004)	20	68 (51-82)	37 (12-115)	No complications 7 knees with extensor lag >30° All grafts that were tensioned tightly in full extension were successful

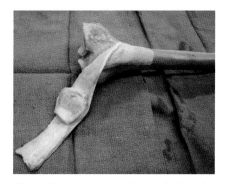

Figure 2 Fresh-frozen EMA including the proximal tibia.

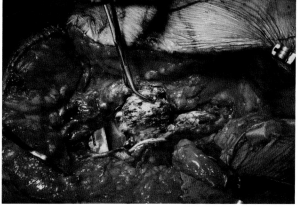

Figure 3 Following a midline arthrotomy, the native patella is shelled out, taking care to preserve the native extensor mechanism.

medial parapatellar or other standard approach to the knee should not be used. The native patella is then shelled out, taking care to fully preserve all surrounding native tissue, which will be used to cover the allograft at the finish of the procedure (**Figure 3**).

Once infection has been ruled out, either an exchange of the modular polyethylene liner is performed or, if required, the prosthetic components are removed and trial revision components are placed (**Figure 4**). If retention of the prosthetic components is planned, the surgeon must ensure that appropriate trial and replacement polyethylene liners are available.

Once thawed, the allograft is prepared on the back table. A small oscillating saw is useful for harvesting the graft and for creation of the tibial bone block. The most proximal cut in the allograft is performed at an approximate 30° angle to create a bevel proximally that resists proximal migration of the graft once locked into a similarly shaped cut in the native proximal tibia (**Figure 5**, *A*). The tibial bone block should measure approximately 2 cm in width and 6 cm in length (**Figure 5**, *B*). A matching trough is then fashioned in the upper end of the tibia (including a back cut of the most proximal end to match the beveled

edge of the graft) using a combination of a small oscillating saw and an osteotome, taking care to maintain a bridge of native tibia proximally of approximately 2 cm. In general, the surgeon starts by making a trough that is slightly smaller than the graft, and then a high-speed burr can be used to slowly enlarge the trough as needed to ensure a snug press-fit. The tibial allograft bone block is then press-fit into the trough; ideally, a bone tamp is required to fully seat the graft secondary to a tight fit. Two or three 16- or 18-gauge wires are then passed around the graft and tightened on the lateral side of the proximal tibia to provide

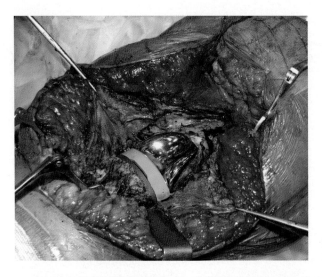

Figure 4 Trial revision component in place.

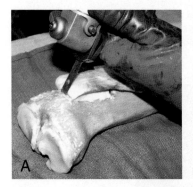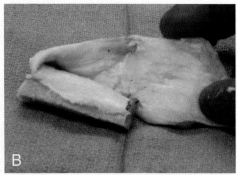

Figure 5 Graft preparation. **A,** A small oscillating saw is used to fashion the graft; note the cut is angled proximally. **B,** The fully prepared tibial bone block, which should measure approximately 2 cm × 6 cm.

adjunctive fixation (**Figure 6,** A). To pass the wires, a drill hole is made on the medial side of the tibia using a bit that is slightly larger than the wire selected, and the wire is passed from medial to lateral. The wire should pass anterior to the stem of the tibial component and may go either through or around the graft. The wires should be tightened on the lateral side, where there is more soft tissue to cover them, to avoid soft-tissue irritation. Although the graft can be fixed with a screw, we prefer wires because the risk of graft fracture is lower and the fixation obtained with wires is usually adequate. If the components are to be revised, the trials can be removed at this point and the revision compo-

nents and final polyethylene liner can be placed now that the graft has been fixed to the tibia.

Next, two heavy nonabsorbable sutures are placed into the quadriceps tendon portion of the allograft in a running, locked fashion to create four strands (**Figure 6,** B). Typically, the graft needs to be trimmed proximally, so that the length of the quadriceps tendon is approximately 5 cm in length. Although this may seem counterintuitive, if the graft is too long proximally, the four strands created will come through the native tissue proximal to the native quadriceps tendon, and suture placed through muscle may not provide as strong a fixation for these critical sutures. If a drain

is desired, it should be placed into the wound at this time.

Next, the leg is fully extended and the four sutures in the allograft are brought underneath the host tissue and through the native quadriceps tendon, as far proximally as possible. The sutures are then tied over the native tissue, tightening the graft in maximal full extension (**Figure 6,** C). Tension on the graft should be such that it is difficult to displace the allograft tendon with a finger (ie, it should be very tight). Once these four sutures are tied, the remaining native tissue should be closed over the allograft with multiple nonabsorbable sutures running through both the native tissue and the allograft to encourage healing between them. In most cases, the entire allograft can be covered with native tissue, except for the most distal portions in the area of the tibial bone block (**Figure 7**).

Wound Closure

Closure of the wound is among the more critical aspects of the procedure. Among the benefits of using an entire EMA is the ability, in most cases, to completely or nearly completely cover the graft with host tissue from the native extensor mechanism. Closure of the subcutaneous tissues over the deep closure and skin is standard.

———————————————————■

■ Postoperative Regimen

Once the wound has been closed completely, a sterile dressing is applied, followed by placement of a plaster splint in the operating room to completely immobilize the extremity. A knee immobilizer is placed over the splint to further ensure that flexion of the knee does not occur. The leg is strictly elevated for the first few post-

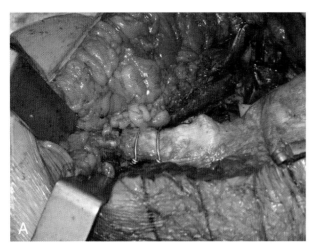

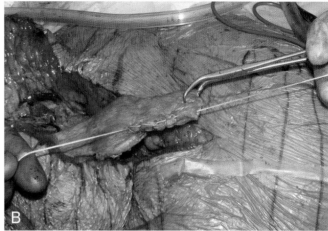

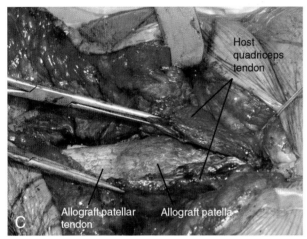

Figure 6 A, The tibial bone block has been press-fit into the native tibia and fixed with two wires for adjunctive fixation. The knots are tightened on the lateral side, where there is more soft-tissue coverage. **B,** Two heavy, nonabsorbable sutures are placed into the allograft quadriceps tendon in a running, locking fashion to create four strands. Note that the allograft quadriceps tendon has been trimmed to approximately 5 cm in length. **C.** With the knee extended, the allograft is tightly tensioned and sewn underneath the native host extensor mechanism. The remaining native soft tissue is then used to completely cover the allograft, with multiple sutures passing between the allograft and host tissue. The Kocher clamps shown are grasping native quadriceps tendon, pulling them toward the patient's foot.

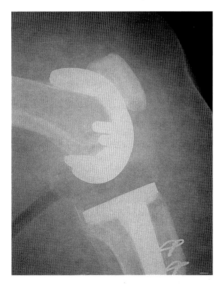

Figure 7 Lateral postoperative radiograph obtained after extensor mechanism allograft reconstruction. Note the bridge of native bone that has been preserved proximally and the bevel in the allograft to help prevent proximal migration or escape of the graft.

operative days, with patients getting out of bed only to use the bathroom and for physical therapy, which consists of gait training with touch-down weight bearing on the extremity until a cast is applied. Isometric quadriceps strengthening exercises are encouraged during the 6-week period of cast immobilization. The deep drain is removed on the second postoperative day (without removal of the surgical dressing), followed by removal of the surgical dressing on the third postoperative day. If wound healing is adequate, a long-leg fiberglass cast is applied to include the foot. Great care must be taken to pad the heel and area around the Achilles tendon to avoid soft-tissue irritation and breakdown. A window in the cast is typically not required but can be incorporated if the

surgeon wants to be able to monitor the wound more closely.

Patients are allowed weight bearing as tolerated in the cast, which is subsequently removed at 3 weeks in the office to allow for the removal of sutures or staples. A new cast is then applied for 3 more weeks. At 6 weeks postoperatively, the cast is removed and a hinged knee brace is applied. Patients are initially allowed a range of motion from full extension to 30° of flexion. Subsequently, the brace is adjusted each week to allow for an additional 10° of active flexion (passive flexion is not permitted), and quadriceps strengthening continues. The brace is discontinued at approximately 3 months postoperatively. Despite the extended period of immobilization and restricted flexion, regaining active flexion is rarely problematic using this regimen, with a recurrent extensor lag being a far more commonly reported complication.

———————■

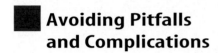

Avoiding Pitfalls and Complications

Many of the potential pitfalls of this procedure can be avoided by meticulous preoperative planning. The surgeon must ensure that replacement polyethylene liners and the necessary trials are available if the prosthetic components are to be retained; a review of the prior surgical note is strongly recommended to make sure that the identity of the implanted components is known. Similarly, appropriate rotation of the implanted components must be ensured if they are to be retained so that any underlying factors that predisposed to extensor mechanism failure are corrected. A thorough perioperative evaluation for infection is likewise required, as implantation of the allograft tissue into an infected bed would lead to recurrent failure. The surgeon must also allow adequate time to identify a right- or left-side allograft as appropriate, as the availability of these allografts can be limited in some areas. Furthermore, obtaining the entire proximal tibia with the EMA is preferred, to ensure an adequately sized bone block on the tibial tubercle.

Intraoperatively, the most critical factors for success include tensioning the allograft tightly in full extension (without flexing the knee or otherwise trialing once the graft has been sewn into place) and coverage of the EMA with as much of the native extensor mechanism as possible to allow for healing of the allograft to native tissue. Fashioning of the trough in the native proximal tibia can be tedious; however, attainment of a good press-fit between the allograft bone block and the trough will ensure adequate strength for healing. Wires used to fix the tibial bone block should always be tightened and crimped on the lateral side of the knee to ensure adequate soft-tissue coverage and avoid irritation beneath the skin. If the components are to be revised, the procedure should proceed in the following sequence: exposure, component removal, insertion of trial revision components, fixation of the allograft into the proximal tibia (including passage of the stainless steel wires) followed by cementing of revision components, and finally proximal fixation of the allograft. If this sequence is not followed, and the final revision components are inserted before fixation of the allograft bone block into the tibia, the surgeon may encounter difficulties in distal fixation, particularly passing the stainless steel wires.

Postoperatively, care must be taken to pad any dressings, splints, and casts adequately to avoid soft-tissue breakdown. Clear communication among the surgeon, patient, and physical therapist is critical so that the postoperative regimen is closely followed to avoid stretching of the allograft tissue.

———————■

Bibliography

Barrack RL, Stanley T, Allen Butler R: Treating extensor mechanism disruption after total knee arthroplasty. *Clin Orthop Relat Res* 2003;416:98-104.

Berger RA, Crossett LS, Jacobs JJ, Rubash HE: Malrotation causing patellofemoral complications after total knee arthroplasty. *Clin Orthop Relat Res* 1998;356356:144-153.

Burnett RS, Berger RA, Della Valle CJ, et al: Extensor mechanism allograft reconstruction after total knee arthroplasty. *J Bone Joint Surg Am* 2005;87(Pt 2Pt 2, Suppl 1)175-194.

Burnett RS, Berger RA, Paprosky WG, Della Valle CJ, Jacobs JJ, Rosenberg AG: Extensor mechanism allograft reconstruction after total knee arthroplasty. A comparison of two techniques. *J Bone Joint Surg Am* 2004;86-A(1212):2694-2699.

Burnett RS, Butler RA, Barrack RL: Extensor mechanism allograft reconstruction in TKA at a mean of 56 months. *Clin Orthop Relat Res* 2006;452:159-165.

Burnett RS, Fornasier VL, Haydon CM, Wehrli BM, Whitewood CN, Bourne RB: Retrieval of a well-functioning extensor mechanism allograft from a total knee arthroplasty. Clinical and histological findings. *J Bone Joint Surg Br* 2004;86(77): 986-990.

Busfield BT, Huffman GR, Nahai F, Hoffman W, Ries MD: Extended medial gastrocnemius rotational flap for treatment of chronic knee extensor mechanism deficiency in patients with and without total knee arthroplasty. *Clin Orthop Relat Res* 2004;428428:190-197.

Crossett LS, Sinha RK, Sechriest VF, Rubash HE: Reconstruction of a ruptured patellar tendon with achilles tendon allograft following total knee arthroplasty. *J Bone Joint Surg Am* 2002;84-A(88):1354-1361.

Della Valle CJ, Sporer SM, Jacobs JJ, Berger RA, Rosenberg AG, Paprosky WG: Preoperative testing for sepsis before revision total knee arthroplasty. *J Arthroplasty* 2007;22(66, Suppl 2)90-93.

Emerson RH Jr, Head WC, Malinin TI: Extensor mechanism reconstruction with an allograft after total knee arthroplasty. *Clin Orthop Relat Res* 1994;303303:79-85.

Jaureguito JW, Dubois CM, Smith SR, Gottlieb LJ, Finn HA: Medial gastrocnemius transposition flap for the treatment of disruption of the extensor mechanism after total knee arthroplasty. *J Bone Joint Surg Am* 1997;79(66):866-873.

Nazarian DG, Booth RE Jr: Extensor mechanism allografts in total knee arthroplasty. *Clin Orthop Relat Res* 1999;367367: 123-129.

Prada SA, Griffin FM, Nelson CL, Garvin KL: Allograft reconstruction for extensor mechanism rupture after total knee arthroplasty: 4.8-year follow-up. *Orthopedics* 2003;26(1212):1205-1208.

Springer BD, Della Valle CJ: Extensor mechanism allograft reconstruction after total knee arthroplasty. *J Arthroplasty* 2008;23(7Suppl 7)35-38.

Coding

CPT Codes		Corresponding ICD-9 Codes	
15738	Muscle, myocutaneous, or fasciocutaneous flap; lower extremity	998	
20680	Removal of implant; deep (eg, buried wire, pin, screw, metal band, nail, rod or plate)	733.81 996.77	996.66 996.78
20900	Bone graft, any donor area; minor or small (eg, dowel or button)	715	733
20902	Bone graft, any donor area; major or large	715	733
27470	Repair, nonunion or malunion, femur, distal to head and neck; without graft (eg, compression technique)	733.81	733.82
27472	Repair, nonunion or malunion, femur, distal to head and neck; with iliac or other autogenous bone graft (includes obtaining graft)	733.81	733.82
29870	Arthroscopy, knee, diagnostic, with or without synovial biopsy (separate procedure)	715	
29880	Arthroscopy, knee, surgical; with meniscectomy (medial AND lateral, including any meniscal shaving)	836	717
29881	Arthroscopy, knee, surgical; with meniscectomy (medial OR lateral, including any meniscal shaving)	836	717

Chapter 37

Prophylaxis for Deep Vein Thrombosis Following Total Knee Arthroplasty

Clifford W. Colwell, Jr, MD
Mary E. Hardwick, MSN, RN

■ Introduction

The 1986 Consensus Development Conference on the Prevention of Venous Thrombosis and Pulmonary Embolism, convened by the National Institutes of Health, first identified major orthopaedic surgery of the lower extremity as being associated with a high risk of venous thromboembolism (VTE). Total knee arthroplasty (TKA) was specifically targeted as a concern for deep vein thrombosis (DVT) and pulmonary embolism (PE), the constituents of VTE. Since this consensus conference, studies in TKA have put the incidence of DVT without any prophylaxis at 40% to 84% and of PE at 1.8% to 7%, with 0.2% to 0.7% of cases being fatal. The use of chemical thromboprophylaxis has significantly decreased mortality, from 0.62% in 1990 to 0.26% in 1998, and has decreased the incidence of DVT to as low as 12%, although this must be balanced with the possibility of bleeding after surgery from the use of anticoagulants. Mechanical devices also have been used and have been found to reduce DVT, but decreased

hospital stays and lack of portability have hindered their use as a single modality. The selection of a prophylactic agent involves balancing the efficacy and the safety of the agent for the individual patient.

With the number of TKAs done annually estimated at more than 500,000 in the United States and more than 1 million in Europe, current choices in prophylaxis have grown in importance and have become significantly more evidence-based since the 1986 conference. The American College of Chest Physicians has published guidelines, updated approximately every 2 to 4 years, for thromboprophylaxis in TKA as well as numerous other orthopaedic procedures. In this meta-analysis approach, a grading system has been developed that rates the information from randomized clinical trials down to cohort trials in establishing guidelines and allows surgeons to practice more data-based medicine. In 2007, the American Academy of Orthopaedic Surgeons (AAOS) published a set of guidelines for the prevention of symptomatic PE following total joint arthroplasty.

In discussing thrombosis, the difference between venous thrombosis and arterial thrombosis needs clarification. Thrombosis in arteries is usually triggered by underlying arteriosclerosis and is composed mainly of platelets that deposit in the sclerotic rough area. A venous thrombosis is composed mainly of clotting proteins, with platelets playing a very minor role. Therefore, the methods used to prevent one type of thrombosis do not necessarily work on the other type of thrombosis. The focus of this chapter is the occurrence of DVT following TKA.

Some studies indicate that proximal DVT is more important than distal DVT in its sequelae and the risk of developing subsequent PE, although distal clot formation is more common following TKA than it is after total hip arthroplasty (THA). Proximal DVT occurs in veins above the knee, from the popliteal vein upward. Because these vessels are larger, the thrombosis is usually more significant and, if dislodged, allegedly could cause a larger PE. Studies have shown that between 20% and 30% of thromboses that originate in the distal veins propagate to proximal veins and can cause PE. Calf vein thrombi are not benign; a high proportion leave residual venous abnormalities, including persistent oc-

Dr. Colwell or an immediate family member serves as a paid consultant for or an employee of Stryker and has received research or institutional support from Stryker. Mary E. Hardwick, MSN, RN, or an immediate family member has received research or institutional support from DePuy, Stryker, Wright Medical Technology, Pancera, and Boehringer-Ingelheim.

clusion and/or venous valvular incompetence, and postthrombotic syndrome develops in 5% of patients after TKA and THA. Therefore, prophylaxis to prevent PE and proximal as well as distal DVT is important. The clinical treatment of distal clots remains an area of controversy.

There are no specific contraindications to the use of DVT prophylaxis; however, the timing of prophylaxis and the selection of a prophylactic agent may need to be adjusted because of concerns related to postoperative bleeding. All patients undergoing TKA are considered to be at high risk for the development of DVT and therefore all patients theoretically require prophylaxis. No definitive clinical signs or symptoms are pathognomonic of DVT; however, patients should be assessed perioperatively and during recovery for any signs or symptoms suggesting VTE (swelling, pain, and change in color). This assessment should lead immediately to more definitive tests, such as duplex ultrasound. Patients should also be educated about clinical signs and symptoms of VTE so that they can report these to their physician.

Genetics and Clotting Factors

Genetic factors, including mutations of factor V Leiden and prothrombin F2 gene mutation *G20210A*, have been reported to increase the risk of VTE in the population. A study of TKA and THA patients indicated that the prothrombin gene mutation *G20210A* was significantly represented in those with symptomatic VTE ($P = 0.0002$). A tendency toward increased risk of VTE was found with factor V Leiden mutation ($P = 0.09$). However, because 90% of the population who had these genetic risk factors

did not have a VTE, general preoperative genotype screening is of questionable value.

Increased levels of the clotting factors factor VIII and fibronectin have been associated with VTE, but these factors have not been examined in relation to orthopaedic surgery patients. A low level of high-density lipoprotein also has been associated with development of VTE, but again, it has not been studied in the orthopaedic surgical patient. Another study reports a positive relationship between plasma cholesteryl ester transfer proteins and increased coagulability in young men, yet whether this would transfer to surgical patients is not known.

Recently, genetic variants of the enzyme that metabolizes warfarin, cytochrome P-450 2C9 (*CYP2C9*), and of a pharmacologic target of warfarin, vitamin K epoxide reductase (*VKORC1*), have been connected to the differences in patients' responses to warfarin doses. One study of this genetic-based dosing in 92 TKA and THA patients proposed an algorithm for warfarin dosing after orthopaedic surgery that took into consideration genetic type, clinical variables, current medication, and preoperative and postoperative laboratory values. Although further study is necessary, a safer, more effective process for initiating warfarin therapy may be developed.

Diagnosis

Doppler duplex ultrasound is a major tool used in both practice and research to detect DVT in patients with joint arthroplasty of the lower extremities as well as DVT in other medical and surgical conditions. Because venous ultrasound is noninvasive, has almost no contraindications, and can be safely used repeatedly, it has become the most widely used test for clinical

detection of symptomatic and asymptomatic DVT. Doppler ultrasound also is used by some surgeons as a screening tool to determine whether any thrombi are present at time of hospital discharge. In several different randomized trials, however, routine screening at discharge has not been found to be an effective strategy.

No standardized documentation procedure exists for Doppler ultrasound that allows central adjudication, so venography is still considered the gold standard for large VTE prophylaxis studies of new anticoagulants if regulated by the U.S. Food and Drug Administration (FDA). Venography is rarely done in clinical practice to detect symptomatic DVT, however, because of the invasiveness and pain of the procedure, the exposure of the patient to radiation and contrast agents, and the cumbersome nature of the test.

Fifty percent of deaths associated with lower extremity orthopaedic surgery are caused by vascular events, and death in these situations can occur within a matter of minutes, making prophylaxis critical. In a patient with symptoms of PE, the D-dimer level is first checked. If the D-dimer test is positive, diagnosis is currently most often done by CT pulmonary angiography, although a few institutions still use ventilation-perfusion lung scans. Lung scan results are categorized as normal, low probability, and high probability. An angiography study is done as follow-up to confirm the PE after a high-probability ventilation-perfusion scan. A study comparing CT pulmonary angiography and ventilation-perfusion lung scans found that the procedures were similarly accurate in diagnosing PE. Either method appears to be acceptable in diagnosing PE; however, a few failures occurred with both screening methods.

Table 1 Anticoagulation Agents Available in the United States

Agent	Type of Drug	Dose	Administration	Site of Action in Clotting Cascade
Enoxaparin	LMWH	30 mg twice per day subcutaneously or 40 mg once per day	Start 12-24 h after surgery	Factor Xa Thrombin
Dalteparin	LMWH FDA-approved only for THA	2,500 units (half dose) subcutaneously 5,000 units (full dose) subcutaneously	Start 4-8 h after surgery with half dose, then full dose once per day	Factor Xa Thrombin
Fondaparinux	Synthetic pentasaccharide	2.5 mg once per day subcutaneously	Start ~6-24 h after surgery	Factor Xa
Warfarin	VKA	2-10 mg orally once per day to maintain INR of 2-2.5	Start 1-12 h before or after surgery	Tissue factor/factor VIIa Factor IXa Factor Xa Thrombin

LMWH = low-molecular-weight heparin, FDA = US Food and Drug Administration, THA = total hip arthroplasty, VKA = vitamin K antagonist, INR = International Normalized Ratio.

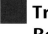

Treatment and Results

Pharmacologic Prophylaxis

Pharmacologic agents used for prophylaxis include unfractionated heparin, low-molecular-weight heparin (LMWH), fondaparinux, and vitamin K antagonists. The drugs in this category are listed in **Table 1**. Some orthopaedic surgeons in the United States use aspirin (acetylsalicylic acid), generally with mechanical devices but occasionally alone. Other products are available in Europe. LMWH, fondaparinux, and warfarin have been demonstrated in randomized trials to be effective in preventing VTE.

The most commonly used category of drugs used worldwide for VTE prophylaxis is LMWH. These drugs are given subcutaneously in different doses with different timing, depending on the particular drug, but do not require laboratory monitoring or dose adjustment. Extensive data have shown that this category of drugs is safe and effective, although concern still exists about related bleeding. Fondaparinux, also given subcutaneously, is a synthetic pentasaccharide

used for prophylaxis. Another drug commonly used is warfarin, a vitamin K antagonist that is given orally. Warfarin is dosed by checking the prothrombin time using the international normalized ratio (INR) to adjust the warfarin dose. The point at which each of these agents provides inhibition in the coagulation cascade is shown in **Figure 1**. Aspirin is prescribed in various doses and often is used as part of a multimodal approach in combination with mechanical devices. Each of these drugs has the potential to cause bleeding.

RESULTS

Randomized clinical trials directly comparing LMWH with adjusted-dose warfarin after TKA using venographic confirmation found the combined rates of DVT were 33% and 48%, respectively (**Table 2**). Major bleeding was slightly higher for LMWH (4.5%) than for warfarin (2.7%).

A randomized clinical trial of fondaparinux compared with enoxaparin 30 mg twice per day in 1,049 patients undergoing TKA with venographic confirmation reported VTE rates of 12.5% and 27.8%, respectively. Proxi-

mal DVTs were reported at 2.4% for fondaparinux and at 5.4% for enoxaparin. Major bleeding, however, was reported as significantly higher (*P* = 0.006) in the fondaparinux group (2.1%) than in the enoxaparin group (0.2%).

The use of adjusted-dose warfarin after TKA was assessed with routine venography in 12 randomized clinical trials; a DVT rate between 25% and 50% was reported. Studies examining the rate of symptomatic VTE when adjusted-dose warfarin was administered found, at 3-month follow-up, a rate of 0.8% with 10 days of prophylaxis and 1.3% with 12 days of prophylaxis. Adjusted-dose warfarin, although an effective method of prophylaxis, is less effective than LMWH or fondaparinux and is more difficult to manage after hospital discharge. Aspirin is a nonsteroidal anti-inflammatory drug that irreversibly inhibits platelets and the aggregation of platelets and vasoconstriction. Aspirin has been reported effective as an antithrombotic agent in heart disease. A meta-analysis of prophylaxis in TKA found a range of DVT reported from 41% to 78% (average, 53%) and a PE

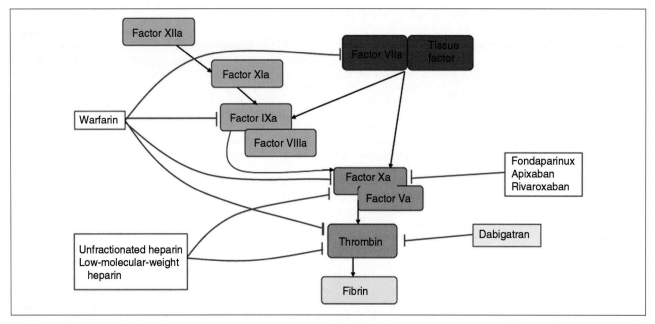

Figure 1 Modified coagulation cascade indicating the point of action for each anticoagulant agent used for prophylaxis. The black arrows denote activation, and the red lines imply inhibition. (Courtesy of S. D. Berkowitz, MD.)

incidence of 11.7% when aspirin was used alone. Use of aspirin alone was not shown to be efficacious in TKA for VTE prophylaxis, with 59% of patients positive for DVT; however, in combination with compression devices, 27% of patients were positive for DVT. The Pulmonary Embolism Prevention trial, an international trial comparing aspirin with placebo, reported decreased DVT and PE in hip fracture patients with aspirin, but aspirin was not superior to placebo in TKA and THA patients.

New oral anticoagulant drugs are currently in clinical trials with FDA oversight before approval. Two of these (apixaban and rivaroxaban) are oral anti-factor Xa drugs, and another (dabigatran) is an oral direct thrombin inhibitor. These drugs have the advantage of being given orally and do not require monitoring of blood levels or adjustment of dosing. Studies of their use for prophylaxis in TKA have produced varied results.

Apixaban was randomized to TKA patients in a double-blind administration of six different doses given either once or twice per day and compared with enoxaparin 30 mg twice per day or open-label warfarin (INR 1.8 to 3.0) for 10 to 14 days of treatment with mandatory venography to determine VTE. Analysis of 856 patients revealed all apixaban groups had lower primary efficacy rates than either comparator, concluding that apixaban in doses of 2.5 mg twice per day or 5 mg once per day had a promising benefit-risk profile for TKA prophylaxis.

In a randomized, double-blind study of 1,833 patients undergoing TKA, rivaroxaban (10 mg once per day) was compared with enoxaparin (40 mg once per day with preoperative dosing), and VTE was demonstrated in 1.0% and 2.6%, respectively. Major bleeding was similar between groups.

A randomized, double-blind study conducted in Europe compared dabigatran 150 or 220 mg once per day with enoxaparin 40 mg once per day after TKA; results reported were a VTE rate of 37.7% for enoxaparin, 36.4% for dabigatran 220 mg, and 40.5% for dabigatran 150 mg, with no difference

in major bleeding. A similar North American study using enoxaparin 30 mg twice per day found a VTE rate of 25% for enoxaparin, a 31% rate for dabigatran 220 mg, and a 34% rate for dabigatran 150 mg, with no difference in bleeding rates. The authors concluded that dabigatran showed inferior efficacy.

Both dabigatran and rivaroxaban have been approved for VTE prophylaxis for TKA in Europe but have not yet been approved in the United States.

TIMING AND DURATION OF DOSING

In Europe, LMWH is routinely started before surgery; however, in North America, LMWH is most often initiated 12 to 24 hours after surgery. The timing of the administration of these agents represents a balance between efficacy and bleeding. For example, fondaparinux was found to increase major bleeding in 3.2% of patients when given within 6 hours of skin closure, compared with 2.1% of patients when administered after more than 6 hours.

Table 2 Results From Major Randomized Controlled Trials Comparing LMWH With Adjusted-Dose Warfarin

Author(s) (Year)	Number of Patients	Prophylactic Agent	Total DVT Events (%)	Proximal DVT Events (%)	Pulmonary Embolism Events (%)
Hull et al (1993)	277	Warfarin	152 (54.9)	34 (12.3)	NA
	258*	LMWH	116 (45.0)	20 (7.8)	NA
RD Heparin Arthroplasty Group (1994)	147	Warfarin	60 (41)	15 (10)	1 (0.6)
	150	LMWH	37 (25)	9 (6)	0
Hamulyak et al (1995)	61	Warfarin	23 (37.7)	6 (9.8)	NA
	65*	LMWH	16 (24.6)	5 (7.7)	NA
Leclerc et al (1996)	211	Warfarin	109 (51.7)	22 (10.4)	3 (1.4)
	206	LMWH	76 (36.9)	24 (11.7)	1 (0.5)
Heit et al (1997)	222	Warfarin	85 (38)	15 (7)	0
	232	LMWH	62 (27)	15 (6)	1 (0.4)
Fitzgerald (2001)	122	Warfarin	72 (59.0)	16 (13.1)	0
	108	LMWH	41 (38.0)	3 (2.8)	0

DVT = deep vein thrombosis, LMWH = low-molecular-weight heparin, NA = not available.
*LMWH was administered once per day; all others were administered twice per day.

The length of time prophylaxis should be continued also has been questioned. In a large epidemiologic study of 26,000 TKA patients, the VTE rate after hospital discharge was 2.1%, but the diagnosis was made a mean of 7 days after discharge, suggesting that the current recommendation of 10 days of prophylaxis is adequate. Another study that examined extending LMWH thromboprophylaxis in TKA patients to postoperative day 28 found the extended treatment did not significantly reduce asymptomatic DVT and symptomatic VTE compared with 7 to 10 days of prophylaxis (17.5% vs 20.8%, respectively). Extended use of warfarin also has been associated with very low rates of readmission for symptomatic VTE in TKA patients. No increase in bleeding was noted with prolonged prophylaxis.

Nonpharmacologic Methods

TYPES OF NONPHARMACOLOGIC PROPHYLAXIS

Mechanical methods, including graduated compression stockings (GCSs), intermittent pneumatic compression (IPC) of the calf or calf and thigh, and venous foot pumps (VFPs), are reported to be effective in combination with early ambulation. One of the problems with these devices is that there is no standardization; therefore, results from a study of one device cannot be applied to another device. Compression devices appear to be effective when used properly; however, fewer data are available for devices than for antithrombotic agents. Two key concerns when using these devices are proper fit and percentage of time used each day. Drawbacks to the use of these devices are that patients find them too warm or uncomfortable to wear; IPC and VFPs require a larger motorized pump, which can be noisy and cumbersome; and the devices have to be disconnected when the patient is ambulating, making compliance an issue for both patient and staff.

RESULTS

The scant data available on GCSs indicate that they provide little or no protection from DVT. A study evaluating use of above-the-knee and below-the-knee GSCs found no reduction of DVT rates with either type of GCS compared with a control group that received no form of prophylaxis. Another study evaluating use of LMWH with GCSs in 97 patients and use of placebo with GCSs in 104 patients reported a 29.9% DVT rate and a 58.7% DVT rate ($P < 0.001$), respectively, and one PE in each group. A further study of GCSs revealed that 98% of the stockings failed to produce the "ideal" pressure gradient from the ankle to the knee.

A 1990 study compared compression boots with aspirin after unilateral TKA (72 patients) and bilateral TKA (47 patients). In unilateral TKA, the study found a 22% DVT rate with compression boots and a 47% DVT rate with aspirin. In bilateral TKA, the study found a 48% DVT rate with compression boots and a 68% DVT rate with aspirin. A comparison of plantar compression and aspirin versus aspirin alone in 132 patients (164 knees) found DVT rates of 27% (22 of 48 patients) and 59% (49 of 83), respectively. Another study compared LMWH (60 patients) with an IPC foot pump (48 patients) and reported 23.9% and 54% DVT rates, respec-

Table 3 Guidelines for Epidural Catheter Use With Anticoagulation Therapy

Prophylactic Agent	Guidelines for Catheter Removal
LMWH	Remove catheter when LMWH effect is minimum (2 h before next injection) Delay LMWH prophylaxis at least 2 h after spinal needle or epidural catheter removal
Fondaparinux	Do not use preoperatively with neuraxial block or with continuous epidural block (lack of safety data)
Warfarin	Continuous epidural should not be used more than 1 to 2 days because of unpredictable anticoagulant effect INR < 1.5 at time of catheter removal

In all patients having spinal puncture or epidural catheter, antithrombotics should be used with caution. Avoid epidural puncture with use of preoperative antithrombotic agents and known bleeding disorders. Delay the start of antithrombotic prophylaxis in a "bloody tap."

LMWH = low-molecular-weight heparin, INR = International Normalized Ratio.

Data from Horlocker TT, Wedel DJ, Benzon H, et al: Regional anesthesia in the anticoagulated patient: Defining the risks (the second ASRA Consensus Conference on Neuraxial Anesthesia and Anticoagulation). *Reg Anesth Pain Med* 2003;28:172-197.

tively. A study comparing two types of pneumatic compression devices—a rapid-inflation, asymmetric compression device (206 patients) and a sequential, circumferential compression device (217 patients)—found 6.9% and 15% DVT rates, respectively. Another study compared LMWH (139 patients) with the use of VenaFlow calf compression devices (Aircast, DJO, Vista, CA) with aspirin (136 patients) and reported 14.1% and 17.8% DVT rates, respectively. A single surgeon reported a 9.3% DVT rate in 856 primary and revision TKAs performed using regional anesthesia and either sequential compression devices or a rapid-inflation asymmetric compression device combined with aspirin.

Recently, a portable compression device has been developed. The portability allows the patient to use the device at home as well as in the hospital and allows the use of the device when the patient is out of bed without disconnecting the device, which increases compliance. In addition, this portable device contains a sensor that

monitors respiratory-related venous phasic flow and times the compression during the expiratory phase when the thoracic pressure is low and the right-heart filling is maximal. No large randomized trials assessing the efficacy of this device in TKA have been published yet. However, a recent multicenter study comparing these portable compression devices with enoxaparin in the THA patients demonstrated a symptomatic PE rate of 1% in both groups.

Epidural Anesthesia and Analgesia

Use of epidural anesthesia has been reported to decrease the incidence of DVT in patients undergoing TKA. One study of 705 TKAs reported a DVT incidence of 48% in patients with epidural anesthesia compared with 64% in patients with general anesthesia.

Another study of 262 TKA patients reported a DVT incidence of 40% with epidural anesthesia and 48% with general anesthesia. However, the use of epidural analgesia by indwelling catheter has created some concerns about the use of anticoagulants after surgery. Initially, the recommendation was to remove the catheter before starting anticoagulation, but this would leave the patient unprotected from VTE for the first few days after surgery. In 2003, the guidelines were changed to accommodate epidural use, but caution and close monitoring are still advised (Table 3).

Guidelines and National Mandates for Prophylaxis

Guidelines for thromboprophylaxis are available to assist in practicing evidence-based medicine. The American College of Chest Physicians released the 8th edition of their antithrombotic and thrombolytic therapy guidelines in 2008. These guidelines are based on current literature reporting on the effectiveness and safety of various types of thromboprophylaxis. The AAOS released guidelines in 2007 for prevention of symptomatic PE in patients undergoing THA or TKA. These guidelines focus on the prevention of symptomatic PE and reduction of bleeding. Most studies with symptomatic PE as the end point were underpowered to evaluate the benefit of prophylaxis. Therefore, these recommendations allow for multiple as well as additive protocols, as no evidence is available that any one protocol is more or less effective.

In the United States, prevention of thrombosis after TKA has been mandated by several regulatory agencies. The Surgical Care Improvement Project (SCIP) Venous Thromboembolism Measures adopted by The Joint Commission state:

• SCIP VTE 1: Surgery patients with recommended venous thromboembolism prophylaxis ordered any time from hospital arrival to anesthesia end time. Recommended prophylaxis options for TKA include:

- ° LMWH
- ° Factor Xa inhibitor (fondaparinux)
- ° Warfarin
- ° IPC devices
- ° VFPs

A combination of aspirin and compression devices for prophylaxis meets the SCIP requirements for acceptable prophylaxis after TKA.

• SCIP VTE 2: Surgical patients who received appropriate venous thromboembolism prophylaxis within 24 hours before anesthesia start time to 24 hours after anesthesia end time. The same agents as above were recommended for TKA prophylaxis.

The SCIP Website also contains tools to assist in achieving these measures, such as a sample order set, a nursing assessment guide, a pocket reminder card, and an education module.

The National Quality Forum released six measures in 2008 that target "the most common preventable cause of hospital death—venous thromboembolism." These measures are directed at all hospital patients, not just surgical patients. The measures include appropriately documented risk of VTE, prescribed and received prophylaxis, and discharge instructions. This project (1) recommends a framework to measure effective screening, prevention, and treatment of persons at risk for VTE/DVT/PE across the continuum of care settings; (2) identifies a statement of organizational policy based on setting of care and scope of services; (3) identifies, endorses, and disseminates a set of key VTE prevention and care characteristics of preferred practices to promote quality care for persons at risk for VTE and works to catalyze their adoption and use; and (4) identifies, develops, pilot tests, and endorses performance measures to evaluate the quality of care for persons at risk for VTE. The measures also include reporting the incidence of potentially preventable VTE.

Conclusions

TKA has become an excellent surgical procedure with long-term pain relief and return to normal function. Risks, however, accompany any major surgical procedure such as TKA, and VTE and its sequelae have been identified as a significant surgical risk. Many different effective prophylaxis regimens are available. The surgeon has the opportunity and responsibility to choose the protocol that gives his or her patient the best risk-benefit ratio. VTE prophylaxis in TKA is a changing field, with new agents and devices currently being tested that will be available in the near future. Physicians should educate themselves about current developments and be willing to adopt new protocols when evidence-based medicine shows that a new modality produces better risk-benefit ratios than older protocols.

Bibliography

American Academy of Orthopaedic Surgeons. AAOS Clinical Guideline on Prevention of Symptomatic Pulmonary Embolism (PE) in Patients Undergoing Total Hip or Knee Arthroplasty. 2007. http://www.aaos.org/news/bulletin/jul07/clinical3.asp. Accessed December 11, 2009.

Anderson DR, Kahn SR, Rodger MA, et al: Computed tomographic pulmonary angiography vs ventilation-perfusion lung scanning in patients with suspected pulmonary embolism: A randomized controlled trial. *JAMA* 2007;298(23):2743-2753.

Bauer KA, Eriksson BI, Lassen MR, Turpie AG; Steering Committee of the Pentasaccharide in Major Knee Surgery Study: Fondaparinux compared with enoxaparin for the prevention of venous thromboembolism after elective major knee surgery. *N Engl J Med* 2001;345(18):1305-1310.

Best AJ, Williams S, Crozier A, Bhatt R, Gregg PJ, Hui AC: Graded compression stockings in elective orthopaedic surgery: An assessment of the in vivo performance of commercially available stockings in patients having hip and knee arthroplasty. *J Bone Joint Surg Br* 2000;82(1):116-118.

Caprini JA, Arcelus JI, Reyna JJ: Effective risk stratification of surgical and nonsurgical patients for venous thromboembolic disease. *Semin Hematol* 2001;38(2, Suppl 5)12-19.

Comp PC, Spiro TE, Friedman RJ, et al; Enoxaparin Clinical Trial Group: Prolonged enoxaparin therapy to prevent venous thromboembolism after primary hip or knee replacement. *J Bone Joint Surg Am* 2001;83-A(3):336-345.

Deguchi H, Fernández JA, Griffin JH: Plasma cholesteryl ester transfer protein and blood coagulability. *Thromb Haemost* 2007;98(6):1160-1164.

Fitzgerald RH, Jr: Preventing DVT following total knee replacement: A review of recent clinical trials. *Orthopedics* 1995; 18(Suppl):10-11.

Geerts WH, Bergqvist D, Pineo GF, et al ; American College of Chest Physicians: Prevention of venous thromboembolism: American College of Chest Physicians Evidence-Based Clinical Practice Guidelines (8th Edition). *Chest* 2008;133 (Suppl 6)S381-S453.

Gelfer Y, Tavor H, Oron A, Peer A, Halperin N, Robinson D: Deep vein thrombosis prevention in joint arthroplasties: Continuous enhanced circulation therapy vs low molecular weight heparin. *J Arthroplasty* 2006;21(2):206-214.

Hamulyák K, Lensing AW, van der Meer J, Smid WM, van Ooy A, Hoek JA: Subcutaneous low-molecular weight heparin or oral anticoagulants for the prevention of deep-vein thrombosis in elective hip and knee replacement? Fraxiparine Oral Anticoagulant Study Group. *Thromb Haemost* 1995;74(6):1428-1431.

Heit JA, Berkowitz SD, Bona R, et al; Ardeparin Arthroplasty Study Group: Efficacy and safety of low molecular weight heparin (ardeparin sodium) compared to warfarin for the prevention of venous thromboembolism after total knee replacement surgery: A double-blind, dose-ranging study. *Thromb Haemost* 1997;77(1):32-38.

Horlocker TT, Wedel DJ, Benzon H, et al: Regional anesthesia in the anticoagulated patient: Defining the risks (the second ASRA Consensus Conference on Neuraxial Anesthesia and Anticoagulation). *Reg Anesth Pain Med* 2003;28:172-197.

Hull R, Raskob G, Pineo G, et al: A comparison of subcutaneous low-molecular-weight heparin with warfarin sodium for prophylaxis against deep-vein thrombosis after hip or knee implantation. *N Engl J Med* 1993;329(19):1370-1376.

Leclerc JR, Geerts WH, Desjardins L, et al: Prevention of venous thromboembolism after knee arthroplasty. A randomized, double-blind trial comparing enoxaparin with warfarin. *Ann Intern Med* 1996;124(7):619-626.

Markel A: Origin and natural history of deep vein thrombosis of the legs. *Semin Vasc Med* 2005;5(1):65-74.

Morris RJ, Woodcock JP: Evidence-based compression: Prevention of stasis and deep vein thrombosis. *Ann Surg* 2004; 239(2):162-171.

Nicolaides AN, Breddin HK, Fareed J, et al; Cardiovascular Disease Educational and Research Trust and the International Union of Angiology: Prevention of venous thromboembolism. International Consensus Statement: Guidelines compiled in accordance with the scientific evidence. *Int Angiol* 2001;20(1):1-37.

RD Heparin Arthroplasty Group: RD heparin compared with warfarin for prevention of venous thromboembolic disease following total hip or knee arthroplasty. *J Bone Joint Surg Am* 1994;76(8):1174-1185.

Robinson KS, Anderson DR, Gross M, et al: Ultrasonographic screening before hospital discharge for deep venous thrombosis after arthroplasty: The post-arthroplasty screening study. A randomized, controlled trial. *Ann Intern Med* 1997;127(6):439-445.

Westrich GH, Haas SB, Mosca P, Peterson M: Meta-analysis of thromboembolic prophylaxis after total knee arthroplasty. *J Bone Joint Surg Br* 2000;82(6):795-800.

White RH, Romano PS, Zhou H, Rodrigo J, Bargar W: Incidence and time course of thromboembolic outcomes following total hip or knee arthroplasty. *Arch Intern Med* 1998;158(14):1525-1531.

Coding

CPT Codes		Corresponding ICD-9 Codes	

Total Knee Arthroplasty

| 27447 | Arthroplasty, knee, condyle and plateau; medial AND lateral compartments with or without patella resurfacing (total knee arthroplasty) | 715
715.80 | 715.16
715.89 |

HCPCS Codes*

Graduated Compression Stockings (GCS)

L8100	Gradient compression stocking, below knee, 18-30 mm Hg, each
L8110	Gradient compression stocking, below knee, 30-40 mm Hg, each
L8120	Gradient compression stocking, below knee, 40-50 mm Hg, each
L8130	Gradient compression stocking, thigh length, 18-30 mm Hg, each
L8140	Gradient compression stocking, thigh length, 30-40 mm Hg, each
L8150	Gradient compression stocking, thigh length, 40-50 mm Hg, each
L8160	Gradient compression stocking, full length/chap style, 18-30 mm Hg, each
L8170	Gradient compression stocking, full length/chap style, 30-40 mm Hg, each
L8180	Gradient compression stocking, full length/chap style, 40-50 mm Hg, each
L8190	Gradient compression stocking, waist length, 18-30 mm Hg, each
L8195	Gradient compression stocking, waist length, 30-40 mm Hg, each
L8200	Gradient compression stocking, waist length, 40-50 mm Hg, each

Intermittent Pneumatic Compression (IPC)

EO675	Pneumatic compression device, high pressure, rapid inflation/deflation cycle, for arterial insufficiency (unilateral or bilateral system)
EO676	Intermittent limb compression device (includes all accessories), not otherwise specified

Venous Foot Pumps (VFPs)

A6451	Moderate compression bandage, elastic, knitted/woven, load resistance of 1.25 to 1.34 foot pounds at 50% maximum stretch, width greater than or equal to three inches and less than five inches, per yard
A6452	High compression bandage, elastic, knitted/woven, load resistance greater than or equal to 1.35 foot pounds at 50% maximum stretch, width greater than or equal to three inches and less than five inches, per yard

*HCPCS codes (supply codes) are separately reportable by the physician when provided in the office setting. If ordered in the hospital or outpatient facility, supply codes are not separately reportable.
CPT copyright © 2010 by the American Medical Association. All rights reserved.
HCPCS copyright ©2010 by the Centers for Medicare and Medicaid Services. All rights reserved.

SECTION 4
Revision Total Knee Arthroplasty
Section Editors
Daniel J. Berry, MD
Jay R. Lieberman, MD

Chapter 38

Overview and Strategies for Revision Total Knee Arthroplasty

William A. Jiranek, MD

John B. Meding, MD

E. Michael Keating, MD

Indications

The indications for revision total knee arthoplasty (TKA) can be divided into four general categories: (1) intractable pain from a clearly definable source, such as prosthetic loosening or component breakage; (2) severe dysfunction of the prosthetic joint, such as ligamentous instability; (3) chronic infection; and (4) impending failure of the implant that, if allowed to fail, would lead to greater morbidity, such as severe and progressive osteolysis.

Revision should be contemplated only after a source of failure of the arthroplasty has been clearly identified and after considering nonsurgical management of the problem.

A review of the Medicare inpatient database indicates that in the population older than 65 years, infection is the most common reason for revision TKA (25%), with loosening second (16%). The national joint registries provide data regarding the overall prevalence of revision surgery as well as the prevalence of each category. Between 1985 and 1999, the Swedish Knee Arthroplasty Register reported a prevalence of revision TKA of between 5% and 6%, with a cumulative 5-year revision risk of 6.4% (N = 44,590 TKAs). In further analysis of these data, specifically revisions (of TKA performed for osteoarthritis) between 1985 and 1999, 40% were performed for implant loosening, 15% for infection, 8% for instability, and 12% for other mechanical causes. The Finnish Arthroplasty Register reported a 15-year survival of TKA performed for osteoarthritis of 80%, with failure defined as revision for any reason. In other words, for those patients who survive 15 years after TKA, 20% will need revision.

Contraindications

Mont and associates reported that the results of revision TKA were more often poor when no clear indication for the arthroplasty failure was identified. This observation has been corroborated by subsequent reports.

Active periprosthetic infection is in most cases a contraindication to revision surgery. A one-stage revision of a knee with an established infection is associated with poorer results than a two-stage revision and should be contemplated only in cases of a very susceptible bacterium, a well-healed wound, and a patient in good health with a good immune system.

In addition, a revision TKA is four times more likely to fail from infection than from other causes. Thus it is very important to rule out sepsis as much as possible before revision through a careful history, serologic tests (C-reactive protein [CRP] level and erythrocyte sedimentation rate [ESR]), and an aspiration of the synovial fluid with analysis of both the cell count and differential, as well as a culture of the fluid. The CRP level and ESR are useful markers of inflammation, but even when taken together, these tests are not 100% accurate. A cell count and differential should always be obtained from the synovial fluid aspirated for culture, to allow interpretation of culture re-

Dr. Jiranek or an immediate family member is a board member, owner, officer, or committee member of the American Association of Hip and Knee Surgeons and The Hip Society; has received royalties from DePuy; and serves as a paid consultant for or is an employee of DePuy. Dr. Meding or an immediate family member has received royalties from Biomet and serves as a board member, owner, officer, or committee member of the American Academy of Orthopaedic Surgeons. Dr. Keating or an immediate family member has received royalties from Biomet; is a member of a speakers' bureau or has made paid presentations on behalf of Biomet and Johnson & Johnson; serves as a paid consultant to Biomet and Johnson & Johnson; has stock or stock options held in Johnson & Johnson; has received research or institutional support from Biomet; and serves as a board member, owner, officer, or committee member of the American Academy of Orthopaedic Surgeons and The Knee Society.

Table 1 Testing Before Revision Total Knee Arthroplasty

Test	Normal Range/Comments
Serologic tests for inflammation/infection	
Peripheral white blood cell count	>4 and <12 × 10⁹ cells/L
Erythrocyte sedimentation rate	<20 mm/h (normal varies by institution)
C-reactive protein level	<0.5 mg/dL
Serologic tests for immune system condition	
Albumin level	>2.5 g/dL
Absolute lymphocyte count	>1,100 cells/mL
Synovial fluid tests	
White blood cell count	<500 cells/mm³ (>2,500 cells/mL, 80% chance of infection per Mason et al)
Differential	<60% neutrophils
Crystal analysis	No urate or calcium pyrophosphate
Culture (consider blood culture bottles to improve yield)	Growth in >1 plate
Polymerase chain reaction testing	Sensitivity better than culture but poor specificity
Radiographic/nuclear tests	
Plain radiographs	New radiolucencies, cement fracture, migration, periosteal elevation Oblique views helpful to demonstrate interface
Bone scan	Will have generalized increased uptake for 24 months following surgery Look for unique areas of increased uptake
Tagged white cell scan (Indium 111)	Increased uptake at the bone-implant interface
CT	Helps to define extent of osteolysis and bone loss
MRI	Some new protocols to define degree of synovial inflammation in cases of polyethylene wear or infection

sults. **Table 1** summarizes the preoperative serologic and radiologic tests used to evaluate the painful knee before revision surgery.

Medical contraindications to surgery are rare and encompass comorbidities that significantly endanger the patient's life or limb during or after surgery. These would include significant cardiac dysfunction (regarded by many cardiologists as an ejection fraction of 20% or less, unstable angina, or critical aortic stenosis) and significant pulmonary dysfunction as evidenced by a FEV₁ (forced expiratory volume in 1 second) less than 50% of pre-

dicted value or a FEV₁/FVC (forced vital capacity) ratio of less than 0.7.

■ Alternative Treatments

Several alternative treatments should be considered for certain categories of problem arthroplasties. In general, a longitudinal evaluation (ie, evaluation at more than one office visit) benefits both the patient and the surgeon.

For patients with mild coronal or sagittal plane ligamentous instability, a trial of proprioceptive training using a knee sleeve may be helpful. A trial of physical therapy also may be beneficial.

For patients with radiographic evidence of loosening, the surgeon should rule out infection by considering the chronology of failure of the arthroplasty, as well as thoroughly analyzing the synovial fluid of that joint. If active infection is present, the patient may be best served by resection arthroplasty followed by reimplantation after the infection has been eradicated. Most radiographically loose knee components are associated with considerable pain, but if the patient is minimally symptomatic, it may be possible to observe the patient for some time, perhaps adding a knee brace for support.

■ Strategies for Successful Revision

Patient Preparation

Relative contraindications that should be corrected before revision TKA is undertaken include nutritional deficiencies, poor dentition, and skin disorders, particularly near the knee. Peripheral vascular disease, both arterial and venous, should be evaluated.

Many studies have shown a significant association between preoperative malnutrition and the development of wound infection in orthopaedic surgery. Most studies have suggested that an albumin level of less than 2.5 g/dL or an absolute lymphocyte count of less than 1,100 cells/mL is associated with a higher risk of postoperative infection. Patients who exhibit these values should have a preoperative nutritional consult and protein supplementation before surgery.

Significant dental decay is associated with higher bacterial counts, which have been implicated in the development of prosthetic infection in published studies. Thus it is reasonable to schedule a dental examination for any patient who has not undergone one during the past year.

A history of recurrent folliculitis or frequent furuncles should prompt an evaluation by a dermatologist and culturing of the skin and nares to rule out colonization with antibiotic-resistant bacteria. This may warrant a preoperative course of antibiotics.

The issue of whether all patients require a preoperative nasal culture is controversial. Some studies have shown a decrease in postoperative infections with a screening program, but other studies have suggested that this is not cost effective. Certainly, if the patient has any history of a previous methicillin-resistant *Staphylococcus aureus* infection, preoperative nasal screening should be performed; if positive, a course of nasal mupericin should be given for 3 days before surgery.

All patients undergoing TKA should be evaluated for peripheral pulses in the lower extremity, but this is particularly important before revision surgery because of the increased surgical time and greater degree of dissection. Any patient with reduced pulses in the lower extremity—particularly those with a history of atherosclerotic cardiovascular disease, vascular injury, or other signs of arterial insufficiency in the lower extremity—should have noninvasive testing to determine ankle-arm pressure ratios. If the ankle indices are 50% less than the arm indices, then referral to a vascular expert should be strongly considered.

The surgeon should consider preoperative referral to a hematologist if the patient has a history of deep vein thrombosis or pulmonary embolism. Other conditions that put the patient at higher than normal risk are active carcinoma, pregnancy, use of oral contraceptive agents, and recent major trauma. The value of screening for variations in humoral coagulation factors has been questioned in some studies and remains controversial. A standard screen includes protein S, protein C, and factor VIII levels, as well as tests for the presence of factor V Leiden and factor II mutations and lupus anticoagulant factor. High-risk patients should not be immediately sent for a vena cava filter. The efficacy of vena cava filters is unclear in joint arthroplasty surgery, and therefore the indications for use of filters are limited. A history of pulmonary embolism despite adequate anticoagulation may be one of the few indications for a vena cava filter. The newer removable filters may decrease the morbidity of the procedure, and many hematologists now recommend against the use of a permanent vena cava filter. Some investigators recommend increasing the duration of prophylaxis for these high-risk patients to 6 weeks.

The patient's hemoglobin level should be evaluated before surgery to determine if there is an existing anemia or if the patient is a candidate for autologous blood donation. A small number of patients (those expected to have significant blood loss [1 to 3 L] during surgery or who start with a hematocrit less than 30% or hemoglobin less than 10 g/dL) are candidates for preoperative erythropoietin therapy, but the anemia should be evaluated and the iron stores should be checked before treatment is begun.

Medical Checklist

Medical checklists have been shown to decrease errors and improve patient outcomes in several situations. Thus, it is helpful to develop a checklist for revision TKA that anticipates patient medical concerns, equipment needs, approaches, components to be revised, bone graft needs, anesthesia requirements, and postoperative management (**Figure 1**). The checklist should be used for every patient, usually at the time the surgery is scheduled. It is helpful to do this in conjunction with templating, and this is best done with protected time well before surgery to allow the procurement of special implants or equipment if needed.

Templating

The goals of templating are as follows:

- Determine the existing alignment and the alignment goals of revision surgery. Long-cassette (36-inch) weight-bearing AP radiographs are helpful for this.
- Radiographically assess the current joint line (too high, too low, or about right) and determine where the new joint line should be. Identifying bony landmarks helps determine the joint line.
- Determine the size of the proposed components and stems.
- Assess the location and size of bone defects to plan for bone graft, metal augments, prosthetic sleeves, and stems.

Surgical Approach

Surgical exposure must be adequate for proper component removal and subsequent replacement without placing the extensor mechanism at risk of damage. Exposure begins with an evaluation of previous incisions about the anterior knee and maintaining the integrity of the skin and soft-tissue envelope. Any notable soft-tissue defects require adequate coverage before revision TKA is performed. Soft-tissue expanders or myocutaneous flaps may

Preoperative Checklist for Revision Total Knee Arthroplasty

Patient name _____

Date and location of surgery _____

Risk factors for surgery

    Age _____

    Body mass index _____

    Albumin/total protein _____

    Hemoglobin _____

    Medical Clearance _____ Appointment Date _____

    Cardiac Clearance _____

Blood management

    Cell saver _____

    Autologous donation _____ # units ____

    Anemia workup _____

Deep vein thrombosis risk factors

    Prior deep vein thrombosis? _____

    Prior pulmonary embolism? _____

    Oral contraceptives? _____

    Ongoing malignancy? _____

    Thrombophilic factors? _____

Dental check in past year? _____

Medical evaluation

    Cardiac risk _____

    Pulmonary risk _____

    Anesthesia risk

        Contraindication for regional _____

        Contraindication for general _____

Surgical approach

    Tibial tubercle osteotomy or turndown necessary? Yes ___ No ___

    Skin condition: Plastic surgery consult? Yes ___ No ___

Equipment needs

    Extraction tools

        Polyethylene tray extractor _____

        Thin flexible osteotomes, punches _____

        Ultrasonic cement removal? _____

    Bone graft options

        Allograft particulate

            Amount _____ Ordered _____

        Allograft bulk

            Femoral head ____ Distal femur ____ Proximal tibia _____

    Sleeve size Femur _____ Tibia _____

    Stem length _____

    Components

        One component: compatible with remaining components?

        Posterior stabilized _____ Semiconstrained _____ Hinge _____

    Cement

        Plain _____ Antibiotic _____

Figure 1 Preoperative checklist for revision total knee arthroplasty.

be indicated. Because the blood supply to the anterior subcutaneous tissues is from medial to lateral, the general rule is that the most lateral skin incision should be used. Even in these cases a standard medial parapatellar approach may be used. Great care must be taken to avoid large lateral skin flaps. Undermining of the skin and subcutaneous tissue should be kept to a minimum. The medial tibial periosteum is released along with the deep medial collateral ligament. A complete synovectomy of the suprapatellar pouch and the medial and lateral gutters along with release of the lateral patellofemoral ligament allows maximal knee flexion and generally gives adequate exposure with patellar eversion. (Note that in many revision TKA cases, patellar eversion is not required.) If the extensor mechanism is still at risk at this point, then exposure may be facilitated with a proximal release of the quadriceps tendon ("quad snip"), a tibial tubercle osteotomy, or, rarely, a V-Y turndown. In all cases, exposure must be adequate to allow component removal while preserving as much bone stock as possible.

Intraoperative Cultures

The surgeon should consider aspirating synovial fluid after the skin incision but before entering the joint. If cultures are sent, obtaining fluid for analysis of cell count and differential allows the surgeon to assess whether a positive result is in fact a false positive. It is often prudent to send intraoperative frozen sections for analysis, and the surgeon should ensure that a pathologist is available to examine these sections.

Instruments/Equipment/Implants

The surgeon should work with the operating room staff to create a set of instruments to be available for all revisions (**Table 2**). Although loose components may be removed with minimal bone loss, removal of well-

fixed components may prove a challenge, especially in the setting of osteolysis (**Figure 2**). The surgeon should have a variety of osteotomes, power and hand-drive bone saws, and cement removal tools immediately available. A Gigli saw may be used to separate the femoral component from the distal femur anteriorly. The bone-prosthesis or cement-prosthesis interface must be completely disrupted before implant removal to minimize bone loss. Patience and meticulous technique are virtues. When a great deal of cement is present in the metaphyseal or diaphyseal bone, special ultrasonic removal devices may be needed. Bone grafting materials may be necessary, depending on an intraoperative assessment of bone quality after component removal. Stems are likely to be needed for most revision TKAs because the recipient bone is usually compromised in revision surgery. Sleeves or cones may be used to provide extra fixation if the metaphyseal bone is significantly compromised. These implants will need to be ordered before surgery. Revision surgery is always associated with some uncertainty, and contingency materials should be available, including tools for removal of broken hardware and for repairing intraoperative fractures and securing bone grafts (**Table 2**). The surgeon should consider what level of varus/valgus and anteroposterior constraint may be required in the revision and should make arrangements for a semiconstrained and perhaps a fully constrained prosthesis to be available.

Most of the major problems in revision surgery occur when a tool or material that is not readily available is needed. These include bone graft products, materials for intraoperative fractures, antibiotic cement, specialized extraction tools, and specialized implants that are not part of the standard revision set.

Occasionally, intraoperative imaging is needed. Similarly, red blood cell

Table 2	Equipment Needs for Revision Total Knee Arthroplasty
Approach equipment	
Osteotomy equipment (oscillating saws, drills, osteotomes)	
Implant removal tools	
Specialized osteotomes (narrow osteotomes, offset osteotomes)	
Gigli saws	
Cement removal tools	
Drills, alligator forceps, taps, ultrasonic tools	
Bone grafting tools	
Reduction clamps, Kirschner wires, small or large fragment sets	

retrieval may be necessary in longer surgeries, when tourniquets cannot be used for the entire procedure. The surgeon should always have the equipment on hand to perform a complete revision even if he or she does not anticipate the need for it.

Anesthesia and Pain Management

Indwelling epidural or peripheral nerve catheters can help manage pain after the large dissection and significant bone and soft-tissue trauma associated with revision surgery. Having anesthesia protocols specifically designed to manage the pain after revision surgery can improve patient outcomes. The protocol should include postoperative pulse oximetry, as well as nursing protocols to allow medication bolus, continuous passive motion machines, and exercise regimens.

Rehabilitation

The hospital should have an organized physical therapy program designed to manage the unique rehabilitation conditions of revision TKA surgery. Special considerations for these patients include weight-bearing status and osteotomy protection.

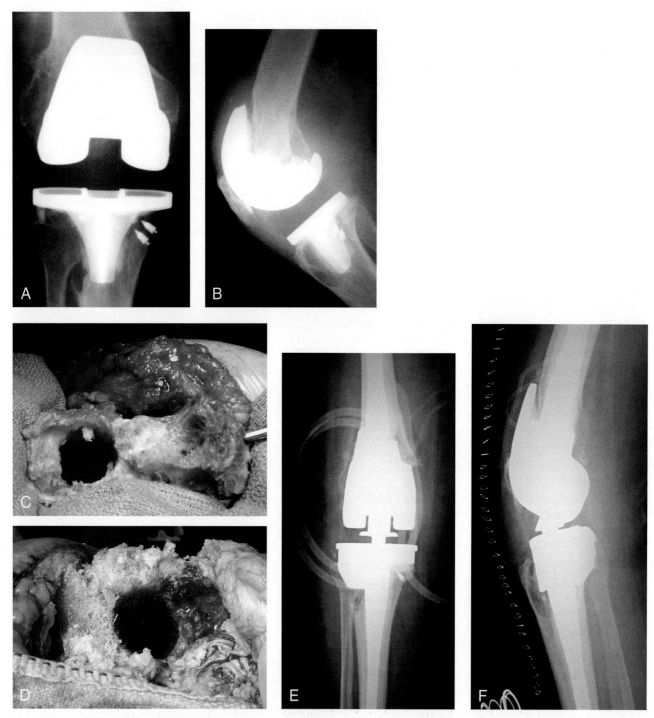

Figure 2 Images of the knee of a 73-year-old woman who presented with implant loosening secondary to severe osteolysis 7 years after a primary TKA. AP (**A**) and lateral (**B**) radiographs obtained at presentation. Intraoperative photographs of the distal femur (**C**) and proximal tibia (**D**) after prosthesis removal and débridement. Note complete loss of the lateral femoral condyle (the surgical instrument in C is pointing to the medial epicondyle) and deficient lateral tibial plateau. AP (**E**) and lateral (**F**) radiographs obtained after revision with a cemented hinged TKA.

■ Bibliography

Bozic KJ, Kurtz SM, Lau E, et al: The epidemiology of revision total knee arthroplasty in the United States. *Clin Orthop Relat Res* 2010;468:45-51.

Fehring TK, Odum S, Griffin WL, Mason JB, Nadaud M: Early failures in total knee arthroplasty. *Clin Orthop Relat Res* 2001;392:315-318.

Koskinen E, Eskelinen A, Paavolainen P, Pulkkinen P, Remes V: Comparison of survival and cost-effectiveness between unicondylar arthroplasty and total knee arthroplasty in patients with primary osteoarthritis: A follow-up study of 50,493 knee replacements from the Finnish Arthroplasty Register. *Acta Orthop* 2008;79(4):499-507.

Mason JB, Fehring TK, Odum SM, Griffin WL, Nussman DS: The value of white blood cell counts before revision total knee arthroplasty. *J Arthroplasty* 2003;18(8):1038-1043.

Mont MA, Serna FK, Krackow KA, Hungerford DS: Exploration of radiographically normal total knee replacements for unexplained pain. *Clin Orthop Relat Res* 1996;331(331):216-220.

Pun SY, Ries MD: Effect of gender and preoperative diagnosis on results of revision total knee arthroplasty. *Clin Orthop Relat Res* 2008;466(11):2701-2705.

Robertsson O: Knee arthroplasty registers. *J Bone Joint Surg Br* 2007;89(1):1-4.

Robertsson O, Dunbar MJ, Knutson K, Lewold S, Lidgren L: The Swedish Knee Arthroplasty Register: 25 years experience. *Bull Hosp Jt Dis* 1999;58(3):133-138.

Robertsson O, Knutson K, Lewold S, Lidgren L: The Swedish Knee Arthroplasty Register 1975-1997: An update with special emphasis on 41,223 knees operated on in 1988-1997. *Acta Orthop Scand* 2001;72(5):503-513.

Robertsson O, Ranstam J: No bias of ignored bilaterality when analysing the revision risk of knee prostheses: Analysis of a population based sample of 44,590 patients with 55,298 knee prostheses from the national Swedish Knee Arthroplasty Register. *BMC Musculoskelet Disord* 2003;4:1.

Chapter 39

Modes of Failure in Total Knee Arthroplasty

Kelly G. Vince, MD, FRCSC

■ Rationale for a System of "Modes of Failure"

Identifying a universal classification system for modes of failure for total knee arthroplasty (TKA) is problematic given that there are multiple paradigms for analyzing failure. Some authors have described TKA failure in terms of symptoms such as pain or giving way. Because these are symptoms and not diagnoses, however, they do not provide the basis for a useful classification system. Other authors have described TKA failure in terms of radiographic signs such as varus positioning or overstuffing, but because these signs do not strictly correspond to a unique diagnosis, they also are not useful as a basis for a classification system. Hybrid systems that include both symptoms and component positioning problems are inconsistent and confusing. In a useful system, each mode of failure should address all aspects of the problem: presenting symptoms, clinical manifestations, required investigations, underlying cause, and treatment. The scheme should include an investigative algorithm of questions, examinations, and studies that would allow the surgeon to classify a problem arthroplasty as a specific mode of failure. The diagnosis of TKA failure may involve confronting the limitations of surgery. Thus, a predetermined diagnostic framework provides structure and may occasionally force the surgeon to face unpleasant conclusions and resist the temptation to invent diagnoses.

A sound diagnosis is essential for successful revision and should define why the arthroplasty has failed; consequently, any classification system must be concise and specific enough to aid in diagnosis. If the pathophysiology (or biomechanics) for a given mode of failure is outlined, this knowledge can be constructively applied to similar patients. Implicit in this approach is the obligation to evaluate each patient systematically and comprehensively. This means there should be a series of diagnostic steps to follow. Also, the classification system must be comprehensive (ie, it must include all possibilities). This approach is consistent with good medical practice, in which the physician collects complete information and evaluates it in the context of a differential diagnosis.

The most useful approach is to work backward, by examining what defines the successful TKA. First, there must be an effective barrier between the patient's knee joint and the outside world to prevent infection in the joint. Adequate muscular power for mobility and stability is necessary, in particular from a connected quadriceps muscle. The joint must be mobile and stable. In addition, the extensor mechanism requires a centrally located patella to function as a fulcrum for the quadriceps. Furthermore, the prosthesis must be solidly attached to the bone and the skeleton and the implants must be intact. If one or more of these standards is not achieved, TKA failure may result. From these standards we arrive at the eight modes of failure, which are (1) infection, (2) extensor mechanism rupture, (3) stiffness, (4) tibiofemoral instability, (5) patellar complications and maltracking, (6) loosening, (7) periprosthetic fracture, and (8) component breakage (**Figure 1**).

Although the main purpose of this classification system is to aid surgeons in the thorough evaluation of patients and the provision of high-quality, consistent care, its benefits extend beyond the operating room. This system also will assist registries and those conducting clinical research to evaluate primary and revision TKAs, with the goal of future improvement.

Dr. Vince or an immediate family member is a member of a speakers' bureau or has made paid presentations on behalf of Zimmer and serves as a paid consultant to or is an employee of Zimmer.

DIAGNOSIS		Patient:		Implant type:			Y/N
1 Infection	Clinical	ESR ( )	Asp. WBC(<2500)	C&S			
	Drainage:						
	Erythema:	CRP ( )	Asp. Diff (<50%)	subcult.			
	Swelling:		% PMN				
2 Extensor mechanism rupture	Extensor lag:	PalpDefect	InsallSalvati	Avulsed	PatFract	QuadsRupt.	
3 Stiffness	ext-flexion	ipsi-hip OK?	CT Tibia	CT Femur	tibial slope:		
					femoral size:		
					fem flex/ext:		
					pat thick:		
4 Tibiofemoral instability	Clinical		CT Tibia	CT Femur	Loose	Y / N	
	VarusValgus arc:				Breakage	Y / N	
	AP (in flexion):				Mech axis:		
	Recurvatum:					deg. Var/Val	
5 Patellar complications & maltracking	Maltrack Y/N	Tilt degrees	Displacement	Pat. Comp	CT Femur	CT Femur	
6 Loosening	Subside?	Radioluc.?	BoneScan	Fluoro	Mech axis:		
						deg. Var/Val	
					CT- osteolysis		
7 Periprosthetic fracture	XR tib:		XR fem:				
8 Component breakage	Instab: Y/N		X-Ray: Y/N				
9 No diagnosis	AP pelvis	LS-Spine	BoneScan	RSD	Pre TKA XR		

Figure 1 Prerevision worksheet for the problem total knee arthroplasty. On the left are eight diagnostic categories or modes of failure. The columns to the right list the tests and data needed to confirm a diagnosis and plan surgery.

History and Physical Examination

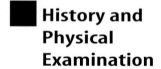

Although the medical history for a problem arthroplasty typically casts a wide net in terms of symptoms, co-morbidities, and causes, the surgeon's questions should be focused and intentional. Approaches differ among clinicians, but in general, an open-ended question is a reliable start; for example, "What is giving you trouble?" or "What is it that we can help you with?" In some situations, this may reveal underlying psychologic or social problems that can exacerbate pain. Each step of the process involves balancing detail with a broad perspective to stay on track. Although the patient's feedback and concerns guide

the analysis to some extent, this alone should not be used to determine diagnosis.

Mode 1: Infection

With most problem arthroplasties, the presenting concern is pain. Because infection may accompany any other diagnosis and because the treatment of infection is distinct, one must first consider sepsis. This is true for the stiff knee as well as the dislocated patella. The obvious radiographic abnormality can be dangerously distracting in a demanding clinical practice. To superbly reconstruct an unstable or loose TKA without recognizing that it was also infected would be tragic.

Diagnostic Steps

After the general questions have been asked, the next line of questioning is specific to the knee, in particular, regarding pain: its temporal course, quality, and location, plus any ameliorative or aggravating effects. Although the symptoms may be experienced at the knee, the problem actually may originate outside the knee joint (eg, an ipsilateral arthritic hip) (**Figure 2**). Listen closely to the patient both for the purposes of diagnosis and to make sure that the patient feels that he or she is being heard.

Infection is unlikely if the patient is not experiencing pain. Nevertheless, it is useful to inquire about how the incision healed, if drainage persisted, or if antibiotics were prescribed for a wound problem. Positive indicators of an aseptic etiology include a low clin-

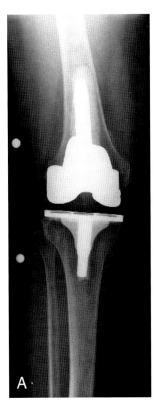
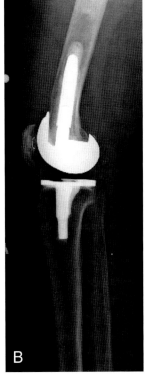
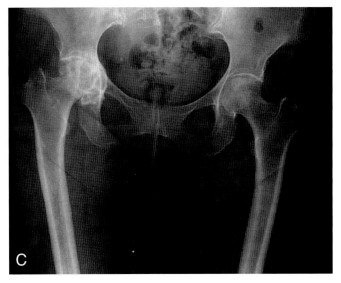

Figure 2 AP (**A**) and lateral (**B**) radiographs taken after an unsuccessful revision of the femoral component only. The patient reported relentless knee pain with an inability to straighten the knee before and after primary surgery, as well as after the single component revision. Had the surgeon "directed" the history more expertly, the hip problem would have been diagnosed. Hip osteoarthritis and a painful stiff hip ipsilateral to the painful TKA are apparent on the radiograph of the pelvis (**C**). Hip arthroplasty resolved the knee symptoms.

ical suspicion of infection, normal peripheral blood tests for erythrocyte sedimentation rate (ESR) and C-reactive protein (CRP) level, and a plausible mechanical explanation for the mode of failure.

When clinical suspicion of infection is high or if the inflammatory markers are elevated, aspiration of synovial fluid for cell count, differential, and culture and sensitivity are mandatory. A synovial fluid cell count above the relatively low threshold of approximately 2,500 white blood cells per mL is highly suspicious for infection in a TKA. Infection is even more likely if the differential indicates more than 50% polymorphonucleocytes. When infection is suspected for any reason, a positive culture (bacteriologic diagnosis) is highly desirable before surgery. It is wise to repeat the aspiration as many as four times, with the patient

off antimicrobial therapy, to establish a bacteriologic diagnosis.

Principles of Treatment
The fundamental concepts guiding treatment of established deep sepsis after TKA are the chronology of the infection, the local and systemic health of the host, and the ability of bacterial colonies to organize themselves into a biofilm on the surface of foreign material. Factors that indicate a positive prognosis for eradicating sepsis and restoring the integrity of the soft-tissue envelope include very recent onset, healthy tissue, a competent host, and an organism that is less likely to form a biofilm. If all of these factors are present, surgical débridement with removal and exchange of modular components may be successful. Although arthroscopic intervention may be useful in septic arthritis

without a prosthesis, this cannot easily be justified in the treatment of an infected arthroplasty.

Biofilms are best treated by removing all foreign material: implants, methylmethacrylate, and allograft. A two-stage reimplantation generally is recommended, including thorough débridement and 6 weeks of antibiotic therapy. Less experience has been reported worldwide with the single-stage exchange of components in the treatment of established sepsis.

——————■

Mode 2: Extensor Mechanism Rupture

The extensor mechanism may rupture at any point between the tibial tuber-

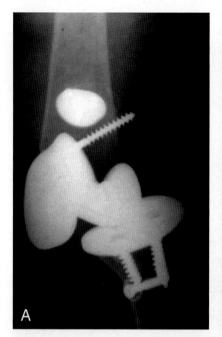 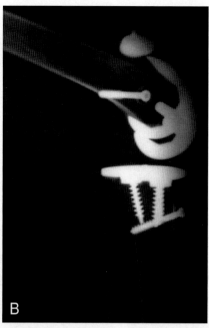

Figure 3 Radiographs of a globally unstable TKA. **A,** AP radiograph shows screws in the tibia and femur indicating a previously unsuccessful attempt to eliminate instability with ligament reconstruction but without revision. Patella alta is apparent. **B,** Lateral radiograph confirms patellar tendon rupture and AP instability of the flexion gap. The extensor mechanism was the last structure holding the arthroplasty together. Once ruptured, the entire TKA became unstable. Investigations demonstrated no infection. Complete revision TKA with rebalanced gaps, constrained implants, and extensor mechanism allograft or arthrodesis is required.

cle and the quadriceps muscle. Along with sepsis, this often is regarded as one of the worst complications in TKA. The extensor rupture either may result from sepsis or induce it, if the rupture leads to wound dehiscence. Infected knees with a ruptured extensor mechanism have classically been treated with arthrodesis, although an extensor allograft as part of a two-stage reimplantation protocol is feasible.

Instability of the knee also may accompany extensor rupture. Without a functioning extensor mechanism, the patient may resort to hyperextension for stability, similar to the polio patient with paralysis at L3-4. This often results in recurvatum and gross instability of the knee. In other cases, the extensor mechanism may have been the last structure holding the arthroplasty together, and global instability ensues when it ruptures (**Figure 3**). Like many other patellar complica-

tions, maltracking and, by implication, internal rotation positioning of the tibial and/or femoral components may be present. Extensor mechanism rupture alone does not necessitate component revision. However, repairing extensor mechanism rupture without correcting any underlying problems will likely fail.

Diagnostic Steps
Extensor mechanism rupture can be suspected even from a telephone conversation with the patient. It is easily confirmed with physical examination if there is mild to complete extensor lag and a radiograph that shows avulsion of the tubercle, new patella alta, displaced transverse fracture of the patella (**Figure 4**), or new patella baja. Defects may be palpable at the site of rupture.

Displaced transverse patellar fractures with a significant lag, especially in a resurfaced patella, are a particular

clinical challenge. In most cases, open reduction and internal fixation should be attempted only once, and then only using cerclage and not tension-band wiring. These cases are better classified as chronic extensor mechanism ruptures rather than patellar fractures.

Principles of Treatment
The extensor mechanism—from the insertion of the Sharpey fibers connecting the patellar ligament to the tubercle, through the tensile collagen fibers of the patellar tendon attached to and through the patella and in turn to the quadriceps tendon, transitioning to quadriceps muscle—is difficult to restore once disrupted. Simple repair is frequently unsuccessful. Therefore, procedures that substitute tissue, most commonly an extensor mechanism allograft, have been developed. Revision arthroplasty is required if concurrent instability is present.

━━━━━━■

■ Mode 3: Stiffness

A stiff TKA often is mistakenly equated with arthrofibrosis, implying that soft-tissue healing (and not surgical technique) is responsible for poor motion. Some knees do scar aggressively and stiffen, although it is difficult to know what percentage of patients are in this category. If the biology of healing alone is responsible for stiffness, revision TKA is not likely to help.

Stiffness is perhaps the most conceptually and technically challenging mode of failure. The cause may be a problem intrinsic to the arthroplasty (eg, component size and position), part of the joint but extrinsic to the arthroplasty (eg, extensor mechanism), or even distant from the joint (eg, ipsilateral arthritic hip joint). Furthermore, conditions outside the musculoskeletal system may be responsible (complex regional pain syndrome

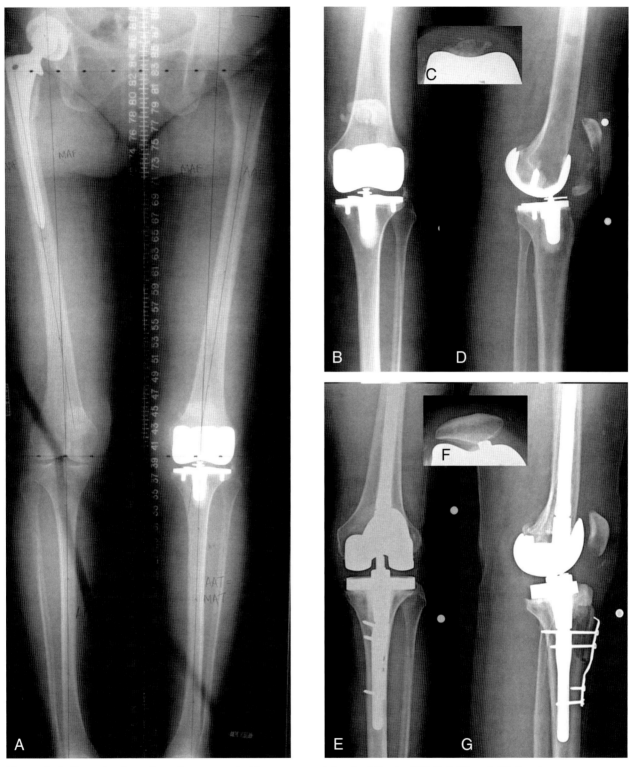

Figure 4 Radiographs of a patient who presented with recurvatum deformity following TKA. **A,** Full-length AP view demonstrates a neutral mechanical axis. **B,** AP view shows the high position of the proximal patellar fragment. **C,** Patellofemoral view shows that the patella is tracking centrally. This indicates satisfactory rotational position of the tibial and femoral implants. **D,** Lateral view demonstrates that the patellar fragments are separated significantly despite several unsuccessful attempts at fixation. Loss of the extensor mechanism resulted in recurvatum deformity, similar to the deformity observed in poliomyelitis patients with weak quadriceps. Revision TKA with extensor mechanism allograft reconstruction was performed to correct the recurvatum deformity and restore extensor power. **E,** Postoperative AP view shows complete revision TKA with a neutral mechanical axis and nonlinked constrained implants. **F,** Patellofemoral view shows a centrally tracking allograft patella. **G,** Lateral view shows the one-third tubular plate used to augment fixation of the allograft tibial tubercle after the initial fixation failed.

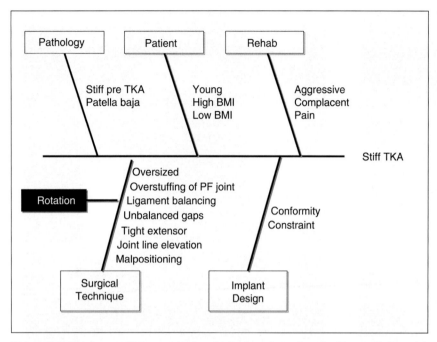

Figure 5 A fish diagram illustrates the factors that have been described in association with the stiff TKA. A recent investigation has added rotation, primarily internal rotation of the tibial component, as a frequent finding in the stiff TKA. BMI = body mass index, PF = patellofemoral.

or spasticity). In most patients, multiple factors contribute to the compromised motion.

If revision for stiffness is contemplated, the knee should be evaluated for the usual triad of symptoms: poor flexion, flexion contracture, and pain. The single most consistent predictor of flexion after TKA is flexion before surgery. The quadriceps muscle, which must elongate to permit motion, may not be able to do so if the knee has not flexed well for an extended period of time. Accordingly, it may not be possible to increase knee arthroplasty flexion if motion in the arthritic knee was poor. Thus, it is important for the patient to have realistic expectations and understand that even if surgery restores normal flexion to the knee joint, the compromised quadriceps muscle will restrict range of motion.

In contrast to limited flexion, a flexion contracture is more easily amenable to surgical correction. With a combination of posterior releases and resection of distal femoral bone, the surgeon can expect to correct flexion contractures of up to 30° during surgery. Larger contractures are more challenging. The difficulty, however, is maintaining the correction in the presence of an extension lag, contractures of the ipsilateral hip, or kyphotic deformity of the spine because any shift of the patient's center of gravity anteriorly is balanced by simultaneous flexed hip and knee posture. Contractures often recur in such situations.

Most patients who report a tight feeling in the knee and lose motion after TKA also experience pain. In evaluating the stiff knee, the surgeon should be wary of using the classical Occam's razor approach to diagnosis, which seeks to identify a single cause. The surgeon who follows this method approaches the stiff knee like a car that won't start and expects success if a single underlying problem can be rectified. A better analogy for the stiff knee, however, would be a one-of-a-kind car

that has never been tested and was exposed to a rust-inducing climate, much like the individual patient's knee that has undergone TKA and is subject to scarring. This car (or knee) may have multiple original problems that need correction. In addition, there may be problems secondary to the "climate." Some factors are causative and others resultant. Scar, for example, may cause an arthroplasty to be stiff, or it may result if the knee has not moved (**Figure 5**).

Diagnostic Steps

A considerable amount of information is necessary if surgeons are to perform the best and most appropriate revision for stiffness as well as predict the results of surgery. If the examination reveals skin hypersensitivity, for example, this would suggest a complex regional pain syndrome. A key response from patients when components are internally rotated is that the knee has "never felt right." Although internal rotation is associated with patellar maltracking, the tight arthroplasty with internal rotation may not flex far enough for the patella to dislocate. Pain, which often is present with tightness, may exacerbate stiffness. Pain and motion may improve if tightness is alleviated and scar tissue is released. However, the longer the knee has been stiff and the more surgeries it has undergone within that period, the less likely it is that the quadriceps will regain elasticity, no matter what else may have been improved by revision.

Physical examination should focus on the hip, the spine, and gait. Knee and hip motion must be quantified, and the surgeon should pay attention to which joints are contracted and if there is spinal kyphosis. Clues for internal rotation positioning of the tibial and femoral components may be apparent; for example, the foot may be externally rotated when the patient sits on the edge of the examination table with the knee flexed, and there may be greater apparent internal rotation of an otherwise normal hip joint on the stiff side. CT, which is useful in planning any revision, should be used to confirm the diagnosis (**Figure 6**).

Lateral radiographs of the stiff knee show the femoral component size relative to the patient's bone; an increase in anterior-posterior diameter creates a tighter flexion gap. A similar effect can result from posterior translation or a flexed position of the component. The size of the tibial base plate (unlike the thickness of the articular polyethylene) is unlikely to restrict motion, although anterior slope, with the posterior component higher, will tighten the joint as it bends. Although a thicker tibial polyethylene is likely to make the knee globally tight, it is not uncommon to see the thinnest tibial inserts in a stiff TKA, suggesting that the initial surgeon struggled with tightness after a conservative proximal tibial resection.

Patellar tracking, which is best assessed on a patellofemoral radiograph, may be difficult to assess in the very stiff knee. Any tendency to lateral tracking suggests internal rotational positioning of tibial and/or femoral components. Consider the patella that would dislocate with flexion: the patient, sensing this, will stop bending before dislocation occurs, and the knee stiffens.

CT is critical in understanding the painful stiff TKA. Internal rotation positioning, especially of the tibial component, is a frequent finding in the stiff knee (**Figure 7**). By considering a comprehensive list of problems and identifying causes first, it is more likely that the revision surgery will be successful.

Principles of Treatment

Surgical exposure is difficult, dangerous, and integral to the treatment of a stiff TKA. Although many surgeons favor a tibial tubercle osteotomy when faced with thick scar, this will not liberate the immobile extensor mechanism. To restore motion, careful atten-

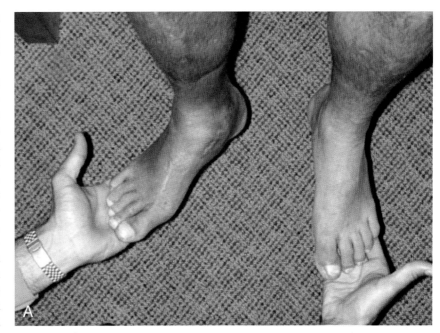

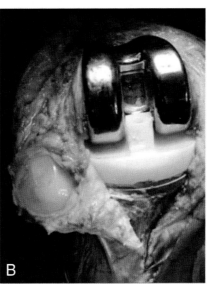

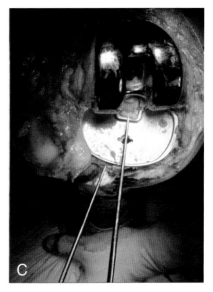

Figure 6 Images of a patient with a failed TKA. **A,** The patient is seated on the examination table with legs extended over the side. Note the internal rotation of the right leg (seen on the left in the figure) caused by an internally rotated tibial component from a failed revision surgery, contributing to patellar maltracking and instability. **B** and **C,** Intraoperative photographs from a second revision surgery. **B,** The tibial tubercle can be seen to the left of the photograph, with the center of the tibial component to the right. **C,** With the polyethylene insert removed, surgical instruments indicate the tubercle on the left and the center of the component on the right. If the patella is to be located between the femoral condyles, the tibial component must line up with the patellar tendon.

tion to detail is necessary, with synovectomy, restoration of the medial and lateral parafemoral gutters, resection of scar on the deep surface of the patellar tendon, separation of the quadriceps from the anterior femur, and a lateral patellar retinacular release.

Alteration of all factors in the stiff TKA away from tightness and in favor

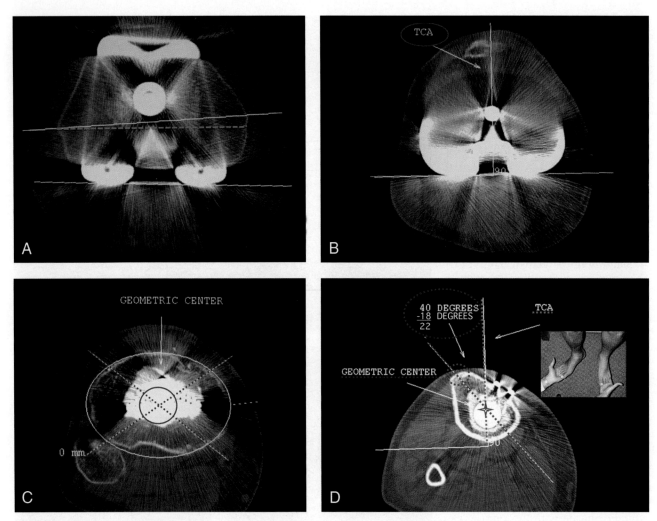

Figure 7 CT scans of the patient shown in Figure 6. A CT protocol provides a practical and validated method for quantifying rotational position of the femoral and tibial components. **A,** One cut through the distal femur at the level of the transepicondylar axis shows the rotation of the femoral component. The white line has been drawn accurately from the lateral epicondyle but inappropriately through the anterior ridge of the medial epicondyle (attachment point of the superficial medial collateral ligament). The dashed red is drawn through the sulcus, or center of the medial epicondyle. Three cuts are required to quantify the rotational position of the tibial component. The first (**B**), at the level of the tibial component, establishes the tibial component angle (TCA). A cut through the tibia immediately below the component (**C**) establishes the geometric center of the proximal tibia. A third, slightly more distal cut through the tibial tubercle (**D**) includes the data from the previous two cuts (TCA and geometric center). A line is drawn from the center of the tibial tubercle through the geometric center of the tibia. The angle subtended by this line and the TCA is the rotational position of the tibial component. Given the asymmetry of the proximal tibia, up to 18° is considered within normal. In this patient, the angle measures 40°, equal to 22° of pathologic internal rotation.

of motion yields the best chance of success. Accordingly, all of the following can be expected to increase flexion and/or extension: correction of internal rotation with improved patellar tracking; reduced thickness of the resurfaced patella; optimal posterior tibial slope; a thinner tibial insert; a smaller femoral component in a non-flexed, non–posterior-translated position; and more tibial and perhaps more distal femoral resection. A simple release of scar or an exchange to a thinner polyethylene has not, in general, proved successful.

Mode 4: Tibiofemoral Instability

Tibiofemoral instability includes instability originating from ligamentous compromise and joint alignment but not secondary to patellar dislocation (mode 5), component loosening (mode 6), periprosthetic fracture (mode 7), or implant breakage (mode 8). The solution to instability is not always a constrained implant and is rarely only a constrained implant (**Figure 8**). Patients may report "instability" if the knee gives out from side to side (varus-valgus) or in the plane of motion of the joint (buckling), or if the flexed knee "comes out of place" while the patient is seated, generally with the tibia subluxating posteriorly under the femoral condyles (relatively larger flexion gap) (**Figure 9**).

Stability in the varus-valgus (frontal) plane requires intact collateral ligaments and a limb alignment that distributes the load over the medial and lateral joint condyles and collateral ligaments. It is useful to compare the extended knee to a four-legged table where the extensor mechanism, posterior capsule, and both collateral structures are necessary for stability. Valgus instability is usually accompanied by a mechanical axis passing through the lateral compartment and plastic deformation of the medial collateral ligament (**Figure 10**). The converse—medial mechanical axis and loss of the lateral stabilizers—occurs with varus instability. Other failures, including loosening, periprosthetic fracture, or prosthetic breakage, may cause instability, but these require a different surgical strategy to restore the articulation.

Spontaneous flexion of the joint, or buckling, results from problems in the extensor mechanism and is best classified as either rupture of the extensor mechanism (mode 2) or maltracking and patellar complications (mode 5). Recurvatum, or hyperextension instability of the knee joint, may occur with or without failure of the extensor mechanism. When instability is the result of neurologic deficits, it may be particularly difficult to achieve stability.

The third category, instability in flexion, may present with a frank pos-

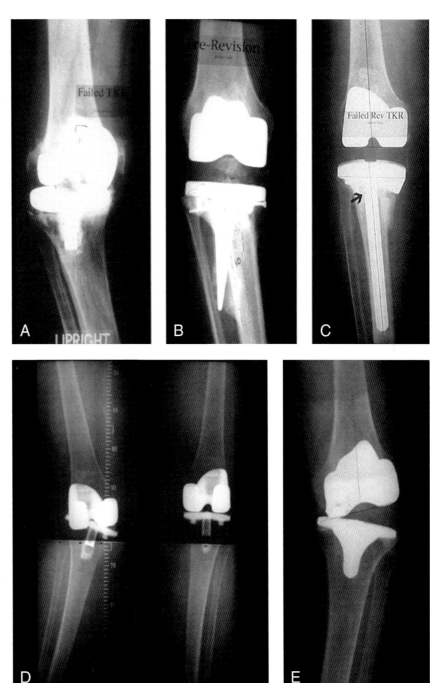

Figure 8 AP radiographs of knees with instability following TKA. **A,** Varus instability resulting from a loose tibial component with subsidence. **B,** Varus instability from medial bone loss. The collateral ligaments are intact. **C,** Instability from component breakage. A custom-fabricated tibial component was used in a single-component revision. Unsupported by bone, it failed at the threaded junction between the baseplate and the stem extension (arrow). **D,** Bilateral AP radiographs at 10-year follow-up of a patient with a cruciate-retaining TKA. The right knee sustained late instability from tibial polyethylene wear and breakage secondary to internal rotation positioning. **E,** True varus instability from failure of the lateral soft-tissue envelope. This is the only case that required a constrained implant. **A** through **D** were revised successfully with reconstitution of ligament tension by bone restoration, solid fixation, balanced gaps, and new components.

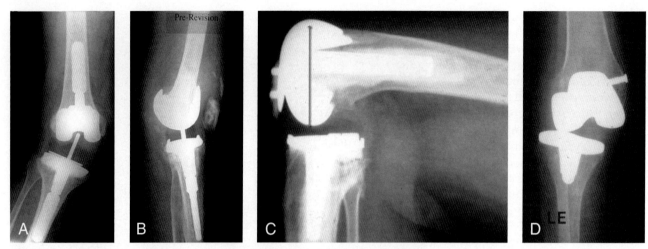

Figure 9 Radiographs of the knees of patients with instability following TKA. **A,** AP view demonstrates coronal plane instability, in this case valgus failure, despite the use of a nonlinked, constrained prosthesis. This highlights the importance of reducing destructive forces by controlling alignment and restoring some soft-tissue integrity. **B,** Lateral view demonstrates instability in the plane of motion, specifically recurvatum deformity as the result of recurrent hyperextension to compensate for a weak quadriceps muscle. **C,** Lateral view with knee flexed to 90° demonstrates early flexion instability following revision TKA that was the result of using a (nonmodular) revision femoral component that fit the residual bone on the distal femur but was too small to restore tension in the collateral ligaments. **D,** AP view demonstrates global instability in a knee with a mobile-bearing TKA that underwent an unsuccessful attempt to stabilize the medial collateral ligament without revision arthroplasty by using a staple.

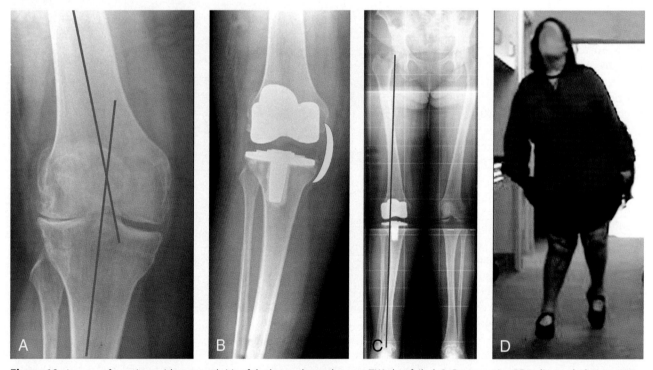

Figure 10 Images of a patient with osteoarthritis of the knee who underwent TKA that failed. **A,** Preoperative AP radiograph demonstrates osteoarthritis with valgus deformity and an apparently intact medial collateral ligament. **B,** AP radiograph obtained after primary TKA. Prototypical valgus instability resulted from imbalance of the medial and lateral collateral ligaments despite apparently reasonable alignment. The medial collateral ligament (yellow crescent) is elongated. **C,** Full-length AP radiograph depicts the mechanical axis (red line) of the limb. Note that it crosses the lateral compartment. The tibial component is aligned in valgus. **D,** Clinical photograph demonstrates the dynamic exacerbation of instability. Note that the patient has shifted her center of gravity over the affected side as a result of weak hip abductors, which contributed to valgus knee instability.

terior dislocation of the tibia under the femur or, more subtly and commonly, with a sense of unease on stairs. Regardless of the severity of the problem, this results from a flexion gap that is relatively larger than the extension gap. Sometimes this results from an arthritic knee with a fixed flexion contracture. If the surgeon has followed a measured resection technique, removing thicknesses of bone equal to the thickness of the metal implant without additional techniques to correct the flexion contracture, a relatively larger flexion gap results. If a modular tibial polyethylene insert is selected to permit full extension, the knee will be unstable in flexion. Conversely, if the insert selected stabilizes the flexed knee, a flexion contracture ensues.

Tibiofemoral instability is a concern in patients with large deformities or instability before surgery, large flexion contractures, and obesity. The obese patient may be at risk because of inherent connective tissue problems or difficulty with surgical exposure. Patients with extra-articular pathology that displaces the center of gravity, alters gait, and dangerously loads the knee also are at increased risk. Accordingly, scoliosis, hip pathology with abductor dysfunction and tibialis posterior ruptures and acquired flatfoot are common among patients with tibiofemoral instability.

Diagnostic Steps
When tibiofemoral instability is accurately diagnosed, revision TKA has the best results of any of the modes of failure. Understanding the patient's experience in such cases is critical, in particular whether the knee is unstable from side to side or if it is buckling. If the knee is buckling, the surgeon should determine whether the extensor mechanism is attached, of normal strength (indicating neurologic compromise), or dislocating.

Physical examination is important. Recurvatum is observable as the pa-

tient walks. Varus-valgus instability should be tested for with the knee in extension and in about 20° to 30° of flexion. This is done not to test for so-called midflexion instability but to eliminate the confounding effect of tight posterior structures that can impart a sense of varus-valgus stability to a joint that lacks collateral integrity. The patient with flexion instability should be asked to sit on the edge of the examination table (with knees flexed to 90°) and slowly extend the knee. Careful observation often will reveal that the flexion gap closes after the quadriceps is activated but before extension occurs. This phenomenon also can be observed by distracting and compressing (like a piston) the flexion gap, with one of the examiner's hands on the tibia and the other on the anterior thigh.

Radiographs should include full-length AP studies obtained prior to any revision, but in particular before revision of the unstable joint. Alignment, which is the most reliable way the surgeon can control varus-valgus forces, is best appreciated on this view. Good-quality, single-leg weight-bearing conventional radiographs show the true magnitude of the instability and other pathology. A loose or broken implant, bone loss, or periprosthetic fracture may mimic ligamentous instability. As with other modes of failure, CT can quantify internal rotation of either the tibia or the femur.

Principles of Treatment
Understanding the type of instability (varus-valgus, recurvatum, flexion, or global) and separating true ligamentous instability from other pathologies are crucial. Instability, especially in the varus-valgus plane, should be conceptualized in terms of the mechanical forces that favor stability (eg, ligamentous integrity or mechanical constraint) versus those that induce instability (eg, eccentric alignment, dynamic gait abnormalities). Simple

restoration or augmentation of stabilizing forces, as with a constrained implant, will eventually fail if "deforming" forces (such as malalignment) persist.

In some cases, the deforming force cannot be diminished, such as with scoliosis or hip abductor dysfunction. It may be helpful to compensate by altering alignment beyond the usual neutral mechanical axis and also maximizing stability. For example, in a patient with valgus instability, a solid plan might include a relative varus mechanical alignment (the line from the center of the hip to the center of the ankle crosses the medial compartment of the knee). Flexion instability usually responds to a larger femoral component or resection of additional distal femur to decrease the imbalance between flexion and extension.

Constrained implants, either non-linked (constrained condylar style) or linked (hinges), are unquestionably useful. These cases, however, require detailed understanding of the type of instability, elimination of the deforming forces, and judicious use of mechanical constraint.

—■

Mode 5: Patellar Complications and Maltracking

Patellar subluxation and dislocation are direct manifestations of maltracking. Other patellar problems, however, such as vertical fractures, component loosening, and destructive wear, also may originate with eccentric tracking. All of these complications share a common origin in positioning of the tibial and/or the femoral components in internal rotation.

Diagnostic Steps
If the joint is mobile, stable in flexion, and stable to varus-valgus forces but collapses in the plane of motion of the

joint, extensor problems are likely. If this occurs during gait, the quadriceps is either not working or not connected. If it occurs with flexion, commonly on stairs or rising from a chair, the extensor probably is maltracking. The patella may even snap over to the lateral side and dislocate with flexion. Alternatively, the patient may be apprehensive and walk with a stiff leg. Some patients will have a chronic, immobile, frank dislocation of the patella with a resultant lump on the lateral knee. CT is particularly helpful for identifying extensor tracking problems. Full revision surgery is the preferred treatment.

Principles of Treatment

Any feature of the arthroplasty that increases the Q angle (valgus alignment and internal component rotation) should be corrected. Prerevision CT is the best guide for repositioning the femoral component at the time of revision, when internal rotation is corrected with a posterolateral augment. Because it lines up under the femur, the position of the tibial component is the best way to bring the tibial tubercle and the attached patella in line with the central femur. Given the larger medial than lateral tibial condyle, alignment on the medial third of the tubercle is the best approximation of the "center" of the proximal tibia and, accordingly, the center of the distal femur.

The chronically dislocated patella is positioned such that the extensor is shortened and contracted. Once the patella is reduced in front of the knee, the contracted quadriceps may not permit much flexion. Even if tibial and femoral component rotation has been corrected, the patella may snap into the shortened, dislocated position with flexion. At times, this will forcefully spin the tibia externally. In such recalcitrant cases, rotational constraint using nonlinked or constrained condylar implants may be required.

Mode 6: Loosening

Loosening, often the first diagnosis considered, is left toward the end of this scheme to ensure a comprehensive evaluation. The relationship between infection and loosening is clear, and was described previously, under failure mode 1. Loosening is most commonly observed 5 or more years after surgery in association with polyethylene wear, particle production, osteolysis, and bone loss. Varus alignment probably is still significant because it increases the load on the medial compartment and accelerates wear. Once bone has been lost to osteolysis, subsidence occurs.

Early loosening is now unusual. It may take the subtle form of failed bone ingrowth in an uncemented prosthesis or collapse of supporting bone under a cemented implant, where either varus alignment has created medial overload or osteoporosis has compromised bone strength. The practice of applying cement only to the cut surface and implanting the keel with a press-fit technique appears to be associated with a slight increase of early loosening. Immunologic pathways that result in loosening are being investigated.

Diagnostic Steps

Most patients with a loose component experience pain with weight bearing even before subsidence makes this diagnosis apparent. Pain often is severe enough that the patient waits a few seconds before taking steps. The pain may diminish slightly after several steps, probably as the prosthesis "settles in," but it recurs with longer excursions. Chronic swelling is typical. Rest pain suggests infection.

Radiographic criteria that confirm loosening are changes in component position and/or circumferential radiolucency. Isotope scanning, equivocal if positive, argues against loosening if negative. CT scans, which are useful for assessing rotation, also can accu-

rately quantify bone loss from osteolysis. Full-length radiographs help plan correction of the usual varus mechanical axis.

Principles of Treatment

Loosening affects the tibial component most frequently, sometimes as the result of varus femoral positioning. It is a mistake to simply re-cement a loose component without correcting alignment. Advanced osteolysis affects all components, commonly with bone loss in the posterior femoral condyles. Because loosening is a common failure mode for revision TKA, fixation at revision should be enhanced over primary technique. Cement is still favored, even in combination with diaphyseal-engaging press-fit intramedullary stems. Porous metal cones are used less to augment missing bone than to provide a reliable transition of interfaces from sclerotic revision bone to porous metal, from porous metal to cement, and from cement to implant.

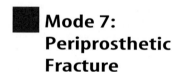

Mode 7: Periprosthetic Fracture

Periprosthetic fractures seem to be increasing, probably as a result of the increased number of arthroplasties in older patients with osteoporosis. Osteolysis exacerbates the problem. Most notches in the supracondylar region are modest and do not result in fracture; however, they may increase risk. Restricted motion also is a problem, so that when a patient falls, the knee quickly reaches maximum flexion and the distal femur yields.

Diagnostic Steps

The diagnosis of supracondylar fracture, if not evident from history and physical examination, will be apparent on radiographs. The usual history of falls should be pursued, but in general these patients are older and sedentary, with poor bone quality. An ipsilateral hip replacement may be problematic, especially above a stemmed, constrained knee replacement, where the forces in play result in a persistent nonunion and the occasional need for a total femur prosthesis.

Principles of Treatment

The supracondylar femur fracture is common and generally is treated with open reduction and internal fixation as opposed to revision. Locking plates or supracondylar nails are favored. Occasionally, extensive bone loss or poor bone quality necessitates revision arthroplasty with a tumor-style prosthesis in the elderly patient. Less commonly, a distal femoral allograft may be used.

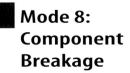

Mode 8: Component Breakage

Breakage of modern components is unusual. The most common occurrence is failure of constrained mechanisms, which often is associated with deviations from a neutral mechanical axis, gait aberration, or internal rotation of components. Rarely, the tibial spine of a posterior stabilized implant may break because of hyperextension or relative hyperextension resulting from a flexed femoral component position and increased posterior tibial slope. Hyperextension may result from loosening and subsidence. Revi-

sion, not just polyethylene exchange, is usually necessary.

Apparent late instability of TKA generally is the result of profound wear, in particular if a tibia was implanted in an internally rotated position. The femoral condyle gradually wears the posterior, lateral polyethylene and eventually slides off the back of the tibia. Broken metal tibial baseplates are usually the aftermath of bone loss from osteolysis, leaving the prosthesis only partially supported.

Diagnostic Steps

Late instability should alert the clinician to the possibility of breakage rather than ligament rupture. Polyethylene breakage may be difficult to recognize radiographically, but it will be apparent on most CT scans.

Principles of Treatment

Complete revision generally is required with correction of the underlying cause of breakage. Polyethylene wear in an otherwise satisfactory arthroplasty after many years is an indication for modular exchange.

No Diagnosis

"No diagnosis," or unexplained pain, can be considered a ninth situation. Surgery performed for pain without a diagnosis is unlikely to yield a satisfactory result. Rather, this is an indication to revisit the diagnostic scheme and ensure that the evaluation has indeed been comprehensive and systematic. Physical examination with repeat attention to the hip, spine, and neurologic etiology is appropriate. A nega-

tive bone scan may be reassuring. Other causes of pain that do not require revision arthroplasty, and thus are not considered true failure, include periarticular neuromas, neuritis, and complex regional pain syndromes.

Summary

The patient with a failed arthroplasty deserves a minimum evaluation consisting of peripheral blood testing for ESR and CRP level. If either is elevated, the arthroplasty should be aspirated and synovial fluid sent for cell count, differential, and culture. The standard radiographic evaluation includes single-leg weight-bearing AP views; single-leg weight-bearing lateral views; patellofemoral views; and full-length views (hip, knee, and ankle on the same image). CT is particularly helpful in preparing for revision TKA.

Ultimately, if the ESR and CRP level are normal, then infection is unlikely. If the affected knee extends fully and flexes beyond 90°, no instability is seen on gait evaluation or in flexion, the patella tracks centrally on the radiographs, and the CT scan is normal, the patient should understand that whatever the problem, it most likely would not improve with additional surgery. Finally, if radiographs obtained before the primary arthroplasty demonstrated minimal arthritic change, the original arthroplasty may have been premature and/or the patient's expectations may have been unrealistic. In such cases, the patient is likely to be similarly dissatisfied after revision surgery.

■ Bibliography

Barrack RL, Schrader T, Bertot AJ, Wolfe MW, Myers L: Component rotation and anterior knee pain after total knee arthroplasty. *Clin Orthop Relat Res* 2001;392:46-55.

Bedard M, Vince K: Stiffness complicating total knee arthroplasty: Computerized tomography (CT) evaluation of rotational positioning of the components—pre and post revision. *Clin Orthop Relat Res,* in press.

Berger RA, Crossett LS, Jacobs JJ, Rubash HE: Malrotation causing patellofemoral complications after total knee arthroplasty. *Clin Orthop Relat Res* 1998;356:144-153.

Costerton JW, Stewart PS: Battling biofilms. *Sci Am* 2001;285(1):74-81.

Daluga D, Lombardi AV Jr, Mallory TH, Vaughn BK: Knee manipulation following total knee arthroplasty. Analysis of prognostic variables. *J Arthroplasty* 1991;6(2):119-128.

Leone JM, Hanssen AD: Management of infection at the site of a total knee arthroplasty. *J Bone Joint Surg Am* 2005;87 (10):2335-2348.

Malo M, Vince KG: The unstable patella after total knee arthroplasty: Etiology, prevention, and management. *J Am Acad Orthop Surg* 2003;11(5):364-371.

Mason JB, Fehring TK, Odum SM, Griffin WL, Nussman DS: The value of white blood cell counts before revision total knee arthroplasty. *J Arthroplasty* 2003;18(8):1038-1043.

Moreland JR: Mechanisms of failure in total knee arthroplasty. *Clin Orthop Relat Res* 1988;226:49-64.

Munjal S, Phillips MJ, Krackow KA: Revision total knee arthroplasty: Planning, controversies, and management—Infection. *Instr Course Lect* 2001;50:367-377.

Ortiguera CJ, Berry DJ: Patellar fracture after total knee arthroplasty. *J Bone Joint Surg Am* 2002;84-A(4):532-540.

Pagnano MW, Hanssen AD, Lewallen DG, Stuart MJ: Flexion instability after primary posterior cruciate retaining total knee arthroplasty. *Clin Orthop Relat Res* 1998;356:39-46.

Park KK, Kim TK, Chang CB, Yoon SW, Park KU: Normative temporal values of CRP and ESR in unilateral and staged bilateral TKA. *Clin Orthop Relat Res* 2008;466(1):179-188.

Parratte S, Pagnano MW: Instability after total knee arthroplasty. *J Bone Joint Surg Am* 2008;90(1):184-194.

Sharkey PF, Homesley HD, Shastri S, Jacoby SM, Hozack WJ, Rothman RH: Results of revision total knee arthroplasty after exposure of the knee with extensor mechanism tenolysis. *J Arthroplasty* 2004;19(6):751-756.

Tharani R, Nakasone C, Vince KG: Periprosthetic fractures after total knee arthroplasty. *J Arthroplasty* 2005;20(4, Suppl 2):27-32.

Vince KG: Revision total knee arthroplasty and arthrodesis of the knee, in Chapman M, ed: *Operative Orthopedics.* Philadelphia, PA, Lippincott, Williams & Wilkins, 2001, pp 2897-2952.

Vince KG, Bedard M: Implanting the revision total knee arthroplasty, in Lotke PA, Lonner J, eds: *Master Techniques in Orthopedic Surgery.* Baltimore, MD, Lippincott, Williams & Wilkins, 2008, pp 203-228.

Vince KG, Nakasone C: Extensor mechanism disruption after total knee arthroplasty, in: Scott WN, ed: *Insall & Scott Surgery of the Knee.* New York, NY, Churchill-Livingstone, 2005.

Vince KG: The stiff TKA, in Harner FF, Vince K, eds: *Knee Surgery.* Baltimore, MD, Lippincott, Williams & Wilkins, Vol 2, 1994, pp 1529-1538.

Vince KG: Why knees fail. *J Arthroplasty* 2003;18(3, Suppl 1):39-44.

Vince KG, Abdeen A, Sugimori T: The unstable total knee arthroplasty: causes and cures. *J Arthroplasty* 2006;21(4, Suppl 1):44-49.

Chapter 40
Revision Total Knee Arthroplasty: Indications and Contraindications

Kevin L. Garvin, MD

Indications

Total knee arthroplasty (TKA) is one of the most successful procedures for patients with osteoarthritis. The vast majority of patients achieve marked relief of symptoms; however, in a small percentage of patients, pain and dysfunction are not improved by surgery or recur after an initial asymptomatic period. Identifying the cause of pain and disability is critical to effective treatment of these patients. If the symptoms are thought to be a result of the TKA, then the etiology of the failure must be identified, because that will determine whether revision surgery is indicated, the specific operation that should be performed, and the likely outcome. The first step in appropriate treatment of a patient with a problematic TKA is performing a thorough preoperative assessment, including a comprehensive history, physical examination, and laboratory and radiologic evaluation.

The most common diagnoses that indicate the need for revision TKA can be divided into two groups, depending on whether the symptoms occur early or late relative to the index knee replacement. Infection and knee insta-

bility are significantly more common causes of early failure, whereas polyethylene wear and component loosening are common causes of late failure. The data are supported by several recent studies. Mulhall and associates evaluated 318 knee revisions and found the most common reason for early failure and subsequent revision surgery was sepsis. Of the failed TKAs, sepsis accounted for 25.4% of early failures but only 6.9% of late failures (defined as those after 2 years). These data were supported by Fehring and associates, who evaluated 440 knee revisions performed within 5 years of the index TKA and found that sepsis was the primary reason for revision in 38% of the knees studied. More common causes of late failure of TKAs requiring revision include polyethylene wear, implant loosening, knee instability, patellofemoral complications, failed inserts, and infection (**Table 1**). Component malrotation and arthrofibrosis also are common causes of failure of TKA and may require revision TKA, but not all patients with these problems are candidates for surgery. The severity of the symptoms, coupled with the complexity of the revision surgery, help the patient and sur-

geon decide when and if surgery is necessary.

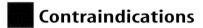

Contraindications

The evaluation of a patient with knee pain and disability following TKA must exclude both local and systemic conditions that may mimic the symptoms of a failed TKA (**Table 2**). Absolute contraindications include problems outside the joint that may mimic problems created by the knee. Uncommon examples of such problems include spinal disease affecting the lumbar nerves to the knee region and also diseases of the hip. A thorough history and physical examination and radiographic tests of the spine, hip, and knee should identify extra-articular sources of symptoms. Other unusual causes of pain about the knee include complex regional pain syndrome, entrapment of the infrapatellar nerve, bursitis, and tendinitis.

Relative contraindications are more difficult for the surgeon to distinguish. Stiffness after TKA is a frustrating problem for the patient and surgeon. Patients with pain because of stiffness after TKA must be evaluated to determine if the prosthetic joint is appropriately placed. Radiographs evaluating restoration of the joint line

Dr. Garvin or a member of his immediate family receives royalties from Biomet and has received research or institutional support from Arthrex, Biomet, Exactech, Stryker, SpineMedica, ESKA Implants, and NIH.

Table 1 Common Causes of Knee Failure Requiring Revision

Authors (Year)	Number of Knees	Causes of Failure (%)*
Sharkey et al (2002)	212	Polyethylene wear (24.1) Loosening (24.1) Instability (21.2) Infection (17.5) Arthrofibrosis (14.6) Malalignment/malposition of components (11.8) Extensor mechanism (6.6) Osteonecrosis of patella (4.2) Periprosthetic fracture (2.8) Patella resurfacing (0.9)
Mulhall et al (2006)	318	Polyethylene wear (41.3) Loosening (41.3) Instability (28.9) Infection (10.4) Malalignment/malposition of components (9.4) Osteolysis (59) Extensor mechanism (1.3)
Bare et al (2006)	295	Polyethylene wear (20.8) Loosening (46.2) Instability (21.8) Infection (26.8) Osteolysis (8.3) Implant breakage (3.4) Metal wear (2.7) Extensor mechanism (patellofemoral failure) (2.3) Periprosthetic fracture (0.5)

*Total adds to >100% because of multiple causes of failure in some patients.

Table 2 Contraindications to Revision Total Knee Arthroplasty

Referred pain (spine/hip)

Infrapatellar saphenous nerve entrapment

Neuromuscular disease

Complex regional pain syndrome

Bursitis

Stress fracture

Tendinitis

Crystalline deposition disease (gout, calcium pyrophosphate deposition disease)

Vascular disease

Fibromyalgia

ported the largest series of patients treated surgically (56 knee revisions in 52 patients) for knee stiffness. Fifty-two of the 56 knees exhibited improvement in range of motion. Another study of 15 patients who underwent revision TKA found that only 10 were satisfied with modest functional improvement.

Pain after TKA also is a relative contraindication for further surgical treatment. A complete evaluation is required to exclude all the possible causes of the pain. In a series of 27 patients managed surgically for persistent pain of unknown etiology, only 11 (41%) had good or excellent results at an average follow-up of 42 months. Furthermore, in 12 of the 27 patients, a problem was diagnosed at the time of revision surgery, and only 3 of those 12 patients (25%) had a successful result.

————————■

Evaluation of the Painful Knee

History

A thorough history and physical examination is critical in evaluating patients for revision TKA (**Table 3**). Pain is one of the more common symptoms in patients with failed TKA, but knee instability, swelling, stiffness, or other symptoms also may be present. Identifying the location and characteristics of pain after TKA is paramount to distinguishing the cause of the failure. Pain located at the knee is more typical of prosthetic joint problems. Pain located in the thigh more likely originates from the hip, although extensor mechanism problems or other diseases of the knee may present with pain at this site as well. Pain that radiates from the spine to the knee and/or below the knee to the foot is unusual for knee joint pathology and more likely represents a spinal origin. Although the location of the pain does not guarantee a specific diagnosis, it

and a CT scan to assess component rotation are necessary to determine appropriate placement of the components. Results of surgery for this group of patients are mixed. Seyler and associates described a comprehensive evaluation and nonsurgical treatment plan for these patients. Of 106 patients (108 knees) in whom the components were appropriately placed, all but one of the patients who presented with stiffness were able to recover without surgical treatment. The comprehensive approach recommended by Seyler and associates included aggressive physical therapy, custom-fit dynamic knee devices to assist with extension and flexion, botulinum toxin injection into the adjacent muscle, and electrical stimulation. Kim and associates re-

Table 3 Evaluation Considerations in the Problematic Total Knee Arthroplasty

Pain

Nature/character

Location/radiation

Exacerbating/relieving activities

Timing

Instability

Nature

Inciting activities

Preoperative/postoperative surgical course

Original indication for surgery

Wound complications/drainage

Presence of an asymptomatic interval

Trauma/injury

Fevers

Effusions

Functional status

Need for medication/assistive devices

Dental procedures

Systemic illnesses

Rehabilitation/physical therapy

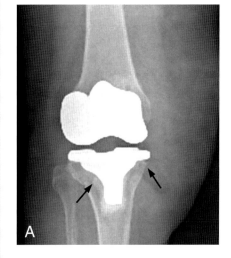
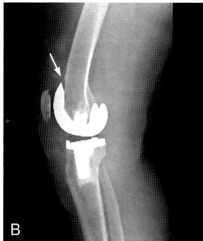
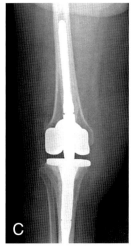
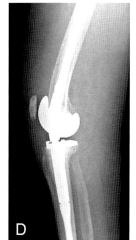

Figure 1 Radiographs of the knee of a 67-year-old woman 1 year after failed treatment for a periprosthetic joint infection. She had been diagnosed with a *Staphylococcus aureus* infection and treated with surgical débridement, component retention, and antibiotics. Bone resorption (arrows) is demonstrated around the tibial component on the AP view (**A**) and around the femoral component on the lateral view (**B**), consistent with infection. AP (**C**) and lateral (**D**) views obtained 1 year after a two-stage reimplantation.

can be highly suggestive. For example, anterior knee pain associated with descending stairs is typical of extensor mechanism problems of the quadriceps, patella, or patellar tendon. Similarly, posterior knee pain can represent hamstring tightness, a large effusion, a popliteal cyst, or soft-tissue impingement.

The timing of pain also can be helpful in arriving at the correct diagnosis. Pain about the knee that is present when the patient first begins to walk is typical after TKA and may last 3 to 4 months after surgery. This "start-up" pain usually occurs within the first several steps and subsides as the patient continues walking. Weight-bearing pain that persists after the first few months is more concerning for me-

chanical problems such as component loosening or instability of the prosthetic joint. Pain associated with activity also is seen on occasion in patients with a well-functioning TKA. This typical and more likely benign pain is associated with vigorous activity or frequent stair climbing and is relieved with rest or nonsteroidal anti-inflammatory drugs (NSAIDs). Significant pain that occurs with even mild activities or that requires narcotics may reflect mechanical knee problems deserving of further investigation.

Of all the types of pain after TKA, pain while the patient is at rest is the most troublesome because it is indicative of an inflammatory problem. Noninfectious inflammatory problems

should eventually ease with a longer interval of rest or NSAIDs. Pain as a result of infection or sepsis normally does not respond to prolonged rest and is rarely relieved by NSAIDs (**Figure 1**). Pain associated with infection may be present from the first few days after surgery; if it is a result of a hematogenous infection, the pain may suddenly occur after the joint is hematogenously seeded. Pain associated with a hematogenous infection will occur within days after the bacteria infect the prosthetic joint.

Multiple symptoms are common in patients with a problematic TKA (Tables 4 and 5). For example, patients with knee stiffness and limited range of motion after TKA commonly report

Table 4 Functional Symptoms Associated With Causes of Total Knee Arthroplasty Failure

Symptom	Diagnosis
Pain with activity but improved or relieved by rest	Synovitis/tendinitis
Pain at night in addition to activity	Inflammation/infection
Pain radiating to or from adjacent joints	Referred pain, consider spine and hip disease
Pain out of proportion to evidence	CRPS
Late pain after asymptomatic interval	Loosening/wear/instability/hematogenous infection
Early pain after surgery	Infection/instability/CRPS/loosening
Effusions	Infection/instability
Fevers	Infection
Giving way	Instability
Pain/difficulty with stairs or rising from seated	Patellofemoral malfunction
Onset of symptoms following dental/colonic/urologic procedure or associated with trophic skin changes or ulcers (venous, diabetic)	Hematogenous infection

CRPS = complex regional pain syndrome.

Table 5 Physical Signs Associated With Causes of Total Knee Arthroplasty Failure

Physical Signs	Diagnosis
Erythema, warmth, drainage, effusion	Infection
Tenderness to palpation of tendon	Tendinitis
Presence of effusion	Infection, soft-tissue impingement, ligamentous imbalance, synovitis
Pain, swelling, stiffness, discoloration, increased skin temperature, hyperhidrosis	CRPS
Presence of scar + Tinel sign	Neuroma
Diminished pulses	Vascular disease/claudication
Poster tibial sag + posterior drawer + 90° quadriceps active test	PCL insufficiency in PCL-retaining TKA
Increased Q angle, patellar apprehension	Patellar subluxation
Audible popping or crepitus with flexion to extension, palpable mass superior to patellar tendon	Patellar clunk, peripatellar fibrosis
Proximal/medial tibia tenderness to palpation	Pes anserine bursitis
Point joint line tenderness to palpation and/or crepitus	Impingement of osteophyte/cement/soft tissue, overhanging implant

CRPS = complex regional pain syndrome, PCL = posterior cruciate ligament, TKA = total knee arthroplasty.

pain anteriorly over the knee but also posteriorly, related to hamstring fatigue and/or tightness. These patients also may report stiffness of the knee that limits their ability to function normally (**Figure 2**). Rising from a chair is not easy for these patients, and walking on a flexed or contracted knee is painful, difficult, and tiring, as they must work hard to maintain an upright position. Bédard and associates performed a CT evaluation of 34 revision TKA candidates who presented with knee stiffness defined as a flexion contracture greater than 15° and/or flexion less than 105°. All 34 knees exhibited some degree of internal rotation on the preoperative CT scan. Postoperatively, the component rotation was improved in the 18 patients with available CT scans ($P < 0.0001$). The knee range of motion improved from 61.4° to 98.1° ($P < 0.0001$).

Patients with knee instability also frequently have multiple symptoms. These patients also may report pain and swelling of the knee, especially if they are active (**Figure 3**).

Physical Examination

The physical examination of the patient should be completed after a thorough history has been obtained. The patient should be examined in shorts

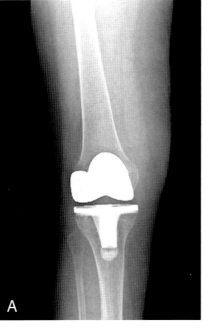
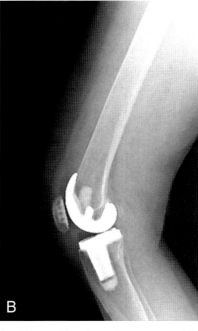

Figure 2 AP (**A**) and lateral (**B**) radiographs of a 63-year-old patient who was treated for osteoarthritis with a routine TKA. The postoperative interval was complicated by slow rehabilitation and stiffness requiring manipulation. Despite manipulation, the stiffness persisted. The patient presented 6 months after surgery with reports of stiffness and pain both anteriorly and posteriorly. The knee range of motion was limited, with a 25° flexion contracture and further flexion to 70°.

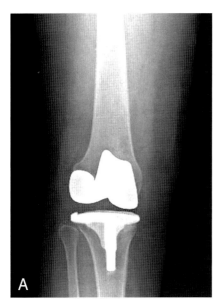
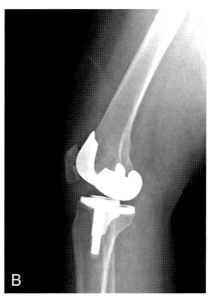
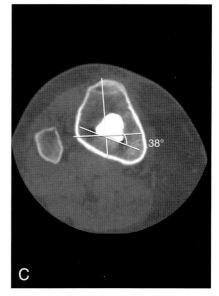

Figure 3 AP (**A**) and lateral (**B**) radiographs of a 52-year-old woman who underwent TKA for osteoarthritis. The patient's early recovery was uneventful, but 3 months postoperatively she reported swelling and giving way of the knee. Physical examination revealed a slight effusion with excellent motion from full extension to flexion greater than 115°. Slight instability was noted with the knee in extension and varus stressing of the knee. A CT scan (**C**) demonstrated that the femur and tibia had a combined internal rotation greater than 30°.

Table 6   Laboratory Evaluation of Symptomatic Total Knee Arthroplasty

WBC count

Frequently normal with infection present

Elevation is significant and suggestive of infection.

Average value with infection present = 8,300/mm³

Erythrocyte sedimentation rate

Nonspecific indicator of inflammation; elevated in inflammatory arthropathies and with infections in other locations

Elevated up to 1 year after surgery; begins declining 1 month after surgery

Continued elevation suggestive of infection

Average value with infection present = 63 mm/h

Value ≥22.5 mm/h should be considered positive for infection

C-reactive protein

Acute phase reactant

Elevated after surgery; normalizes in 2 to 4 weeks

Continued elevation suggestive of infection

Value ≥13.5 mg/L should be considered positive for infection.

Knee aspiration

Cultures, cell count, protein, and glucose should be measured.

Gram stain of little value

Use of antibiotics before aspiration is a major cause of false-negative results.

Wait more than 2 weeks after stopping antibiotics before performing aspiration; if on recent antibiotic, repeat aspiration may be indicated.

WBC >2,500/mm³ or with >60% polymorphonuclear leukocytes strongly indicative of infection

Increased protein and decreased glucose suggestive of infection

Metal debris or polyethylene fragments may indicate wear.

WBC = white blood cell.

or a gown, allowing inspection of both limbs and the spine. The opposite limb, if normal, is useful as a baseline for comparison. Gait and muscle tone should be assessed, and the patient should be examined for scars and deformity at this time. The knee and adjacent areas are palpated and assessed for tenderness, swelling, or an effusion. The adjacent tendons and bursae should be palpated. The range of motion of the knee should be full and smooth. Comparing the range of motion with that of the normal, contralateral limb helps identify subtle flexion contractures or loss of flexion. Lateral patellar tracking, grinding that emanates from the patellofemoral joint, or a patellar clunk will be evident during the range-of-motion testing. Ligamentous testing for instability is performed with the knee in extension, at midflexion, and at 90°. A thorough neurovascular examination should be completed, including skin sensation, proprioception, muscle strength, and reflexes. A check of pulses, capillary refill, the presence or absence of hair, and other trophic changes completes the examination.

Laboratory Evaluation

Laboratory studies are particularly useful in evaluating a symptomatic TKA for possible infection (**Table 6**). The principal laboratory values used in this evaluation are the white blood cell count, C-reactive protein level, and erythrocyte sedimentation rate. Additionally, laboratory analysis of knee aspiration fluid, including culture, cell count, glucose, and protein, is of great utility. Aspiration analysis can also be effective in identifying a mechanical etiology such as wear.

Imaging Evaluation

The radiologic evaluation of a symptomatic TKA begins with standard weight-bearing AP and lateral views and a Merchant view to assess component positioning and fixation. **Table 7** lists the radiographic studies that are useful for assessing the symptomatic

Table 7 Radiographic Evaluation of Symptomatic Total Knee Arthroplasty

All views

Alignment of components relative to each other

Alignment of components relative to respective anatomic and mechanical axes

Presence of radiolucent lines at prosthesis-bone interface or prosthesis-cement interface

Fractures

AP view of the knee

Femoral component in 4° to 7° of valgus

Tibial component perpendicular to the long axis of the tibia

Medial and lateral joint spaces equivalent

Lateral view of the knee

Femoral component parallel to long axis of femur and posterior aspect of anterior flange flush with underlying anterior cortex

Tibial component with a posterior slope of 0° to 10° and positioned centrally or posteriorly on tibia

Patellar height of 10 to 30 mm

Merchant view

Patella within femoral groove

No patellar maltracking or subluxation

Weight-bearing AP of entire lower extremity

Adequate limb alignment

Ipsilateral ankle or hip pathology

Stress views

AP and varus/valgus stability

Weight-bearing lateral flexion/extension views

No change in femorotibial contact point

TKA. Additional studies, including fluoroscopy, CT, ultrasound, and nuclear medicine scans, may be useful, depending on the etiologies that are being considered. MRI has traditionally been of little value in evaluating TKA because of extensive metal artifact; however, newer MRI technology allows clinically relevant diagnostic information to be obtained. **Table 8** lists relevant imaging studies and pertinent findings associated with common mechanisms of TKA failure.

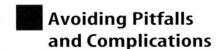

Avoiding Pitfalls and Complications

Surgical treatment is contraindicated for patients who have pain without an underlying diagnosis (eg, infection, instability, mechanical loosening). On the other hand, the evaluating surgeon should use the resources necessary to investigate the cause of a patient's pain. Failure to thoroughly evaluate a patient who has pain secondary to a problem with a TKA also is a pitfall.

Table 8   Common Imaging Findings Associated With Total Knee Arthroplasty Failure

Loosening

Most commonly involves tibial component

Any radiolucency >2 mm or that is progressive

Radiolucent line extending under entire prosthesis

Change in component position on sequential studies

Cement cracking or fragmentation

Fluoroscopic view with X-ray beam placement tangential to interface helpful in diagnosis

Increased uptake on bone scan sensitive but not specific

Polyethylene wear

More common at patellar and tibial components

Asymmetrically narrowed joint spaces; more pronounced on weight-bearing radiographs

Synovitis and bone resorption seen on radiographs and CT scans

Infection

Resorption at interfaces, periosteal reaction, soft-tissue swelling

Negative nuclear white blood cell scan excludes infection with good certainty

Incongruent results of dual bone and nuclear white blood cell scan indicates likely infection

Malrotation/malposition of components

Most easily assessed with CT

Patellofemoral malfunction

Presence of patellar fracture

Patella baja may indicate quadriceps tendon tear vs scarring of the patella inferiorly

Patella alta may indicate patellar tendon rupture

Fluoroscopy useful for evaluating patellar tracking and identifying subluxation

Instability

Varus/valgus stress views useful in diagnosing collateral ligament instability

Femorotibial contact position more anterior in flexion than extension on lateral weight-bearing radiograph may indicate PCL instability

Complex regional pain syndrome

Osteopenia on conventional radiographs

Increased uptake on all phases of three-phase bone scan

PCL = posterior cruciate ligament.

Bibliography

Bare J, MacDonald SJ, Bourne RB: Preoperative evaluations in revision total knee arthroplasty. *Clin Orthop Relat Res* 2006; 446:40-44.

Bédard M, Vince KA, Dunbar M: Abstract: Stiffness complicating total knee arthroplasty: Computerized tomography (CT) evaluation of rotational positioning of the components—Pre and post revision. The Knee Society and the American Association of Hip and Knee Surgeons Combined Specialty Day Meeting, Las Vegas, NV, 2009.

Dennis DA, Berry DJ, Engh G, et al: Revision total knee arthroplasty. *J Am Acad Orthop Surg* 2008;16:442-454.

Fehring TK, Odum S, Griffin WL, Mason JB, Nadaud M: Early failures in total knee arthroplasty. *Clin Orthop Relat Res* 2001;392:315-318.

Haidukewych GJ, Jacofsky DJ, Pagnano MW, Trousdale RT: Functional results after revision of well-fixed components for stiffness after primary total knee arthroplasty. *J Arthroplasty* 2005;20:133-138.

Kim J, Nelson CL, Lotke PA: Stiffness after total knee arthroplasty: Prevalence of the complication and outcomes of revision. *J Bone Joint Surg Am* 2004;86:1479-1484.

Math KR, Scheider R: Imaging of the painful TKR, in Scuderi GR, Tria, AJ Jr, Insall JN, eds: *Surgical Techniques in Total Knee Arthroplasty.* New York, NY, Springer Verlag, 2002, pp 351-367.

Mont MA, Serna FK, Krackow KA, Hungerford DS: Exploration of radiographically normal total knee replacements for unexplained pain. *Clin Orthop Relat Res* 1996;331:216-220.

Mulhall KJ, Ghomrawi HM, Scully S, Callaghan JJ, Saleh KJ: Current etiologies and modes of failure in total knee arthroplasty revision. *Clin Orthop Relat Res* 2006;446:45-50.

Nelson CL, Kim J, Lotke PA: Stiffness after total knee arthroplasty. *J Bone Joint Surg Am* 2005;87(Suppl 1):264-270.

Seyler TM, Marker DR, Bhave A, et al: Functional problems and arthrofibrosis following total knee arthroplasty. *J Bone Joint Surg Am* 2007;89(Suppl 3):59-69.

Sharkey PF, Hozack WJ, Rothman RH, Shastri S, Jacoby SM: Insall Award paper: Why are total knee arthroplasties failing today? *Clin Orthop Relat Res* 2002;404:7-13.

Sofka CM, Potter HG, Figgie M, Laskin R: Magnetic resonance imaging of total knee arthroplasty. *Clin Orthop Relat Res* 2003;406:129-135.

Coding

CPT Code		Corresponding ICD-9 Codes	
	Revision Total Knee Arthroplasty		
27446	Arthroplasty, knee, condyle and plateau; medial OR lateral compartment	715 715.80	715.16 715.89

CPT copyright © 2010 by the American Medical Association. All rights reserved.

Chapter 41

Revision Total Knee Arthroplasty: Extensile Surgical Approaches

Bassam A. Masri, MD, FRCSC
Donald S. Garbuz, MD, FRCSC
Muhyeddine Al-Taki, MD

Indications

Exposure in revision total knee arthroplasty (TKA) can be challenging, especially in the multiply revised knee. The exposure might be compromised by scar tissue that limits the range of motion, prevents eversion or mobilization of the patella, and predisposes the patellar tendon to iatrogenic avulsion. Several approaches can be used to expose the knee, and the appropriate choice is imperative to successful completion of the procedure.

A more extensile approach, such as the quadriceps snip, quadriceps turndown, or tibial tubercle osteotomy, is indicated in several situations. One indication is when a standard parapatellar approach fails to adequately and safely expose the joint for extraction of the prosthetic components, preparation of the bony surfaces, and insertion of the trial implant followed by the definitive new components. Another indication is if the knee cannot

be passively flexed to 100° to 110° with the patient under anesthesia. In these cases, the surgeon should anticipate the potential need for one of the extensile approaches to avoid causing iatrogenic avulsion of the patellar tendon or placing the definitive components in a suboptimal position. It is also imperative to respect and maintain the vascular supply of the patella and the skin flaps to avoid catastrophic complications. Another important indication for extensile exposure is the presence of retained hardware or cement within the medullary canal of the tibia. For such cases, an extended tibial tubercle osteotomy is invaluable.

Contraindications

When selecting the best extensile exposure for revision TKA, the surgeon should consider various factors that may favor one approach over another.

For example, if quadriceps strength is more important to the patient than range of motion, then a quadriceps turndown with a V-Y lengthening of the quadriceps tendon should not be considered. Similarly, if the proximal tibial bone stock is compromised, a tibial tubercle osteotomy should not be considered. With any of these techniques, the surgeon must keep in mind that, particularly in the setting of previous multiple operations and possibly multiple incisions, raising wide flaps and ignoring the vascularity of the skin will pose challenges to wound healing and ultimately to the knee reconstruction (**Figure 1**). For this reason, great care needs to be taken with patients with peripheral vascular disease or those who have had previous radiation treatments, and with elderly patients with diabetes. Skin flaps should be kept thick and any undue undermining of the skin should be avoided. Moreover, extensive approaches that reduce the vascular supply to the patella should be avoided unless absolutely necessary to minimize the risk of osteonecrosis and subsequent fracture of the patella.

Dr. Masri or an immediate family member serves as a board member, owner, officer, or committee member of the Canadian Orthopaedic Association and has received research or institutional support from Stryker. Dr. Garbuz or an immediate family member serves as a paid consultant for or is an employee of Zimmer and has received research or institutional support from Zimmer. Neither Dr. Al-Taki nor any immediate family member has received anything of value from or owns stock in a commercial company or institution related directly or indirectly to the subject of this chapter.

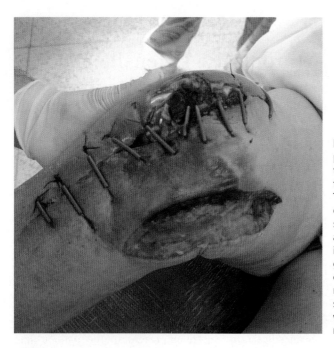

Figure 1 Clinical photograph of a multiply operated knee that underwent a TKA through a standard anterior incision. After a secondary débridement and irrigation, the surgeon was unable to close the wound, so a relaxing medial incision was made, which resulted in massive necrosis.

terior cruciate ligament, if present, is released. A posterior capsular release is initiated by resecting some of the obvious scar tissue at this stage. The polyethylene liner is removed early during the procedure, which also makes the exposure easier. Gradually, as the tibia is subluxated and the implants are extracted, exposure becomes easier and, in a large number of cases, an extensile exposure can be avoided altogether. In a few situations, extensile exposures are unavoidable.

————————■

Results

Results for extensile approaches are summarized in **Table 1**. A study that compared the functional outcome of the various extensile approaches in revision TKA showed that when a quadriceps snip was done, patients had better functional outcome, as reflected by a higher Knee Society score postoperatively, than did patients who had a quadriceps turndown or a tibial tubercle osteotomy, who had roughly equal functional outcomes. These results are confounded, however, by the fact that patients who had a quadriceps turndown or an osteotomy had lower preoperative scores. It is therefore difficult to ascertain whether the lower scores are related to the exposure or to the lower preoperative scores. Nevertheless, patients can be expected to have good functional outcome after a quadriceps snip approach if the knee reconstruction is otherwise satisfactory. Results from two 16-patient studies showed a slightly better functional outcome with the quadriceps snip versus the more extensile quadriceps turndown.

The tibial tubercle osteotomy has undergone modifications that have significantly improved its outcomes. In the past, a short tibial tubercle osteotomy was used, which was associated with fracture of the tibial tubercle or avulsion of the tubercle fragment,

Alternative Treatments

Several deep capsular incisions can be used to access the knee joint. These capsular incisions are made either medial or lateral to the patella and can be accessed through almost any skin incision. In general, the most lateral but still usable skin incision that requires the least amount of undermining should be used to preserve the vascularity of the skin flaps. In addition, when an extensile exposure is required, the one that poses the lowest risk of complications for a particular patient should be considered. For example, a patient with extension lag preoperatively, in whom a quadriceps snip does not provide sufficient exposure, might be better served by a tibial tubercle osteotomy than a quadriceps turndown procedure. On the other hand, a patient with suboptimal proximal tibial bone stock and no extension lag might do better with a quadriceps turndown approach if more conservative releases do not provide satisfactory access. Extensile approaches have their own unique po-

tential complications, and they should not be overused. The surgeon should always start with a medial patellar arthrotomy and excise the scar tissue from the medial and lateral gutters to bring the medial and lateral flaps back to what they would have looked like at the time of the primary TKA. The lateral patellofemoral ligament should be released, and the scar tissue adhering the patellar tendon to the proximal tibia should be released, taking extreme care not to detach the patellar tendon from its insertion on the tibia. The safe dissection zone can be easily ascertained from the lateral radiograph by measuring the distance between the anterior rim of the tibial component and the proximal edge of the tibial tubercle. After this scar is released, the lateral rim of the tibia is carefully exposed, and the patella is subluxated laterally. Any attempts to evert the patella in the revision setting, in our opinion, may lead to more harm than good. In fact, exposure is not always facilitated by everting the patella, and the senior author (B.A.M.) does not evert the patella even in primary TKA. In case of stiffness, the knee is gently flexed and the tight pos-

Table 1 Results of Extensile Surgical Approaches in Total Knee Arthroplasty

Author(s) (Year)	Number of Knees	Approach	Mean Patient Age in Years (Range)	Mean Follow-up (Range)	Results
Trousdale et al (1993)	16	Quadriceps turndown	66 (51-81)	30 months (12-53)	HSS knee scores: 2 excellent, 10 good, 2 fair, 2 poor Mean active ROM, 4°-85° Weaker (statistically significant) active extension vs contralateral normal knee Weaker (statistically insignificant) active extension vs contralateral replaced knee
Whiteside (1995)	136	TTO	(34-88)	2 years	Mean postoperative ROM, 93.7° (range, 15°-140°) No TTO nonunions 2 avulsion fractures 2 postoperative extension lag (was present preoperatively)
Garvin et al (1995)	16	Quadriceps snip	65 (50-73)	30 months (2-4 years)	Postoperative HSS knee score: 10 patients excellent, 6 good 30° mean increase in ROM (14 of 16 patients) Significantly decreased peak torque vs contralateral nonreplaced knee No significant difference in peak torque vs contralateral replaced knee
Barrack et al (1998)	60	31 quadriceps snip 14 quadriceps turndown 15 TTO	NR	2-4 years	Quadriceps snip: KSS 97 preoperatively, 134 postoperatively; postoperative extension lag 0.9° Quadriceps turndown: KSS 78 preoperatively, 117 postoperatively; postoperative extension lag, 4.5° TTO: KSS 77 preoperatively, 117 postoperatively; postoperative extension lag, 1.5°

HSS = Hospital for Special Surgery, ROM = range of motion, TTO = tibial tubercle osteotomy, NR = not reported, KSS = Knee Society score.

leading to severe functional deficits. The modern modification of the tibial tubercle osteotomy was introduced by Whiteside, who stressed the importance of a long osteotomy (at least 8 cm) and fixation with wires instead of screws. This modification has led to a significantly lower incidence of fracture and avulsion of the tibial fragment. In 1995, Whiteside reported on 136 patients in whom this modified tibial osteotomy was performed. Only

two had avulsion fractures, and another two had an extension lag that had been present preoperatively.

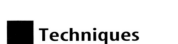

■ Techniques

Skin Incision and Superficial Dissection

With any revision TKA, because of the presence of previous incisions, the

placement of the skin incision is crucial. If there is only one previous incision and it is reasonably close to the midline of the knee, it should be used regardless of whether it is the surgeon's preferred incision. Slight deviations from a previous incision may leave narrow skin islands and can risk wound-edge necrosis or necrosis of the skin bridge and subsequent wound slough. In the case of multiple parallel incisions, the most lateral usable incision should be used because most of the blood supply to the skin of the knee comes from the medial side, and any excessively medialized incisions, particularly when more lateral incisions are present, can devascularize a part of the knee and lead to skin necrosis. If there are previous transverse or oblique incisions, the new incision should intersect them at a right angle, which will substantially reduce the risk to the skin. After the skin incision is made, dissection should be deepened to and through the underlying fascia. If skin flaps are to be raised, this should be done in a subfascial manner to avoid injury to the transverse vessels that run between the fascia and the skin. This applies to all extensile and nonextensile exposures at the time of revision TKA.

Resection of Scar Tissue

With all extensile exposures, a medial parapatellar arthrotomy is required for initial exposure. The difference between this exposure for a revision TKA and for a previously unoperated knee is that in the revision setting, there is scar tissue that tethers the medial and lateral tissue flaps. Also, the patellar tendon typically is adhered to the underlying proximal tibia with scar tissue. If these two issues are addressed early in the procedure, the need for extensile exposure can be minimized.

After a standard medial parapatellar arthrotomy is performed, the medial edge of the cut quadriceps tendon is gently grasped with two Kocher forceps. The edge between the scar tissue and the native tendon and muscle is identified. Dissection then proceeds in that plane to restore the tendon and muscle to their original thickness. Typically, after the edge of the scar tissue is released, the remainder of the dissection can proceed in a blunt manner, using the finger as a dissector; small tethered areas may require a sharp release. This allows the thick scar tissue in the medial gutter to be

resected and thins the tissues in the medial gutter substantially. Next, a similar dissection is performed in the lateral gutter proximal to the patella. Distal to the patella, the patellar tendon typically is covered in scar and is tethered to the underlying tissues. With great care, the interval between the native patellar tendon and the underlying scar tissue is determined. Using a sharp scalpel, this interval is developed, thus separating the scar from the tendon. The scar tissue is then resected. A Hohmann retractor is placed along the lateral tibial plateau, just lateral to the patellar tendon, and the scar tissue that tethers the lateral retinacular area to the lateral femoral condyle is cut with scissors. This allows the patella to be retracted laterally and inferiorly and takes the tension off the patellar tendon. No attempt should be made to evert the patella as this is not necessary and is in fact potentially dangerous at this stage. This also gives improved exposure to the anterior portion of the lateral tibial plateau. The final step of the dissection is to release the scar tissue off the anterior part of the lateral tibial plateau and to expose the implant-bone junction. A medial release of a magnitude appropriate to the deformity is performed, and the posterior cruciate ligament, if present, is resected. The tibia is externally rotated and, if there is a modular polyethylene liner, the liner is removed. This frees up space within the knee and greatly simplifies exposure. If the rest of the knee still cannot be exposed safely and sufficient flexion cannot be obtained without potentially compromising the patellar tendon, or if there is another indication for an extensile exposure as already mentioned, the extensile exposure can proceed at this stage.

Quadriceps Snip

The quadriceps snip is attributed to Insall and was first described as a transverse incision in the quadriceps tendon. It was later modified to an

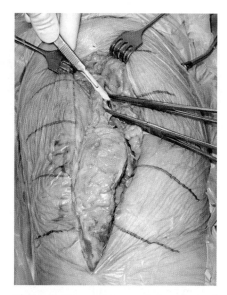

Figure 2 The quadriceps snip is performed along the line of the scalpel as shown.

oblique (45°) incision, extending from the medial aspect of the quadriceps tendon distally to its lateral aspect proximally in continuity with the standard medial parapatellar approach (**Figure 2**). The snip typically is made 6 to 10 cm superior to the proximal pole of the patella. The advantages of the oblique incision are that it avoids the lateral superior genicular artery, which supplies the patella, and that its direction is in line with the vastus lateralis muscle fibers. Recently, some authors have described making the quadriceps snip at a 45° angle pointing proximal to distal, as this facilitates extending the incision to a formal quadriceps turndown should the snip not provide enough exposure. A quadriceps snip can be combined with lateral retinacular release, which helps mobilize the patella and facilitates its lateral dislocation, thereby improving exposure.

The quadriceps snip has several advantages. It is easy to perform and it spares the vascular supply to the patella. It has no significant detrimental effect on the functional outcome of the procedure; multiple studies have shown no association with postoperative extensor mechanism weakness or knee extensor lag. Moreover, the postoperative rehabilitation protocol for a revision TKA does not need to be modified after a quadriceps snip procedure.

The quadriceps snip, with or without a lateral retinacular release, provides adequate exposure in knees with mild to moderate stiffness. In knees with severe limitation of flexion, the quadriceps snip can be extended to a quadriceps turndown procedure or combined with a tibial tubercle osteotomy as noted above in the Indications section. Alternatively, the surgeon may proceed directly to one of these exposures based on preoperative planning. At the end of the procedure, the snip is repaired using two or three interrupted sutures at the site of the snip and multiple interrupted sutures closing the quadriceps tendon in a side-to-side manner. The side-to-side repair provides much of the strength of the closure.

One complication that has been reported is delayed rupture of the quadriceps tendon. This is a serious complication and should be addressed promptly with a robust repair of the quadriceps tendon.

Quadriceps Turndown

Converting a medial parapatellar arthrotomy to a quadriceps turndown is quite straightforward. An incision is made from the apex of the medial parapatellar incision and is extended laterally along the lateral side of the patella (**Figure 3**); this is Insall's modification of the procedure described by Coonse and Adams, which serves to spare the inferior lateral genicular artery. A quadriceps turndown provides fast and almost complete exposure and access to the knee joint in the setting of moderate to severe stiffness. It also allows a V-Y lengthening of the tendon at the time of closure to increase the potential range of motion. This is done at the expense of quadriceps strength, however, and the patient should be warned ahead of time

that a substantial extensor lag will be the consequence of this maneuver. Typically, low-demand patients who value range of motion more than strength will accept this. Nevertheless, it is valuable to clearly discuss and document this before the procedure to avoid misunderstandings. At the end of the procedure, the quadriceps should be repaired with heavy sutures, but the lateral retinaculum is left open to improve patellar tracking. The repair should be such that the knee flexes to around 90° with acceptable tension on the sutures. Lengthening the quadriceps in excess of that results in unacceptable extensor lag. An extension lag up to 10° is considered the norm after this procedure.

When a turndown procedure is used, the postoperative rehabilitation schedule is modified. Continuous passive motion from 0° to 30° is allowed immediately after surgery, and this is increased by 5° every day until the point at which the repair comes under tension as noted intraoperatively. Active flexion and passive extension are allowed, but active extension is delayed until postoperative week 4 to 6, at which time the tendon is expected to be healed.

In addition to the expected extensor lag, a potential problem after a quadriceps turndown is transection of the superior lateral genicular artery, which further contributes to devascularization of the patella and the extensor mechanism, with the potential for patellar osteonecrosis.

Tibial Tubercle Osteotomy

If the medullary canal of the tibia needs to be exposed for the removal of retained hardware or cement, or if an extensor lag is to be avoided at all costs, a quadriceps turndown approach should be avoided. In these situations, a tibial tubercle osteotomy can be used. The osteotomy provides adequate exposure, can be securely fixed, and does not necessitate the al-

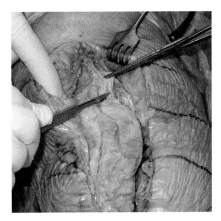

Figure 3 The quadriceps turndown is performed along the line of the scalpel as shown.

tered rehabilitation protocol needed after a turndown approach.

A transverse osteotomy inclined superiorly is made 8 cm distal to the upper border of the tibial tubercle (**Figure 4, A**). The osteotomy is then carried proximally, medial to the tibial tubercle and along the tibial crest. The lateral part of the osteotomy is completed from within the tibia using a curved 0.5-in osteotome to preserve the lateral muscular attachment to the bony fragment. Proximally, a transverse osteotomy is made, using a reciprocating saw just proximal to the insertion of the patellar tendon. This creates a shelf for the osteotomy fragment to butt against proximally, and allows the fragment to key into its bed securely, thus increasing the stability of the repair at the end of the procedure (**Figure 4, B**). The well-vascularized muscle-bone flap is reflected laterally together with the patellar tendon and patella, thereby fully exposing the knee joint. To avoid a fracture of the tibia at the end of the osteotomy due to a stress-riser effect, it is imperative to use a stem for the tibial component that extends beyond the distal extent of the osteotomy. Careful preoperative planning to ensure the availability of an adequate stem length is crucial. After trialing the components and before mixing

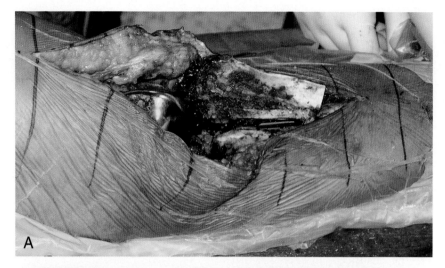

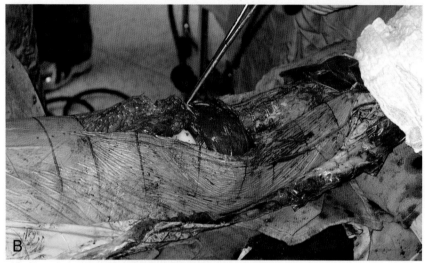

Figure 4 The tibial tubercle osteotomy. **A,** The osteotomy fragment should be at least 8 cm in length and hinged on its lateral side. **B,** Closure of a tibial tubercle osteotomy using wires. In this case, a medial gastrocnemius flap was added to cover the proximal tibial allograft, which was used for the reconstruction of a massive tibial defect.

the cement, three wires are inserted into the medullary canal of the tibia at the site of the osteotomy, from medial to lateral. These wires are then passed through the medullary canal of the tibia behind the stem. Going behind the posterior tibial cortex (ie, all the way around the tibia) is avoided to prevent neurovascular injury. Another drill hole is then made through the tibial tubercle itself, and the most proximal wire is passed through this drill hole from within the medullary canal of the tibia, at a 45° angle, to further resist the forces that tend to

drive the fragment proximally during flexion. The remaining two wires are passed through two drill holes in the lateral part of the tibia but not through the osteotomy fragment. Once the implants are inserted and the osteotomy fragment is closed, the wires are tightened around it. Ideally, these wires

 Video 41.1 Tibial Tubercle Osteotomy. Robert B. Bourne, MD; Cecil Rorabeck, MD (6 min)

should also pass at a 45° angle. Postoperatively, a standard rehabilitation protocol is allowed, with full weight bearing and unrestricted active range of motion.

Wound Closure

The tourniquet is deflated and hemostasis is secured before closure. In the case of a quadriceps turndown, suturing the tendon with heavy sutures is also done with the tourniquet deflated to assess proper muscle and tendon tension. Over- and underlengthening of the quadriceps mechanism is thus avoided. For a tibial tubercle osteotomy, the knee is maximally flexed and the fixation of the bone fragment is double checked. A suction drain is placed, and the capsule is securely closed using interrupted No. 1 absorbable polyglycolic acid sutures. Routine subcutaneous and skin closure is then performed.

Postoperative Regimen

Patients receive antibiotics for 24 hours. The drain is removed on the first postoperative day and the dressing is changed. Weight bearing as dictated by the bony reconstruction is allowed in all patients, and active extension is permitted except for those patients who had a quadriceps turndown procedure, in which case it is delayed for 4 to 6 weeks. Patients are followed up according to the practice routine of the individual surgeon and facility.

Avoiding Pitfalls and Complications

Knee range of motion should be assessed with the patient under anesthesia before starting the operation as well as after dissecting all accessible scar tissue. It is very important to determine whether the knee will do well with a standard approach, will need a quadriceps snip, or will need a more extensile approach such as a quadriceps turndown or an extended tibial tubercle osteotomy. Typically, this is determined before the operation, during preoperative planning; however, if there is any doubt about the ability to expose the knee using a standard approach, consideration should be given to an extensile exposure. In most cases, a quadriceps snip is sufficient, and the quadriceps turndown should be reserved for very few cases. The vascularity of the skin flaps is a poten-

tial issue, and using the techniques discussed previously will minimize the risk. The quadriceps tendon and the tendon snip should be repaired very carefully to avoid the potential rupture of the quadriceps tendon, a reported complication of this technique. When a quadriceps turndown is performed, too much lengthening should be avoided as it leads to an unacceptably large extensor lag postoperatively. Also, aggressive rehabilitation should be avoided to prevent a rupture of the quadriceps tendon.

With the tibial tubercle osteotomy, careful attention to every step in the technique minimizes the risk of complications, which include neurovascular injury if wires are passed posterior

to the tibia, superior migration if fixation is not secure, and fracture of the osteotomy fragment if it is cut too thin or too short or if too many drill holes are made in it. The knots from the wires can be painful, and the patient should be warned about this ahead of time. Finally, as with any complex knee exposure, if there is inadequate skin cover for a primary closure, a rotational gastrocnemius flap and skin grafting should be considered, and the opinion of a plastic surgeon should be sought as a part of the preoperative workup.

———————■

Bibliography

Arsht SJ, Scuderi GR: The quadriceps snip for exposing the stiff knee. *J Knee Surg* 2003;16(1):55-57.

Barrack RL: Specialized surgical exposure for revision total knee: Quadriceps snip and patellar turndown. *Instr Course Lect* 1999;48:149-152.

Barrack RL, Smith P, Munn B, Engh G, Rorabeck C: The Ranawat Award: Comparison of surgical approaches in total knee arthroplasty. *Clin Orthop Relat Res* 1998;356:16-21.

Clarke HD: Tibial tubercle osteotomy. *J Knee Surg* 2003;16(1):58-61.

Denham RA, Bishop RE: Mechanics of the knee and problems in reconstructive surgery. *J Bone Joint Surg Br* 1978;60-B(3): 345-352.

Garvin KL, Scuderi G, Insall JN: Evolution of the quadriceps snip. *Clin Orthop Relat Res* 1995;321:131-137.

Hendel D, Weisbort M: Modified lateral approach for knee arthroplasty in a fixed valgus knee—the medial quadriceps snip. *Acta Orthop Scand* 2000;71(2):204-205.

Insall JN: Surgical approaches to the knee, in Insall JN, Windsor RE, Scott WN, Kelly MA, Aglietti P, eds: *Surgery of the Knee*, ed. 2. New York, NY, Churchill Livingstone, 1993, pp 135-148.

Kelly MA: Patellofemoral complications following total knee arthroplasty. *Instr Course Lect* 2001;50:403-407.

Lahav A, Hofmann AA: The "banana peel" exposure method in revision total knee arthroplasty. *Am J Orthop* 2007;36(10): 526-529, discussion 529.

Laskin RS: Ten steps to an easier revision total knee arthroplasty. *J Arthroplasty* 2002;17(4, Suppl 1):78-82.

Mendes MW, Caldwell P, Jiranek WA: The results of tibial tubercle osteotomy for revision total knee arthroplasty. *J Arthroplasty* 2004;19(2):167-174.

Parker DA, Dunbar MJ, Rorabeck CH: Extensor mechanism failure associated with total knee arthroplasty: Prevention and management. *J Am Acad Orthop Surg* 2003;11(4):238-247.

Ritter MA, Herbst SA, Keating EM, Faris PM, Meding JB: Patellofemoral complications following total knee arthroplasty: Effect of a lateral release and sacrifice of the superior lateral geniculate artery. *J Arthroplasty* 1996;11(4):368-372.

Rosenberg AG: Surgical technique of posterior cruciate sacrificing, and preserving total knee arthroplasty, in Rand JA, ed: *Total Knee Arthroplasty,* New York, NY, Raven Press, 1993, pp 115-153.

Scott RD, Siliski JM: The use of a modified V-Y quadricepsplasty during total knee replacement to gain exposure and improve flexion in the ankylosed knee. *Orthopedics* 1985;8(1):45-48.

Stiehl JB, Anouchi Y, Dennis DA, et al: Symposium: Revision total knee replacement. *Contemp Orthop* 1995;30(3):249-266.

Trousdale RT, Hanssen AD, Rand JA, Cahalan TD: V-Y quadricepsplasty in total knee arthroplasty. *Clin Orthop Relat Res* 1993;286:48-55.

Whiteside LA: Exposure in difficult total knee arthroplasty using tibial tubercle osteotomy. *Clin Orthop Relat Res* 1995; 321:32-35.

Younger AS, Duncan CP, Masri BA: Surgical exposures in revision total knee arthroplasty. *J Am Acad Orthop Surg* 1998; 6(1):55-64.

 ## Video Reference

Bourne RB, Rorabeck CH: Video. *Tibial Tubercle Osteotomy.* Video clip from Bourne RB, Rorabeck CH: *Extensile Exposure Techniques,* in Ries MD, ed: *Surgical Techniques in Orthopaedics: Revision Total Knee Arthroplasty.* DVD. Rosemont, IL, American Academy of Orthopaedic Surgeons, 2004.

	Coding			
CPT Code			**Corresponding ICD-9 Codes**	
27447	Arthroplasty, knee, condyle and plateau; medial AND lateral compartments with or without patella resurfacing (total knee arthroplasty)		715 715.80	715.16 715.89

CPT copyright © 2010 by the American Medical Association. All rights reserved.

Chapter 42

Revision Total Knee Arthroplasty: Management of Osteolysis

William L. Griffin, MD

Indications

Approximately 22% of revision total knee arthroplasties (TKAs) are performed for polyethylene wear and osteolysis. TKA designs are a much harsher environment for polyethylene than the more congruent total hip designs. The wear debris generated from polyethylene wear in TKA has historically occurred in the form of pitting and delamination at the articular surface secondary to polyethylene fatigue failure from high contact stresses. When pitting and delamination occur, the wear debris generated tends to be large and therefore not as bioactive or as likely to incite an osteolytic reaction as submicron-size particles (**Figure 1**). With the introduction of modular tibial trays and the potential for abrasive backside wear creating submicron-size polyethylene debris, osteolysis has become a more common cause of failure in TKAs. The amount of debris generated from backside wear is determined by the following factors: the extent of micromotion, the surface roughness of the tibial base plate, and the resistance of the polyethylene insert to abrasive wear (**Figure 2**).

Osteolysis may be difficult to detect and is usually underestimated on plain radiographs. Routine follow-up radiographs should include AP and lateral views. If osteolysis is suspected, oblique views can be used to better evaluate the medial and lateral femoral condyles (**Figure 3**). Accelerated polyethylene wear and the subsequent development of periprosthetic osteolysis can initiate a variety of failure mechanisms, including aseptic loosening, periprosthetic fracture, component fracture, catastrophic polyethylene failure, or recurrent painful effusions, all of which may be indications for revision surgery (**Figure 4**).

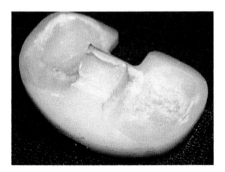

Figure 1 Photograph of a retrieved polyethylene insert shows pitting and delamination.

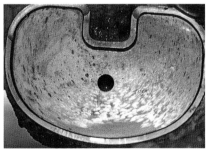

Figure 2 Intraoperative photograph of a tibial tray shows burnishing caused by backside micromotion and wear.

Contraindications

Revision surgery for polyethylene wear and osteolysis may not be indicated in patients with small asymptomatic lesions that do not jeopardize the stability of the implants. In addition, older patients who have become less active or are poor surgical candidates because of medical comorbidities might be better managed with periodic serial radiographic evaluation, with intervention only when failure has occurred.

Dr. Griffin or an immediate family member serves as a board member, owner, officer, or committee member of the Charlotte Surgery Center; has received royalties from DuPuy; is a member of a speakers' bureau or has made paid presentations on behalf of DuPuy; serves as a paid consultant to or is an employee of DuPuy; has received research or institutional support from DuPuy, Smith & Nephew, and Zimmer; owns stock or stock options in Johnson & Johnson; and has received nonincome support (such as equipment or services), commercially derived honoraria, or other non–research-related funding (such as paid travel) from DuPuy.

Alternative Treatments

Proper timing and treatment of accelerated wear and arresting the osteolytic process with bone-preserving and low-morbidity methods are paramount to preventing more severe wear-related complications.

Treatment can range from close observation with serial radiographs for smaller, stable lesions in less active patients to revision surgery with either a polyethylene insert exchange and synovectomy or a full component revision. The extent of bone loss secondary to osteolysis, the fixation of the components, and the track record of the TKA design dictate the best treatment option.

Modular polyethylene insert exchange should be limited to those patients with well-aligned, stable implants that have a good locking mechanism and for which modern replacement polyethylene inserts are

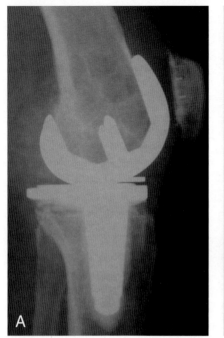 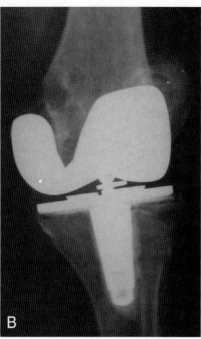

Figure 3 Radiographs of a knee with osteolysis of the medial femoral condyle. **A,** Lateral view. **B,** Oblique view demonstrates osteolysis and lack of femoral bony support.

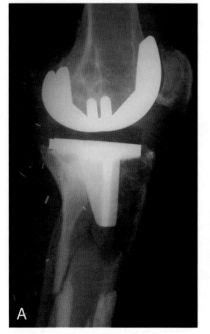 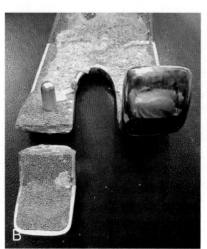 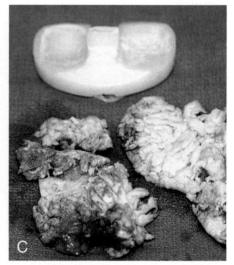

Figure 4 Osteolysis-initiated TKA failures. **A,** Lateral radiograph shows a knee with a periprosthetic fracture secondary to osteolysis. **B,** Photograph of a retrieved femoral component that fractured secondary to osteolysis of the posterior femoral condyle and loss of support. **C,** Photograph of a retrieved polyethylene insert with broken locking tab. Excised synovial tissue from the knee is also shown; note the hypertrophic synovitis.

Table 1 Results of Polyethylene Insert Exchange and Full Component Revision for Osteolysis

Authors (Year)	Number of TKAs	Mean Age in Years (Range)	Mean Follow-up in Months	Revision Rate (%)
Polyethylene Insert Exchange				
Engh et al (2000)	22	68 (43-90)	90	27
Babis et al (2002)	24	66 (35-83)	54	33
Griffin et al (2007)	68	68 (41-85)	44	16
Maloney et al (unpublished)*	22	NA	40	0
Full Component Revision				
Suarez et al (2008)	122	65.7	35	11
Burnett et al (2009)	28	NA	48	14

NA = not available.

* Maloney WJ, Callaghan JJ, Taylor SG, Clohisy JC: Liner exchange and bone grafting for osteolysis and wear following total knee arthroplasty. Presented at closed meeting of The Knee Society, October 2008.

available. Insert exchange with component retention may result in a quicker recovery, decreased blood loss, decreased cost, and better bone stock preservation compared with a complete revision.

Full component revision is indicated when there is component fracture, poor alignment, impending or definite loosening, or a poorly functioning TKA. In a review of 22 cases treated with isolated polyethylene exchange, Engh and associates identified a higher failure rate in patients who developed severe wear and lysis within 5 years of the index TKA. They recommended full component revision for patients who developed early wear and osteolysis. Early failure due to wear and lysis may be an indicator of several patient and implant variables that are associated with excessive wear, such as poor alignment, polyethylene gamma irradiated in air,

poor component design, or a high-activity patient. It is important to try to identify these risk factors as part of the decision-making process when choosing between isolated polyethylene exchange and full component revision surgery.

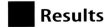

■ Results

Polyethylene Insert Exchange
Early studies on modular polyethylene tibial insert exchange for osteolysis were unfavorable. Some studies reported a failure rate greater than 27% within 5 years when the polyethylene exchange was performed because of advanced wear.

More recent studies using polyethylene not sterilized by gamma irradiation in air have produced more favorable results, with failure rates

ranging from 0% to 16% at mid-term follow-up (**Table 1**). These studies also demonstrated no significant progression of the osteolysis-induced bone loss when the defects were treated with either bone grafting or cement fillers.

Of note, the femoral component was more susceptible than the tibial component to loosening after isolated insert exchange. The stem on the tibial component seems to provide some additional protection, as the osteolysis rarely extends down to the tip of the tibial stem.

Full Revision
There is little information in the literature regarding full component revision performed specifically for osteolysis and wear. At my institution, 122 knees were revised for osteolysis with full component revision; at a mean follow-up of 3 years, 13 (11%)

had failed. In a comparable study with 4-year follow-up, 4 (14%) of the 26 knees revised for osteolysis had failed.

———————◼

◼ Technique

Preoperative Planning

Prior to revision for osteolysis, the patient should be evaluated to rule out the possibility of infection, and the extent of bone loss should be evaluated radiographically to determine the amount of bone remaining for reconstruction. Infection can be reliably ruled out based on a clinical history and physical examination, combined with an aspiration for cell count and cultures, an erythrocyte sedimentation rate, and C-reactive protein level.

Assessment of bone loss due to osteolysis usually can be accomplished with plain radiographs. Good-quality AP and lateral views of the knee along with oblique views of the femoral component provide enough information for surgical planning, with the understanding that the amount of bone loss is generally underestimated by radiographs. If questions remain regarding the extent of bone loss, a CT scan with metal subtraction techniques can provide a more accurate assessment of the defects that will be encountered at the time of surgery.

Exposure

The knee should be exposed through the prior knee incision with a standard medial parapatellar arthrotomy, as described in chapter 1. If additional old incisions are present, the most lateral incision should be used, to preserve blood supply to the anterior skin flaps. Minimal incisions that provide limited exposure are strongly discouraged. Revision surgery for osteolysis with potential significant bone loss requires excellent visualization to inspect and test the components for secure fixation and to inspect the bone for osteolytic defects. Adequate expo-

sure also avoids the need for excessive retraction force, which can lead to fractures of the weakened epicondyles or tibial tubercle.

Instruments/Equipment/Implants Required

A full range of revision instruments is required for component removal and for reconstruction. Oscillating microsaws and cement removal equipment should be available for removing well-fixed components.

Procedure

The first step is to remove the polyethylene insert. (The knee should be checked for motion within the locking mechanism before removal.) This creates more space and takes tension off the tibial tubercle. The next step is a complete synovectomy. This decreases the particulate burden within the knee and also provides improved exposure.

Using a hemostat as a probe and preoperative radiographs for guidance, the bone around the prosthesis is palpated to check for bony defects behind the components. In particular, the posterior femoral condyles should be assessed for bone loss, as this is an important area of support for the femoral component. The components are then stressed to determine if they remain solidly fixed to the bone. Rather than impacting the components with a mallet, a torque force should be applied and the bone-cement-prosthesis interface should be inspected closely for motion and extrusion of blood. If any motion is detected, the component should be revised.

If the components remain well fixed and have adequate bony support, then an isolated polyethylene insert exchange can be considered. If significant ligamentous instability is present, with a mismatch between the flexion and extension gaps, an incompetent posterior cruciate ligament with a posterior cruciate ligament–retaining design, or varus/valgus instability requiring additional con-

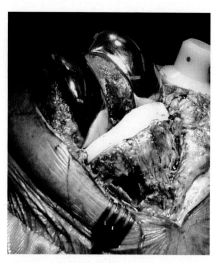

Figure 5 Intraoperative photograph shows an osteolytic lesion exposed through a window in the medial tibial plateau.

straint, then the components should be revised, even if they are well fixed. Trial inserts are used to assess the ligamentous balance of the knee. Usually an insert one or two sizes thicker than the original polyethylene is required to achieve stability.

Accessible bone defects should be débrided and packed with morcellized bone graft or filled with doughy cement using a Toomey syringe (**Figure 5**). No data are available to guide the surgeon regarding the use of cement augmentation or morcellized bone graft to treat osteolytic lesions. In general, for younger patients, who are more likely to require repeat revision surgeries in the future, it makes sense to use bone graft in an attempt to restore bone stock. In elderly, more sedentary patients, who are less likely to require a revision, cement augmentation of osteolytic defects provides immediate stability and no concerns about bone graft resorption (**Figure 6**). Another consideration is whether the osteolytic defect is contained or uncontained. With an uncontained bone defect, it is difficult to keep the morcellized bone graft within the lesion. Bone particles dislodged from the defect can create an abrasive slurry, potentially accelerating wear.

For this reason, cement augmentation may be the better option for uncontained bone defects, particularly in older patients. Both techniques have performed well at limited follow-up.

If full component revision is required because of loosening, impending failure, or instability, extensive bone loss should be anticipated (**Figure 7**). As mentioned earlier, radiographs underestimate the amount of bone loss in cases of osteolysis.

Bone defects can be treated in several ways. Small contained defects can be treated with morcellized allograft or metal augments. Larger uncontained defects can be treated with metal augments, cones or sleeves, or structural allografts. The degree of implant constraint should be tailored to the individual case. In revisions for osteolysis, the implants used should be at least posterior cruciate–substituting and should have the ability to provide varus/valgus support for an incompetent collateral ligament or to act as an internal splint for a weakened epicondyle. Stems should be used to bypass stress risers and to provide additional support for more constrained constructs.

Postoperative Regimen

The postoperative protocol for a TKA revised for osteolysis is the same for as a standard TKA, with a few caveats. Previous incisions and extensive soft-tissue dissections for synovectomy and exposure put the revised TKA at risk for wound healing problems and hematomas. Holding motion for 1 to 2 days to allow the soft tissues to recover therefore may be prudent in some cases.

Revisions for osteolysis are also associated with bone damage, which may weaken the epicondyles and their ligamentous attachments, or the tibial

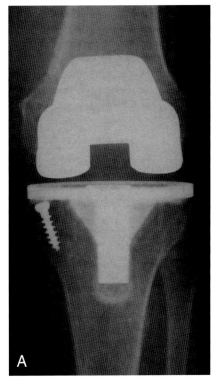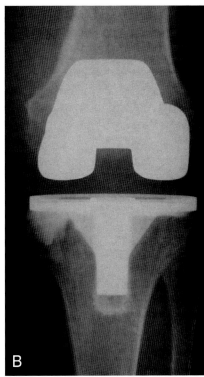

Figure 6 Radiographs of a knee revised for osteolysis of the medial tibial plateau. **A,** Preoperative AP view shows a well-fixed, well-aligned TKA. **B,** Postoperative AP radiograph shows the new polyethylene insert and cement augmentation of the osteolytic defect.

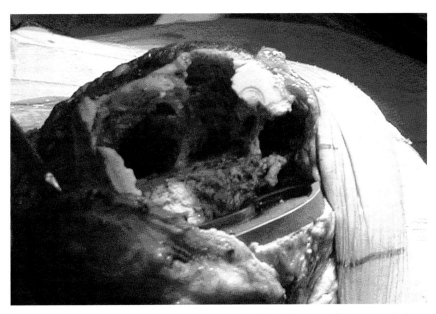

Figure 7 Intraoperative photograph shows extensive bone loss secondary to osteolysis.

tubercle, putting varus-valgus stability and the extensor mechanism at risk. Protected weight bearing for 4 to 6 weeks is recommended when con-

cern exists for fracture of the compromised bone.

Avoiding Pitfalls and Complications

The primary pitfall encountered with revision surgery for osteolysis is preoperative underestimation of bone loss. Attempting an isolated polyethylene insert exchange in patients with inadequate bony support of the components can lead to early failure. In addition, not having the appropriate equipment to deal with unexpected large structural bone defects also will lead to poor results. Preparing for worst-case scenarios is particularly important when revising TKAs for polyethylene wear and osteolysis.

———————■

Bibliography

Babis GC, Trousdale RT, Morrey BF: The effectiveness of isolated tibial insert exchange in revision total knee arthroplasty. *J Bone Joint Surg Am* 2002;84-A(1):64-68.

Burnett RS, Keeney JA, Maloney WJ, Clohisy JC: Revision total knee arthroplasty for major osteolysis. *Iowa Orthop J* 2009; 29:28-37.

Engh GA, Koralewicz LM, Pereles TR: Clinical results of modular polyethylene insert exchange with retention of total knee arthroplasty components. *J Bone Joint Surg Am* 2000;82(4):516-523.

Engh CA Jr, Sychterz CJ, Young AM, Pollock DC, Toomey SD, Engh CA Sr: Interobserver and intraobserver variability in radiographic assessment of osteolysis. *J Arthroplasty* 2002;17(6):752-759.

Fehring TK, Murphy JA, Hayes TD, Roberts DW, Pomeroy DL, Griffin WL: Factors influencing wear and osteolysis in press-fit condylar modular total knee replacements. *Clin Orthop Relat Res* 2004;428(428):40-50.

Griffin WL, Fehring TK, Pomeroy DL, Gruen TA, Murphy JA: Sterilization and wear-related failure in first- and second-generation press-fit condylar total knee arthroplasty. *Clin Orthop Relat Res* 2007;464:16-20.

Griffin WL, Scott RD, Dalury DF, Mahoney OM, Chiavetta JB, Odum SM: Modular insert exchange in knee arthroplasty for treatment of wear and osteolysis. *Clin Orthop Relat Res* 2007;464:132-137.

Suarez J, Griffin W, Springer B, Fehring T, Mason JB, Odum S: Why do revision knee arthroplasties fail? *J Arthroplasty* 2008;23(6, Suppl 1):99-103.

Wasielewski RC, Parks N, Williams I, Surprenant H, Collier JP, Engh G: Tibial insert undersurface as a contributing source of polyethylene wear debris. *Clin Orthop Relat Res* 1997;345(345):53-59.

Whiteside LA, Katerberg B: Revision of the polyethylene component for wear in TKA. *Clin Orthop Relat Res* 2006;452: 193-199.

Coding		
CPT Codes		**Corresponding ICD-9 Codes**
Revision Total Knee Arthroplasty, One Component		
27486	Revision of total knee arthroplasty, with or without allograft; one component	996.6
Revision Total Knee Arthroplasty, Multiple Components		
27487	Revision of total knee arthroplasty, with or without allograft; femoral and entire tibial component	996.6

Chapter 43

Revision Total Knee Arthroplasty: Removing the Well-Fixed Implant

Peter F. Sharkey, MD
Wadih Y. Matar, MD, MSc, FRCSC

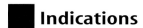 **Indications**

The burden of revision total knee arthroplasty (TKA) is projected to increase markedly over the next decade. The indications for TKA revisions are numerous and most commonly include infection, malalignment, malpositioning, instability, periprosthetic fracture, stiffness, and aseptic loosening. Removal of well-fixed implants during revision surgery is often necessary, and it is critically important that the orthopaedic surgeon use optimal techniques when removing a prosthesis before proceeding with the revision arthroplasty.

The principles of removing a well-fixed implant consist of obtaining excellent surgical exposure and then removing the implant with minimal loss of bone and without injury to ligaments, neurovascular structures, and the extensor mechanism. Iatrogenic bone loss or soft-tissue compromise can complicate the procedure and

negatively impact the results of revision arthroplasty.

Contraindications

The decision to proceed with revision TKA is made in concert with the patient and is subject to the same contraindications as a primary TKA (eg, a limb with vascular compromise). The overall condition of the patient is of prime importance; the patient's nutritional status and general medical condition should be optimized before proceeding with the revision arthroplasty. If this cannot be achieved, the patient should not be offered revision TKA. The soft tissues about the knee should be assessed. If findings are concerning, preoperative evaluation by a plastic surgeon for consideration of gastrocnemius flaps or use of a soft-tissue expander before proceeding with the planned revision TKA may be valuable.

Other contraindications include active infection in the presence of extensor mechanism incompetence.

Alternative Treatments

When revision is contraindicated, alternative treatments may be considered. These include lifelong suppressive antibiotic treatment, fusion, or amputation.

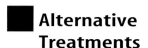

Technique

Preoperative Planning

Significant preoperative planning is important for a successful revision TKA. Before proceeding with surgery, it is critical that a specific reason for revision surgery be established and supported by objective physical, laboratory, and imaging findings, because revision for unexplained pain is rarely successful. Preoperative planning involves careful evaluation of the radiographs and records to identify the manufacturer, type, and size of the present implant. This process can be facilitated with old surgical records or

Dr. Sharkey or an immediate family member serves as a board member, owner, officer, or committee member for Physician Recommended Nutriceuticals and the American Association of Hip and Knee Surgeons; has received royalties from Stryker and Stelkast; serves as a paid consultant to or is an employee of Stryker; has received research or institutional support from Surgical Monitoring Associates, Stryker, and Stelkast; and owns stock or stock options in Cross Current, Physician Recommended Nutriceuticals, CardoMedical, and Knee Creations. Neither Dr. Matar nor any immediate family member has received anything of value from or owns stock in a commercial company or institution related directly or indirectly to the subject of this chapter.

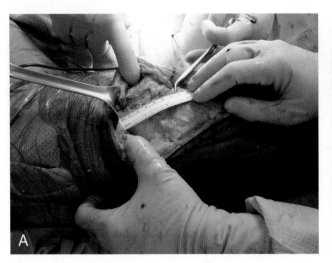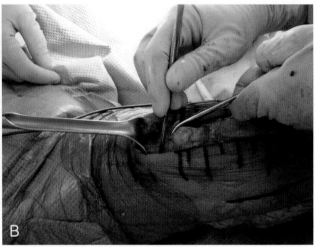

Figure 1 Quadriceps snip procedure. **A,** The medial parapatellar arthrotomy is extended proximally through the quadriceps tendon and at a level 5 to 7 cm proximal to the superior patellar pole. **B,** An oblique snip is made in the fibers of the vastus lateralis.

a review of the implant labels from the index procedure. The surgical notes should be examined for any intraoperative problems encountered during the index procedure, such as soft-tissue disruption. If the old surgical notes are not available and the surgeon cannot identify the implant from radiographs, we recommend comparing the radiographs to an implant atlas or showing them to manufacturers' representatives or other orthopaedic surgeons for identification. This is especially important when dealing with modular stemmed implants and hinged components.

Radiographs also should be examined for areas of osteolysis and bone loss as well as for overall limb and component alignment, joint line position, and component loosening. A CT scan may be used to better delineate the areas of bone loss and to assess component rotation.

Instruments and Equipment Required

The specific extraction instruments for the present implant, if they exist, should be available, in addition to the usual equipment needed for implant removal. Standard implant removal equipment includes, but is not limited to, osteotomes, various saws (Gigli

and power saws), burrs, metal-cutting disks, punches, and ultrasonic tools for cement removal.

Setup/Exposure

On the day of the surgery, the patient should be reexamined under anesthesia to assess knee stability and range of motion. More important, before preparing and draping is completed, the surgeon should carefully assess the knee for previous incisions and determine if an old incision can and should be used. When multiple parallel incisions are present, to minimize the chance of skin necrosis, we routinely use the most lateral incision possible because most of the vascular supply originates medially. In addition, more recent incisions should be favored because collateral circulation will have had less opportunity to develop. In exceptional circumstances, a sham incision can be considered, but in practice this is rarely necessary. It is important to note that so-called minimally invasive incisions do not have a role in the revision setting; a 20- to 25-cm incision often is required to visualize the knee optimally and perform the revision procedure safely.

The patient is placed in the supine position on the operating room table as for a primary TKA, and tourniquet

control is used when possible. A foot bump is placed under the calf muscle, allowing the limb to rest with minimal support with the knee at near-maximal flexion. The knee is usually approached through a standard medial parapatellar arthrotomy, and extensor mechanism tenolysis and synovectomy are usually performed. This routine exposure often is sufficient for a straightforward revision procedure; however, some revisions (eg, those performed for infection, stiffness, or for removal of a stemmed implant) may be more complicated and necessitate a more extensile exposure with proximal or distal exposure enhancement techniques.

The options for increasing exposure proximally include a quadriceps snip (**Figure 1**) or V-Y quadricepsplasty. Both techniques allow for lengthening of the extensor mechanism in a very stiff knee; with the V-Y lengthening procedure, however, weight bearing and flexion should be restricted postoperatively to allow the quadricepsplasty to heal properly. Even with these restrictions, an extensor lag is still a common residual finding. With a quadriceps snip, on the other hand, the patient can follow a standard postoperative protocol, including full range of motion and immediate full weight bearing.

Distal exposure can be enhanced with a tibial tubercle osteotomy. A tibial tubercle osteotomy should be considered for removal of a long-stemmed component. In all these techniques, protecting the patellar tendon and its insertion is of paramount importance. A headed pin can be placed through the tendon insertion if the surgeon believes that the tendon is at risk of avulsion.

Following the standard arthrotomy, cautery is used to perform careful dissection around the implant to expose the bone-cement interface for a cemented prosthesis and the bone-implant interface for an uncemented prosthesis. We also routinely perform a complete synovectomy, using sharp dissection, and reestablish the medial and lateral gutters. The patellar implant usually is dissected with the patella everted and extensor mechanism subluxated laterally. This should be done carefully to avoid an avulsion of the patellar tendon. If patellar eversion is required but is very difficult, the surgeon can use one of the above-mentioned enhancement techniques to improve visualization.

Procedure

UNSTEMMED COMPONENTS

Surgeons should not attempt to remove a component until the exposure is optimized and the implant interface is completely identified. The tibial polyethylene component is usually removed first, allowing better exposure of both femoral and tibial implants and lowering the tension on the soft tissues. The removal technique to be used depends on the particular locking mechanism of the polyethylene insert, as some inserts are fixed to the baseplate with a clip or a screw. Ordering the proper instruments preoperatively facilitates this task. Most polyethylene inserts can be removed by inserting a narrow osteotome between the polyethylene and the tibial base-

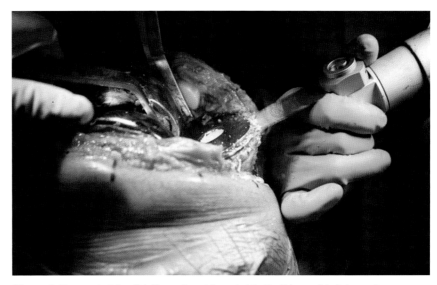

Figure 2 Removal of the tibial baseplate. A broad, thin, flexible saw blade is used to separate the undersurface of the tibial baseplate from the underlying cement. In areas unreachable with a saw, straight, thin osteotomes are used to complete the separation.

plate and levering out the insert, but some designs have a reinforcing metal pin in the post that may require removal before the insert can be levered out. A saw can be used to cut the polyethylene post, exposing the pin, which then can be removed with pliers.

When the tibial baseplate requires removal, we favor removing it before addressing the femoral component because the retained femoral implant will protect the bone when the retractors are placed against the distal femur to subluxate the tibia anteriorly. The retractor rests on the metal implant instead of the native osteoporotic bone. With the proximal tibia well exposed, a lateral finger retractor is used to subluxate the patella laterally. The undersurface of the tibial baseplate is then freed from the bone or cement using a combination of an oscillating saw blade and straight osteotomes. A broad, thin, flexible saw blade is first used at the visualized cement-implant interface on the undersurface of the tibial implant (**Figure 2**). Caution must be exercised to protect the surrounding soft tissues, particularly the patellar tendon. The posterior aspect

of the tibial implant must be visualized to avoid plunging posteriorly toward the neurovascular structures. The posterior and posterolateral areas of the cement-implant interface usually are not accessible with the saw because the central peg of the implant is in the way. A 0.25- or 0.5-in straight osteotome is used from a medial to lateral direction to complete the separation of the cement from the implant. Once the undersurface is freed, the tibia is subluxated anteriorly and the knee is hyperflexed to allow removal of the tibial component without it catching or being impeded by the femoral component. If the surgeon anticipates that the removal path of the tibial implant will be hindered by the femur, the femoral implant can be removed before removal of the tibial implant. The femoral bone can be protected from retractors by preparing a "sponge cushion." Most unstemmed tibial baseplates can be removed with the gentle use of a slap hammer extraction device or with a punch. Excessive force should be avoided, as this may lead to an iatrogenic fracture or bone loss of the osteopenic proximal tibia. The surgeon should remove the implant by using forces directed perpendicular to

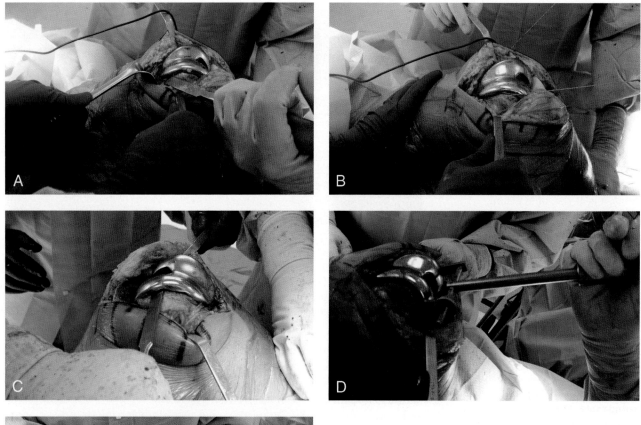

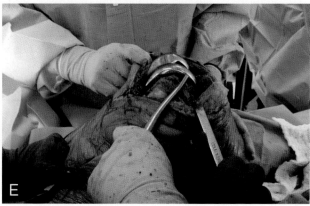

Figure 3 Removal of the femoral component. **A,** A 0.5-in osteotome is used to create a slot for insertion of a Gigli saw between the cement and the proximal flange of the femoral prosthesis on the anterior aspect of the distal femur. **B,** The surgeon must continuously pull up firmly against the implant with the Gigli saw to avoid migration of the saw blade into the bone, causing excessive bone loss. **C,** Osteotomes are used from both the medial and lateral sides, parallel to the undersurface of the femoral implant. The femoral implant is removed gently with the use of an extraction device (**D**) or by using light taps with a punch (**E**). Asymmetric implant removal should be avoided, as it may cause the implant to wedge and result in bone fracture.

the center of the tibial plate as much as possible to avoid making the component tilt and wedge in the cement mantle. If the implant does not dislodge easily, osteotomes are used again. Broad osteotomes can be stacked to facilitate removal of a well-fixed implant. Usually this technique results in little bone damage; however, care must be taken to avoid tibial plateau fracture during stacking. The surgeon should avoid using excessive force or levering

the implant with the osteotome, as this may lead to fracture. After the implant is removed, a burr and cement grabber combination is used to remove cement from the metaphyseal tibia. Alternatively, the cement mantle can be removed with small curved osteotomes, placing the curvature toward the cement mantle. Standard reverse curets commonly used in revision hip arthroplasty or ultrasonic equipment also may be helpful.

The femoral component is addressed only after excellent visualization of its bone-cement-prosthesis interface has been achieved. The component removal can be performed by using a 0.5-in osteotome to create a slot between the cement and the proximal flange of the femoral prosthesis on the anterior aspect of the distal femur (**Figure 3,** *A*). Once the slot is created, a Gigli saw is introduced through the slot to free up the under-

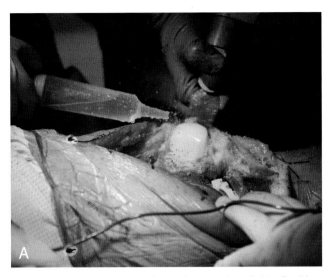 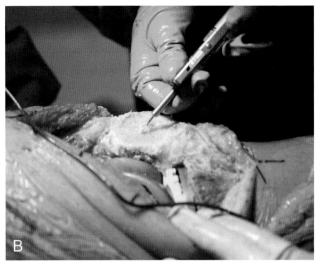

Figure 4 Removal of the patellar implant. **A,** A broad, thin, flexible saw blade can be used to remove an all-polyethylene patellar component with little bone loss. **B,** A pencil-tip burr is used to remove the sawed-off polyethylene pegs and cement from the patellar bone.

surface of the anterior femoral component from the underlying cement (or bone, if the implant is uncemented). While using the Gigli saw, the surgeon must continuously pull up firmly against the implant with the saw to avoid excessive bone loss (**Figure 3,** *B*). A combination of curved, narrow osteotomes is then used to debond the cement from the undersurface of the femoral condyles and around the pegs of the femoral implant if any are present. Once again, the surgeon should be careful to protect the posterior neurovascular structures; good visualization is needed to avoid overly deep osteotome insertion. The osteotomes are used from both the medial and lateral sides, parallel to the undersurface of the implant (**Figure 3,** *C*). Transverse use of the osteotomes across both condyles should be avoided, as this may risk crushing of the underlying bone as the trochlear groove directs the osteotome into the bone. Once the debonding of the implant is completed, the femoral implant can be removed gently by hand or by light tapping with an extraction device (**Figure 3,** *D*) or punch (**Figure 3,** *E*). Asymmetric force should be avoided when removing the implant, as this may cause wedging, which can fracture the

bone. Once the implant is removed, cement can be removed from the distal femur using the techniques described for the tibia. It may not be necessary to remove well-fixed cement unless infection is present or the cement interferes with proper placement of the new implant.

Revising the patellar implant should be done cautiously, as this may result in thin osteopenic patellar bone that is recalcitrant to reconstruction. Surgeons should consider not revising well-fixed patellar implants that have minimal wear. The ease of patellar implant removal depends greatly on the implant design. All-polyethylene patellar buttons usually can be removed by using a broad, thin, flexible saw blade at the bone-cement interface (**Figure 4,** *A*). The pegs are sawed off, and the remaining cemented plugs are then removed using a pencil-tip burr (**Figure 4,** *B*). Metal-backed patellar implants are more difficult to remove. A metal-backed and well-fixed patellar component is best removed using a diamond cutting wheel to cut the implant free of bone and fixation pegs. The pegs generally can be left in the remaining patellar bone, and a new all-polyethylene patellar implant can be cemented around them. Alterna-

tively, if the pegs need to be removed, such as in cases of infection, this can be accomplished by using a pencil-tip burr.

Uncemented TKA implants can be removed using a procedure similar to that described previously; however, instead of working at the implant-cement interface, the surgeon works at the implant-bone interface. Of note, some uncemented tibial trays made with trabecular metal have two pegs that can be severed from the baseplate by cutting them with a large, broad osteotome. This should be done carefully in osteopenic bone, as the osteotome can push the whole tibial implant posteriorly through the proximal tibial bone. An alternative and safer method is to cut the pegs with a thin oscillating saw blade.

STEMMED COMPONENTS

Removing long-stemmed components is often challenging and requires careful preoperative planning. Implant extraction should start with removal of the polyethylene insert. If the insert is of the semiconstrained or hinged type, it should be disassembled using the manufacturer's recommended technique and instruments for that particular design. Tapered cemented stems usually have a smooth surface, which facilitates their removal from the cement. If a stem offset device is present, however, its irregular shape may interface with the cement in a manner that makes removal very difficult. The offset mechanism may need to be exposed via a bone window. Once the component is removed, cement is subsequently removed using techniques similar to those described for cemented total hip arthroplasty. If the stem is well fixed or if it is of the uncemented variety, however, it may be advantageous to disassemble the stem from the articular component to allow access to the stem-cement or stem-bone interface, greatly facilitating its removal. Some manufacturers' designs allow for disassembly of the stem from the articulating part of the implant, whereas in others, a metal-cutting burr or diamond disk may be needed to separate the stem from the articulating part of the implant. Knowledge of the design nuances of a particular implant is critical, and having the appropriate instruments can make the surgeon's job much easier. Once exposed, the well-fixed stem is removed with the use of burrs, osteotomes, trephine reamers, or ultrasonic tools. Some manufacturers produce specialized stem-extraction tools.

On occasion, an osteotomy may be required to remove a well-fixed stem. A tibial tubercle osteotomy can be performed to remove the difficult well-fixed tibial stem. This is performed by making an 8- to 10-cm–long x 1- to 1.5-cm–thick osteotomy of the tibial tubercle with the help of a saw and broad osteotomes. The surgeon must be careful not to disrupt the lateral soft tissues so that the osteotomy can be hinged on this tissue-preserving blood supply to the osteotomized bone. Furthermore, by maintaining the lateral soft-tissue sleeve, the osteotomy is easier to reattach. Once the osteotomy is made, access to the tibial stem is

easy, and the stem can be removed with osteotomes and burrs. Closure of the osteotomy can be achieved with a variety of methods using either screws or multiple wires and cables.

———————————■

■ Postoperative Regimen

Postoperative activity restrictions should be tailored to intraoperative assessment of soft-tissue quality, knee range of motion, and the exposure method used. If the arthrotomy closure is secure and little tension is placed on the repair with flexion, no restrictions are needed and aggressive physical therapy can be pursued; however, revision TKA often has the associated challenge of poor tissue quality and limited preoperative range of motion. In this situation, the surgeon should inspect the arthrotomy suture line and note the amount of flexion possible without jeopardizing the repair. Flexion should be limited postoperatively to a degree consistent with this intraoperative finding. If a quadriceps snip is performed, no additional precautions need to be instituted. If a V-Y lengthening is performed, however, no range of motion should be allowed for the first 2 weeks after surgery. After this period, the motion allowed should again be titrated to the intraoperative assessment. A knee immobilizer is necessary for all ambulation for 6 weeks after surgery. Likewise, if a tibial tubercle osteotomy is performed, the surgeon must carefully judge the quality of repaired bone and the rigidity of fixation. In general, after tibial tubercle osteotomy, no motion is allowed for the first 2 weeks following surgery. Then, gentle range-of-motion exercises are allowed, but only by a skilled therapist aware of the patient's complex situation. Again,

just as with V-Y lengthening, immediate weight bearing is allowed, but a knee immobilizer must be used during ambulation for the first 6 postoperative weeks.

———————————■

■ Avoiding Pitfalls and Complications

Successful TKA revision depends on proper preoperative planning. Patients should be properly assessed and the indications for revision well established; infection as a cause of failure needs to be considered in all cases. Furthermore, the surgeon should ensure that all equipment that could possibly facilitate performance of the procedure is available before surgery.

Intraoperatively, the key principle is to obtain excellent exposure and avoid insufficient incisions. Compromise of soft-tissue structures, bone loss, and fractures may be avoided by gentle and optimal use of extraction instruments. Furthermore, it is of prime importance to protect the extensor mechanism and avoid avulsion of the patellar tendon by using the techniques outlined previously. All components should be debonded carefully to minimize bone loss and should be removed gently; excessive force should be avoided at all times, as it may lead to iatrogenic fracture of osteopenic bone. Whenever TKA components are removed, a substantial amount of bone, cement, metal, and polyethylene debris is generated. These particles are inflammatory and may cause third-body wear of the revision components. Copious irrigation and covering of exposed soft tissue and bone with moistened sponges prevents the inadvertent retention of unwanted debris in the knee joint.

———————————■

■ Bibliography

Dennis DA: Removal of well-fixed cementless metal-backed patellar components. *J Arthroplasty* 1992;7(2):217-220.

Firestone TP, Krackow KA: Removal of femoral components during revision knee arthroplasty. *J Bone Joint Surg Br* 1991;73(3):514-515.

Garvin KL, Scuderi G, Insall JN: Evolution of the quadriceps snip. *Clin Orthop Relat Res* 1995;321:131-137.

Ghanem E, Parvizi J, Burnett RS, et al: Cell count and differential of aspirated fluid in the diagnosis of infection at the site of total knee arthroplasty. *J Bone Joint Surg Am* 2008;90(8):1637-1643.

Klein GR, Levine HB, Hartzband MA: Removal of a well-fixed trabecular metal monoblock tibial component. *J Arthroplasty* 2008;23(4):619-622.

Kurtz SM, Ong KL, Schmier J, et al: Future clinical and economic impact of revision total hip and knee arthroplasty. *J Bone Joint Surg Am* 2007;89(Suppl 3):144-151.

Sharkey PF, Homesley HD, Shastri S, Jacoby SM, Hozack WJ, Rothman RH: Results of revision total knee arthroplasty after exposure of the knee with extensor mechanism tenolysis. *J Arthroplasty* 2004;19(6):751-756.

Sharkey PF, Hozack WJ, Rothman RH, Shastri S, Jacoby SM: Insall Award paper: Why are total knee arthroplasties failing today? *Clin Orthop Relat Res* 2002;404:7-13.

Whaley AL, Trousdale RT, Rand JA, Hanssen AD: Cemented long-stem revision total knee arthroplasty. *J Arthroplasty* 2003;18(5):592-599.

Whiteside LA, Ohl MD: Tibial tubercle osteotomy for exposure of the difficult total knee arthroplasty. *Clin Orthop Relat Res* 1990;260:6-9.

Coding

CPT Codes		Corresponding ICD-9 Codes	
Revision Total Knee Arthroplasty			
27487	Revision of total knee arthroplasty, with or without allograft; femoral and entire tibial component	996.4 996.77 715	996.6 996.78
Removal of Prosthesis When Done Separately From Revision*			
27488	Removal of prosthesis, including total knee prosthesis, methylmethacrylate with or without insertion of spacer, knee	996.4 996.77	996.6 996.78

*If prosthesis removal is done at the same time as the revision, it is included in the revision.
CPT copyright © 2010 by the American Medical Association. All rights reserved.

Chapter 44

Revision Total Knee Arthroplasty: Patellar Treatment

R. Stephen J. Burnett, MD, FRCSC
Robert L. Barrack, MD

Indications

The patella is frequently the last component addressed at the time of revision total knee arthroplasty (TKA), and therefore it is often neglected. Many studies on revision TKA do not even address the method of patellar treatment. Many patients who undergo a revision TKA will have had anterior knee pain or other symptoms preoperatively, and therefore the extensor mechanism and patellofemoral tracking should be evaluated carefully. Poor extensor mechanism function following revision TKA is a leading cause of persistent pain, limited function, and a compromised result.

Contraindications

Contraindications to revision of the patellar component at the time of revision TKA include concurrent infection of the TKA, lack of availability of appropriate patellar implants and instrumentation, and a patient who is medically unfit to undergo revision surgery. Isolated failure of the patellar component should alert the surgeon to seek a cause for the failure, such as femoral or tibial component internal malrotation, and to perform further investigations. In a patient with a painful TKA and anterior knee pain with a resurfaced patella, the cause of the anterior knee pain (component malposition, osteonecrosis, aseptic loosening, or occult periprosthetic fracture) must be determined before considering a revision procedure. In a patient with an extensor lag, the etiology of the extensor mechanism disruption must be determined preoperatively and a plan developed to reconstruct the extensor mechanism and not just the patella at the time of revision.

Alternative Treatments

Alternatives to revision of the patellar component include retention, if the component is well fixed, or resection arthroplasty of the patella, if insufficient bone remains for component revision (**Figure 1**). There is substantial dispute in the literature regarding the results of a resection arthroplasty of the patella, which has been variously called patellaplasty, patellar resection arthroplasty, patellar component resection, and patellar bony shell. In this procedure, the patella is contoured to remove sharp or eccentric bone edges and to facilitate central patellar tracking within the femoral trochlea. Although the procedure is done frequently, in our experience, the results are often unpredictable; patellar fragmentation, lateral subluxation of the remnant, and persistent anterior knee pain may be seen. It appears that patients treated with isolated patellar resection arthroplasty are more likely to have continuing pain and require reoperation compared with patients who had concomitant revision of the tibial and femoral components. Patellar component resection without reimplantation is a reasonable approach for patients with markedly compromised patellar bone stock; however, persistent anterior knee pain may be expected approximately one third of the time.

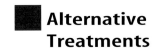

Dr. Burnett or an immediate family member serves as a paid consultant to or is an employee of Smith & Nephew. Dr. Barrack or an immediate family member serves as a board member, owner, officer, or committee member of the American Association of Hip and Knee Surgeons and the American Orthopaedic Association; has received royalties from Smith & Nephew; and has received research or institutional support from Medtronic Sofamor Danek and Smith & Nephew.

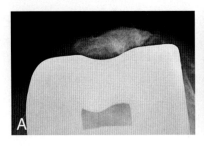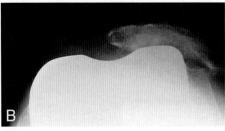

Figure 1 Axial views after patellar resection arthroplasty show normal tracking of the retained shell (**A**) and lateral maltracking and fragmentation (**B**).

Table 1 Results of Patellar Treatment in Revision Total Knee Arthroplasty

Author(s) (Year)	Number of Knees	Procedure	Mean Patient Age (Range)	Mean Follow-up (Range)	Results/Conclusions
Buechel (1991)	7	Iliac crest bone graft	NR	75.4 months (24-125)	Good to excellent results in 6/7.*
Barrack et al (1998)	113	21 resections of patellar component with retention of bony shell 92 retained patellar components	2.5 years (2-4)	NR	Resection of patellar component with retention of a bony shell was associated with problems including stairs, satisfaction, and return to activities.
Barrack et al (2000)	73	34 well-fixed components retained 39 revised	69	36 months (24-54)	No difference in KSS scores, SF-36, satisfaction
Hanssen (2001)	9	Impaction grafting into a patellar shell covered by a tissue flap	66 (45-76)	37 months (24-55)	Case series. Technique of impaction grafting into a patellar shell covered by a tissue flap. Simple to perform, does not require sophisticated instrumentation or a long learning curve. An important addition to the options for patellar treatment.
Leopold et al (2003)	40	Isolated patellar revision	63 (32-79)	5 years (2-11)	15 failed; 8 of these required a total of 12 additional operations. Elements of the implant design and component alignment contributed to the patellar component failure. In 25 that did not fail, mean HSS score at final follow-up was 87.
Lonner et al (2003)	202	Retained all-polyethylene patellar components	71 (19-83)	7 years (2-14)	21 had anterior knee pain. Inferior results when the patellar component has been gamma irradiated in air.
Nelson et al (2003)	20	Resurfacing with trabecular metal patellar shell	70 (38-83)	23 months (12-35)	Good or excellent results in 17/20.

NR = not reported, KSS = Knee Society score, SF-36 = Short-Form 36, TKA = total knee arthroplasty, HSS = Hospital for Special Surgery score.
 * Patellar shell must not be fractured and must be of sufficient quality to accept screw purchase; extensor mechanism must be in continuity.

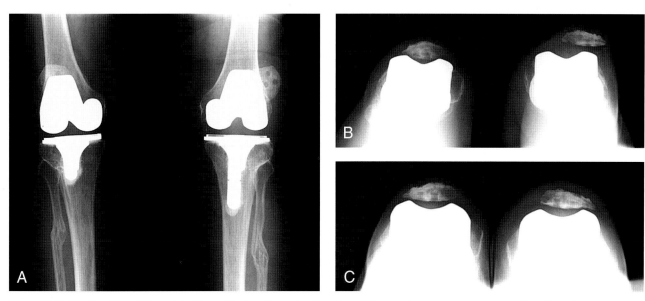

Figure 2 Isolated revision of the patella. The patient had lateral maltracking of the patella secondary to a malpositioned patellar component, as shown on the preoperative AP (**A**) and axial (**B**) radiographs. The rotation of the tibial and femoral components was normal on preoperative CT scan. **C,** Postoperative axial view following an isolated patellar revision demonstrates central patellar tracking.

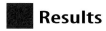 ## Results

Table 1 lists details for the studies summarized below.

Isolated Patellar Revision

Leopold and associates found that isolated patellar revision, with or without concurrent lateral retinacular release, was associated with a high rate of reoperation and complications and a relatively low rate of success. This procedure, while occasionally necessary, is rarely performed (**Figure 2**). When considering an isolated patellar revision, the surgeon must evaluate the etiology of the patellar component failure.

Retaining a Well-Fixed Component

The results of retaining a well-fixed patellar component in revision TKA when residual bone is thin and prone to fracture with component removal have been favorable. The fact that the component is not worn at the time of revision indicates that the extensor mechanism is probably reasonably well balanced, and this probably also explains why retained components continue to do well subsequent to the revision procedure. Lonner and associates noted that failures due to loosening or wear were related to whether the polyethylene component had been gamma irradiated in air, which was associated with oxidation and failure of the patellar implant. A manufacturing mismatch is acceptable with most contemporary component designs, provided that the patellar component articulates properly and that the extensor mechanism tracking is neutral.

Resection Arthroplasty of the Patella

Barrack and associates compared 21 knees that had a shell of bone left during revision TKA because of inadequate residual patellar bone with 92 knees that had a patellar component in place after revision TKA. Although the consensus of recent studies of patellar resection arthroplasties is that retaining a shell of bone is an acceptable alternative, the authors found a relatively high incidence of persistent symptoms, lateral patellar sublux-

ation, and fragmentation. These outcomes appear to be suboptimal and have led other authors to seek alternative approaches for these patients.

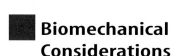 ## Biomechanical Considerations

The patella acts as a dynamic fulcrum to transmit the forces generated by the extensor mechanism through the knee, and it may be responsible for providing up to a 50% increase in knee extension. The contraction of the quadriceps mechanism has been associated with contact pressures exceeding 6.5 times body weight at the patellofemoral joint. It has been proposed that anterior knee pain following TKA may in fact be secondary to altered biomechanics at the patellofemoral joint. Increased patellofemoral joint forces are present with increased degrees of flexion, which is one measure of success in TKA outcome. It has been shown that higher flexion concentrates forces on the superolateral and medial facets of the patella. The resurfaced patella has been reported to be subjected to increased strain and decreased tensile strength by as much as 30% to 40%. The decreased thickness of bone, combined with osteopenia, may predispose the resurfaced patella to fracture. This may be worsened when combined with a lateral retinacular release, which may devascularize the extensor mechanism. Thus, multiple biomechanical factors may contribute to patellar component or host bone stresses in association with a TKA.

Techniques

Preoperative Planning

Before selecting a treatment method for a problematic patella in TKA, the surgeon should focus on femoral and tibial component rotation, as incorrect rotation may be the primary reason for failure of the patellar implant. Careful preoperative planning, effective intraoperative decision making, and availability of specialized implants, instruments, and bone grafting techniques will optimize patellar revision options. During the planning process, implant stability and the type of existing implants should be evaluated. Remaining host bone stock should be assessed, as management of a deficient patella with poor remaining bone stock is particularly challenging.

Surgical Considerations

EXPOSURE

The first priority in the treatment of the patella in revision TKA is to avoid extensor mechanism disruption in the form of either a patellar tendon avulsion or patellar fracture. This begins with the surgical approach to the knee. Eversion of the patella is necessary to assess the status of the patellar implant and to proceed with the definitive treatment. This should be accomplished in a careful, sequential man-

ner. The patella should not be immediately everted while flexing the knee past 90°, as is often possible in a primary TKA. The gutters should be cleared of adhesions, particularly on the lateral side. The patella should be placed under tension with a laterally directed retractor while adhesions are released, starting with the patellofemoral ligament. We recommend placing a headed pin through the patellar tendon just proximal to the tibial tubercle before flexing the knee, to act as a stress reliever and minimize the risk of avulsion. This also focuses the surgeon's attention on the patellar tendon insertion so that inadvertent avulsion is less likely. Once the adhesions have been completely released down to the periphery of the lateral tibial plateau and between the proximal tibia and patellar tendon down to the level of the insertion of the tibial tubercle, an attempt can be made to evert the patella while gently flexing the knee. Externally rotating the knee and foot helps to further reduce the tension on the patellar tendon during knee flexion. Complete eversion of the patella is rarely required for exposure, and the patella may be partially everted or slid laterally (without complete eversion) to provide similar exposure with less stress on the extensor mechanism. If undue tension on the patellar tendon insertion is still apparent with attempted patellar eversion or patellar slide, an alternative surgical approach should be considered. The options include a rectus snip with or without a lateral release, partial or complete V-Y quadricepsplasty, or tibial tubercle osteotomy. The vascular supply to the patella and the risk of osteonecrosis must be considered when selecting one of these alternative exposures.

EXTENSOR MECHANISM CONSIDERATIONS

After the patella has been everted, the interface between the patellar component and the underlying bone must be

everted. Frequently this interface is obscured by overlying fibrous tissue/meniscus. This should be circumferentially removed and the interface examined. An osteotome can be placed under the patellar component to determine if it can be levered out; however, levering on a thin patellar remnant may cause iatrogenic injury or fracture and should be avoided if the component appears well fixed. Occasionally, a component that appears well fixed radiographically will prove to be loose when tested in this manner. If the patella is not loose radiographically or at intraoperative testing, a decision must be made as to whether there are other indications for removal of the component.

After a definitive method of patellar treatment has been elected, the final surgical consideration is ensuring optimal tracking of the extensor mechanism. This is equally important regardless of the method of patellar treatment elected. The major methods of optimizing tracking include attaining appropriate rotation of the prosthesis and external rotation of the femoral and tibial components. This is most reliably obtained in the revision situation by aligning the femoral component with the epicondyles. Internal rotation of the tibial component should be avoided. Generally, alignment of the midportion of the tibial component just medial to the midpoint of the tibial tubercle will position the component appropriately. If the extensor mechanism does not track centrally, the femoral and tibial component rotation should be carefully reassessed with these landmarks in mind, as the magnitude of the combined internal rotation of the implants has been shown to be directly proportional to the degree of patellar maltracking on radiographs. In one study of patellar dislocation in TKA, patellar tracking improved only after soft-tissue realignment in combination with revision of malaligned or loose components. Although revision significantly improved active knee extension and Knee Society scores, two thirds of the patients had residual disabilities and pain.

Certain extremes of component positioning can place undue stress on the extensor mechanism. If the anterior flange of the femoral component is flexed so that the flange is not flush with the femoral cortex, this will increase the forces on the extensor mechanism during knee flexion. Elevation of the joint line will produce a similar effect. If a very thick tibial polyethylene tibial insert is used and there is undue stress on the extensor mechanism with knee flexion, the position of the patella relative to the joint line should be carefully assessed. The joint line is normally approximately 1.5 to 2.0 cm above the fibular head, and in extension, the inferior pole of the patella should be approximately 2 cm proximal to the surface of the tibial insert (range, 1 to 4 cm on lateral radiograph). If a thick tibial insert is necessary to obtain stability in extension and results in a relative patellar baja, consideration should be given to using distal femoral augments and a thinner tibial insert to effectively lower the joint line.

TREATMENT-SPECIFIC CONSIDERATIONS
Once the patellar component has been adequately exposed and its fixation status has been assessed, a decision must be made regarding the optimal method of treatment of the patella. If removal of the femoral component is elected, there are certain surgical technique considerations. The patellar component should be stabilized with care, usually with towel clips through the quadriceps and patellar tendons, to avoid clipping and tension at the insertion of these tendons onto the patella. If the remaining patellar component bone is overly thick (>15 mm), it may be possible to simply take a saw and undercut the pegs of the component, but this is rarely feasible. A well-fixed all-polyethylene patellar compo-

nent, however, can still be removed by placing a saw blade right at the implant-bone interface and sawing off the polyethylene from the pegs. The cement and pegs may then be removed with narrow sharp osteotomes or a pencil-tipped burr, with care being taken not to fragment the residual patellar bone. Well-fixed polyethylene cemented pegs can be efficiently removed by drilling the center of the peg with a sharp drill bit; this should be performed with caution, to avoid perforation through the anterior cortex and further stress-riser creation in the patella. This technique will remove the polyethylene from the cement, and the cement may then be removed with sharp curets and small osteotomes, again with care being taken not to fragment the bone.

When a metal-backed component is removed, it is usually easier to first remove the polyethylene from the metal. Cemented metal-backed components are carefully removed with osteotomes around the periphery. The most difficult component to remove is the bone-ingrown metal-backed component. A diamond-wheel cutting tool is used to side-cut the lugs at the junction of the baseplate. If the revision is for an aseptic diagnosis, leaving the well-fixed lugs in place and cementing the revision component over the host bone and lugs has been described. Certain metal-backed patellar component designs are extremely difficult to remove without loss of significant patellar bone. In this situation, sectioning the metal baseplate has been suggested as a method of minimizing the risk of patellar fracture during component removal. Metal-backed patellar components should be removed when the components show significant polyethylene wear, component malposition, or extensive underlying osteolysis. If the component is metal-backed and does not have these characteristics, then it may be reasonable to maintain the implant if the

tracking and geometry of the components are suitable.

The most commonly selected options for treating the patella in revision TKA are to leave a well-fixed patellar component in place (used in 30% to 50% of knees) or to revise the patellar component to one that is specific for the revision component being implanted. After patellar component removal, the residual bone may not be sufficient to allow implantation of a standard three-peg patellar component. Generally, if 10 mm or more of bone is remaining throughout the patella, adequate implant fixation may be obtained with an all-polyethylene onlay cemented implant. When less than 10 mm of bone remains, the options include using a special biconvex revision component, leaving the residual bone unresurfaced, using a "crossed Kirschner wire" technique to reinforce a cemented central-peg patella, impaction grafting using a bone graft contained in a synovial pouch, a trabecular metal patella that has both bone and soft-tissue ingrowth potential, and using the so-called gull-wing osteotomy. Finally, occasionally a patient with a TKA will have had a prior patellectomy. Surgical considerations for these various scenarios are described below.

Treatment Options
ISOLATED REVISION OF A FAILED PATELLAR COMPONENT
The patient who presents with a failed patellar component in association with a TKA should be evaluated carefully. The temptation to proceed with an isolated revision of the patellar component should be undertaken with caution, as this procedure is associated with poor results in a substantial percentage of cases, likely secondary to unrecognized component malrotation. If the decision is made to proceed, the patient should be counseled that despite this being an isolated patellar revision (or "smaller" surgical procedure), the complication

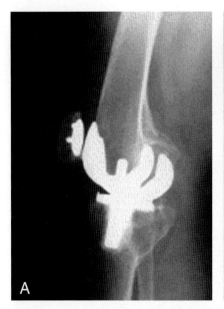 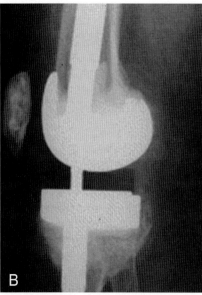

Figure 3 Revision TKA in a knee with a metal-backed patellar component and adequate bone. **A,** Lateral radiograph demonstrates a well-fixed metal-backed patellar component and the adequate bone (>10 mm) to support a revision component. Because of the poor track record of metal-backed components and the presence of sufficient residual bone, revision to a cemented all-polyethylene component was performed. **B,** Postoperative lateral view.

rate and patient satisfaction after surgery are often disappointing for both patient and surgeon.

A thorough evaluation should be performed to search for a primary mode of failure or extensor/component malalignment. A careful clinical history and physical examination and serial radiographs should be obtained. Radiographs obtained before the index arthroplasty are useful to assess the preoperative tracking of the native patella. If patellar maltracking, subluxation, or dislocation is present, the axial rotation of the tibial and femoral components should be evaluated on a CT scan. If the combined measurements of the components represent an abnormal degree of internal rotation, revision of the femoral and/or tibial components to restore extensor mechanism tracking and create patellofemoral stresses closer to normal will be required.

RETAINING A WELL-FIXED PATELLAR COMPONENT

Retaining a patellar component that is not loose has several distinct advantages, including eliminating the risk of patellar fracture during component removal, retaining the maximal patellar bone stock and thus minimizing the risk of subsequent patellar fracture, decreased surgical time, and elimination of the additional component expense. There are several prerequisites to retention of a well-fixed component. First, the fixation must be verified both on the preoperative radiographs and at the time of surgery. Any component with evidence of loosening or significant osteolysis should be removed, and if infection is present, the component and underlying cement should be removed. If the component has gross evidence of surface damage, it should also be revised. If the patellar component is well fixed, minimally damaged, and tracks well, it must be geometrically compatible with the femoral component in order to be retained. This is usually the case, as most patellar components are symmetric domes that are compatible with the trochlear flange of the vast majority of femoral components.

Retaining a well-fixed metal-backed patellar component is contro-

versial. Rarely, a metal-backed component will accept a new polyethylene insert, and an exchange procedure may be performed for wear. More commonly, if significant wear occurs, the femoral component becomes damaged and burnished, metallosis occurs, and a complete revision of all components is necessary. Nonetheless, the etiology of patellar polyethylene wear should be sought, and component rotation and/or extensor mechanism malalignment should be suspected and investigated. Most metal-backed patellar components have had a relatively high failure rate. For this reason alone, some authors have recommended revision of all metal-backed patellar components at the time of revision surgery. If the residual bone is sufficiently thick so that at least 10 mm of bone will remain after removal of a metal-backed component, then revision to a cemented all-polyethylene component is preferable (**Figure 3**). If, however, the metal-backed component is well fixed, the residual bone is already <10 mm in thickness, and there has not been substantial wear, removal of such a metal-backed component is probably not advisable (**Figure 4**).

When a component is revised, adequate bone for interdigitation of cement must be present so that early loosening does not occur. The resurfaced patella should be a consistent thickness, and it has been suggested that a caliper be used to ensure that the thickness of the patella is within 2 mm by medial, lateral, proximal, and distal measurements. In many cases, the residual patellar bone is deficient and is not amenable to implantation of a standard three-peg patellar component, so the deficient patellar bone must be managed.

TECHNIQUES FOR TREATING THE DEFICIENT PATELLA

In our experience, approximately 10 mm of residual patellar bone is necessary to provide adequate support for

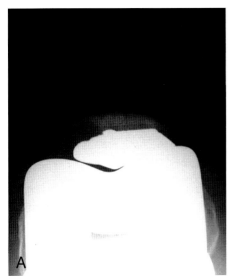
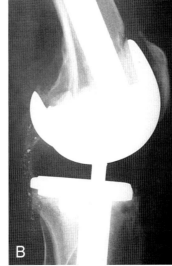
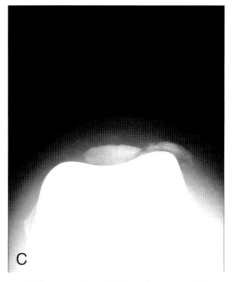

Figure 4 Revision TKA in a knee with a metal-backed patellar component and insufficient bone. **A,** Preoperative axial view shows a well-fixed uncemented metal-backed patellar component. Removal of this component resulted in a thin remaining patella, which went on to fragment and elongate, as shown in postoperative lateral (**B**) and axial (**C**) views.

implantation of a patellar component. If the patella is more than 10 mm thick but has a large central concavity, we prefer to use a component such as a biconvex patellar implant (**Figure 5**) versus a standard three-peg component. A biconvex patellar component may be considered when as little as 5 mm of central bone remains, provided there is adequate peripheral support of the implant. A biconvex reamer is used to implant the component. We remove any remaining fibrous tissue with the reamer, as well as 1 to 2 mm of underlying bone. This type of component requires that some degree of cancellous bone be present to allow for interdigitation of bone cement. When only a cortical shell is present with or without fracture, we perform simple component removal without reinsertion of another component as a treatment option or consider using a porous metal revision patellar component.

Impaction Grafting
The technique and results of impaction grafting for severe patellar bone loss encountered during revision TKA have been reported (**Table 1**). The restoration of host bone stock is per-

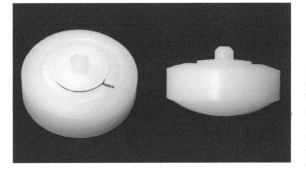

Figure 5 Biconvex revision all-polyethylene patella (Smith & Nephew, Memphis, TN). A biconvex patellar design is a useful option with thin remaining central patellar bone and an intact supporting rim.

formed using cancellous bone graft. The graft is tightly impacted into the patellar defect, which is then covered with a tissue flap created from peripatellar fibrotic tissue or free tissue obtained from the suprapatellar pouch (**Figure 6**). The short-term results of this procedure show better pain and function scores than reported for previous series of resection arthroplasty of the patella. Meticulous technique is important for obtaining a successful result with this procedure. Retention of the pseudomeniscus of scar tissue and most of the parapatellar fibrotic tissue on the undersurface of the quadriceps tendon and on the periphery of the remaining rim should be preserved. The tissue at the periph-

ery of the patella is elevated from proximal to distal, leaving the pedicle at the distal insertion on the patella. Multiple nonabsorbable 0 sutures are used to close the pouch, which is then filled with bone graft (local femoral autograft or cancellous allograft). The graft is impacted to produce a height of 25 to 30 mm of newly grafted patella. The bone graft then compression molds against the femoral trochlea, and a normal postoperative rehabilitation protocol is followed. One complication of this technique that we have seen is early escape of bone graft from the patellar shell, with subsequent heterotopic bone deposition in the soft tissues of the capsule and the posterior aspect of the patellar tendon.

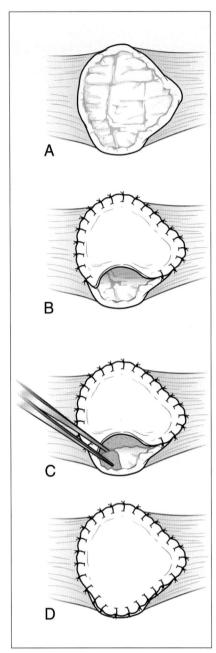

Figure 6 Impaction grafting for severe patellar bone loss. **A,** The patellar shell. Severe loss of patellar bone stock has left only the anterior cortex, variable amounts of the patellar rim, and an irregular cavitary surface to the remaining patellar bone. **B,** Peripheral suture fixation of the tissue flap into the patellar rim and surrounding peripatellar fibrous tissue. **C,** Insertion of the cancellous bone graft into the purse-string opening of the tissue flap–patellar shell construct. **D,** After final impaction of bone graft into the patellar defect, the opening of the tissue flap is closed with additional sutures to provide a watertight closure to contain the bone graft.

Kirschner Wire Fixation

Some authors have described using crossed Kirschner wires (**Figure 7**) to provide reinforcement fixation and support for cementing a central-peg patellar component in place when a cortical shell of bone is encountered during revision TKA. This technique has been used in small case series with good clinical results.

PATELLECTOMY

The most difficult situation to address is the absence of the patella. A high percentage of patients with a patellectomy experience extensor weakness, extensor lag, and difficulty with activities that involve the patellofemoral joint, such as stair climbing. For these reasons, performing a patellectomy at the time of revision TKA is rarely recommended.

TREATING THE KNEE THAT HAS UNDERGONE A PRIOR PATELLECTOMY

When performing a TKA in a knee that has undergone a previous patellectomy, several procedures may be considered in patients with severely compromised function to attempt to restore the lever arm that the patella provides. General indications include an extensor lag greater than 10° to 15°, extensor weakness, and functional giving way. Although not routinely encountered, this clinical problem has recently received attention with the use of tissue-ingrowth patellar components.

One method that attempts to reestablish some of the mechanical advantages of the patella is "tubularization" of the residual extensor mechanism. This technique is illustrated in **Figure 8**.

Another technique that has been described involves sewing a 2.5-cm × 1-cm–thick iliac crest bone graft into a subsynovial pouch in the previous anatomic position of the patella (**Figure 9**). Seven knees in six patients were treated with such an autografting technique and followed for a mean of 75.4 months (range, 24 to 125 months). Good or excellent results were reported in six of seven knees; all but one achieved painless extension.

A third option is to attempt attachment of a component to the soft tissue of the extensor mechanism; however, simply sewing an all-polyethylene component to the undersurface of the extensor mechanism has resulted in generally unsatisfactory results. This approach has been modified to include suturing a porous metal baseplate into position at the desired location of the patella in the quadriceps tendon. Studies have documented that extensive fibrous ingrowth can occur, attaching the porous metal device via soft-tissue fixation; however, the durability of this construct has not been established. We do not recommend suturing a porous metal implant into a patellectomized extensor mechanism and have observed early failures with this technique.

PORUS METAL PATELLAR REVISION IMPLANTS

When a thin shell of patella remains, an all-polyethylene patella can be cemented into a porous metal revision patellar base (**Table 1**). The porous metal base is first sutured into the remaining host–patellar bone shell and adjacent soft tissue. A recent study reported qualitative results that compare favorably with patellar resection arthroplasty in this setting. Results with the use of a porous metal patellar component depend on the presence of remaining host patellar bone, and we find this a useful technique in selected patients (**Figure 10**). When this technique is used without some remaining patellar bone stock, however, the results are very poor (**Figure 11**), and thus we do not recommend this technique in patients who have undergone prior patellectomy and/or have no remaining host patellar bone stock.

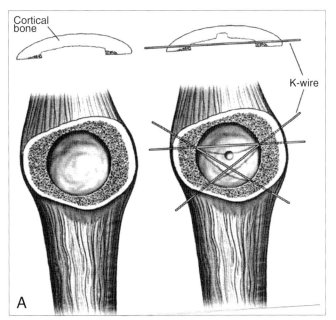

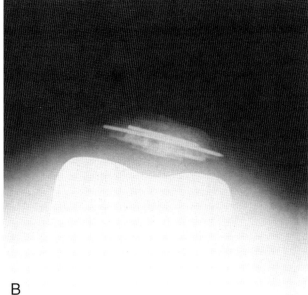

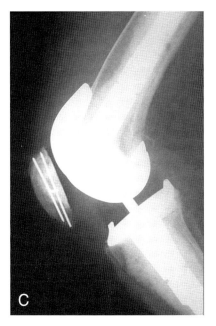

Figure 7 The crossed Kirschner wire (K-wire) technique. Schematic (**A**) and postoperative sunrise (**B**) and lateral (**C**) radiographs show the reconstruction with K-wires and a cemented polyethylene implant. (Panel A is reproduced with permission from Barrack RL, Burnett R: Managing the patella in revision total knee arthroplasty, in Berry DJ, Trousdale RT, Dennis D, Paprosky W, eds: *Revision Total Hip and Knee Arthroplasty.* Lippincott, Williams & Wilkins, 2005.)

◼ Postoperative Regimen

Communication with the patient, nursing staff, and physical therapist is important to ensure that all partici-pants understand the postoperative therapy plan following a patellar revision surgery. All patients should be considered for thromboembolic pro-phylaxis with the use of an American Academy of Orthopaedic Surgeons or American College of Chest Physicians protocol. All patients should receive preemptive, intraoperative, and post-operative multimodal pain control us-ing a protocol for revision TKA sur-gery. We use a drain in all revision TKA procedures. A compression dressing is applied over the knee, and

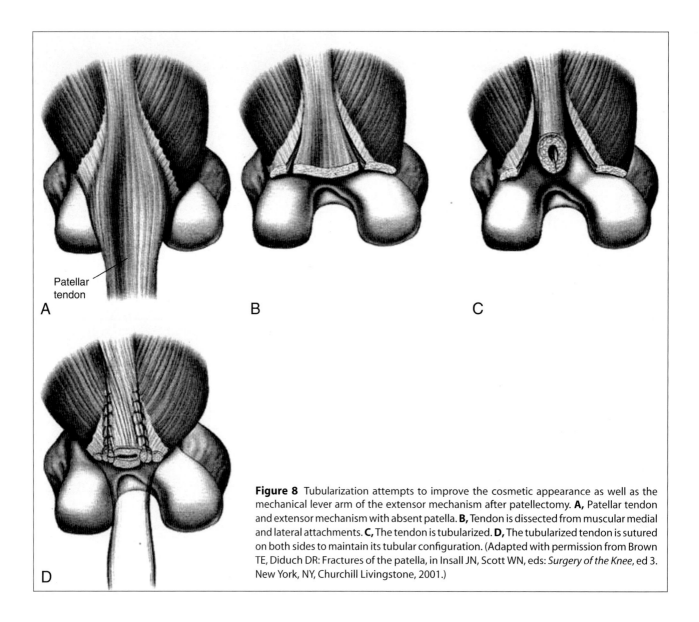

Figure 8 Tubularization attempts to improve the cosmetic appearance as well as the mechanical lever arm of the extensor mechanism after patellectomy. **A,** Patellar tendon and extensor mechanism with absent patella. **B,** Tendon is dissected from muscular medial and lateral attachments. **C,** The tendon is tubularized. **D,** The tubularized tendon is sutured on both sides to maintain its tubular configuration. (Adapted with permission from Brown TE, Diduch DR: Fractures of the patella, in Insall JN, Scott WN, eds: *Surgery of the Knee*, ed 3. New York, NY, Churchill Livingstone, 2001.)

we recommend the use of long-leg compression stockings combined with sequential compression devices such as full-length devices or foot pumps. If continuous passive motion is available, it may be used following surgery. Routine postoperative prophylactic intravenous antibiotics are continued until intraoperative culture results are negative. Mobilization with physical therapy the day of or the day

following surgery is routine, allowing full weight bearing. Bracing is not usually necessary, unless a reconstruction of the extensor mechanism has been performed. AP and lateral radiographs are obtained postoperatively. An axial view of the patella is not performed until 6 weeks postoperatively.

Avoiding Pitfalls and Complications

Treatment of the patella in revision TKA is a challenging procedure with potential complications, and techniques continue to evolve. Considerations at the time of surgery include patient factors, fixation of the implant, host bone stock, tibial and femoral

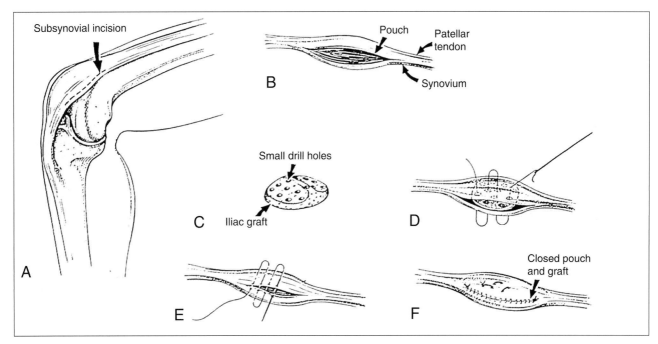

Figure 9 Iliac crest bone grafting procedure for patients with a prior patellectomy, in which a 2.5-cm × 1-cm–thick iliac crest bone graft is sewn into a subsynovial pouch in the previous anatomic position of the patella. **A,** A subsynovial incision is made along the border of the patellar tendon–synovial junction at the level of the original patella. **B,** A 3-cm x 3-cm pouch is developed between the synovial layer and the patellar tendon. **C,** The bone graft, with 2.5-mm holes spaced 5 mm apart. **D,** The predrilled bone graft is sutured into the subsynovial pouch. **E,** The pouch is closed with a running suture. **F,** The bone graft is stabilized completely in the closed subsynovial pouch. (Adapted with permission from Buechel FF: Patellar tendon bone grafting for patellectomized patients having total knee arthroplasty. *Clin Orthop Relat Res* 1991;271:72-78.)

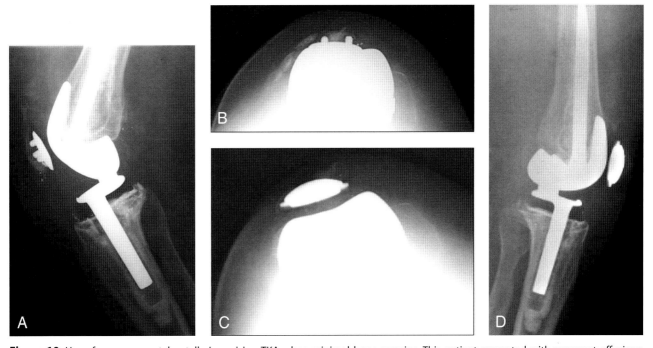

Figure 10 Use of a porous metal patella in revision TKA when minimal bone remains. This patient presented with recurrent effusions, squeaking, and anterior knee pain, possibly related to the rotating-hinge TKA. Preoperative lateral (**A**) and sunrise (**B**) views. Postoperative sunrise (**C**) and lateral (**D**) views obtained 14 months following patellar revision demonstrate an ingrown porous metal patella. The patient's anterior knee pain had resolved.

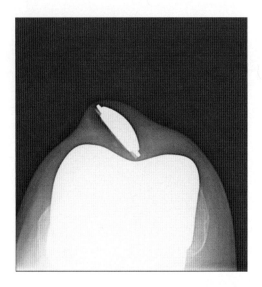

Figure 11 Use of a porous metal patella sewn into the extensor mechanism in a knee with no remaining bone stock. At 14 months, the patient returned for pain with associated erosion of the implant through the extensor mechanism into the subcutaneous tissues, as shown on this axial view. The implant was removed with no extensor mechanism complications.

component rotation, and avoiding further damage to the patella and its blood supply during reconstruction. The importance of carefully assessing femoral and tibial component position and rotation before addressing the patella cannot be overstated. Performing a patellar component revision with underlying tibial and/or femoral component malposition or malrotation is all but doomed to failure.

————■

Bibliography

Barrack RL, Matzkin E, Ingraham R, Engh G, Rorabeck C: Revision knee arthroplasty with patella replacement versus bony shell. *Clin Orthop Relat Res* 1998;356:139-143.

Barrack RL, Rorabeck C, Partington P, Sawhney J, Engh G: The results of retaining a well-fixed patellar component in revision total knee arthroplasty. *J Arthroplasty* 2000;15(4):413-417.

Barrack RL, Schrader T, Bertot AJ, Wolfe MW, Myers L: Component rotation and anterior knee pain after total knee arthroplasty. *Clin Orthop Relat Res* 2001;392:46-55.

Buechel FF: Patellar tendon bone grafting for patellectomized patients having total knee arthroplasty. *Clin Orthop Relat Res* 1991;271(271):72-78.

Eisenhuth SA, Saleh KJ, Cui Q, Clark CR, Brown TE: Patellofemoral instability after total knee arthroplasty. *Clin Orthop Relat Res* 2006;446:149-160.

Garcia RM, Kraay MJ, Conroy-Smith PA, Goldberg VM: Management of the deficient patella in revision total knee arthroplasty. *Clin Orthop Relat Res* 2008;466(11):2790-2797.

Hanssen AD: Bone-grafting for severe patellar bone loss during revision knee arthroplasty. *J Bone Joint Surg Am* 2001;83-A(2):171-176.

Hanssen AD, Pagnano MW: Revision of failed patellar components. *Instr Course Lect* 2004;53:201-206.

Kelly MA: Patellofemoral complications following total knee arthroplasty. *Instr Course Lect* 2001;50:403-407.

Leopold SS, Silverton CD, Barden RM, Rosenberg AG: Isolated revision of the patellar component in total knee arthroplasty. *J Bone Joint Surg Am* 2003;85-A(1):41-47.

Lonner JH, Mont MA, Sharkey PF, Siliski JM, Rajadhyaksha AD, Lotke PA: Fate of the unrevised all-polyethylene patellar component in revision total knee arthroplasty. *J Bone Joint Surg Am* 2003;85-A(1):56-59.

Maheshwari AV, Tsailas PG, Ranawat AS, Ranawat CS: How to address the patella in revision total knee arthroplasty. *Knee* 2009;16(2):92-97.

Malo M, Vince KG: The unstable patella after total knee arthroplasty: Etiology, prevention, and management. *J Am Acad Orthop Surg* 2003;11(5):364-371.

Nelson CL, Lonner JH, Lahiji A, Kim J, Lotke PA: Use of a trabecular metal patella for marked patella bone loss during revision total knee arthroplasty. *J Arthroplasty* 2003;18(7, Suppl 1):37-41.

Parvizi J, Seel MJ, Hanssen AD, Berry DJ, Morrey BF: Patellar component resection arthroplasty for the severely compromised patella. *Clin Orthop Relat Res* 2002;397:356-361.

Rorabeck CH, Mehin R, Barrack RL: Patellar options in revision total knee arthroplasty. *Clin Orthop Relat Res* 2003;416: 84-92.

Coding

CPT Code		Corresponding ICD-9 Codes	
	Revision Total Knee Arthroplasty, Patellar Component		
27486	Revision of total knee arthroplasty, with or without allograft; one component	996.40 996.42 996.45	996.60 996.43 996.66

CPT copyright © 2010 by the American Medical Association. All rights reserved.

Chapter 45

Conversion of Failed Unicompartmental Knee Arthroplasty to Total Knee Arthroplasty

James Benjamin, MD

■ Indications

In the properly selected patient, unicompartmental knee arthroplasty (UKA) can be an excellent option for the management of degenerative arthritis in the knee. The resurgence of interest in UKA and its use in younger and more active patients undoubtedly will result in an increase in UKA revisions in the future. Currently, the most common indication for revision of UKA to total knee arthroplasty (TKA) is mechanical failure, which is reported to be the reason for revision in 22% to 100% of cases. This is usually the result of polyethylene wear (**Figure 1**) or implant loosening (**Figure 2**). Progression of arthritis in adjacent compartments is the second leading cause for revision, occurring in 19% to 48% of cases. Other modes of failure leading to revision are ligament instability and medial tibial bone collapse. These variations in failure mechanisms probably are related to technical factors, indication, and the type of UKA being revised.

Although mechanical failure can be diagnosed routinely on clinical and radiographic examination, it is important to rule out other causes of failure,

such as septic arthritis or pain referred to the knee from the hip or lumbar spine. Subtle femoral component loosening can be difficult to diagnose on standard radiographs, and bone scans often are helpful in this setting. Technetium Tc 99m bone scan will demonstrate increased uptake for up to 1 year after the initial procedure even in well-fixed UKAs, but asymmetric uptake between the femoral and tibial component is indicative of failure of fixation (**Figure 3**).

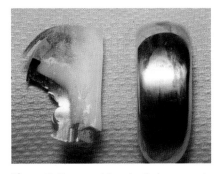

Figure 1 Catastrophic polyethylene wear in a retrieved unicompartmental knee arthroplasty implant.

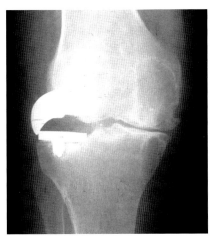

Figure 2 AP radiograph demonstrates failure of implant fixation after unicompartmental knee arthroplasty.

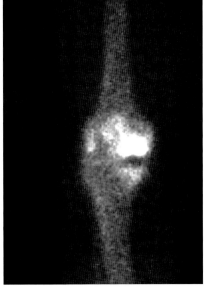

Figure 3 Technetium Tc 99m bone scan shows asymmetric uptake indicative of femoral component loosening in a unicondylar knee arthroplasty.

Dr. Benjamin or an immediate family member is a member of a speakers' bureau or has made paid presentations on behalf of DePuy and serves as a paid consultant to or is an employee of DePuy.

Table 1 Results of Revision of Unicompartmental Knee Arthroplasty to Total Knee Arthroplasty

Authors (Year)	Number of Knees	Mean Patient Age in Years (Range)	Mean Follow-up in Years (Range)	Mean Time to Revision in Months (Range)	Clinical Results	Percentage of Knees in Which Augments Were Used
Barrett and Scott (1987)	29	62 (40-76)	4.6 (2-10)	47 (4-113)	66% good/excellent	52
Padgett et al (1991)	21	(49-76)	(2-10)	(8-96)	76% good/excellent HSS	76
Gill et al (1995)	30	67 (57-87)	3.8 (2-9)	80 (24-96)	78/68 KSS	77
Levine et al (1996)	31	72 (49-88)	3.8 (2-9)	62 (7-107)	91/81 KSS	45
McAuley et al (2001)	32	59 (35-73)	4.4 (2-10)	67 (9-204)	89/81 KSS	69
Johnson et al (2007)	77	66	6.9 (1-15)	NR	77% good/excellent Bristol score	NR
Saldanha et al (2007)	36	66 (52-76)	2 (0.2-9)	60 (2-228)	86/78 KSS	22
Aleto et al (2008)	32	66 (41-90)	2.3	68 (4-240)	88/72 KSS	81
Dudley et al (2008)	68	NR	NR	NR	NR	43

HSS = Hospital for Special Surgery score, KSS = Knee Society scores (functional score/prosthesis score), NR = not reported.

 Contraindications

Primary revision of UKA to TKA is contraindicated in cases of chronic sepsis or acute infection with resistant organisms. These cases are best managed with a two-stage revision.

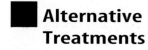 **Alternative Treatments**

Some authors have reported revision of a failed UKA to another UKA. This alternative often is not feasible, however, and it may be contraindicated in cases in which degenerative changes have progressed in other compart-

ments, bone stock has been lost, or implant failure has resulted in metal-on-metal articulation and significant metallic synovitis and staining of the articular cartilage.

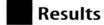 **Results**

Most published series report good results with revision of UKA to TKA. Using various knee rating systems, authors report 66% to 77% good to excellent results following revision. In series reporting Knee Society scores, functional scores range from 78 to 91 and prosthesis scores range from 68 to 81. Most of these reports are from short- to intermediate-term follow-up

and should be interpreted with caution. Although some authors report that revision UKA results are comparable to those of primary TKA, these claims may not be entirely accurate. Even in series with short- to intermediate-term follow-up, a significant incidence of early re-revision occurs and the results of the revision of UKA to TKA actually may be compared more accurately with results of revision TKA (**Table 1**).

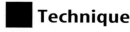 **Technique**

Surgical Exposure

Surgical exposure can be obtained with the use of a standard parapatellar approach. Extensile approaches such as quadriceps snip, quadriceps turn-down, or tibial tubercle osteotomy rarely are required, but, as in any revision, the surgeon should be familiar with at least one method of extensile exposure to the knee. Other surgical approaches, such as the subvastus and midvastus approaches, can be used, but they are not recommended because they are not extensile and may limit exposure.

Instruments/Equipment/ Implants Required

Revision instruments often are required to facilitate implant removal. The use of thin osteotomes and careful technique help to mobilize the host-implant interface and minimize the loss of bone stock during implant removal. Revision of a UKA to a TKA often can be performed with a "primary" TKA implant, but this depends on the type of UKA being revised and the reason for revision. UKA implants that require large tibial bone resections or implants that fail because of tibial loosening or tibial bone collapse often will require the use of metal tibial augments, bone grafts, or stems, so it is prudent to have a revision TKA system available in case augments or stem extensions are required.

Component Alignment

FEMORAL COMPONENT

Coronal alignment of the femur can be obtained easily using intramedullary guides, but care must be taken to avoid overresection distally. Because the distal femoral resection usually is based off the intact condyle, it is important to remember that, in primary arthroplasty, the resection of the distal lateral femoral condyle is thinner than that of the distal medial condyle. This is especially notable in valgus knees. Because most UKAs are medial, referencing the resection depth off the lateral femoral condyle will result in excessive bone resection and elevation of the joint line. This error will be magnified if progression of arthritis in the lateral compartment is the reason for revision. One way to avoid this problem is to pin the distal cutting block before removal of the femoral component (**Figure 4**). Femoral component sizing also can be difficult because of the posterior medial bone defect present after removal of the prosthesis, since most sizing guides reference the posterior femoral condyles and the anterior cortex. Preoperative templating and intraoperative sizing should be done before removal of the femoral component.

Rotational alignment of the femoral component is one of the biggest challenges surgeons face during revision of UKA to TKA, but it can be achieved using several techniques. Gap balancing using the cut surface of the proximal tibia ignores the pre-existing posterior femoral defect. Surgeons familiar with this technique can use their primary TKA work flow to determine femoral rotation. Those who routinely use a measured resection technique still can use anatomic referencing, but posterior condylar referencing usually is not a viable option. The recommended technique to determine femoral rotation is to use either the epicondylar axis or the AP axis, depending on the surgeon's experience and preference (**Figure 5**).

TIBIAL COMPONENT

Intramedullary or extramedullary instrumentation can be used with equal accuracy for tibial alignment, but the depth of resection should be based off

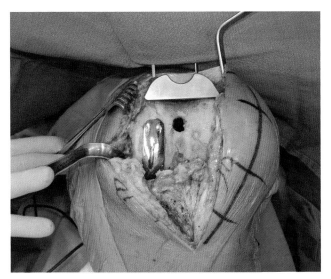

Figure 4 Intraoperative photograph demonstrates placement of a distal femoral cutting block before removal of the femoral component.

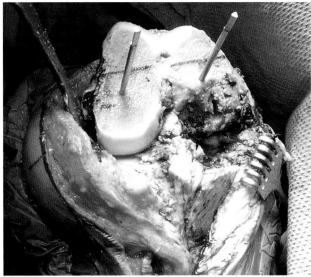

Figure 5 Intraoperative photograph shows the use of the epicondylar axis to determine femoral component rotation.

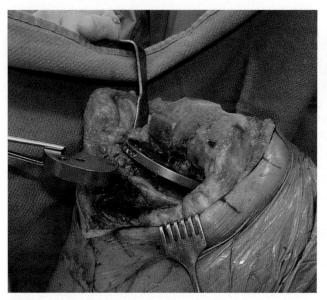

Figure 6 After trialing to determine tibial component rotation, bone preparation for augments can be performed.

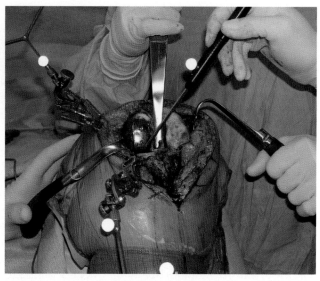

Figure 7 Intraoperative photograph depicting the use of computer-assisted surgery during revision of a UKA to a TKA. Landmark registration is performed before the removal of implants.

the nonimplanted side to avoid over-resection. Regardless of the defect present after removal of the prosthesis, a standard resection guide should be used rather than a stepped or mediolaterally sloped guide that is designed to prepare the tibia to accept an augment. A small variation in the rotational alignment of these cutting guides can result in significant varus-valgus malalignment. Regardless of their shape, augments allow no rotational variability of the tibial tray. Trialing should be performed with a primary nonaugmented tibial trial to allow rotational freedom of the tibial implant. Once tibial rotational alignment has been determined, the tibial defect can be contoured to accept an augment, often with less bone resection than originally anticipated (Figure 6).

Computer-Assisted Surgery

Computer-assisted surgery (CAS) is another option for revision of a UKA to a TKA and has been an excellent application, in my experience. Anatomic landmark registration can be performed before implant removal, and bone resection can be planned

and executed independently of the bone defects present. Surgeons using a measured resection work flow can determine femoral size and rotation without being influenced by bone defects present after implant removal. Those using a gap-balancing work flow can use their standard techniques to determine femoral component rotation (**Figure 7**).

Management of Bone Defects

In many revisions, the existing bone defects do not require formal augmentation. Clinical series report revision without augmentation in 19% to 78% of cases (**Table 1**). These results are highly dependent on the type of implant being revised and the cause of the failure leading to revision. Defects smaller than 5 mm and partial defects usually can be managed using cement without compromising the outcome of the procedure. Larger defects may require augmentation; the use of augments on the tibial side often predicates the use of a stem extension on the tibial component. A paucity of objective clinical and biomechanical evidence exists regarding the length and style of stem, but available data seem

to indicate that if tibial augments are required, a cemented stem at least 70 mm in length should be used. The use of uncemented metaphyseal stems is not recommended because they have been associated with early failure in revision TKA series. If uncemented stems are used, they should be long enough to engage the diaphysis of the tibia.

Augmentation may be required on the femur posteromedially depending on the amount of bone loss, but this is relatively rare. The use of augments on the femoral side usually dictates that the implant is cruciate-substituting in design. A single augment on the femoral side (eg, a 4-mm posterior medial augment) does not necessarily require a femoral stem. If multiple augments are used on the femoral component or if the augments are 8 mm or larger, the use of a stem is recommended, using the same guidelines as on the tibial side.

Bone grafting is seldom required because the defects usually are uncontained and are of a size that can be managed easily with cement and metal augments. Small cavitary defects can be managed with morcellized autograft obtained from bone resected during the revision surgery.

Cruciate-Retaining Versus Cruciate-Substituting (Posterior Stabilized) Implants

Although several series have reported good results revising UKA to TKA with the use of cruciate-retaining implants, many of these studies are from institutions that preferentially use this style of implant. The average reported thickness of polyethylene inserts used in revision UKA series is 11.3 to 13.7 mm, with ranges from 8 to 25 mm, suggesting that, in most cases, the reconstruction resulted in an elevation of the joint line or significant tibial resection that was inconsistent with the preservation of a functional posterior cruciate ligament. The choice of a cruciate-retaining versus posterior stabilized implant ultimately is the surgeon's decision and depends on his or her ability to achieve a reconstruction that is balanced in both the coronal and the sagittal plane. If the polyethylene thickness is greater than 10 mm or femoral augmentation is needed, the surgeon should consider using a posterior stabilized knee design (**Figure 8**).

Wound Closure

Wound closure is identical to that of a primary TKA and depends on the surgeon's preference. I use a deep wound drain in these cases.

Postoperative Regimen

Postoperative management of UKA is no different from that after primary TKA with regard to deep vein thrombosis prophylaxis, wound management, and rehabilitation.

Avoiding Pitfalls and Complications

The biggest pitfall in any revision procedure is underestimating the complexity and requirements of the operation. The surgeon should assume that a revision prosthesis, augments, and stems will be required and have them available at the time of surgery. It is always better to be overprepared than to lack the implants required to perform the procedure properly. The surgeon should take additional time to mobilize the implant-host interface before removing the prosthesis. Because of the small size of the UKA implants, it is easy to disimpact them with a mallet and bone tamp; however, doing so often results in an unnecessary loss of bone stock.

The surgeon must avoid overresection of the distal femur or proximal tibia. The resection level should be referenced from the intact condyle/plateau. Caution should be exercised when determining the rotation of the femoral component. The AP axis and epicondylar axis can be used for rota-

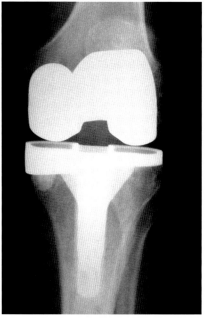

Figure 8 AP radiograph demonstrates the use of posterior stabilized TKA with a tibial augment and cemented stem extension in a knee that was revised from a UKA to a TKA.

tional alignment, but the posterior condylar axis cannot be used. Gap-balancing techniques that reference the femoral component rotation relative to the tibial resection are an excellent option in these cases. The tibia should not be prepared for augmentation until after component rotation has been determined during trialing. Augments do not permit any rotational freedom of the tibial tray, and having to redo this step can result in unnecessary and excessive bone resection.

Bibliography

Aleto TJ, Berend ME, Ritter MA, Faris PM, Meneghini RM: Early failure of unicompartmental knee arthroplasty leading to revision. *J Arthroplasty* 2008;23(2):159-163.

Barrett WP, Scott RD: Revision of failed unicondylar unicompartmental knee arthroplasty. *J Bone Joint Surg Am* 1987; 69(9):1328-1335.

Dudley TE, Gioe TJ, Sinner P, Mehle S: Registry outcomes of unicompartmental knee arthroplasty revisions. *Clin Orthop Relat Res* 2008;466(7):1666-1670.

Gill T, Schemitsch EH, Brick GW, Thornhill TS: Revision total knee arthroplasty after failed unicompartmental knee arthroplasty or high tibial osteotomy. *Clin Orthop Relat Res* 1995;321:10-18.

Johnson S, Jones P, Newman JH: The survivorship and results of total knee replacements converted from unicompartmental knee replacements. *Knee* 2007;14(2):154-157.

Levine WN, Ozuna RM, Scott RD, Thornhill TS: Conversion of failed modern unicompartmental arthroplasty to total knee arthroplasty. *J Arthroplasty* 1996;11(7):797-801.

McAuley JP, Engh GA, Ammeen DJ: Revision of failed unicompartmental knee arthroplasty. *Clin Orthop Relat Res* 2001;392:279-282.

Padgett DE, Stern SH, Insall JN: Revision total knee arthroplasty for failed unicompartmental replacement. *J Bone Joint Surg Am* 1991;73(2):186-190.

Saldanha KA, Keys GW, Svard UC, White SH, Rao C: Revision of Oxford medial unicompartmental knee arthroplasty to total knee arthroplasty—Results of a multicentre study. *Knee* 2007;14(4):275-279.

Coding				
CPT Codes			**Corresponding ICD-9 Codes**	
20680	Removal of implant; deep (eg, buried wire, pin, screw, metal band, nail, rod or plate)		996.40	993.66
20985	Computer-assisted surgical navigational procedure for musculoskeletal procedures; imageless (List separately in addition to code for primary procedure)		996.40	996.60
27447	Arthroplasty, knee, condyle and plateau; medial AND lateral compartments with or without patella resurfacing (total knee arthroplasty)		996.40	996.60

CPT copyright © 2010 by the American Medical Association. All rights reserved.

Chapter 46

Revision Total Knee Arthroplasty: Cemented and Uncemented Stems

Thomas Parker Vail, MD

Introduction

The increasing number of primary total knee arthroplasty (TKA) procedures being performed in the United States has been accompanied by an increase in the number of complex revision TKAs. Infection and mechanical loosening remain the most common indications for revision TKA. Managing complicated revision situations requires a stable mechanical construct designed to address ligamentous instability, bone loss, and poor bone quality. When present, the cancellous bone in the proximal tibia is uniquely designed to transmit load, with an elastic modulus that is 30 times less than that of cortical bone and a three-dimensional architecture demonstrating a high degree of anisotropy secondary to its variable geometry. The proximal cancellous bone is capable

of transferring 80% of axial load from the tibial plateau to the distal cortex. When this is absent, the remaining cortical rim is required to bear substantially greater load, perhaps more than can be expected without additional implant support in the form of cemented or uncemented stems.

Stems have been developed to provide supplemental fixation, additional bone-implant contact surface area, and internal structural support that can extend from the joint line to the diaphysis of the femur or tibia. There are several clear indications for using a stem in conjunction with knee joint revision, including obesity, osteoporosis, the need for increased articular constraint, periarticular bone loss requiring grafting, and the correction of deformity with wedges or metallic augments. Ligamentous instability requiring articular constraint leads to

increased shear at the articular prosthesis-bone interface that can be diminished by using a stem. Specific bone-loss situations where stem use is appropriate include condylar defects requiring bone graft, cement and screw augmentation, wedges, or blocks greater than 4 mm. Other indications include large contained metaphyseal bone defects, cortical bone defects, and metaphyseal or periarticular diaphyseal fractures. In considering the type of stem to implant, the surgeon must understand how a stem will fit the local anatomy, whether the stem should engage the diaphysis, and whether the function of the stem would be enhanced or potentially harmed by extending the fixation surface area through use of cement.

———————————■

Dr. Vail or an immediate family member is a board member, owner, officer, or committee member of the American Association of Hip and Knee Surgeons, the American Board of Orthopaedic Surgery, The Hip Society, and The Knee Society; has received royalties from DePuy; serves as a paid consultant for or is an employee of DePuy; has received research or institutional support from Johnson & Johnson, Medtronic, Musculoskeletal Transplant Foundation, National Institutes of Health, AIOD-Assn Intl l'Osteosynthese Dynamique, Aleeva Medical, American College of Sports Medicine Foundation, American Orthopaedic Society for Sports Medicine, AO Foundation, Arthritis Foundation, Arthrocare Corporation, Arthroscopy Association of North America, Canadian Academy of Sports Medicine, Columbia University Deafness Research Foundation, DePuy, Hacettepe University, Harold K.L. Castle Foundation Histogenics Corporation, International Spinal Injection Society, ISTO Technologies, March of Dimes Birth Defects Foundation, Musculoskeletal and Skin NIH, National Institute of Dental and Craniofacial Research, North American Spine Society, North Shore-Long Island Jewish Health Systems, Novo Nordisk, Orthologic Corporation, Orthopaedic Research and Education Foundation, Orthopaedic Trauma Association, Scios, Scoliosis Research Society, Spinal Kinetics, SpinalMotion, Spine Solutions, Stryker Corporation, Stryker Howmedica Osteonics, Synthes, TissueLink Medical, TranS1, UC Berkeley United Health Group Company, University of Minnesota, University of Texas at Dallas, Wisconsin Alumni Research Foundation, and Zimmer; and owns stock or stock options in Pivot Medical.

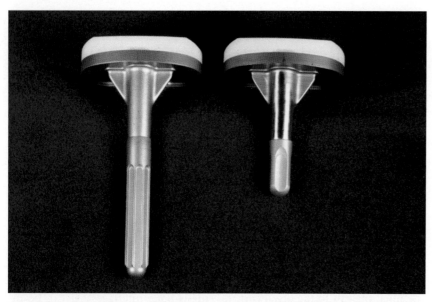

Figure 1 An uncemented and a cemented stem attached to a tibial tray. The uncemented stem on the left has a larger diameter with flutes designed to engage the endosteal bone, providing torsional stability. The cemented stem on the right shows a typical shape that is more rounded. The cemented stem is designed to provide some macro interlock of cement without creating any sharp edges that would concentrate stress in the cement mantle.

Cemented Versus Uncemented Stems: General Considerations

Whether or not to use cement around the stem (**Figure 1**) remains largely a function of surgeon discretion and experience applied to specific clinical needs. In general, uncemented, or press-fit, stems are better suited for use in patients with better overall bone quality and a diaphyseal dimension that is not oversized (not >18 mm), regardless of age. Nevertheless, certain situations favor the use of one type of stem over the other. Additionally, the techniques for implantation of a cemented or an uncemented stem are different and merit specific attention. Whether or not one chooses cement, the stem is meant to augment the joint construct, not dictate the position of the articulating components. This concept is particularly relevant when using longer stems in the presence of extra-articular deformity.

When the position of a stem is altered by a deformity or the anterior femoral bow or tibial varus bow, there is a risk that the stem position could incorrectly dictate the position of the tibial or femoral component. Techniques for avoiding such pitfalls are important for successful restoration of knee function.

Uncemented Stems

Indications and Contraindications
Uncemented stems are relatively uncomplicated to implant, are easy to remove, and are compatible with either intramedullary or extramedullary instrument systems. A press-fit stem works nicely as an internal strut when fractures are present and does not introduce the possibility of cement extravasation into the fracture site. Recent experience seems to suggest that cementing into the metaphysis and

extending the uncemented stem to the diaphysis are important factors in achieving success and durability with uncemented stems.

Revisions for infection are commonly associated with bone loss and instability, thus requiring a stem. The choice of a cemented or an uncemented stem relates more to weighing the advantage of infection prophylaxis afforded by the use of antibiotic-impregnated bone cement versus the ease of removing an uncemented stem in the event of recurrent infection. Despite a success rate better than 90% with two-stage reimplantation protocols, some surgeons feel uncomfortable cementing a stem at the time of reimplantation because of the risk of postoperative repeat infection in the setting of more virulent organisms or a compromised host.

An uncemented stem provides extended bone-implant contact, but it does not provide fixation to the bone in the way that cement or porous surfaces integrate with bone. The lack of true bone fixation may be a long-term drawback for uncemented stems. Another potential downside of an uncemented stem is that the stem may not accommodate extra-articular deformity or retained hardware. An uncemented stem is meant to contact the endosteum and engage the diaphysis of the femur or tibia, while at the same time maintaining a fixed valgus relationship (generally between 5° and 7°) on the femoral side and posterior slope (0° to 5°) on the tibial side. To accommodate an unusual anatomic pattern such as an exaggerated femoral or tibial bow or diaphyseal-metaphyseal offset, it may be necessary to choose a cemented stem or an offset uncemented stem that allows adjustment of the femoral valgus angle or posterior tibial slope.

Another downside of an uncemented stem is apparent when the diameter of the diaphyseal bone is quite large because of cortical bone loss and endosteal expansion, which is often

Table 1 Results of Revision Total Knee Arthroplasty With Uncemented Stems

Authors (Year)	Number of Knees	Mean Patient Age in Years (Range)	Mean Follow-up (Range)	Results
Bertin et al (1985)	53	(<40-84)	18 months (6-48)	9% unsatisfactory because of pain
Barrack et al (1999)	78	NA	36 months (24-48)	End-of-stem pain: 11% femur, 14% tibia
Shannon et al (2003)	63	66 (38-85)	5.75 years (2-10)	16% loose
Barrack et al (2004)	143	70	60 months (24-84)	Less pain with slotted than solid stem
Mahoney and Kinsey (2006)	22	NA	1 year	Satisfactory restoration of joint line 1 revision at 3 years
Peters et al (2005)	50	68 (35-90)	36 months (24-96)	No loosening 1 patient with thigh pain

NA = not available.

seen with age-related bone remodeling or osteoporosis. In this situation, to engage the endosteum of the femur or tibia, the diameter of an uncemented stem would necessarily be quite large. A long, large-diameter stem in combination with osteopenia may increase the chance for end-of-stem pain. This combination of anatomic features may be better managed with a cemented stem.

Results

There are a few reported series of press-fit stems at short- to medium-term follow-up (**Table 1**). Despite admonitions regarding early loosening of uncemented stems when used in conjunction with constrained liners, the published results are reasonably good. The concern is that the early good results may yield to later difficulties or may not compare to the longer-term follow-up available on cemented stems. The reason for that concern is the consistent reporting of radiolucent lines around the uncemented stems (**Figure 2**). The radiolucency may portend earlier failure, but this remains to be elucidated. Engagement of the di-

aphysis, rather than placing a stem short of the diaphysis, may create a more stable and durable uncemented stem construct.

Technique

SETUP/EXPOSURE

The exposure of the knee when using an uncemented stem is no different from the exposure for any revision TKA procedure. At times it can be difficult to find the medullary canal of the femur or tibia if there has been prior trauma resulting in obstruction of the canal with bone or retained cement from the prior TKA. Establishing the entry point to the canal is very important, as it will to some extent establish the initial valgus angle of the intramedullary guides. An excessively medial entry point will bias the joint line into varus, and a lateral entry point will create a valgus joint line (**Figure 3**). The varus or valgus alignment of the intramedullary guides is critically important, as the intramedullary guide set into the diaphysis will be the point of reference for the joint-line resection angle and the translation of the articular portion of the

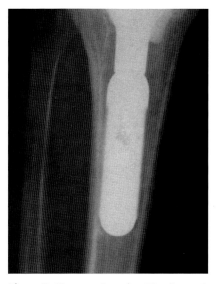

Figure 2 Close-up view of an AP radiograph of an uncemented stem 4 years after implantation reveals a radiolucent line between the stem and the endosteal cortex of the tibia.

TKA components. Thus, it is important to be aware of any excessive anterior femoral bow, varus tibial bow, or extra-articular deformity. Long radiographs allow visualization of deformity, assessment of the anatomic and mechanical axis, and initial implant size estimation. Preoperative planning

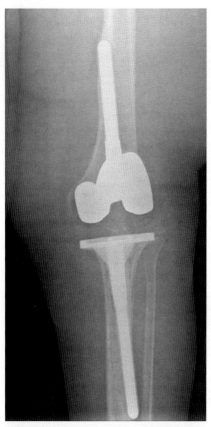

Figure 3 Weight-bearing AP radiograph of a TKA in a left knee demonstrates the relationship of the stem angle to the joint-line position. The lateral entry point on the femoral side creates a valgus femoral component position, and the tip of the stem has penetrated the femoral cortex. Likewise, the medial entry point on the tibial side has created a varus component position, with the tip of the tibial stem exiting the tibial cortex. The resulting joint line is not parallel to the mechanical axis.

from those radiographs can minimize the risk of error.

INSTRUMENTS/EQUIPMENT/IMPLANTS REQUIRED

Although either intramedullary or extramedullary instrument systems can be used when implanting an uncemented stem, it is more common to use intramedullary guide systems. Instrumentation includes diaphyseal reamers for stem preparation and articular surface cutting blocks that reference off either the reamers or the intramedullary rods. Deformities such as unusual offsets or angles will require a stem system that includes a variety of stem angles, offset stems, stem diameters, and stem lengths.

PROCEDURE

Stem preparation can start on either the femoral or tibial side. However, the algorithm for revision TKA most commonly starts with tibial preparation to establish the flexion gap, followed by femoral preparation to match the extension gap with the flexion gap.

Starting with the tibia, the diaphysis is reamed with progressively increasing diameters of medullary reamers until the endosteum is engaged. The medullary reamer, or a medullary guide, is then used as the axial reference to cut a perpendicular tibial joint line. It is very important that the intramedullary guide engages the diaphysis and that the surgeon accounts for the tibial bow to avoid creating a varus joint-line resection. The position of the intramedullary guide can be checked with surface landmarks. Ideally, the intramedullary guide passes through the medial third of the tibial tubercle and the center of the ankle. This position will ensure that the stem and the intramedullary guide are colinear with the mechanical axis. Once the joint surface is cut, the surgeon must determine that the articular portion of the prosthesis covers the proximal tibial surface. If there is a conflict between the position of the diaphyseal stem and the articular surface portion of the tibial component, then it may be necessary to consider an offset stem. Once a stem exceeds a length of 100 mm, in most cases the diaphysis will be engaged by the reamer or the stem. This contact between the diaphysis and the stem should be recognized to avoid component malposition caused by the diaphyseal engagement. Press-fit stems offer the option of varying amounts of posterior slope, generally between 0° and 5°. Once chosen, the posterior slope is dictated by the stem-surface locking mechanism. The correct choice of angle will be driven by the desire to optimize the prosthesis kinematics and balance the flexion and extension gaps.

The femoral side preparation is similar to the tibial side. The diaphysis is reamed progressively, generally with hand reamers rather than power reamers to avoid creating excessive heat when reaming. The entry point of the reamer on the femoral side is at the medial edge of the intercondylar notch, just above the roof of the notch distally. Once the diaphysis is engaged by the reamers or the intramedullary guides, the joint-line cuts will be made using blocks that fit over the intramedullary guide. Given the presence of the anterior femoral bow, it is very common to find that the intramedullary guide sits slightly more anterior than desired at the joint line. To avoid placing the femoral component too far anterior such that the anterior flange of the component does not contact the anterior distal femoral cortex, it may be necessary to choose a stem option that allows variability in selecting the distance between the anterior flange of the femoral component and the stem attachment onto the articular portion of the femoral prosthesis. It is also necessary to choose the valgus angle of the stem relative to the articular portion of the component before beginning the articular cuts. The femoral valgus angle options generally range between 3° and 9° for most implant systems. As mentioned relative to the tibial component positioning, individual anatomy or deformity may necessitate choosing various amounts of valgus, bowed stems, and offset stems. A slotted stem design creates a more flexible stem tip that can displace slightly during implantation to accommodate a tight or bowed medullary canal. Decisions regarding size, offset, bow, and length are made largely through templating of radiographs and preoperative planning.

Once the stems are prepared and the articular cuts are made in the operating room, it is extremely important to implant trial components to determine that the component position relative to the stem and relative to the bone is satisfactory. If the trial tray and stem construct will not easily seat, then the canal needs to be reexamined to be sure that there is no retained cement or neocortex that is preventing the stem from sliding down the canal. In some cases, the only way to seat the construct is to switch to an offset stem. To avoid any surprises, this should be done before opening and constructing the final implants. An intraoperative radiograph is not routinely required with trials in place, but it can be helpful when component position or stem alignment is in question.

When using uncemented stems, the articular interfaces are most often cemented (unless a completely uncemented knee design is chosen). It is generally recommended that the cement contact around the implant be extended into the metaphysis of the bone. The cement will generally cover the housing on the prosthesis, where the stem attaches to the articular portion of the implant. Extending the cement into the metaphysis creates a more stable implant-bone composite. End-of-stem pain has been reported in the presence of uncemented diaphyseal stems. In one study using solid fluted cobalt-chrome stems, there was an 11% incidence of end-of-stem pain on the femoral side (7 of 66) and 14% incidence on the tibial side (7 of 50). In a series of 143 revision TKAs, the incidence of end-of-stem pain was significantly lower with the slotted tibial stem (5 of 62 stems [8%]) when compared with solid cobalt-chrome stems (36 of 112 stems [32%]). Slot closure was not a risk factor for developing end-of-stem pain. Patients with end-of-stem pain were more likely to be only somewhat satisfied or dissatisfied

with their overall pain relief compared with patients without such pain.

Finally, the use of a "dangle" stem has been attributed to Insall. The dangle stem is press-fit into the diaphysis of the femur or tibia to provide a larger surface area for load transfer. No attempt is made to create cortical contact. The dangle-stem technique is indicated for osteoporosis, notching, or similar situations in which the stem provides an internal strut for weakened bone but no large structural defect or instability pattern is present.

———————■

■ Cemented Stems

Indications and Contraindications

The cemented stem is the gold standard in terms of performance and outcome in stemmed TKA. Cemented stems have a proven track record of performance, durability, and absence of radiolucencies at up to 10 years. Cement allows the surgeon to extend the fixation surface area around the length of the stem. In addition, bone cement can be used as a delivery vehicle for antibiotics. A cemented construct has been described as the ultimate "custom composite" technology because the cement mantle around the rigid metal stem allows the surgeon some ability to accommodate anatomic variability. Because the cemented stem does not "engage" the diaphysis, there is room to adjust the stem position relative to the confines of the endosteal bone (**Figure 4**).

An advantage of a cemented stem is that it does not engage the diaphysis and is generally shorter than an uncemented stem. A potential disadvantage is that the technique of implanting a cemented stem does not rely on the diaphysis to act as a guide for positioning of the stem within the bone. In other words, unless landmarks other than the diaphysis (typically the joint-line cuts) are used to determine

the appropriate component position, it is more likely that a prosthesis with a cemented stem might be placed in an undesired degree of varus, valgus, flexion, or extension.

Although the enhanced fixation surface is an advantage of cemented stems, it is also a potential disadvantage. The extended fixation surface makes a cemented stem more difficult to extract from the bone than an uncemented stem. As stated previously, this may be an issue when an unanticipated revision is required because of infection or because the bearing surfaces need to be changed when increased constraint is indicated at the time of revision. An additional concern is that the cemented fixation of the stem to the diaphysis may stress-shield the periarticular bone. The bone behind the anterior flange of the femoral component seems to be particularly vulnerable to this phenomenon.

Cement is not appropriate when no cancellous bone is present. Because bone cement derives its fixation by functioning as a grout within the interstices of the cancellous bone structure, the fixation will be compromised if the cancellous bone is absent. This situation arises when a prior loose stem has eroded or polished the endosteal bone. Likewise, extraction of a well-fixed cemented stem can often cause damage to the endosteum of the bone, making it impossible to use a cemented stem a second time. In such cases, a fluted, slotted uncemented stem is more likely to achieve primary stability than a cemented stem by engaging the endosteum in the diaphyseal bone. Finally, cement may also be difficult to use when one is dealing with a bone defect or periarticular fracture, such as a supracondylar femur fracture. In these cases, it is very difficult to contain the extravasation of the bone cement into the fracture site or outside of the canal of the femur or tibia into the soft tissues.

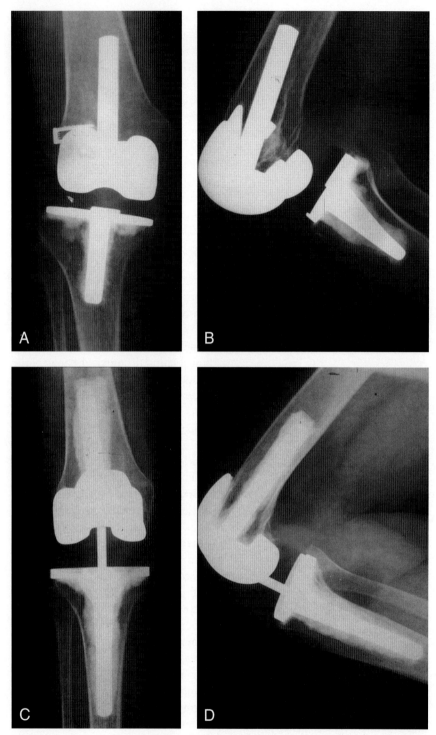

Figure 4 Preoperative AP (**A**) and lateral (**B**) views of an unstable cruciate-retaining TKA with a varus joint line. AP (**C**) and lateral (**D**) radiographs obtained 4 years after revision surgery show a joint line perpendicular to the mechanical axis, with cemented stems well integrated into the cancellous bone of the tibial and femoral metaphysis.

Results

Numerous reports have indicated satisfactory results with cemented stems up to 10 years after surgery. Radiolucent lines are rare, and failures correlate with infection and aseptic loosening. Results are also related to the degree of bone loss and ligamentous compromise at the time of revision surgery (**Table 2**).

Technique

SETUP/EXPOSURE

The setup and exposure of the knee when using a cemented stem is the same as for an uncemented stem. However, the extra-articular deformity and metaphyseal-diaphyseal relationships are less important because the cemented stem will be shorter and will not engage the diaphysis of the bone. Templating is still important to determine that the stem will not inadvertently contact or penetrate the cortex when positioning the articular portion of the knee component.

INSTRUMENTS/EQUIPMENT/IMPLANTS REQUIRED

The basic difference in technique in contrast to placing uncemented stems is that the joint-line cuts are made before stem preparation when using cemented stems. The stem preparation is done using the joint line as the guide to stem position by reaming the stem opening through the joint-line blocks. Cemented stems require cement restrictors. Some surgeons prefer to use a cement gun to fill the canal with cement starting at the cement restrictor and filling to the joint line. Most commonly, cemented stems are placed using intramedullary technique on the femoral side and extramedullary technique on the tibial side. However, intramedullary technique can be used on both sides of the joint without consequence.

PROCEDURE

As with any revision, the tibia is generally prepared first to establish the

Table 2 Results of Revision Total Knee Arthroplasty With Cemented Stems

Authors (Year)	Number of Knees	Mean Patient Age in Years (Range)	Mean Follow-up in Years (Range)	Results
Fehring et al (2003)	113 (107 cemented, 95 press-fit stems)	NA	≥2	93% of cemented stems stable; 71% of press-fit stems stable (Knee Society scoring system)
Whaley et al (2003)	38	67 (39-83)	10.1 (2-17.3)	96.7% survivorship
Mabry et al (2007)	73	73 (50-90)	10.2 (2-15)	5-year survivorship, 98% 10-year survivorship, 92%

NA = not available.

flexion gap. The tibial cut is made using either intramedullary or extramedullary guides. Once the joint-line cut is made, a tibial baseplate trial is placed onto the cut surface, positioned optimally relative to rotation and translation, and then fixed with pins. The canal is then reamed through a guide on the tibial baseplate trial to create the space for the stem. The stem opening should be created 2 to 4 mm larger than the outer diameter of the cemented stem to allow a 1- to 2-mm cement mantle around the stem, and it should be reamed far enough away from the joint line to allow 1.5 to 2.0 cm of cement mantle at the tip of the stem. The length of the stem is chosen to be long enough to bypass any defect or engage healthy cancellous bone beyond the limits of the damage created by the implant being revised.

Femoral preparation also is performed by preparing the joint-line cuts first. Once the joint-line cuts are made, the femoral stem preparation is completed by drilling through the femoral block with the same considerations regarding diameter and length mentioned regarding the tibial component preparation. As with the uncemented stem preparation, trialing of the components is essential to determine that the components fit, seat fully, and maintain the appropriate relationship with the joint line and the cut surfaces of the bone. As with the uncemented

stem procedure, an intraoperative radiograph can be helpful to define the component position if there is uncertainty during the trial reduction. Standard cement technique is used, with retrograde filling using a cement gun, cement restrictors, control of the surgical field to minimize lamination of blood or debris into the cement, and cement pressurization to achieve interdigitation of cement within the cancellous bone. In addition, any neocortex present within the diaphysis that is left over from bone remodeling should be removed. The cement needs access to cancellous bone to achieve optimal interdigitation and fixation (**Figure 5**).

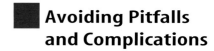

Postoperative Regimen

The postoperative regimen is not based upon the use of a stem, but rather the stability of the overall construct and the condition of the soft tissues. Generally, weight bearing is restricted for at least several weeks after surgery. The length of restrictions will depend on the condition of the bone, the extent of bone grafting required, and the patient's ability to comply. The presence of a stem is an indicator of complexity but does not drive the postoperative recommendations.

Avoiding Pitfalls and Complications

The use of a stem (especially a press-fit stem) tends to move the femoral component anteriorly. Therefore, an offset stem should be considered to decrease the distance between the stem and the anterior flange. Care with the placement of the canal entry hole will also help prevent anteriorization of the anterior flange of the femoral component.

Placing a free saw blade, a ruler, or a stylus along the anterior cortex through the femoral AP cutting guide before making the anterior cut can aid in positioning the femoral component along the anterior femoral cortex. This strategy will help to avoid both excessive offset of the anterior femoral flange and a large flexion gap caused by an anteriorly translated femoral component.

The effect of the tibial or femoral bow should be assessed by templating preoperatively to anticipate potential impingement during implantation. Templating is also important in TKA after tibial osteotomy or trauma, where alterations in the normal anatomy may preclude the use of standard stems or off-the-shelf components without customized offsets.

The surgeon should be aware of the possibility of reaming through the anterior femoral cortex with straight,

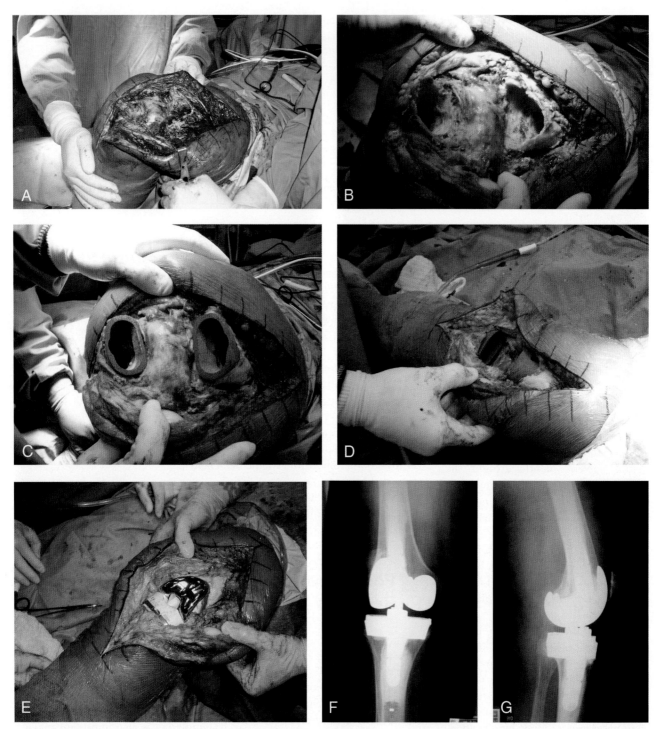

Figure 5 Cemented or uncemented stems can be used to support metaphyseal sleeves or blocks used to reconstruct areas of bone loss. In this case, cemented stems have been used to support a porous metal tibial sleeve. The sequence of events in stem preparation involves satisfactory exposure of the knee and removal of components, definition of the bone defect, filling of the metaphyseal bone defect with allograft or metallic augmentation, and placement of a stemmed component with trials. **A,** Extensile exposure of the knee, demonstrating significant metaphyseal defects in both the femur and the tibia. **B,** Closer magnification shows extensive metaphyseal bone loss on both the femoral and tibial sides of the joint. **C,** Flexion view with metal porous sleeves in place used to manage large metaphyseal defects and reestablish the joint line. **D,** Intraoperative extension view with porous sleeves in place shows how the joint line is brought down from the femur and up from the tibia to decrease the extension gap. **E,** Trial components with stems in place allow the surgeon to evaluate the ligamentous stability at the construct. AP (**F**) and lateral (**G**) radiographs of the knee demonstrate use of metaphyseal sleeves combined with short cemented stems.

rigid reamers designed for femoral stem implantation. In a bowed femur, the "line of trajectory" of the stem and the reamer should be assessed to establish a safe reaming depth.

Trial components with appropriate-length stems should be used intraoperatively. Trialing will ensure that the components will seat properly and that the stem has not forced the articular portion of the implant into a less than optimal position.

Uncemented stems may be optimized by cementation in the metadiaphysis as well as the articular interface to achieve optimal primary implant stability.

The importance of good cement technique—the use of restrictors, retrograde filling, pressurization, and removing any penetrated neocortex left from the prior implant—cannot be overemphasized. The surgeon should not try to cement into sclerotic or smooth bone.

Bibliography

Barrack RL, Rorabeck C, Burt M, Sawhney J: Pain at the end of the stem after revision total knee arthroplasty. *Clin Orthop Relat Res* 1999;367:216-225.

Barrack RL, Stanley T, Burt M, Hopkins S: The effect of stem design on end-of-stem pain in revision total knee arthroplasty. *J Arthroplasty* 2004;19(7 suppl 2):119-124.

Bertin KC, Freeman MA, Samuelson KM, Ratcliffe SS, Todd RC: Stemmed revision arthroplasty for aseptic loosening of total knee replacement. *J Bone Joint Surg Br* 1985;67(2):242-248.

Channer MA, Glisson RR, Seaber AV, Vail TP: Use of bone compaction in total knee arthroplasty. *J Arthroplasty* 1996;11(6):743-749.

Fehring TK, Odum S, Olekson C, Griffin WL, Mason JB, McCoy TH: Stem fixation in revision total knee arthroplasty: A comparative analysis. *Clin Orthop Relat Res* 2003;416:217-224.

Jazrawi LM, Bai B, Kummer FJ, Hiebert R, Stuchin SA: The effect of stem modularity and mode of fixation on tibial component stability in revision total knee arthroplasty. *J Arthroplasty* 2001;16(6):759-767.

Mabry TM, Vessely MB, Schleck CD, Harmsen WS, Berry DJ: Revision total knee arthroplasty with modular cemented stems: Long-term follow-up. *J Arthroplasty* 2007;22(6 Suppl 2):100-105.

Mahoney OM, Kinsey TL: Modular femoral offset stems facilitate joint line restoration in revision knee arthroplasty. *Clin Orthop Relat Res* 2006;446:93-98.

Musgrave DS, Glisson RR, Graham RD, Guilak F, Vail TP: Effects of coronally slotted femoral prostheses on cortical bone strain. *J Arthroplasty* 1997;12(6):657-669.

Nakasone CK, Abdeen A, Khachatourians AG, Sugimori T, Vince KG: Component alignment in revision total knee arthroplasty using diaphyseal engaging modular offset press-fit stems. *J Arthroplasty* 2008;23(8):1178-1181.

Peters CL, Erickson J, Kloepper RG, Mohr RA: Revision total knee arthroplasty with modular components inserted with metaphyseal cement and stems without cement. *J Arthroplasty* 2005;20(3):302-308.

Shannon BD, Klassen JF, Rand JA, Berry DJ, Trousdale RT: Revision total knee arthroplasty with cemented components and uncemented intramedullary stems. *J Arthroplasty* 2003;18(7 suppl 1):27-32.

Vince KG, Long W: Revision knee arthroplasty: The limits of press fit medullary fixation. *Clin Orthop Relat Res* 1995;317:172-177.

Whaley AL, Trousdale RT, Rand JA, Hanssen AD: Cemented long-stem revision total knee arthroplasty. *J Arthroplasty* 2003;18(5):592-599.

Coding				
CPT Codes			**Corresponding ICD-9 Codes**	
27487	Revision of total knee arthroplasty, with or without allograft; femoral and entire tibial component	996.40 996.42	996.60 996.43	

CPT copyright © 2010 by the American Medical Association. All rights reserved.

Chapter 47

Revision Total Knee Arthroplasty: Bone Loss Management Using Cancellous Grafts

Charles L. Nelson, MD

 ## Indications

Cancellous bone grafts are one option for managing bone loss encountered during revision total knee arthroplasty (TKA) (**Figure 1**). Cancellous bone grafts can be used to address both contained and uncontained defects. Wire mesh permits conversion of partially uncontained defects to contained defects.

Bone defects noted at the time of revision TKA frequently are irregular. Because cancellous bone grafts can be impacted into irregular defects, these grafts can be useful in restoring bone stock and stability without significant removal of host bone. Sacrifice of good-quality host bone often is required when preparing a defect to properly fit a contoured bulk allograft or factory-assembled metal augment.

 ## Contraindications

Active infection is the primary contraindication to the use of cancellous bone grafts during revision TKA. In addition, if insufficient bone is present

to achieve initial implant stability, cancellous bone graft cannot be used as the primary method of managing bone loss during TKA revision. Large circumferential, uncontained, segmental bone defects may require a megaprosthesis or bulk allograft prosthesis composite to obtain satisfactory initial stability.

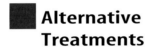

 ## Alternative Treatments

Alternative techniques for the management of bone loss during TKA revision include the use of cement (with or without screw augmentation), bulk allografts, metallic augments, or a more distal resection than usual, with thicker polyethylene. No technique is appropriate for all cases; however, cancellous bone grafts offer several advantages over other techniques. Cancellous bone grafts allow reconstitution of bone stock and are incorporated more rapidly and completely than are bulk allografts. Bulk allografts may heal to host bone and may be associated with a few millime-

ters of creeping substitution; however, these grafts remain permanently nonviable. Bulk allografts, metal augments, and megaprostheses provide a rigid substrate that substitutes for bone loss and facilitates initial prosthetic stability.

 ## Results

Tight impaction of morcellized cancellous or corticocancellous allograft with cement has a long history of use during revision total hip arthroplasty on both the acetabular and femoral sides. Only a few short- to intermediate-term series have evaluated this technique in the setting of revision TKA, however (**Table 1**). To my knowledge, the earliest reports of the use of impacted morcellized bone graft for bone loss during revision TKA were from Whiteside, who described this technique in combination with a stemmed, uncemented total knee prosthesis.

Lotke and associates reported their experience using impaction bone grafting with cement fixation and wire mesh for large contained bone defects. In a series of 42 consecutive revision TKAs for which impaction bone grafting was required for large bone defects, no cases of aseptic loosening had occurred at a mean 3.8-year follow-up.

Dr. Nelson or an immediate family member is a member of a speakers' bureau or has made paid presentations on behalf of Zimmer; serves as a paid consultant for or is an employee of Zimmer; and is a board member, owner, officer, or committee member for the J. Robert Gladden Society.

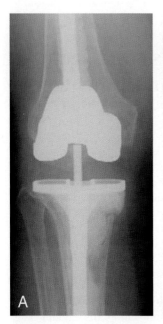
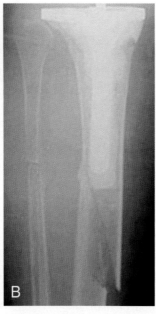
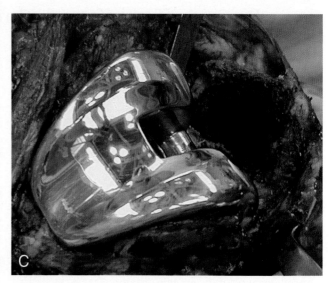

Figure 1 Impaction grafting and metal augment was used in this patient with a loose tibial prosthesis associated with a periprosthetic fracture. Preoperative AP (**A**) and oblique (**B**) radiographs of the right knee and tibia. **C**, Intraoperative photograph demonstrates marked metallosis with contained and uncontained bone loss. (Reproduced with permission from Beharrie AW, Nelson CL: Impaction bone-grafting in the treatment of a periprosthetic fracture of the tibia. *J Bone Joint Surg Am* 2003;85:703-707.)

Table 1 Results of Revision Total Knee Arthroplasty With Impaction Grafting

Author(s) (Year)	Number of Knees	Mean Patient Age (Range)	Mean Follow-up (Range)	Results
Whiteside and Bicalho (1998)	62	71 (57-91)	NR	82.6% pain free 22% complication rate (14 reoperations) 2 patients revised for aseptic loosening Histologic analysis of reoperations demonstrated new bone formation with progressive maturation with increase in time from surgery.
Heyligers et al (2001)	11	75 (62-87)	22 months (3-48)	100% good results No loosening or graft resorption
Lonner et al (2002)	17	68 (59-79)	NR	KSS improved from 47 to 95 FS improved from 48 to 73 No mechanical loosening Complications: 1 deep infection, 1 traumatic periprosthetic fracture at 8 months postoperatively, 1 surgery for patellar clunk
Lotke et al (2006)	42	69.5 (38-81)	3.8 years (2-6.5)	KSS improved from 57 to 90 FS improved from 52 to 80 No mechanical loosening High complication rate: 2 deep infections, 2 patellar clunk syndromes, 2 late traumatic periprosthetic fractures

NR = not reported, KSS = Knee Society knee score, FS = Knee Society function score.

The Knee Society knee scores in these patients improved from a mean of 57 (out of 100) to a mean of 90, and the Knee Society function scores improved from a mean of 52 (out of 100) to 80. Complications developed in 6 patients, including two infections, two patellar clunk syndromes, and two late traumatic periprosthetic fractures.

Technique

Setup/Exposure

The procedure and the surgical site are confirmed and marked before entry into the surgical theater. Following administration of preoperative antibiotics and induction of anesthesia, the patient is placed supine on the surgical table.

Procedure

After exposure, the implant is removed, taking care to protect neurovascular structures, the extensor mechanism, and key ligamentous supports. Recognition and protection of bone stock important to the stability and function of the definitive reconstruction is a key element of implant removal. Use of oscillating and reciprocating saws allows debonding of the prosthesis from host bone or cement without levering against deficient host bone and may facilitate removal with better bone preservation. Adjacent structures must be protected during this procedure, taking into account the entire excursion of the saw blade.

After removal of the implants, membranous tissue, and cement (if present), an assessment of bone stock is made. Use of a curet or small burr facilitates conservative débridement of membranous tissue, cement, and necrotic bone. An intramedullary guide or rod placed down the tibia is helpful in establishing tibial alignment. When small or large contained tibial defects are present, the use of cancellous bone grafts is an excellent technique. A ce-

ment restrictor with a central guide rod is placed 2 to 3 cm below the point at which the tibial stem of the tibial component is anticipated to rest. Corticocancellous bone chips are packed tightly above the cement restrictor using cannulated bone tamps. After placement of more bone graft into the canal, cannulated smooth diaphyseal reamers or broaches are used to pack bone graft centripetally around the canal. Using proximal bone tamps, bone graft is packed tightly into the proximal tibia (**Figure 2,** *A*). An intramedullary stem trial prevents bone graft from entering the intramedullary canal during cancellous bone graft impaction. With uncontained bone defects, the surgeon may choose to use impaction grafting for contained areas of bone loss and a metal augment for uncontained areas (**Figure 2,** *B* through *D*). Alternatively, stainless steel wire mesh can be cut manually and contoured to overlap from a contained to an uncontained area of bone loss, thereby creating a contained defect. The wire mesh is then attached to host bone with small screws, circumferential wire or cable, or a combination of these devices.

A tibial trial implant maintains compression on the impacted cancellous bone graft during femoral preparation. I prefer to use a stem augment in all cases of revision TKA with sufficient bone loss to perform impaction grafting, although good results were reported using primary components in one small series with short follow-up.

The key aspect of femoral preparation is achieving the desired femoral alignment and rotation with an appropriate-size implant at the normal joint line. Use of long-stem trials or intramedullary guides allows establishment of good alignment in the absence of notable extra-articular deformity. The meniscal scar, if present and identifiable, represents the best estimate of the original joint line. Additional landmarks that help to identify the

original joint line include the inferior pole of the patella and the medial or lateral femoral epicondyle. I prefer to use distal femoral augments against a stable platform to ensure accurate and reproducible establishment of the joint line with both the femoral trial and the final component. Once a stable platform is achieved against one or both distal femoral condyles, cancellous bone grafts are impacted into areas of contained bone loss, as described earlier for impaction cancellous bone grafting of the tibia. For areas of uncontained bone loss, wire mesh can be used to achieve containment of impacted cancellous grafts (**Figure 3**).

After femoral and tibial preparation and with trial components in place, knee range of motion, stability, and patellar tracking are assessed, and the appropriate size and style of tibial insert is selected. Cement mixing is begun and the femoral and tibial implants are cemented into place.

Wound Closure

After cement polymerization and assessment of final knee range of motion, stability, and patellar tracking, wound closure is performed according to the surgeon's preference, in layers. My preference is to initiate closure of the quadriceps tendon and extensor layer in 90° of flexion, starting with anatomic repair across the superomedial aspect of the patella using interrupted No. 1 braided absorbable sutures. The Scarpa fascia and the subcutaneous layer are then closed with interrupted 2-0 braided absorbable sutures. The skin is then closed with staples.

Postoperative Regimen

The appropriate postoperative protocol for weight bearing following revi-

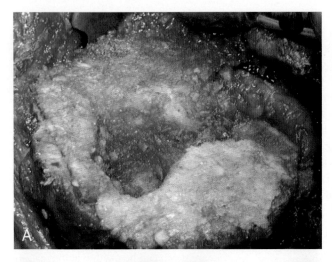

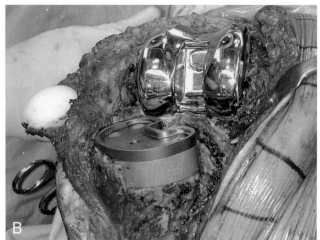

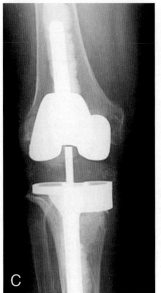

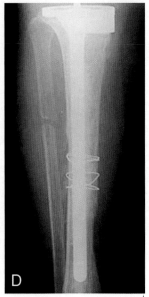

Figure 2 Images of the knee shown in Figure 1. **A,** Intraoperative photograph depicts the defect after débridement of metal debris, membranous tissue, and nonviable bone and after impaction bone grafting. **B,** Intraoperative photograph demonstrates the use of a block metal augment to manage the uncontained medial tibial defect in this patient. An augment was chosen instead of mesh because minimal host-bone sacrifice was needed to accommodate the augment. Postoperative AP (**C**) and oblique (**D**) radiographs. (Panels A, C, D reproduced with permission from Beharrie AW, Nelson CL: Impaction bone-grafting in the treatment of a periprosthetic fracture of the tibia. *J Bone Joint Surg Am* 2003;85:703-707.)

sion TKA with impaction bone grafting is controversial. The regimen used for the initial series of impaction bone grafting during revision total hip arthroplasty included a 6- to 12-week period of protected weight bearing. Subsequent series with shorter follow-up allowed weight bearing as tolerated immediately following surgery, and in fact, some authors believe that weight bearing and stress on the impacted cancellous grafts are important to promote incorporation of bone graft. I have allowed my patients to bear weight as tolerated immediately following surgery in most cases. In the only series describing this technique

used in knees with primary knee components without revision stems, however, the authors prescribed protected weight bearing for up to 3 months. In the setting of periprosthetic fracture, or if concern about initial stability or diaphyseal bone quality is present, an initial course of protected weight bearing is warranted.

My postoperative regimen with regard to range of motion and rehabilitation is the same as for other revision TKA procedures. In most cases, continuous passive motion is instituted in the postanesthesia care unit and is advanced as tolerated. Patients are instructed to perform isometric quadri-

ceps sets as early as possible and to attempt active straight-leg raises. Gentle range of motion and conditioning are then advanced under the supervision of a physical therapist.

Avoiding Pitfalls and Complications

Revision TKA, particularly in the presence of massive bone loss, is associated with a high complication rate. The key surgical principles for preventing complications are avoidance

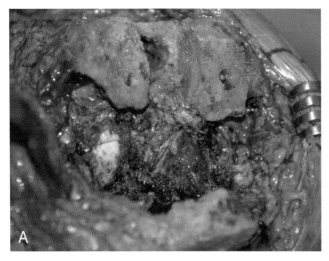

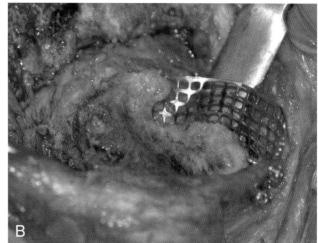

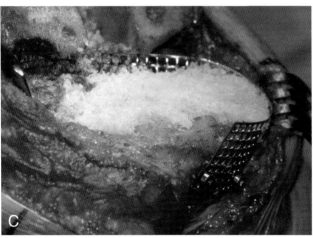

Figure 3 Intraoperative photographs depict the use of stainless steel wire mesh to convert an uncontained defect to a contained defect. **A,** Metallosis and uncontained bone loss following removal of a total knee prosthesis. **B,** Conversion of the uncontained medial tibial defect to a contained defect using contoured stainless steel wire mesh and screws. **C,** Impaction bone grafting into the tibia with wire mesh containing graft. (Reproduced with permission from Lonner JH, Lotke PA, Kim J, Nelson C: Impaction grafting with wire mesh for uncontained defects in revision TKA. *Clin Orthop Relat Res* 2002; 404:145-151.)

of nerve or vascular injury, protection of the extensor mechanism, and prevention of periprosthetic infection or fracture. An atraumatic surgical approach that respects skin vascularity and provides excellent visualization and protection of important structures is paramount in avoiding these complications. Preoperative antibiotics, good sterile technique, and reasonably efficient surgery are important measures for minimizing the risk of infection. When bone stock is severely compromised, special care must be exercised to avoid tibial tubercle avulsion and periprosthetic fractures of the femur or tibia during bone impaction or trial reduction. Using a pro- phylactic wire or cable before impaction is helpful, particularly on the femoral side, when concern about fracture or fracture propagation is present.

Bibliography

Beharrie AW, Nelson CL: Impaction bone-grafting in the treatment of a periprosthetic fracture of the tibia: A case report. *J Bone Joint Surg Am* 2003;85:703-707.

Gie GA, Linder L, Ling RSM: Impacted cancellous allograft and cement for revision total hip arthroplasty. *J Bone Joint Surg Br* 1993;75:14-21.

Heyligers IC, van Haaren EH, Wuisman PI: Revision knee arthroplasty using impaction grafting and primary implants. *J Arthroplasty* 2001;16:533-537.

Insall JN, Dorr LD, Scott RD, Scott WN: Rationale of the Knee Society clinical scoring system. *Clin Orthop Relat Res* 1989; 248:13-14.

Lonner JH, Lotke PA, Kim J, Nelson C: Impaction grafting and wire mesh for uncontained defects in revision knee arthroplasties. *Clin Orthop Relat Res* 2002;404:145-151.

Lotke PA, Carolan GF, Puri N: Impaction grafting for bone defects and revision knee arthroplasty. *Clin Orthop Relat Res* 2006;446:99-103.

Sloof TJ, Schimmel JW, Buma P: Cemented fixation with bone grafts. *Orthop Clin North Am* 1993;24:667-672.

Suárez-Suárez MA, Murcia A, Maestro A: Filling of segmental bone defects in revision knee arthroplasty using morcellized bone grafts contained within a metal mesh. *Acta Orthop Belg* 2002;68:163-167.

Toms AD, McClelland D, Chua L, et al: Mechanical testing of impaction bone grafting in the tibia: Stability and design of the stem. *J Bone Joint Surg Br* 2005;87:656-663.

Ullmark G, Obrant KJ: Histology of impacted bone-graft incorporation. *J Arthroplasty* 2002;17:150-157.

Whiteside LA: Cementless reconstruction of massive tibial bone loss in revision total knee arthroplasty. *Clin Orthop Relat Res* 1989;248:80-86.

Whiteside LA, Bicalho PS: Radiologic and histologic analysis of morcellized allograft in revision total knee replacement. *Clin Orthop Relat Res* 1998;357:149-156.

Coding

CPT Codes		Corresponding ICD-9 Codes	
Removal of Total Knee Implant			
27488	Removal of prosthesis, including total knee prosthesis, methylmethacrylate with or without insertion of spacer, knee	996.40 996.43	996.42 996.60
Prophylactic Treatment of Knee			
27495	Prophylactic treatment (nailing, pinning, plating, or wiring) with or without methylmethacrylate, femur	996.40 996.43	996.42 996.60
Bone Graft			
20900 20902	Bone graft, any donor area; minor or small (eg, dowel or button) Bone graft, any donor area; major or large	996.40 996.43 996.40 996.43	996.42 996.60 996.42 996.60

Revision Total Knee Arthroplasty: Bone Loss Management Using Structural Grafts

David Backstein, MD, MEd, FRCSC
Allan E. Gross, MD, FRCSC
Oleg Safir, MD, MEd, FRCSC
Joseph B. Aderinto, MD, FRCS (Tr and Orth)

■ Indications

The management of bone loss encountered at the time of revision total knee arthroplasty (TKA) can be challenging. Etiologies of bone loss include infection, stress shielding, aseptic loosening, and periprosthetic fracture. Bone loss also can be iatrogenic, occurring during the process of implant removal or débridement for infection. Defects can be categorized as contained or uncontained. Uncontained defects can be further categorized as circumferential or noncircumferential. Small contained defects can be managed with impacted morcellized bone graft or cement, and small uncontained defects on the tibial and femoral sides can be managed with metallic blocks or wedges and the use of thicker than usual polyethylene. Large defects associated with the loss of metaphyseal bone and compro-

mised support of the prosthesis are more challenging to treat and may require structural allografts.

Structural allografts are used to reconstruct bone defects that are beyond the scope of morcellized bone, cement, or augments. They can be used to treat segmental femoral or tibial defects larger than 20 mm, which is the extent to which most metallic augments are effective. Circumferential defects up to 45 mm may be manageable with augments and thick polyethylene liners. Tibial circumferential defects larger than 45 mm require structural allograft. Massive circumferential uncontained defects can be managed with an allograft-prosthesis composite that consists of stemmed tibial or femoral components cemented to corresponding allograft, which in turn is stabilized to host bone.

Structural allograft restores bone stock, which can be advantageous in

young, active patients who may require future revision surgery. For older, less active patients, in whom bone stock restoration is a lower priority, endoprosthetic replacement may be more appropriate.

The lack of a universally accepted bone defect classification system makes comparisons difficult when evaluating treatment options. For example, Engh's classification categorizes bone loss into three groups, based on the severity of the bone deficiency encountered during revision surgery (**Table 1**). A classification system developed by the Mount Sinai Group is used when communicating about and describing specific cases of bone loss around TKAs. In this system, contained bone loss is defined as a lesion that is surrounded by an intact cortical rim of bone. Bone loss is considered uncontained when no surrounding cortical sleeve is present (**Table 2**).

In summary, factors that influence decision making about reconstructive options include defect size and location, patient age and activity level, associated comorbidity, and the patient's ability to comply with a rehabilitation regimen. Our primary indication for the use of structural allografts is the

Dr. Backstein or an immediate family member is a member of a speakers' bureau or has made paid presentations on behalf of Stryker and Zimmer and serves as a paid consultant for or is an employee of Stryker and Zimmer. Dr. Gross or an immediate family member has received royalties from Zimmer; is a member of a speakers' bureau or has made paid presentations on behalf of Zimmer; serves as a paid consultant for or is an employee of Zimmer; and is a board member, owner, officer, or committee member of the Canadian Orthopaedic Association, The Knee Society, and The Hip Society. Neither of the following authors nor any immediate family member has received anything of value from or owns stock in a commercial company or institution related directly or indirectly to the subject of this chapter: Dr. Safir and Dr. Aderinto.

Table 1 Anderson Orthopaedic Research Institute Bone Defect Classification

Type	Severity of Bone Deficiency Encountered During Revision Surgery
1	Minor femoral or tibial defects with intact metaphyseal bone, not compromising the stability of a revision component
2	Damaged metaphyseal bone. Loss of cancellous metaphyseal femoral or tibial bone requiring reconstruction (cement fill, prosthetic augment, or bone graft) to provide stability of the revision component A: Defects in one femoral or tibial condyle B: Defects in both femoral or tibial condyles
3	Deficient metaphyseal segment compromising a major portion of either the femoral condyle or tibial plateau, occasionally associated with collateral or patellar ligament detachment

Reprinted with permission from Engh GA: Bone defect classification, in Engh GA, Rorabeck CH, eds: *Revision Total Knee Arthroplasty*. Baltimore, MD, Lippincott Williams & Wilkins, 1997, pp 63-120.

Table 2 Mount Sinai Hospital Bone Defect Classification

Type	Type of Bone Loss	Description
1	No notable loss of bone stock	There may be erosion of the endosteal bone, but no involvement of the cortex. There has been no migration of the primary component and bone is largely intact.
2	Contained loss of bone stock with cortical thinning	The canal is widened, but there is still an intact cortical sleeve.
3	Uncontained (segmental) loss of bone stock involving <50% of medial and/or lateral condyle	Uncontained bone loss represents less than 50% of medial and/or lateral femoral and/or tibial condyle and is less than 15 mm deep.
4	Uncontained (segmental) loss of bone stock >50% of medial and/or lateral condyle	Uncontained bone loss represents more than 50% of medial and/or lateral femoral and/or tibial condyle and is more than 15 mm deep.

Reproduced with permission from Safir O, Gross AE, Backstein D: Management of bone loss: Structural grafts in revision total knee arthroplasty, in Brown TE, Cui Q, Mihalko WM, Saleh KJ, eds: *Arthritis and Arthroplasty: The Knee—Expert Consult*. Philadelphia, PA, Saunders Elsevier, 2009, pp 212-220.

presence of large uncontained bone defects that lie outside the range of metal augments or thicker polyethylene.

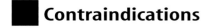

Contraindications

Several contraindications are specific to the use of allograft bone. The success of the allograft requires stable union to host bone; therefore, local or systemic conditions that impair graft union to host bone can be considered contraindications. For example, previous irradiation of the surgical field can compromise the union of allograft to host bone. Smoking should be discouraged until the allograft has united because it may impair graft incorporation. Consideration also should be given to the patient's ability to complete and comply with rehabilitation after surgery, because protected weight bearing is mandatory until radiographic evidence of healing at the allograft–host bone junction is present; such healing usually occurs by 3 months, but it can take longer.

Alternative Treatments

Distal femoral or proximal tibial endoprostheses are alternatives to structural allografts. They have been used for tumor reconstruction for many years, and their use in the setting of severe bone loss has increased recently for reconstruction in revision knee surgery because of the availability of off-the-shelf modular systems. Their principal advantages over allograft and allograft-implant composites include a less technically complex reconstruction and more rapid rehabilitation, because weight bearing usually can be commenced at an earlier stage. These implants do not restore bone stock, however; instead, they compromise diaphyseal bone, thus making revision surgery more complex. In our opinion, their use is therefore more appropriate in older, lower-demand patients and for reconstruction after tumor excision.

Knee arthrodesis is another option for the treatment of catastrophic TKA failure; however, this treatment often is associated with a poorer functional outcome than TKA revision. Despite this drawback, fusion remains a viable option in patients who are not good candidates for reconstructive procedures using allograft or an endoprosthesis, such as patients with persistent and recalcitrant infection or extensor mechanism failure.

Results

Structural allografts have been effective in the reconstruction of both large contained defects and massive uncon-

Table 3 Results of Structural Allograft for Revision TKA

Authors (Year)	Number of Knees	Procedure	Mean Patient Age (Range)	Complications	Survivorship at Mean Follow-up
Stockley et al (1992)	20	Structural allografts and morcellized bone	69.4 (37.9-83.3)	0 nonunions 2 graft fractures 3 infections	85% at 4.2 years
Harris et al (1995)	14	Allograft-prosthesis composites	67 (37-82)	0 nonunions 1 infection	93% at 43 months
Mow and Wiedel (1996)	15	Contained and uncontained defects	63 (26-85)	No nonunions, infections, or graft fractures	80% at 47 months
Ghazavi et al (1997)	30	Allograft-prosthesis composites and large structural allografts	65.8 (24-89)	1 nonunion 3 infections 1 graft fracture	67% at 5 years
Engh et al (1997)	30	Femoral head and allograft-prosthesis composites	70 (43-86)	No nonunions, infections, or graft fractures	100% at 50 months
Clatworthy et al (2001)	52	Allograft-prosthesis composites and large structural allografts	68 (24-85)	2 nonunions 4 infections 1 graft fracture	92% at 5 years; 72% at 10 years
Backstein et al (2006)	61	Allograft-prosthesis composites and large structural allografts	73.4 (26-92)	1 nonunion 4 infections 2 graft fractures	79% at 5.4 years
Engh and Ammeen (2007)	46	Femoral head allograft for tibia defects	67 (39-86)	0 nonunions 2 infections 0 graft fractures	91% at 10 years

tained defects encountered at the time of revision TKA. Most reported series have shown good clinical results, and early outcomes have been promising, with 5-year survivorship ranging from 67% to 92% (**Table 3**). Graft union rates generally are high, and the rate of nonunion is less than 4%. The incidence of other graft-related complications has been variable. Graft fracture rates range from 0% to 10%. Graft revascularization resulting in resorption is a recognized complication that can lead to graft collapse and implant migration. Although resorption rates of up to 8% have been reported in earlier studies, more recent studies demonstate this to be an inconsistent finding. In studies that include patients who underwent revision for any reason, infection rates range from 0% to 15%. In a recent study, we reported on 68 structural allografts used for re-

vision of 61 TKAs performed at our institution. At 5.4-year follow-up, graft survivorship was 85%, with a graft union rate greater than 98%.

■ Techniques

Setup/Exposure

Preoperative planning includes a review of the following radiographs: AP (**Figure 1**, *A*) and lateral views of the knee, a skyline patella view, and AP long-leg weight-bearing views. CT can be useful in detecting defects that cannot be visualized clearly on radiographs because of overlying implants (**Figure 1**, *B*). The extent of bony deficiency is assessed, and the level of proposed tibial and femoral resections is determined. If an allograft-implant composite is to be used, an allograft of

similar or smaller diameter than the host's own bone should be selected because a graft-implant composite that is too large will preclude closure of the soft tissues. Too large an allograft may be an even greater problem during the second stage of a two-stage revision for infection, when contracture of the soft-tissue envelope occurs between stages. In such cases, consultation with a plastic surgeon with expertise in rotational gastrocnemius flaps and use of a skin graft may be required to achieve wound closure (**Figure 2**).

The patient is positioned supine on the operating table; care should be taken to ensure that pressure areas are protected adequately. A tourniquet is placed on the proximal thigh. When skin graft may be needed or sufficiently proximal placement of the tourniquet cannot be achieved because of patient habitus, a sterile tour-

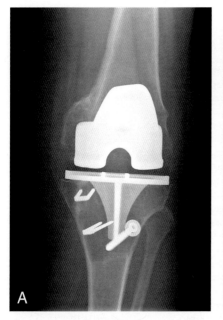 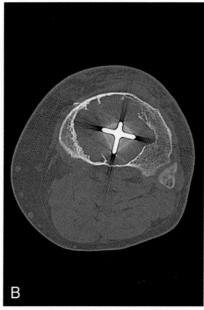

Figure 1 Images of a patient with a loose TKA. **A,** AP radiograph demonstrates signs of osteolysis. **B,** CT scan demonstrates a significant defect of the proximal tibia.

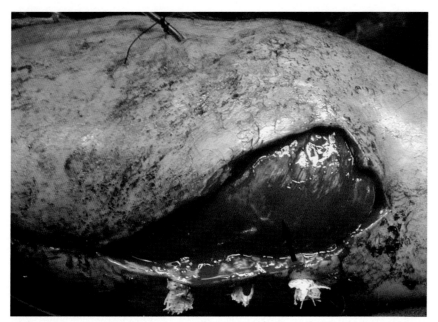

Figure 2 Photograph demonstrates a gastrocnemius flap (arrow) used to cover a wound after a staged revision TKA for infection.

to accommodate a tibial allograft composite, a tibial tubercle osteotomy is performed so the tubercle can be reattached to the allograft. All nonviable bone, tissue, and cement are removed to delineate the bone defects, which are then measured. Infected TKAs are revised in two stages. In the first stage, the implants are removed, infected tissue is débrided, and an antibiotic-impregnated cement spacer is inserted. In the second stage, reimplantation is performed with structural allograft once infection has been eradicated. Our practice is to perform frozen section at the second stage, with a neutrophil count of 5 or fewer per high-power field considered to be consistent with absence of infection when combined with normal serologic markers.

Allograft Selection

It is important to ensure that the appropriate allograft is available before commencing the procedure. Tissue is ordered from a bank accredited by the American Association of Tissue Banks. Our bone bank takes radiographs of all allograft bones. During preoperative planning, host defects are quantified using radiographs and CT. Allograft tissue is then selected based on the size and shape of the donor tissue. In general, we prefer to select anatomically similar tissue, using a femoral allograft for a femoral defect and tibial bone for a tibial defect. Bone graft tissue should be of high quality and not osteoporotic.

Instruments/Equipment/ Implants Required

A variety of modular tibial and femoral implants with variable stem lengths and augments of various sizes should be available to the surgeon. In addition, prostheses with varying degrees of constraint are required. Allograft bone is harvested under sterile conditions according to the protocol of the American Association of Tissue Banks, frozen at –70°C, and irradiated (25,000 Gy). Using a second team to

niquet should be used, which can be removed intraoperatively to gain more proximal exposure. Ideally, a midline skin incision is used, incorporating the incision of the prior exposure where possible. A medial parapatellar approach is performed routinely, but in select cases, a tibial tubercle osteotomy, quadriceps snip, or quadriceps turndown can be used to improve exposure. If tibial resection below the level of the tibial tuberosity is planned

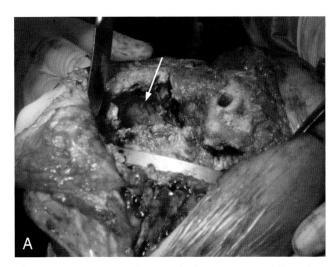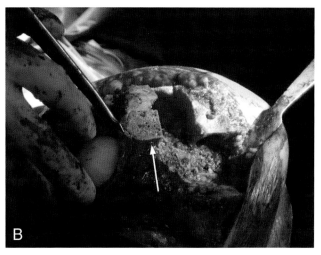

Figure 3 Intraoperative photographs depict a structural allograft press-fit into a bony defect without supplementary fixation. **A,** A segmental, uncontained defect in the lateral femoral condyle (arrow). **B,** A femoral metaphysis structural allograft (arrow) is press-fit into the defect in the distal femur without need for hardware fixation.

prepare the allograft on a sterile back table helps to reduce operating time.

Procedure

Our routine procedure is to first establish the level of the tibia platform, and then determine the size and position of the femoral component to balance the flexion gap with a 12- to 14-mm trial polyethylene insert. The distance between the joint line and the tip of the fibula can be measured on radiographs of the contralateral knee and used as a guide for the level of the joint line. If the contralateral knee has been replaced previously, the joint line can be estimated as being 1.5 cm proximal to the tip of the fibula or 2.5 cm distal to the medial epicondyle. After the trial stemmed implants are inserted and the flexion and extension gaps are balanced, the size of the bone defect is determined.

SEGMENTAL ALLOGRAFTS

Large uncontained defects outside the range of most augments (>20 mm) can be treated with segmental, structural allografts. After the tibial or femoral canal has been reamed so that the stem will fit tightly, freshening cuts are made to the available host bone. The defects are then assessed and quanti-

fied. Irregular defects are fashioned into more regular rectangular or square configurations, trying to preserve as much host bone as possible. This is done with a reciprocating saw, either freehand or using standard revision TKA guides. The bone defects are then measured with a ruler to determine length and depth. On a separate allograft table, donor bone of similar shape and dimension is fashioned. Ideally, allograft from the anatomic site corresponding to that of the defect is used. Femoral allograft is preferred for femoral defects, and tibial graft is preferred for tibial defects. If such bone is not available, high-quality femoral heads from a man or a premenopausal woman may be used.

Graft of matching geometric shape and size is crafted on the allograft preparation table. Initially, an allograft that is larger than the defect is prepared. The allograft is then taken to the recipient knee and assessed for fit. It usually is necessary to trim the graft down to the appropriate size and shape in a process that may require several comparisons between allograft and defect and repeated trips between the allograft preparation table and operating table. The process is much the same if a femoral head is used; how-

ever, exact contouring may be more prolonged because the bone initially is not the same anatomic shape. The required instruments include oscillating and reciprocating saws, a scalpel, a rongeur, and a bone cutter. A burr may be required to fine-tune the shape of the host defect to the shape of the graft.

Cases of massive osteolysis caused by polyethylene wear may produce large contained or uncontained defects. When combinations of contained and uncontained defects are present, a stable press-fit of the graft into the bony defect can be achieved, and in such cases supplementary fixation is not required (**Figure 3**). In our experience, this type of fit is more likely to occur when the defect lies between two columns of host bone, or between host bone and the articulating surface of a stemmed prosthesis. In such instances, the absence of fixation may confer an advantage by preventing the creation of stress risers associated with the use of screws.

When supplementary fixation of the allograft is required, the allograft is first placed in the defect and temporarily secured with Kirschner wires. Trial implants are inserted, and then definitive fixation of the allograft is

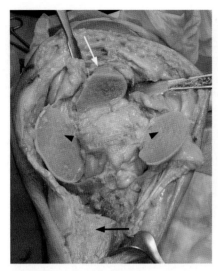

Figure 4 A cadaveric demonstration of bone defects. A medial tibial metaphyseal defect (black arrow) and massive bone loss of the femur (white arrow) are seen. The femoral medial and lateral epicondyles are indicated by the black arrowheads.

achieved using screws and washers. It is important that the trial components be in place before fixation of the graft occurs so that impingement of fixation hardware with the definitive components can be avoided. Stemmed components are always used, because they protect the structural allograft from excessive stress.

ALLOGRAFT-IMPLANT COMPOSITES

For large bone deficiencies such as circumferential, uncontained defects involving more than 20 mm of the femur or 30 mm to 40 mm of the proximal tibia, an allograft-prosthesis composite can be used.

When the distal femur is to be replaced with a femoral allograft-prosthesis composite, the epicondyles attached to the collateral ligaments are detached from the host distal femur so they can be reattached to the allograft. After removal of components, all nonviable bone, tissue, and cement are removed and the bone defects are delineated. The femoral epicondyles are retained if possible with preservation of the attached collateral ligaments. (Figure 4).

A step or oblique cut is made in the host bone at the proposed level of graft fixation to provide rotational stability. The longer limb of the step cut is fashioned on the host side if at all feasible, to preserve as much bone as possible. For a very large host femoral diaphysis, the allograft can be fitted into the host bone in a telescoping manner.

On the back table, either proximal tibial or distal femoral allograft is prepared, depending on the location of the defect.

Tibial Allograft-Implant Composite

The tibial allograft is cut to the appropriate length based on measurements made in the host knee after clearance of all cement and nonviable tissue. It is advisable to prepare the graft slightly longer than the measured defect initially so it can be trimmed down to the appropriate size. The canal is reamed to accept a tightly fitting stem in the host bone that will bypass the host-graft junction by at least 5 cm. The ultimate height of the joint line is determined based on radiographic measurements, with a goal of achieving a similar level as the opposite (healthy) knee, or approximately 1 cm above the level of the fibula. Step or oblique cuts are fashioned at the end of the graft to complement those in the host bone, positioned in a way that ensures correct rotational alignment, so the extensor mechanism tracks satisfactorily. While the allograft is still on the side table, standard revision jigs are used to make the proximal tibial allograft cuts. Next, the trial stemmed components are inserted into the allograft. Rotation of the allograft is determined using the patella and extensor mechanism as a guide. A trial implant is inserted into the allograft and trial reduction and range of motion of the knee is conducted. The tibial allograft rotation is chosen so as to allow the patella to track smoothly and without patellar tilt or dislocation. Once the appropriate rotation has been selected, a mark is made using a pen or methylene blue dye on the host tibia for later alignment of the definitive allograft-implant composite.

Femoral Allograft-Implant Composite

The host canal is reamed to accept a well-fitting stem that will bypass the host-graft junction by at least 5 cm. The distal femoral allograft is prepared by removing the graft epicondyles and placing nonabsorbable sutures through the bone tunnels made in the former positions of the epicondyles (Figure 5, A). These tunnels are made on the side table using a drill bit. Heavy nonabsorbable sutures are then passed, with the ends left free and held with a snap. The ends are left long and are used for later attachment of the host epicondyles to their associated collateral ligaments once the graft has been implanted. While still on the side table, standard revision jigs are used to make the distal femoral allograft cuts.

Next, the trial stemmed components are inserted into the allograft (Figure 5, B). The chosen stem size should provide a tight fit in the host canal. The trial composites are press-fit into host bone and the flexion gap is balanced by adjusting tibial height and femoral component size. The extension gap is balanced by progressively shortening the proximal end of the femoral allograft at the step cut until full extension is achieved. The definitive prosthesis is then cemented to the allograft on the back table. As mentioned previously, it is important to avoid using an implant-allograft composite that is too large, because it could compromise soft-tissue coverage at the time of wound closure.

Implantation

A fundamental principle of allograft-implant composite surgery is to use uncemented fixation in the host bone and cemented fixation in the allograft. Once the allografts have been sized appropriately and implantation is about to occur, the graft is cleansed

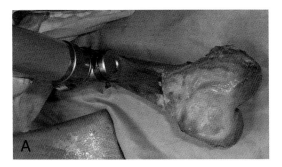
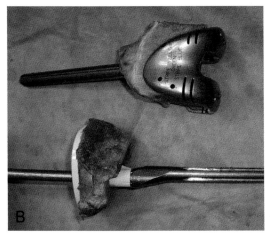
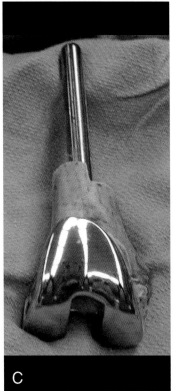
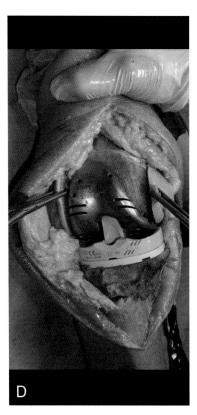

Figure 5 Preparing and implanting a femoral allograft-implant composite. **A,** A distal femoral allograft. The allograft is trimmed down to the appropriate size and shape using measurements from the host defect. **B,** The trial components are inserted into the allograft. **C,** Allograft-implant composite illustrating cementation of implant into the graft with uncemented fixation to the host. **D,** Intraoperative photograph demonstrating the distal femoral and proximal tibial allograft inserted into the host bone. The epicondyles are attached to the allograft.

and dried thoroughly. The implant is cemented into the dry allograft bone on the side table using antibiotic-impregnated cement. A low prophylactic dose of antibiotic should be used; we prefer to use cement with antibiotic added by the manufacturer. Once the cement has cured, the stems are inserted into the host bone in a press-fit manner. Stems are not cemented into the host diaphysis; stability is achieved by press-fit (**Figure 5,** *C* and *D*). Ideally, the cement is confined to the metaphyseal interface between the allograft and the prosthesis. Cementation of the diaphyseal part of the stems is avoided because this would make future revision more difficult. In addition, cement extrusion into the interface between host and allograft absolutely must be avoided because it will prevent union at the graft-host junction.

The stems of the prosthesis-allograft composite are inserted into the host bone, with stability at the host-allograft junction achieved by the press-fit of the prosthesis stem, and the step or oblique cut providing rotational stability. An oblique cut can be used as an alternative to a step cut, but this provides less stability. Morcellized autograft and allograft bone are then packed around the graft-host junction site. A cortical strut allograft may be used to augment stability on the femoral side. Placement of a cortical strut usually is not possible on the tibial side because of limited soft-tissue coverage; however, no further fixation generally is needed on this side. If any concern exists regarding stability, cortical screws can be used for supplementary tibial fixation. In our opinion, plates should not be used because multiple drill holes can stimu-

late rapid vascularization, increasing the risk of graft resorption and fracture.

Host epicondyles are then attached to the femoral allograft using the sutures that were placed previously. The host epicondyles are tied down to the allograft-implant composite with the knee at 90° of flexion, maximally tensioning the attached collateral ligaments. Any remnants of distal femoral host bone with soft-tissue attachments are wrapped around the distal femoral allograft and the allograft-host junction with cerclage wires.

Decision making about implant constraint is based on intraoperative assessment of stability. If the collateral ligaments are functioning well, then a posterior stabilized implant is favored over devices of greater constraint to prevent excessive stress transfer to the allograft-host junction. Should signif-

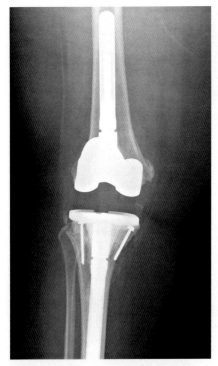

Figure 6 AP radiograph of a knee 5 months after revision TKA, demonstrating tibial implant–allograft composite. Radiographic evidence of host-graft union is present.

icant instability exist, however, further constraint is added with a higher post. A rotating-hinge knee prosthesis may be required, but it can lead to increased forces at the allograft-host junction, so we generally avoid using these prostheses in our practice.

Wound Closure
A single suction drain is placed deep to the retinaculum in close proximity to the prosthesis. For parapatellar approaches, the quadriceps tendon and retinaculum are closed with a combination of interrupted and continuous absorbable sutures. Continuous ab-

sorbable sutures are placed in the subcutaneous tissue to assist apposition of the wound edges and obliterate dead space, and the skin is closed with wound clips. If the tibial tubercle was osteotomized for the approach, it is reduced and secured with a screw using a lag technique or intraosseous wires. If a quadriceps turndown was performed, the quadriceps tendon is repaired with a nonabsorbable suture.

Postoperative Regimen

Range-of-motion exercises are encouraged within 48 hours. If a quadriceps turndown or tibial tubercle osteotomy has been performed, then active extension is restricted for 6 weeks. Weight bearing is not permitted until 8 weeks postoperatively; then, partial weight bearing can commence. Full weight bearing is allowed once evidence of graft union, which takes approximately 3 months, is present (**Figure 6**).

Avoiding Pitfalls and Complications

The importance of preoperative planning cannot be overemphasized. Preoperative radiographs provide crucial information about implant size, stem length, host bone resection level, and allograft size. The knee should be examined for previous surgical incisions

and the presence of soft-tissue contracture. The multiply operated knee is at high risk of wound complications, and soft-tissue handling must be well planned and meticulously performed. A plastic surgery consultation is advised if problems with wound closure are anticipated. Although supplementary fixation of segmental grafts for noncircumferential defects often requires screws to achieve satisfactory stabilization, drilling of the graft should be kept to a minimum to reduce the risk of graft revascularization, resorption, and collapse. Extrusion of cement into the interface at the graft-host junction is to be avoided because it will impair graft union. If a distal femoral allograft-implant composite is used, then correct rotational alignment is crucial to avoid maltracking of the extensor mechanism. It is important, therefore, that matching step cuts are fashioned in the correct position.

Postoperatively, protection of the graft from full weight bearing must be reinforced strongly to both patients and physical therapists to avoid graft collapse or fixation failure. Although early range of motion is imperative to prevent stiffness, a minimum of 6 to 8 weeks is needed before weight bearing is permitted.

Acknowledgment

The authors would like to thank Dr. Yona Kosashvili for his assistance with the cadaveric surgery for this chapter.

Bibliography

Backstein D, Safir O, Gross A: Management of bone loss: Structural grafts in revision total knee arthroplasty. *Clin Orthop Relat Res* 2006;446:104-112.

Clatworthy MG, Ballance J, Brick GW, Chandler HP, Gross AE: The use of structural allograft for uncontained defects in revision total knee arthroplasty: A minimum five-year review. *J Bone Joint Surg Am* 2001;83:404-411.

Engh GA, Ammeen DJ: Use of structural allograft in revision total knee arthroplasty in knees with severe tibial bone loss. *J Bone Joint Surg Am* 2007;89:2640-2647.

Engh GA, Herzwurm PJ, Parks NL: Treatment of major defects of bone with bulk allografts and stemmed components during total knee arthroplasty. *J Bone Joint Surg Am* 1997;79:1030-1039.

Fawcett K, Barr AR: *Tissue Banking*. Arlington, VA, American Association of Blood Banks, 1987, pp 97-107.

Ghazavi MT, Stockley I, Yee G, Davis A, Gross AE: Reconstruction of massive bone defects with allograft in revision total knee arthroplasty. *J Bone Joint Surg Am* 1997;79:17-25.

Harris AI, Poddar S, Gitelis S, Sheinkop MB, Rosenberg AG: Arthroplasty with a composite of an allograft and a prosthesis for knees with severe deficiency of bone. *J Bone Joint Surg Am* 1995;77:373-386.

Mow CS, Wiedel JD: Structural allografting in revision total knee arthroplasty. *J Arthroplasty* 1996;11:235-241.

Stockley I, McAuley JP, Gross AE: Allograft reconstruction in total knee arthroplasty. *J Bone Joint Surg Br* 1992;74:393-397.

Coding

CPT Codes		Corresponding ICD-9 Codes	
Removal of Total Knee Implant			
27488	Removal of prosthesis, including total knee prosthesis, methylmethacrylate with or without insertion of spacer, knee	996.40 996.43	996.42 996.60
Prophylactic Treatment of Knee			
27495	Prophylactic treatment (nailing, pinning, plating, or wiring) with or without methylmethacrylate, femur	996.40 996.43	996.42 996.60
20900	Bone graft, any donor area; minor or small (eg, dowel or button)	996.40 996.43	996.42 996.60
20902	Bone graft, any donor area; major or large	996.40 996.43	996.42 996.60
Bone Graft			
20900	Bone graft, any donor area; minor or small (eg, dowel or button)	996.40 996.43	996.42 996.60
20902	Bone graft, any donor area; major or large	996.40 996.43	996.42 996.60

Chapter 49

Metal Augments for Bone Loss in Revision Total Knee Arthroplasty

Robert T. Trousdale, MD
Daniel J. Berry, MD

▪ Indications

Bone loss of greater or lesser severity is a feature of almost all revision total knee arthroplasties (TKAs). Effective management of bone loss is essential for reestablishing appropriate implant and limb alignment and achieving good implant support and durable fixation. Multiple methods for managing bone loss are available, including filling the bone deficiency with cement, cement reinforcement with screws, bone reconstruction with cancellous allograft or autograft bone, bone reconstruction with bulk allograft, filling the defects with metal augments or highly porous metal cones, and resecting the defects and filling them with a larger implant or tumor prosthesis. Most surgeons use each of these strategies in different circumstances and with specific patterns of bone loss. Other methods are discussed in chapters 46, 47, and 48; this chapter focuses on the use of metal augments to fill bone defects.

Metal augments can be divided into two types: (1) augments dedicated to a specific implant that are designed to fill a femoral or tibial segmental bone defect with a metal wedge or block that attaches directly to the prosthesis, and (2) metaphyseal cones or sleeves that are designed to fill contained cavitary and/or combined cavitary and segmental metaphyseal defects. These cones or sleeves can be dedicated to a specific implant design or may be independent of a specific implant. Porous cones not only provide a means of filling metaphyseal bone defects but also may enhance implant fixation by providing an uncemented interface with biologic ingrowth potential between the cone or sleeve and the metaphyseal bone.

Block or wedge metal augments are most commonly used to fill small- to medium-sized segmental defects of the distal or posterior femur or proximal tibia. Most surgeons use these augments when defects are between 5 and 15 mm in depth and extend over most of the width of one femoral condyle or one half of the tibia. These metal augments are simple and quick to use and do not carry the risk of resorption that is associated with bone grafts. It is important to note, however, that these augments do not restore bone. They effectively provide support for the prosthesis and at the same time allow restoration of implant alignment and joint line position.

In contrast, metaphyseal cones or sleeves typically are used to manage bone loss when there is a large cone-shaped deficiency in the metaphysis. Most such defects consist of some combination of cavitary and segmental bone loss. Cones and sleeves can be used to fill the bone deficiency, provide enhanced support for the implant, and provide the option for biologic fixation of the construct in the metaphyseal portion of the femur or tibia.

Metal augments are almost always used in combination with implant stems, either cemented or uncemented. The stems help to off-load stress from the implant and implant interfaces in areas of damaged and deficient bone.

———————▪

▪ Contraindications

Metal block or wedge augments are contraindicated when defects are so small that placing even a very thin augment would require removal of more bone than is justified. In most cases,

Dr. Trousdale has received royalties from DePuy, Wright Medical Technology, and Ortho Development and serves as a paid consultant to or is an employee of DePuy and Wright Medical Technology. Dr. Berry has received royalties from DePuy and has received research or institutional support from DePuy.

Table 1 Results of Metal Augments in Revision Total Knee Arthroplasty

Authors (Year)	Number of Patients	Type of Augment	Mean Follow-up (Range)	Mean Patient Age in Years (Range)	Mean Clinical Result at Follow-up	Radiographic Status at Follow-up
Jones et al (2001)	15	Femoral tibial attached cones with hinges	2 years (27-71 months)	63 (33-83)	Knee Society score: 76.5	Revisions for loosening: 0
Patel et al (2004)	102	Modular metal augments	7 years (5-11)	69 (41-87)	Survival: 92%	Nonprogressive radiolucent line: 14%
Radnay and Scuderi (2006)	9	Femoral and tibial tantalum cones	10.2 months (5-14)	NR	Repeat revisions: 0	All osteointegrated
Meneghini et al (2008)	15	Tibial tantalum cones	34 months (24-47)	68.1	Knee Society score: 85	All osteointegrated
Long and Scuderi (2009)	16	Tibial tantalum cones	31 months (24-38)	66 (48-83)	Repeat revisions for aseptic loosening: 0	All osteointegrated

NR = not reported.

very small defects can be filled with cement or small amounts of cancellous bone graft. Metal block or wedge augments typically are limited in thickness to 15 mm or less. Larger-thickness segmental bone defects may require a different strategy such as structural allograft, a porous metal metaphyseal cone, or a tumor prosthesis.

Metal cones and sleeves usually are contraindicated when the bone loss pattern does not allow a stable interference fit to be obtained between the cone or sleeve and the host bone. This can occur when segmental bone loss extends too far proximally in the femoral metaphysis or too far distally in the tibial metaphysis.

Rather than restoring bone, metal augments, cones, and sleeves replace bone with metal. Therefore, bone grafting methods may be the better option when bone reconstitution is highly desirable, such as in some younger patients. Metal cones and sleeves can be difficult to remove because they not only fill the metaphysis but also usually gain substantial metaphyseal fixation. This should be considered in situations such as reimplantation after infection, because future failure as a result of infection is a major concern.

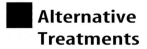

Alternative Treatments

The main alternative to metal block augments or wedges on the tibia is deeper tibial resection with use of a thicker polyethylene insert. This strategy is reasonable when only a few additional millimeters of tibia would be resected. With more substantial resection, the tibia is smaller in diameter at the point of resection and the required polyethylene thickness also can become excessive. On the femur, deeper resection adversely affects the joint line position and knee kinematics.

Another alternative for either the femur or the tibia is to use cement, cement and screws, bulk autograft or allograft, or impaction grafting. Cement or cement and screws may be satisfactory in very small defects or very low demand older patients, but for most patients, metal augments provide better construct support. When used in defects of appropriate size, metal augments are usually faster and easier to use than bone grafts and hence are preferred by many surgeons. Certain segmental condylar defects, particularly those in the femur, have a geometry or size that is not ideal for filling with a metal augment; in such cases, a bone graft may be preferred. However, this decision must be balanced with the knowledge that bone grafts are at risk for resorption and must heal to the host bone to be successful.

The main alternatives to metaphyseal sleeves or cones for a metaphyseal defect are cement, impacted cancellous bone graft, or bulk structural bone graft. Cement may be used to fill such defects when they are small and the cancellous bone remaining in the metaphysis allows for good cement interdigitation, and in some older low-demand patients. Of the alternatives mentioned, impacted cancellous allograft has the best potential to reconstitute living host bone and may be preferred in some young patients with favorable host biology for bone healing. Bulk structural grafts are the most versatile option because they can be contoured to fit most defects. Therefore, they may be the preferred method

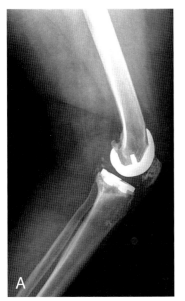 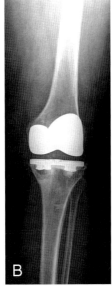 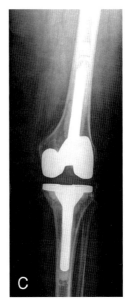 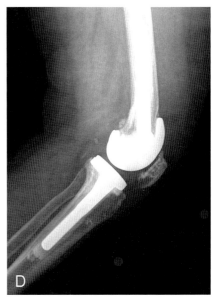

Figure 1 Images of a patient who presented with failed total knee arthroplasty (TKA) and posterior condylar bone loss as a result of osteolysis. Preoperative lateral (**A**) and AP (**B**) radiographs show the bone loss. AP (**C**) and lateral (**D**) radiographs obtained after revision demonstrate the use of metal block augments to replace the deficient bone of the posterior femoral condyles.

when defect geometry or size is not optimal for a metaphyseal cone or sleeve. Bulk grafts are the most time-consuming to prepare and the most difficult to fix to host bone. Porous metaphyseal sleeves and cones can be quite expensive, which may be an important consideration in some cases.

Results

Successful early and midterm results following revision TKA using conventional block and wedge augments in minor segmental defects have been reported; only a few results have been published for large metal cones used in revision TKA (**Table 1**). One study reported good short-term results with a mean follow-up of 10 months for both femoral and tibial trabecular metal cones. In this series, the core components had been cemented in every case and either a press-fit or cemented stem extension was used for additional fixation. At early follow-up, favorable results were documented in 9 of 10 knees, with apparent osseoin-

tegration of the bone against the femoral and tibial cones. Another study reviewed the results of 15 patients who had tibial cones placed in large tibial defects. The patients were followed for 24 to 38 months, and all tibial augments showed obvious osseointegration. Although the early results appear promising, further studies with longer follow-up are required to verify the durability of results with these metal cones.

Techniques

The surgical technique and type of metal augment used to repair bone deficiency depends on the location and size of the defect. Small distal femoral defects, posterior femoral defects, and medial and lateral tibial defects are handled easily with metal augments (**Figure 1**) Most knee systems have cutting guides to facilitate bone preparation, although many experienced knee surgeons use a freehand technique. The bony defect is first contoured with a saw or a burr to match

the augment. Then the component trials are used with trial augments to achieve good bony contact (**Figure 2**).

Large metaphyseal defects can be managed with metaphyseal metal augments (**Figure 3**). The two main types are augments that are attached to the implant with a taper and augments that are completely independent of the implant. Both types typically are covered with a porous surface that facilitates bony ingrowth to the metaphyseal sleeve or cone. Each type has advantages and disadvantages. Metaphyseal bone defects that are centrally located on the femur or tibia are handled easily with the type of metaphyseal sleeve that attaches to the implant because the sleeve is centrally located on the femur or tibial component. Femoral or tibial metaphyseal defects that are located medial, lateral, anterior, or posterior may be more easily treated with a detached cone.

If a noncentral defect is present and an attached sleeve is used, a fair amount of intact bone must be removed to fill the defect and obtain stability. The detached metaphyseal cone augments can be shifted in different

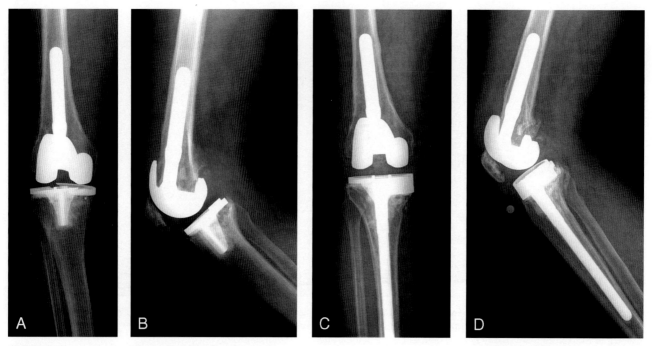

Figure 2 Images of a patient who presented with moderate medial segmental bone loss of the tibia and failed TKA. Preoperative AP (**A**) and lateral (**B**) radiographs show the bone loss. AP (**C**) and lateral (**D**) radiographs taken after reconstruction demonstrate the use of metal tibial augment to replace deficient bone of the proximal medial tibia.

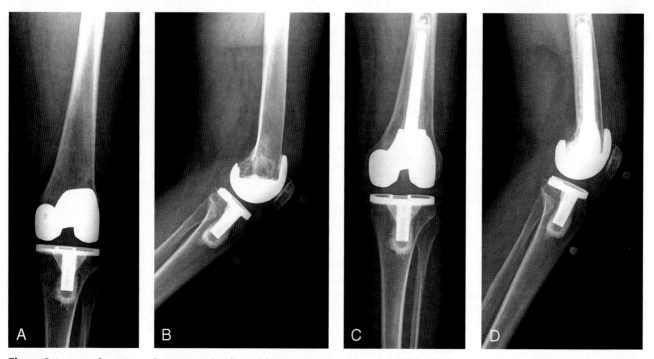

Figure 3 Images of a patient who presented with notable cavitary and segmental distal femoral bone loss as a result of osteolysis. Preoperative AP (**A**) and lateral (**B**) radiographs show the bone loss. AP (**C**) and lateral (**D**) radiographs taken after reconstruction show the use of a highly porous metal metaphyseal cone for the femur.

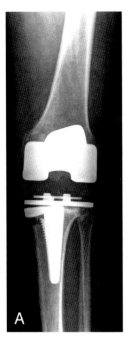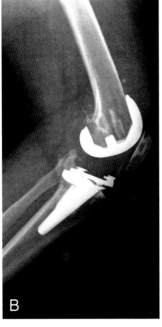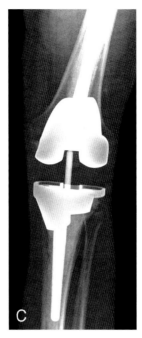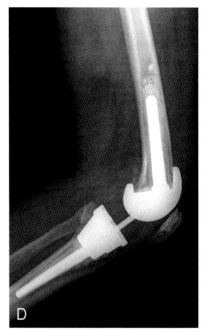

Figure 4 Images of a patient who presented with marked cavitary and segmental tibial metaphyseal bone loss. Preoperative AP (**A**) and lateral (**B**) radiographs show the bone loss. AP (**C**) and lateral (**D**) radiographs taken after reconstruction demonstrate the use of a porous metal metaphyseal cone for the tibia.

directions to facilitate bony contact and minimize further bone removal. Both techniques are fairly straightforward. The attached sleeve augments have broach systems that allow the surgeon to broach up to a large enough implant to achieve both axial and rotational stability. Trial femoral or tibial implants with metaphyseal sleeve trials are used to ensure that proper joint mechanics have been obtained prior to final implantation. The sleeves typically are used without cement between the porous surfaces and the metaphyseal bone, and the distal femur and proximal tibial component interfaces are cemented. Press-fit or cemented stems also are used to provide further stability while ingrowth occurs into the sleeve (**Figure 4**).

Detached cones usually are placed using a burr to freshen and contour the defect and trials and to ensure good bony contact and stability. These augments have a very high coefficient of friction and typically provide very good stability. Trial implants should be used meticulously to ensure that

the final femur and tibial components are properly positioned with the augment in place. Occasionally, the augment may need to be modified intraoperatively to achieve proper fit with the final implant; augments are constructed from highly porous materials that can be contoured with a burr. Cement, bone graft, or bone graft substitutes can be placed at the distal femur or proximal tibia cone–bone junction to prevent cement from interdigitating between the augment and the bony metaphyseal surface. When metaphyseal cones are used, implant stems may be press-fit or cemented; the distal femur and proximal tibia interfaces typically are cemented (**Figure 5**).

![decorative rule]

Avoiding Pitfalls and Complications

When preparing the bone to receive a metal augment, unnecessary bone removal should be avoided. Optimizing

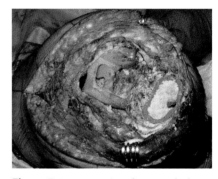

Figure 5 Intraoperative photograph shows tantalum augments in the femur and tibia. Note that bone graft has been placed about the tibial cone.

the host bone contact with porous surfaces and achieving adequate bony support and support of metal augments is important. Before final implantation, trials should be used and intraoperative radiographs should be obtained to verify that the augments are not forcing implants into an undesirable position. When shaping bone for defects, the surgeon should shape cortical bone with a burr or saw to avoid iatrogenic fracture. For metaphyseal cones and sleeves used in an uncemented mode, the surgeon should strive to gain both axial and rotational stability to facilitate bony ingrowth. For uncemented cones, the surgeon should seal the interface between the cone and bone with bone graft, bone graft substitute, or cement to keep the cement away from the host bone–augment interface.

Bibliography

Jones RE, Skedros JG, Chan AJ, Beauchamp DH, Harkins PC: Total knee arthroplasty using the S-ROM mobile-bearing hinge prosthesis. *J Arthroplasty* 2001;16(3):279-287.

Long WJ, Scuderi GR: Porous tantalum cones for large metaphyseal tibial defects in revision total knee arthroplasty: A minimum 2-year follow-up. *J Arthroplasty* 2009;24(7):1086-1092.

Meneghini RM, Lewallen DG, Hanssen AD: Use of porous tantalum metaphyseal cones for severe tibial bone loss during revision total knee replacement. *J Bone Joint Surg Am* 2008;90(1):78-84.

Patel JV, Masonis JL, Guerin J, Bourne RB, Rorabeck CH: The fate of augments to treat type-2 bone defects in revision knee arthroplasty. *J Bone Joint Surg Br* 2004;86(2):195-199.

Radnay CS, Scuderi GR: Management of bone loss: Augments, cones, offset stems. *Clin Orthop Relat Res* 2006;446:83-92.

Coding

CPT Code		Corresponding ICD-9 Codes	
27487	Revision of total knee arthroplasty, with or without allograft; femoral and entire tibial component	996.40 996.42 996.44	996.41 996.43 996.45

Chapter 50

Revision Total Knee Arthroplasty: Constraint Level

Douglas A. Dennis, MD
Derek R. Johnson, MD
Raymond H. Kim, MD

■ Introduction

One of the leading causes of failure in total knee arthroplasty (TKA) is instability, which accounts for up to 25% of failures. Revision TKA in the presence of instability often requires increasing the level of implant constraint. Various levels of prosthetic constraint are available. Each constraint level requires the competency of certain native anatomic structures and has unique benefits as well as potential disadvantages.

Five types of instability may exist following TKA: symmetric extension instability (recurvatum), asymmetric (varus-valgus) extension instability, symmetric flexion instability, asymmetric flexion instability, and global (multiplanar) instability.

Symmetric Extension Instability (Recurvatum)

Recurvatum is rare following TKA in patients with normal neuromuscular control unless significant technical er-

rors occurred intraoperatively. Patients with neuromuscular disorders are susceptible to recurvatum because of a weakened extensor mechanism, which causes the individual to hyperextend the knee to stabilize it during gait. This ultimately leads to attenuation of the posterior capsule and collateral ligaments, leaving the knee extremely unstable in extension. Common intraoperative technical errors resulting in recurvatum include overresection of the distal femur, resulting in an excessive extension gap width, or selection of a tibial component of insufficient thickness.

Management of recurvatum is difficult. Three primary approaches are available for treatment. The first is to reduce the extension gap width by lowering the joint line using distal femoral augmentation, leaving the patient with a slight flexion contracture. However, in the patient with significant quadriceps weakness, single-leg stance may be difficult if the degree of residual flexion contracture is too great. A second approach is to transfer

the femoral origin of the medial and lateral collateral ligaments proximally and posteriorly. This causes the collateral ligament complex to tighten sooner during extension and prevents hyperextension. The final approach is to use a rotating-hinge prosthesis with an extension stop. Although a hinged prosthesis places increased stress on both the implant's constraining mechanism and the fixation interface, this level of constraint may be required to prevent hyperextension in patients with significant quadriceps weakness.

Asymmetric (Varus-Valgus) Extension Instability

Asymmetric (varus-valgus) extension instability is more common than symmetric extension instability (recurvatum). It is often associated with significant preoperative deformity and may be secondary to technical errors in ligament balancing, asymmetric bone resection, iatrogenic intraoperative ligament injury, or ligament failure following the surgical procedure.

Asymmetric errors in soft-tissue balancing can occur from either underrelease or overrelease of the tighter concave side of a knee deformity. Undercorrection of a fixed varus deformity is the most common cause of postoperative varus-valgus instability and results in varus malalignment and subsequent lateral laxity. Over time,

Dr. Dennis or an immediate family member serves as a board member, owner, officer, or committee member of The Knee Society and The Hip Society; has received royalties from DePuy; is a member of a speakers' bureau or has made paid presentations on behalf of DePuy; serves as a paid consultant to or is an employee of DePuy; and has received research or institutional support from DePuy. Dr. Kim or an immediate family member has received research or institutional support from DePuy. Neither Dr. Johnson nor any immediate family member has received anything of value from or owns stock in a commercial company or institution related directly or indirectly to the subject of this chapter.

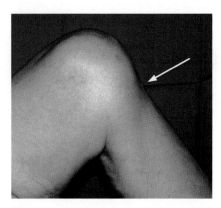

Figure 1 Clinical photograph of a knee with an unstable posterior cruciate ligament (PCL)-retaining total knee arthroplasty (TKA) demonstrates a posterior sag sign (arrow) due to posterior tibial subluxation.

ligament imbalance leads to asymmetric contact stresses with subsequent polyethylene wear, increased lateral ligament laxity, and eventual failure requiring revision surgery in some cases. Similarly, undercorrection of a fixed valgus deformity leads to asymmetric lateral polyethylene wear, worsening valgus deformity, and medial collateral ligament laxity. Conversely, overrelease of medial structures in cases of fixed varus deformity or excessive release of lateral soft-tissue structures in cases of fixed valgus deformity will result in asymmetric extension instability.

Errors in bone resection also may lead to asymmetric extension instability. This often occurs in conjunction with inadequate soft-tissue release. For instance, a varus tibial or femoral resection with respect to the mechanical axis of the limb, coupled with an inadequate medial release, may give the impression that the limb is well balanced in extension when in fact the medial structures remain tight and the limb is left in residual varus alignment with joint line obliquity, which typically results in eventual ligament attenuation.

Iatrogenic collateral ligament injury is rare. It most commonly occurs inadvertently with a saw during resection of the proximal tibia or the poste-

rior femoral condyles. It also may result from overly aggressive ligament retraction or from application of excessive tension when testing ligamentous balance. Although iatrogenic injury can occur in any patient, it is more common in obese patients. If discovered intraoperatively, primary repair using a Krackow-type suture technique with or without autogenous allograft or synthetic tendon augmentation is required. An implant that provides increased coronal plane constraint is recommended in these cases to protect the intraoperative ligament repair.

Symmetric Flexion Instability

Symmetric flexion instability is an underrecognized yet frequent cause of persistent pain and poor outcome following TKA. It is associated with an enlarged flexion gap due to an undersized femoral component, resection of the tibia with excessive posterior slope, or failure of the posterior cruciate ligament (PCL) in PCL-retaining TKA designs. An additional cause is initial underresection of the distal femur, resulting in a tight extension gap, and subsequent selection of a tibial polyethylene bearing thickness that is too thin to provide adequate flexion gap stability. Patients with flexion instability without dislocation often report myriad symptoms, including recurrent effusions, giving way, difficulty ascending or descending stairs, or diffuse periretinacular or pes anserine bursal pain.

Dislocation after TKA is uncommon. Occasionally, it occurs after PCL failure in PCL-retaining TKA designs; rarely, it occurs after PCL-substituting (posterior stabilized) TKA. In PCL-substituting designs, dislocation most commonly occurs in deep flexion when a varus stress is applied to the knee (figure-of-4 position) in subjects who have undergone release of the popliteus tendon and lateral collateral ligament to correct a preoperative valgus deformity.

It can be difficult to diagnose flexion instability clinically because of the subtleness of the instability. Radiographs typically reveal well-aligned, well-fixed implants, and the knee is often stable in lesser degrees of flexion. Occasionally, a classic posterior tibial sag sign (**Figure 1**) will be seen, but it is observed only in cases with marked symmetric flexion instability and PCL insufficiency. More commonly, this condition is best diagnosed by detection of excessive anterior-posterior laxity. This is assessed with the patient seated with the knee flexed and the foot either dangling from the side of the examination table or resting lightly on the floor.

Asymmetric Flexion Instability

Asymmetric instability in flexion most commonly results from errors in soft-tissue balancing or malrotation of the femoral component. Patients with this type of instability most commonly report insecure limb stability during flexion activities (eg, stair climbing, transfers) and may have associated arthrofibrosis if significant femoral component internal rotation is present. As with asymmetric extension instability, errors in soft-tissue balancing may result from either under- or overrelease of the tighter concave side of a knee deformity. Inadequate medial release may lead to lateral laxity in flexion. Likewise, inadequate lateral release in a valgus knee may lead to medial laxity in flexion. These patients present with medial- or lateral-side laxity in both flexion and extension; both problems may be treated as described earlier.

Understanding which anatomic structures provide medial and lateral stability of the flexion gap can lessen the risk of asymmetric flexion instability resulting from overrelease of soft-tissue stabilizing structures. Medial stability in flexion is provided primarily by the superficial medial collateral ligament, and lateral stability requires integrity of the lateral collateral ligament and popliteus tendon. Preservation of these structures during soft-tissue balancing, when possible, will lessen the incidence of asymmetric flexion stability.

Placement of the femoral component in internal rotation or excessive external rotation will create asymmetric flexion instability. The best method for determining correct femoral component rotation and subsequent coronal plane stability in flexion is debated. Many surgeons use a measured-resection technique in which bone landmarks (femoral epicondyles, anterior-posterior axis, posterior condylar axis) are used alone or in combination to determine femoral component rotation. Advocates of this technique recommend placement of the femoral component parallel to the transepicondylar axis, perpendicular to the anterior-posterior axis, or externally rotated approximately 3° to 4° relative to the posterior condylar axis. Other surgeons prefer a gap-balancing technique in which the femoral component is positioned parallel to the proximal tibia resection with equal collateral ligamentous tension. We believe that a gap-balancing technique results in more reproducible flexion stability. The measured-resection technique is less reliable because the surgeon cannot precisely identify critical bone landmarks reproducibly when deciding correct femoral component rotation. Patients with flexion instability secondary to substantial femoral component malrotation require revision of the femoral component to address the issue.

Global Instability
Global instability can result from a combination of the instability patterns discussed previously. Laxity in both the coronal and sagittal planes is present, typically occurring throughout the entire range of flexion. Global instability typically results from damage of multiple ligamentous and capsular structures and is often associated with substantial periarticular bone loss.

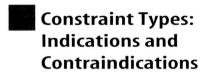

Constraint Types: Indications and Contraindications

When revising an unstable TKA, it is imperative to adhere to the fundamental principles of revision surgery, including restoring the joint line, attaining good alignment, reconstructing bone defects, and creating a well-balanced and stable knee in both flexion and extension while using the least amount of prosthetic constraint necessary to attain adequate stability. Less constraint minimizes fixation stresses and the subsequent risk of loosening and lessens loads on the constraining mechanism of the implant. The levels of prosthetic constraint available in TKA designs (from least to most constrained) are (1) PCL-retaining, (2) PCL-substituting, (3) varus-valgus constrained (VVC) or unlinked constrained designs, and (4) hinged or linked constrained designs.

PCL-Retaining TKA
PCL-retaining implants are the least constrained TKA implants available. The advantages of PCL-retaining implants include less bone resection and possibly improved proprioception due to retention of neural mechanoreceptors within the PCL. PCL-retaining designs provide minimal intrinsic stability, however, and rely on good-quality bone with intact collateral ligament structures, as well as an intact and well-tensioned PCL. For these reasons, PCL-retaining designs are not often used in revision TKA, where bone and soft-tissue deficiencies are common. The most common revision TKA situations in which PCL-retaining implant designs have been successful are in patients who have had a well-functioning PCL-retaining implant for many years that failed because of polyethylene wear and in patients with a failed unicompartmental knee arthroplasty (UKA) being revised to a TKA. Revision with a PCL-retaining design is likely to fail in patients with preoperative flexion instability or a nonfunctional PCL; failure rates in these patients are as high as 40% at 5 years.

PCL-Substituting TKA
PCL-substituting designs provide more constraint to anterior-posterior translation than do PCL-retaining designs, but they provide minimal increase in varus-valgus or rotational constraint. These implants require slightly more bone resection to allow for the cam-spine mechanism of the femoral component. The cam-spine mechanism provides posterior femoral translation through engagement of the femoral cam and tibial post and eliminates the technical aspects of balancing the PCL. PCL-substituting designs have a relatively short spine height and lax coronal fit within the intercondylar box of the femoral component, so, as with PCL-retaining designs, an intact medial and lateral collateral ligament complex is a prerequisite for these designs to be used in revision TKA. Because most patients requiring revision TKA have intact collateral ligament structures, PCL-substituting designs are most commonly used in revision TKA. Although PCL-substituting designs provide anterior-posterior constraint, they cannot overcome a loose flexion gap, and dislocation is possible if the flexion gap is not symmetric and balanced to the width of the extension gap (**Figure 2**).

Unlinked VVC Designs
The next level of increased prosthetic constraint used in revision TKA is the unlinked VVC TKA. These implants provide significantly more varus-valgus and rotational constraint than do

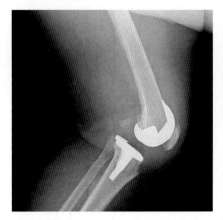

Figure 2 Lateral radiograph of a knee with a dislocated PCL-substituting TKA.

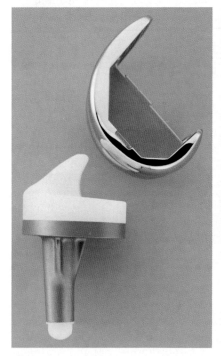

Figure 3 Photograph of varus-valgus constrained TKA components. (Courtesy of DePuy Orthopadics, Warsaw, IN.)

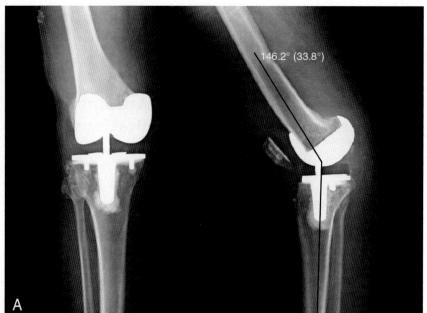

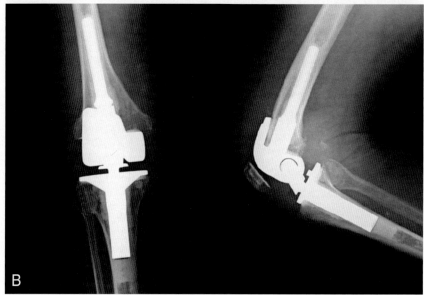

Figure 4 Images of a patient with recurvatum and global instability that developed as a result of poliomyelitis and substantial secondary quadriceps weakness. **A,** AP (left) and lateral (right) radiographs obtained before revision surgery. **B,** AP (left) and lateral (right) radiographs of the same patient after revision to a rotating-hinge prosthesis.

PCL-substituting designs. The taller spine and tighter coronal fit within the intercondylar box of VVC femoral components provide stability in cases of laxity of the medial or lateral collateral ligamentous structures. In contrast to hinge TKA designs, the femoral and tibial components are not mechanically linked (**Figure 3**). If the medial collateral ligament is completely incompetent, VVC designs will

ultimately fail due to excessive stresses encountered by the spine-cam mechanism. The taller spine in VVC designs, like the spine in PCL-substituting designs, cannot overcome severe flexion instability, and the potential for posterior dislocation remains if the flexion space is not balanced ap-

propriately. An additional potential disadvantage of VVC designs is increased stress at the fixation interface, which may lead to premature implant loosening. Recently, rotating-platform (mobile-bearing) unlinked VVC TKA designs have been introduced that offer the potential advantage of lessening stresses at both the spine-cam mechanism and the fixation interface. Longer-term experience is needed with these new prosthetic devices to confirm their potential benefits in reduction of constraint and fixation stresses.

Linked-Hinge Constrained Designs

A linked-hinge prosthesis is the most constrained TKA design currently used in revision TKA. Although the VVC designs have been very effective in most cases of revision for substantial instability, a linked-hinged TKA design should be considered when one or both collateral ligaments are totally incompetent or in patients demonstrating extreme flexion instability. Additional indications for linked-hinge designs include severe posterior capsular insufficiency with uncontrolled hyperextension (**Figure 4**) and elderly patients with osteopenia and severely comminuted supracondylar femoral fractures. As noted previously, uncontrolled hyperextension is most commonly observed in patients with paralytic conditions with marked quadriceps weakness in which the patient repeatedly hyperextends the knee to stabilize the limb during the stance phase of gait with resulting posterior capsular attenuation. Elderly patients with severely comminuted supracondylar fractures above a TKA can be managed with a distal femoral–replacing rotating-platform hinge prosthesis that provides immediate knee stability and eliminates the need for fracture healing (**Figure 5**). Patients with massive osteolysis, particularly of the distal femur, often lose collateral ligament integrity because of osteolytic bone loss of the osseous ligament attachments. These cases may require reconstruction with a distal femoral allograft and can benefit from selection of a hinged prosthesis to substitute for the absence of the collateral ligaments. Despite the improved stability provided, linked-hinge

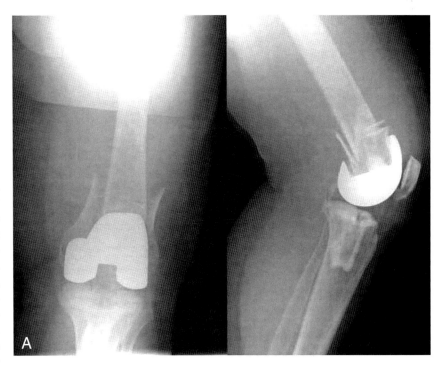

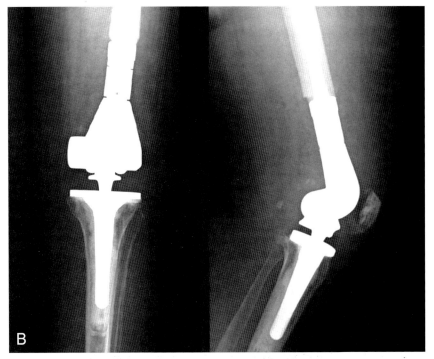

Figure 5 Images of a patient with osteoporosis and a supracondylar periprosthetic femur fracture. **A,** AP (left) and lateral (right) radiographs obtained before revision surgery. **B,** AP (left) and lateral (right) radiographs of the same patient after revision to a rotating-hinge prosthesis.

TKAs (especially fixed-hinge implants) have had an inferior track record, with increased rates of loosening, recurrent instability, prosthetic failure, extensor lag, chronic pain, and infection. Therefore, they should be used only when stability cannot be achieved with a VVC design. However,

Table 1 Results of Revision Total Knee Arthroplasty With Constrained Devices

Authors (Year)	Number of Knees	Level of Constraint in Revision	Mean Patient Age in Years (Range)	Mean Follow-up in Years (Range)	Results
Pagnano et al (1998)	25 unstable CR knees	22 PS 3 PCR	65 (35-77)	3.1 (2.1-6.5)	1 of 22 PS knees with recurrent instability 2 of 3 CR knees with recurrent instability
McAuley et al (2001)	32 failed UKAs	25 PCR 4 PS 3 UKA	59 (35-73)	4.5 (2-10)	0 cases of instability upon conversion from UKA
Jones et al (2001)	13 failed hinge 17 failed PS or VVC	Hinge	66 (33-83)	4.1 (2-6.2)	0 rerevisions 1 radiolucent line along anterior flange of femur
Nazarian et al (2002)	207 revisions, all causes	VVC	67 (43-84)	4.2 (2-6.2)	3 cases of recurrent instability 8 cases of aseptic loosening
Mabry et al (2007)	70 knees with aseptic failure	PS	73 (50-90)	10.2 (1.3-21.8)	5 rerevisions for loosening 2 rerevisions for sepsis 0 rerevisions for instability
Deehan et al (2008)	72 failed TKAs	Hinge	69	10 (3-18)	90% 10-year survival 5 deep infections 5 patients with extensor lag > 5°

CR = cruciate-retaining, PS = posterior stabilized (posterior cruciate ligament [PCL]-substituting), PCR = PCL-retaining, UKA = unicondylar knee arthroplasty, VVC = varus-valgus constrained, TKA = total knee arthroplasty.

as previously discussed with VVC implants, rotating-platform linked-hinge devices are most commonly selected because of the lower stresses incurred by the implant and fixation interfaces due to the presence of bearing mobility.

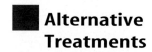

Alternative Treatments

In patients with mild instability or those who are too medically unstable to undergo revision surgery, either custom or off-the-shelf hinged knee braces may be used to increase stability. Physical therapy focusing on quadriceps and hamstring strengthening also may be beneficial in patients with only mild instability.

Results

PCL-Retaining TKA

As previously discussed, the situations in which revision TKA with PCL-retaining designs is successful are limited to patients who have had a well-functioning PCL-retaining TKA for several years that failed because of polyethylene wear, and knees being revised from a UKA to a TKA. In one study, PCL-retaining designs were successful at 5-year follow-up in nearly 80% of revisions from UKA to TKA (**Table 1**).

PCL-Substituting Designs

Because intact collateral ligament structures are present in most patients requiring revision TKA, PCL-substituting designs are most commonly used in the revision setting. In one series, 19 of 22 knees converted to

PCL-substituting designs for flexion instability had marked pain relief, and only one had recurrent instability at 3 years (**Table 1**). Other series have shown similar results, with 80% to 90% success rates at follow-up greater than 10 years reported for revision to PCL-substituting TKA.

Unlinked VVC Designs

Excellent results with various unlinked VVC designs in revision TKAs have been reported by several authors. One series reported on 33 constrained condylar revisions and observed 72% good or excellent results with only a 9% failure rate (**Table 1**). Similar results, with success rates of 70% to 94%, have been reported in series from other authors at more than 5 years of follow-up.

Linked-Hinge Constrained Designs

Although early results with fixed linked-hinge designs were discouraging, more recent studies, with newer designs incorporating bearing mobility, have shown promising results. One study reported 30 patients with 100% survivorship at 24- to 74-month follow-up (**Table 1**). In a series of 72 salvage revision TKA procedures with a rotating-hinge prosthesis, survival analysis showed 90% implant survival at 10 years.

Technique

To achieve a successful outcome in revision TKA, a detailed, stepwise approach must be used. Our recommended sequence in performing a revision TKA is surgical exposure, component removal, establishing the tibial platform, assessing stability, balancing the flexion gap, equalizing the extension gap to the flexion gap, prosthesis selection, implant fixation, and wound closure.

Exposure

In general, it is preferable to use the same incision that was used for the initial TKA. If multiple skin incisions are present, however, it is important to use the most lateral skin incision to avoid large lateral skin flaps that may have compromised oxygen levels and reduced wound-healing capacity. Meticulous soft-tissue dissection and handling is imperative. A medial parapatellar arthrotomy is most commonly used because of its extensile capabilities for dealing with challenges found in the revision setting. This approach allows use of the rectus snip (**Figure 6**), V-Y quadricepsplasty, or an extended tibial tubercle osteotomy if necessary to improve access to the knee joint.

Component Removal

Multiple instruments are available for component removal, including osteotomes, power saws, Gigli saws, disimpaction punches, and component-specific extraction devices. A thin, narrow oscillating saw (**Figure 7**) is used to divide the implant-bone or implant-cement interface initially. Once a division is begun, it is completed with thin osteotomes. After complete division of the interface, the components are easily removed with disimpaction devices (**Figure 8**). All remaining cement can then be removed with osteotomes or power burrs. Great care is taken during this process to preserve bone and avoid iatrogenic fracture.

Establishing the Tibial Platform

The tibial platform is addressed initially because it affects both the flexion and extension gaps. Intramedullary or extramedullary cutting guides may be used to create a platform perpendicular to the mechanical axis of the tibia. Minimizing bone resection is

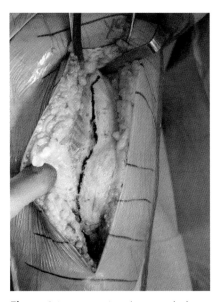

Figure 6 Intraoperative photograph shows the arthrotomy line for a rectus snip.

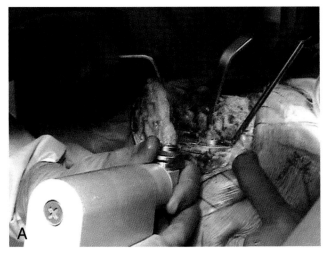
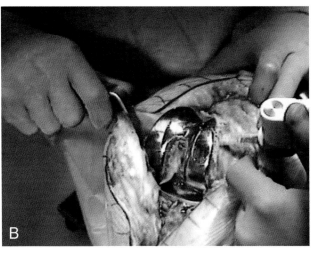

Figure 7 Component removal. **A,** Use of an oscillating saw for tibial component removal. **B,** Use of an oscillating saw for femoral component removal.

Table 2 Treatment Options for Flexion-Extension Gap Imbalance

	Extension satisfactory	Extension tight	Extension loose
Flexion satisfactory	No changes	Resect posterior osteophytes Increase distal femoral resection Posterior capsular release	Augment or bone graft distal femur
Flexion tight	Decrease femoral component size Consider PCL-substituting implant Increase posterior tibial slope	Increase tibial resection Select thinner tibial component	Augment distal femur + use smaller femoral component
Flexion loose	Increase femoral component size + posterior femoral augmentation	Increase distal femoral resection Increase femoral component size + posterior femoral augmentation	Increase tibial component thickness

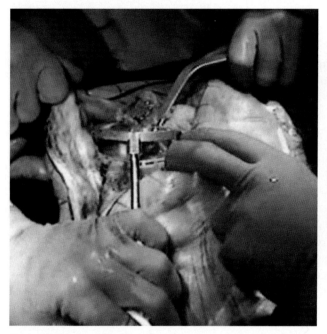
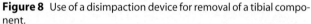

Figure 8 Use of a disimpaction device for removal of a tibial component.

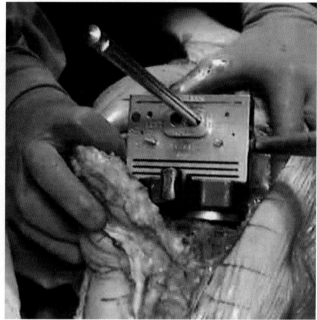

Figure 9 Use of a spacer block to set the femoral rotation parallel to the tibial resection.

essential. This is done by resecting no more than 1 or 2 mm from the highest point of the most prominent tibial condyle and using cement (with or without screws), augments, or bone graft as needed to manage residual bone defects.

Assessing Stability

Once a stable tibial platform is created, it is necessary to assess the flexion and extension gaps. It is important to assess the medial-lateral symmetry of each gap as well as the balance of the flexion versus the extension gap. Several combinations of extension gap tension versus flexion gap tension may be encountered in revision TKA (**Table 2**), and different treatment solutions should be selected based on the extension-flexion relationship that is present.

Establishing the Flexion Gap

Once a stable tibial platform has been established and the gaps have been assessed, the flexion gap is established. If the flexion gap is looser than the extension gap, a larger femoral component with posterior femoral augments is used. If the flexion gap is tighter than the extension gap, a smaller femoral component is needed. Proper rotation of the femoral component is necessary to obtain a rectangular flexion gap and to improve patellar tracking. In the revision setting, the intercondylar (anterior-posterior) and posterior condylar axes are no longer available to assist in determination of proper femoral component rotation. Therefore, we recommend placing the femoral component parallel to the transepicondylar axis or parallel to the proximal tibia resection (**Figure 9**), with each collateral ligament equally tensioned (gap-balancing technique). With the knee flexed 90°, we apply traction on the foot to tension the collateral ligaments and then rotate the cutting guide so that the posterior condylar cuts are parallel to the already established tibial platform. The transepicondylar axis is then used as a secondary check to establish proper rotation.

Equalizing the Extension Gap to the Flexion Gap

After the flexion gap is established, the surgeon next needs to equalize the extension gap to the flexion gap. This is accomplished by adjustment of the femoral component either proximally, by performing additional resection of the distal femur, or, more commonly, by lowering the joint line by application of distal femoral augmentations to the revision femoral component. Reestablishing the joint line as close to the anatomic level as possible is necessary to achieve optimal stability and joint kinematics. The joint line typically falls 30 mm distal to the medial epicondyle and 25 mm distal to the lateral epicondyle. Additional anatomic landmarks that may be used to locate the joint line are the level of the old meniscal scar, one finger width above the fibular head, or one finger width below the inferior pole of the patella.

Prosthesis Selection

Once balanced flexion and extension gaps have been established and efforts to restore the joint line have been completed, the appropriate type of implant must be selected. Again, it is important to realize that the long-term durability of the prosthetic components and fixation interface is inversely proportional to the level of prosthetic constraint. For this reason, it is important to always use the least

constrained components necessary to provide adequate stability.

Unless obvious collateral ligament instability is present, initial trialing should be performed with a PCL-substituting design. As previously stated, a PCL-retaining design is considered only in revision of a failed UKA or in elderly patients who have enjoyed many years of good function with a PCL-retaining prosthesis that failed due to polyethylene wear. If adequate stability is present in full extension, midflexion, and 90° of flexion, a PCL-substituting TKA is selected. If inadequate stability is apparent when trialing with a PCL-substituting design, most commonly in mid or late flexion, a more constrained VVC design should be used.

Rarely, a linked constrained design is necessary. We typically reserve use of these devices for patients with severe posterior capsular insufficiency and recurvatum, or for patients with an absent medial collateral ligament complex. This is most often determined preoperatively rather than intraoperatively.

Component Fixation

A review of the results of revision TKA clearly demonstrates improved results with the use of diaphysis-engaging intramedullary stems. The literature has suggested that press-fit and cemented stems provide similar success at midterm follow-up. Recent reports at longer term follow-up, however, have demonstrated better fixation with cemented stems than with press-fit stems. We especially favor cemented stems for patients with significant osteopenia and capacious canals or patients with deformity in which a press-fit stem would alter condylar implant position. The recent development of metaphyseal sleeves and trabecular metal augments has allowed fixation of the prosthesis to host bone in situations in which cement or massive allografts would have been necessary in the past.

Wound Closure

Prior to wound closure, tourniquet release is necessary to assess patellar tracking and ensure adequate hemostasis. The wound is closed in layers over a drain. In the event of excessive skin tightness, particularly over the proximal tibia, rotation of a medial gastrocnemius flap may be required to prevent ischemic necrosis.

Postoperative Regimen

Early mobilization is recommended for all patients to minimize postoperative complications associated with inactivity, such as thromboembolic disease, ileus, urinary retention, and pneumonia. Multimodal thromboembolic prophylaxis, including chemical and mechanical prophylaxis, is recommended. Weight-bearing status is individualized depending on the quality of host bone and security of the fixation obtained intraoperatively.

Avoiding Pitfalls and Complications

Revision TKA is associated with an increased risk of complications such as infection, iatrogenic bone loss, extensor mechanism complications, and recurrent instability. Accordingly, the surgeon should have a heightened awareness for the possibility of these complications.

Infection is perhaps the most problematic complication following revision TKA. Efficient surgery and meticulous surgical technique are critical for minimizing the risk of this complication; in addition, we routinely perform a synovectomy and thorough irrigation and débridement of the soft tissues during revision surgery. It is also reasonable to consider the use of commercially prepared antibiotic-impregnated bone cement in all revision surgery to minimize the risk of infection.

Iatrogenic bone loss during implant removal is another problematic complication. Loss of host bone may put native anatomic structures such as the collateral ligaments at risk and may make obtaining stable fixation of the implant to host bone difficult. It is imperative to be patient when removing implants. It is best to initially divide the implant-cement interface, rather than the cement-bone interface, because it is more bone preserving. After the component is removed, the cement can then be more precisely removed under direct vision. The entire interface should be released before attempting disimpaction of the implant.

Extensor mechanism complications can be devastating in the revision setting. These complications often occur during exposure. It is often necessary to perform a lateral reti-nacular release during exposure to mobilize the extensor mechanism and avoid complications. A headed pin may be placed through the patellar ligament into the tibial tubercle to avoid iatrogenic avulsion to the ligament insertion. A quadriceps snip may be performed to enhance the exposure if access to the joint is difficult.

In addition to intraoperative complications, postoperative patellofemoral symptoms are common after revision. Appropriate implant rotation is critical for patellofemoral function. Centering the tibial tray over the middle third of the tibial tubercle and rotating the femoral component so that it is parallel to the tibial component with the collateral ligaments equally tensioned and parallel to the transepicondylar axis is a reproducible technique for ensuring appropriate patellar tracking.

Finally, recurrent instability is another possible complication in revision surgery. Following the surgical techniques outlined in this chapter—reestablishing the joint line, creating a tibial platform perpendicular to the long axis of the tibia, balancing the flexion and extension gaps, maintaining proper femoral component rotation, and increasing constraint when necessary—will avoid this complication in most circumstances. The history and preoperative evaluation also are key in avoiding recurrent instability. Understanding the cause of instability in the index procedure will allow the surgeon to better address instability during the revision surgery. In addition, it is important to recognize patients with neuromuscular conditions or collagen vascular disorders that cause them to be more prone to develop instability. In these patients, it may be necessary to use a more constrained design, such as a VVC or linked-hinge design, despite the fact that there is apparent stability with a less constrained implant during the revision.

Bibliography

Babis GC, Trousdale RT, Morrey BF: The effectiveness of isolated tibial insert exchange in revision total knee arthroplasty. *J Bone Joint Surg Am* 2002;84-A(1):64-68.

Deehan DJ, Murray J, Birdsall PD, Holland JP, Pinder IM: The role of the rotating hinge prosthesis in the salvage arthroplasty setting. *J Arthroplasty* 2008;23(5):683-688.

Fehring TK, Valadie AL: Knee instability after total knee arthroplasty. *Clin Orthop Relat Res* 1994;299:157-162.

Jones RE, Barrack RL, Skedros J: Modular, mobile-bearing hinge total knee arthroplasty. *Clin Orthop Relat Res* 2001;392: 306-314.

Mabry TM, Vessely MB, Schleck CD, Harmsen WS, Berry DJ: Revision total knee arthroplasty with modular cemented stems: long-term follow-up. *J Arthroplasty* 2007;22(6, Suppl 2):100-105.

McAuley JP, Engh GA: Constraint in total knee arthroplasty: When and what? *J Arthroplasty* 2003;18(3, Suppl 1):51-54.

McAuley JP, Engh GA, Ammeen DJ: Revision of failed unicompartmental knee arthroplasty. *Clin Orthop Relat Res* 2001; 392:279-282.

Nazarian DG, Mehta S, Booth RE Jr: A comparison of stemmed and unstemmed components in revision knee arthroplasty. *Clin Orthop Relat Res* 2002;404:256-262.

Pagnano MW, Hanssen AD, Lewallen DG, Stuart MJ: Flexion instability after primary posterior cruciate retaining total knee arthroplasty. *Clin Orthop Relat Res* 1998;356:39-46.

Parratte S, Pagnano MW: Instability after total knee arthroplasty. *J Bone Joint Surg Am* 2008;90(1):184-194.

Scuderi GR: Revision total knee arthroplasty: How much constraint is enough? *Clin Orthop Relat Res* 2001;392:300-305.

Vince KG, Abdeen A, Sugimori T: The unstable total knee arthroplasty: Causes and cures. *J Arthroplasty* 2006;21(4, Suppl 1):44-49.

Waslewski GL, Marson BM, Benjamin JB: Early, incapacitating instability of posterior cruciate ligament-retaining total knee arthroplasty. *J Arthroplasty* 1998;13(7):763-767.

Chapter 51

Revision Total Knee Arthroplasty: Hinged Implants

Henry D. Clarke, MD

◼ Indications

Early in the development of total knee arthroplasty (TKA), hinged implants of a variety of designs were used with mediocre results. Many of those failures, however, were due in large part to poor prosthesis design, early surgical techniques, and the complex nature of the cases in which these devices were typically used. Indeed, many of these early designs constituted a simple hinge that essentially ignored the patellofemoral compartment. Consequently, with the development of total condylar–type resurfacing prostheses that achieved excellent early results, the use of hinged knee implants rapidly fell out of favor in primary TKA. Indeed, in orthopaedic adult reconstruction, these devices were largely relegated to a footnote in the history of TKA, although they continued to be used in orthopaedic oncology. New protocols for adjuvant chemotherapy and radiation improved attempts at limb salvage and prompted the need for better reconstructive options following segmental bone resection about the knee. Improved designs of hinged implants were developed that allowed segmental replacement of the distal femur and

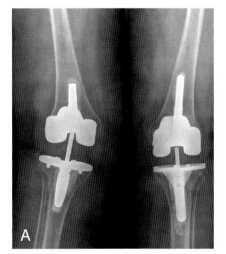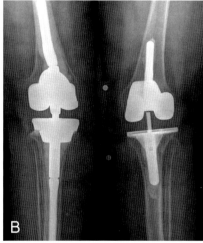

Figure 1 Images of a patient who underwent bilateral TKA with constrained but unlinked condylar prostheses. Valgus deformity developed on the right side due to complete incompetence of the medial soft-tissue stabilizers. In this case, the constrained unlinked prosthesis did not provide enough stability and failed. **A,** Preoperative weight-bearing AP radiograph demonstrates the valgus deformity. **B,** Weight-bearing AP radiograph of the same patient after revision of the right knee with a condylar hinged prosthesis.

proximal tibia. In many cases, some of the desirable features of resurfacing prostheses were incorporated into these segmental replacement prostheses, such as an anatomic trochlear groove to accommodate the native or resurfaced patella. In addition, the simple hinge concept was abandoned and mobile bearings were incorporated in most designs to improve the kinematics and functional outcomes.

Improved results with these second-generation hinged implants led to the reexamination of the use of these devices in revision TKA as the problems encountered became more complex. It was clear that, over time, the complexity of some revisions challenged the capabilities of constrained but unlinked prosthetic designs (**Figure 1**). Current indications for the use of hinged implants in nononcologic TKA include segmental bone loss due to infection, trauma, osteolysis, or iatrogenic causes; complete failure of one or both of the medial or lateral liga-

Dr. Clarke or an immediate family member is a board member, owner, officer, or committee member of the American Academy of Orthopaedic Surgeons and has received research or institutional support from Stryker.

mentous stabilizers; and inability to balance the flexion and extension gaps. In most cases of flexion and extension gap mismatch, loss of control of the flexion space poses the biggest problem. In this circumstance, where the tibia falls away from the femur in flexion, use of a constrained but unlinked prosthesis may provide adequate medial and lateral stability but can lead to dislocation in flexion.

Contraindications

Relative contraindications to the use of a hinged prosthesis in complex TKA include soft-tissue compromise that will result in wound healing problems. In these cases, staged or simultaneous plastic surgery procedures, such as tissue expanders or muscle transfers, should be considered. Compromise of the extensor mechanism represents another relative contraindication. Both patellar fractures and tendon ruptures should be addressed with additional reconstructive techniques at the time of revision TKA, as lack of active knee extension will limit functional results. Similarly, neurologic or vascular compromise of the extremity is a relative contraindication, as these also limit the potential functional results and increase the risk of early failure. In addition, inadequate remaining femoral bone stock may prevent the use of a hinged knee prosthesis. The most common scenario in which this is encountered is when the patient has an ipsilateral long-stemmed hip component that would prevent adequate fixation of the hinged knee prosthesis. In some of these cases, a complete femoral replacement may be required, especially if the hip replacement has also failed or is at risk of failure. Finally, in these patients with complex failed TKAs, the presence of a suppressed or chronically infected total joint arthroplasty elsewhere in the body represents a rel-

ative contraindication to revision of a failed TKA with a hinged prosthesis because of the risk of hematogenous seeding. When possible, other joint infections should be eradicated before proceeding with revision of the TKA.

Distinct from the relative contraindications reviewed above, acute or chronic infection of the involved knee or ipsilateral hip represents the only absolute contraindication to revision of the failed TKA with a hinged prosthesis. In these cases, two-stage reconstruction of the infected joints should be performed with an antibiotic-impregnated spacer. In some cases, removal of the entire femur with the infected hip and knee should be considered.

Alternative Treatments

At one end of the spectrum, in patients with less challenging problems, significant bone loss may be managed successfully with structural bone grafts or massive metal augments in conjunction with unlinked, constrained prostheses. Alternatively, use of an allograft-prosthesis composite rather than reconstruction with a segmental replacement-type hinged prosthesis may be considered. More active patients and those with longer projected remaining life spans may be the best candidates for these alternative reconstructive methods of managing bone loss. Similarly, in patients with ligamentous incompetence rather than complete failure of the medial or lateral stabilizing structures or with mild asymmetry in the flexion-extension gap balance, constrained but unlinked knee prostheses may be successfully used in revision TKA. In some cases, reconstruction or repair of the collateral ligaments may be undertaken in conjunction with the use of these constrained but unlinked prosthetic de-

vices. In general, the least constraint possible should be considered.

At the other end of the spectrum are those patients with extremely complex knee problems in conjunction with other local problems (eg, soft-tissue compromise, loss of the extensor mechanism, neurologic compromise) or systemic conditions that preclude attempts at reconstruction with a hinged prosthesis. In these extreme cases, knee fusion is often challenging because of the extent of the bone loss, and above-knee amputation must be considered.

Results

The use of hinged prostheses in revision TKA is associated with high rates of complications; however, these problems largely reflect the complexity of the cases in which these devices are used (**Table 1**). In certain centers, especially in Germany, hinged prostheses have been used extensively in primary TKA with long-term results similar to those obtained with resurfacing-type condylar prostheses. Common complications seen in the revision setting at midterm follow-up include infection (~15%), aseptic loosening (~15%), patellar complications (~13% to 22%), and prosthetic component breakage (~5% to 10%). Furthermore, although patient satisfaction rates are high postoperatively, likely due to significant improvements in pain, only modest functional gains may be noted.

Technique

Setup/Exposure

The patient is positioned supine on a standard operating table with a tourniquet high on the thigh. Before preparing the patient, it is helpful to eval-

Table 1 Results of Hinged Prostheses Used in Total Knee Arthroplasty

Authors (Year)	Number of Knees	Primary or Revision TKA	Mean Patient Age in Years (Range)	Mean Follow-up (Range)	Results
Böhm and Holy (1998)	69	Primary	70 (46-89)	50 months (21-101)	5.2% revision rate
Westrich et al (2000)	24	9 primary 15 revision	63 (16-91)	33 months (21-62)	12.5% complication rate 0% reoperation rate
Jones et al (2001)	16	1 primary 15 revision	63 (33-83)	47 months (27-71)	12.5% reoperation rate
Springer et al (2001)	69	12 primary 58 revision	72 (46-89)	75.2 months (24-199)	27% reoperation rate
Utting and Newman (2004)	30	Revision	75.7 (61-87)	3 years (0.5-9.3)	20% deep infection 7% prosthetic breakage
Pour et al (2007)	44	3 primary 41 revision	71.8 (55-88)	4.2 years (2-8)	31.8% revision rate at 5 years

uate the ligamentous stability of the knee with the patient under anesthesia. Gross incompetence of the collateral structures with no distinct end point confirms the decision to proceed with a hinged implant. Preoperative antibiotics should be administered within 1 hour of the incision and before the tourniquet is inflated.

When possible, a prior vertical anterior midline incision should be used. However, it is imperative to consider the placement of prior incisions. In general, a single prior vertical or curvilinear incision should be used, even if it is offset from the midline. Short curvilinear incisions should be incorporated into a new incision and may be brought back toward the midline by extending the incision proximally and distally as required. It is imperative to avoid creation of parallel vertical incisions. When prior incisions are too far medial or lateral, a new vertical incision may be made, but skin bridges of at least 5 cm should be maintained, especially over the area of the tibial tubercle, where skin tension may be tight.

The optimal exposure is gained in these difficult cases by starting with a medial parapatellar arthrotomy. This arthrotomy is familiar to most surgeons and is quite versatile. If difficulties with exposure are encountered later in the case, it may be extended with a quadriceps snip or tibial tubercle osteotomy. Before proceeding with these extensile options, however, a series of other steps should be performed to optimize the standard exposure. After the arthrotomy is performed, the fibrotic scar tissue from the suprapatellar region should be excised. Then, the medial and lateral gutters should be reestablished with an electrocautery device or a scalpel. The remnants of the infrapatellar fat pad and peripatellar scar tissue should then be excised. Next, the medial subperiosteal dissection is continued to the posteromedial corner of the tibia, elevating the fibers of the deep medial collateral ligament from the tibial insertion. The knee is gently flexed and the patella is subluxated from the field of view. The tibia is then subluxated and externally rotated out from underneath the femur while the subperiosteal dissection is continued around the posteromedial corner of the tibia, releasing the insertion of the semimembranosus (**Figure 2**). This maneuver will allow sufficient expo-

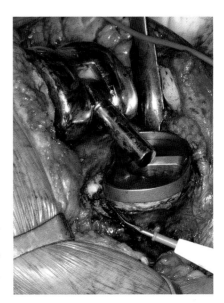

Figure 2 Exposure of the proximal tibia with a medial tibial peel.

sure to gain full access to the proximal tibia to remove the old component and prepare for the new prosthesis. If there is difficulty flexing the knee, or if there is unacceptable tension on the extensor mechanism, a quadriceps snip should be performed with little reservation at this point. Alternatively, when the knee is extremely stiff and less than 70° to 80° of flexion has been

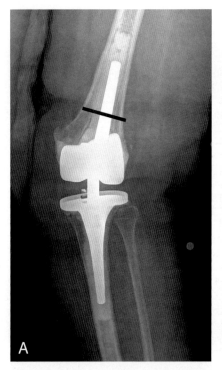
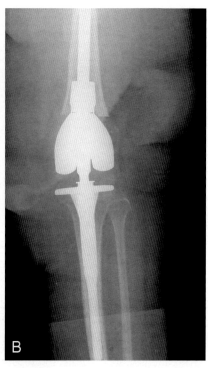

Figure 3 Images of a patient with a failed condylar-type hinge with evidence of loosening of the femoral component and medial ligament incompetence. **A,** Weight-bearing AP radiograph of the left knee. An approximate resection level has been marked (black line) after evaluating the femoral component and additional body options in the segmental system selected for use. **B,** AP radiograph obtained intraoperatively of the distal femoral segmental replacement prosthesis in place.

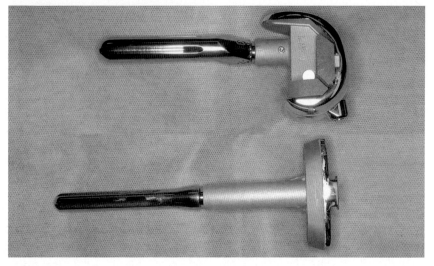

Figure 4 Example of a condylar-type hinge with femoral and tibial augments used to fill bone defects and correct component position to balance the flexion and extension gaps.

obtained despite these maneuvers, it is preferable to proceed with a tibial tubercle osteotomy. In most cases requiring a hinge for massive bone loss or ligamentous instability, exposure usually is not difficult because of the underlying pathology.

Instruments/Equipment/Implants Required

In these complex cases, preoperative planning is critical to ensure that all required prosthetic parts are available along with bone graft options and metal augments. Lateral, Merchant, and weight-bearing AP views of the involved knee, as well as a hip-to-ankle view, provide important information for determining approximate resection levels and body-stem options to restore limb length and alignment (**Figure 3, A**). The full-length view also facilitates identification of other hardware in the limb that may compromise proximal and distal fixation options.

Currently, numerous hinged knee prosthesis options exist. These devices can be divided into two broad categories: segmental replacement-type hinges that allow replacement of large bone defects of the distal femur or proximal tibia, where ligamentous insufficiency is a by-product of the massive bone loss (**Figure 3, B**); and condylar-type resurfacing hinges for use in patients in whom the bone stock is adequate for use of a less constrained unlinked device yet there is complete incompetence of the soft-tissue stabilizers on the medial or lateral sides, or a massive flexion gap is present (**Figure 4**). In general, condylar-type resurfacing hinged knee prostheses are more likely to be used in the less complex revisions, and the segmental replacement-type hinged prostheses in the most severe cases, where both bone loss and ligament dysfunction are encountered.

When selecting a specific prosthesis, it is helpful to consider those design features that appear to be important to the success of contemporary hinged devices. These include load-bearing condyles, rather than load bearing through the axle or hinge of the prosthesis; side-specific femoral components with an anatomic trochlear groove; and revisability of the hinge or bearing, as these parts have

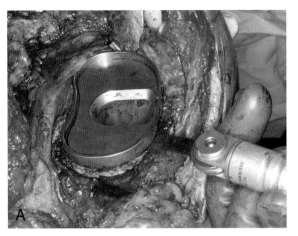
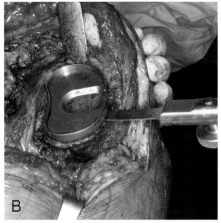
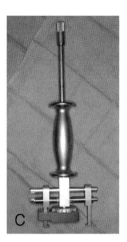

Figure 5 Removing a failed implant. **A,** A nitrogen-powered microsaw is used to open up the interface between the prosthesis and cement. **B,** Flexible osteotomes are used after the initial plane has been developed with the nitrogen-powered microsaw. **C,** A slap hammer used for component extraction.

been prone to failure in past designs. Regardless of the specific system chosen, it is important to verify that the full range of augments, prostheses, and stem options are available. It is also helpful to be familiar with the different body, stem, and extension segments that are standard in the system selected. Even when preoperative templating has been performed, unanticipated scenarios that require adjustments to be made to the surgical plan are often encountered. It is also important to ensure that tools are available for removal of the prior implants. These include a powered microsaw to work at the prosthesis-bone interfaces, flexible osteotomes, and a component removal slap hammer (**Figure 5**). In these revision cases, antibiotic-impregnated cement should be used. Tobramycin at a dose of 1.2 g per batch of cement is a good choice, unless the patient has an underlying allergy to this antibiotic.

Procedure

Once adequate exposure has been obtained, the next step, before removing the old implants, should be to mark a provisional line perpendicular to the epicondylar axis of the femoral component on the anterior aspect of the distal femur. This line, which approx-

imates a proximal extension of the AP axis, or the Whiteside line, will serve as a rotational reference for determining rotation of the new femoral component. In addition, at this time it is helpful to mark an approximate resection level on the distal femur that is based on the preoperative templating and measured from the distal aspect of the femoral condyles (**Figure 6**). Old components are then removed, and all cement and bony debris are removed with curets and rongeurs. Next, the bone loss is evaluated. If at this point the decision is confirmed to proceed with a segmental replacement–type hinged implant, the soft tissues are released from the distal femur, beginning posteriorly in the intercondylar notch. The entire dissection occurs in the subperiosteal plane. The cruciate ligaments and scar tissue are excised from the notch and then the capsule is dissected from the posterior femur. This is begun at the back of the notch with the electrocautery device and then continued medially and laterally with a blunt periosteal elevator. The electrocautery device is then used to release the collateral ligaments and capsule from the medial and lateral condyles. It is helpful to have an assistant pull up on the distal femur using a T-handle or other device placed in the

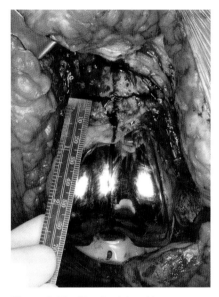

Figure 6 The AP axis of the old component is marked on the anterior femur for use as a rotational landmark at the time of trial component insertion. Any adjustments may be made relative to this guide as required. Also marked is an approximate horizontal resection level, based on the available prosthesis and body-segment lengths.

canal. The origins of the medial and lateral heads of the gastrocnemius muscle must then be elevated from the posterior femur using the electrocautery device. Finally, with a curved retractor placed posterior to the femur, the distal femoral cut is made at the predetermined level.

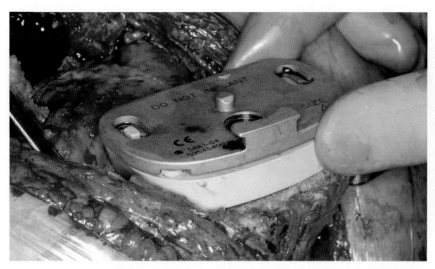

Figure 7 Trialing the tibial component. A mark is made on the proximal tibia that approximates the junction of the medial and middle thirds of the tibial tubercle. This mark is used as the rotational landmark for the tibial component and is particularly helpful in cases of proximal tibial bone loss.

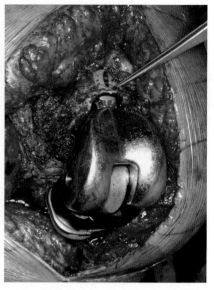

Figure 8 The trial components of a distal femoral segmental replacement hinge are evaluated to ensure that the flexion gap is adequately filled.

Before the reconstructive phase of the procedure begins, it is helpful to ream the femoral and tibial canals by hand to size for the stem extensions. Next, reconstruction begins. First, a flat tibial plateau surface is created by removing minimal bone or selecting an appropriate wedge or block. Alignment of the tibial surface perpendicular to the mechanical axis of the tibia is verified with a spacer block and extramedullary drop rod. The tibial component is then sized, and rotation is set relative to the junction of the medial and middle thirds of the tibial tubercle (**Figure** 7). The metaphyseal area of the tibia is prepared with reamers and punches specific to the system selected. The trial component is then impacted, along with the longest trial stem available in the system selected that has the diameter determined during the hand reaming. This helps ensure alignment, as long as the tibia does not have a distal deformity. Later, stem size and length can be adjusted depending on whether cemented or uncemented fixation is used. The trial femoral component is then assembled with the core prosthesis, any predetermined body segments, and the stem extension in the width determined during the intramedullary hand reaming. The femoral component is inserted, and rotation is set relative to the mark placed on the anterior femur before removing the original implant. Any needed adjustments are made relative to this mark based on the preoperative and intraoperative assessment of any malrotation of the prior component. The locking pin or axle is then inserted into the trial components along with the polyethylene insert that is estimated to be the best fit to fill the flexion gap (**Figure** 8). The knee is then brought into extension and the extension gap is evaluated. Gross hyperextension generally should be avoided even though many systems have an extension stop, as this prevents constant impingement on the stop. If the flexion gap is adequately filled but the knee grossly hyperextends, additional body segments may be added to move the joint line more distally. In some cases where the knee cannot fully extend, additional bone resection may be required. It is helpful to be familiar with the incremental increase in body lengths in the system being used. When the flexion space is grossly loose compared to the extension space, the polyethylene insert size may be increased and body segments removed to allow the femoral component to be moved more proximally; this will prevent residual flexion contracture. However, there is a limit to how proximally the joint line can be elevated, and it is preferable to avoid producing impingement of the patella on the tibial component, except where severe patellar infera existed preoperatively. Alternatively, upsizing the femoral component will better fill the flexion gap and minimize elevation of the joint line; however, in most segmental replacement systems, the number of femoral component sizes is limited.

The soft-tissue stabilizers may be so attenuated that essentially unlimited lengthening occurs. In these cases, it may be impossible to prevent hyperextension except via the extension stop. Similarly, it may be impossible to prevent the tibia from falling away from the femur in flexion. In these situations, it is important to increase the polyethylene thickness and elevate the joint line until it is impossible for the tibia to completely disengage from the femur, even if some distraction occurs. In general, distraction should not exceed about 75% of the "jump height" of the femoral-tibial hinge mechanism, or dislocation may occur. Overall lengthening of the limb may occur in these cases, and patients should be counseled preoperatively. Although the absolute lengthening that is tolerated by the neurovascular structures about the knee is unknown, the peroneal nerve is more tethered at the knee than is the sciatic nerve at the hip. Therefore, less overall lengthening is tolerated at the knee. Consequently, lengthening the leg at the knee by more than about 20 to 30 mm should be approached very cautiously.

Once the final trial components have been assembled, patellar tracking should be evaluated. If subluxation or maltracking occurs, rotation of the femoral and tibial components must be verified and adjusted if necessary before performing a lateral patellar release. Once proper component position and rotation has been set and patellar tracking has been optimized, the component alignment and stem length may be assessed with an intraoperative AP radiograph (**Figure 3**, *B*). The real components are then assembled.

When resurfacing hinges are used to address ligamentous incompetence, the body of the prosthesis may have adequate bone support to allow the use of uncemented stems. In these cases, long diaphyseal-engaging uncemented stems may be used. When the body of the prosthesis has little host bone contact, or when segmental replacement components are used, however, cemented stems should be considered. When cemented stems are used, the canals are prepared by placing cement restrictors at the appropriate depths. The canals are then lavaged and packed to keep them dry until cement is inserted. Antibiotic-impregnated cement is introduced in a retrograde fashion using a cement gun and then pressurized to optimize the mantle. In most cases, it is helpful to

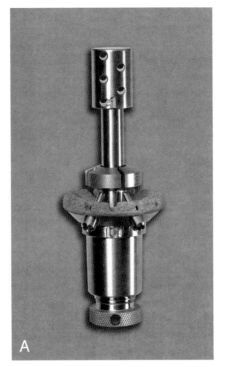
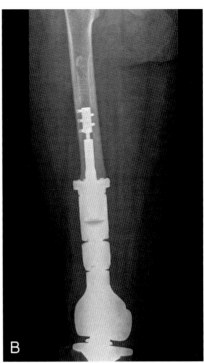

Figure 9 A compression osseointegration device may be used for gaining intramedullary fixation and represents an alternative to conventional cemented or uncemented stems, especially when the length of available canal is limited. **A,** Intramedullary spindle and housing of a compression osteointegration device. **B,** AP radiograph obtained 1 year after implantation of a compression osteointegration device used for fixation of a distal femoral segmental replacement hinged knee prosthesis.

cement the components separately; the tibia is cemented first. Pressure should be maintained on each component as the cement hardens to prevent the component from being pushed back out by the hardening cement. In addition to the use of uncemented and cemented stems for gaining diaphyseal fixation, compression osteointegration appears to hold promise. This technique uses a short spindle that is inserted into the canal and is fixed in place with multiple transcortical pins (**Figure 9**). Next, compression is applied to the bone-prosthesis interface through the spindle to promote bone ingrowth into the porous coating that is in contact with the cortical bone of the distal femur or proximal tibia. The prosthetic parts are then attached to the end of the spindle apparatus through a coupling taper. These compression devices can be used when the

available medullary canal is too short to allow the use of conventional stems because of prosthetic components above or below the knee, and in cases of massive loss of the diaphyseal bone.

Once the final components have been implanted, the polyethylene insert is selected and the locking pin, screw, or axle is inserted into the hinge mechanism and tightened.

When a condylar-type resurfacing hinge is used, the tibial preparation is similar to that described earlier. The femoral preparation is more like the preparation for a standard constrained unlinked femoral component, however, with the only real difference being that the depth and width of the intercondylar resection will be greater because the hinge mechanism is larger than the cam-and-post mechanism of a constrained unlinked device. In these cases, posterior and distal augments are used on the femoral components to help restore distal joint line position, posterior condylar offset, and rotation. Because the femur is more constrained by the bony anatomy in these cases, there is less flexibility in the positioning of the femoral component to help balance the flexion and extension gaps; still, the same principles apply.

Wound Closure

The arthrotomy (and quadriceps snip, if performed) is closed with interrupted braided absorbable No. 0 sutures over an intra-articular drain. The subcutaneous layer is then closed with interrupted braided absorbable 2-0 sutures, followed by staples in the skin. In cases with friable skin, 2-0 monofilament nonabsorbable sutures are used in a vertical mattress fashion instead of staples. A sterile dressing consisting of nonadherent gauze, absorbent pads, cast padding, and a toe-to-thigh 6-in elastic bandage is then applied.

Postoperative Regimen

When skin closure is tight or the skin is friable, an immobilizer is used to prevent flexion until adequate early skin healing is confirmed at 1 to 3 days. When a tibial tubercle osteotomy has been performed, a brace is used for 6 weeks until radiographic union occurs. A continuous passive motion machine typically is not used, but physi-cal therapy begins on postoperative day 1 and continues twice a day until the patient is discharged from the hospital. Weight bearing with a walker or crutches is encouraged as tolerated for 2 to 3 weeks postoperatively, at which time the patient transitions to the use of a cane. In most cases, physical therapy is continued for 6 to 8 weeks on an outpatient basis.

Postoperative pain management includes an oral nonsteroidal anti-inflammatory agent, short- and long-acting narcotic pain medications, and femoral and sciatic peripheral nerve blocks. The sciatic nerve blocks are not started until the patient is awake in the recovery room and distal function of the tibial and peroneal branches has been documented.

All patients are treated with 28 days of postoperative chemical venous thromboembolic prophylaxis, and intermittent pneumatic compression devices are used during the hospital stay. Prophylactic antibiotics are continued for 24 hours postoperatively in all patients.

Avoiding Pitfalls and Complications

Failure to gain adequate exposure in these difficult cases ultimately may lead to injury to the extensor mechanism and/or malpositioning of the femoral and tibial components. Use of extensile exposures is encouraged and ultimately improves the efficiency of the procedure.

The desired rotation of the femoral component should be marked before bone resection and removal of the prior implant. In addition, before removing the old femoral implant, an approximate resection level can be marked on the distal femur that is based on the preoperative assessment of the core prosthesis and the body segments that are likely to be used. This resection level is based on a measurement from the distal aspect of the prosthesis (**Figures 3** and **7**).

During attempts to balance the flexion and extension gaps, it is important to verify that the femoral component does not dislocate from the tibial component. If this occurs (typically in flexion), adjustments to the size and position of the femoral component are required, as described previously.

When a tibial tubercle osteotomy is used to facilitate exposure, it is important to remember to pass the three 18-gauge wires through the tibial metaphysis before insertion of a cemented or uncemented stem. At the time of implantation of the final components, the wires are pushed to the back of the tibial canal after the canal is lavaged and dried; if the stem is to be cemented, the canal is then filled with cement in a retrograde fashion. The final prosthesis is then inserted. This anchors the wires in the cement posterior to the stem and eliminates the difficult task of having to drill though the cement mantle and avoid the stem extension.

Bibliography

Böhm P, Holy T: Is there a future for hinged prostheses in primary total knee arthroplasty? A 20-year survivorship analysis of the Blauth prosthesis. *J Bone Joint Surg Br* 1998;80:302-309.

Harrison RJ Jr , Mihir M, Thacker MM, Pitcher JD, Temple HT, Scully SP: Distal femur replacement is useful in complex total knee arthroplasty revisions. *Clin Orthop Relat Res* 2006;446:113-120.

Jones GB: Total knee replacement: The Walldius hinge. *Clin Orthop Relat Res* 1973;94:50-57.

Jones RE, Skedros JG, Chan AJ, Beauchamp DH, Harkins PC: Total knee arthroplasty using the S-ROM mobile-bearing hinge prosthesis. *J Arthroplasty* 2001;16:270-287.

Lettin AFW, Deliss LJ, Blackburne JS, Scales JT: The Stanmore hinged knee arthroplasty. *J Bone Joint Surg Br* 1978;60: 327-332.

O'Donnell RJ: Compressive osseointegration of modular endoprostheses. *Curr Opin Orthop* 2007;18:590-603.

Pour AE, Parvizi J, Slenker N, Purtill JJ, Sharkey PF: Rotating hinged total knee replacement: Use with caution. *J Bone Joint Surg Am* 2007;89:1735-1741.

Springer BD, Hanssen AD, Sim FH, Lewallen DG: The kinematic rotating hinge prosthesis for complex knee arthroplasty. *Clin Orthop Relat Res* 2001;392:283-291.

Utting MR, Newman JH: Customised hinged knee replacements as a salvage procedure for failed total knee arthroplasty. *Knee* 2004;11:475-479.

Westrich WH, Mollano AV, Sculco TP, Buly RL, Laskin RS, Windsor R: Rotating hinge total knee arthroplasty in severely affected knees. *Clin Orthop Relat Res* 2000;379:195-208.

Coding

CPT Codes		Corresponding ICD-9 Codes	
27446	Arthroplasty, knee, condyle and plateau; medial OR lateral compartment	715	715.16
		715.80	715.89

CPT copyright © 2010 by the American Medical Association. All rights reserved.

Indications

Knee arthrodesis remains an important salvage technique for complex problems of the knee such as severe trauma, chronic infection, or failed total knee arthroplasty (TKA). Technical advances in intramedullary fixation have increased fusion rates dramatically, to the extent that resection arthroplasty has been eliminated as a long-term solution for chronic problems. Simple resection leaves patients with significant instability that must be splinted or braced indefinitely; however, temporary resection is still indicated in the setting of two-stage débridement and reconstruction for chronic knee infection. Although late reconstruction with TKA is successful in more than 90% of patients, arthrodesis still may be required in certain cases.

The patient should be made aware of the functional expectations following knee arthrodesis. The greatest disadvantage of knee arthrodesis is the resultant complete stiffness. With the knee fused in extension, walking is effective and generally smooth, but sitting can be difficult, especially in areas with limited leg room such as movie theaters, sports stadiums, and airplanes. Most older patients require a cane or walker for community ambulation.

In general, patients adapt their activity level to the knee fusion. Automobile driving is not a problem, particularly if the car has an automatic transmission. Most patients avoid sitting in theater seats unless an aisle seat can be reserved. Household chores pose special problems, but most patients are able to bend to reach the floor as a result of stretching of the hamstrings and hypermobility of the lumbar spine. Patients with knee arthrodeses have engaged in virtually every type of sport or recreational activity, including tennis, golf, bowling, baseball, handball, and even horseback riding; however, no patient has been known to attempt snow skiing.

Primary Arthrodesis

With the increasing success rates of TKA, primary arthrodesis of the arthritic knee has become an uncommon operation; however, it remains an attractive or at least a reasonable option in several settings. The first indication is a young patient with severe trauma to the knee joint complicated with chronic sepsis and extensor mechanism loss. The second indication is a neuropathic Charcot joint, where the limb may be asensate and the patient has very poor control of knee function because of severe spinal cord involvement or a myelopathic process. Other indications for primary arthrodesis include treatment of primary malignant bone tumors using augments such as autologous grafts or vascularized fibular transplants, or situations in which inadequate motor function exists to maintain stability in extension, such as in chronic poliomyelitis syndrome. Knee arthrodesis has been shown by numerous authors to be durable in the long term even if interposing grafts are needed. For virtually all other circumstances, primary arthrodesis has been displaced by TKA. The functional outcome is significantly inferior with arthrodesis. Most older patients will require ambulatory aids such as a cane or crutches, and the lifestyle compromise for some patients may be severe.

Secondary Arthrodesis

The most common current indication for knee arthrodesis is chronic sepsis following TKA in a patient who is not a candidate for reimplantation. Typically, these patients are type B or C hosts. Type A hosts have normal, vascularized soft tissues and normal immune status. Type B hosts have significant local and systemic factors that impair the normal immune processes. Local factors include chronic lymphedema, major vessel disease, venous

Dr. Stiehl or an immediate family member has received royalties from Zimmer, Blue Ortho, SAS, and Orthotool LLC; is a member of a speakers' bureau or has made paid presentations on behalf of Zimmer; serves as a paid consultant for or is an employee of Zimmer; and holds stock or stock options in Blue Ortho, SAS, and Orthotool LLC.

stasis, extensive scarring, and radiation fibrosis. Systemic factors include malnutrition, malignancy, extremes of age, hepatic or renal failure, diabetes mellitus, and alcohol abuse. Type C hosts are sufficiently fragile that they might not survive aggressive treatment. Type B and C hosts have a higher risk of infection recurrence, especially when combined with extensor mechanism problems such as patellar tendon rupture. Patients in whom a periprosthetic infection is unlikely to be cured include those with chronic malnutrition with decreased serum albumin and protein, multiple organism infections, chronic infections with persistent signs of inflammation, or life-threatening infections from methicillin-resistant *Staphylococcus aureus* or vancomycin-resistant *Enterococcus*. A recent study has shown chronic sepsis with resistant organisms is likely to recur in at least 50% of patients following two-stage débridement and reimplantation. Careful judgment is needed when treating each patient, and close consultation with an infectious disease specialist is required to balance the risk of long-term antibiotic treatment or suppressive antibiotic therapy against the surgical choices of fibrous resection arthroplasty, total knee reimplantation, arthrodesis, or, occasionally, amputation.

Contraindications

Contraindications to knee arthrodesis include situations in which healing of the fusion and soft tissues may not occur, such as patients with chronic osteomyelitis, poor soft-tissue coverage, or severely impaired vasculature. In patients with a poor vascular supply, not only may arthrodesis be contraindicated, but the success of flap coverage also may be limited.

Results

Several fixation techniques have been shown to result in a successful knee arthrodesis, including standard external fixation frames, Ilizarov technique with small-wire fixation, double-plate fixation, and intramedullary nailing. In severe cases, allografts or vascularized fibular grafts have been used to treat bone defects to promote fusion (**Table 1**).

External Fixation

One report has shown 100% solid fusion using an anterior unilateral frame for arthrodesis. Another series demonstrated fusion in 20 of 21 knees when an Ilizarov-type fixation was used. This contrasts with the 40% to 80% success rate of earlier methods that used the Charnley compression technique. Inadequate stability probably explained these high failure rates.

Complications of arthrodesis reported in the literature include delayed union, recurrence of infection, wound healing problems, stress fracture, reflex sympathetic dystrophy, and partial peroneal nerve palsy. Complication rates have ranged from 38% to 50% in selected series. Peroneal nerve palsy has been noted by multiple authors, and no obvious explanation is offered other than that stretching of the peroneal nerve may result from positioning of the knee during the surgical procedure. Most of the reported peroneal nerve palsies resolved over time, and in no case was direct surgical trauma identified as the cause.

Intramedullary Nail

The Wichita Fusion Nail (Stryker Orthopaedics, Rutherford, NJ) is a significant improvement over older methods. Compression at the fusion site is optimal with the turnbuckle bolt, and midterm experience has been excellent, with a 100% fusion rate in a recent series.

Techniques

Setup/Patient Positioning

For all methods of knee arthrodesis, the patient is positioned supine on the operating table or with a pelvic bump if anterograde intramedullary nail insertion is planned. The entire lower extremity is prepared and draped in standard fashion; if a proximal nail entry site is chosen, draping should include the hip joint. A sterile tourniquet is used during the initial exposure to minimize blood loss. The surgeon must plan in advance for the chosen fixation method, which may include an external fixation system, compression bone plates, or various intramedullary nailing systems.

Procedure

EXPOSURE

The standard exposure is an anterior midline incision or an incision that follows an older incision. Flaps are made that avoid undermining subcutaneous tissues. Typically, the extensor mechanism, including the patella and patellar tendon, is removed. During exposure, the surgeon must be wary of dissection that will damage neurovascular structures. As with total knee revision, a safe margin is the posterior cortex of the proximal tibia. A sharp bone instrument such as a pointed Hohmann retractor may be used to define this junction for posterior exposure (**Figure 1**). The posterior surface of the distal femoral condyles is relatively safe and may be stripped under direct visualization. The lateral fibula and lateral collateral ligament of the knee define the position of the peroneal nerve at the knee joint. Adequate soft-tissue mobilization allows the joint surfaces to be positioned for fixation.

GENERAL PRINCIPLES

To obtain successful fusion, standard concepts of primary bone healing apply. The ends of the distal femur and proximal tibia should be flat, with

Table 1 Results of Knee Arthrodesis

Authors (Year)	Number of Knees	Technique	Etiology	Fusion Rate (%)	Complications
Stiehl and Hanel (1993)	8	IM nail with dynamic compression plate	Chronic knee infection	100	1 rod perforation 1 peroneal nerve palsy 1 nonunion 1 reinfection
Hak et al (1995)	36	ExFix	Infected TKAs, loose TKA	75	14 nonunions 6 pin-tract infections 5 delayed unions 1 stress fracture through pin tract 1 amputation for persistent infection
Arroyo et al (1997)	21	IM nail	16 knee tumors 5 failed TKAs	90	3 stress fractures 3 peroneal nerve palsy 1 superficial wound infection 1 reflex sympathetic dystrophy
Kuo et al (2005)	3	Dual locking compression plates	Infected TKAs	100	None noted
Bargiotas et al (2006)	12	IM nail	Infected TKAs	83	1 amputation 1 nail breakage
McQueen et al (2006)	44	IM nail (Wichita Fusion Nail, Stryker)	Failed TKAs	100	20% major: 6 delayed unions 3 deep infections 2 fractures
Salem et al (2006)	21	Ilizarov frame	Chronic knee infection	95	9 (43%; 3 required redébridement)
Mabry et al (2007)	85	61 ExFix 24 IM rods	Infected TKA	ExFix: 67 IM rod: 96	ExFix: 3 infections IM rod: 2 infections

IM = intramedullary; ExFix = external fixator, TKA = total knee arthroplasty.

well-vascularized bone. This is particularly true when intercalated allograft is used, as union relies on incorporation from the host side only. Maximum bone apposition is sought. In the case of chronic sepsis or osteomyelitis, all necrotic or nonviable tissues must be excised.

Stiehl and Hanel noted that an optimal amount of shortening for clearance of the shoe on gait swing through ambulation was 1.5 to 2.5 cm. Patients would choose shoe lift adjustments to this level.

Several fixation methods are presented here. For most, some form of compression arthrodesis is applied, such as external fixation clamps, crossed screws, or compression bone plates. The Wichita Fusion Nail incorporates a compression function into its design, which includes a turnbuckle. Optimal bone apposition may require some planning and will require surface cuts in the intramedullary axis if long nails are used. A typical solution is to use conventional jigs as applied in primary TKA.

EXTERNAL FIXATION

The most stable construct is a double-frame technique in which two or three threaded pin groups are applied proximally and distally in sound cortical bone of the femur and tibia. Optimum apposition with a degree of compression is desired. Meticulous pin-site care is necessary, and the development of foci of osteomyelitis may be associated with long-term pin use. Patients are best kept non–weight bearing or partial weight bearing for 3 to 5 months.

DOUBLE-PLATE FIXATION

This technique uses two broad AO dynamic compression plates with 10 to 18 holes (average, 12 holes). Bone

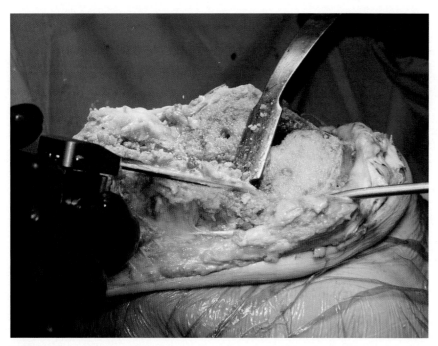

Figure 1 Standard technique is used to cut the proximal tibial surface perpendicular to the axis of the tibial shaft.

cuts are made such that the normal femorotibial valgus of 7° is restored. One plate is placed anteromedially, and the other is placed anterolaterally. Careful contouring of the plates is usually needed. The patella may be osteotomized and applied to the anterior surface of the femur and tibia as a graft. In the presence of sepsis, a two-stage technique is required, with arthrodesis performed after 8 weeks of antibiotic treatment. Postoperative management includes a long-leg cast until the fusion is solid, which may take 5 to 6 months. Recently, authors have reported using this method with a locking compression plate in difficult cases.

INTRAMEDULLARY NAIL FIXATION

Several different rod configurations have been developed, with particular advantages noted for each. This technique is particularly valuable if a long interposing allograft is required, as rigid fixation of the graft is essential for union. The procedure is done using fluoroscopic guidance, and it is important to have the imaging machine placed such that the nail insertion can be visualized all the way down the leg, to be sure that the distal aspect of the rod remains within the bone. After exposure, the knee implant is removed or the previously débrided infected knee is assessed, and the fusion site is prepared. At this point, an incision is made over the greater trochanter and the gluteus medius muscle is split to expose the piriformis fossa. An entry site is created in the piriformis fossa, and a guidewire is passed into the proximal femur down to the knee joint. The bone surfaces may then be cut, using the axis of the guide pin to create maximally abutting surfaces. Anterograde reaming of the femur is done over the guidewire. Generally, this can be done to 12 or 13 mm, which is the nominal size of the tibial reaming and provides a suitable nail size for strength. The guide pin is passed down the tibia under fluoroscopic control to make certain that the center of the ankle joint is reached. Depending on the nail used, one may overream 0.5 mm on the tibial side and 1 mm on the femoral side. The

dimensions of the nail are determined on the basis of the tibial size. The length of the nail is based on guide pin measurement from the tip of the greater trochanter to a point 2 cm above the ankle joint. The bowed fusion nail is then carefully inserted over the guide pin down to the knee joint and passed across to the tibia while an assistant holds the bone ends in apposition. The anterior bow of the femoral shaft determines the position of the nail and tends to direct the nail out the most anterior cortex of the distal femur. Insertion into the tibia must be assessed carefully to prevent perforation and to ensure distal positioning about 2 cm above the ankle joint. The proximal end of the nail should be within 1 cm of the tip of the greater trochanter. At this point, adjunct fixation may be considered. A 10-hole medial AO neutralization plate, crossed cancellous screws, or proximal and distal locking screws in the nail may be considered. Additional bone graft or bone graft substitutes may be added to the fusion site. Postoperatively, no external splints or casts are needed, but the patient must be non–weight bearing for 6 to 10 weeks, depending on the progression of healing. This shortened immobilization could be considered an advantage over double plating or external fixators.

Video 52.1 Arthrodesis of the Knee Utilizing Intramedullary Nailing. Steven Incavo, MD; Todd Havener, MD (4 min)

AUTHOR'S PREFERRED TECHNIQUE: INTRAMEDULLARY NAIL (MCQUEEN TECHNIQUE)

Although other devices may be used, my preference is to use the Wichita Fusion Nail (**Figure 2**), a unique intramedullary nail that can be assembled and compressed in situ. This nail has relatively short femoral and tibial segments that are fixed with interlocking screws at each end. Reaming is done using fixed-dimension reamers (**Figure 3**). Adjustment of tibial placement allows for eventual engagement of a tibial locking segment with a matching female side in the femoral nail, secured by a turnbuckle nut that engages and creates longitudinal compression on tightening (**Figure 4**). The particular advantage of this system is that excellent compression of the fu-

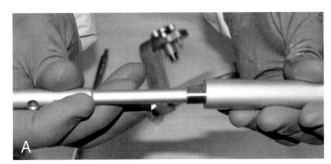
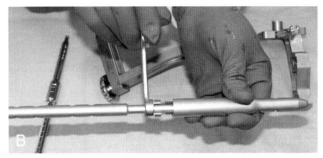

Figure 2 Photographs of the Wichita Fusion Nail. **A,** Engagement of the tibial and femoral components of the Wichita Fusion Nail require insertion of the tibial bolt into the femoral side. **B,** Note placement of the "turnbuckle" nut that secures and provides compression of the fusion site.

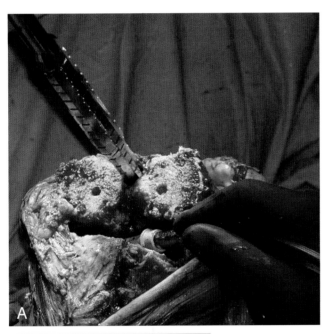
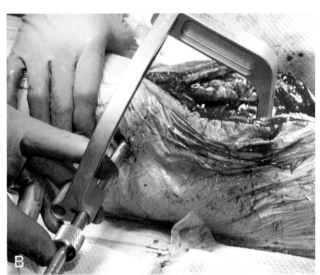
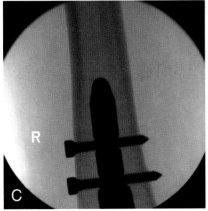

Figure 3 Femoral preparation for knee arthrodesis using the Wichita Fusion Nail. **A,** An intramedullary reamer is used. **B,** An outrigger applied to the Wichita femoral rod allows for lateral percutaneous insertion of the proximal interlocking screws. **C,** Fluoroscopic view shows optimal positioning of the femoral rod before placement of fusion compression. The screws extend through the nail and engage both cortices of the bone.

sion site is possible and blood loss is minimal, which can be a problem if intramedullary reaming is needed. Another important advantage is that the Wichita Fusion Nail is relatively short compared with other intramedullary nails and therefore can be removed without taking down the fusion site. McQueen and associates advise cutting the tibial component at the smaller dimension through a window for removal and state that the femoral component is short enough that removal can be done in a straightforward manner without disturbing the fusion site (**Figure 5**).

Wound Closure

Wound closure requires that soft tissues be reapproximated without excessive tension. This may be problematic, as typical leg shortening after failed TKA creates significant redundant tissue. Debulking of soft tissues and removal of the patella may be helpful. Wound healing problems are rare, however, because the wound is held rigidly in one position. Because wound débridement may lead to oozing from the soft tissues, a wound drain may be preferable for the first 24 hours after the procedure.

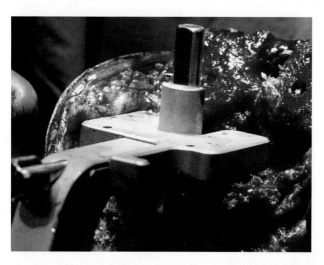

Figure 4 Tibial preparation for knee arthrodesis using the Wichita Fusion Nail. An outrigger applied to the tibial rod places the device at the appropriate position for interlocking. Note the beveled surface of the proximal bolt; this engages a female hole in the femoral nail.

Postoperative Regimen

With any of the compression fusion techniques, the extremity must be kept strictly non–weight bearing for the initial 6 to 12 weeks, or longer for intercalated allografts. Most authors recommend casts or splints with plate fixation. With intramedullary fixation, no external immobilization or splint is needed. For most patients, only sedentary activities with transfer techniques are allowed. Partial weight

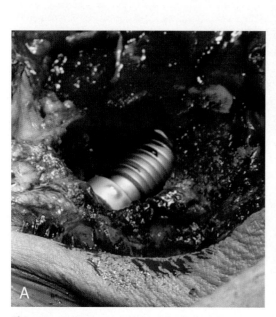
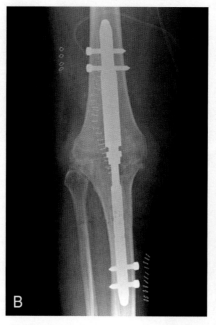
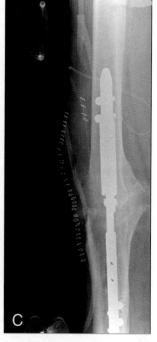

Figure 5 Final placement of the intramedullary fusion nail. **A,** The turnbuckle nut is engaged through a small window that is created when the fusion site is prepared. Postoperative AP (**B**) and lateral (**C**) radiographs show excellent placement of the fusion nail and correct placement of screws in the interlocking holes.

bearing may begin at 6 to 12 weeks depending on the progression of healing and quality of the fixation. Full weight bearing is allowed when union is confirmed.

———————■

Avoiding Pitfalls and Complications

With chronic sepsis after TKA, a staged reconstruction seems appropriate, with a delay of 6 to 8 weeks combined with appropriate adjunctive antibiotic therapy. The choice of nail does not seem to affect fusion rates, but certain advantages and disadvantages are associated with each particular nail. The simple bowed femoral nail allows straightforward anterograde insertion but carries the possibility of migration, bone perforation,

and proximal femoral fracture if reaming is inadequate. Adjunct fixation such as crossed cancellous screws or a neutralization bone plate may be needed at the fusion site. The addition of interlocking screws can add rotational stability at the fusion site.

Chronic sepsis before knee arthrodesis remains a controversial topic. Salem and associates noted a high fusion rate with the Ilizarov hybrid fixation but noted several refractures and problems that required additional surgical procedures. Mabry and associates reported in the largest series to date a fusion rate of 96% with intramedullary fusion, with recurrent infection in 8% of cases compared with an external frame fixation fusion rate of 67% with a 5% infection rate. The authors concluded that the choice between an intramedullary nail and external fixator requires balancing the risks of each technique, with the most

difficult cases of highly resistant organisms in compromised patients being treated with the external fixator. However, Bargiotas and associates were successful with intramedullary fusion in 10 of 12 knees, of which 6 had methicillin-resistant *S aureus* infections.

Recently, investigators have discussed the possibility of late takedown of fusions after failed TKA. In general, patients have been satisfied with this approach, with most stating that they would consider having the operation again if offered. All series have reported very high complication rates exceeding 50%, however, and for this reason, patients must be selected carefully and realistic expectations should be emphasized.

———————■

Bibliography

Arroyo JS, Garvin KL, Neff JR: Arthrodesis of the knee with a modular titanium intramedullary nail. *J Bone Joint Surg Am* 1997;79(1):26-35.

Bargiotas K, Wohlrab D, Sewecke JJ, Lavinge G, Demeo PJ, Sotereanos NG: Arthrodesis of the knee with a long intramedullary nail following the failure of a total knee arthroplasty as the result of infection. *J Bone Joint Surg Am* 2006;88(3):553-558.

Barton TM, White SP, Mintowt-Czyz W, Porteous AJ, Newman JH: A comparison of patient based outcome following knee arthrodesis for failed total knee arthroplasty and revision knee arthroplasty. *Knee* 2008;15(2):98-100.

Benson ER, Resine ST, Lewis CG: Functional outcome of arthrodesis for failed total knee arthroplasty. *Orthopedics* 1998;21(8):875-879.

Cameron HU, Hu C: Results of total knee arthroplasty following takedown of formal knee fusion. *J Arthroplasty* 1996;11(6):732-737.

Green DP, Parkes JC II , Stinchfield FE: Arthrodesis of the knee: A follow-up study. *J Bone Joint Surg Am* 1967;49(6):1065-1078.

Hak DJ, Lieberman JR, Finerman GA: Single plane and biplane external fixators for knee arthrodesis. *Clin Orthop Relat Res* 1995;316(316):134-144.

Hessmann M, Gotzen L, Baumgaertel F: Knee arthrodesis with a unilateral external fixator. *Acta Chir Belg* 1996;96(3):123-127.

Kim YH, Kim JS, Cho SH: Total knee arthroplasty after spontaneous osseous ankylosis and takedown of formal knee fusion. *J Arthroplasty* 2000;15(4):453-460.

Kuo AC, Meehan JP, Lee M: Knee fusion using dual platings with the locking compression plate. *J Arthroplasty* 2005; 20(6):772-776.

Mabry TM, Jacofsky DJ, Haidukewych GJ, Hanssen AD: Comparison of intramedullary nailing and external fixation knee arthrodesis for the infected knee replacement. *Clin Orthop Relat Res* 2007;464:11-15.

MacDonald JH, Agarwal S, Lorei MP, Johanson NA, Freiberg AA: Knee arthrodesis. *J Am Acad Orthop Surg* 2006;14(3): 154-163.

McQueen DA, Cooke FW, Hahn DL: Knee arthrodesis with the Wichita Fusion Nail: An outcome comparison. *Clin Orthop Relat Res* 2006;446:132-139.

Salem KH, Keppler P, Kinzl L, Schmelz A: Hybrid external fixation for arthrodesis in knee sepsis. *Clin Orthop Relat Res* 2006;451:113-120.

Stiehl JB, Hanel DP: Knee arthrodesis using combined intramedullary rod and plate fixation. *Clin Orthop Relat Res* 1993; 294(294):238-241.

Wolf RE, Scarborough MT, Enneking WF: Long-term followup of patients with autogenous resection arthrodesis of the knee. *Clin Orthop Relat Res* 1999;358(358):36-40.

■ Video Reference

Incavo SJ, Havener T: Video. *Arthrodesis of the Knee Utilizing Intramedullary Nailing.* Video clip from *Arthrodesis of the Knee Utilizing Intramedullary Nailing.* Houston, TX, 2003.

Coding			
CPT Code		**Corresponding ICD-9 Codes**	
Knee Arthrodesis			
27580	Arthrodesis, knee, any technique	714.0 733.16 996.66	715.16 905.4

CPT copyright © 2010 by the American Medical Association. All rights reserved.

Chapter 53

Overview and Indications for Articular Cartilage Restoration

Brian J. Cole, MD, MBA
Cecilia Pascual-Garrido, MD
Robert C. Grumet, MD

Introduction

The treatment of articular cartilage lesions in the knee remains a challenge. Studies have shown that up to 66% of knees have a chondral lesion at the time of arthroscopy, but many of these lesions are partial-thickness injuries, and they are generally asymptomatic. The natural history of these chondral lesions is largely unknown. Clinical experience suggests that, because of the poor vascular supply in articular cartilage and its limited capacity for repair, chondral lesions are likely to deteriorate with time and can progress to a symptomatic joint condition. Early intervention for symptomatic chondral defects often is recommended to restore force distribution and joint congruity and, most important, to reduce pain and improve function.

The goals of surgical intervention are to improve symptoms and restore joint function, thereby allowing patients to return to their desired activity level. To select the most appropriate surgery to meet these goals, each case should be considered on an individual basis through careful consideration of the patient's history, physical examination, copathologies, activity level, and expectations.

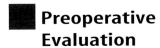

Preoperative Evaluation

History

The decision to treat a chondral lesion begins with a thorough discussion with the patient about the dysfunction in the affected knee. The clinical presentation of chondral defects is highly variable, from asymptomatic with minimal limitations to significant pain, swelling, and functional disability.

As in any evaluation, patients should be asked about the location and quality of the pain, as well as activities that provoke or improve symptoms. Reports of achy discomfort, effusions, mechanical symptoms, or pain with weight bearing suggest a symptomatic chondral defect. Pain with prolonged sitting, stair climbing, or kneeling suggests a cartilage defect on the patella or femoral trochlea. Discomfort that is localized to the medial or lateral joint line is more suggestive of a chondral lesion on the femoral condyle or tibial plateau. The patient's clinical response to previous nonsurgical interventions, including nonsteroidal anti-inflammatory drugs (NSAIDs), physical therapy, and intra-articular corticosteroid or viscosupplementation injections, should be assessed. Any previous surgery must be reviewed thoroughly, including surgical findings documented in surgical notes or intraoperative photographs. Noting the time from surgery and any symptomatic relief gained from the procedure helps determine the subsequent surgical procedures, which may differ from the index treatment. The choice of additional surgical intervention often can be affected significantly by the type of surgery that previously was done and the findings of that surgery.

Finally, a realistic and comprehensive understanding of the patient's desired activity level and expectations is critical to any decision to treat a symptomatic chondral defect.

Physical Examination

Physical examination should begin with an evaluation of the patient's gait.

Dr. Cole or an immediate family member has received royalties from Arthrex and Stryker; serves as a paid consultant to or is an employee of Genzyme, Zimmer, DePuy, Arthrex, Carticept, and Regentis; and has received research or institutional support from Arthrex, DePuy, Zimmer, and Genzyme. Neither of the following authors or any immediate family member has received anything of value from or owns stock in a commercial company or institution related directly or indirectly to the subject of this chapter: Dr. Pascual-Garrido and Dr. Grumet.

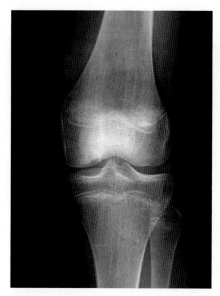

Figure 1 AP view of a left knee in a skeletally immature patient. Note the lucency in the bone on the lateral side of the medial condyle, which is consistent with an OCD lesion.

Information about limb-length discrepancy, alignment, varus or valgus thrust, and any associated muscular weaknesses or avoidance patterns (eg, Trendelenburg, foot drop, quadriceps avoidance) can be appreciated by watching the patient walk. General inspection of the affected limb should include evaluation of alignment and the location of any previous incisions. Any muscle atrophy or swelling should be assessed and compared with the unaffected extremity. Palpation of the knee can locate the specific area of pain and any associated warmth or effusion. The specific location of the pain may help to localize the area of the cartilage defect. For example, patients with classic osteochondritis dissecans (OCD) may experience tenderness on the anteromedial aspect of the knee. Patients with femoral condylar defects may experience tenderness over the defect on the medial or lateral side of the knee. This tenderness is best appreciated with the knee in flexion. In addition to chondral injury with joint line or condylar tenderness, the possibility of associated meniscal pathology should be considered. Me-

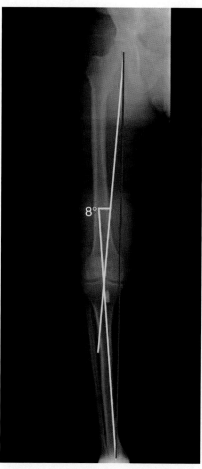

Figure 2 Full-length weight-bearing AP radiograph of a patient with varus alignment of the knee. The red line extends from the center of the hip to the center of the ankle and is consistent with the weight-bearing axis of the knee joint. Normally, this line should pass near the center of the knee. In varus malalignment, the center passes through the medial compartment. The yellow lines indicate the degree of correction required with a high tibial osteotomy to restore neutral alignment and protect the medial joint should cartilage restoration procedures be indicated.

niscal tenderness, however, typically is more posterior along the joint line than tenderness associated with cartilage defects. Range of motion should be assessed by extending and flexing the knee as far as possible. (Normal range of motion is 1° to 2° of extension and 125° to 135° of flexion.) Special tests can be used to evaluate for associated pathologies such as ligamen-

tous insufficiency or concomitant meniscal deficiency. Evaluation and management of these associated pathologies is essential to restore normal joint kinematics and improve the likelihood of successful surgical intervention.

Imaging Studies

Plain radiographs and MRI are the most useful investigations in the assessment of chondral lesions and associated pathologies. Plain radiographs, including bilateral weight-bearing AP, non–weight-bearing lateral, bilateral weight-bearing PA in 45° of flexion, and sunrise views, are obtained in all patients with a suspected cartilage lesion, because each projection provides specific information. The AP and notch views are useful in evaluating for the presence of joint space narrowing, osteophyte formation, and involvement of more than one compartment. Chondral defects can be seen on some views if the lesion is deep enough to compromise the underlying bone, such as an OCD lesion. The notch view may be particularly helpful in evaluating for a suspected OCD lesion because these lesions tend to be in the posterolateral aspect of the medial femoral condyle (**Figure 1**). The sunrise view is useful in evaluating the position of the patella within the trochlear groove (lateral tilt) as well as the integrity of the patellofemoral joint (joint space narrowing) in knees with suspected patellofemoral lesions that may require a tibial tubercle osteotomy. Finally, all views should be reviewed for an associated loose body in the knee joint.

Malalignment should be assessed radiographically with weight-bearing full-length AP radiographs (**Figure 2**). Failure to correct malalignment has been implicated in the failure of cartilage restoration procedures. Varus alignment causes the load-bearing axis to shift to the inside, causing increased load on the medial compartment of the knee. For knees with medial compartment lesions, high tibial osteotomy should be considered to "off load" the medial knee after the cartilage restoration procedure. Alternatively, valgus alignment shifts the load bearing axis to the lateral knee. Valgus malalignment can be corrected to a neutral alignment with a distal femoral osteotomy. To analyze load distribution, a line is drawn from the center of the hip to the center of the ankle on the full-length weight-bearing radiographs (**Figure 2**). The point of intersection at the joint line is the weight-bearing axis of the extremity. In normally aligned limbs, the weight-bearing axis should pass approximately through the center of the knee joint. To determine the degree of correction necessary to achieve neutral alignment, a line is drawn from the center of the hip to the desired point of weight-bearing on the joint line. A second line is drawn from the center of the tibiotalar joint to the same point on the joint line. The angle subtended by these two lines is the required degree of correction to achieve neutral alignment (**Figure 2**).

MRI with or without contrast enhancement will provide additional information about the extent and position of articular cartilage disease. T1- and T2-weighted, 3D, and spoiled gradient-echo (SPGR) images have been reported to be very sensitive in detecting articular cartilage defects. A new technique, delayed gadolinium-enhanced MRI of cartilage can evaluate the glycosaminoglycan content within the cartilage, which may have implications for longitudinal evaluations of the injured cartilage. MRI also can evaluate the location, number, size, and depth of the defects and the condition of the subchondral bone and the surrounding and opposing surface cartilage (Figure 3). Associated pathologies of the meniscus, ligaments, and other anatomic structures can be analyzed to substantiate the physical examination and history.

Diagnostic Arthroscopy

Diagnostic arthroscopic examination can be used in selected patients to obtain additional information for the decision-making process, including a definitive diagnosis, the extent of associated pathologies, and the condition of the opposing cartilage surface. In some patients, arthroscopic lavage or débridement can be used as palliative treatment. If autologous chondrocyte implantation (ACI) is thought to be an appropriate treatment, a biopsy sample also can be taken at the time of arthroscopy. At the time of this writing, a biopsy sample can be cryopreserved for up to 2 years.

Patients with a history of previous surgical intervention may require a diagnostic arthroscopic examination if arthroscopic images are unavailable to assess the integrity of the cartilage lesion and supporting structures, or if enough time has passed since the surgery that the chondral defect may have changed or new injuries may have occurred. During arthroscopy, care should be taken to assess the location, depth, size, and degree of containment of the chondral defect to determine the appropriate treatment. The zone of damaged cartilage often extends well beyond the most visible aspects of the chondral defect, which must be considered in the context of surgical decision making.

——————————■

■ Decision-Making Principles

The appropriate management of articular cartilage lesions in the knee should focus on patient-specific and lesion-specific variables, which individualizes treatment and avoids "linear thinking." Several potential causes of knee pain exist and many chondral defects are well tolerated and not associated with any symptoms. Thus,

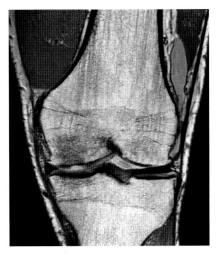

Figure 3 T1-weighted coronal MRI of a chondral defect of the medial femoral condyle. The size, depth, and location of the chondral lesion can be evaluated more accurately with MRI than with radiographs. Additional information may be gained about any associated pathology (ligamentous or meniscal deficiency) and the quality of the bone underlying the chondral lesion. This lesion is well-contained and solitary, with associated bony edema under the lesion.

careful consideration of alternative sources of knee pain is important.

Patient-Specific Factors

A patient's chronologic age often is cited as a relative indication or contraindication to nonarthroplasty solutions for cartilage injury. It is the patient's physiologic age, however, that is more appropriate for determining eligibility. Physiologic age correlates with the patient's activity level and physical demands more closely than does chronologic age and therefore better determines the appropriate treatment of a specific cartilage lesion. Active, high-demand patients may require more aggressive intervention, such as an osteochondral autograft or allograft or ACI, earlier in the treatment algorithm than less active patients. The primary relevance of chronologic age is that the older the patient is at the time of presentation, the longer they have been living with asymptomatic disease and the greater

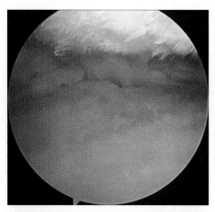

Figure 4 Arthroscopic view obtained during a diagnostic arthroscopic examination of a patient with medial joint pain shows evidence of significant meniscal deficiency in addition to chondral disease. This patient underwent an osteochondral allograft and concomitant meniscal transplant.

the likelihood that biologic restoration will not be feasible.

The patient's history and symptoms also are important preoperative considerations. The location of the pain may help determine whether a cartilage lesion is clinically significant. For example, a patient with anterior knee pain and a cartilage lesion on the medial femoral condyle that is evident on MRI should be evaluated for a patellofemoral etiology to explain the symptoms. Weight-bearing pain along the joint line may be more indicative of a symptomatic cartilage lesion on the weight-bearing portion of the femoral condyle or tibial plateau rather than a patellofemoral lesion. Patients with cartilage lesions typically describe activity-related effusions in the joint. Finally, any previous treatments and their results should be noted.

Perhaps the most important factors in preoperative decision making are the patient's goals for, concerns about, and expectations of surgical intervention. Clarifying these issues during the preoperative discussion is critical for achieving a successful outcome from the patient's perspective. Specific issues to be discussed include the patient's desired activity level, results of previous surgical procedures, and the

predicted marginal improvements expected from additional procedures. Patients often express concerns about the continued progression of the cartilage lesion if surgical treatment is delayed and whether it is safe to remain active despite symptoms. Given the knowledge from existing literature, we educate patients with asymptomatic defects about symptoms that may develop and, as such, often delay treatments in some settings until proper indications exist.

Lesion-Specific Factors

The appropriate intervention for a specific cartilage lesion also is guided by specific characteristics of the defect such as size, location, number, and bone quality. Large lesions (more than 2 to 3 cm²), for example, are better treated with osteochondral allograft or ACI, whereas small lesions typically are best treated with marrow-stimulation techniques or osteochondral autograft transplantation. Lesion location must be evaluated as well. Patellofemoral lesions, for example, may be difficult to treat with allograft or autograft procedures because of the contour of the patella and trochlea. The bone quality under the lesion and condition of the opposing cartilage surface may guide treatment options and help predict the outcome. Defects with bone loss may require bone grafting procedures or necessitate an allograft or autograft procedure. In addition, defects for which MRI indicates significant subchondral edema may require solutions that involve the subchondral bone (ie, osteochondral allograft) rather than surface treatment (ie, ACI).

Additional Considerations

Additional copathologies, such as malalignment and ligamentous or meniscal deficiency, should be evaluated and considered in treatment decisions because they can affect the outcome of the cartilage procedure. Varus or valgus malalignment should be corrected

with a high tibial osteotomy or distal femoral osteotomy, respectively, either before or at the time of the cartilage procedure. Similarly, deficient anterior or posterior cruciate ligaments should be reconstructed either before or at the time of the cartilage procedure because ligamentous laxity can increase the shear stress across the affected cartilage surface. Finally, careful examination and discussion with the patient about previous procedures, including meniscectomy, may necessitate further investigation. When the cartilage lesion is in the same compartment as the deficient meniscal tissue, it may be difficult to discern which pathology is contributing to the symptoms. In such a situation, diagnostic arthroscopy performed to evaluate the integrity of the meniscus can be a critical component in preoperative planning (**Figure 4**). Significant meniscal deficiency may warrant concomitant meniscal transplantation.

The final factor to consider when planning cartilage restoration procedures is the potential for future procedures. The treatment chosen should not rule out options for future treatment if the proposed procedure fails to relieve the symptoms. With this principle in mind, the least destructive and least invasive treatment necessary to alleviate the patient's symptoms and restore joint function should be done first. More extensive treatments should be reserved as potential "salvage" operations if symptoms persist.

■ Treatment

Indications

Indications for the surgical treatment of cartilage lesions include a symptomatic lesion that affects the patient's ability to participate in activities at his or her desired level and that has failed to improve with nonsurgical measures (activity modification, NSAIDs, injec-

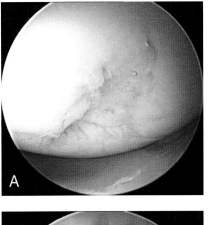
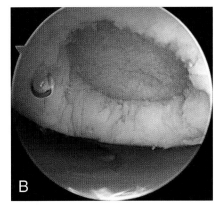
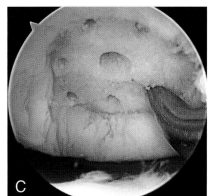
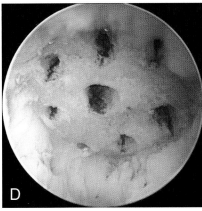

Figure 5 Arthroscopic views of a marrow stimulation procedure. **A**, A focal cartilage defect is seen on the femoral condyle. **B**, The diseased cartilage is removed, taking care to create vertical borders around the lesion. **C,** A sharp awl is used to perforate the subchondral bone. **D**, Fat droplets and blood are released from the perforations. The pluripotent marrow elements will create a fibrin clot in the defect, which will mature into a reparative fibrocartilage.

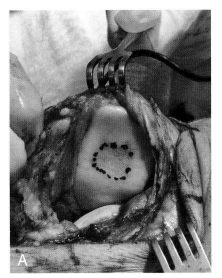
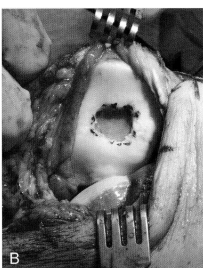
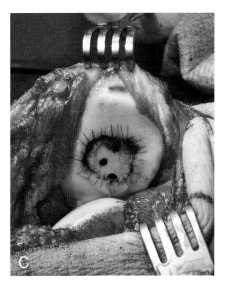

Figure 6 Intraoperative photographs of an autologous chondrocyte implantation procedure. **A**, The chondral lesion on the patella is marked by the purple dashed line. **B**, The diseased cartilage has been removed with sharp ring curets. **C**, A patch has been sewn in position over the defect, sealed with fibrin glue, and filled with cultured chondrocytes.

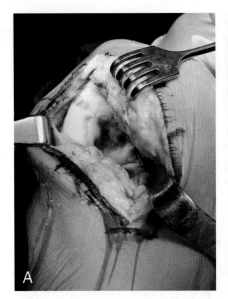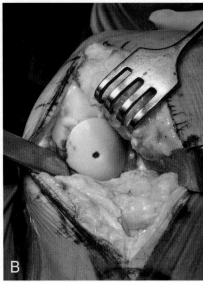

Figure 7 Intraoperative photographs of an osteochondral allograft procedure. **A**, A large osteochondral defect is seen in the lateral femoral condyle. **B,** After preparation of the defect, the osteochondral allograft was placed in the defect site. It is shown in position.

tions). A successful outcome is more likely when the lesion seen on radiographs, MRI, or arthroscopy correlates with the patient's symptoms.

Contraindications

Relative contraindications to surgical treatment of cartilage lesions include copathology or comorbidity that could preclude an outcome that meets the patient's expectations. A body mass index (BMI) greater than 30 may be associated with less clinical improvement because of the higher contact forces in patients with a high BMI. Any malalignment or ligamentous or meniscal deficiency should be corrected either before or at the time of the cartilage procedure. Finally, relatively poor outcomes may be seen in bipolar lesions or cartilage injuries on opposing surfaces, such as the femoral condyle and tibial plateau.

Treatment Algorithm

The treatment options for articular cartilage lesions can be divided into palliative, reparative, and restorative procedures. Palliative procedures, including débridement and lavage, are done primarily for symptomatic relief and have little potential for cartilage regeneration. Reparative techniques, including marrow stimulation or microfracture, perforate the subchondral plate of the chondral defect to promote formation of a fibrin clot and migration of stem cells to the area (**Figure 5**). These pluripotent stem cells then create a reparative fibrocartilage tissue. Finally, restorative procedures such as osteochondral grafting and ACI (**Figure 6**) use osteochondral autografts or allografts (**Figure 7**) or cultured chondrocytes to replace or restore the native hyaline articular cartilage surface.

Our treatment algorithm for reparative and restorative procedures is shown in Figure 8. A systematic approach to choosing the best treatment for articular lesions should include a thorough evaluation of the patient- and lesion-specific variables in an effort to determine the least invasive and most effective treatment that will alleviate these patients' symptoms, meet their expectations, and allow them to return to their desired level of activity.

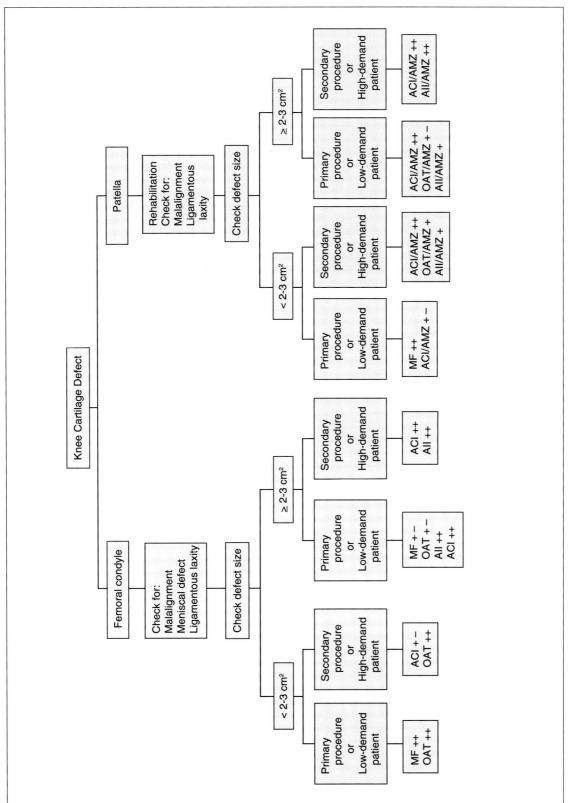

Figure 8 Treatment algorithm for cartilage injury. The decision points of the algorithm include the articular surface involved, concomitant pathology, lesion size, previous treatments, and the activity demand of the patient. Each arm of the algorithm concludes with competing procedures that have relative consideration. ++ = strong consideration. + = moderately strong consideration, + – = less strong consideration, + – = less strong consideration, ACI = autologous chondrocyte implantation, OAT = osteochondral autograft transplantation; AMZ = anteromedialization of the tibial tubercle. (Reproduced from Lewis PB, Nho SJ, Colton AE, Cole BJ: Overview and first-line treatment, in Cole BJ, Busam ML, eds: *Surgical Management of Articular Cartilage Defects in the Knee.* Rosemont, IL, American Academy of Orthopaedic Surgeons, 2009, p 10.)

■ Bibliography

Curl WW, Krome J, Gordon ES, Rushing J, Smith BP, Poehling GG: Cartilage injuries: A review of 31,516 knee arthroscopies. *Arthroscopy* 1997;13(4):456-460.

Fox JA, Kalsi RS, Cole BJ: Update on articular cartilage restoration. *Tech Knee Surg* 2003;2(1):2-17.

Gobbi A, Francisco RA, Lubowitz JH, Allegra F, Canata G: Osteochondral lesions of the talus: Randomized controlled trial comparing chondroplasty, microfracture, and osteochondral autograft transplantation. *Arthroscopy* 2006;22(10): 1085-1092.

Gomoll AH, Kang RW, Chen AL, Cole BJ: Triad of cartilage restoration for unicompartmental arthritis treatment in young patients: Meniscus allograft transplantation, cartilage repair and osteotomy. *J Knee Surg* 2009;22(2):137-141.

Gross AE, Shasha N, Aubin P: Long-term followup of the use of fresh osteochondral allografts for posttraumatic knee defects. *Clin Orthop Relat Res* 2005;435:79-87.

Higgins L: Patient evaluation, in Cole B, Malek M, eds: *Articular Cartilage Lesions: A Practical Guide to Assessment and Treatment.* New York, NY, Springer, 2004, pp 13-22.

McCulloch PC, Kang RW, Sobhy MH, Hayden JK, Cole BJ: Prospective evaluation of prolonged fresh osteochondral allograft transplantation of the femoral condyle: Minimum 2-year follow-up. *Am J Sports Med* 2007;35(3):411-420.

Muscolo DL, Ayerza MA, Aponte-Tinao LA, Abalo E, Farfalli G: Unicondylar osteoarticular allografts of the knee. *J Bone Joint Surg Am* 2007;89(10):2137-2142.

Rue JP, Yanke AB, Busam ML, McNickle AG, Cole BJ: Prospective evaluation of concurrent meniscus transplantation and articular cartilage repair: Minimum 2-year follow-up. *Am J Sports Med* 2008;36(9):1770-1778.

Shapiro F, Koide S, Glimcher MJ: Cell origin and differentiation in the repair of full-thickness defects of articular cartilage. *J Bone Joint Surg Am* 1993;75(4):532-553.

Yoshioka H, Stevens K, Hargreaves BA, et al: Magnetic resonance imaging of articular cartilage of the knee: Comparison between fat-suppressed three-dimensional SPGR imaging, fat-suppressed FSE imaging, and fat-suppressed three-dimensional DEFT imaging, and correlation with arthroscopy. *J Magn Reson Imaging* 2004;20(5):857-864.

Chapter 54

Arthroscopy for Osteoarthritis of the Knee

Matthew J. Matava, MD

Indications

Since the emergence of arthroscopic instrumentation and techniques in the 1970s, many investigators have studied the role of arthroscopy in the treatment of osteoarthritis of the knee. The goals of treatment are to reduce or eliminate pain and improve function. Available evidence has shown that this procedure is indicated for the symptomatic treatment of mechanical locking and catching caused by the presence of joint debris, loose bodies, painful osteophytes, hypertrophic synovitis, and meniscal tears in patients with degenerative arthritis unresponsive to nonsurgical treatment.

A complete radiographic series of the knee, including 45° flexion weight-bearing radiographs (**Figure 1**, *A* and *B*), should be obtained in all patients to assess the extent of arthrosis present. The presence of chondrocalcinosis often is indicative of meniscal and possibly articular degeneration (**Figure 1**, *C*). Long-cassette radiographs of the lower extremities are useful to assess the mechanical axis (**Figure 1**, *D* and *E*), although they are not routinely obtained unless an osteotomy is contemplated. Unfortunately, plain radiographs have been shown to have only a

moderately strong correlation with the actual degree of articular cartilage degeneration. MRI, although helpful in diagnosing the presence of cartilaginous loose bodies or meniscal pathology, is not mandatory if the patient's history, physical examination, and plain radiographs suggest a mechanical etiology for symptoms. In fact, MRI can be counterproductive because the surgeon who sees a meniscal tear on MRI may assume it is the cause of the patient's symptoms when in fact the patient's pain is due to osteoarthritis alone.

Arthroscopic débridement can be effective in at least temporarily alleviating symptoms in patients whose general medical condition prohibits more aggressive surgery such as knee arthroplasty. Arthroscopy of the knee may be useful in patients whose symptoms are localized to the medial or lateral compartment, as an adjunct to either a proximal tibial or distal femoral osteotomy, respectively; to treat associated joint pathology before realignment of the mechanical axis (**Figure 2**); or to assess the condition of the opposite compartment (**Figure 3**). Similarly, arthroscopy can be used to determine the degree of arthrosis in the remaining asymptomatic compart-

ments in patients contemplating unicompartmental knee arthroplasty.

Arthroscopy for knee osteoarthritis can be technically challenging because joint contractures often are associated with osteoarthritis. Therefore, the surgeon must be technically proficient in knee arthroscopy before undertaking this operation for this particular condition.

———————————————■

Contraindications

Arthroscopic débridement of the osteoarthritic knee is contraindicated in patients who report pain as their only symptom without mechanical locking or catching. Other relative contraindications to this procedure include obesity, malalignment of the involved lower extremity, markedly restricted range of knee motion (>15° flexion contracture, <90° of flexion), and ligamentous instability. Patients with advanced arthrosis also are more effectively treated with knee arthroplasty rather than arthroscopy because of the limited success rate in this patient cohort (**Figure 4**). Obviously, any type of surgical intervention is contraindicated if symptoms can be effectively managed with nonsurgical means or if the patient's medical condition precludes general anesthesia.

———————————————■

Dr. Matava or an immediate family member serves as a paid consultant to or is an employee of ISTO Technologies and Schwartz Biomedical and has received research or institutional support from Breg, Axial Biotech, Biomet, Cerapedics, K2M, Medtronic, Midwest Stone Institute, Smith & Nephew, Stryker, Synthes, Wright Medical Technology, Wyeth, and Zimmer.

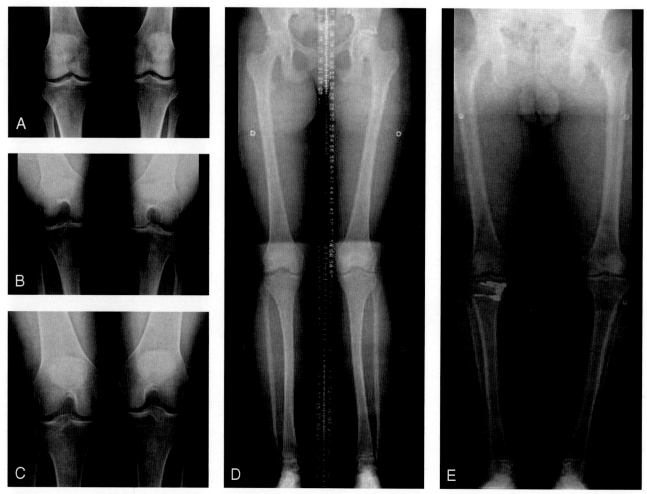

Figure 1 Knee radiographs. **A,** Weight-bearing AP radiographs of both knees in full extension. **B,** 45° flexion weight-bearing PA radiographs of the same patient. Note the decreased medial joint space of the right knee evident on this view. **C,** PA weight-bearing radiograph showing chondrocalcinosis of the medial and lateral menisci of both knees. Long-cassette AP radiographs of both lower extremities demonstrate genu valgum of the left knee in one patient (**D**) and genu varum of the left knee in another patient (**E**).

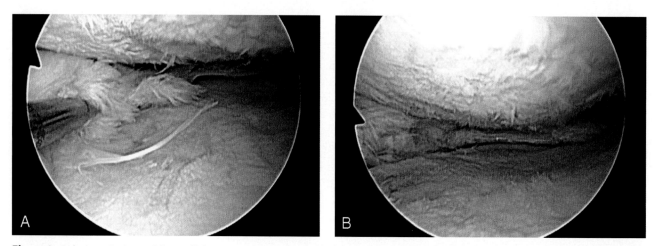

Figure 2 Arthroscopic views of the medial compartment performed before a concurrent proximal tibial osteotomy. **A,** Degenerative meniscal tear and osteoarthritis of the medial compartment. **B,** Medial compartment after partial meniscectomy and chondroplasty of the medial femoral condyle.

Alternative Treatments

Nonsurgical treatment of osteoarthritis of the knee includes maintenance of ideal body weight with weight loss if necessary, avoidance of high-impact activities, lower limb strengthening, and use of unloader braces in patients whose arthritis is limited to either the medial or lateral compartment. Inexpensive, off-the-shelf knee orthoses also have been shown to be effective in improving proprioception and relieving knee pain.

Acetaminophen, nonsteroidal anti-inflammatory drugs, and nonnarcotic pain medications are a mainstay of nonsurgical treatment and are used as appropriate for the degree of pain. Narcotic pain medications have a limited role because of the associated side effects and potential for addiction with chronic use. Injectable medications, such as corticosteroids, can be effective in temporarily relieving pain, but injections should be limited to no more than three per year. Injectable hyaluronic acid substitutes also have been shown to be effective in the treatment of pain associated with mild to moderate osteoarthritis of the knee. These agents typically require a series of three to five injections and can be repeated at 6-month intervals. Neither corticosteroid nor hyaluronic acid injections are effective for the elimination of mechanical symptoms, and they are less effective in more advanced disease. Patients with advanced arthrosis with pain as the primary symptom are better treated with either an osteotomy (indicated for younger, heavier, more active patients) or knee arthroplasty (unicompartmental or total).

Results

Long-term results of this procedure are difficult to predict because success

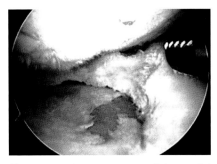

Figure 3 Arthroscopic view of the medial compartment of a right knee demonstrates significant arthrosis of the tibial plateau in a patient scheduled to undergo a distal femoral osteotomy. Advanced degenerative changes of the contralateral compartment are present. Such changes are a contraindication to a realignment osteotomy.

rates are extremely variable, with a tendency to deteriorate over time (Table 1). Factors associated with at least short-term success include symptoms of short duration, localized arthritic degeneration, the presence of mechanical symptoms, normal mechanical alignment of the lower extremity, minimal signs of radiographic degeneration, and normal body weight. Although approximately two thirds of patients have at least short-term (1- to 2-year) relief of symptoms, it is unclear why some patients maintain this improvement, some have no improvement, and some are actually made worse by the procedure. Multiple studies have observed that poor results correlate with older age, chronic symptoms, multicompartment disease, advanced arthritis, severe malalignment, chondrocalcinosis, and obesity. Patients with lower preoperative activity levels, pending litigation, and workers' compensation claims also tend to have limited improvement with arthroscopic débridement. Limited data are available to support procedures that purport to result in the stimulation of fibrocartilage formation, such as abrasion arthroplasty or microfracture, over simple joint lavage and débridement alone.

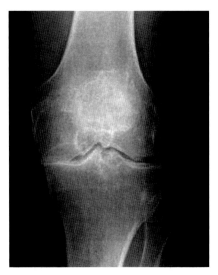

Figure 4 AP radiograph of a left knee indicates advanced osteoarthritis.

Technique

Setup and Instruments/Equipment Required

As with any surgical procedure, the surgeon should develop a routine to avoid missing any relevant pathology. Familiarity with the different types of arthroscopes commonly used is imperative, and more than one of each type should be available in the event that damage occurs to one of them (typically, to the optical lens at the tip). Related to this is the need for various arthroscopic basket forceps (straight and curved), graspers, rotary shavers (straight and curved varieties), and burrs. Curved and narrow (3.5-mm) shavers are extremely helpful in the navigation of tight compartments of the knee, especially the medial compartment in older men. Satisfactory joint distension is mandatory to maintain proper hemostasis to optimize the viewing. This can be regulated by an increase in intra-articular fluid pressure, use of epinephrine in the fluid, or inflation of a tourniquet. I prefer to use lactated Ringer solution because of its more favorable physiologic profile compared to normal saline.

Table 1 Results of Arthroscopic Débridement for Osteoarthritis of the Knee

Author(s) (Year)	Number of Knees	Mean Patient Age in Years (Range)	Minimum Follow-Up	Success Rate	Predictors of Failure
Edelson et al (1995)	29	58 (39-79)	2 years	81%	NR
Harwin (1999)	204	62.1 (32-88)	2 years	63%	Prior surgery, angular deformity, older age
Wai et al (2002)	14,391	62.4 (50-92)	1 year	NR; 9.2% required TKA within 1 year	Age ≥70 years
Moseley et al (2002)	202	53.6 (41-65)	2 years	No difference in Knee-Specific Pain Scale between arthroscopic lavage, débridement, or placebo surgery	NR
Fond et al (2002)	36	64.8 (50-82)	2 years	2-year: 89% 5-year: 69%	Longer duration of symptoms, tricompartmental disease, flexion contracture >10°, preoperative HSS score <22
Dervin et al (2003)	126	61.7 (43-75)	2 years	44%; Significantly greater improvement with medial joint-line pain, a positive Steinmann test, and an unstable meniscal tear	Arthritis severity
Miller et al (2004)	81	49 (40-70)	2 years	94%	Less improvement with bipolar lesions and lesions >400 mm²
Harrison et al (2004)	121	43.7 (30-55)	Mean 7.9 years	60%	Obesity
Aaron et al (2006)	110	61.7 (18-70)	2 years	65%	Severe arthritis, limb malalignment, genu valgum, joint space <2 mm
Kuraishi et al (2006)	25	66 (44-81)	1 year	92%	Femoral-tibial angle <166°
Spahn et al (2006)	156	51.6 (37-69)	47 months	29%	Arthritis >24 months, obesity, smoking, medial tibial osteophytes, medial joint space <5 mm, absence of effusion, absence of synovitis, presence of crystal deposits, deep tibial cartilage defect, need for subtotal/total meniscectomy

NR = not reported, TKA = total knee arthroplasty, HSS = Hospital for Special Surgery.

A tourniquet is applied to the proximal thigh and the patient is positioned supine with the end of the operating table flexed 90°. The thigh is held stationary in a leg holder, suspending the extremity with the knee at the level of the surgeon's umbilicus. The contralateral limb should be supported with the hip flexed and abducted and the knee resting in a flexed, supported position. This position reduces the strain on the anterior hip joint and the femoral nerve that can occur if the healthy limb is unsupported over the end of the operating table. A sequential compression pump or compression stocking is recommended for the contralateral limb, to reduce the risk of deep vein thrombosis (**Figure 5**).

Procedure

PORTAL PLACEMENT

All portals are created with a #11 scalpel through just the skin and subcutaneous tissue. A blunt trochar is used for synovial penetration. A superomedial portal is created at the junction of the superior pole of the patella and patellofemoral joint. The knee is passively flexed to 90°, and the anterolateral and anteromedial portals are similarly created. These portal incisions are made with the blade facing superiorly and directed at a 45° angle from midline through the fat pad toward the intercondylar notch. In general, the anteromedial portal is positioned approximately 5 to 10 mm more proximal than the anterolateral portal. I prefer to treat each pathologic process as it is viewed, to most efficiently complete the surgical procedure without making redundant passes through the knee. Therefore, all three standard knee portals are made at the beginning of the procedure so that instrumentation (probe, shaver, and basket forceps) can be inserted into the joint as needed.

ARTHROSCOPIC ASSESSMENT

A 30° arthroscope is placed in the anterolateral portal with the fluid inflow through the arthroscopic cannula to "blow away" any joint material (eg, cartilaginous debris, synovium) that may impair the viewing. The suprapatellar pouch is examined to determine accurate placement of the outflow cannula and to remove any synovial hypertrophy or loose bodies that frequently are found here (**Figure 6**). It is important not to débride healthy synovium because this will merely increase the amount of bleeding postoperatively.

The entire patellar articular surface can be viewed by simply sweeping the arthroscope from medial to lateral. Alternatively, if the knee is particularly "tight," the surgeon can manually translate the patella from side to side with his or her free hand while holding the arthroscope stationary in the trochlear groove. A 70° arthroscope can be used for a more direct view to better evaluate the articular surface, if necessary.

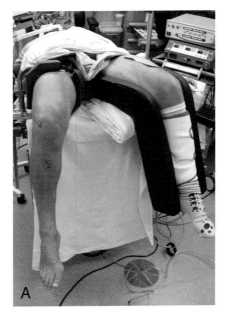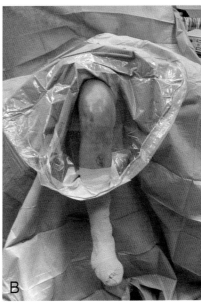

Figure 5 Setup for arthroscopic examination of a right knee.

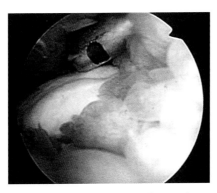

Figure 6 Arthroscopic view shows a loose body in the suprapatellar pouch. Note the presence of associated synovitis. The outflow cannula is evident in this view; its patency should be confirmed at the beginning of the procedure.

The arthroscope should next be directed posteriorly and withdrawn slightly to evaluate the relationship of the patella to the trochlear groove. The knee should be moved slowly from extension to flexion while the groove is evaluated for any signs of cartilaginous wear. At this point, the superiormost aspects of both femoral condyles should be visible. Osteophytes along the medial or lateral femoral condyle typically are left alone unless specifically symptomatic. A hypertrophic and inflamed medial plica

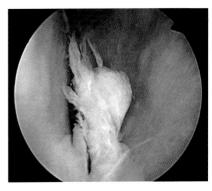

Figure 7 Arthroscopic view shows a displaced meniscal fragment in the medial gutter.

has been implicated as a cause of chondral wear and should be resected.

The medial and lateral gutters should be examined fully because loose bodies and synovial hypertrophy often are present here as well (**Figure 7**). Osteophytes may make navigation of the medial and lateral gutters difficult. The popliteal tendon is at the inferiormost portion of the lateral gutter and can be seen descending through the popliteal hiatus. This is a common location for small loose bodies. These can be brought into view by gently pressing on the posterolateral aspect of the knee to "flush" them out.

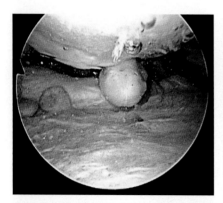

Figure 8 Arthroscopic view shows an osteochondral loose body and degenerative meniscal tear in the medial compartment of the right knee.

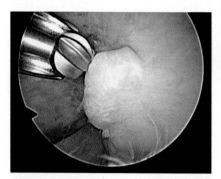

Figure 10 Arthroscopic view of a knee shows an arthroscopic burr débriding an intercondylar notch osteophyte of the left lateral femoral condyle.

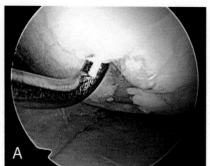

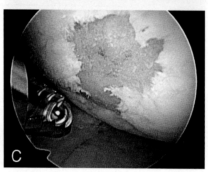

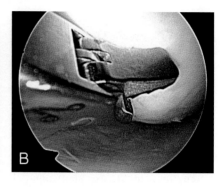

Figure 9 Arthroscopic views of a knee with a chondral defect of the left medial femoral condyle. Such defects are often larger than is immediately apparent. **A,** The lesion is probed to reveal an unstable cartilage flap. **B,** A basket forceps is used to débride unstable portions of cartilage. **C,** The full extent of the lesion following débridement.

Any fibrotic synovium or capsule obliterating the medial or lateral gutter can be resected through either the superior or anterior portal using a suction shaver, basket forceps, or bipolar ablative device.

The knee is placed in approximately 20° of flexion and 10° of external rotation as a valgus force is applied to the leg with the patient's foot locked onto the surgeon's hip or anterior pelvis to allow examination of the medial compartment (**Figure 8**). The medial meniscus should be probed from both the superior and inferior surfaces to assess its stability, determine the presence of any tears, and to make sure there are no loose bodies entrapped between it and the tibial plateau. Moving the knee into near-full extension can improve viewing of the posterior

horn and root (frequently torn in this patient population) in a tight knee. External pressure on the posteromedial aspect of the knee can help deliver the posterior horn into view. Meniscal tears should be débrided back to a stable peripheral rim. Meniscal repair typically is not feasible in patients with associated degenerative arthrosis. The medial femoral condyle and tibial plateau are evaluated for any cartilaginous lesions. Loose cartilage flaps are débrided with a basket forceps or shaver back to stable hyaline cartilage, if possible (**Figure 9**). Areas of exposed bone can be treated with either microfracture or abrasion arthroplasty for localized, circumscribed lesions. Chapter 58 provides a detailed discussion of these techniques. These procedures have limited efficacy for advanced cartilaginous wear. In addition, they necessitate restricted weight bearing and continuous passive knee motion, which can significantly lengthen the period of postoperative rehabilitation. Patients with isolated osteoarthritis of the medial compartment may benefit from release of the medial capsule and deep

medial collateral ligament. This so-called arthroscopic medial release extends superiorly from the midline of the suprapatellar pouch, inferiorly to the upper margin of the medial meniscus, and anteriorly to the medial margin of the patella.

The arthroscope is moved into the intercondylar notch to remove any hypertrophic synovitis or loose bodies that often are found between or adjacent to the cruciate ligaments. Notch stenosis can act as a mechanical impediment to knee extension and cause erosion of the anterior cruciate ligament with resulting reflex inhibition of the quadriceps muscle. The result is painful instability of the knee with flexion contracture. Notch stenosis should be treated with a notchplasty, removing all hypertrophic bone impinging on the cruciate ligaments or tibial spine (**Figure 10**).

The arthroscope should then be moved to the lateral compartment by positioning the knee at approximately 20° of flexion with internal rotation and a varus load applied. Once in the lateral compartment, the surgeon should carry out a systematic evalua-

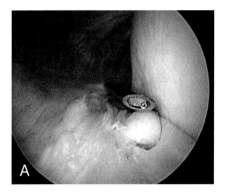 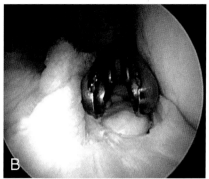 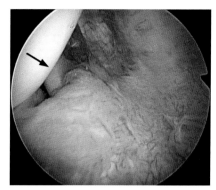

Figure 11 Arthroscopic views of a right knee with an osteochondral loose body lying posterior to the medial meniscus. **A,** 70° arthroscopic view of the posteromedial compartment of the right knee shows the loose body. **B,** Grasping forceps are placed through a posteromedial portal to remove the loose body.

Figure 12 70° arthroscopic view of the posterolateral compartment of the right knee. The arrow indicates the right popliteal tendon.

tion starting with the posterior horn of the lateral meniscus. The popliteal hiatus should then be probed superiorly and inferiorly and inspected for any occult loose bodies, especially under the synovial fold adjacent to the undersurface of the lateral meniscus. The midbody of the lateral meniscus should be evaluated for any tears by moving the camera laterally and aiming the arthroscope inferiorly. This maneuver is facilitated by a rotating motion so as not to damage the articular surface of the lateral femoral condyle. Switching the arthroscope to the anteromedial portal and placing the instruments in the anterolateral portal can facilitate excision of far posterior root tears, which are often difficult to reach from an anteromedial working portal. The anterior horn of the lateral meniscus also is a common location for degenerative meniscal tears that are vertically oriented in line with their fibers. The use of left and right curved forceps can facilitate excision of these tears. The articular surface of the lateral femoral condyle and tibial plateau also should be evaluated. This is done by holding the camera stationary and aiming the arthroscope superiorly while moving the knee from near-full extension to 100° of flexion.

The posteromedial and posterolateral compartments should both be examined from the contralateral ante-

rior portals by traversing through the intercondylar notch with the knee at 90° of flexion. The arthroscopic cannula with a blunt trochar is introduced through the anterolateral portal, posteriorly and inferiorly along the medial wall of the intercondylar notch, under the posterior cruciate ligament, and into the posteromedial compartment. A 70° arthroscope connected to the camera will provide an excellent view of the posterior aspect of the medial femoral condyle, confirm the presence of any loose bodies, rule out a displaced meniscal flap, and reveal how much of the meniscus remains after débridement (**Figure 11**). If a loose body or other pathology is identified, the surgeon must be prepared to make an accessory posteromedial portal for access. This portal is created by first transilluminating the skin over the posteromedial corner of the knee with the light from the arthroscope. An 18-gauge spinal needle is then inserted into the compartment 2 cm above the medial joint line, just posterior to the medial femoral condyle. A longitudinal skin incision is made with a #11 scalpel, with care taken to avoid both the saphenous nerve and vein. A sharp trochar is then advanced through this incision to puncture the posteromedial capsule under direct observation. Operating

instruments can then be inserted as necessary.

The posterolateral compartment can be entered in the same fashion as the posteromedial compartment but is typically easier to reach. With the knee in 90° of flexion, the blunt trochar and cannula are placed in the anteromedial portal and directed posterolaterally along the medial wall of the lateral femoral condyle above the anterior cruciate ligament until a giving-way sensation is perceived, indicating successful navigation through the intercondylar notch (**Figure 12**). From this view, the posterolateral compartment is similarly evaluated for loose bodies or displaced meniscal fragments. If necessary, a posterolateral portal is created in a similar fashion to the posteromedial portal.

Wound Closure

The portals can be closed with interrupted absorbable or nonabsorbable sutures or staples. A drain is not necessary unless an extensive synovectomy has been done. Local anesthetic (10 to 20 mL of 0.5% bupivacaine) is injected intra-articularly and into the portal sites, and a sterile dressing is applied with a compressive wrap. A cold compression unit can be very helpful to reduce the amount of postoperative swelling. The dressing can be removed after 72 hours, when showering over the wound is allowed; however, underwater submersion should be avoided for at least 10 days or until the portals have healed.

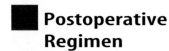

Postoperative Regimen

Patients are allowed to be fully weight bearing on the involved lower extremity immediately after surgery; crutches are used only as needed. However, if a microfracture procedure or abrasion arthroplasty is done, the patient is kept non–weight bearing for 6 weeks, with use of continuous passive motion for 6 hours per day.

A focused physical therapy regimen is prescribed, emphasizing knee range of motion, quadriceps and hamstring strengthening, and patellar mobilization. Cold compression is help-ful in the early postoperative period to prevent swelling, which is common following an extensive synovectomy. Electrical stimulation to the vastus medialis also is beneficial to prevent quadriceps atrophy. Progression to a stationary cycle for range of motion and aerobic conditioning usually is possible within the first 2 to 3 weeks. A graduated return to low-impact, light sports activities can be anticipated within 6 weeks from the time of surgery.

Avoiding Pitfalls and Complications

Patients (especially older men) with osteoarthritis of the knee often have very tight medial and lateral compartments that can make access difficult. This situation, compounded by the presence of osteoporosis often seen in older patients, demands that caution be exercised when applying a valgus force to the joint. Overly aggressive force can lead to rupture of the medial collateral ligament or, worse, a fracture of the femur or tibia. Iatrogenic ligamentous injury or fracture is less common with varus stress.

Corticosteroids should not be injected intraoperatively because this is strongly associated with the development of a deep infection after knee arthroscopy. Use of mechanical prophylaxis intraoperatively and aspirin postoperatively may be beneficial to reduce the risk of deep vein thrombosis common in this patient population after knee surgery. A permissive physical therapy regimen instituted soon after surgery is recommended to avoid the potential for permanent knee stiffness.

Bibliography

Aaron RK, Skolnick AH, Reinert SE, Ciombor DM: Arthroscopic débridement for osteoarthritis of the knee. *J Bone Joint Surg Am* 2006;88(5):936-943.

Dervin GF, Stiell IG, Rody K, Grabowski J: Effect of arthroscopic débridement for osteoarthritis of the knee on health-related quality of life. *J Bone Joint Surg Am* 2003;85-A(1):10-19.

Edelson R, Burks RT, Bloebaum RD: Short-term effects of knee washout for osteoarthritis. *Am J Sports Med* 1995;23(3): 345-349.

Fond J, Rodin D, Ahmad S, Nirschl RP: Arthroscopic debridement for the treatment of osteoarthritis of the knee: 2- and 5-year results. *Arthroscopy* 2002;18(8):829-834.

Gibson JN, White MD, Chapman VM, Strachan RK: Arthroscopic lavage and debridement for osteoarthritis of the knee. *J Bone Joint Surg Br* 1992;74(4):534-537.

Goldman RT, Scuderi GR, Kelly MA: Arthroscopic treatment of the degenerative knee in older athletes. *Clin Sports Med* 1997;16(1):51-68.

Harrison MM, Morrell J, Hopman WM: Influence of obesity on outcome after knee arthroscopy. *Arthroscopy* 2004;20 (7):691-695.

Harwin SF: Arthroscopic debridement for osteoarthritis of the knee: Predictors of patient satisfaction. *Arthroscopy* 1999; 15(2):142-146.

Hunt SA, Jazrawi LM, Sherman OH: Arthroscopic management of osteoarthritis of the knee. *J Am Acad Orthop Surg* 2002; 10(5):356-363.

Kirkley A, Birmingham TB, Litchfield RB, et al: A randomized trial of arthroscopic surgery for osteoarthritis of the knee. *N Engl J Med* 2008;359(11):1097-1107.

Kuraishi J, Akizuki S, Takizawa T, Yamazaki I, Matsunaga D: Arthroscopic lateral meniscectomy in knees with lateral compartment osteoarthritis: A case series study. *Arthroscopy* 2006;22(8):878-883.

León HO, Blanco CE, Guthrie TB, Martínez OJ: Intercondylar notch stenosis in degenerative arthritis of the knee. *Arthroscopy* 2005;21(3):294-302.

Lyu SR: Arthroscopic medial release for medial compartment osteoarthritis of the knee: The result of a single surgeon series with a minimum follow-up of four years. *J Bone Joint Surg Br* 2008;90(9):1186-1192.

Miller BS, Steadman JR, Briggs KK, Rodrigo JJ, Rodkey WG: Patient satisfaction and outcome after microfracture of the degenerative knee. *J Knee Surg* 2004;17(1):13-17.

Moseley JB, O'Malley K, Petersen NJ, et al: A controlled trial of arthroscopic surgery for osteoarthritis of the knee. *N Engl J Med* 2002;347(2):81-88.

Ogilvie-Harris DJ, Fitsialos DP: Arthroscopic management of the degenerative knee. *Arthroscopy* 1991;7(2):151-157.

Richmond JC: Surgery for osteoarthritis of the knee. *Rheum Dis Clin North Am* 2008;34(3):815-825.

Spahn G, Mückley T, Kahl E, Hofmann GO: Factors affecting the outcome of arthroscopy in medial-compartment osteoarthritis of the knee. *Arthroscopy* 2006;22(11):1233-1240.

Wai EK, Kreder HJ, Williams JI: Arthroscopic débridement of the knee for osteoarthritis in patients fifty years of age or older: Utilization and outcomes in the Province of Ontario. *J Bone Joint Surg Am* 2002;84-A(1):17-22.

Coding

CPT Codes		Corresponding ICD-9 Codes	
29874	Arthroscopy, knee, surgical; for removal of loose body or foreign body (eg, osteochondritis dissecans fragmentation, chondral fragmentation)	714.0 711.96	715.0 716.6
29875	Arthroscopy, knee, surgical; synovectomy, limited (eg, plica or shelf resection) (separate procedure)	714.0 719.96	715.0
29876	Arthroscopy, knee, surgical; synovectomy, major, two or more compartments (eg, medial or lateral)	714.0 719.96	715.0
29877	Arthroscopy, knee, surgical; debridement/shaving of articular cartilage (chondroplasty)	714.0 717.6	715.0
29879	Arthroscopy, knee, surgical; abrasion arthroplasty (includes chondroplasty where necessary) or multiple drilling or microfracture	714.0 717	715.0
29880	Arthroscopy, knee, surgical; with meniscectomy (medial AND lateral, including any meniscal shaving)	714.0 717.1	715.0 717.41
29881	Arthroscopy, knee, surgical; with meniscectomy (medial OR lateral, including any meniscal shaving)	714.0 717.1	715.0 717.41
29882	Arthroscopy, knee, surgical; with meniscus repair (medial OR lateral)	714.0 717.1	715.0 717.41
29883	Arthroscopy, knee, surgical; with meniscus repair (medial AND lateral)	714.0 717.1	715.0 717.41
29884	Arthroscopy, knee, surgical; with lysis of adhesions, with or without manipulation (separate procedure)	714.0 717.1	715.0 717.41
29885	Arthroscopy, knee, surgical; drilling for osteochondritis dissecans with bone grafting, with or without internal fixation (including debridement of base of lesion)	714.0 717.1	715.0 717.41

Chapter 55

Autologous Chondrocyte Implantation

Andreas H. Gomoll, MD
Tom Minas, MD, MS

Indications

Autologous chondrocyte implantation (ACI) is indicated for the treatment of medium to large full-thickness focal defects of the articular cartilage (**Figure 1**). Because of the invasiveness of the procedure, ACI is indicated mainly for the treatment of large lesions, generally those larger than 4 cm^2. ACI is approved by the U.S. Food and Drug Administration (FDA) for lesions located on the femoral condyles and the trochlea. Patellar and tibial plateau lesions are being treated using ACI as an off-label procedure. Ideally, the lesion is contained, thus providing a stable rim of intact cartilage to support the periosteal sutures. Defects that extend deep into the subchondral bone occasionally require staged or concomitant bone grafting.

Most chondral defects other than those caused by acute trauma, such as anterior cruciate ligament (ACL) tear or patellar dislocation, are associated with other intra-articular comorbidities that induce or increase abnormal forces on the articular cartilage and lead to accelerated degeneration. Examples of such comorbidities include malalignment, patellar maltracking, and ligamentous or meniscal insufficiency. Coronal plane malalignment and patellar maltracking shift the load-bearing axis, resulting in local overload and accelerated degeneration of the articular surface. Ligamentous insufficiency, most commonly of the ACL, increases shear forces in the knee joint and contributes to chondral wear. Meniscal insufficiency resulting from subtotal meniscectomy increases contact stresses by up to 300% in the respective compartment and predictably is associated with the development of osteoarthritis. Unless these conditions are corrected in staged or concomitant procedures, cartilage repair is doomed to fail in the short to mid term.

ACI involves a two-stage procedure and an extended postoperative rehabilitation, and this must be discussed carefully with the patient and the patient's family to establish reasonable expectations and provide an overview of the projected postoperative course. This discussion should include the need for limited weight bearing, the use of crutches and a continuous passive motion (CPM) device, the length and extent of rehabilitative exercises, the estimated time to return to activities (daily living and athletic), and potential complications.

Contraindications

Lower extremity malalignment, ligamentous or patellar instability, loss of

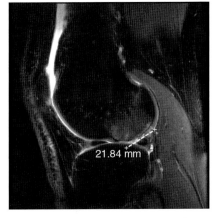

Figure 1 Fat-suppressed proton density–weighted MRI demonstrates a chondral defect in the medial femoral condyle. Note the near-complete absence of cartilage in the defect area and the underlying high signal intensity, representing edema of the subchondral bone.

Dr. Gomoll or an immediate family member is a member of a speakers' bureau or has made paid presentations on behalf of Arthrex and Genzyme; serves as a paid consultant to or is an employee of Genzyme, Tigenix, Arthrex, and Mentice; and has received research or institutional support from Genzyme and ConforMIS. Dr. Minas or an immediate family member is a member of a speakers' bureau or has made paid presentations on behalf of Genzyme and ConforMIS; serves as a paid consultant to or is an employee of Genzyme; has received research or institutional support from Genzyme and ConforMIS; and owns stock or stock options in ConforMIS.

motion, and meniscal insufficiency are not absolute contraindications to ACI, but they require careful preoperative assessment and staged or concomitant treatment. A history of active or recent infection, inflammatory arthritis, or significant medical comorbidities and the inability to follow a complex postoperative rehabilitation protocol are contraindications to ACI.

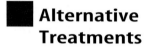

Alternative Treatments

Alternative treatments include nonsurgical management options, such as physical therapy, activity modification, weight loss, injections, and oral anti-inflammatory medications. If nonsurgical measures fail to alleviate symptoms, minimally invasive surgical options directed at the cartilage defect should be explored first, including débridement and lavage. Marrow stimulation techniques, such as microfracture, recently have been found to increase the failure rate of subsequent ACI by a factor of 3. Although useful for the treatment of small lesions, marrow stimulation techniques should not be seen as a necessary first step before ACI for the treatment of large lesions.

Results

The results of ACI have been documented in multiple large-cohort studies (**Table 1**), with good to excellent results in more than 80% of patients with lesions of the femoral condyles and in more than 70% of patients with patellofemoral lesions. Several studies have compared ACI with other cartilage repair modalities such as microfracture and osteochondral autograft transfer. Historically, no significant differences in results have been demonstrated

among these three techniques for small defects. Recently, however, a randomized controlled trial comparing microfracture and ACI demonstrated significantly better histologic and functional outcomes with ACI.

Techniques

Patient Positioning

The patient is positioned supine on a standard operating table with a thigh tourniquet. For the arthroscopic cartilage biopsy, we use either a lateral post or a thigh holder; no post is used during reimplantation. A leg positioning device helps to stabilize the knee in hyperflexion, however, especially when treating posterior lesions of the femoral condyle. The lower leg is prepared into the field to just above the ankle to allow harvesting of the periosteal patch just distal to the pes anserine insertion.

Procedure

ARTHROSCOPIC CARTILAGE BIOPSY

A diagnostic arthroscopy is performed to evaluate the defect and assess the joint for any potential articular comorbidities, such as ligamentous instability, patellar maltracking, or meniscal deficiency. Ligamentous instability should be corrected either at this time or during the chondrocyte implantation. Significant meniscal deficiency should be noted and treated with meniscal transplantation if necessary. The number, size, and location of chondral defects are noted. The opposing articular surface must be evaluated thoroughly for a bipolar (kissing) lesion. The quality and thickness of the surrounding articular cartilage are assessed to determine whether the lesion is contained or uncontained; whether a rim of healthy cartilage is available for periosteal suturing; and whether an uncontained chondral injury will require suturing through adjacent synovium, small drill holes, or bone anchors. The posterior extent of

the lesion is critical, because it could complicate access for suturing at the time of arthrotomy.

If the defects are found to be suitable for ACI, a full-thickness cartilage biopsy is removed with a sharp gouge from the superolateral aspect of the intercondylar notch or the medial aspect of the trochlea. A side-to-side twisting motion of the gouge or curet will remove the desired biopsy more precisely while protecting against unwanted slippage (**Figure 2, A**). We have found it helpful to leave one end of the biopsy attached so that it can be grasped more easily (**Figure 2, B**). The biopsy should measure approximately 5 mm wide by 10 mm long and weigh 200 to 300 mg. After removal from the joint, the biopsy is placed directly in sterile transport medium and shipped for cell culturing. At the culturing facility, the cartilage matrix is digested enzymatically, and the approximately 200,000 to 300,000 cells contained within are grown to approximately 12 million cells per 0.4 mL of culture medium per implantation vial. Up to four vials can be obtained through standard culture. Additional vials for multiple and very large defects require additional cell passage.

AUTOLOGOUS CHONDROCYTE IMPLANTATION

Exposure

For isolated lesions of the femoral condyles, a limited medial or lateral parapatellar arthrotomy is used. Multiple and larger lesions require more extensile approaches, including standard parapatellar or subvastus approaches. Adequate exposure is critical, and it may become necessary to mobilize the meniscus by incising the coronary ligament and taking down the intermeniscal ligament, with subsequent repair at the end of the procedure. Tibial plateau lesions frequently require take-down and subsequent repair of the anterior horn insertion of the respective meniscus for exposure. Correct placement of retractors is cru-

Table 1 Results of Autologous Chondrocyte Implantation

Author(s) (Date)	Number of Knees	Defect Type	Mean Patient Age in Years (Range)	Mean Follow-up (Range)	Results
Brittberg et al (1994)	23	16 femoral lesions 7 patellar lesions	(14-48)	39 months	14/16 femoral lesions with good/excellent results, 5/7 patellar grafts failed
Peterson et al (2000)	94	25 femoral lesions 19 patellar lesions 18 OCD lesions 16 concomitant ACL reconstructions 15 multiple lesions	(15-51)	4 years	Good/excellent results in: 24/25 patients with femoral lesions 11/19 patients with patellar defects treated with concomitant realignment 16/18 OCD lesions 12/16 with concomitant ACL reconstruction 9/15 with multiple lesions
Micheli et al (2001)	50	Knee, all locations	36 (19-53)	> 36 months	94% graft survivorship at 36 months postoperatively
Minas (2001)	107	Knee, all locations	(13-58)	> 12 months	Overall 87% improvement, 13% failure (defined as lack of improvement or objective graft failure)
Peterson et al (2003)	58	OCD knee	26.4 (14-52)	5.6 years	91% good or excellent results 93% patient satisfaction
Mithöfer et al (2005)	20 patients	Knee, all locations	"Adolescents"	47 months	96% good or excellent results 60% return to athletic activity levels equal to or greater than before injury
Minas and Bryant (2005)	45	Patellofemoral defects	37.5 (15-55)	46 months	71% good or excellent results
Rosenberger et al (2008)	56 patients	Knee, all locations	48.6 (45-60)	4.7 years	4.9% failure rate in non–workers' compensation patients; 81% of patients would again undergo ACI
Minas et al (2009)	321	Knee, all locations	35.2 (13-60)	55 months	Failure rate of ACI increased from 8% to 26% in knees that previously had undergone marrow stimulation

OCD = osteochondritis dissecans, ACL = anterior cruciate ligament, ACI = autologous chondrocyte implantation.

cial, especially in limited incisions. We routinely place a bent Hohmann retractor into the femoral notch, displacing the patella to the contralateral side. A Z retractor or rake retractor is helpful in controlling the peripheral soft tissues.

Defect Preparation
Careful defect preparation is crucial for the success of the procedure. The defect must be cleaned of all degenerated tissue to achieve a stable rim with vertical shoulders (**Figure 3**, *A*). This step is performed by first outlining the defect with a fresh scalpel down to the subchondral plate. The degenerated cartilage is then débrided with small ring or conventional curets, taking as much of the surrounding cartilage as necessary to remove all unstable or undermined cartilage (**Figure 3**, *B*). If this removal would transform a contained lesion into an uncontained lesion, however, a small rim of degenerated cartilage should be retained to sew into, rather than using bone tunnels or suture anchors. During débridement, which must include the zone of calcified cartilage, it is essential to maintain an intact subchondral plate. Significant bleeding from the marrow cavity underneath the plate results in migration of a mixed stem-cell population into the chondral defect, in addition to the end-differentiated chondrocytes grown in vitro; it also has the potential for compromising the mechanical integrity of the

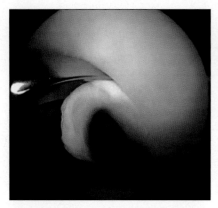

Figure 2 Arthroscopic view of a cartilage biopsy being harvested from the superolateral aspect of the intercondylar notch.

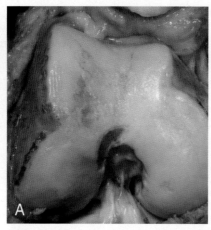

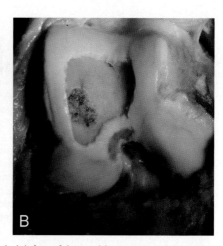

Figure 3 Defect preparation. **A,** A large chondral defect of the trochlea is exposed through a concurrent tibial tubercle osteotomy for anteromedialization. The previous cartilage biopsy site can be seen in the superolateral aspect of the intercondylar notch. **B,** The prepared defect. The minimal bleeding seen at the defect bed will be controlled with epinephrine-soaked sponges. Note the abnormal-appearing subchondral bone in the area of a previous microfracture in the lateral aspect of the prepared defect.

patch as a result of increased pressure from a significant bleed, which could lead to cell leakage. Minor punctate bleeding is encountered frequently but usually can be controlled with thrombin- or epinephrine-soaked sponges, fibrin glue, or electrocautery. Once a healthy defect bed is prepared, it is then measured in length and width or outlined with a sterile marking pen and tracing paper, such as glove packaging paper, to create a template. The template should be oversized by 1 to 2 mm in all dimensions to allow for shrinkage of the periosteum after harvest.

Periosteal Patch Harvest

The most accessible site for harvesting periosteum is the medial proximal tibia just distal to the insertion of the pes anserine, because more proximally, fibers of the sartorius blend with the periosteum, resulting in a low-quality graft. The arthrotomy incision can be extended distally or a separate, smaller incision can be made centrally over the medial surface of the proximal tibia, starting 2 to 3 cm inferior to the pes anserine insertion. The subcutaneous fat is incised superficially, and further dissection with Metzenbaum scissors exposes the tibial periosteum. A wet sponge can be used to gently sweep away loose areolar tissue. The periosteal patch is now outlined according to the template, and the superficial surface and orientation of the patch are marked with a pen. A fresh scalpel blade is used to sharply divide the periosteum, which is then mobilized with a small, sharp periosteal elevator (**Figure 4,** *A*). The patch should be removed from its bony bed very gently to avoid ripping. The periosteum is pulled upward with nontoothed microforceps as it is removed from the tibia with gentle push-pull and side-to-side motions of the periosteal elevator. After the patch has been harvested, it should be spread out on a moist sponge to prevent desiccation and shrinkage. If a tourniquet has been used, it can be deflated at this point for the remainder of the procedure.

Patch Fixation, Integrity Testing, and Fibrin Glue Sealing

Minor bleeding from the defect bed is not uncommon, especially after the tourniquet has been deflated; usually it can be controlled with epinephrine and thrombin, fibrin glue, or electrocautery. Once the defect is completely dry, the periosteal patch is retrieved from the back table and placed over the defect, with the cambium layer facing the defect bed. The periosteum is unfolded gently and stretched with nontoothed forceps; if the patch is obviously oversized, it can be trimmed carefully at this time, preserving a small rim of 1 to 2 mm. Suturing is performed with 6-0 Vicryl suture (Ethicon, Somerville, New Jersey) on a P-1 cutting needle that has been immersed in mineral oil or glycerin for better handling. The sutures are placed through the periosteum and then the articular cartilage, exiting approximately 3 mm from the defect edge, everting the periosteal edge slightly to provide a better seal against the defect wall. The knots are tied on the patch side, seated below the level of the adjacent cartilage (**Figure 4,** *B*). Interrupted sutures initially are placed on each side of the patch (at 3, 6, 9, and 12 o'clock), adjusting the tension of the patch after each suture and trimming the periosteum as needed to obtain a patch that is neither so loose that it sags into the defect nor so tight that it would cut out of the sutures. Additional sutures are placed between the initial sutures circumferentially to close the gaps. An opening wide enough to accept an angiocatheter to

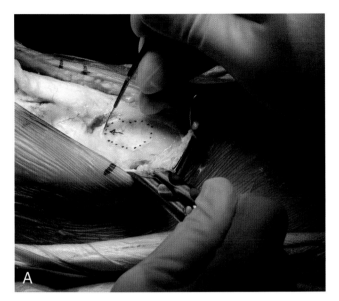
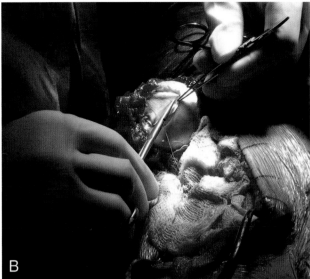

Figure 4 Periosteal patch harvest and fixation. **A,** A periosteal patch is harvested from the proximal tibia (template in place). **B,** A patch is sutured over a defect with multiple interrupted sutures.

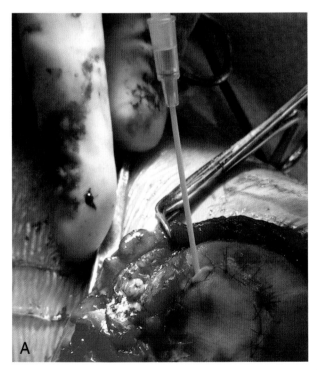
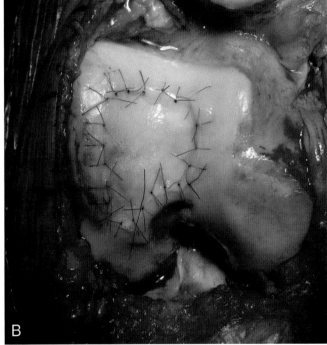

Figure 5 Chondrocyte implantation. **A,** Cells are injected into a defect from the 12 o'clock position. **B,** The final appearance of the defect in the patient shown in Figure 3 after the patch has been sutured in place.

inject the chondrocytes is left in the most superior aspect of the periosteal patch. The suture line is waterproofed with fibrin glue and then tested for water tightness by slowly injecting saline into the covered defect with a tu-

berculin syringe and plastic 18-gauge angiocatheter. Any leakage should be addressed with additional sutures or fibrin glue as needed. The saline is re-aspirated to prepare the defect for chondrocyte implantation.

Chondrocyte Implantation

The vials containing the chondrocytes are removed from the shipping container. The cells are resuspended and sterilely aspirated with a tuberculin syringe through an 18-gauge or larger needle. Smaller-gauge needles can damage the cells. The needle is then removed and replaced with a flexible, plastic 18-gauge 2-in angiocatheter. The angiocatheter is introduced into the defect through the residual opening in the periosteal patch (**Figure 5, A**). As the angiocatheter is withdrawn slowly, cells are injected until the defect is filled with fluid. One or two additional sutures and fibrin glue are then used to close the injection site (**Figure 5, B**).

Wound Closure

We minimize the use of intra-articular drains to avoid damaging the periosteal patch. When a drain is used, it should be used without suction and placed with care to position the tubing away from the defect. The wound is closed in layers, and a soft dressing is applied to the knee. Prophylactic intravenous antibiotics are administered for 24 hours after surgery.

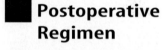

■ Postoperative Regimen

Arthroscopic Cartilage Biopsy

Generally, patients can be returned rapidly to their baseline activity level because of the low morbidity and minimal invasiveness of arthroscopic cartilage biopsy. Patients use crutches for 2 to 5 days for comfort. Occasionally, physical therapy is required for quadriceps shutdown, stiffness, or persistent swelling.

Autologous Chondrocyte Implantation

In general, tissue maturation after ACI is divided into three phases—proliferation, transition, and remodeling—and the rehabilitation protocol is tailored to these phases. During the first phase (proliferation, weeks 1 to 6), the implant is vulnerable to shear and compression forces, and the focus of rehabilitation is protecting the graft. Patients are instructed to maintain touch-down weight bearing on two crutches and to use CPM for 6 to 8 hours per day for 6 weeks after surgery. The exercise protocol is determined by the defect location: patients with condylar defects are allowed full range of motion, whereas those with patellofemoral defects are limited to passive extension to protect the graft. Likewise, CPM is advanced as tolerated to 90° in patients with condylar lesions, but held at 40° in those with patellofemoral defects. To prevent arthrofibrosis, patients are instructed to dangle the leg over the side of the bed at least 3 to 5 times a day to achieve 90° of flexion by 3 weeks. During the second phase (transition, weeks 7 to 12), patients gradually progress to full weight bearing at 2 to 3 months and begin closed-chain strengthening exercises, depending on the size and location of the lesion(s). The third phase (remodeling, weeks 13–) includes a slow return to activities of daily living, and additional strengthening and proprioceptive exercises are added to the regimen. Patients are restricted from in-line impact activities such as running for 12 to 18 months and from cutting sports for at least 18 months.

■ Avoiding Pitfalls and Complications

Complications include not only the standard risks associated with open knee surgery, such as superficial and deep wound infection, deep vein thrombosis and pulmonary embolism, arthrofibrosis, and neurovascular damage, but also risks specific to the ACI procedure. The overall need for second-look arthroscopy ranges from 25% to 50%. Graft delamination causes painful catching or locking of the knee and is best managed by sharp excision of the unstable portions of the graft. Treatment of the resultant defect depends on the size and location: marginal defects may be left alone, small defects may be treated with microfracture, and very large defects may be treated with repeat ACI. Complete delaminations should be removed with no attempt at suture repair, which has been uniformly unsuccessful. Graft delamination was described in five of the seven failures that occurred in the first 100 ACI procedures in a Swedish series; the other two failures resulted from central degeneration. Late-onset, painful catching presenting between 4 and 9 months postoperatively is associated with hypertrophy of the periosteal patch and occurs in up to 35% of cases. Initial treatment is activity restriction. If the condition is unresponsive to nonsurgical measures, arthroscopic evaluation is recommended. The most common appearance of hypertrophy of the periosteal patch is superficial periosteal fibrillation, followed by edge overlapping. Onion-skinning is a full-thickness periosteal loosening or delamination in situ, in which the underlying ACI is intact. Rarely, a large asymmetric lumping of the periosteum occurs, a condition that has been termed *mounding*. Hypertrophic patch material can be débrided by sharp excision with a protected arthroscopic shaver, which generally results in the resolution of symptoms.

Significant intra-articular adhesions are uncommon except when periosteal grafts have been taken from the intra-articular part of the distal femur, a technique that has been associated with intra-articular fibrosis and, rarely, heterotopic ossification in the quadriceps muscle. Other risk factors for arthrofibrosis are a history of keloid wound healing after surgery and concomitant tibial tubercle osteotomy. Adhesions are best released with arthroscopic electrocautery and shaving, followed by gentle manipulation. It is important to ensure that the grafts are free of adhesions, because they otherwise may delaminate at the time of manipulation.

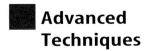

Advanced Techniques

Bone Deficiency

Osteochondral lesions deeper than 6 to 8 mm frequently require staged or concomitant bone grafting. The depth of the lesion should be assessed preoperatively, ideally by CT arthrography. Autologous bone graft can be obtained from the proximal tibia or distal femur. A small cortical window is made, and multiple cylinders of cancellous bone are removed with several passes of an osteochondral autograft transplantation system harvester or angled curet at different angles. The defect bed is prepared by removing all degenerated cartilage and fibrous tissue. The often sclerotic underlying bone is débrided with a burr, and the bed is perforated with a small drill, Kirschner wire, or microfracture pick to stimulate bleeding. The cancellous bone is morcellized and then compacted into the defect with a bone tamp. If performed concomitantly with ACI, the bone graft is covered with a periosteal patch, with the cambium layer facing away from the bone. Subsequently, standard ACI is performed as outlined above. If performed in a staged fashion, ACI should be delayed for 6 to 9 months to permit the cancellous bone graft to harden and form a new subchondral bone plate. This hardening also minimizes bleeding when preparing the defect site before cell implantation.

Special Considerations for Patellofemoral and Tibial Defects

Treatment of patellofemoral defects is complicated by the convexity and concavity of the articular surfaces. In trochlear defects, the concave mediolateral curvature is best reconstituted by oversizing the periosteum in the mediolateral direction by several millimeters. Alternating sutures are then placed on the superior and inferior margins of the defect, and tension is adjusted while the work is performed from the medial to the lateral side. If suturing begins centrally, the trochlea may be flattened, resulting in central chondropenia, potential early breakdown, and resultant failure. Patellar ACI has unique technical considerations for the correction of malalignment or instability, and, as with the suturing technique for trochlear defects, the suturing of the periosteal patch in patellar ACI must reproduce the contour of the patella. This is done most easily by oversizing the periosteal patch in the mediolateral direction, starting the suturing at the apex of the median ridge and alternating from side to side, as when pitching a tent.

The exposure of tibial defects requires a take-down of the ipsilateral meniscus, which covers much of the tibial plateau. Access to the lateral compartment is achieved easily through a lateral arthrotomy, and incision of the intermeniscal ligament and the coronary ligament while retracting the meniscus laterally as the knee is hyperflexed and internally rotated. Only rarely does it become necessary to remove the bony origin of the posterolateral ligamentous structures from the lateral epicondyle to gain posterolateral exposure. The medial tibial plateau is not accessed as easily, however, and all but small anterior lesions require routine take-down of the medial epicondyle–medial collateral ligament complex. A prefitted unloader brace routinely is used postoperatively for 6 months after ACI of bipolar tibiofemoral lesions.

Bibliography

Bentley G, Biant LC, Carrington RW, et al: A prospective, randomised comparison of autologous chondrocyte implantation versus mosaicplasty for osteochondral defects in the knee. *J Bone Joint Surg Br* 2003;85(2):223-230.

Brittberg M, Lindahl A, Nilsson A, Ohlsson C, Isaksson O, Peterson L: Treatment of deep cartilage defects in the knee with autologous chondrocyte transplantation. *N Engl J Med* 1994;331(14):889-895.

Horas U, Pelinkovic D, Herr G, Aigner T, Schnettler R: Autologous chondrocyte implantation and osteochondral cylinder transplantation in cartilage repair of the knee joint: A prospective, comparative trial. *J Bone Joint Surg Am* 2003;85-A(2): 185-192.

Knutsen G, Engebretsen L, Ludvigsen TC, et al: Autologous chondrocyte implantation compared with microfracture in the knee: A randomized trial. *J Bone Joint Surg Am* 2004;86-A(3):455-464.

Micheli LJ, Browne JE, Erggelet C, et al: Autologous chondrocyte implantation of the knee: Multicenter experience and minimum 3-year follow-up. *Clin J Sport Med* 2001;11(4):223-228.

Minas T: Autologous chondrocyte implantation for focal chondral defects of the knee. *Clin Orthop Relat Res* 2001;(391, Suppl):S349-S361.

Minas T, Bryant T: The role of autologous chondrocyte implantation in the patellofemoral joint. *Clin Orthop Relat Res* 2005;436:30-39.

Minas T, Gomoll AH, Rosenberger R, Royce RO, Bryant T: Increased failure rate of autologous chondrocyte implantation after previous treatment with marrow stimulation techniques. *Am J Sports Med* 2009;37(5):902-908.

Mithöfer K, Minas T, Peterson L, Yeon H, Micheli LJ: Functional outcome of knee articular cartilage repair in adolescent athletes. *Am J Sports Med* 2005;33(8):1147-1153.

Peterson L, Minas T, Brittberg M, Lindahl A: Treatment of osteochondritis dissecans of the knee with autologous chondrocyte transplantation: Results at two to ten years. *J Bone Joint Surg Am* 2003;85-A(Suppl 2):17-24.

Peterson L, Minas T, Brittberg M, Nilsson A, Sjögren-Jansson E, Lindahl A: Two- to 9-year outcome after autologous chondrocyte transplantation of the knee. *Clin Orthop Relat Res* 2000;374:212-234.

Rosenberger RE, Gomoll AH, Bryant T, Minas T: Repair of large chondral defects of the knee with autologous chondrocyte implantation in patients 45 years or older. *Am J Sports Med* 2008;36(12):2336-2344.

Saris DB, Vanlauwe J, Victor J, et al: Characterized chondrocyte implantation results in better structural repair when treating symptomatic cartilage defects of the knee in a randomized controlled trial versus microfracture. *Am J Sports Med* 2008;36(2):235-246.

Coding

CPT Codes		Corresponding ICD-9 Codes	
Autologous Chondrocyte Implantation			
27412	Autologous chondrocyte implantation, knee	717.8 718 905.6	717.7 732.7
Arthroscopic Knee Débridement			
29877	Arthroscopy, knee, surgical; debridement/shaving of articular cartilage (chondroplasty)	717.8 715	717.7

CPT copyright ©2010 by the American Medical Association. All rights reserved.

Chapter 56
Osteochondral Autograft Transplantation

William Bugbee, MD
Simon Görtz, MD

Indications

Osteochondral grafting as a means of biologic resurfacing of osteoarticular lesions has a long history of clinical success. Osteochondral autograft transplantation entails transplanting structurally complete osteochondral cylinders from relatively less-weight-bearing areas of the knee into articular cartilage defects. This technique is most appropriate for small, focal lesions of the femoral condyles, especially those with associated subchondral abnormalities, such as a bone cyst or an intralesional osteophyte. Autologous plugs also are a potential salvage option, as in situ fixation for a delaminating osteochondritis dissecans lesion (International Cartilage Repair Society [ICRS] grades II-IV). Advantages of autologous grafts are their immediate availability, relatively low cost, and nonantigenic and osteogenic behavior, which reliably leads to osteointegration. The use of multiple plugs (mosaicplasty) in large lesions (>3 cm²) has been described by multiple authors; however, this method remains technically challenging and its utility is intrinsically limited by donor tissue volume.

Contraindications

Osteochondral autograft transplantation is not advised for reciprocal bipolar ("kissing") lesions or for lesions presenting with a lack of containment or substantial subchondral bone loss, which might lead to loss of fixation and graft failure. Persistent impairment of the mechanical or biologic milieu of the knee joint is considered a contraindication to all cartilage repair procedures. These categorical contraindications include uncorrected ligamentous instability, meniscal deficiency, and axial malalignment of the lower extremity, as well as the presence of inflammatory or crystal-induced arthropathy or any unexplained global synovitis of the knee.

Alternative Treatments

The maximal surface area of an autologous osteochondral graft is limited by donor volume to medium-sized lesions, especially in a previously injured or operated knee. The suitability of tissue quality and overall joint topography must be critically assessed preoperatively because increasing lesion size is a relative contraindication for the use of autologous osteochondral grafts. Larger, contained chondral lesions can be treated with autologous chondrocyte implantation or osteochondral allografting. Allografts are particularly useful in the treatment of conditions with marked osseous involvement or loss of containment, such as high-grade osteochondritis dissecans, osteonecrosis, and posttraumatic defects. None of these restorative procedures should be considered an alternative to prosthetic arthroplasty in individuals with symptoms, age, and activity levels appropriate for prosthetic replacement.

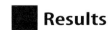

Results

The published long-term results of autologous osteochondral grafting (**Table 1**) are similar to those of com-

Dr. Bugbee or an immediate family member serves as a board member, owner, officer, or committee member of AAOS Biologics Committee; has received royalties from Smith & Nephew and Zimmer; serves as a paid consultant to or is an employee of Arthrex, DePuy, Smith & Nephew, Zimmer, and the Joint Restoration Foundation; and has received research or institutional support from Depuy. Neither Dr. Görtz nor any immediate family member has received anything of value from or owns stock in a commercial company or institution related directly or indirectly to the subject of this chapter.

Table 1 Selected Outcomes of Osteochondral Autografting in the Knee

Authors (Year)	Number of Knees	Site of Lesion	Mean Patient Age in Years (Range)	Mean Follow-up (Range)	Outcome
Outerbridge et al (2000)	18	Femur	27	7.6 years (2-14.6)	81% high functional level
Jakob et al (2002)	52	Femur		37 months (24-56)	92% improved knee function
Hangody and Füles (2003)	740	597 femur 118 PFJ 25 tibia	NR	NR	Femoral lesions: 92% good/excellent PFJ lesions: 87% good/excellent Tibial lesions: 79% good/excellent
Chow et al (2004)	30	Femur	44.6	45.1 months	83% good/excellent
Karataglis et al (2006)	37	Femur and PFJ	31.9 (18-48)	36.9 months (18-73)	87% high functional level
Marcacci et al (2007)	30	Femur	29.3	7.0	77% good/excellent

PFJ = patellofemoral joint, NR = not reported.

parable cartilage repair techniques, with good to excellent outcomes reported in 77% to 92% of patients at a mean follow-up of up to 10 years. In general, femoral condyle grafts performed best, followed by tibial grafts and grafts of the patellofemoral joint. However, surgical technique varies considerably across these studies with regard to donor-site selection and graft number, size, and delivery (arthroscopic versus open). Further confounding the analysis, these studies generally have a high percentage (up to 85%) of concomitant surgery (anterior cruciate ligament reconstruction, realignment procedures, and meniscal surgeries), inconsistently reported lesion location and size, and variable outcome measures. Postoperative complications such as hemarthrosis and donor-site morbidity were reported in up to 8% and 12% of patients, respectively, and a revision rate of up to 10% and a reoperation rate for graft-related symptoms of up to 25% were reported. On both follow-up MRI and second-look arthroscopy, grafts appeared to be mechanically durable, and donor sites were reliably filled in with fibrocartilagenous repair tissue.

Technique

Exposure

The patient is positioned supine to allow full flexion of the knee. A tourniquet is recommended to assist with intraoperative visualization. A leg or foot holder can help position and maintain the leg in 70° to 100° of flexion during open procedures. The technique can be done through a standard arthrotomy, a mini-arthrotomy, or arthroscopically. Even in arthroscopic approaches, graft harvest from the trochlea almost always necessitates a mini-incision, and the surgeon should be prepared for conversion to a standard arthrotomy because certain locations, such as the posterior femoral condyle, may be difficult to access with less invasive approaches, and perpendicularity in graft harvest and placement might be hard to achieve.

After the entire knee joint has been inspected and the adequacy of the tissue at the potential donor sites has been validated, the lesion is accessed, probed, and measured, and a corresponding graft match is established. In current practice, donor plugs from 4 to 12 mm are used, depending on the technique and instrumentation system used and the size of the chondral lesion. We advocate medium-sized

trochlear plugs, optimally harvested through the same ipsilateral incision. We also recommend beginning the procedure with the graft harvest to ensure availability of a suitable graft before creating a recipient tunnel. A fallback option should be available, such as a bone graft substitute or an osteochondral allograft.

Graft Harvest

Proprietary instrument systems generally provide a hollow-core instrument for graft harvest. Under direct observation, an appropriate-size T-handle recipient harvester (**Figure 1**, *A*) is tapped perpendicular to the articular surface of the far ipsilateral margin of the trochlea, just proximal to the sulcus terminalis, to a minimal depth of 8 mm. The actual depth depends on the extent of subchondral involvement of the lesion being treated. It is of paramount importance to check the harvesting device from several angles after introduction to make sure it is perpendicular before advancing it farther. Once tapped, the harvester chisel is removed by rotating the driver to amputate the graft (**Figure 1**, *B*). The functional length of the graft is measured and the recipient socket is fashioned to provide a secure press-fit circumferentially and to be deep enough to easily accommodate the length of the plug.

Graft Placement

Depending on the instrument system used, the recipient socket is prepared using either a coring device or drill. Traditional systems usually use a tubular coring device. Using the same technique described above but using a T-handle harvester with a slightly smaller circumference, the recipient socket is created. Again, the harvester must be introduced absolutely perpendicularly, the circumference of the recipient tunnel should ensure a secure press-fit, and the depth of the tunnel should be equal to or greater than the donor plug length. Drilling the recipient site might produce a more precise socket depth than using a coring device. With either method, the recipient socket should be measured for accuracy. The bony portion of the plug can be rasped down to the desired depth measurement if necessary. After verifying the length of the donor graft, the graft is then transplanted into the recipient site with the donor insertion guide (**Figure 2**, *A*), which has a beveled edge that dilates the cartilage layer to create a tight press-fit. The last 1 mm of impaction should be done by lightly tapping a bone tamp over the cartilaginous cap. The bone tamp should be oversized or placed offset (**Figure 2**, *B*) to avoid countersinking a graft that is slightly shorter than the tunnel.

Multiple Grafts

If multiple grafts are required, the process can be repeated until a reasonable tissue fill is achieved in the lesion, but careful spacing of the plugs is essential. A 2-mm bone bridge between recipient sockets is recommended to help achieve and maintain a secure press-fit. The resulting voids on the articular surface should fill with fibrocartilage. Careful planning of the graft harvest site geometry is essential. To avoid premature amputation of the graft during harvest, the osseous portions should not intersect. This can be most problematic with longer grafts obtained in areas of the knee where there is high curvature, such as the posterior femoral condyle. Finally, to prevent fracture of the wall of the re-

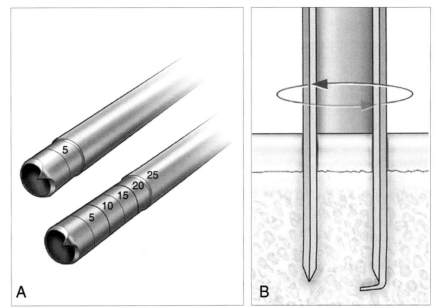

Figure 1 Drawings illustrating graft harvest. **A,** The appropriate-size graft cutter is introduced. **B,** The plug is harvested via a twisting (clockwise and counterclockwise) motion of the cutter. (Reproduced with permission from Levy A, Meier SW: Osteochondral autograft replacement, in Cole BJ, Malek M, eds: *Articular Cartilage Lesions.* New York, NY, Springer-Verlag, 2004, pp 76-77.)

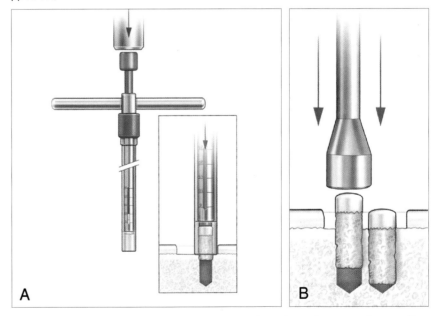

Figure 2 Drawings illustrating placement of the graft. **A,** The graft is inserted perpendicularly into the defect. **B,** Final seating of the graft is achieved by gentle tapping with an oversized tamp. (Reproduced with permission from Levy A, Meier SW: Osteochondral autograft replacement, in Cole BJ, Malek M, eds: *Articular Cartilage Lesions.* New York, NY, Springer-Verlag, 2004, pp 76-77.)

cipient tunnel, each plug transfer should be completed before proceeding with additional recipient sockets.

Following the grafting process, surface congruity is confirmed and the joint is put through a range of motion to ensure graft stability and lack of impingement.

Wound Closure

The knee is closed in a standard fashion over a drain after irrigation of the joint and inspection for loose bodies.

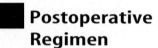

Postoperative Regimen

Patients are kept on crutches and partial weight-bearing restriction for 3 to 4 weeks. Isometric quadriceps strengthening and early range of motion are encouraged unless additional reconstructive procedures have been done that would alter the rehabilitation plan. Closed-chain exercises are introduced at 4 weeks. The return to weight bearing is gradual, and patients return to full daily activities by 3 to 4 months.

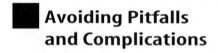

Avoiding Pitfalls and Complications

Correct selection and implantation of donor plugs are essential to accurately recreate the topographic anatomy of the recipient site, to minimize risk of donor-site morbidity and graft failure,

and to optimize outcomes. Recent reports have demonstrated that traditional donor sites of the distal trochlea and intercondylar notch do bear significant weight, which can theoretically contribute to increased donor-site morbidity. The lateral trochlea appears the most involved in loading, followed by the intercondylar notch and distal medial trochlea. Because of its load-bearing demands, the lateral trochlea has thicker articular cartilage, making it the favored graft source of most surgeons. Because the lateral trochlea is wider than the medial side, larger plugs can be taken from it, starting proximal to the sulcus terminalis, where the contact pressures of the lateral trochlea are lowest. Plugs taken from the far medial and lateral margins of the femoral trochlea, just proximal to the sulcus terminalis, appear to provide the most accurate reconstruction of the surface anatomy of central lesions in the weight-bearing portion of either femoral condyle. Smaller grafts (4 or 6 mm) from the lateral intercondylar notch also can provide precise matches to similar lesions; however, significant inaccuracies are noted when the lateral intercondylar notch grafts are increased to 8 mm. Although all traditional donor sites have less cartilage thickness than common recipient sites, this discrepancy is most profound between the lateral intercondylar notch and the weight-bearing portion of the femoral condyles. In addition, the concave central intercondylar notch grafts do not match the topography of the convex femoral condyles, and their harvest jeopardizes the integrity of the trochlear subchondral bone, which might be responsible for the higher in-

cidence of anterior knee pain reported in some studies. In general, matching articular geometry becomes more difficult and the potential for donor-site morbidity increases with larger grafts.

Biomechanical studies have confirmed that optimal-size, level-seated plugs experience nearly normal joint contact pressures in situ. Results also showed that slightly countersunk grafts and angled grafts with the highest edge placed flush to neighboring cartilage demonstrated fairly normal contact pressures. On the other hand, elevated angled grafts increased contact pressures as much as 40%, making them biomechanically disadvantageous. There is general consensus that it is more favorable to leave a graft slightly countersunk than elevated with respect to the neighboring cartilage. We thus advise making the recipient tunnel slightly longer than the graft to avoid leaving the graft proud or subjecting it to undue insertion forces in an effort to bury an oversized graft.

Hemarthrosis, ostensibly due to bleeding from the donor site, is the most common postoperative complication after autologous grafting. Retrofilling of the created defects has been recommended to reduce the risk of this complication and, in turn, donor-site morbidity. Using the plugs removed from the recipient sockets carries the risk of displacement because of their small size relative to the donor voids. Osteobiologic bone-substitute plugs that correspond to the diameters of commercial coring devices are available for this purpose.

Bibliography

Ahmad CS, Cohen ZA, Levine WN, Ateshian GA, Mow VC: Biomechanical and topographic considerations for autologous osteochondral grafting in the knee. *Am J Sports Med* 2001;29(2):201-206.

Bartz RL, Kamaric E, Noble PC, Lintner D, Bocell J: Topographic matching of selected donor and recipient sites for osteochondral autografting of the articular surface of the femoral condyles. *Am J Sports Med* 2001;29(2):207-212.

Bobic V: Autologous osteo-chondral grafts in the management of articular cartilage lesions. *Orthopade* 1999;28(1):19-25.

Chow JC, Hantes ME, Houle JB, Zalavras CG: Arthroscopic autogenous osteochondral transplantation for treating knee cartilage defects: A 2- to 5-year follow-up study. *Arthroscopy* 2004;20(7):681-690.

Hangody L, Füles P: Autologous osteochondral mosaicplasty for the treatment of full-thickness defects of weight-bearing joints: Ten years of experimental and clinical experience. *J Bone Joint Surg Am* 2003;85(Suppl 2):25-32.

Jakob RP, Franz T, Gautier E, Mainil-Varlet P: Autologous osteochondral grafting in the knee: Indication, results, and reflections. *Clin Orthop Relat Res* 2002;401:170-184.

Karataglis D, Green MA, Learmonth DJ: Autologous osteochondral transplantation for the treatment of chondral defects of the knee. *Knee* 2006;13(1):32-35.

Koh JL, Kowalski A, Lautenschlager E: The effect of angled osteochondral grafting on contact pressure: A biomechanical study. *Am J Sports Med* 2006;34(1):116-119.

Koh JL, Wirsing K, Lautenschlager E, Zhang LO: The effect of graft height mismatch on contact pressure following osteochondral grafting: A biomechanical study. *Am J Sports Med* 2004;32(2):317-320.

Marcacci M, Kon E, Delcogliano M, Filardo G, Busacca M, Zaffagnini S: Arthroscopic autologous osteochondral grafting for cartilage defects of the knee: Prospective study results at a minimum 7-year follow-up. *Am J Sports Med* 2007;35(12): 2014-2021.

Miniaci A, Tytherleigh-Strong G: Fixation of unstable osteochondritis dissecans lesions of the knee using arthroscopic autogenous osteochondral grafting (mosaicplasty). *Arthroscopy* 2007;23(8):845-851.

Outerbridge HK, Outerbridge RE, Smith DE: Osteochondral defects in the knee: A treatment using lateral patella autografts. *Clin Orthop Relat Res* 2000;377:145-151.

Thaunat M, Couchon S, Lunn J, Charrois O, Fallet L, Beaufils P: Cartilage thickness matching of selected donor and recipient sites for osteochondral autografting of the medial femoral condyle. *Knee Surg Sports Traumatol Arthrosc* 2007; 15(4):381-386.

Coding				
CPT Codes			**Corresponding ICD-9 Codes**	
27416	Osteochondral autograft(s), knee, open (eg, mosaicplasty) (includes harvesting of autograft[s])		716.60 717.7	716.66 718.00
29866	Arthroscopy, knee, surgical; osteochondral autograft(s) (eg, mosaicplasty) (includes harvesting of the autograft[s])		718.01 716.60 717.0 717.2	718.02 716.66 717.1 717.3

Chapter 57

Osteochondral Allograft Transplantation

Bert Mandelbaum, MD
Simon Görtz, MD
William Bugbee, MD

Indications

Fresh osteochondral allografts, because of their compound osteoarticular nature, are uniquely suited to treat a wide spectrum of articular cartilage pathologies, especially those seen in conditions that present with an osseous deficiency. Osteochondral allograft transplantation can be considered as the primary treatment for purely chondral defects when the size of the defect poses a relative contraindication for other treatments, especially defects that involve a loss of containment or bone involvement 6 to 10 mm deep. Allografts also have proved valuable in knee salvage when other cartilage-resurfacing procedures, such as microfracture, autologous chondrocyte implantation (ACI), and osteochondral autologous plug transfer, have failed.

Conditions most suitable for allografting include osteochondritis dissecans (OCD) **(Figure 1)**, osteonecrosis, and posttraumatic defects. Other indications include selected multifocal or bipolar lesions that occur in isolated, unicompartmental patellofemoral or tibiofemoral arthrosis in patients of an age and activity level not optimally suited for partial or total knee arthroplasty. If a meniscus is absent, it can be replaced as part of a compound graft attached to its correlating tibial plateau, avoiding many of the size-match and fixation pitfalls associated with isolated meniscal allograft transplantation. The advantage of an allogeneic graft source is that even large and complex lesions can be resurfaced by reintroducing orthotopically appropriate, mature hyaline cartilage, with the fixation issue predictably relegated to bone-to-bone healing.

Contraindications

Although bipolar and multicompartmental allografting has been moderately successful in younger individuals, allografting should not be considered an alternative to prosthetic arthroplasty in patients who have advanced multicompartment arthrosis and whose age and activity levels are appropriate for prosthetic replacement. Other relative contraindications to the allografting procedure include uncorrected ligamentous instability, meniscal insufficiency, or contributory axial malalignment of the limb, which should be corrected before or at the time of allografting to optimize the biomechanical environment. The presence of inflammatory disease, crystal-induced arthropathy, or unexplained global synovitis generally represents a contraindication to cartilage repair procedures.

Alternative Treatments

Small- to medium-sized osteochondral lesions may be suitable for autologous grafting techniques such as osteochondral autograft transplantation (chapter 56) or autologous chondrocyte im-

Dr. Mandelbaum or an immediate family member is a member of a speakers' bureau or has made paid presentations on behalf of Tigenix; serves as a paid consultant for or is an employee of DePuy, Genzyme, Regeneration Technologies, Smith & Nephew, Stryker, Zimmer, Tigenix, and ONI; has received research or institutional support from DePuy, Genzyme, and Smith & Nephew; owns stock or stock options in ONI; and has received nonincome support (such as equipment or services), commercially derived honoraria, or other non–research-related funding (such as paid travel) from Arthrex. Dr. Bugbee or an immediate family member serves as a board member, owner, officer, or committee member for the AAOS Biologic Implants Committee and Advanced Biohealing; has received royalties from Smith & Nephew; serves as a paid consultant for or is an employee of Arthrex, DePuy, Smith & Nephew, Zimmer, and the Joint Restoration Foundation; and has received research or institutional support from OREF. Neither Dr. Görtz nor any immediate family member has received anything of value from or owns stock in a commercial company or institution related directly or indirectly to the subject of this chapter.

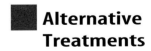

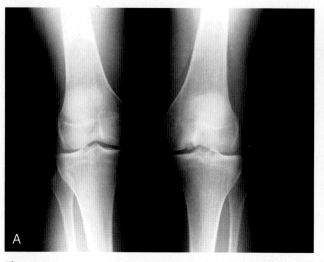
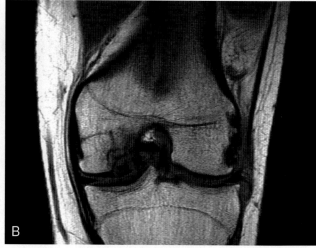

Figure 1 Images of a 17-year-old girl with OCD in the left knee. **A,** AP weight-bearing radiograph displays a large lesion in classic position in the lateral aspect of the medial femoral condyle. **B,** Coronal MRI of the same patient documents a fragmented and displaced International Cartilage Repair Society (ICRS) grade IV OCD lesion and subchondral bone edema.

plantation (chapter 55), which have yielded good outcomes in well-contained, unipolar lesions. Although a "sandwich" modification to the ACI procedure has been described to treat significant bony deficiencies, the results of this technique have not been individually reported. Overall, lesions that meet the inclusion criteria for osteochondral allografting often are poorly suited for other cartilage restoration procedures, especially for revision. None of these restorative procedures should be considered an alternative to prosthetic arthroplasty in an individual whose symptoms, age, and activity level are appropriate for prosthetic replacement.

When realignment osteotomy to correct axial malalignment is being considered along with an osteochondral allograft and the osteotomy site is juxtaposed to the allograft site, a staged procedure is advised to avoid jeopardizing the microvascularity of the recipient bone bed. Patients who gain satisfactory symptomatic relief from an osteotomy alone may not require further surgical intervention but should be followed closely for signs of disease progression.

Results

The use of osteochondral transplants in biologic reconstruction of the knee joint has a long-standing clinical history internationally, and it has evolved into a mainstay of clinical practice in the United States over the last quarter century. Traditionally, allograft outcomes reported in the literature have been compounded by a high percentage of salvage cases because of the lack of suitable treatment alternatives. In patients with matched indications, however, the results of osteochondral allografting compare favorably with those of other cartilage restoration procedures, with consistent reports of good to excellent outcomes in more than 80% of patients at up to 14-year follow-up (**Table 1**). Retrieval studies have demonstrated that viable chondrocytes are present and mechanical properties of the collagen matrix are maintained many years after transplantation.

Techniques

Setup/Exposure
The patient is positioned supine with a proximal thigh tourniquet. A leg or foot holder is helpful in accessing the lesion by positioning and maintaining the leg in 70° to 100° of flexion. A standard midline incision is made from the center of the patella to the tip of the tibial tubercle. For most femoral condylar lesions, a minimal anterior approach is sufficient, and eversion of the patella is not necessary. The skin incision is elevated subcutaneously, either medially or laterally, to the patellar tendon, ipsilateral to the location of the lesion. A retinacular incision is then made from the superior aspect of the patella inferiorly, incising the fat pad without disrupting the anterior horn of the meniscus or damaging the articular surface. Once the joint capsule and synovium have been incised and the joint has been entered, retractors are placed medially and laterally, taking care to protect the cruciate ligaments and articular cartilage in the notch. The knee is then flexed or extended to the degree of flexion required to present the lesion to be treated into the arthrotomy site (**Figure 2**). Excessive degrees of flexion

Table 1 Results of Osteochondral Allograft Transplantation in the Knee

Author(s) (Year)	Site of Lesion	Diagnosis/ Indication	Number of Patients	Mean Follow-up in Years (Range)	Outcome
McDermott et al (1985)	Knee	Trauma	50	3.8	76% successful
Garrett (1986)	Femur	OCD	17	(2-9)	94% good/excellent
Beaver et al (1992)	Knee	Trauma	92	14.0	63% survivorship
Ghazavi et al (1997)	Knee	Trauma	126	7.5	85% survivorship
Chu et al (1999)	Knee	Multiple	55	6.2	84% good/excellent
Gross et al (2005)	Femur	Trauma	60	10.0	85% survivorship
Emmerson et al (2007)	Femur	OCD	69	5.2	80% good/excellent
McCulloch et al (2007)	Femur	Multiple	25	3.9	84% successful
Williams et al (2007)	Femur	Multiple	19	4.0	79% successful
LaPrade et al (2009)	Femur	Multiple	23	3.0	91% good/excellent

OCD = osteochondritis dissecans.

limit the ability to mobilize the patella. The lesion then is inspected and palpated with a probe to determine its extent, margins, and maximal size. If the lesion is posterior or very large, the meniscus may have to be detached and reflected, leaving a small cuff of tissue adjacent to the anterior attachment of the meniscus for reattachment at closure.

Procedure

The two commonly used techniques for the preparation and implantation of osteochondral allografts are the dowel technique and the shell graft technique. Each technique has advantages and disadvantages.

The dowel technique, which is similar in principle to autologous osteochondral transfer systems, is optimal for contained condylar lesions between 15 and 35 mm in diameter. Fixation generally is not required because of the stability achieved with the press-fit of the dowel. One disadvantage of this technique is that many lesions, such as very posterior femoral, tibial, patellar, and trochlear lesions,

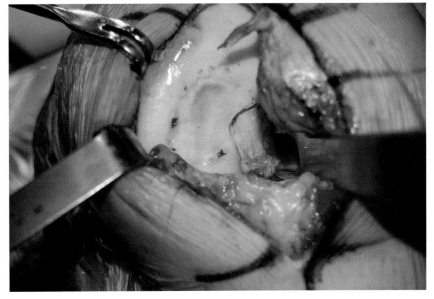

Figure 2 Intraoperative photograph of the same patient shown in Figure 1, demonstrating a large ICRS grade IV OCD lesion in the classic position in the lateral aspect of the medial femoral condyle with displacement of a fragmented loose body into the intercondylar notch. The fragment bed has been outlined with a surgical marker.

are not conducive to the use of a circular coring system. In addition, ovoid lesions require more normal cartilage to be sacrificed at the recipient site to accommodate the circular donor plug.

Shell grafts are technically more difficult and typically require fixation. Depending on the technique used, however, less normal cartilage may need to be sacrificed than in the dowel technique. Certain lesions also are

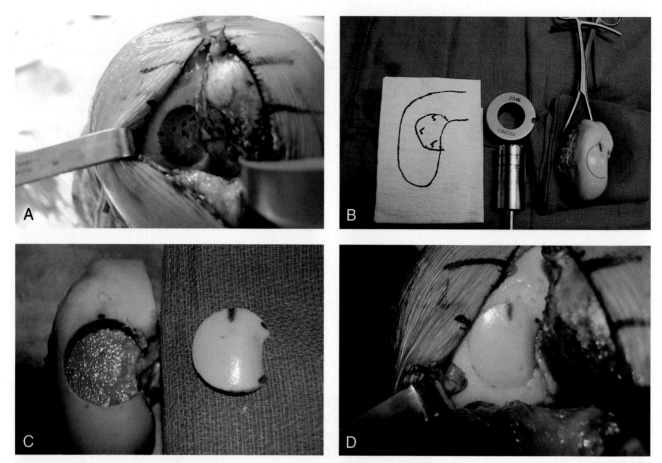

Figure 3 Preparation and implantation of a dowel allograft. **A**, The graft bed has been prepared using a core reamer. Areas of subchondral sclerosis have been perforated with a Kirschner wire to invite active bleeding into the graft site. Note the margin of the intercondylar notch and the shallow resection level. **B**, Left to right, a basic surgical map reflecting graft depth in three of four quadrants (with the fourth falling into the intercondylar notch); a 27.5-mm-diameter saw guide with corresponding tube saw; and a bone clamp holding an allograft condyle before amputation of the cored graft portion. **C**, En face view of the allograft condyle (left) and the removed graft portion (right). Note the ink marks identifying graft orientation and intersection with the intercondylar notch. **D**, The seated dowel allograft in orthotopic position after fixation with two bioabsorbable chondral darts. Note the restoration of the articular surface and the condylar contour, without signs of impingement.

more suitable for shell allografts because of their location.

DOWEL ALLOGRAFT

Several similar proprietary instrumentation systems currently are available for the preparation and implantation of dowel allografts up to 35 mm in diameter. After the size of the lesion is determined using a sizing guide dowel, a guidewire is driven into the center of the lesion, perpendicular to the curvature of the articular surface. The size of the proposed graft then is determined with sizing dowels; overlapping dowels (in a "snowman" configuration) may deliver the best fit.

The remaining articular cartilage is scored, and a core reamer is used to remove the scored cartilage and at least 3 to 4 mm of subchondral bone (**Figure 3**, *A*). In deeper lesions, fibrous and sclerotic bone is removed to a healthy, bleeding osseous base. More extensive lesions should be curetted by hand and packed with morcellized autologous bone graft. The guide pin then is removed, and circumferential depth measurements are taken of the prepared recipient site.

The corresponding orthotopic location of the recipient site then is identified on the graft. The graft is placed in a graft holder (or held se-

curely with bone-holding forceps). A saw guide then is placed in the appropriate position and alignment, again perpendicular to the articular surface, and an appropriately sized tube saw is used to core out the graft under irrigation. Before removing the graft dowel from the condyle, an identifying mark is made to ensure proper orientation (**Figure 3**, *B*). Once the graft cylinder is amputated with an oscillating saw and removed, depth measurements, which were taken from the recipient, are transferred to the bony portion of the graft. The graft then is cut with an oscillating saw and trimmed with a rasp to the appropriate thickness in all four quadrants. The deep edges of the bone plug can be chamfered with a rongeur and bone rasp (**Figure 3**, *C*). Often, this step must be done multiple times to ensure precise thickness, preferably refashioning the graft rather than the recipient site and optimally keeping the allograft and host cartilage moist throughout the procedure.

The graft then is irrigated copiously with high-pressure lavage to remove marrow elements and debris. The recipient site can be dilated using a slightly oversized tamp to prevent excessive impact loading of the articular surface when the graft is inserted. At this point, any remaining osseous defects are bone grafted. The allograft is then inserted by hand in the appropriate rotation. If a line-to-line fit exists, the graft often can be seated with gentle manual pressure or by using the appositional joint surface as a fulcrum while gently cycling the knee through a range of motion. Alternatively, a cupped mallet can be used to gently tamp the graft into place until it is flush, again minimizing any mechanical insult to the articular surface of the native and the graft tissue.

Once the graft is seated, a determination is made about whether additional fixation is required. Typically, bioabsorbable pins are used, particularly if the graft is large or has an exposed edge within the notch (**Figure 3**, *D*). Sometimes the graft needs to be trimmed in the notch region to prevent impingement. The knee is then moved through a complete range of motion to confirm that the graft is stable and that there is no catching or soft-tissue obstruction noted. At this point, the wound is irrigated copiously. If no further adjunct procedures are planned, routine closure is performed.

Video 57.1 Allograft Osteochondral Transplantation: Dowel Allograft. William Bugbee, MD; Ronald A. Navarro, MD (8 min)

SHELL ALLOGRAFT

After exposure has been achieved as described earlier, the defect is assessed, and the circumference of the lesion is marked with a surgical pen. An attempt is made to create a geometric shape for which a shell graft can be handcrafted while minimizing the sacrifice of normal cartilage. A No. 15 scalpel blade is used to demarcate the lesion, and sharp ring curets are used to remove all tissue inside this mark. With motorized burrs and sharp curets, the defect is then débrided down to a depth of 4 to 5 mm. Deep cystic defects are curetted by hand and later bone grafted. The allograft is fashioned freehand. Initially it is helpful to oversize the graft slightly and remove excess bone and cartilage carefully as necessary through multiple trial fittings (**Figure 4**, *A*). If deep bone loss is present in the defect, more bone can be left on the graft and the defect can be grafted with cancellous bone before graft insertion (**Figure 4**, *B*). The graft is placed flush with the articular surface. The need for fixation depends on the degree of inherent stability. Bioabsorbable pins typically are used when fixation is required (**Figure 4**, *C*), but compression screws can be used as an alternative. Wound irrigation and routine closure are done as described previously.

Postoperative Regimen

Patients are allowed full range of motion postoperatively, unless the requirements of additional reconstructive procedures alter the rehabilitation plan. Although range-of-motion exercises and quadriceps strengthening generally are introduced early, toe-touch–only weight bearing is continued for at least 8 weeks, ultimately depending on radiographic evidence of incorporation (**Figure 5**). At 4 weeks,

patients are assigned closed-chain exercises such as cycling. Progressive weight bearing as tolerated usually is allowed at 3 months, and patients are permitted to return to recreation and sports when functional rehabilitation is complete, usually at 6 months. Typically, braces are not used, unless the grafting involves the patellofemoral joint, in which case flexion is limited to less than 45° for the first 4 to 6 weeks. If bipolar tibial femoral grafts are used, an unloader or range-of-motion brace can be used to prevent excessive stress on the grafted surfaces.

Avoiding Pitfalls and Complications

Graft Selection

In current practice, small-fragment, fresh osteochondral allografts are not matched according to human leukocyte antigen type or blood group between donor and recipient, and no immunosuppression is used. Instead, the allografts are matched to recipients based on size alone. Preoperatively, the knee is sized using an AP radiograph with a standardized magnification marker. A measurement of the medial-lateral dimension of the tibia is then made, just below and parallel to the joint surface. The measurement is adjusted accurately for magnification, and the tissue bank compares it with direct measurements on the donor tibial plateau. A match is considered acceptable within a tolerance of ± 2 mm; it should be noted, however, that anatomy varies significantly. Particularly in OCD, the pathologic condyle typically is larger, wider, and flatter; therefore, a larger donor allograft generally should be used. In general, it is technically less challenging to fit an allograft that is too large into a small recipient condyle than vice versa because of radius of curvature. The surgeon ultimately is responsible for in-

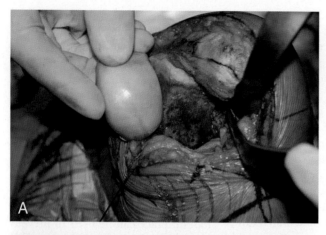
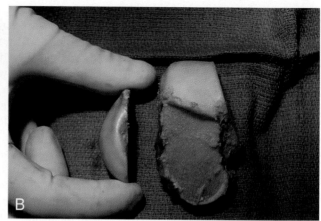
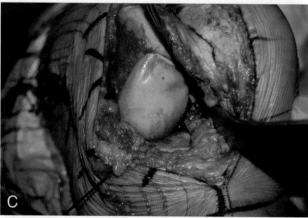

Figure 4 Implantation of a shell allograft. **A**, The shell allograft is displayed next to a massive osteonecrotic femoral condyle lesion, showing the resection level from the sulcus terminalis to the posterior condyle. The subchondral bone has been perforated to invite active bleeding into the graft site. **B**, The shell allograft has been prepared. The complete weight-bearing area of an allograft femoral condyle has been removed. Note the thickness of the graft aimed at restoring bone loss secondary to osteonecrosis. **C**, The shell graft rests in situ after fixation with bioabsorbable devices, displaying restoration of orthotopic osteoarticular anatomy.

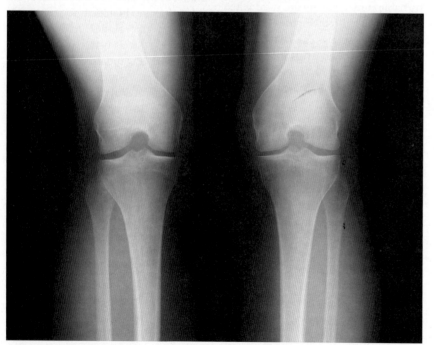

Figure 5 AP weight-bearing radiograph 3 months after dowel osteochondral allograft for OCD of the left medial femoral condyle. Note complete osseous incorporation of the graft, with radiographic evidence of maintained joint space.

specting the tissue intended for transplantation, optimally before beginning the actual procedure. This inspection should include affirmation of the site, size, and integrity of the tissue, as well as its packaging and the adequacy of its storage and refrigeration.

Disease Transmission

The recovery, processing, and testing of donor tissue follow guidelines established by the American Association of Tissue Banks. Strict and consistent adherence to tissue banking standards and the quality control of transplantation protocols safeguard but do not guarantee acceptable tissue for implantation. Osteochondral allograft tissue cannot be sterilized, but it is procured aseptically, a process that reduces but does not eliminate the risk of graft contamination. Isolated cases of allograft-associated bacterial infections have been reported. As with most procedures, infection may become apparent days to weeks after surgery. Deep infection should be distinguished from superficial infection through physical examination findings and a joint aspiration. Deep infection involving the allograft should be treated immediately with removal of the allograft because the fresh tissue may be either the source of the infection or a nidus for a recurrence. Patients should be informed of this risk preoperatively and counseled to look for signs of infection before and after discharge from the hospital.

Allograft Failure

Failure of the allograft procedure can occur because of nonunion or late fragmentation and graft collapse. Although healing of the graft-host interface occurs reliably, particularly with smaller grafts, the degree of revascularization appears to be variable. Fragmentation and collapse typically occur in areas of unvascularized allograft bone. Because it serves merely as an osteoconductive scaffold for healing to the host by creeping substitution, which is a rate-limited process, the portion of transplanted bone should be minimized as much as possible without compromising the stability of the graft as warranted by the clinical situation. Doing so also will minimize the potential antigenic burden of marrow elements possibly remaining in the transplanted spongiosa. Patients with graft collapse typically present with new-onset pain or mechanical symptoms. Radiographs may show joint space narrowing, cysts, or sclerotic regions. MRI can help rule out contributory concomitant joint pathology in the differential diagnosis of postoperative symptoms. Depending on the status of the knee joint, the treatment options include observation, removal of the fragmented portion of the graft, repeat allografting, or conversion to arthroplasty.

Bibliography

Beaver RJ, Mahomed M, Backstein D, Davis A, Zukor DJ, Gross AE: Fresh osteochondral allografts for post-traumatic defects in the knee: A survivorship analysis. *J Bone Joint Surg Br* 1992;74(1):105-110.

Chu CR, Convery FR, Akeson WH, Meyers M, Amiel D: Articular cartilage transplantation: Clinical results in the knee. *Clin Orthop Relat Res* 1999;360:159-168.

Emmerson BC, Görtz S, Jamali AA, Chung C, Amiel D, Bugbee WD: Fresh osteochondral allografting in the treatment of osteochondritis dissecans of the femoral condyle. *Am J Sports Med* 2007;35(6):907-914.

Garrett JC: Treatment of osteochondral defects of the distal femur with fresh osteochondral allografts: A preliminary report. *Arthroscopy* 1986;2(4):222-226.

Ghazavi MT, Pritzker KP, Davis AM, Gross AE: Fresh osteochondral allografts for post-traumatic osteochondral defects of the knee. *J Bone Joint Surg Br* 1997;79(6):1008-1013.

Görtz S, Bugbee WD: Allografts in articular cartilage repair. *J Bone Joint Surg Am* 2006;88(6):1374-1384.

Görtz S, Bugbee WD: Fresh osteochondral allografts: Graft processing and clinical applications. *J Knee Surg* 2006;19(3):231-240.

Gross AE, Shasha N, Aubin P: Long-term followup of the use of fresh osteochondral allografts for posttraumatic knee defects. *Clin Orthop Relat Res* 2005;435:79-87.

Jamali AA, Hatcher SL, You Z: Donor cell survival in a fresh osteochondral allograft at twenty-nine years: A case report. *J Bone Joint Surg Am* 2007;89(1):166-169.

LaPrade RF, Botker J, Herzog M, Agel J: Refrigerated osteoarticular allografts to treat articular cartilage defects of the femoral condyles: A prospective outcomes study. *J Bone Joint Surg Am* 2009;91(4):805-811.

McCulloch PC, Kang RW, Sobhy MH, Hayden JK, Cole BJ: Prospective evaluation of prolonged fresh osteochondral allograft transplantation of the femoral condyle: Minimum 2-year follow-up. *Am J Sports Med* 2007;35(3):411-420.

McDermott AG, Langer F, Pritzker KP, Gross AE: Fresh small-fragment osteochondral allografts: Long-term follow-up study on first 100 cases. *Clin Orthop Relat Res* 1985;197:96-102.

Williams RJ III , Ranawat AS, Potter HG, Carter T, Warren RF: Fresh stored allografts for the treatment of osteochondral defects of the knee. *J Bone Joint Surg Am* 2007;89(4):718-726.

Williams SK, Amiel D, Ball ST, et al: Analysis of cartilage tissue on a cellular level in fresh osteochondral allograft retrievals. *Am J Sports Med* 2007;35(12):2022-2032.

Video Reference

Navarro R, Bugbee W: Video. *Allograft Osteochondral Transplantation: Dowel Allograft.* Video clip from *Autograft/Allograft Osteochondral Transplantation*, Orthopaedic Learning Center, American Academy of Orthopaedic Surgeons, Rosemont, IL, 2007.

Coding

CPT Codes		Corresponding ICD-9 Codes	
Osteochondral Allograft of the Knee			
27415	Osteochondral allograft, knee, open	732.7 718.0	716.66 905.6

CPT copyright © 2010 by the American Medical Association. All rights reserved.

Chapter 58

The Microfracture Technique

J. Richard Steadman, MD
Karen K. Briggs, MPH
William G. Rodkey, DVM

Introduction

Microfracture is a tissue repair technique that relies on a "marrow-stimulation" strategy, but it does not replace tissue. For tissue to regenerate, cells must be present. The creation of controlled "microfractures" through the subchondral bone promotes the release of undifferentiated marrow-based pluripotential stem cells and growth factors. A marrow clot, or "super clot," is formed at the base of the prepared chondral lesion. From this marrow clot, the versatile stem cells proliferate and differentiate into cells that have the morphologic features of chondrocytes, and they produce a cartilaginous repair tissue that fills the chondral defect.

Indications

Full-thickness articular cartilage defects of the knee rarely heal without surgical intervention. Because articular cartilage lacks an inherent ability to heal spontaneously, these lesions can be difficult to treat and often become irreversible, with the eventual development of profound arthritis if no adequate therapeutic intervention is implemented. The microfracture technique has been shown to be an effective arthroscopic treatment of full-thickness chondral lesions of the knee. The microfracture technique has many advantages, including a relatively low procedural cost, technical simplicity, and an extremely low rate of associated morbidity. In addition, treating a lesion with microfracture places no limitations on future treatment.

Factors to consider when contemplating microfracture include patient age, acceptable biomechanical alignment of the knee, activity level, and the patient's expectations of the procedure and willingness to accept the extensive rehabilitation protocol. Advanced age is not always a contraindication; however, patient age older than 60 years is a relative contraindication for microfracture, even if the patient meets all other criteria, because patients older than 60 years may find it difficult to use crutches and properly perform the required rigorous rehabilitation. Our previous studies have shown that patients younger than 35 years with acute lesions show greater improvement than older patients, but older patients still demonstrate clinically meaningful improvement.

Large lesion size is not a contraindication for microfracture. In previous studies, we have shown that large acute lesions respond well to microfracture; however, lesions smaller than 400 mm² tend to respond better to microfracture than lesions larger than 400 mm², although the difference is not statistically significant.

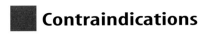

Contraindications

The most important factor to consider when contemplating microfracture for

Dr. Steadman or an immediate family member has received research or institutional support from Arthrex, Ossur, Smith & Nephew, and Genzyme and owns stock or stock options in Regeneration Technologies and Regen Biologics. Ms. Briggs or an immediate family member serves as a paid consultant to or is an employee of IBalance; serves as an unpaid consultant to Regen Biologics; and has received research or institutional support from Smith & Nephew, Ossur, and Genzyme. Dr. Rodkey or an immediate family member serves as a paid consultant to or is an employee of Regen Biologics; has received research or institutional support from Ossur, Regen Biologics, Smith & Nephew, Arthrex, and Genzyme; owns stock or stock options in Johnson & Johnson and Regen Biologics; and has received nonincome support (such as equipment or services), commercially derived honoraria, or other non–research-related funding (such as paid travel) from Regen Biologics.

a degenerative lesion is axial alignment. Correct axial alignment is crucial to the success of the procedure, and axial malalignment is a contraindication. Other contraindications to microfracture include global degenerative osteoarthrosis or cartilage surrounding the lesion that is too thin to establish a perpendicular rim that can hold the marrow clot (**Figure 1**). Other specific contraindications include systemic immune-mediated disease, disease-induced arthritis, or cartilage disease.

Factors that may affect the outcome of surgery include the patient's activity level and expectations of surgery, which should be determined preoperatively. If patient expectations do not match the reported outcomes of microfracture, the procedure may be contraindicated.

Alternative Treatments

A recent study compared the outcomes of autologous chondrocyte implantation (ACI) with microfracture in 40 patients. At 2-year follow-up, both groups showed significant improvement on the Lysholm Knee Scoring Scale, particularly in pain, with no difference in Lysholm scores between the groups; however, the microfracture group showed more improvement in the Short Form-36 Health Survey (SF-36) physical component score. The authors theorized that this difference may have occurred because microfracture is a single arthroscopic procedure, whereas ACI requires two procedures, one arthroscopic and one open. This study also found age to be a predictor of improvement with microfracture. It also identified activity level and lesion size as predictors of clinical results. Histologic evaluations showed no differences between the groups. Based on these results and other studies (**Table 1**) that show microfracture outcomes to be similar to those of ACI, we believe that microfracture should be the recommended initial treatment for isolated chondral defects.

Results

Studies have shown microfracture to be a safe and effective method to treat

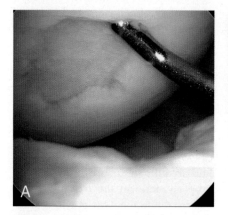
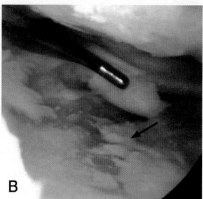

Figure 1 Arthroscopic views of full-thickness articular cartilage defects of the knee. **A**, A cartilage defect with an adequate rim height to hold the marrow clot. **B**, A degenerative cartilage lesion with no rim of cartilage (arrow).

Table 1 Results of Microfracture

Authors (Year)	Number of Knees	Type of Lesion	Patient Age in Years (Range)	Mean Follow-up (Range)	Lysholm Score	Tegner Score
Steadman et al (2003; *Arthroscopy*)	71	Traumatic lesions	(13-45)	(7-17 years)	89	6
Steadman et al (2003; *J Knee Surg*)	25	Full-thickness chondral lesions in NFL players	(22-36)	4.5 years (2-13)	90	9
Knutsen et al (2004)	40	Traumatic lesions	(18-45)	2 years	76	4
Miller et al (2004)	81	Degenerative knees	49 (40-70)	2.6 years (2-5)	83	4.5
Sterett and Steadman (2004)	33	Varus malalignment and chondral lesions	51 (34-72)	45 months (24-80)	78	5

NFL = National Football League.

cartilage defects of the knee. In 2003, the first long-term outcomes study on the microfracture technique was published. This study followed 72 patients younger than 45 years at the time of surgery for an average of 11 years after microfracture, with the longest follow-up being 17 years. The follow-up rate was 95%. Patients reported reduced pain and swelling at postoperative year 1. Both factors continued to decrease at year 2, and the clinical improvements were maintained over the study period. Most patients indicated good to excellent results on the SF-36 and Western Ontario and McMaster Universities (WOMAC) scoring systems at final follow-up. The study identified age as the only independent predictor of Lysholm score improvement. Patients older than 35 years did not improve as much as patients younger than 35 years ($P = 0.048$); nonetheless, both groups showed improvement. In summary, we found that arthroscopically performed microfracture for isolated full-thickness chondral defects in patients younger than 45 years of age led to significant improvement, as measured by the Lysholm scoring system. Given the pain relief ($P < 0.001$), improvement in function ($P < 0.01$), and lack of perioperative complications seen in these patients, we recommend that the arthroscopically performed microfracture procedure be the initial treatment for traumatic full-thickness chondral defects of the knee.

In a study of the outcomes of microfracture in 25 active National Football League (NFL) players, 76% of players returned to play during the next football season. After returning to play, those same players played an average of 4.6 additional seasons. All players had reduced symptoms and improved function. Most of the players who did not return to play had preexisting degenerative changes of the knee.

A study of the outcomes of microfracture in degenerative knees at 2-year follow-up found improvement in function and reduced symptoms. Proper surgical technique, including removal of the sclerotic bone, and patient compliance with a well-defined rehabilitation program were critical factors in this population. Lysholm scores improved from 54 to 83, and the mean Tegner Activity Scale score at follow-up was 4.5. Factors that were associated with less improvement on the Lysholm scale included bipolar lesions, lesions larger than 400 mm², and knees with absent menisci. Repeat arthroscopy was reported in 15.5% of these patients. Failures, as defined by revision microfracture or total knee arthroplasty, were documented in 6% of the patients. These results confirm excellent short-term outcomes. We will continue to follow these patients to determine how long the results last.

Evaluation

History and Physical Examination

Patients with articular defects may have pain, swelling, stiffness, and mechanical symptoms. Point tenderness over a femoral condyle or tibial plateau is a useful finding but in itself is not diagnostic. If compression of the patella elicits pain, this finding may be indicative of a patellar or trochlear lesion. Physical diagnosis can be difficult and elusive at times, especially if only an isolated chondral defect is present.

Imaging

Long weight-bearing radiographs are used to assess angular deformity and joint space narrowing of the knee, which are possible indicators of articular cartilage loss. Axial alignment is determined by drawing a line from the center of the head of the femur to the center of the tibiotarsal joint and assessing the load-bearing line within the knee joint. Standard AP and lateral radiographs of both knees, as well as weight-bearing views with the knees flexed to 30° or 45°, also are obtained. The patellofemoral joint also is evaluated with patellar views. In patients suspected of having chondral lesions, MRI is used to review sequences specific for articular cartilage.

Techniques

Setup/Portal Placement

Three portals are made for the inflow cannula, the arthroscope, and the working instruments. A thorough diagnostic arthroscopic examination of the knee is performed. Although a tourniquet generally is not used during the microfracture procedure, the arthroscopic fluid pump pressure is varied to control bleeding. Microfracture itself should be the final intra-articular procedure, to avoid the loss of visualization that occurs when blood and fat droplets enter the knee joint and to prevent the marrow clot from being dislodged.

Preparation of the Lesion

After assessing the full-thickness articular cartilage lesion, all remaining unstable cartilage is removed from the bone. A hand-held curved curet and a full radius resector can be used to remove the loose or marginally attached cartilage back to a stable rim of cartilage (**Figure 2, A**). The calcified cartilage layer that remains as a cap on many lesions must be removed, usually with a curet (**Figure 2, B**). Complete removal of this calcified cartilage layer is integral to a successful outcome following microfracture, according to basic science studies, but equally important is maintaining the integrity of the subchondral plate. This preparation of the cartilage lesion

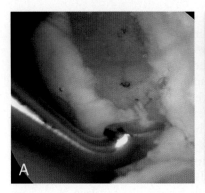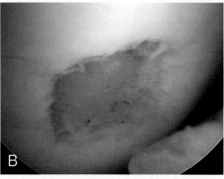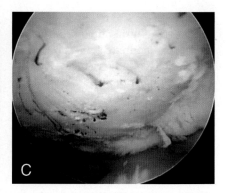

Figure 2 Arthroscopic views show preparation of the lesion. **A**, A curved curet is used to remove loose or unstable cartilage back to a stable rim. **B**, A prepared defect before microfracture. The calcified cartilage was removed and the edge of the lesion is perpendicular to the subchondral bone so the clot will pool and adhere. **C**, A motorized burr has been used to remove the sclerotic bone in the chronic cartilage lesion; punctate bleeding is seen.

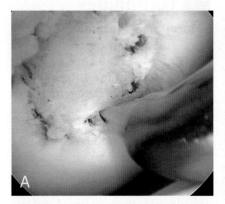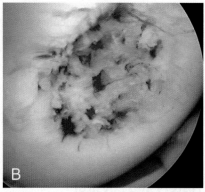

lease of fat droplets and blood from the microfracture holes. Microfracture creates a rough surface on the subchondral bone that allows the marrow clot to adhere more easily, meanwhile maintaining the integrity of the subchondral plate for joint surface shape.

 Video 58.1 Microfracture in the Knee. J. Richard Steadman, MD; Erol Yoldas, MD (4 min)

Figure 3 Arthroscopic views show the microfracture procedure. **A**, Microfracture holes are created at the edge of the defect. The holes are made close together but should not break into one another. This process is continued until the defect is full of holes. **B**, After the completion of microfracture, a rough surface is noted in the bed of the defect. This surface is not shaved because the rough surface improves adherence of the clot.

creates a stable, perpendicular edge of healthy, well-attached, viable cartilage surrounding the defect and serves as a pool that helps contain the marrow clot as it forms.

When treating a chronic cartilage lesion with microfracture, a motorized burr is used to remove the sclerotic bone until punctate bleeding is seen (**Figure 2, C**). This preparation is based on the process described for abrasion arthroplasty. After the bleeding appears uniformly over the surface of the lesion, a microfracture procedure can be performed.

Procedure

After preparation of the lesion, multiple holes, or "microfractures," are made in the lesion with awls. The awls should be perpendicular to the bone as they are advanced. A 90° awl is used for the patella if an angle cannot be created to accommodate the 45° awl. It is important that the 90° awl be advanced manually, without the use of a mallet. Microfracture holes are made first around the edge of the defect and then in the center (**Figure 3**). The holes are made close together, but not so close that one breaks into another, damaging the subchondral plate between them. When the appropriate depth (approximately 2 to 4 mm) has been reached, fat droplets can be seen coming from the marrow cavity. When all the holes have been made, the fluid pressure is reduced to verify the re-

Postoperative Regimen

The postoperative rehabilitation program for microfracture requires special consideration. The size and location of the cartilage defect affect the rehabilitation protocol; however, use of a continuous passive motion (CPM) machine (or equivalent) and 6 to 8 weeks of crutch-assisted touch-down weight bearing form the basis of the program. When patients undergo other intra-articular procedures concurrently with microfracture, the rehabilitation program may be customized as necessary. Many possible variations of the rehabilitation program exist; two of the main protocols are described here (**Table 2**).

We prescribe cold therapy for all patients postoperatively. Our experience and observations indicate that cold helps control pain and inflammation, and most patients report that the cold provides overall postoperative pain relief. Cold therapy usually is used for 1 to 7 days postoperatively, but it can be used throughout the rehabilitation period.

We commence CPM immediately in the recovery room. The initial range of motion is determined by the location of the defect and can be increased as tolerated by the patient. The CPM machine usually is set at 1 cycle per minute, but the rate can be varied based on patient preference and comfort. Many patients tolerate use of the CPM machine at night. We have observed that for those who do not, intermittent CPM during the day probably is just as beneficial. Regardless of when the CPM machine is used, the goal is to have the patient in the CPM machine for 6 to 8 hours out of every 24 hours. If the patient is unable to use the CPM machine, then instructions are given for passive flexion and extension of the knee for 500 repetitions 3 times per day. We encourage patients to gain full passive range of motion of the injured knee as soon as possible after surgery.

We prescribe crutch-assisted touch-down weight-bearing ambulation for 6 to 8 weeks, depending on the size of the lesion. For most patients, 6 to 8 weeks seems to be adequate for limited weight bearing; however, for patients with small lesions (<1 cm diameter), weight bearing may begin a few weeks earlier. Patients with lesions of the patellofemoral joint treated by microfracture are allowed to bear weight as tolerated in their brace 2 weeks after surgery.

Patients with lesions on the femoral condyles or tibial plateaus rarely use a brace during the initial postoperative period; however, when the pa-

tient becomes more active and the postoperative swelling has resolved, we prescribe an unloading type of brace. All patients with patellofemoral lesions who have been treated with microfracture must use a brace set at 0° for 6 to 8 weeks. This brace limits the compression of the regenerating surfaces of the trochlea or patella. We allow passive motion with the brace removed, but otherwise the brace must be worn at all times. The brace is removed for CPM and replaced following CPM.

We begin mobilization immediately after surgery, with an emphasis on range of motion of the knee, patella, and patellar tendon. Patients are allowed touch-down weight bearing, placing 20% of their body weight on the injured leg while standing. Patients then begin using a stationary bike without resistance and a deep-water exercise program 1 to 2 weeks after microfracture. The deep-water exercises include the use of a flotation vest for deep-water running. It is imperative that the foot of the injured leg not touch the bottom of the pool during this exercise. Patients progress to

full weight bearing after about 8 weeks and begin more vigorous biking with increasing resistance. They also begin knee flexion exercises at approximately the same time. An elastic resistance band is added to the exercise regimen at about 12 weeks. A detailed description has been published of how to use the band and the exercises that accompany it. We have observed that the achievement of predetermined maximal levels for sets and repetitions of elastic resistance band exercises is an excellent indicator for the beginning of weight training. We permit the use of free or machine weights when the patient has achieved the early goals of the rehabilitation program but not before 16 weeks after microfracture. We strongly emphasize the importance of proper technique when beginning a weight training program. The decision to return to sport is based on several factors, including clinical examination, the size of the patient, the sport involved, and the size of the lesion. We usually recommend that patients refrain from returning to sports that involve pivot-

Table 2 Key Points for Rehabilitation Following Microfracture

Lesions of the Femoral Condyle or Tibial Plateau

Immediate continuous passive motion 8 hours daily for 8 weeks at 1 cycle/min with the knee flexed 30° to 70°

No brace

Touch-down (20% to 30%) crutch walking for 8 weeks

Stationary bike (light resistance) starts 2 weeks postoperatively

Deep water exercise starts 2 weeks postoperatively

After 8 weeks, full weight bearing and active range of motion

No cutting, turning, or jumping for at least 4 to 9 months, depending on the patient; time may be longer for competitive or larger patients

Patellofemoral Lesions

Immediate continuous passive motion 8 hours daily for 8 weeks at 0° to 50° of knee flexion

Brace locked at 0°; full weight bearing at 2 weeks

Stationary bike (light resistance) starts 2 weeks postoperatively

Water program (no impact) starts 2 weeks postoperatively

After 8 weeks, walking with a brace is begun

Treadmill at 7° incline starting at 12 weeks postoperatively

Biking and water program; intensity increased at 8 to 12 weeks

Elastic resistance program with 0° to 30° knee bends starting at 12 weeks postoperatively

ing, cutting, or jumping until at least 4 to 9 months after microfracture.

For patients with patellofemoral joint lesions, we carefully observe the joint angles at the time of arthroscopy to determine where the defect comes into contact with the patellar facet or the trochlear groove. These angles are avoided during strength training for approximately 4 months. Stationary biking is allowed 2 weeks postoperatively, with increased resistance added 8 weeks after microfracture. At 12 weeks after microfracture, the exercise program is the same as that used for femorotibial lesions.

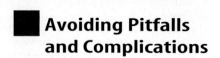

Avoiding Pitfalls and Complications

Patient selection, including management of patient expectations and compliance with rehabilitation, is crucial to success. Neutral or near-neutral alignment is necessary for the micro- fracture procedure to succeed. In addition, performing an adequate microfracture is more difficult in chronic degenerative chondral lesions because of the eburnated bone and bony sclerosis with thickening of the subchondral plate. When preparing the lesion, the height of the surrounding rim of cartilage must be sufficient to hold the clot in place. Finally, appropriate rehabilitation is crucial to the success of the microfracture technique.

Bibliography

Bellamy N, Buchanan WW, Goldsmith CH, Campbell J, Stitt LW: Validation study of WOMAC: A health status instrument for measuring clinically important patient relevant outcomes to antirheumatic drug therapy in patients with osteoarthritis of the hip or knee. *J Rheumatol* 1988;15(12):1833-1840.

Briggs KK, Steadman JR, Hay CJ, Hines SL: Lysholm score and Tegner activity level in individuals with normal knees. *Am J Sports Med* 2009;37(5):898-901.

Frisbie DD, Morisset S, Ho CP, Rodkey WG, Steadman JR, McIlwraith CW: Effects of calcified cartilage on healing of chondral defects treated with microfracture in horses. *Am J Sports Med* 2006;34(11):1824-1831.

Frisbie DD, Oxford JT, Southwood L, et al: Early events in cartilage repair after subchondral bone microfracture. *Clin Orthop Relat Res* 2003;407:215-227.

Frisbie DD, Trotter GW, Powers BE, et al: Arthroscopic subchondral bone plate microfracture technique augments healing of large chondral defects in the radial carpal bone and medial femoral condyle of horses. *Vet Surg* 1999;28(4): 242-255.

Hagerman GR, Atkins JA, Dillman C: Rehabilitation of chondral injuries and chronic degenerative arthritis of the knee in the athlete. *Oper Tech Sports Med* 1995;3:127-135.

Irrgang JJ, Pezzullo D: Rehabilitation following surgical procedures to address articular cartilage lesions in the knee. *J Orthop Sports Phys Ther* 1998;28(4):232-240.

Johnson LL: The sclerotic lesion: Pathology and the clinical response to arthroscopic abrasion arthroplasty, in Ewing JW, ed: *Articular Cartilage and Knee Joint Function: Basic Science and Arthroscopy*. New York, NY, Raven Press, 1990, pp 319-333.

Knutsen G, Engebretsen L, Ludvigsen TC, et al: Autologous chondrocyte implantation compared with microfracture in the knee: A randomized trial. *J Bone Joint Surg Am* 2004;86-A(3):455-464.

Kocher MS, Steadman JR, Briggs KK, Sterett WI, Hawkins RJ: Reliability, validity, and responsiveness of the Lysholm knee scale for various chondral disorders of the knee. *J Bone Joint Surg Am* 2004;86-A(6):1139-1145.

Lysholm J, Gillquist J: Evaluation of knee ligament surgery results with special emphasis on use of a scoring scale. *Am J Sports Med* 1982;10(3):150-154.

Mankin HJ: The response of articular cartilage to mechanical injury. *J Bone Joint Surg Am* 1982;64(3):460-466.

Miller BS, Steadman JR, Briggs KK, Rodrigo JJ, Rodkey WG: Patient satisfaction and outcome after microfracture of the degenerative knee. *J Knee Surg* 2004;17(1):13-17.

Ohkoshi Y, Ohkoshi M, Nagasaki S, Ono A, Hashimoto T, Yamane S: The effect of cryotherapy on intraarticular temperature and postoperative care after anterior cruciate ligament reconstruction. *Am J Sports Med* 1999;27(3):357-362.

Steadman JR: The microfracture technique, in Feagin J, Steadman JR, eds: *The Crucial Principles in Care of the Knee.* Philadelphia, PA, Lippincott Williams & Wilkins, 2008.

Steadman JR, Briggs KK, Rodrigo JJ, Kocher MS, Gill TJ, Rodkey WG: Outcomes of microfracture for traumatic chondral defects of the knee: Average 11-year follow-up. *Arthroscopy* 2003;19(5):477-484.

Steadman JR, Miller BS, Karas SG, Schlegel TF, Briggs KK, Hawkins RJ: The microfracture technique in the treatment of full-thickness chondral lesions of the knee in National Football League players. *J Knee Surg* 2003;16(2):83-86.

Steadman JR, Rodkey WG, Briggs KK: Microfracture to treat full-thickness chondral defects: Surgical technique, rehabilitation, and outcomes. *J Knee Surg* 2002;15(3):170-176.

Sterett WI, Steadman JR: Chondral resurfacing and high tibial osteotomy in the varus knee. *Am J Sports Med* 2004;32(5):1243-1249.

Tegner Y, Lysholm J: Rating systems in the evaluation of knee ligament injuries. *Clin Orthop Relat Res* 1985;198(198):43-49.

Video Reference

Steadman JR, Yoldas E: Video. Microfracture in the knee. Video clip from Microfracture for DJD of the knee, in Cole BJ, ed: *Surgical Techniques in Orthopaedics: Cartilage Restoration of the Knee.* DVD. Rosemont, IL, American Academy of Orthopaedic Surgeons, 2003.

Coding

CPT Codes		Corresponding ICD-9 Codes	
Microfracture Repair			
29879	Arthroscopy, knee, surgical; abrasion arthroplasty (includes chondroplasty where necessary) or multiple drilling or microfracture	716.66 717.9	716.96 732.7
Autologous Chondrocyte Implantation			
27412	Autologous chondrocyte implantation, knee	716.66 717.8 732.7	716.96 717.9 905.6

Chapter 59

Meniscal Transplantation

E. Lyle Cain, Jr, MD

Indications

The meniscus protects the articular cartilage of the knee by providing shock absorption, stress distribution, and protection from excess loads during normal functional activities. Despite a trend toward more aggressive repair attempts for meniscal injuries, meniscal deficiency is frequently encountered by the knee surgeon. The minimal amount of meniscal tissue required to maintain articular cartilage homeostasis has not been demonstrated definitively; however, it has been well documented for more than 50 years that long-term arthritic chondral and bony changes occur in the postmeniscectomy knee.

Surgical indications for meniscal transplantation are controversial. Some authors advocate meniscal replacement for any active patient without normal meniscal protection, to lessen the likelihood of future chondral wear. Unfortunately, it currently is not possible to accurately predict which patients will suffer cartilage degeneration as a result of meniscal deficiency. Therefore, allograft meniscal transplantation currently is indicated

for patients with pain in the meniscus-deficient compartment and relatively intact articular cartilage after meniscectomy. It also may be indicated for patients with focal chondral defects if the chondral lesion is treated with an appropriate articular cartilage resurfacing procedure and any concurrent malalignment or instability is corrected. Although there are no definitive age limits, 50 years generally is regarded as the upper limit at which meniscal transplantation should be considered for highly active patients with minimal arthritis. In some patients, concomitant anterior cruciate ligament (ACL) and medial meniscal deficiency may require combined ACL reconstruction and meniscal allograft replacement to correct significant anteromedial rotatory instability.

Contraindications

Contraindications to meniscal transplantation include articular cartilage loss in the involved compartment that cannot be treated with cartilage restoration (eg, diffuse chondral wear), un-

corrected malalignment, ligamentous instability, systemic inflammatory disease (rheumatoid arthritis), and infection.

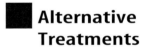

Alternative Treatments

Alternative treatment includes nonsurgical treatment of the symptoms associated with the postmeniscectomy knee, such as nonsteroidal anti-inflammatory drugs, bracing, and/or injections. Surgical procedures include techniques to decrease the pressure or loads across the articular cartilage of the involved compartment (high tibial osteotomy) and partial knee replacement (unicompartmental arthroplasty). New technology currently in development and research includes artificial meniscal replacement with a bioengineered meniscal scaffold or synthetic meniscus.

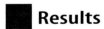

Results

Several authors have reported good and excellent results at up to 14 years after allograft meniscal transplantation (**Table 1**). Outcomes generally are better in patients with normal ar-

Dr. Cain or an immediate family member has received royalties from Biomet; is a member of a speakers' bureau or has made paid presentations on behalf of Genzyme and Biomet; and has received research or institutional support from Biomet and Stryker.

Table 1 Results of Meniscal Transplantation

Author(s) (Year)	Number of Patients	Number/Type of Grafts	Concurrent Procedures	Mean Follow-up (Range)	Results/Comments
Milachowski et al (1989)	20	6 fresh-frozen 16 freeze-dried	21 ACL reconstruction	14 months	Both groups showed decrease in size at second-look arthroscopy Fresh-frozen better than freeze-dried
Noyes and Barber-Westin (1989)	82	96 fresh-frozen irradiated allografts	51 ACL reconstruction	(2-5 years) (67 grafts)	Overall, 58% failed (56/96), 9% healed, 31% partially healed Grafts fixed only at the posterior horn attachment
Garrett (1993)	43	16 fresh 27 cryopreserved	24 ACL reconstruction 13 osteotomy	(2-7 years)	20/28 grafts intact at second-look arthroscopy Graft type had no effect 2/32 failed with grade 3 chondral wear, 6/11 failed with grade 4 chondral wear
Rath et al (2001)	18	22	11 ACL reconstruction 1 osteotomy	5.4 years	All patients had improved function and decreased pain 8/22 failures Allografts repopulated with fewer cells than natural meniscus
Wirth et al (2002)	23	6 deep-frozen meniscal allografts 17 lyophilized meniscal allografts	23 ACL reconstruction 19 MCL advancement	14 years	Deep-frozen grafts better MRI and arthroscopy demonstrated graft shrinkage
van Arkel and de Boer (2002)	57	63	2 ACL reconstruction 21 ACL-deficient knees	5 years	13/63 failures, primarily in instability, ACL deficiency Graft survival: 76% lateral, 50% medial, 67% medial and lateral
Sekiya et al (2003)	28	31	31 ACL reconstruction	2.8 years	90% near-normal or normal IKDC scores and Lachman stability scores No radiographic joint-space narrowing
Graf et al (2004)	9	Medial meniscus graft	8 ACL reconstruction 1 osteotomy	9.7 years	7/9 near-normal or normal IKDC scores 6/8 active in recreational sports 1 failure due to infection
Verdonk et al (2005)	96	100	17 HTO	7.2 years	Graft failure: 11/39 (28%) medial, 10/61 (16%) lateral Survival rates at 10 years: 74% medial, 70% lateral, 83% with HTO
van der Wal et al (2009)	57	63	NR	13.8 years	Graft failure: 8/23 medial (35%), 10/40 (25%) lateral, overall 29% IKDC and KOOS decreased over time, maintained functional improvement

ACL = anterior cruciate ligament, HTO = high tibial osteotomy, IKDC = International Knee Documentation Committee, KOOS = Knee injury and Osteoarthritis Outcome Score, NR = not reported.

ticular cartilage surfaces and are poor in patients with grade 4 articular cartilage loss in the involved compartment. Concurrent procedures to treat chondral deficiency, ligamentous instability, or malalignment also affect the outcome.

━━━━━━━━■

■ Techniques

Instruments/Equipment/ Implants Required

The instruments, equipment, and implants required are a radiographic marker of known size (I use 25 mm), graft preparation board, drill guide, bits, coring reamer, and an accurately sized allograft meniscus.

Appropriate allograft meniscal size is critical for the best surgical fit and to provide maximal chondral protection (**Figure 1**). Graft sizing can be based on plain radiographs, MRI, or CT, but most authors advocate plain radiographs with magnification markers to accurately size the native tibial plateau (**Figure 2**). A cadaver meniscus up to 10% larger than the native meniscus is considered acceptable; however, undersizing (smaller than the native me-

niscus) should be avoided because of the difficulty of properly implanting a small allograft at the native root attachment sites.

Procedure

The patient is placed supine with the involved leg either draped free or placed in a leg holder. The knee is examined arthroscopically, and any remaining meniscal tissue in the involved compartment is resected. The peripheral 1 to 2 mm of meniscocapsular attachment is left intact, and the capsule is gently abraded to provide a bleeding surface to aid meniscal healing. Any coexisting pathology is treated with chondral débridement, loose body removal, ligament reconstruction, or realignment.

The surgical technique varies depending on which compartment (medial or lateral) is being treated. Medial meniscal replacement requires the use of two individual bone plugs for the anterior and posterior horns to avoid the tibial attachment of the ACL. Lateral transplantation is most easily done with a "keyhole" technique, with a bone bridge connecting the anterior and posterior horns of the meniscus.

MEDIAL MENISCAL TRANSPLANTATION

Medial meniscal transplantation generally is done using individual bone plugs for the anterior and posterior horn attachments to avoid injury to the ACL tibial insertion. Some authors have advocated a keyhole technique that makes graft placement easier by resecting a few fibers of the medial ACL insertion footprint.

Using a commercial ACL drill guide, metal guidewires are placed into the anterior horn and posterior horn root attachments (**Figure 3**, *A*).

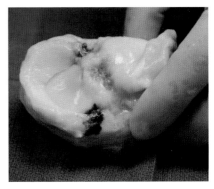

Figure 1 Photograph of an allograft proximal left tibia with medial and lateral menisci. The anterior and posterior root attachments of the medial meniscus are marked with methylene blue to assist with preparation.

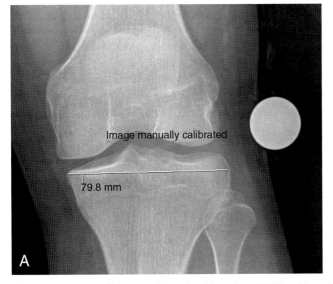
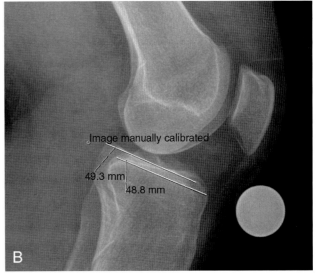

Figure 2 Meniscal graft size is determined based on AP (**A**) and lateral (**B**) radiographs of the knee with a 25-mm magnification marker. Tibial plateau measurements are made using digital imaging software with calibration.

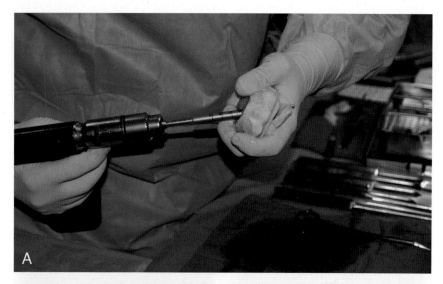

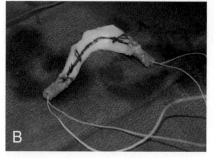

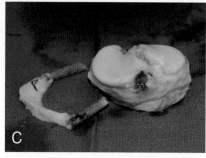

Figure 3 Medial meniscal graft preparation. **A,** A cylindrical reamer 9 mm in diameter is used to prepare meniscal bone plugs at the root attachments. **B,** Final graft preparation with heavy suture placed through bone plugs to assist with passage and fixation. Methylene blue lines mark the dorsal surface of the graft. **C,** Bone plugs are marked *A* for anterior or *P* for posterior orientation.

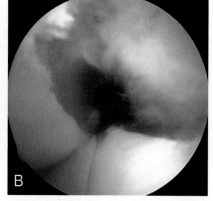

Figure 4 Arthroscopic preparation of the knee for medial meniscal transplantation. **A,** The meniscal remnant is excised and the synovium is rasped to provide a healing surface. A portion of the meniscocapsular attachment is retained to prevent capsular disruption. **B,** To assist with graft passage, femoral notchplasty is performed by removing a portion of the medial intercondylar wall.

Careful dissection is mandatory to avoid inadvertent release of the root attachment during preparation. An 8- to 9-mm bone plug is fashioned at each attachment site of the allograft with a coring reamer on a power drill; the dorsal surface is completed carefully by hand to avoid meniscal damage. A heavy No. 2 suture is placed through each bone plug and woven through the meniscal root to provide plug fixation after graft placement (**Figure 3,** *B*). The dorsal surface of the meniscus is marked with methylene blue to assure proper graft orientation and prevent flipping of the meniscus during implantation (**Figure 3,** *C*). Arthroscopic preparation of the knee begins with meniscal remnant excision and synovial rasping to provide a healing surface (**Figure 4,** *A*). A small medial femoral condyle notchplasty improves visualization for posterior tunnel placement and graft passage (**Figure 4,** *B*). The posterior root insertion is marked with electrocautery, and a guidewire is placed from the proximal tibia into the root attachment site using an ACL drill guide. The allograft bone plugs generally are prepared with a 9-mm-diameter coring reamer, and the tunnel at each root attachment site is reamed to 10 mm for ease of bone plug passage. A passing suture is placed at the midbody region of the graft to help reduce the graft after bone plug placement.

A medial arthrotomy is made from the anteromedial arthroscopy portal to approximately 2 cm distal to the joint line. The allograft is carefully placed in the knee with the posterior horn root attachment passed through the medial intercondylar notch into the posterior tunnel with the aid of a wire suture shuttle or Hewson suture passer. A probe may be used to assist with positioning of the plug in the tunnel. In some cases, a posteromedial incision is made to assist with graft passage and inside-out suture fixation. With valgus stress applied to the knee, the passing suture is used to re-

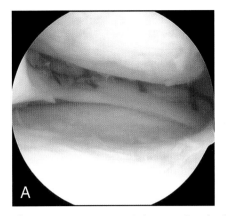

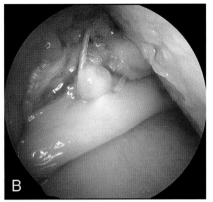

Figure 5 Placing the medial meniscal graft. All-inside suture repair generally includes six to eight sutures placed in the posterior meniscus from the posterior horn to the midbody portion (**A**) and inside-out sutures placed from midbody to the anterior horn and tied extracapsularly through the arthrotomy incision (**B**).

Figure 6 Photograph of an allograft lateral meniscus transplant prepared for keyhole technique with anterior and posterior root attachments connected by a bone bridge.

duce the meniscus into proper position. The passing suture can be passed with a Beath pin through the posteromedial capsule. The knee is moved through a complete arc of motion to allow the meniscus to find the anatomic position on the proximal tibia, and the anterior horn attachment site is marked with electrocautery. A 10-mm tunnel is reamed over a guidewire through the anterior incision under direct visualization for placement of the anterior horn bone. Multiple meniscal sutures are placed with either an inside-out or all-inside meniscal repair technique, depending on surgeon preference. I prefer an all-inside suture technique for the posterior meniscus from the posterior horn to the midbody portion, with inside-out sutures placed from midbody to the anterior horn and tied extracapsularly through the arthrotomy incision (**Figure 5**).

LATERAL MENISCAL TRANSPLANTATION

Preparation for lateral meniscal transplantation begins with a minimal notchplasty of the lateral femoral condyle to allow easy graft passage and improve visualization. A trough is made between the anterior and posterior horn attachment sites with a high-speed burr in preparation for keyhole placement. The meniscal allograft is prepared with a commercial ACL drill guide that separates the meniscus from the tibial plateau with a small cylinder of bone attaching the horns of the meniscus (**Figure 6**). Maintaining the meniscal root attachments is critical to the proper function of the transplanted meniscus. The prepared donor meniscus should slide easily into a keyhole notch in the recipient tibia. A small lateral parapatellar arthrotomy is made from the inferior surface of the patella to the proximal tibia, and a portion of the retropatellar fat pad is excised to improve visualization. Through the lateral incision, a drill guide is used to place a guidewire from the tip of the posterior horn insertion and align the guidewire to the anterior horn attachment site, with arthroscopic viewing from the anteromedial portal. A 10-mm solid reamer (for a 9-mm prepared allograft bone cylinder) is placed over the guidewire and stopped just before it exits the posterior tibial cortex, producing a 10-mm tunnel approximately 1 cm distal to the articular surface. The tunnel is dilated using the appropriately sized keyhole dilator, and two traction suture holes are drilled using an ACL drill guide. Peripheral traction sutures from the anterior and posterior horns of the allograft are pulled through the drill holes, and the meniscus is gently placed into the keyhole and impacted to the back of the tunnel at the posterior cortex. The traction sutures are tied over a bone bridge along the proximal tibia as additional fixation to prevent the bone plug from dislodging from the keyhole.

Wound Closure

The wound is closed with absorbable suture in the retinaculum and subcutaneous tissue. The skin is closed with running subcuticular suture, and adhesive skin closure strips are applied. An intra-articular drain generally is not used, although a drain can be placed in the anterior incision if there is significant bone bleeding.

■

■ Postoperative Regimen

Postoperative rehabilitation is performed in four stages that coincide with the timing of tissue healing (**Table 2**). Return to full activity generally is allowed at 6 months after surgery, depending on individual sport requirements.

■

Table 2 Postoperative Rehabilitation Following Meniscal Transplantation

Phase	Weeks	Goals	Treatment
I (immediate postoperative phase)	1–2	Reduce swelling, inflammation, and pain Gradually increase range of motion Reestablish patellar mobility Restore voluntary quadriceps control Protect healing tissues	Cryotherapy, elevation, and compression Knee immobilizer (sleeping in brace) Toe-touch weight bearing (< 25% of weight) CPM machine 2 to 4 hours per day Full passive knee extension with gradual progression to 90° of flexion
II (protection phase)	3–8	Gradually restore range of motion (flexion) Maintain full passive extension Progress weight bearing Restore quadriceps muscle strength	Bracing is continued (sleeping in brace weeks 3–6) Weight bearing increases to 50% at week 3, 75% at week 4, and full weight bearing at week 6 Pool exercises are started at week 6 Patient is allowed to use a bicycle at week 6
III (moderate protection phase)	9–12	Normalize strength and proprioception Protect tissue healing	Hamstrings and gastrocnemius-soleus muscle stretching Strengthening exercises Low-impact walking program Swimming Lateral step-ups Wall squats (not deep) Progressive proprioception training
IV (minimal protection)	13–22	Increase strength, power, and endurance	Begin gradual return to function

Avoiding Pitfalls and Complications

Pitfalls and intraoperative complications can occur at several points throughout the procedure, including graft selection/sizing, graft preparation, recipient site preparation, and graft placement and fixation.

Improper graft selection can be disastrous. Potential problems include a too-small graft that is impossible to place properly; an oversized graft that fails to resist shear and compression forces; and, at worst, a graft that is incorrectly labeled as to whether it is from a right or left extremity. The surgeon must pay careful attention to detail and be closely involved in the graft selection process, including confirming proper measurement and graft identification before surgery. I typically remove the allograft meniscus from its packaging and examine it closely before starting any portion of the procedure.

The most common complication during graft preparation is avulsion of the meniscal root attachment site, which may make it impossible to place the graft with bone plugs. An implanted meniscal graft without bony root attachments is similar biomechanically to a meniscus-deficient knee and may not provide any protective function. Careful graft preparation with adequate exposure of the meniscal root sites will prevent this complication.

During recipient site preparation, improper root placement may lead to iatrogenic damage to the articular surface of the tibia by reaming a trough in the weight-bearing portion of the tibial plateau. Graft placement and reduction can be the most challenging part of the procedure. Adequate notch widening, tension suture placement, and accessory incisions may help with graft insertion. Placement of the knee in relative extension (20° to 30° of flexion) with a valgus stress applied will make medial meniscal reduction easier; the figure-of-4 varus stress position is easier for lateral meniscal placement.

Meniscal suturing and fixation can be accomplished with a standard inside-out two-incision technique or with all-inside arthroscopic devices. I prefer an all-inside meniscal repair device (FasT-Fix, Smith & Nephew, Andover, MA) for the posterior horn because of ease of fixation while avoiding dissection around medial or lateral neurovascular structures, but other devices are available, and the choice of device depends on surgeon preference. The most common complication during meniscal fixation is injury to the saphenous nerve medially or the peroneal nerve laterally. The anterior horn and midbody are easily approached through the arthrotomy, and sutures are easily tied over the anterior capsule.

■ Bibliography

Alhalki MM, Howell SM, Hull ML: How three methods for fixing a medial meniscal autograft affect tibial contact mechanics. *Am J Sports Med* 1999;27(3):320-328.

Garrett JC: Meniscal transplantation: A review of 43 cases with 2 to 7 year follow-up. *Sports Med Arthrosc Rev* 1993;1: 164-167.

Graf KW Jr, Sekiya JK, Wojtys EM: Long-term results after combined medial meniscal allograft transplantation and anterior cruciate ligament reconstruction: Minimum 8.5-year follow-up study. *Arthroscopy* 2004;20(2):129-140.

Kelly BT, Potter HG, Deng XH, et al: Meniscal allograft transplantation in the sheep knee: Evaluation of chondroprotective effects. *Am J Sports Med* 2006;34(9):1464-1477.

Milachowski KA, Weismeier K, Wirth CJ: Homologous meniscus transplantation: Experimental and clinical results. *Int Orthop* 1989;13(1):1-11.

Noyes FR, Barber-Westin SD: Irradiated meniscus allografts in the human knee: A two to five year follow-up. *Orthop Trans* 1989;19:417.

Paletta GA Jr, Manning T, Snell E, Parker R, Bergfeld J: The effect of allograft meniscal replacement on intraarticular contact area and pressures in the human knee: A biomechanical study. *Am J Sports Med* 1997;25(5):692-698.

Rath E, Richmond JC, Yassir W, Albright JD, Gundogan F: Meniscal allograft transplantation: Two- to eight-year results. *Am J Sports Med* 2001;29(4):410-414.

Rodeo SA, Seneviratne A, Suzuki K, Felker K, Wickiewicz TL, Warren RF: Histological analysis of human meniscal allografts: A preliminary report. *J Bone Joint Surg Am* 2000;82(8):1071-1082.

Sekiya JK, Giffin JR, Irrgang JJ, Fu FH, Harner CD: Clinical outcomes after combined meniscal allograft transplantation and anterior cruciate ligament reconstruction. *Am J Sports Med* 2003;31(6):896-906.

Szomor ZL, Martin TE, Bonar F, Murrell GA: The protective effects of meniscal transplantation on cartilage: An experimental study in sheep. *J Bone Joint Surg Am* 2000;82(1):80-88.

van Arkel ER, de Boer HH: Survival analysis of human meniscal transplantations. *J Bone Joint Surg Br* 2002;84(2):227-231.

van der Wal RJ, Thomassen BJ, van Arkel ER: Long-term clinical outcome of open meniscal allograft transplantation. *Am J Sports Med* 2009;37(11):2134-2139.

Verdonk PC, Demurie A, Almqvist KF, Veys EM, Verbruggen G, Verdonk R: Transplantation of viable meniscal allograft: Survivorship analysis and clinical outcome of one hundred cases. *J Bone Joint Surg Am* 2005;87(4):715-724.

Wirth CJ, Peters G, Milachowski KA, Weismeier KG, Kohn D: Long-term results of meniscal allograft transplantation. *Am J Sports Med* 2002;30(2):174-181.

Coding

CPT Codes		Corresponding ICD-9 Codes	
Meniscus Repair			
29882	Arthroscopy, knee, surgical; with meniscus repair (medial OR lateral)	836.0 717.1 717.3	836.1 717.2 717.4
29883	Arthroscopy, knee, surgical; with meniscus repair (medial AND lateral)	836.0 717.1 717.3	836.1 717.2 717.4
ACL Repair			
29888	Arthroscopically aided anterior cruciate ligament repair/augmentation or reconstruction	717.83	844.2

CPT copyright © 2010 by the American Medical Association. All rights reserved.

Chapter 60
High Tibial Osteotomy

David Backstein, MD, MEd, FRCSC
Allan E. Gross, MD, FRCSC
Oleg Safir, MD, MEd, FRCSC
Joseph B. Aderinto, MD, FRCS(Tr and Orth)

Indications

Although the frequency of high tibial osteotomy (HTO) for unicompartmental arthritis of the knee has declined since its initial description in 1958, several indications still exist for the procedure. HTO currently is used most commonly for isolated medial compartment osteoarthritis of the knee with varus tibiofemoral alignment in a young and physically active patient. A preoperative range of motion arc of at least 90° with less than 15° flexion contracture is recommended because some loss of motion is common after HTO. Additionally, candidates must have adequate bone stock to allow effective fixation and early range of motion. Because osteoporosis reduces bone mass and may preclude solid fixation, we limit HTO to men younger than 65 years and women younger than 60 years.

The goal of HTO is to reduce the forces passing through the diseased tibiofemoral compartment of the knee by altering the angular alignment of the lower limb to preferentially load the relatively normal nondiseased compartment. Realignment of the proximal tibia can be achieved with medial opening wedge, lateral closing wedge, or dome osteotomy of the proximal tibia. Medial opening wedge osteotomies and lateral closing wedge osteotomies are more often described in the literature than is dome osteotomy, and therefore they are the focal points of this chapter.

Other indications for HTO include osteonecrosis and adult osteochondritis dissecans of the medial femoral condyle in young, active individuals. For each of these clinical entities, unloading of the affected condyle can result in significant improvement in pain and function. Valgus-producing HTO also can be performed at the time of autologous chondrocyte implantation or osteochondral grafting of cartilaginous defects to off-load the involved compartment.

HTO for lateral compartment arthritis and a valgus deformity is far less commonly performed than is HTO for medial osteoarthritis. Knees with lateral tibiofemoral compartment disease resulting in a mild valgus deformity of less than 12° potentially can be treated with HTO. Varus HTO to treat valgus intra-articular deformity risks the creation of an oblique joint line, however, particularly with larger angular corrections; therefore, distal femoral varus osteotomy is the preferred realignment procedure in such cases because these knees tend to have a superolateral tilt to the joint line (**Figure 1**). Medial closing wedge osteotomy or lateral opening wedge osteotomy of the tibia tends to worsen this obliquity. Furthermore, most valgus deformities are associated with a hypoplastic lateral femoral condyle, so a femoral osteotomy corrects the problem more directly.

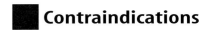

Contraindications

HTO performed to unload a varus knee requires that the medial compartment be involved in isolation.

Dr. Backstein or an immediate family member is a member of a speakers' bureau or has made paid presentations on behalf of Stryker, Sanofi-Aventis, and Zimmer and serves as a paid consultant for or is an employee of Stryker and Zimmer. Dr. Gross or an immediate family member serves as a board member, owner, officer, or committee member of the Musculoskeletal Transplant Foundation; is a member of a speakers' bureau or has made paid presentations on behalf of Zimmer; and serves as a paid consultant for or is an employee of Zimmer. Neither of the following authors nor any immediate family members has received anything of value from or owns stock in a commercial company or institution related directly or indirectly to the subject of this article: Dr. Safir and Dr. Aderinto.

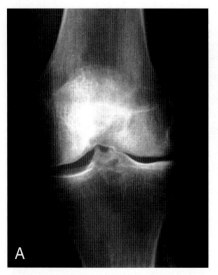 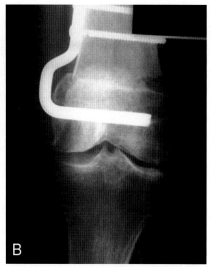

Figure 1 AP radiographs of a knee with lateral osteoarthritis and valgus deformity before (**A**) and after (**B**) distal varus femoral osteotomy.

Moderate to severe lateral compartment arthritis as well as significant and symptomatic patellofemoral changes are considered contraindications. Mild or moderate patellofemoral changes on radiographs without significant symptoms often are considered acceptable for HTO.

HTO is contraindicated in patients with an arc of motion less than 90°, a flexion deformity greater than 15°, and maximal flexion less than 90° to 100°. For varus deformity correction of less than 15°, we prefer a medial opening wedge osteotomy. For deformities of 15° to 20°, we use lateral closing wedge osteotomies, which have a lower risk of nonunion because of apposition and compression of the bone. A fixed varus deformity greater than 20° may require osteotomies both proximal and distal to the joint to achieve correction. Another option for severe deformity is osteotomy and gradual correction using an external fixator such as an Ilizarov or Taylor frame. Inflammatory arthritis, which affects the entire joint in a congruous manner, also is considered a contraindication for this operation. A high adductor moment (varus thrust) is associated with relatively poor results and recurrence of varus deformity after

HTO. Obesity has been shown to be a risk factor for early failure of HTO, so obese patients should be encouraged to lose weight before surgery.

Good bone quality is required for rigid fixation, which is a critical component of the HTO procedure. Without good fixation, early range of motion is impossible, and results are thus compromised. Certain other patient factors also must be taken into consideration. Rehabilitation after HTO is quite arduous, and patients who do not have the capability of completing the extensive rehabilitative effort required are not considered to be candidates. Because a moderate degree of overcorrection is associated with better long-term survivorship of HTOs, the patient must be willing to accept an extremity with a valgus appearance.

Alternative Treatments

Before considering any surgical procedure, patients with mild or early unicompartmental varus osteoarthritis may benefit from the use of orthoses. Valgus force–producing knee braces

and laterally wedged foot inlays have been shown to reduce the knee adductor moment during the gait cycle and may have a role in reducing knee pain and improving function, despite an absence of data proving their effectiveness. (Neither of these treatments is in accordance with the American Academy of Orthopaedic Surgeons' Clinical Practice Guideline *The Treatment of Osteoarthritis [OA] of the Knee*, available at http://www. aaos.org/research/guidelines/GuidelineOAKnee.asp.)

Alternatives to HTO for the management of isolated arthritis of the medial compartment of the knee include unicompartmental knee arthroplasty (UKA) and total knee arthroplasty (TKA). Factors to consider when determining the best treatment option include the patient's chronologic and physiologic age, activity level, occupation, capacity to rehabilitate, and arthritis pattern. Physiologically young, active, and high-demand patients with true unicompartmental medial osteoarthritis are ideal candidates for HTO. A similar pattern of osteoarthritis in patients who are older and more sedentary may better be suited to UKA in our opinion. Although UKA is susceptible to wear and loosening and is less capable of withstanding heavy loads than is HTO, it permits a more rapid recovery and rehabilitation than HTO. Older, low-demand patients with unicompartmental arthritis are candidates for either UKA or TKA, whereas TKA is more suitable for patients with multicompartmental arthritis.

Results

Numerous scoring systems have been used to define the clinical outcomes of HTO, and failure has been variably defined, making direct comparison of results among studies difficult (**Table 1**). Undercorrection and excessive overcorrection both are associated

Table 1 Results of High Tibial Osteotomy

Author (Year)	Number of Knees	Procedure	Mean Patient Age in Years (Range)	Mean Follow-up in Years (Range)	Complications	Criteria for Failure	Survivorship Rate
Coventry (1965)	22	Lateral closing wedge HTO	(35-72)	NR	0 nonunion 2 infection 1 peroneal nerve palsy	Results less than satisfactory	81% at minimum 1 year
Harris and Kostuik (1970)	36	Lateral closing wedge HTO for varus knees Medial closing wedge HTO for valgus knees	52 (34-78)	(1-6)	0 nonunion 3 infection 2 peroneal nerve palsy	Results less than good	72% at 1 to 6 years
Insall et al (1984)	95	Lateral closing lateral wedge HTO	60 (30-83)	8.9 (5-15)	1 nonunion 0 infection 0 peroneal nerve palsy	Results less than good	97% at 2 years 85% at 5 years
Healy and Riley (1986)	25	Lateral closing wedge HTO	60 (39-67)	5.5 (2-14)	0 nonunion 1 infection 0 peroneal nerve palsy	Results less than good	92% at 2 years 88% at 5 years 80% at 9 years
Hernigou et al (1987)	93	Opening wedge HTO	60 (43-77)	11.5 (10-13)	0 nonunion 2 infection 1 peroneal nerve palsy	Results less than good	90% at 5 years 45% at 10 years
Holden et al (1988)	51	Lateral closing wedge HTO	41 (23-50)	10 (5-13)	0 nonunion 0 infection 1 peroneal nerve palsy	Results less than good	70% at 10 years
Hutchison et al (1999)	292	Lateral closing wedge HTO	NR	≥2	1 nonunion 0 infection 1 peroneal nerve palsy	Conversion to TKA	83% at 10 years
Naudie et al (1999)	106	94 lateral closing wedge HTOs 12 dome osteotomies	55 (16-76)	14 (10-22)	6 nonunion 10 infection 2 peroneal nerve palsy	Conversion to TKA	73% at 5 years 51% at 10 years 39% at 15 years 30% at 20 years
Majima et al (2000)	26	Lateral closing wedge HTO	59.5 (47-70)	12 (10-15)	0 nonunion 0 infection 0 peroneal nerve palsy	Results less than fair	91% at 1 year 61% at 10 years
Akizuki et al (2008)	118	Lateral closing wedge HTO	NR	16.4 (16-20)	2 nonunion 1 infection 5 peroneal nerve palsy	Conversion to TKA or HSS score <70	99.3% at 5 years 97.6% at 10 years 90.4% at 15 years

HTO = high tibial osteotomy, TKA = total knee arthroplasty, HSS = Hospital for Special Surgery score, NR = not reported.

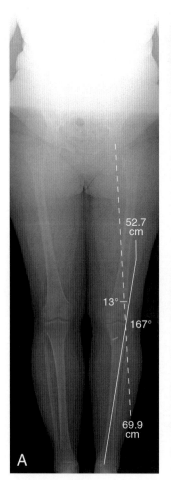

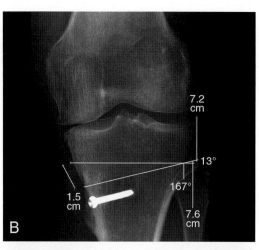

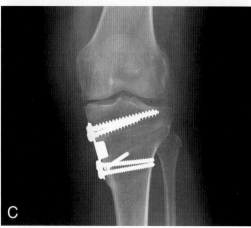

Figure 2 Radiographic templating prior to a medial opening wedge high tibial osteotomy to correct varus deformity. **A**, The mechanical axis of the femur (dashed line) is drawn from the center of the femoral head through the 62% coordinate on the tibial plateau. The mechanical axis of the tibia (solid line) is drawn from the tibiotalar joint through the 62% coordinate. The angle where the lines intersect is the angle of correction needed—in this case, 13°. **B**, Calculation of the 15-mm wedge height for the medial opening wedge high tibial osteotomy. **C**, AP weight-bearing radiograph obtained after a medial opening wedge high tibial osteotomy.

with poor results. The incidence of nonunion is low, occurring in fewer than 2% of knees in most studies, and the risk of peroneal nerve injury ranges from 0% to 5.5% when a lateral closing wedge osteotomy is used.

Studies of HTO for medial tibiofemoral compartment osteoarthritis have shown good or excellent results in 85% to 90% of knees at 5-year follow-up. Several authors have reported 10-year results of HTO that include survivorship rates ranging from 58% to 80%. In a carefully selected group of patients younger than 50

years, survivorship at 15-year follow-up was 60%. With TKA defined as an end point, another study reported a 10-year rate of survival of 90% for HTO when the alignment was corrected to 8° to 16° of anatomic valgus, and a survival rate of only 80% when alignment fell outside this range.

Patella infera (patella baja) has been commonly reported after both opening and closing wedge HTO. This phenomenon is thought to result from postoperative contracture of the patellar tendon. Protracted rehabilitation programs with prolonged immobiliza-

tion likely are contributing factors. With the use of contemporary rigid fixation techniques and more rapid rehabilitation, patella infera has become less common.

Technique

Preoperative Planning
Full-length weight-bearing AP radiographs of the lower limbs, including the hips, ankles, and knees, are required to establish the mechanical axis, anatomic axis, and point of intersection of the weight-bearing line at the joint line. Opinions differ about the best way to calculate the osteotomy correction angle, but most authors agree that some overcorrection of the deformity is required. In the normal knee, physiologic alignment results in a mechanical tibiofemoral angle of 0°. Even in nonpathologic situations, however, the weight-bearing line often passes through the medial tibial plateau, resulting in transmission of approximately 60% of force through the medial joint space and 40% through the lateral joint space.

After correction, the weight-bearing line should pass through the 62% coordinate of the tibial articular surface (with the medial border of the tibial articular surface defined as 0% and the lateral border as 100%), resulting in preferential loading of the lateral tibiofemoral compartment.

The angular correction is calculated by drawing a line from the center of the femoral head to the 62% coordinate of the tibia at the knee (**Figure 2**, *A*). A second line is then drawn from the center of the tibiotalar joint to the 62% coordinate. The angle between the first and the second lines represents the angle of correction required. Some authors advocate the use of the lateral border of the lateral tibial spine as a landmark for the optimal point of intersection of the weight-bearing line after correction. Others aim to achieve

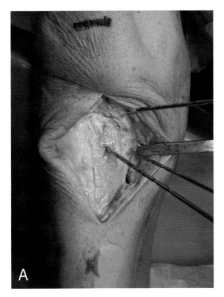 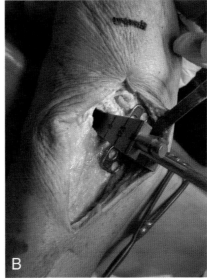 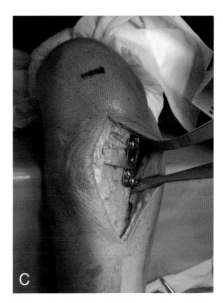

Figure 3 Cadaveric photographs demonstrate a medial opening wedge high tibial osteotomy. **A**, A proximal guide pin is inserted parallel to the joint line. Two distal osteotomy guide pins are inserted in an inferomedial-to-superolateral direction. The lateral ends of all pins are approximately 1 cm from the lateral cortex of the tibia and 1.5 cm distal to the joint line. **B**, A specially calibrated wedge is tapped into the osteotomy after the osteotome is removed, until the desired degree of correction is achieved. A plate is then inserted. **C**, Screws are inserted into the osteotomy plate for fixation. The graft is inserted into the defect created by the osteotomy.

a specific value for postoperative alignment based on values of the anatomic or mechanical axis. For closing wedge osteotomy, the size of the wedge can be measured directly from properly magnified radiographs once the amount of angular correction required is determined (**Figure 2**, *B*). The precise size of the wedge should be measured on radiographs; rule-of-thumb estimations (such as 1 mm of resection is equivalent to 1° of correction) are discouraged (**Figure 2**, *C*).

Patient Positioning

The patient is positioned supine on a radiolucent table to allow intraoperative imaging of the hip, knee, and ankle with a fluoroscope, which is located on the opposite side of the table from the extremity to be operated on. Prophylactic antibiotics are administered intravenously. After exsanguination of the leg, a tourniquet is applied to the proximal thigh and inflated. The skin is prepared from the proximal thigh to and including the foot, which is wrapped in a transparent bag to facilitate location of the center of the ankle

when assessing alignment later in the procedure. If an iliac crest autograft is to be harvested, the overlying skin is prepared and draped accordingly. A sandbag or wedge is placed beneath the distal femur so that the knee is flexed to approximately 45°.

Medial Opening Wedge Osteotomy

EXPOSURE

The approach to the proximal tibia is made through a longitudinal midline incision that extends from the level of the upper border of the tibial tuberosity distally for 10 to 15 cm. The incision should be positioned so that it could be used easily for TKA at a later date. The deep dissection is made between the medial border of the patellar tendon and the pes anserinus, which is reflected subperiosteally from the tibia by sharp dissection and retracted posteriorly. The superficial part of the medial collateral ligament is then elevated from the medial tibia to expose the underlying bone, and a Hohmann retractor is placed around the posteromedial border of the tibia to protect

the vessels. Another Hohmann retractor is placed over the anterior border of the tibia deep to the patellar tendon, to protect the patellar tendon.

Procedure

With the knee in extension, a single pin is drilled from medial to lateral under fluoroscopic guidance, parallel and 1.5 cm distal to the joint line. Next, using the jig provided by most implant manufacturers, two osteotomy guide pins are drilled in an inferomedial-to-superolateral direction, beginning above the level of the tibial tubercle. All pins should stop approximately 1 cm from the lateral cortex of the tibia to avoid fracture of the lateral tibial plateau (**Figure 3**, *A*). Pin position should be confirmed fluoroscopically. An osteotome is then inserted along the inferior side of the two guide pins and advanced to within 1 cm of the lateral cortex. Fluoroscopy is again used to confirm the position of the osteotome. The osteotome is removed, and a specially calibrated wedge is tapped into the osteotomy. The wedge is inserted until the desired

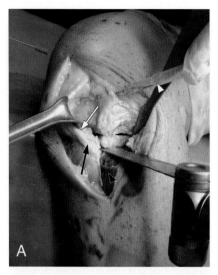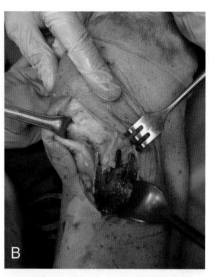

Figure 4 Cadaveric photographs demonstrate a lateral closing wedge high tibial osteotomy. **A**, The tibial tuberosity is osteotomized, keeping a distal bone hinge (black arrow). The proximal transverse osteotomy is made at the level of the patellar tendon insertion, parallel to the joint line. The distal oblique osteotomy is then made distally, at the desired distance from the transverse osteotomy. The white arrow indicates the patellar tendon. The black arrowhead indicates the reflected anterior compartment muscles. The white arrowhead indicates the needle in the knee joint. **B**, The osteotomy is fixed with two offset staples.

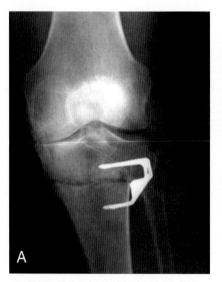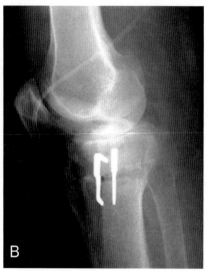

Figure 5 AP (**A**) and lateral (**B**) postoperative radiographs depict the results of a lateral closing wedge high tibial osteotomy fixed with two staples.

degree of correction is achieved. We use an osteotomy plate that comes with specially calibrated wedges of various sizes that match the size of the base of the osteotomy (**Figure 3**, *B*) and provide immediate mechanical support. The plate is then fixed proximally with large-fragment cancellous screws and distally with cortical screws. Small degrees of correction (up to 10°) can be managed with the osteotomy plate alone; however, larger defects require some form of bone grafting. Options include tricortical wedges of iliac crest autograft, synthetic bone graft substitute, and al-

lograft. The graft is packed into the defect created by the osteotomy (**Figure 3**, *C*).

Lateral Closing Wedge Osteotomy

EXPOSURE

A longitudinal midline skin incision is made anteriorly, extending distally from the joint line for approximately 10 cm. The incision is designed to be reused easily should a TKA become necessary at a later date. The patellar tendon is identified, and the fascia overlying the anterior compartment is opened with an arc-shaped incision. Subperiosteal dissection of the dorsiflexors exposes the lateral tibial cortex while protecting the arterial bifurcation and the peroneal nerve. The fibular side of the tibiofibular joint is carefully excised with osteotomes. The medial and lateral aspects of the patellar tendon are well exposed and protected. The tibial tuberosity is osteotomized in a lateral to medial direction, keeping a distal bone hinge. The tubercle is elevated 2 to 3 mm to allow access to the tibia for the closing wedge osteotomy. A blunt retractor is then placed around the posterior border of the tibia.

Procedure

The proximal transverse osteotomy is made at the level of the patellar tendon insertion, parallel to the joint line. The tibial tubercle osteotomy allows inferior displacement of the patellar tendon, so that the osteotomy can be made more distal without the risk of intra-articular fracture, and also provides stronger bone for fixation (**Figure 4**, *A*). Our clinical and radiographic results have confirmed less patellar tendon shortening from contracture with this technique than with more proximal osteotomies. After excision of the wedge, the medial cortex is broken gently and the osteotomy is fixed with two offset staples (**Figure 4**, *B*, and **Figure 5**). The tubercle is then allowed to fall back to an anatomic position and usually covers the osteotomy site as a living bone graft.

Intraoperative Determination of Angular Correction

The weight-bearing line can be determined intraoperatively by centering a radiopaque rod or diathermy wire over the center of the femoral head, using the image intensifier for confirmation. The distal end of the rod is placed over the center of the tibiotalar joint, and placement is again confirmed with the image intensifier. The position of the rod or diathermy wire over the center of the knee gives the position of the weight-bearing axis. The objective is to overcorrect the varus deformity by establishing a weight-bearing axis that passes through the 62% coordinate of the tibial articular surface.

Wound Closure

Subcutaneous layers are closed with nonabsorbable suture. The skin is closed over a drain with wound staples or an absorbable subcuticular suture. WIth lateral closing wedge osteotomies, the fascia of the anterior compartment is left open to prevent the development of compartment syndrome.

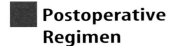

Postoperative Regimen

After undergoing either a medial opening wedge osteotomy or a lateral closing wedge osteotomy, the patient is instructed to remain non–weight-bearing until early evidence of healing of the osteotomy is present, usually at 6 to 8 weeks postoperatively. Range-of-motion and isometric quadriceps exercises are initiated 7 to 10 days postoperatively. At 6 weeks, partial weight bearing and light resisted exercises usually are begun. If radiographic and clinical evidence of union is apparent, full weight bearing usually is allowed by 10 to 12 weeks postoperatively.

Avoiding Pitfalls and Complications

Correct patient selection is crucial to the success of this procedure; it is important that significant disease is limited to one compartment. In addition to full-length weight-bearing radiographs, we recommend including at least the following radiographic views to determine the extent of arthritis: weight-bearing AP and lateral radiographs, 30° flexed-knee views, and skyline views of the patella. If uncertainty remains, knee MRI or arthroscopy can be used for confirmation.

When performing the osteotomy, the surgeon should avoid leaving a too-wide medial hinge for a lateral closing wedge or a too-wide lateral hinge for a medial opening wedge, because this increases the risk of fracture propagation into the tibial articular surface should the osteotomy need to be opened for deformity correction.

For the lateral closing wedge technique, we recommend making the osteotomy at the level of the tibial tuberosity, where an abundance of can-cellous bone is present, to reduce the risk of nonunion. Maintaining a periosteal hinge and irrigating the site copiously also are recommended to avoid thermal injury when cutting bone.

Regardless of the technique used, undercorrection should be avoided because it has been associated with relatively poor survival results. On the other hand, excessive overcorrection can lead to overloading of the lateral compartment, accelerating the onset of lateral compartment osteoarthritis. Excessive overcorrection also might be unacceptable cosmetically. In addition, it will lead to an increase in the Q angle and can result in patellar maltracking.

When a closing lateral wedge osteotomy is performed, the tendency to reduce the normal posterior tibial slope should be avoided. This tendency occurs because of a natural proclivity to remove more bone from the anterior, better visualized portion of the tibia than from the posterior half. Reducing the tibial slope can pose a problem for anterior cruciate ligament–deficient knees in particular. Likewise, in opening wedge osteotomies, there is a tendency to increase the posterior slope; therefore, we recommend placing the plate and the wide portion of its block as posterior as possible.

Acknowledgment

The authors would like to thank Dr. Yona Kosashvili for his assistance with the cadaveric surgery portion of this chapter.

Bibliography

Akizuki S, Shibakawa A, Takizawa T, Yamazaki I, Horiuchi H: The long-term outcome of high tibial osteotomy: A ten- to 20-year follow-up. *J Bone Joint Surg Br* 2008;90(5):592-596.

Coventry MB: Osteotomy of the upper portion of the tibia for degenerative arthritis of the knee: A preliminary report. *J Bone Joint Surg Am* 1965;47:984-990.

Coventry MB, Ilstrup DM, Wallrichs SL: Proximal tibial osteotomy: A critical long-term study of eighty-seven cases. *J Bone Joint Surg Am* 1993;75(2):196-201.

Dowd GS, Somayaji HS, Uthukuri M: High tibial osteotomy for medial compartment osteoarthritis. *Knee* 2006;13(2): 87-92.

Harris WR, Kostuik JP: High tibial osteotomy for osteo-arthritis of the knee. *J Bone Joint Surg Am* 1970;52(2):330-336.

Healy WL, Riley LH Jr : High tibial valgus osteotomy: A clinical review. *Clin Orthop Relat Res* 1986;209:227-233.

Hernigou P, Medevielle D, Debeyre J, Goutallier D: Proximal tibial osteotomy for osteoarthritis with varus deformity: A ten to thirteen-year follow-up study. *J Bone Joint Surg Am* 1987;69(3):332-354.

Holden DL, James SL, Larson RL, Slocum DB: Proximal tibial osteotomy in patients who are fifty years old or less: A long-term follow-up study. *J Bone Joint Surg Am* 1988;70(7):977-982.

Hutchison CR, Cho B, Wong N, Agnidis Z, Gross AE: Proximal valgus tibial osteotomy for osteoarthritis of the knee. *Instr Course Lect* 1999;48:131-134.

Insall JN, Joseph DM, Msika C: High tibial osteotomy for varus gonarthrosis: A long-term follow-up study. *J Bone Joint Surg Am* 1984;66(7):1040-1048.

Jackson JP: Osteotomy for osteoarthritis of the knee. *J Bone Joint Surg Br* 1958;40-B:826.

Jones R: Direct and indirect orthotic management of medial compartment osteoarthritis of the knee. *Gait Posture* 2006; 24:S141-S142.

Lindenfeld TN, Hewett TE, Andriacchi TP: Joint loading with valgus bracing in patients with varus gonarthrosis. *Clin Orthop Relat Res* 1997;344:290-297.

Majima T, Yasuda K, Katsuragi R, Kaneda K: Progression of joint arthrosis 10 to 15 years after high tibial osteotomy. *Clin Orthop Relat Res* 2000;381:177-184.

Marti RK, Verhagen RA, Kerkhoffs GM, Moojen TM: Proximal tibial varus osteotomy: Indications, technique, and five to twenty-one-year results. *J Bone Joint Surg Am* 2001;83-A(2):164-170.

Naudie D, Bourne RB, Rorabeck CH, Bourne TJ: The Install Award: Survivorship of the high tibial valgus osteotomy. A 10- to -22-year followup study. *Clin Orthop Relat Res* 1999;367:18-27.

Prodromos CC, Andriacchi TP, Galante JO: A relationship between gait and clinical changes following high tibial osteotomy. *J Bone Joint Surg Am* 1985;67(8):1188-1194.

Ritter MA, Fechtman RA: Proximal tibial osteotomy: A survivorship analysis. *J Arthroplasty* 1988;3(4):309-311.

Sprenger TR, Doerzbacher JF: Tibial osteotomy for the treatment of varus gonarthrosis: Survival and failure analysis to twenty-two years. *J Bone Joint Surg Am* 2003;85-A(3):469-474.

Williams A, Natasa D: Osteotomy in the management of knee osteoarthritis and of ligamentous instability. *Curr Orthop* 2006;20:112-120.

Wright JM, Crockett HC, Slawski DP, Madsen MW, Windsor RE: High tibial osteotomy. *J Am Acad Orthop Surg* 2005; 13(4):279-289.

Coding

CPT Codes		Corresponding ICD-9 Codes	
Tibial Osteotomy			
27705	Osteotomy; tibia	715 733.81	715.16 736.9
Unicompartmental Knee Arthroplasty			
27446	Arthroplasty, knee, condyle and plateau; medial OR lateral compartment	715 715.80	715.16 715.89
Total Knee Arthroplasty			
27447	Arthroplasty, knee, condyle and plateau; medial AND lateral compartments with or without patella resurfacing (total knee arthroplasty)	715 715.80	715.16 715.89
Application of Cast			
29405	Application of short leg cast (below knee to toes);	715 821.20 823.30	715.16 823.00 823.80
29425	Application of short leg cast (below knee to toes); walking or ambulatory type	715 821.20 823.30	715.16 823.00 823.80
29435	Application of patellar tendon bearing (PTB) cast	715 821.20 823.30	715.16 823.00 823.80

HCPCS Codes	
Graduated Compression Stockings (GCS)	
L8100	Gradient compression stocking, below knee, 18-30 mm hg, each
L8110	Gradient compression stocking, below knee, 30-40 mm hg, each
L8120	Gradient compression stocking, below knee, 40-50 mm hg, each
L8130	Gradient compression stocking, thigh length, 18-30 mm hg, each
L8140	Gradient compression stocking, thigh length, 30-40 mm hg, each
L8150	Gradient compression stocking, thigh length, 40-50 mm hg, each
L8160	Gradient compression stocking, full length/chap style, 18-30 mm hg, each
L8170	Gradient compression stocking, full length/chap style, 30-40 mm hg, each
L8180	Gradient compression stocking, full length/chap style, 40-50 mm hg, each
L8190	Gradient compression stocking, waist length, 18-30 mm hg, each
L8195	Gradient compression stocking, waist length, 30-40 mm hg, each
L8200	Gradient compression stocking, waist length, 40-50 mm hg, each
Intermittent Pneumatic Compression (IPC)	
EO675	Pneumatic compression device, high pressure, rapid inflation/deflation cycle, for arterial insufficiency (unilateral or bilateral system)
EO676	Intermittent limb compression device (includes all accessories), not otherwise specified
Venous Foot Pumps (VFPs)	
A6451	Moderate compression bandage, elastic, knitted/woven, load resistance of 1.25 to 1.34 foot pounds at 50% maximum stretch, width greater than or equal to three inches and less than five inches, per yard
A6452	High compression bandage, elastic, knitted/woven, load resistance greater than or equal to 1.35 foot pounds at 50% maximum stretch, width greater than or equal to three inches and less than five inches, per yard

HCPCS copyright © 2010 by the Centers for Medicare and Medicaid Services. All rights reserved.

HPCPS (supply codes) are separately reportable by the physician when provided in the office setting. If ordered in the hospital or outpatient facility, supply codes are not separately reportable.

Chapter 61

Distal Femoral Osteotomy

Kenneth A. Krackow, MD

Indications

Because of the success of tibial osteotomy in the treatment of isolated medial compartment arthritis and varus deformity, the concept was expanded to the management of valgus deformity with lateral compartment arthrosis of the knee. Although varus proximal tibial osteotomy corrected the valgus deformity, abnormal downward and medial sloping of the knee joint line often resulted, making the distal femur a more desirable location for the osteotomy. Because valgus deformity is much less common than varus deformity, the literature and experience regarding distal femoral osteotomy (DFO) are much less extensive.

Some consider distal femoral and proximal tibial osteotomies for arthrosis outdated operations that are of only historical interest or very rarely indicated, but I do not agree. An increasing number of patients with knee arthritis are young (35 to 60 years) and may live many more decades. Osteotomy is the conservative, and perhaps more reasonable, alternative to total knee arthroplasty (TKA) or unicondylar knee arthroplasty for individuals of relatively high activity with

this life expectancy. TKA has a projected survivorship of 15 to 20 years, even in older patients with lower activity levels. Even considering the 5% to 10% of patients who do not live 15 to 20 years, a large number of TKA patients can be expected to require revision.

The primary indication for DFO is knee joint arthritis that involves primarily the lateral compartment in association with valgus deformity. Other considerations include patient age and activity goals that make TKA a less desirable option. In my practice, this typically is 60 years or younger or, in patients with higher activity levels, 65 years or younger. The ideal patient for DFO is 60 years of age or younger with a reasonable body build and a fair-to-good activity level; has arthritic changes localized primarily to the lateral compartment with a valgus deformity; and reports pain after reasonable activity, such as walking an extended distance, at the end of the day, or with specific higher activity levels.

Contraindications

DFO generally is contraindicated in patients with inflammatory arthritis

(such as rheumatoid or crystalline), even if the radiographic appearance is that of osteoarthrosis. DFO also is contraindicated in patients with marked ligamentous instability of the knee, flexion contracture of more than 15°, or tricompartmental degenerative disease. Coexisting patellofemoral degeneration, symptoms, and malalignment have been cited as contraindications to DFO, but I have had success in treating these with simultaneous lateral patellar release, medial tibial tubercle osteotomy, and occasionally lateral patellar facetectomy. In my experience, patients with extremely sensitive joints (such as to touch or weight bearing) usually are poor candidates for either tibial or femoral osteotomy.

The difficulty of performing TKA after a DFO has been suggested as a reason to avoid osteotomy. Often, however, TKA after DFO is no more difficult than primary TKA and usually is less difficult than after high tibial osteotomy. Partial plate or screw removal may be necessary to allow use of alignment instrumentation during TKA after DFO. Leaving at least the side plate in place or bypassing it with the femoral component stem lessens the chance of fracture, although such a fracture after partial or even complete plate removal is uncommon. DFO may actually be beneficial to subsequent TKA because it places the limb in approximately neutral align-

Dr. Krackow or an immediate family member has received royalties from Stryker; serves as a paid consultant for or is an employee of Stryker; and has received research or institutional support from Stryker.

Table 1 Results of Distal Femoral Osteotomy for Lateral Compartment Arthritis

Authors (Year)	Number of Patients (Knees)	Mean Follow-up in Years (Range)	Results	Conversion to TKA
Kosashvili et al (2010)	31 (33)	15 (10-25)	10 (30%) excellent/good 2 fair 5 poor	16 (48.5%)
Backstein et al (2007)	36 (38)	10 (3-20)	24 (63%) excellent/good 3 fair 3 poor	8 (21%)
Wang and Hsu (2005)	30 (30)	8 (5-14)	25 (83%) satisfactory 2 fair	3 (10%) 10-yr survival 87%
Aglietti and Menchetti (2000)	17 (17)	9 (5-16)	13 (76%) excellent/good 3 fair	1 (6%)
Mathews et al (1998)	21 (21)	3 (1-8)	7 (33%) satisfactory – HSS 12 (57%) satisfactory – KSCR	5 (24%)
Finkelstein et al (1996)	20 (21)	11 (8-20)	13 (62%) "successful" 1 patient died	7 (35%) 10-yr survival 64%
Edgerton et al (1993)	23 (24)	8 (5-11)	17 (71%) excellent/good 3 fair 1 poor	3 (13%)

HSS = Hospital for Special Surgery; KSCR = Knee Society Clinical Rating; TKA = total knee arthroplasty.

ment, which avoids major collateral ligament balancing, ligament advancement, or use of a more constrained prosthesis than is ideal for a younger, more active patient. Although the results of TKA after DFO are reported to be inferior to those of primary TKA, the comparison is not valid. A patient with a DFO probably has had long-standing pain and deformity, indicating more severe degenerative disease, joint destruction, and deformity than most candidates for primary TKA.

Alternative Treatments

Alternative treatments of osteoarthritis of the lateral compartment of the knee include nonsurgical measures, unicompartmental TKA, and tricompartmental TKA. In addition to the common nonsurgical measures such as weight loss and activity modification, a medial heel wedge or an unloader brace may relieve symptoms. Unicompartmental TKA may be appropriate for an older patient with isolated lateral compartment symptoms, whereas tricompartmental TKA may be needed for a patient with diffuse symptoms and evidence of arthritis in the medial or patellofemoral compartments.

A simple method for determining if DFO will be effective is to apply an offset cast on the affected leg. A short-leg fiberglass cast is made with the ankle in neutral or very slight calcaneus. Next, half of a 4- to 6-in roll of casting material is wound away from the full roll. The remaining half roll is placed at the plantar surface but out to the medial edge of the heel of the cast. The remaining half roll of cast material is used to fix the protruding half roll against the plantar-medial aspect of the heel. This creates a clear, firm medial offset prominence that, with weight bearing, generates a varus moment at the knee. To assess the effect, the patient simply walks around the office, or the cast can be worn out of the office for minutes, hours, or even overnight. Typically, the response is very clear—improvement, great improvement, or no significant improvement. DFO is unlikely to be effective in a patient who does not have a clearly positive result. If DFO is indicated, it should be done as soon as possible to avoid the risk of progressive degeneration of the knee joint.

Results

Excellent or good results have been reported after DFO in 30% to 83% of knees, with 10-year survival rates from 64% to 87% (**Table 1**). Percentages of patients requiring TKA after DFO also are variable, ranging from 10% to almost 50%, depending partially on the length of follow-up. One recent report noted that TKA can be expected to be necessary in about half of patients at approximately 15 years after DFO. The variability of these reported outcomes reflects the variations in patient selection, surgical techniques, postoperative alignment achieved, and length of follow-up in the various studies.

Technique

Preoperative Planning

Long weight-bearing lower extremity radiographs are preferable for preoperative planning because they allow assessment of the degree of deformity and determination of the involved compartments, information that is useful for planning the location of the osteotomy (femur or tibia, or possibly both) and the angular degree of the osteotomy. The amount of overall deformity should be measured and compared with neutral mechanical alignment. The femoral and tibial joint line angles should be compared with anatomic normal values and with the typical cut angles made for TKA, such as 0° perpendicular tibial cuts and 5° to 7° valgus femoral cuts. This assesses how much of the overall deformity is due to the femoral side versus the tibial side.

If a large proportion of the deformity is on the tibial side or the deformity is severe, performing all the correction in the femur presents potential problems. Extreme rotation of the epicondylar axis into a "varus position" may place the medial collateral ligament origin excessively cephalad, leading to extension tightness on the medial side and making flexion-extension balancing during future TKA problematic. Such extreme situations may require both femoral and tibial osteotomies.

A gapping of the medial compartment is common in knees with valgus deformity because of attenuation of the medial collateral ligament from the tension placed on it over the years of severe deformity. Correction to neutral alignment, and especially overcorrection to a few degrees of varus alignment, eliminates the gapping of the medial compartment. The angular amount of this gapping, anywhere from 1° to 5°, will be evident in the measurement of deformity on the long weight-bearing lower extremity radiograph as the knee is distracted. Because the patient will likely not have medial gapping when standing after varus correction, the estimated angle of the medial gapping should not be included in the total angle of deformity and the planned correction or overcorrection is possible.

As with a valgus tibial osteotomy, the usual goal with varus DFO is to overcorrect by 2° to 4°. In preoperative planning, one must consider that it is always easier and better to create a smaller angle of osteotomy first and increase it, rather than start too large and attempt to decrease it. Once a too-large angle has been created, removing bone at the apex of the osteotomy to lessen the correction angle creates a lateral bone gap that eliminates the stabilizing effect of the lateral soft tissues.

Instruments/Equipment/Implants Required

This technique uses a 90° adult hip blade plate rather than a 95° condylar blade plate because the medial-based wedge resection at this level of the femur creates a step-off, which better fits the obvious step-off at the blade of the 90° plate than the gentle curve of the 95° plate. Step-offs vary from 10 to 20 mm, in 5-mm increments, and blade lengths range from 40 to 70 mm.

Three or more 1/8-in (3.2-mm) Steinmann pins are used, two as saw guides and one to mark the location of the distal cut. At least two of the next smaller size (7/64-in [2.8-mm]) Steinmann pins also are used. I use the foil packaging of a scalpel blade to make a template. A Bovie cord is run from the center of the hip to the center of the ankle to check that the traverse point over the knee is as desired. The accuracy of the osteotomy is assessed after resection and bone approximation using the Steinmann pins and image-intensified fluoroscopy. Use of the fluoroscope is absolutely necessary during the Bovie cord assessment of the correction. All placements of the pins and use of the saw can be done without image control, but it should be available.

Setup/Patient Positioning

The patient is positioned on a radiolucent table so that the hip center can be seen. A folded bed sheet is placed under the surgical-side buttock, and a tourniquet is placed as proximal as possible on the thigh. The skin is prepared from the edge of the tourniquet to the toes, and routine draping is done.

Procedure
EXPOSURE

Either a midline or slightly medial incision is marked 10 to 12 cm above the patella to the level of the joint line. The surgeon stands on the patient's side opposite the involved extremity. With the tourniquet inflated, a subvastus exposure is made without making an arthrotomy. With the knee flexed, the hip is flexed slightly and externally rotated (figure-of-4 position).

In the proximal half of the wound, over the quadriceps muscle, a deep fascia lies just below the subcutaneous fat. This fascia is incised and retracted medially and anterolaterally to reveal the vastus medialis obliquus muscle (**Figure 1**, *A*). The distal medial edge of muscle connecting to the superior medial patella is separated from the knee joint capsule. A cobra hip retractor can be used at this point, reaching over the distal femur and under the quadriceps tendon.

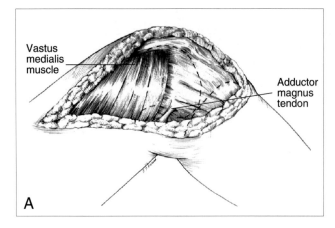

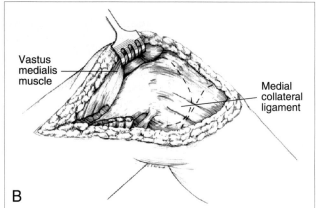

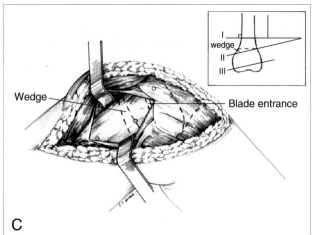

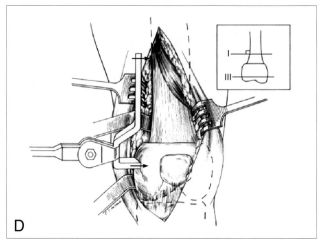

Figure 1 Exposure for distal femoral osteotomy (DFO). **A,** Initial exposure. The vastus medialis obliquus muscle lies over the distal medial femur and the knee joint deep to the capsule. **B,** Medial distal femoral bone. **C,** Pin and wedge locations are indicated. **D,** Blade plate with step-off for fixation of distal femoral element.

The quadriceps muscle more proximally is freed from the overlying fascia at the posterior medial aspect of the dissection with cutting cautery, leaving 1 cm or more of quadriceps muscle attached to the fascia and the linea aspera. This incision is directed toward the slightly posterior but definitely medial aspect of the femoral shaft. Care is taken here not to cut a perforating vessel so deep that the lateral end retracts back and through the fascia, becoming particularly difficult to control.

As the medial aspect of the distal femoral shaft is exposed (**Figure 1**, *B*), the cobra retractor can be moved and placed over the femoral shaft at the more proximal extent of dissection.

This entire dissection is carried as far proximal as necessary to accommodate placement of the side plate, including the length of the wedge of bone to be resected (**Figure 1**, *C*).

At the distal aspect of the wound, the subcutaneous tissue is cleared from the medial knee capsule. With the knee flexed, it is easy to feel the distal aspect of the medial femoral condyle. The medial epicondyle also is palpable, providing excellent assessment of the position for the blade to enter without using the image intensifier. The blade position will be determined by palpation of the distal medial femoral joint surface. Its entry point is anterior to and about at the level of the medial femoral epicon-

dyle. The distal cut will then be located approximately 2.0 cm proximal to the surface of the blade, which again is entering just above the epicondyle. This 2.0-cm thickness is located so as to put as much bone as possible between the blade and the osteotomy cut (**Figure 1**, *D*).

DETERMINING THE OSTEOTOMY LEVEL
A sharp ¼-in osteotome is used to perforate the medial cortex at the entry point for the seating chisel. The seating chisel is used to start its entry for only approximately 1 cm in a roughly anteromedial to posterolateral direction. The osteotome is used first, because seating chisels have a tendency to slide before they enter, missing the

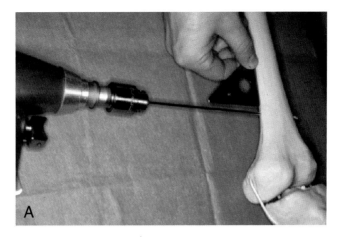

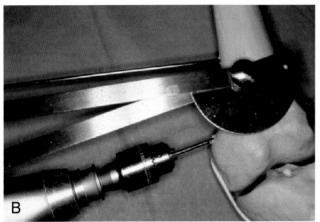

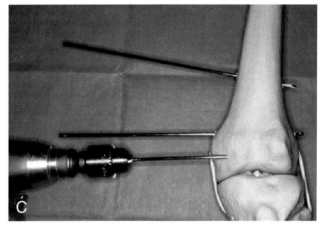

Figure 2 Initial placement of pins for the three-pin technique for DFO is demonstrated on a Sawbones model. **A,** Pin I is placed proximal to the osteotomy and perpendicular to the femoral shaft. **B,** Pin II is placed at the level of the distal cut for the osteotomy wedge and is angled the amount of the planned osteotomy. **C,** Pin III is placed distal and anterior to pin II, out of the way of the blade placement and parallel to pin II.

initially chosen point. The entry to the medial bone is relatively anterior for two reasons. First, the femoral shaft meets the distal femur in a relatively anterior position, and the femoral condyles extend farther posteriorly. Second, entering anteriorly allows the blade to be directly slightly posterior, as it will be moving laterally. This "external rotation" of the entire blade plate is necessary so that the side plate ultimately fits properly against the femoral shaft.

The level of the osteotomy is measured to be equal to the distance from the underside of the blade to the very beginning of the side plate at its straight extent, just proximal to the step-off. Thus, the maximal amount of bone is between the blade and the os-

teotomy for maximal strength of fixation. The goal is a complete wedge resection without trying to dovetail the proximal shaft into the distal fragment because this does not provide total contact. The level of the distal cut for the osteotomy wedge is marked with the cautery.

With the level of the osteotomy determined, the periosteum at that site is elevated anterior and posterior as far to the lateral aspect of the distal femur as possible. A blunt Hohmann retractor can be placed along the posterior cortex, and a 1.0-cm-wide malleable retractor is particularly convenient to use over the anterior bone. Its malleability allows it to be bent so that the amount of periosteal stripping is minimized. A similar malleable retractor

can be used posteriorly instead of the Hohmann. Before placing either form of posterior retractor, a pulled-out gauze sponge can be inserted for more soft-tissue protection.

"THREE-PIN" OSTEOTOMY TECHNIQUE
The next step is the "three-pin technique," which evolved from experience with the Dwyer calcaneal osteotomy. Using the metal triangles commonly supplied with blade plating instrumentation, the first ⅛-in pin (pin I) is placed from medial to lateral, perpendicular to the femoral shaft, and clearly proximal to any anticipated level for the proximal cut of the resected wedge (**Figure 2,** *A*). This pin, as the other two will be, is placed completely through the far lateral cor-

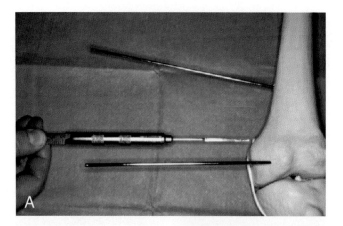

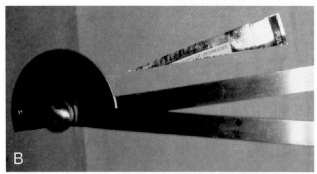

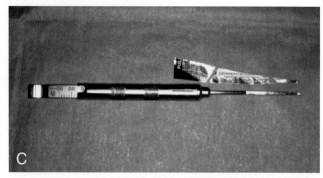

Figure 3 Templating the osteotomy. **A,** The thickness of the bone (the resulting wedge resection) is measured with a depth gauge. **B,** A foil template representing the angle of the osteotomy is made from a scalpel blade cover. **C,** The thickness of the wedge is marked on the foil and the foil template is cut. The larger end of the triangle (the "tail") is cut off and used to mark the level of the proximal cut.

tex. This permits each pin to be removed and the identical path to be measured by a depth gauge or retraced by easy placement of a ⁷/₆₄-in pin.

A sterile goniometer is opened to the initial angle estimated for the osteotomy wedge, and its cephalad limb is held parallel to the first pin (pin I). Then, pin II is held parallel to the distal limb of the goniometer and drilled into the medial femur at the desired point marked for the start of the distal cut of the wedge (**Figure 2**, *B*). Pin II is drilled through the lateral cortex; this pin indicates the line or level of cutting for the distal aspect of the wedge to be resected.

Pin III is placed parallel to pin II, anterior and distal to it and out of the way of the entry point for the seating chisel (**Figure 2**, *C*).

Pin II is removed, and a depth gauge is used to measure the thickness of the bone at the hole created by the pin (**Figure 3**, *A*). The sterile foil from a scalpel blade envelope is smoothed and straightened, and the angle of the osteotomy to which the goniometer is opened is transferred to the foil (**Figure 3**, *B*). The foil is cut, yielding a triangle with an apex angle equal to that of the proposed osteotomy (**Figure 3**, *C*). The larger end (the "tail") of this triangle is cut off, roughly approximating the curve of the medial femur, and this piece can later be conveniently held against the medial cortex to show the entry level for the proximal saw cut.

The distal cut is next. Pin I, the most proximal pin, is removed. Pin II was removed when the thickness of the femur was measured with the depth gauge. Pin III remains and functions as a saw guide for the distal cut (**Figure 4**).

The wedge resection is made using a thin saw blade long enough to cut through the far lateral cortex. The first step is to cut through the distal medial resection line previously drawn on the medial aspect of the femur. It is important to cut the line just a few millimeters deep. This cut is made without regard for the angle, but rather just to create a straight opening into the bone so that the saw blade can be directed exactly parallel to pin III. Again, pin III is kept in place and serves as a saw guide, accurately directing the distal cut. After completing most of the distal cut, through and toward the lateral femoral cortex, the tail of the template is used to mark the level of the proximal cut.

Pin III is removed, as it will be in the way of the saw making the proximal cut just as pin I was in the way for the distal cut.

The path of pin I, placed perpendicular to the femoral shaft and proximal to the level of the osteotomy, is used as the saw guide to create the proximal cut. Originally, ⅛-in pins were used; now, the path of pin I is easily reestablished by inserting a ⁷⁄₆₄-in Steinmann pin.

The osteotomy cuts are made almost all the way through the lateral cortex; an "incomplete" cut, one that leaves the far cortex truly intact, is not appropriate for most wedge osteotomies. At some point in clearing the wedge resection, the far cortex will crack.

An important step in a successful osteotomy is the trimming of the cortical bone as well as some cancellous bone so that accurate approximation of the cortical edges as well as all aspects of the cut surfaces is achieved. To maintain optimal stability with no additional shortening, a triangular, not trapezoidal, resection is required. This can be accomplished by first taking the saw resection to within 2 to 4 mm of the lateral cortex, then "opening," or exaggerating, the osteotomy. A straight, narrow osteotome is used to perforate the far cortex. Then the distal femur is gently rotated and the

tibia is moved laterally to crack the far lateral cortex. Finally, the far edges are smoothed with a saw or very sharp osteotomes, so that the surfaces approximate perfectly. Leaving residual lateral bone medial to the lateral cortex leads to an incomplete osteotomy and produces overcorrection.

Pins I and III, used as saw guides, are now used both to check the angle of correction and to ensure that no rotational deformity has been produced. When the osteotomy is closed according to preoperative planning, pins I and III should be parallel (**Figure 5**, *A*).

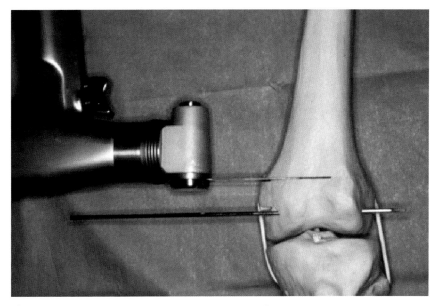

Figure 4 Making the proximal cut using pin III as a guide.

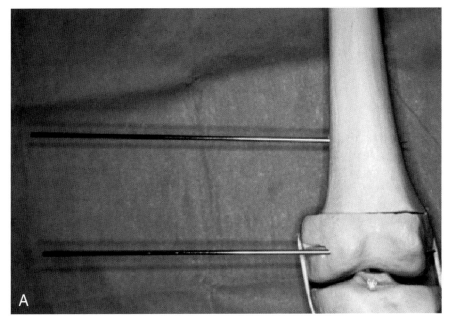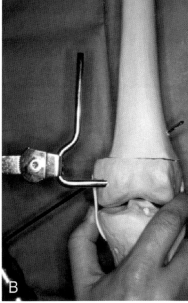

Figure 5 Osteotomy approximation and fixation. **A,** After approximating the cut edges of bone, pin I is parallel to pin III. Pin I was used to direct the proximal cut. Together, pins I and III allow assessment of proper correction and maintenance of rotation. **B,** The blade plate is placed without the use of the seating chisel. Note the oblique Steinmann pin stabilizing the bones.

ASSESSING THE ACCURACY OF THE OSTEOTOMY

After the osteotomy is satisfactorily completed, it is temporarily stabilized with an oblique Steinmann pin. Then a Bovie cord is centered over the femoral head under fluoroscopy and stretched to the visual center of the ankle. The C-arm is then used to see the point where the cord crosses the knee. The goal is to have the cord cross the medial compartment of the knee at the predetermined level, generally one third to one half of the way across the medial compartment. During this assessment, the person holding the Bovie cord over the center of the ankle should be exerting compression from the tibia to the femur, so that the contact at the knee mimics weight bearing.

If the crossing point of the cord is not correct, then the osteotomy is adjusted. If the wedge was underresected, a little more medial bone is shaved away, typically from the proximal osteotomy cut. Starting with a conservative resection makes it less likely that an excessive varus alignment will be present. If excessive varus does result, lateral bone can be removed, converting the resection into a trapezoidal one, to achieve the correct angle and have complete contact along the osteotomy and maximal interfragmentary stability. An alternative may be to add bone graft at the lateral aspect; however, because the osteotomy is made from the medial side, stability may not be optimal.

PLACING THE BLADE PLATE

Once the osteotomy has been completed to a satisfactory degree of accuracy, the last task is placing the blade plate (**Figure 5**, *B*). In the very early stages of the osteotomy, a seating chisel was placed into the distal aspect of the femur to create a trough or perforation. This perforation is exposed, and the chosen hip blade plate, held by the appropriate instrument, is inserted into the perforation. I strongly advise that the blade plate enter slightly anterior to the medial epicondyle and be directed slightly posteriorly, while maintaining a proper varus-valgus and flexion-extension relationship to the femoral shaft, so that the side plate lies properly on the bone. Otherwise, the anterior edge of the side plate tends not to touch the femoral shaft cortex, although the posterior edge of the plate does. As a result, as the side plate is screwed flat to the bone, the femoral condyles and joint line are likely to rotate externally. This rotation can be prevented by using an oblique crossing screw; however, fixation will not be optimal unless the side plate is flat against the medial femoral cortex.

The osteotomy is reduced and is temporarily fixed in proper varus-valgus and flexion-extension alignment with a 1/8-in (3.2-mm) Steinmann pin. While an assistant supports this position, the surgeon drives the blade into the distal aspect of the femur, adjusting its position so that the side plate lies perfectly along the medial cortex of the distal femur. Because the procedure is being done on the medial side of a valgus knee, the bone is relatively osteopenic from underloading and the distal element of the osteotomy is relatively large, so placing the blade in adequate bone is not difficult with the use of the preliminary path made by the seating chisel. Blade plating is significantly easier, in fact, if one is not a "slave" to the seating chisel!

An extreme step-off at the level of the osteotomy is not needed, as would be the case in a larger wedge resection. The magnitude of the step-off can be estimated by drawing the wedge resection on the radiograph and making a cut-out pattern after closing the osteotomy. With this technique, it is relatively simple to use a blade plate with a smaller step-off and pull the shaft to the side plate, centralizing it over the distal femoral bone.

WOUND CLOSURE

The wound is closed in routine manner with suction drainage. A Jones dressing is applied, with medial and lateral plaster splints extending just past the midpoint of the calf.

———————————■

■ Postoperative Regimen

Although this technique provides good early stability of the osteotomy, the overall strength of fixation is largely determined by bone quality and other factors such as proportional obesity of the patient and the weight of the extremity. Knee immobilizer braces are not particularly effective for support above the knee because of the soft intervening flesh and the fact that they do not extend adequately, if at all, above the region to be protected.

Different patient populations may require very different postoperative regimens. At one extreme, morbidly obese patients with particularly soft bone are treated with relatively firm Jones dressings changed weekly; the patients are kept nonambulatory, being transferred only from bed to wheelchair to commode for 4 to 6 weeks. This is a rare example, but it is important to note the special concerns in these patients. Nonunion in a very obese patient may not be manageable. The first chance is the best chance, with the largest amount and best quality of bone available. These patients are usually younger than the ideal TKA patient, and the salvage surgery required may be TKA using a highly constrained distal femoral-replacing prosthesis.

At the other extreme, some patients require no external stabilization, especially when they have strong bone and excellent fixation. Others may use standard knee immobilizers, making sure they are snug at the distal thigh and do not fall to the ankle. After the first 2 weeks, bracing is removed several times per day to perform gentle active and passive flexion. Weight bearing is advanced fairly quickly from 2 weeks of toe-touch to medium partial weight bearing at about 3 weeks to weight bearing as tolerated after 4 to 6 weeks, if there is no sign of any loosening or other compromise of fixation.

The most important consideration at this stage is healing of the osteotomy, not muscle strength or range of motion. The operation is essentially, if not actually, extra-articular, and regaining or even improving range of motion is not a significant issue.

———————————————■

Avoiding Pitfalls and Complications

Although some early descriptions of DFO reported frequent complications such as knee stiffness requiring manipulation, delayed union and nonunion, infection, and fixation failure, these complications have become infrequent with current techniques. Most complications can be avoided with careful attention to patient selection and surgical technique.

Patient selection is critical to the success of this procedure. The offset cast test can help identify patients who will benefit from a DFO. Patients with excessive pain and sensitivity at the knee and patients with rheumatoid arthritis are not good candidates for DFO.

During preoperative planning, both tibial and femoral deformities should be measured, because they contribute to the overall malalignment. Any medial gapping that exaggerates the deformity must be considered in planning the osteotomy to avoid overcorrection.

During the surgical procedure, several points should be remembered. First, any extreme alteration of the epicondylar axis should be avoided, as this may complicate future TKA. After making the osteotomy cuts, the Bovie cord technique can be used to identify the traverse point of the hip-ankle line. After the osteotomy is reduced, the blade plate can be inserted with the seating chisel. The distal femoral condylar area is a relatively large target. Keeping maximal bone thickness between the osteotomy and the blade enhances the strength of the fixation. When the plate is placed, the side plate should not pull the shaft into external rotation; the blade of the blade

plate should be angled anteromedial to posterolateral, with care taken as it approaches the medial femur.

Postoperatively, if the fixation needs more protection because of osteopenia and obesity, the patient's activities are severely restricted—bed to chair, or even to wheelchair. In general, the patient's activity and stress on the fixation should not get ahead of the healing. Knee immobilizers do not provide significant external stability. They are at best reminders and can produce an unwanted moment acting at the osteotomy site that can result in fixation failure. If a knee immobilizer is used, it should be kept high at the osteotomy site and not allowed to fall to the ankle.

If conversion to a TKA is required after a DFO, removal of the entire blade risks fracture because the bone may be weakened by the screw holes and the osteopenia from the plate. If possible, the whole blade plate should be left in place. Otherwise, the blade plate can be cut at its angle to the side plate. Also, one can burr through the plate with a carbide bit to accommodate femoral component fixation lugs. A stemmed femoral component could even be considered.

———————————————■

Bibliography

Aglietti P, Menchetti PP: Distal femoral varus osteotomy in the valgus osteoarthritic knee. *Am J Knee Surg* 2000;13(2):89-95.

Backstein D, Morag G, Hanna S, Safir O, Gross A: Long-term follow-up of distal femoral varus osteotomy of the knee. *J Arthroplasty* 2007;22(4, suppl 1):2-6.

Edgerton BC, Mariani EM, Morrey BF: Distal femoral varus osteotomy for painful genu valgum: A five-to-11-year follow-up study. *Clin Orthop Relat Res* 1993;288(288):263-269.

Finkelstein JA, Gross AE, Davis A: Varus osteotomy of the distal part of the femur: A survivorship analysis. *J Bone Joint Surg Am* 1996;78(9):1348-1352.

Healy WL, Anglen JO, Wasilewski SA, Krackow KA: Distal femoral varus osteotomy. *J Bone Joint Surg Am* 1988;70(1):102-109.

Jackson JP, Waugh W: Tibial osteotomy for osteoarthritis of the knee. *J Bone Joint Surg Br* 1961;43-B:746-751.

Kosashvili Y, Safir O, Gross A, Morag G, Lakstein D, Backstein D: Distal femoral varus osteotomy for lateral osteoarthritis of the knee: A minimum ten-year follow-up. *Int Orthop* 2010;34(2):249-254.

Krackow KA, Hales D, Jones L: Preoperative planning and surgical technique for performing a Dwyer calcaneal osteotomy. *J Pediatr Orthop* 1985;5(2):214-218.

Martens M, De Rycke J: Facetectomy of the patella in patellofemoral osteoarthritis. *Acta Orthop Belg* 1990;56(3-4):563-567.

Mathews J, Cobb AG, Richardson S, Bentley G: Distal femoral osteotomy for lateral compartment osteoarthritis of the knee. *Orthopedics* 1998;21(4):437-440.

McDermott AG, Finklestein JA, Farine I, Boynton EL, MacIntosh DL, Gross A: Distal femoral varus osteotomy for valgus deformity of the knee. *J Bone Joint Surg Am* 1988;70(1):110-116.

Nelson CL, Saleh KJ, Kassim RA, et al: Total knee arthroplasty after varus osteotomy of the distal part of the femur. *J Bone Joint Surg Am* 2003;85-A(6):1062-1065.

Paulos LE, O'Connor DL, Karistinos A: Partial lateral patellar facetectomy for treatment of arthritis due to lateral patellar compression syndrome. *Arthroscopy* 2008;24(5):547-553.

Phillips MI, Krackow KA: Distal femoral varus osteotomy: Indications and surgical technique. *Instr Course Lect* 1999;48: 125-129.

Wang JW, Hsu CC: Distal femoral varus osteotomy for osteoarthritis of the knee. *J Bone Joint Surg Am* 2005;87(1):127-133.

Coding

CPT Codes		Corresponding ICD-9 Codes	
Femoral Osteotomy			
27448	Osteotomy, femur, shaft or supracondylar; without fixation	736.41	736.42
27450	Osteotomy, femur, shaft or supracondylar; with fixation	715.15 736.41 715.15	736.42
Total Knee Arthroplasty			
27447	Arthroplasty, knee, condyle and plateau; medial AND lateral compartments with or without patella resurfacing (total knee arthroplasty)	736.41 715.15	736.42
Unicompartmental Knee Arthroplasty			
27446	Arthroplasty, knee, condyle and plateau; medial OR lateral compartment	736.41 715.15	736.42
Knee Cast			
29405	Application of short leg cast (below knee to toes);	736.41	736.42
29425	Application of short leg cast (below knee to toes); walking or ambulatory type	715.15 736.41 715.15	736.42
Heel Wedge			
29740	Wedging of cast (except clubfoot casts)	736.41 715.15	736.42

Anterior Cruciate Ligament Reconstruction: Overview of Anatomy, Biomechanics, and Indications for Surgery

James R. Andrews, MD
Steven W. Meisterling, MD

■ Introduction

The anterior cruciate ligament (ACL) is the most commonly injured ligament in the knee requiring surgical treatment. More than 200,000 ACL injuries are estimated to occur annually in the United States, and more than 100,000 ACL reconstructions are done each year. The initial cost of ACL reconstructions in the United States exceeds $2 billion annually, and evidence exists that the number of these procedures is increasing. It is estimated that 70% of ACL injuries occur through noncontact mechanisms, and the remaining 30% result from direct contact with another player or object. Noncontact injuries often are associated with deceleration coupled with cutting, pivoting, or side-stepping maneuvers.

■ Anatomy and Biomechanics

The ACL originates on the medial surface of the lateral femoral condyle, runs obliquely across the knee joint from posterolateral to anteromedial, and then inserts into a broad area of the central tibial plateau. A vascularized connective tissue separates the ligament into two distinct bundles, the anteromedial (AM) and the posterolateral (PL) bundle, each of which has a distinct origin site on the femur and insertion site on the tibia. The AM and PL bundles change alignment as the knee moves from extension to flexion. When the knee is at 0° of flexion, the femoral insertion sites are oriented vertically and the bundles are parallel. As the knee moves into 90° of flexion, the femoral insertion sites become horizontally aligned. This change in alignment causes the two

bundles to twist around each other and become crossed (**Figure 1**). With knee flexion, the AM bundle tightens, whereas with extension or internal/external tibial rotation, the PM bundle tightens. The AM bundle is believed to control anterior movement of the tibia, and the PL bundle controls rotation.

The double-bundle anatomy of the ACL was first described in 1938, but it was not until anatomic and biomechanical studies confirmed the importance of the anatomic and functional differences between the two bundles of the ACL that "double-bundle" reconstruction techniques were developed in an attempt to provide a more anatomic reconstruction and restore more rotational stability. There are several technical variations of these double-bundle techniques—one or two tibial or femoral tunnels, autograft or allograft, and different graft tensioning methods. These techniques and their outcomes are described in later chapters.

In addition to the structural stabilizing function of the ACL, it also is believed to provide a stabilizing function through a neurologic feedback mechanism. Mechanoreceptors on the ACL have been described as relaying joint position information, which is involved in muscular stabilization of the joint.

Dr. Andrews or an immediate family member serves as a paid consultant to or is an employee of Biomet Sports Medicine, Bauerfeind, Theralase, and MiMedx; and serves as an unpaid consultant to Arthrotek. Neither Dr. Meisterling nor any immediate family member has received anything of value from or owns stock in a commercial company or institution related directly or indirectly to the subject of this chapter.

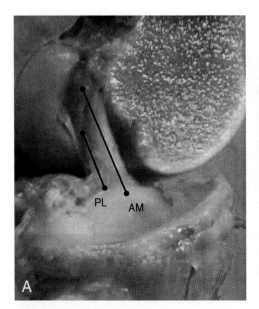

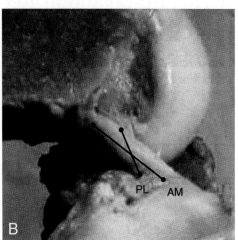

Figure 1 Crossing pattern of the anteromedial (AM) and posterolateral (PL) bundles. **A,** With the knee in extension, the AM and PL bundles are parallel. **B,** With the knee in flexion, the AM and PL bundles are crossed. (Reproduced with permission from Starman JS, Ferretti M, Järvelä T, Buoncristiani A, Fu FH: Anatomy and biomechanics of the anterior cruciate ligament, in Prodromos CC, ed: *The Anterior Cruciate Ligament: Reconstruction and Basic Science.* Philadelphia, PA, Saunders Elsevier, 2008, pp 3-11.)

Indications for and Timing of ACL Reconstruction

The most obvious indication for ACL reconstruction is the potential for reestablishment of normal knee biomechanics to provide adequate stability and pain-free function for a return to preinjury levels of activity, whether at the professional or recreational level of sports participation. Although we routinely reconstruct the ACL in young, active patients, skeletally immature and older patients require a different approach; we tend to be less aggressive in the latter patient populations. There is no real upper age limit for ACL reconstruction. The decision should be based on activity level, degree of instability, and desire to continue vigorous physical activity. ACL reconstruction is indicated for athletically active older patients who require stability for their activities, whether they are work related or sports related. In less active patients without reports of instability, a nonsurgical protocol can be considered. Skeletally immature patients who are less than 1 year from skeletal maturity and in whom the physeal lines are

blurred usually can be treated as adults with a definitive reconstruction procedure; however, if the physes are completely open, bone–patellar tendon–bone grafts should be avoided, a soft-tissue graft should be used, and a femoral physeal-sparing procedure should be considered. The indications, contraindications, and techniques for ACL reconstruction in skeletally immature patients are discussed in detail in chapter 69.

A delay in reconstruction or failure to reconstruct the ACL can cause several other problems; the ACL-deficient knee is a well-recognized clinical entity. Left untreated, a torn ACL can lead to anterior laxity, rotary instability, and meniscal tears. O'Donoghue's "unhappy triad" of ACL and medial collateral ligament tears combined with a medial meniscal tear has long been recognized; however, more recently, it has been suggested that the meniscal tear is a result of chronic ACL deficiency rather than a component of the original injury. Despite these findings, the timing of ACL reconstruction remains a matter of controversy. Earlier studies indicated better functional results when reconstruction was delayed at least 3 weeks. The rationale for delayed ACL reconstruction is to provide time

for preoperative rehabilitation to regain normal knee range of motion, eliminate swelling, and regain leg control; however, a prospective, randomized study of 69 patients with acute ACL tears treated with early (average, 9 days after injury) or delayed (average, 85 days after injury) reconstruction found similar long-term clinical results, but early treatment conferred certain benefits. Patients in the early surgery group returned to full activity 1 to 3 months earlier than those in the delayed surgery group. Early reconstruction also was beneficial in treating concurrent injuries. More than 90% of patients in the early group had meniscal tears, and nearly 60% of these tears could be repaired during ACL reconstruction surgery. In the 69% of patients in the delayed group who had meniscal tears, less than a third (27%) of the tears could be repaired.

Some authors suggest delaying ACL reconstruction in adolescents with open physes. Waiting until the femoral and tibial physes are closed allows an anatomic reconstruction, but it also may increase the rate of additional knee injuries, particularly in adolescents who do not comply with activity restrictions. A recent study of 70 adolescent athletes determined that patients whose treatment was delayed for more than 12 weeks had a significant increase in the number and severity of medial meniscal tears, as well as higher grade lateral compartment injuries and chondral injuries. An earlier study, however, found no evidence that delayed ACL reconstruction increased the rate of additional knee injuries in adolescents with open physes. Advocates of both early and delayed ACL reconstruction emphasize that neither protocol is appropriate for all patients and that the decision to delay reconstruction must be individualized. Bottoni, an early advocate of delayed reconstruction, noted that "we have learned that it is not so much the timing of the surgery, but the condition of the knee before surgery that is important."

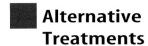

Contraindications

Contraindications to ACL reconstruction are few, mainly active infection and limited knee range of motion. Other suggested contraindications include partial tears (>50% of the ACL intact) that cause no functional instability and isolated complete tears in patients with low activity levels. Some authors consider the following to be relative contraindications: obesity (body mass index >30), varus malalignment unless corrected by high tibial osteotomy, poor patient motivation, symptomatic arthritis, and complex regional pain syndrome.

Alternative Treatments

Alternatives to reconstruction include physical therapy and bracing. Nonsurgical treatment historically has been recommended to patients with sedentary occupations and low activity de-

mands and patients who are older than 40 years. However, a recent review of 36 patients with nonsurgically managed partial ACL tears, all of whom were younger than 45 years (average age, 28 years), found that only 3 of the tears (8%) progressed to full tears and none of the patients had a meniscal injury during an average 42-month follow-up. The nonsurgically managed group lost an average of 2 points on the Marx Activity Scale, compared with a 4-point loss in a control group of 935 patients who had reconstructive surgery for complete ACL tears. Suggested criteria for nonsurgical management include an isolated ACL injury (no meniscal or other ligamentous injury), no recurrent episodes of giving way, no knee pain, and no recurrent effusions.

Results

Results of specific procedures are discussed in their respective chapters, but overall reported success rates range from 70% to 95%. It is difficult to state definitively a success rate for ACL reconstruction, partly because the definition of "success" differs widely among patients. The professional athlete and the low-demand older patient have very different expectations about the performance of their reconstructed knee. A recent study of 27 National Basketball Association players who had ACL reconstructions found that 6 (22%) did not return to professional competition, and 12 of the remaining 21 players had a decrease of more than 1 point in their player efficiency rating. An earlier study reported that only about half of patients who had reconstruction within 3 months of injury were able to return to their previous or higher levels of activity. Among patients with late reconstruction (more than 3 months after injury), only 37% returned to preinjury or higher levels of activity. Current literature indicates that revision ACL reconstruction is re-

quired in from 3% to 25% of patients because of unsatisfactory outcomes (loss of motion, locking, instability, effusion, and pain) or graft failure.

Complications

Complications of specific reconstruction procedures are discussed in their respective chapters, as are complications related to poor technique such as inaccurate tunnel placement or graft tensioning. Common general complications associated with ACL reconstruction regardless of technique include loss of extension (arthrofibrosis), recurrent instability, patellofemoral pain, infection, neurovascular complications, and osteoarthritis. Rates of knee stiffness or loss of motion have been reported at between 10% and 35%; anterior knee pain, between 4% and 56%; recurrent instability, approximately 10%; infection, less than 1%; nerve injury (saphenous nerve), as high as 88%; and vascular injury, less than 1%. Radiographic evidence of osteoarthritis has been reported in 79% to 90% of patients as few as 7 years after surgery.

Summary

With the current high success rates and low complication rates, ACL reconstruction is indicated for almost any patient in whom knee instability prohibits activities of daily living, vocational activities, or sports activities. Several choices exist concerning timing, technique, graft, fixation, and rehabilitation, and these are discussed in detail in subsequent chapters. As our understanding of the anatomy and function of the ACL increases, the specific procedure may be individualized to the patient's unique anatomy, injury pattern, and degree of laxity.

■ Bibliography

Adachi N, Ochi M, Uchio Y, Iwasa J, Ryoke K, Kuriwaka M: Mechanoreceptors in the anterior cruciate ligament contribute to the joint position sense. *Acta Orthop Scand* 2002;73(3):330-334.

Bottoni CR, Liddell TR, Trainor TJ, Freccero DM, Lindell KK: Range of motion following reconstruction using autograft hamstrings: A prospective, randomized clinical trial of early versus delayed reconstructions. *Am J Sports Med* 2008;36: 656-662.

Busfield BT, Kharrazi FD, Starkey C, Lombardo SJ, Seegmiller J: Performance outcomes of anterior cruciate ligament reconstruction in the National Basketball Association. *Arthroscopy* 2009;25(8):825-830.

Chhabra A, Starman JS, Ferretti M, Vidal AF, Zantop T, Fu FH: Anatomic, radiographic, biomechanical, and kinematic evaluation of the anterior cruciate ligament and its two functional bundles. *J Bone Joint Surg Am* 2006;88(Suppl 4):2-10.

Flik KR: What is your preferred nonoperative treatment protocol for acute ACL injuries in patients who do not wish to undergo surgery? Bach BR, Verman NN, eds: *Curbside Consultation of the ACL: 29 Clinical Questions.* Thorofare, NJ, Slack Inc, 2008, pp 187-188.

Getelman MH, Friedman MJ: Revision anterior cruciate ligament reconstruction surgery. *J Am Acad Orthop Surg* 1999; 7(3):189-198.

Kjaergaard J, Faunø LZ, Faunø P: Sensibility loss after ACL reconstruction with hamstring graft. *Int J Sports Med* 2008; 29(6):507-511.

Lawrence JT, Agrawal N, Ganley TJ: Anterior cruciate ligament rupture in patients with significant growth remaining: What is the risk to the meniscus and cartilage when treatment is delayed? The American Orthopaedic Society for Sports Medicine. http://www.sportsmed.org. Accessed March 16, 2010.

Laxdal G, Kartus J, Ejerhed L, et al: Outcome and risk factors after anterior cruciate ligament reconstruction: A follow-up study of 948 patients. *Arthroscopy* 2005;21(8):958-964.

Lind M, Menhert F, Pedersen AB: The first results from the Danish ACL reconstruction registry: Epidemiologic and 2 year follow-up results from 5,818 knee ligament reconstructions. *Knee Surg Sports Traumatol Arthrosc* 2009;17(2):117-124.

Marx RG, Stump TJ, Jones EC, Wickiewicz TL, Warren RF: Development and evaluation of an activity rating scale for disorders of the knee. *Am J Sports Med* 2001;29(2):213-218.

Mauro CS, Irrgang JJ, Williams BA, Harner CD: Loss of extension following anterior cruciate ligament reconstruction: Analysis of incidence and etiology using IKDC criteria. *Arthroscopy* 2008;24(2):146-153.

O'Donoghue DH: The unhappy triad: Etiology, diagnosis and treatment. *Am J Orthop* 1964;6:242-247.

Sanders B, Rolf R, McClelland W, Xerogeanes J: Prevalence of saphenous nerve injury after autogenous hamstring harvest: An anatomic and clinical study of sartorial branch injury. *Arthroscopy* 2007;23(9):956-963.

Woods GW, O'Connor DP: Delayed anterior cruciate ligament reconstruction in adolescents with open physes. *Am J Sports Med* 2004;32(1):201-210.

Chapter 63

Anterior Cruciate Ligament Reconstruction: Overview of Evaluation and Technical Pearls

Mark D. Miller, MD
Jennifer A. Hart, MPAS, PA-C

■ Evaluation

Physical examination of the anterior cruciate ligament (ACL)–injured knee should include a thorough evaluation of the knee, including observation, range-of-motion testing, palpation, and stability testing. The two most important tests for ACL evaluation are the Lachman test and the pivot-shift, or jerk, test. Many descriptions of these tests are available. Our technique is described here.

The Lachman test is best done with the patient supine, with hands on the chest (which forces the patient to lie down completely), and with a rolled-up pillow under the knee to be examined (**Figure 1**, *A*). The examiner places the hand that is closest to the patient's head on the thigh to stabilize it and also to assess the patient's relaxation. The examiner encourages the patient to relax by rocking the knee while distracting him or her. The other hand is placed around the tibia with the thumb close to the lateral joint line. Once the patient is relaxed, the tibia is firmly and deliberately pulled anteriorly, and the displace-

ment and presence or absence of an end point are assessed. If objective results are desired, an instrumented Lachman test can be conducted using a KT-1000 arthrometer (MEDmetric, San Diego).

We prefer what we call the "fly-fishing technique" for the pivot-shift test (**Figure 1**, *B*). With the patient supine, the foot ipsilateral to the knee to be examined is secured in the examiner's axilla with the leg in full extension, leaving the examiner's hands free to evaluate the knee. Both hands are placed around the leg at the level of the proximal tibia, and as the knee is flexed, a fluid valgus and rotational force is applied to the knee, much as if casting a line when fly-fishing.

Imaging evaluation should always include plain radiographs to evaluate for bony pathology. Weight-bearing flexion PA radiographs are routinely recommended, especially if there is suspicion of degenerative joint disease. Although arthritis is not a contraindication for ACL reconstruction, it is helpful to know how much joint space narrowing has occurred when counseling patients. Other findings on plain radiographs include a small

avulsion fracture of the proximal lateral tibial plateau just below the joint line (Segond or lateral capsular sign) that is reliably associated with an ACL tear (**Figure 2**, *A*). MRI is not always required to make the diagnosis, but it can show disruption of the continuity of the ACL fibers, anterior displacement of the tibia in relation to the femur (what radiologists call a drawer sign), and the classic bone contusion pattern (seen in about 60% of cases) (**Figure 2**, *B* through *D*).

■ Graft Selection

Hamstring grafts have become more popular than patellar tendon grafts over the last several years; however, each graft has its place. We have informally developed a set of patient criteria for these two graft choices (**Table 1**). Other grafts, including quadriceps tendon grafts (with or without bone) and allografts, also are used frequently for ACL reconstruction. The literature suggests that clinical results with allografts are similar to those with autografts, but we believe autografts provide more consistent results.

Dr. Miller or an immediate family member has received nonincome support (such as equipment or services), commercially derived honoraria, or other non-research-related funding (such as paid travel) from Miller Orthopaedic Research & Education and has received royalties from Saunders/ Mosby-Elsevier and Lippincott Williams & Wilkins. Ms. Hart or an immediate family member has received nonincome support (such as equipment or services), commercially derived honoraria, or other non-research-related funding (such as paid travel) from Saunders/Mosby-Elsevier.

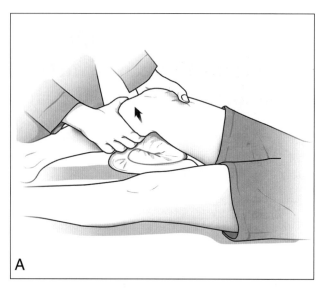

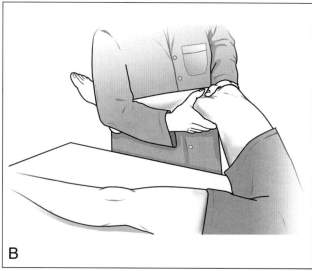

Figure 1 Clinical tests for ACL evaluation. **A**, The Lachman test. **B**, The pivot-shift test.

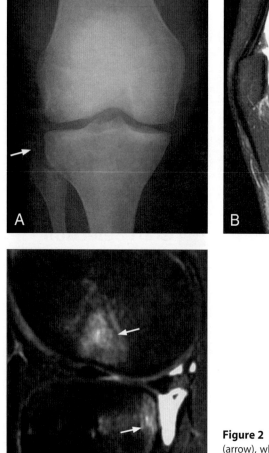

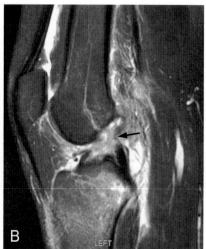

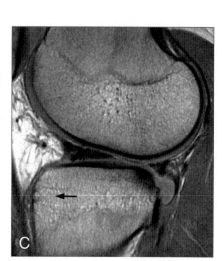

Figure 2 Imaging evaluation of the ACL. **A**, AP radiograph demonstrates a Segond fracture (arrow), which is frequently associated with an ACL tear. Classic appearance of an ACL tear (arrows) on T2-weighted MRI includes disruption of the ACL fibers (**B**), anterior translation of the tibia (**C**), and evidence of contusion (**D**).

Table 1 Patient Factors in Graft Selection for Anterior Cruciate Ligament Reconstruction

Patellar Tendon Graft

Football players (American football)

Hyperlaxity

Young male athletes

Ballet dancers, gymnasts

Martial arts

Sprinters, hurdlers

"High-profile" athletes

Revision of prior hamstring graft

Hamstring Graft

Prior anterior knee pain/patellar surgery

Patellar chondrosis

Inadequate patellar tendon width

People who need to kneel frequently

Older patients

Athletes who participate in jumping sports

Patients with cosmesis concerns

Revision of prior patellar tendon graft

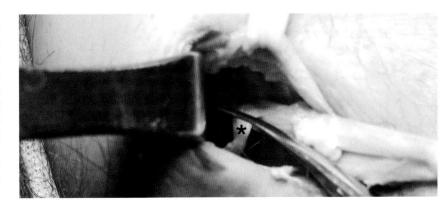

Figure 3 Intraoperative photograph shows the common semitendinosus attachment(s) to the gastrocnemius (asterisk). Failure to free this may result in graft amputation.

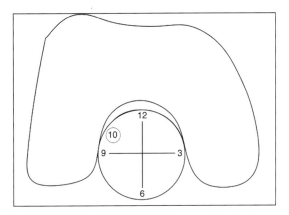

Figure 4 Cross-sectional drawing shows the 10:00 to 10:30 position that is now favored for drilling the femoral tunnel in a right knee. This results in a more horizontal tunnel.

Technical Pearls

Graft Harvest

Extreme care must be taken when harvesting grafts for ACL reconstruction. Specific techniques for harvesting various grafts are described in other chapters in this section; a few technical points are described here.

When harvesting bone–patellar tendon–bone grafts, we prefer to begin with an 11- or even 12-mm–wide graft at the distal pole of the patella. The fiber orientation narrows at the tibial tubercle, so this typically results in a 10-mm graft. Electrocautery can be used when outlining the patellar cuts so that a 10-mm plug can be harvested. At the tibial tubercle, saw cuts can be almost vertical and can go deep, but at the patella they must be more oblique and precise. (The saw is advanced until it "gives"—about 10 mm.) Likewise, an osteotome can be used more aggressively on the tibia

than the patella; it should never be used to lever from the sides for the patella. Bone grafting of the patellar defect is routine. We prefer to pack it with the bone that collects in the flutes of a fully threaded drill bit during tibial drilling.

When harvesting hamstring grafts, it is helpful to recognize that the orientation of the semitendinosus and gracilis is almost horizontal near the insertion, particularly with the knee flexed, and that they lie 5 to 7 mm distal to the medial joint line. Once they are isolated beneath the sartorial fascia, they must be completely freed of any soft-tissue attachments before harvesting. It is routine for the semitendinosus to have at least one, and often two, thick bands that attach to the medial head of the gastrocnemius (**Figure 3**), and these must be freed before using a tendon stripper.

Tunnel Placement

Other aspects of the surgical reconstruction, such as graft preparation, débridement and notchplasty, and placement of the tibial and femoral tunnels are discussed in subsequent chapters, but one change in technique deserves mention here—the preferred location for the femoral tunnel. Most surgeons now favor a lower, more horizontal, femoral tunnel placement, at the 10 o'clock or 10:30 position in a right knee and at 1:30 or 2 o'clock in a left knee (**Figure 4**), believing that this will better control rotation. This can be accomplished with a transtibal technique through a medial tibial tunnel or with an accessory medial portal. It is critical to recognize that the knee must be hyperflexed if an accessory medial portal is used. The graft should not be passed through the medial portal, but a passing suture should be retrieved through the tibial tunnel before passing the graft. For single-bundle reconstructions, most surgeons still favor a 1- to 2-mm backwall after femoral tunnel placement. We find that offset guides are helpful in achieving this consistently.

Graft Fixation

For soft-tissue fixation, our research has shown that suspensory fixation may result in slightly more tunnel osteolysis than double cross-pin fixation, but results are similar. For tibial fixation of soft-tissue grafts, we prefer an expanding sleeve interference screw device and a simple staple for backup. For patellar tendon fixation, metal interference screws still are the gold standard, and we routinely use a 7- × 20-mm screw for the femur and a 9- × 20-mm screw for the tibia because the tibial bone is less dense.

Double-Bundle ACL Reconstruction

Although some biomechanical and even early clinical studies have shown that there may be an advantage to double-bundle reconstructions, this procedure may introduce new technical challenges and complications that may outweigh its potential benefits. Another concern is that the use of additional grafts (often allografts) brings added disadvantages. One of the most crucial aspects of double-bundle reconstruction is defining the landmarks for tunnel location, and these have not been universally agreed upon. Long-term clinical studies will ultimately determine if more-horizontal femoral tunnel placement or double-bundle reconstruction will improve results with ACL reconstruction.

Bibliography

Baumfeld JA, Diduch DR, Rubino LJ, et al: Tunnel widening following anterior cruciate ligament reconstruction using hamstring autograft: A comparison between double cross-pin and suspensory graft fixation. *Knee Surg Sports Traumatol Arthrosc* 2008;16(12):1108-1113.

Brandser EA, Riley MA, Berbaum KS, el-Khoury GY, Bennett DL: MR imaging of anterior cruciate ligament injury: Independent value of primary and secondary signs. *AJR Am J Roentgenol* 1996;167(1):121-126.

Chhabra A, Diduch DR, Blessey PB, Miller MD: Recreating an acceptable angle of the tibial tunnel in the coronal plane in anterior cruciate ligament reconstruction using external landmarks. *Arthroscopy* 2004;20(3):328-330.

Golish SR, Baumfeld JA, Schoderbek RJ, Miller MD: The effect of femoral tunnel starting position on tunnel length in anterior cruciate ligament reconstruction: A cadaveric study. *Arthroscopy* 2007;23(11):1187-1192.

Harner CD, Honkamp NJ, Ranawat AS: Anteromedial portal technique for creating the anterior cruciate ligament femoral tunnel. *Arthroscopy* 2008;24(1):113-115.

Howell SM, Gittins ME, Gottlieb JE, Traina SM, Zoellner TM: The relationship between the angle of the tibial tunnel in the coronal plane and loss of flexion and anterior laxity after anterior cruciate ligament reconstruction. *Am J Sports Med* 2001;29(5):567-574.

Jackson DW, Gasser SI: Tibial tunnel placement in ACL reconstruction. *Arthroscopy* 1994;10(2):124-131.

Jonsson T, Althoff B, Peterson L, Renström P: Clinical diagnosis of ruptures of the anterior cruciate ligament: A comparative study of the Lachman test and the anterior drawer sign. *Am J Sports Med* 1982;10(2):100-102.

Kim SJ, Kim HK: Reliability of the anterior drawer test, the pivot shift test, and the Lachman test. *Clin Orthop Relat Res* 1995;317:237-242.

Kustos T, Bálint L, Than P, Bárdos T: Comparative study of autograft or allograft in primary anterior cruciate ligament reconstruction. *Int Orthop* 2004;28(5):290-293.

Liu SH, Osti L, Henry M, Bocchi L: The diagnosis of acute complete tears of the anterior cruciate ligament: Comparison of MRI, arthrometry and clinical examination. *J Bone Joint Surg Br* 1995;77(4):586-588.

Loh JC, Fukuda Y, Tsuda E, Steadman RJ, Fu FH, Woo SL: Knee stability and graft function following anterior cruciate ligament reconstruction: Comparison between 11 o'clock and 10 o'clock femoral tunnel placement. 2002 Richard O'Connor Award paper. *Arthroscopy* 2003;19(3):297-304.

Zeiss J, Paley K, Murray K, Saddemi SR: Comparison of bone contusion seen by MRI in partial and complete tears of the anterior cruciate ligament. *J Comput Assist Tomogr* 1995;19(5):773-776.

Chapter 64

Anterior Cruciate Ligament Reconstruction: Overview of Technique Choices and Complications

Rick W. Wright, MD

Introduction

Significant advances have been made in the surgical reconstruction of the anterior cruciate ligament (ACL) over the past 20 years. With these advances has come an increased expectation of favorable outcomes. Currently, the success rate for surgical reconstruction of the ACL is greater than 90%.

Since the 1980s, when appropriate tunnel placement on the femur and tibia was determined, most reconstruction techniques have proved to be successful. Surgeons must make two significant decisions when performing ACL reconstruction: the approach (open, rear entry, endoscopic, single bundle, double bundle) and the graft type (patellar, hamstring, or quadriceps tendon autograft; or Achilles, patellar, hamstring, anterior tibial, or posterior tibial tendon allograft).

Reconstruction Approach

Rear-entry or two-incision reconstruction was the method of choice in the early days of ACL reconstruction. Although it continues to have proponents who appreciate the ability to place the graft down the wall on the femur, endoscopic or one-incision reconstructions are now more common. A systematic review of endoscopic compared with rear-entry ACL reconstruction demonstrated no significant differences in pain, rehabilitation, strength, range of motion, anterior-posterior laxity, or clinical outcome. Surgeons should choose the technique with which they are most comfortable or the one they have been trained to perform.

Graft Choice

Graft choice remains somewhat controversial but ultimately depends on surgeon experience and preference. The graft chosen must have structural properties similar to the ACL, allow reasonable fixation, and incorporate appropriately. Fortunately, these parameters apply to a variety of grafts. Systematic reviews evaluating hamstring and patellar tendon autografts demonstrated minimal clinically significant differences between the two graft types. Hamstring tendons were associated with slightly increased anterior-posterior laxity, and patellar tendon grafts were associated with increased kneeling pain, but beyond this, no dramatic differences were noted. A third autograft choice is the quadriceps tendon. This is less commonly chosen than hamstring and patellar tendons, but it has demonstrated good clinical results and minimal donor-site morbidity.

Less evidence exists regarding allograft versus autograft ACL reconstruction outcomes. No randomized trials have been conducted to answer this question. The current evidence in this area is level 2 and 3 cohort and case-control studies, which indicate no difference in patient-based outcomes, functional outcomes, or anterior-posterior laxity. There does appear to be a trend toward increased graft failure with allografts. Recent unpublished data presented by the Multicenter Orthopaedic Outcomes Network (MOON) indicate a higher failure rate in young active patients who have allograft reconstructions than in those who have autograft reconstructions. Until additional data become available, allograft use should be limited in younger patients.

Dr. Wright or an immediate family member has received research or institutional support from Biomet, Breg, Cerapedics, Medtronic, Smith & Nephew, Stryker, Wright Medical Technology, Wyeth, Axial Biotech, Midwest Stone Institute, Synthes Spine, and K2M.

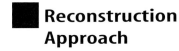

Single- Versus Double-Bundle Reconstruction

Recently, double-bundle ACL reconstruction has become popular. In this technique, the two major bundles of the ACL, the anteromedial and posterolateral, are reconstructed. Although single-bundle reconstructions have in general been very successful, a small subset of patients are unable to return to play or have less than successful results with single-bundle reconstructions. The single-bundle reconstruction technique has been demonstrated to control anterior-posterior laxity, but it may not control rotation completely. Biomechanical testing of the double-bundle reconstruction technique has suggested that it may improve knee kinematics, but overall clinical outcomes, including revision rates, have not been demonstrated to be improved. Additional studies are necessary to determine if improved outcomes justify the increased technical difficulty of the double-bundle technique.

Skeletally Immature Patients

ACL injuries in skeletally immature patients continue to become more prevalent as more children participate in organized sports at younger ages. ACL injuries in this age group typically require either activity limitation until skeletal maturity or ACL reconstruction using physeal protective measures. The results of ACL reconstructions in skeletally immature patients have been difficult to interpret because of flaws in the studies, including small numbers of patients, inclusion of older adolescents, failure to separate results by sex of patient, and lack of methodical evaluation of limb-length inequality. The adolescent growth spurt typically occurs in boys at 12.5 years and in girls at 10.5 years. Thus, reported procedures that include patients more than 2 years older than these ages may not have any relevant risk remaining to physes. Bone age or other objective measures of skeletal maturity remain the most accurate way to assess potential growth remaining. A variety of technical approaches to ACL reconstruction in skeletally immature patients has been described. In general, these are soft-tissue grafts that either spare the physis or minimize the trauma to the physis. Details of these approaches are outlined in chapter 69.

Complications

Potential complications of ACL reconstruction include graft failure, range-of-motion deficits, deep vein thrombosis, infection, nerve injury, and additional surgery. A recent systematic review of reconstructions with hamstring and patellar tendon autografts demonstrated a mean failure rate of 3.7% (range, 1.5% to 5.7%). A recently published study analyzing the MOON cohort demonstrated an overall 2.9% failure rate at 2-year follow-up, which was identical to the ACL tear rate of the opposite normal knee during those 2 years. The systematic review demonstrated no nerve injuries or deep vein thromboses and a 0.8% infection rate. An iatrogenic injury to the infrapatellar branch of the saphenous nerve resulting in lateral knee cutaneous numbness is a recognized risk of ACL reconstruction, especially when the hamstrings or patellar tendon is harvested as an autograft. A lower rate of additional surgery has been demonstrated in patients with an ACL-reconstructed knee compared with those treated nonsurgically, with a recent review demonstrating that 14.7% of those treated nonsurgically required additional surgery. Loss of extension has been suggested as the most common complication following ACL reconstruction. Typically, this loss of extension can be prevented by having the patient regain a full range of knee motion before surgery, ensuring proper tunnel placement, especially the tibial tunnel, and instituting an appropriate rehabilitation that includes early work on extension.

It has been estimated that the rate of ACL graft failure after reconstruction ranges from 0.7% to 8%. Three broad categories of graft failure have been described: (1) technical surgical errors, (2) graft incorporation failure, and (3) trauma. Technical errors at the time of surgery are believed to be the most common source of recurrent pathologic laxity requiring revision reconstruction. These errors include improper femoral and tibial tunnel placement, inadequate notchplasty, inappropriate graft tensioning or fixation, and inadequate graft tissue. The timing of ACL reconstruction failure can be an indicator of the etiology of the recurrent instability. Failure within 6 months after reconstruction usually indicates technical surgical failure or graft incorporation failure. Failure later than 1 year after reconstruction with an intervening period of knee stability and appropriate function indicates a traumatic etiology.

Revision ACL Reconstruction

A consistent belief among sports medicine orthopaedic specialists is that even with attention to surgical detail with a well-thought-out preoperative plan, the results of revision ACL reconstructions do not approach those of routine primary reconstructions; however, little direct evidence exists to support this claim. Most revision

ACL reconstruction studies have focused on techniques rather than assessment of outcomes and have consisted of level 4 retrospective case series with no control group or comparison to primary ACL reconstructions. Recently, the MOON group published 2-year outcome results from the first year of their prospective longitudinal cohort of ACL reconstructions. This study demonstrated a 15% reoperation rate in revision ACL reconstructions. In addition, although Short Form-36 scores improved significantly for both the physical and mental component summaries, they did not achieve the levels noted in studies involving primary reconstructions. Thus, to involve enough patients to develop level 1 evidence about the outcomes of revision reconstruction compared with primary reconstruction, a multisurgeon, multicenter prospective longitudinal cohort is needed. For that reason, the Multicenter ACL Revision Study (MARS) group has been developed to investigate these issues.

Later chapters in this book provide much more in-depth information regarding the issues presented in this overview. Details regarding the technical issues involved in a variety of ACL reconstruction techniques are provided and should help orthopaedic surgeons determine the approaches and techniques with which they will be most comfortable.

———————■

■ Bibliography

Biau DJ, Tournoux C, Katsahian S, Schranz PJ, Nizard RS: ACL reconstruction: A meta-analysis of functional scores. *Clin Orthop Relat Res* 2007;458:180-187.

Biau DJ, Tournoux C, Katsahian S, Schranz PJ, Nizard RS: Bone-patellar tendon-bone autografts versus hamstring autografts for reconstruction of anterior cruciate ligament: Meta-analysis. *BMJ* 2006;332(7548):995-1001.

Dunn WR, Lyman S, Lincoln AE, Amoroso PJ, Wickiewicz T, Marx RG: The effect of anterior cruciate ligament reconstruction on the risk of knee reinjury. *Am J Sports Med* 2004;32(8):1906-1914.

George MS, Dunn WR, Spindler KP: Current concepts review: Revision anterior cruciate ligament reconstruction. *Am J Sports Med* 2006;34(12):2026-2037.

George MS, Huston LJ, Spindler KP: Endoscopic versus rear-entry ACL reconstruction: A systematic review. *Clin Orthop Relat Res* 2007;455:158-161.

Gottlob CA, Baker CL Jr, Pellissier JM, Colvin L: Cost effectiveness of anterior cruciate ligament reconstruction in young adults. *Clin Orthop Relat Res* 1999;367:272-282.

Miller MD: Revision cruciate ligament surgery with retention of femoral interference screws. *Arthroscopy* 1998;14(1):111-114.

Noyes FR, Barber-Westin SD: Revision anterior cruciate ligament reconstruction: Report of 11-year experience and results in 114 consecutive patients. *Instr Course Lect* 2001;50:451-461.

Noyes FR, Barber-Westin SD: Revision anterior cruciate surgery with use of bone-patellar tendon-bone autogenous grafts. *J Bone Joint Surg Am* 2001;83-A(8):1131-1143.

Petsche TS, Hutchinson MR: Loss of extension after reconstruction of the anterior cruciate ligament. *J Am Acad Orthop Surg* 1999;7(2):119-127.

Salmon LJ, Pinczewski LA, Russell VJ, Refshauge K: Revision anterior cruciate ligament reconstruction with hamstring tendon autograft: 5- to 9-year follow-up. *Am J Sports Med* 2006;34(10):1604-1614.

Saperstein AL, Fetto JF: The anterior cruciate ligament-deficient knee: A diagnostic and therapeutic algorithm. *Orthop Rev* 1992;21(11):1297-1305.

Spindler KP, Kuhn JE, Freedman KB, Matthews CE, Dittus RS, Harrell FE Jr: Anterior cruciate ligament reconstruction autograft choice: Bone-tendon-bone versus hamstring: Does it really matter? A systematic review. *Am J Sports Med* 2004;32(8):1986-1995.

Spindler KP, Wright RW: Clinical practice: Anterior cruciate ligament tear. *N Engl J Med* 2008;359(20):2135-2142.

Wright RW, Dunn WR, Amendola A, et al: MOON Cohort: Anterior cruciate ligament revision reconstruction: Two-year results from the MOON cohort. *J Knee Surg* 2007;20(4):308-311.

Wright RW, Dunn WR, Amendola A, et al: Risk of tearing the intact anterior cruciate ligament in the contralateral knee and rupturing the anterior cruciate ligament graft during the first 2 years after anterior cruciate ligament reconstruction: A prospective MOON cohort study. *Am J Sports Med* 2007;35(7):1131-1134.

Zelle BA, Vidal AF, Brucker PU, Fu FH: Double-bundle reconstruction of the anterior cruciate ligament: Anatomic and biomechanical rationale. *J Am Acad Orthop Surg* 2007;15(2):87-96.

Chapter 65

Graft Choices for Anterior Cruciate Ligament Reconstruction: Bone–Patellar Tendon–Bone Graft

Bernard R. Bach, Jr, MD
Dana P. Piasecki, MD

Indications

Isolated anterior cruciate ligament (ACL) reconstruction is indicated in patients with clinical evidence of knee instability and a desire to continue performing cutting/pivoting activities. The specific indications for bone–patellar tendon–bone (BTB) reconstructions are relative and are dictated largely by surgeon preference. Given the objective evidence that these grafts provide superior stability to the knee with minimal donor-site morbidity with more aggressive postoperative rehabilitation protocols, we prefer this graft over other available options. In younger, highly active patients, the reliable incorporation of autograft tissue is preferable to allografts because of the issues that accompany the latter (risk of disease transmission, slower incorporation of allografts). In older patients (over 30 years of age), allografts are preferable because of the easier postoperative recovery and reduced donor-site morbidity.

Contraindications

ACL reconstruction should not be done before patients regain full motion and quadriceps strength, nor is it indicated in low-demand patients who do not wish to perform cutting/pivoting activities or those who will not comply with postoperative rehabilitation. Reconstruction also is contraindicated in patients with significant limb malalignment or secondary stabilizer deficiency if these are not corrected concomitantly. BTB autografts should not be harvested from patients with patellar tendon abnormalities (history of rupture, prior graft harvest), with patellofemoral instability or maltracking, or with particularly narrow tendons.

Alternative Treatments

Alternatives to ligament reconstruction include avoidance of cutting/pivoting activities or, in patients who participate in these activities infrequently, the use of functional bracing. Alternatives to BTB grafts include soft-tissue only grafts (hamstring autografts or allografts) and bone–soft tissue grafts (quadriceps autograft or allograft, Achilles tendon allograft).

Results

Modern endoscopic ACL reconstruction produces excellent outcomes in most patients (Table 1). Differences in mean instrumented side-to-side laxity measurements have been reported as negligible in 70% to 95% of patients after reconstruction, with more than 90% participating in vigorous cutting/pivoting activities. Overall satisfaction with a willingness to undergo the surgery again also is reported by more than 90% of patients. Several large retrospective and prospective series have demonstrated 80% to 90% good to excellent outcomes after 3 to 10 years of follow-up using the classic BTB autograft, with additional reports demonstrating similar outcomes using BTB allograft, hamstring autograft, and Achilles tendon allograft. Nonetheless, BTB grafts appear to provide superior improvements in postoperative instrumented laxity measure-

Dr. Bach or an immediate family member has received research or institutional support from Smith & Nephew, DJ Orthopedics, MioMed Orthopaedics, Athletico, Ossur, Arthrex, and Scheck & Siress. Neither Dr. Piasecki nor any immediate family member has received anything of value from or owns stock in a commercial company related directly or indirectly to the subject of this chapter.

Table 1 Results of ACL Reconstruction With Bone–Patellar Tendon–Bone Graft

Author(s) (Year)	Number of Knees	Mean Patient Age (Range)	Graft Type	Mean Follow-up (Range)	Outcomes	Failure Rate
Bach et al (1998)	97	26 years (12-53)	BTB autograft	(5 to 9 years)	>90% good to excellent results <3 mm side-to-side differences in 70%	0%
Peterson et al (2001)	60	25 years (14-49)	30 BTB autograft 30 allograft	63 months (55 to 78)	No differences in outcome (90% good to excellent) or instrumented laxity (<3 mm in 70%)	3.3% in both groups,
Beynnon et al (2002)	56	29 years (18-46)	28 BTB autograft 28 hamstring autograft	39 months (36 to 57)	No subjective or functional differences Mean instrumented laxity 4.4 mm for hamstring graft versus 1.1 for BTB graft Decreased knee flexion strength in hamstring patients	0%
Bach et al (2005)	60	41 years (18-61)	BTB allograft	51 months	>80% good to excellent results: <3 mm side-to-side differences in 95%	0%

BTB = bone–patellar tendon–bone.

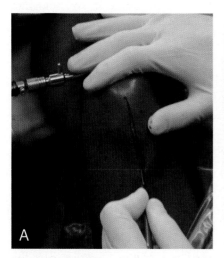 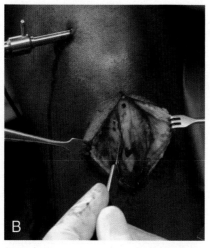

Figure 1 Graft harvest for ACL reconstruction. **A,** The incision is made from the inferior pole of the patella to the medial aspect of the tibial tubercle. **B,** Harvesting the graft.

ments when compared with soft-tissue grafts and with minimal morbidity.

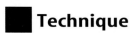

Technique

Patient Positioning and Setup

Surgery is done with the patient supine and following administration of preoperative antibiotics and a general anesthetic. Before definitive positioning, the injured knee is carefully examined under anesthesia to grade ACL insufficiency and assess potential secondary restraint compromise. A padded tourniquet is then placed on the surgical thigh, which is stabilized in a leg holder. The nonsurgical limb is supported in an obstetric stirrup, the lumbar spine is flexed to protect the femoral and common peroneal nerves, and the surgical limb is prepared and draped. If a pivot shift is appreciated during the examination under anesthesia, we proceed with graft preparation before diagnostic arthroscopy. If the knee does not demonstrate a definitive pivot, a thorough diagnostic arthroscopy is done before harvesting the autograft (or thawing the allograft).

Graft Harvest

The autograft is harvested with the knee in flexion to maintain tension on the patellar tendon. A 6- to 8-cm longitudinal incision is made, aligned with the medial border of the tendon (**Figure 1,** *A*), extending from the inferior pole of the patella to the medial aspect of the tibial tubercle. Skin flaps are raised, and the paratenon is carefully divided longitudinally to expose the underlying tendon. The centers of the inferior pole of the patella and tibial tubercle are then marked, and the width of the tendon is measured to confirm that a 10-mm graft can be accommodated. To create the bone plugs, the dimensions (10 mm wide × 25 mm long) are measured and score marks are made with a knife at the inferior pole of the patella and proximal tibial tubercle. Full-thickness division of the tendon is done with a scalpel in line with the fibers of the tendon and on either side of the 10-mm central-third graft (**Figure 1, B**). An oscillating saw with a 10-mm blade is then used to cut the bone plugs. When obtaining the tibial plug, the saw blade is angled roughly 45° to the midline to preserve tubercle bone on either side of the graft, creating a plug that is triangular on cross section. The patella is cut in a similar fashion, although the blade of the saw is angled more vertically (roughly 60°) to create a more trapezoidal graft to reduce the risk of perforating the subchondral bone. Additional care must be taken not to violate the superior pole during patellar plug harvest or to allow bone cuts to cross each other at the plug corners because stress risers in these locations may lead to iatrogenic fracture. Following completion of the bone cuts, both plugs are gently pried loose with an osteotome, the tendinous portion is dissected free of the fat pad, and the graft is then transported to the back table by the operating surgeon to reduce the likelihood of it being dropped.

 Video 65.1 Patellar Tendon Harvest for ACL Reconstruction. J.W. Thomas Byrd, MD (4 min)

If an allograft is used, we prefer a fresh-frozen, nonirradiated or low-dose–irradiated, whole or hemi patellar tendon–bone graft, sized relative to the patient's height. Once thawed, the graft is positioned by an assistant with the patella proximal and the tibial tubercle distal (the same orientation as would be seen during an autograft har-

vest). An identical sequence of steps is then undertaken as described for autograft harvest.

Final fashioning of the autograft or allograft is done with a rongeur such that 10 × 10 × 25-mm bone plugs are created. If one plug is appreciably shorter than the other, we recommend using the shorter plug for the tibial side to help alleviate potential graft-tunnel mismatch. Using a 0.62-inch Kirschner wire, two holes are drilled parallel to the cortical surface and perpendicular to the long axis of whichever bone plug is designated for tibial tunnel fixation; a traction suture is placed through each hole. The patellar tendon length is measured and noted, and a marking pen is used to mark the bone-tendon junction of each plug, as well as the cortical margin of the plug intended for tibial-side fixation. The graft is then wrapped in a clearly marked lap sponge and placed in a secure location on the back table.

Diagnostic Arthroscopy

An initial diagnostic arthroscopy is always done using a superomedial outflow portal and standard inferolateral (IL) viewing and inferomedial (IM) instrumentation portals. In the case of allograft reconstruction, these portals are created through individual portal incisions, but when autograft patellar tendon grafts are harvested first, the IL and IM portals can be created within the graft harvest incision. Careful attention is paid to the articular surfaces, meniscal status, and the presence or absence of loose bodies.

Intercondylar Notch Exposure and Preparation

To maximize visualization and subsequent instrumentation of the intercondylar notch, we routinely débride the innermost portion of the fat pad. With the arthroscope in the IL portal, a large shaver is introduced through the IM portal and used to resect the fat pad from the intercondylar notch anteromedially along the medial gutter,

including the medial plica sheet and shelf. The arthroscope is then repositioned laterally, and the fat pad is further excised to the lateral condylar margin with the shaver placed in the IM portal. Once visualization of the notch is maximized in this way, the ACL stump and status of the posterior cruciate ligament (PCL) can be assessed easily.

Intercondylar notch preparation begins with a "soft-tissue notchplasty." The ACL stump and remnant tissue along the lateral wall are morcellized with arthroscopic scissors and an elevator, and the fragments are removed with a large shaver and radiofrequency ablation. Once this is complete, the posterior wall of the notch and lateral border of the PCL, in addition to the osseous tibial insertion of the ACL, should be visible and easily probed.

A bony notchplasty is then made with a curved ¼-inch osteotome introduced through the IM portal. A width of bone is removed from the anteromedial portion of the lateral femoral condyle such that roughly 1 cm of space is created between the PCL and the lateral wall following resection (**Figure 2, A**). Bone fragments are removed with a grasper. When an autograft is used, the fragments are saved for later grafting of the patellar and tibial donor sites. A spherical burr is used to continue the resection of the lateral wall from anterior to posterior, gently contouring the roof and superolateral corner of the notch so that instead of a pointed Gothic arch shape, it has a more squared corner, resembling a Roman arch (**Figure 2, B**). In practice, more bone is removed posteriorly than anteriorly. An adequate notchplasty improves both visualization and instrumentation of the notch, greatly facilitating later anatomic positioning of the femoral tunnel with a transtibial technique.

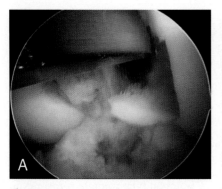
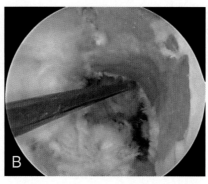

Figure 2 Bony notchplasty. **A,** The bony notchplasty is initiated with an osteotome. **B,** The completed notchplasty should have a distinct superolateral corner and a back wall that can be hooked easily with a probe. The squared superolateral corner of the finished notch resembles a Roman arch.

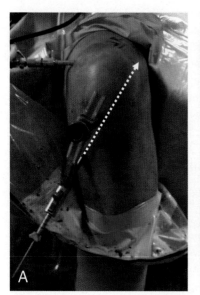
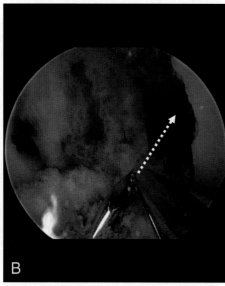

Figure 3 Creating the tibial tunnel in a left knee. **A,** The tibial aimer is inserted through an accessory IM portal, which allows a more horizontal orientation of the guide pin. Note the oblique angle that the pin makes relative to the joint line in the coronal plane, with the tip of the pin pointing roughly to the 1:30 position. (In a right knee, the pin would point to the 10:30 position.) **B,** The guide pin is drilled through the center of the ACL tibial insertion. Note that the low-angled trajectory of the aimer (dashed arrow) creates a pin trajectory that is low on the lateral wall of the notch, facilitating later transtibial drilling of the femoral tunnel.

Tibial Tunnel

Following notch preparation, the tibial tunnel is created. An accessory transpatellar tendon portal is first established roughly 1 cm lateral and distal to the IM portal, through which the tibial aimer is introduced. The more lateral position of this portal relative to the IM portal allows increased external rotation of the aimer to facilitate an oblique orientation of the resulting tibial tunnel. Additionally, the portal's more distal location helps position the aimer's external trocar farther from the joint line, resulting in a longer tibial tunnel and thereby reducing the likelihood of graft-tunnel mismatch. A spinal needle is first used to localize this accessory portal, through the patellar tendon (or autograft harvest defect) and just above the joint line. The ability to translate the needle off the tibial articular surface confirms that the position is not too distal. The tip of the tibial drill guide, set at an angle equal to the length of the graft's patellar tendon plus 10 (N+10), is then introduced through this accessory IM portal. We typically use an elbow guide, positioning the tip of this guide 3 to 4 mm posterior and slightly lateral to a point midway between the two tibial spines and along the posterior margin of the anterior horn of the lateral meniscus. The elbow of the guide should lie along a line connecting the center of the tibial insertion of the native ACL and the desired location on the femur. The external trocar of the drill guide is then seated on the outer tibia, either through an accessory incision (allograft) or the graft harvest site (autograft).

Once the tip of the guide is placed appropriately within the joint and the extra-articular drill sleeve is firmly apposed to the tibial metaphysis, a final external check of alignment can be made by evaluating the angle the guide makes to the vertical. This angle should correspond to the 1:30 position for a left knee (**Figure 3,** *A*) or the 10:30 position for a right knee, with the center of the patella denoted as 12:00 on a clock face. If placement is adequate, a 3/32-inch Steinmann pin is drilled through the drill guide into the joint. If the guide is positioned appropriately, the tip of the pin should penetrate the joint midway between the two spines and along the posterior margin of the anterior horn of the lateral meniscus. The trajectory of the pin should be to a 1:30 position (in a left knee) along the lateral wall of the notch (**Figure 3,** *B*). The drill guide is then removed, and the knee is brought into extension to confirm that the pin does not inappropriately impinge on the roof of the notch (ie, that it is not placed too anterior). If the pin position is deemed adequate, the knee is brought back into flexion, and the pin is gently tapped into the femur, both to confirm an adequate trajectory and to secure it for tunnel reaming. An 11-mm cannulated reamer is then passed over the pin to ream the tibial tunnel. The tibial tunnel is over-reamed by 1 mm to reduce the likelihood of delaminating the soft tissue of the graft during later passage. Following intra-articular perforation, fluid inflow is clamped to facilitate collection of tunnel reamings that drain through the tibial tunnel and are saved on the back table for grafting of autograft harvest sites. Once soft tissue is cleared from the tunnel entrance with a shaver, a chamfer reamer and hand rasp are used to bevel the posterolateral corner of the tunnel to further facilitate transtibial instrumentation and subsequent positioning of the femoral tunnel. A shaver placed retrograde through the tibial tunnel also can be used for this purpose. This eliminates the ledge of cortical bone on the posterior portion of the tunnel that would otherwise necessitate extending the knee to properly position the femoral offset aimer.

Femoral Tunnel

The femoral tunnel is created through a transtibial approach. A 7-mm offset aimer is introduced retrograde through the tibial tunnel. The lip of the guide is placed along the posterior wall of the notch, and its handle is externally rotated to bring the inserted pin to an even lower position along the lateral wall (**Figure 4, *A***). If the notch was prepared adequately and the tibial tunnel was positioned appropriately, this guide should allow placement of a pin at the 1:30 position in a left knee (10:30 in a right knee) on the wall of the notch. Excessive force should not be required to position the offset guide appropriately. If it is necessary to lever the aimer over the back of the tibial tunnel or posterior intercondylar notch, the trajectory of subsequent pin placement may be too posterior and could result in compromise of the posterior wall. Likewise, an inability to obtain the 1:30 position

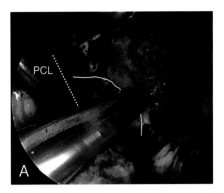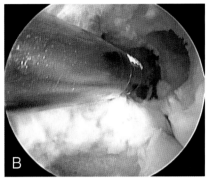

Figure 4 Creating the tibial tunnel in a right knee. **A,** A 7-mm offset guide is inserted through the tibial tunnel and externally rotated to place the femoral tunnel guide pin low on the wall of the notch. Note the angle the guide and pin make relative to the PCL. (The dotted line marks the lateral margin of the PCL, which is being retracted with a probe; the solid line marks the edge of the posterior notch.) **B,** Appearance of the completed femoral tunnel. Note the anatomic position of the tunnel, spanning the 1:00 to 3:00 position.

in a left knee or the 10:30 position in a right knee may compromise rotational stability by positioning the femoral tunnel too vertically. If additional beveling of the posterior aspect of the tibial tunnel or additional notchplasty does not allow for an adequate femoral tunnel position, we advise creating an accessory anteromedial (AM) portal just distal to the standard IM portal, through which the aimer and pin/reamer assembly can be more easily and correctly positioned on the femoral side. Once this is positioned appropriately, a 3/32-inch Steinmann pin is drilled into the femur through the guide to a depth of 30 to 35 mm. A 10-mm cannulated reamer is then inserted and used to create a 5- to 8-mm-deep footprint for the femoral tunnel. Because the offset guide positions the pin 7 mm anterior to the posterior "over the top" cortex, a 10-mm reamer (5-mm radius) will leave 2 mm of bone at the posterior wall if these steps are performed correctly. Withdrawing the reamer after this initial reaming allows a probe to be used through the IM portal to confirm that the posterior wall remains intact or, if the wall is compromised, to allow repositioning of the pin before definitive tunnel reaming. If the trajectory of reaming is satisfactory, the reamer can be advanced over the wire to a tunnel depth

of 30 to 35 mm and then removed with the wire (**Figure 4, *B***). A secondary contouring of the lateral wall of the notch often is done at this point to remove excess bone anterior to the entrance of the femoral tunnel for ease of later graft passage and fixation. Final inspection of the femoral tunnel is made by passing the arthroscope retrograde through the tibial tunnel, allowing final confirmation that the posterior wall is intact, that there is no intratunnel blowout, and that a small rim of posterior cortex remains.

Graft Passage and Fixation

Once soft tissue is cleared from the metaphyseal entrance of the tibial tunnel, the graft is taken from the back table and the femoral bone plug is pushed through the tunnel into the joint with a graft pusher; the cancellous surface of the plug is oriented anteriorly and the cortex posteriorly. With the arthroscope in the IL portal, a curved hemostat is introduced through the IM portal to receive the bone plug and direct it into the femoral tunnel entrance (a "push-in" technique). Once the plug is inserted roughly two thirds of the way in, the curved hemostat is used to dilate the plug–femoral tunnel interface at the 11 o'clock position. A flexible nitinol wire is introduced through the IM por-

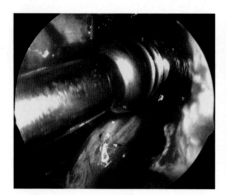

Figure 5 Femoral fixation with an interference screw. Note that the screw is inserted parallel to the axis of the graft to avoid screw divergence or graft transection.

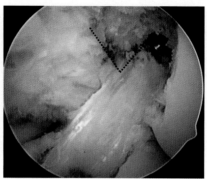

Figure 6 Final graft position in a left knee. Note the anatomic relationship of this single-bundle graft relative to the normal tibial insertion, the wall of the notch, and the PCL. The normal space between the PCL and ACL at the roof of the notch is recreated (dotted lines), and the reconstructed femoral insertion extends from the 1:00 to the 3:00 position. (This would be from 9:00 to 11:00 in a right knee.)

tal into this interface and advanced until the pin bottoms out in the depth of the socket. A blunt graft pusher is then used to tamp the plug to a flush position with the tunnel entrance, at which time the tibial end of the graft should be inspected for possible graft-tunnel mismatch. If significant protrusion of the tibial plug exists at this point, the femoral plug can be recessed up to 10 mm farther into the femoral tunnel to still allow 15 mm of overlap with an interference screw. If the mismatch is only minimal, the plug is left flush with the femur and fixed with a 7 × 25-mm metal interference screw, threaded over the nitinol wire (**Figure 5**). During screw insertion, care must be taken to thread the screw along a line colinear with the long axis of the plug to avoid inadvertent divergence or graft laceration. This is easier to do if an assistant hyperflexes the knee during screw insertion. Once the end of the screw is flush with the notch, the screwdriver is removed and the graft is cycled to remove creep. The knee is then brought into extension to confirm the absence of roof impingement and, if graft position is adequate, the arthroscope is removed for tibial fixation.

Tibial fixation is done with the knee axially loaded in extension to prevent overconstraining of the joint. Before fixation, the tibial bone plug is externally rotated 180° with a curved hemostat so that the cortical portion of the graft, once posterior, is now facing anteriorly and in the coronal plane. The terminal portion of the bone plug is checked to be sure it is not incarcerated on the inner rim of the tunnel (preventing adequate tensioning of the graft), and a 9 × 20-mm metal interference screw is then introduced over a nitinol wire into the interface between the plug and anterior aspect of the tunnel. Providing a cortical surface for screw interdigitation and impacting the cancellous portion of the bone plug to the posterior margin of the tunnel will maximize pullout strength. Having the tibial screw anterior also prevents ligament abrasion on the tip of the screw during knee flexion if there is some advancement of the screw beyond the tendoosseous interval. After full insertion of the screw, Lachman and pivot-shift tests are performed as a final confirmation of knee stability. Final graft appearance is then confirmed arthroscopically and should mirror the normal ACL anatomy with respect to its tibial and femoral insertions. An anatomically placed graft will mimic

the normal triangle of space between the ACL and PCL (**Figure 6**). In autograft reconstructions, bone graft collected from the BTB preparation and tibial and femoral tunnel reamings are packed into the distal patellar and tibial tubercle defects before closure.

Wound Closure

When an autograft is used, the central patellar tendon defect is loosely approximated with the knee in flexion to minimize shortening of the extensor mechanism. The paratenon is then closed over the tendon, followed by interrupted dermal sutures and a running subcuticular stitch. Simple sutures are used for portal closure, and local anesthetic (0.5% bupivicaine) is routinely injected into the joint and all incisions.

——————————■

■ Postoperative Regimen

All patients are placed in a hinged, drop-lock knee brace at the time of surgery. They begin immediate active range-of-motion exercises and are encouraged to bear weight as tolerated with the brace locked in extension. To protect the donor site, autograft reconstructions are braced for 6 weeks postoperatively, but bracing can be discontinued in allograft patients at 7 to 10 days. Closed-chain strengthening is initiated as soon as patients can bear weight comfortably on the surgical limb. A strong emphasis is placed on achieving full knee extension rapidly, with supervised patellar mobilization, passive range of motion, and prone heel hangs. At 6 weeks, motion (typically 0° to 120° or more) and closed-chain strengthening are advanced. Jogging is permitted at 8 weeks; agility, plyometric, and sport-specific activities at 3 months; and a return to sport in 4.5 to 6 months. We encourage ACL functional bracing during cutting/pivoting activities until 1 year after surgery.

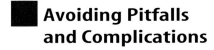

Avoiding Pitfalls and Complications

Careful attention to detail is of paramount importance for a successful ACL reconstruction. This applies to all portions of the procedure, but the greatest potential for error occurs during tunnel placement. With use of the described landmarks, the surgeon should be able to consistently place the tibial tunnel in an anatomic position; however, several factors demand focus when positioning the femoral tunnel through a transtibial technique. We recommend that extra time be taken to expose the lateral intercondylar notch and to confirm that the tibial tunnel is adequately oblique to ensure that the femoral tunnel is created at the 1:30 (in a left knee) or 10:30 (in a right knee) position. It also is recommended that sagittal orientation of the femoral tunnel guide pin be closely monitored to prevent posterior wall blow-out. Reaming or rasping the posterior lip of the tibial tunnel helps to orient this pin safely, reducing the risk of the femoral tunnel violating the posterior femoral cortex. If a proper femoral tunnel position and orientation cannot be obtained with a transtibial technique, the femoral tunnel can be drilled through the IM (or accessory AM) portal. If the described technique is carefully followed, portions of both the PL and AM bundles can be reconstructed with a well-positioned single-bundle graft, eliminating both the Lachman and pivot-shift tests and producing consistently excellent clinical results with a low failure rate.

Bibliography

Bach BR Jr, Aadalen KJ, Dennis MG, et al: Primary anterior cruciate ligament reconstruction using fresh-frozen, nonirradiated patellar tendon allograft: Minimum 2-year follow-up. *Am J Sports Med* 2005;33:284-292.

Bach BR Jr, Levy ME, Bojchuk J, Tradonsky S, Bush-Joseph CA, Khan NH: Single-incision endoscopic anterior cruciate ligament reconstruction using patellar tendon autograft: Minimum two-year follow-up evaluation. *Am J Sports Med* 1998;26:30-40.

Bach BR Jr, Tradonsky S, Bojchuk J, Levy ME, Bush-Joseph CA, Khan NH: Arthroscopically assisted anterior cruciate ligament reconstruction using patellar tendon autograft: Five- to nine-year follow-up evaluation. *Am J Sports Med* 1998;26:20-29.

Beynnon BD, Johnson RJ, Fleming BC, et al: Anterior cruciate ligament replacement: Comparison of bone-patellar tendon-bone grafts with two-strand hamstring grafts. A prospective, randomized study. *J Bone Joint Surg Am* 2002;84:1503-1513.

Chang SK, Egami DK, Shaieb MD, Kan DM, Richardson AB: Anterior cruciate ligament reconstruction: Allograft versus autograft. *Arthroscopy* 2003;19:453-462.

Kleipool AE, Zijl JA, Willems WJ: Arthroscopic anterior cruciate ligament reconstruction with bone-patellar tendon-bone allograft or autograft: A prospective study with an average follow up of 4 years. *Knee Surg Sports Traumatol Arthrosc* 1998;6:224-230.

Levitt RL, Malinin T, Posada A, Michalow A: Reconstruction of anterior cruciate ligaments with bone-patellar tendon-bone and achilles tendon allografts. *Clin Orthop Relat Res* 1994;303:67-78.

Otto D, Pinczewski LA, Clingeleffer A, Odell R: Five-year results of single-incision arthroscopic anterior cruciate ligament reconstruction with patellar tendon autograft. *Am J Sports Med* 1998;26:181-188.

Peterson RK, Shelton WR, Bomboy AL: Allograft versus autograft patellar tendon anterior cruciate ligament reconstruction: A 5-year follow-up. *Arthroscopy* 2001;17:9-13.

Shaieb MD, Kan DM, Chang SK, Marumoto JM, Richardson AB: A prospective randomized comparison of patellar tendon versus semitendinosus and gracilis tendon autografts for anterior cruciate ligament reconstruction. *Am J Sports Med* 2002;30:214-220.

Shelbourne KD, Gray T: Results of anterior cruciate ligament reconstruction based on meniscus and articular cartilage status at the time of surgery: Five- to fifteen-year evaluations. *Am J Sports Med* 2000;28:446-452.

Spindler KP, Warren TA, Callison JC Jr, Secic M, Fleisch SB, Wright RW: Clinical outcome at a minimum of five years after reconstruction of the anterior cruciate ligament. *J Bone Joint Surg Am* 2005;87:1673-1679.

■ Video Reference

Byrd JWT: Video. *Patellar Tendon Harvest for ACL Reconstruction*. Video clip from Basic Principles in Endoscopic ACL Reconstruction: Patellar Tendon Autograft, in Johnson DJ, ed: *Surgical Techniques in Orthopaedics: Anterior Cruciate Ligament Reconstruction*. DVD. Rosemont, IL, American Academy of Orthopaedic Surgeons, 2002.

Coding

CPT Codes		Corresponding ICD-9 Codes	
Anterior Cruciate Ligament Repair			
29888	Arthroscopically aided anterior cruciate ligament repair/augmentation or reconstruction	717.83 717.84	717.84 844.2
Additional Procedure Codes Referenced in This Chapter			
29870	Arthroscopy, knee, diagnostic, with or without synovial biopsy (separate procedure)	715	733
20900	Bone graft, any donor area; minor or small (eg, dowel or button)	715	733
20902	Bone graft, any donor area; major or large	715	

CPT copyright © 2010 by the American Medical Association. All rights reserved.

Chapter 66

Graft Choices for ACL Reconstruction: Hamstring Graft

Champ L. Baker, Jr, MD
Champ L. Baker III, MD

 ## Indications

Hamstring (semitendinosus and gracilis) autografts have become an increasingly popular choice for anterior cruciate ligament (ACL) reconstruction because of their excellent biomechanical properties, improved fixation, and minimal harvest-site morbidity. Quadrupled hamstring tendons are our preferred autograft in patients with a history of patellar tendinitis, patellofemoral pain or instability, or extensor mechanism surgery or injury. For individuals whose occupations or lifestyles require kneeling, hamstring grafts may be preferable to bone–patellar tendon–bone autografts. Hamstring grafts also are preferred in patients with open physes.

Contraindications

An absolute contraindication to the use of a hamstring autograft is a previous hamstring harvest. Relative contraindications include generalized ligamentous laxity and previous hamstring injury. Hamstring autografts should not be used in athletes such as competitive sprinters who require high peak knee flexion torque because terminal flexion weakness persists with these grafts.

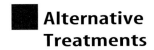 ## Alternative Treatments

Excellent clinical results have been achieved with a variety of both autograft and allograft tissues. Alternative autograft choices include bone–patellar tendon–bone and quadriceps tendon grafts. Allograft choices include bone–patellar tendon–bone, Achilles tendon, hamstring tendon, anterior tibialis tendon, and posterior tibialis tendon grafts.

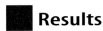 ## Results

Earlier studies and meta-analyses detailing results of hamstring autograft ACL reconstructions typically included older fixation methods and graft constructs with double-stranded grafts. These studies concluded that ACL reconstruction with hamstring grafts resulted in inferior clinical outcomes compared to reconstructions with bone–patellar tendon–bone autografts. More recently, multiple randomized controlled trials comparing outcomes of ACL reconstruction with quadrupled hamstring grafts and with bone–patellar tendon–bone autografts have concluded that the grafts provide equivalent clinical and functional outcomes at follow-up. Reconstruction with quadrupled hamstring grafts provides a high rate of good and excellent clinical outcomes, a low rate of graft failure, and minimal graft harvest morbidity (**Table 1**).

Technique

Patient Positioning and Anesthesia

The patient is positioned supine on the operating room table. Typically, general anesthesia is administered, but a spinal anesthetic with concurrent intravenous sedation is an acceptable alternative. An examination under anesthesia is done on both the surgical and nonsurgical extremities to evaluate and document range of motion, varus/valgus instability, an-

Dr. Champ Baker, Jr, or an immediate family member serves as a board member, owner, officer, or committee member of the American Orthopaedic Society for Sports Medicine; serves as an unpaid consultant to Arthrex; and owns stock or stock options in Arthrex. Dr. Champ Baker III or an immediate family member serves as an unpaid consultant to Arthrex.

Table 1 Results of ACL Reconstruction Using Quadrupled Hamstring Grafts

Author(s) (Year)	Number of Knees	Fixation	Mean Patient Age in Years (Range)	Mean Follow-up (Range)	Results
Feller and Webster (2003)	34	Femoral: EndoButton (Smith & Nephew Endoscopy, Mansfield, MA) Post-tibial: Acufex fixation (Smith & Nephew Endoscopy)	26.3	36 months	Cincinnati 93.7 IKDC 37% normal; 56% nearly normal; 7% abnormal
Gobbi et al (2003)	80	Femoral: EndoButton Tibial: Fastlok (Neoligaments, Leeds, England)	28	36 months (24-52)	Noyes 88 Lysholm 91 Tegner 6.5 IKDC: 72 normal/nearly normal; 7 abnormal; 1 severely abnormal
Prodromos et al (2005)	139	Femoral: EndoButton Tibial: Screw and washer	Skeletally mature	54.4 months (24-104)	KT-1000: Full stability Noyes 94 Lysholm 94.5 SANE 90
Lidén et al (2007)	37	Soft-headed interference screws	29 (15-59)	86 months (68-114)	Lysholm 90 Tegner 6 IKDC: 50% normal/nearly normal; 50% abnormal/ severely abnormal
Pinczewski (2007)	90	Titanium cannulated interference screws	24 (13-52)	10 years	IKDC: 97% normal or nearly normal Lysholm 91% good or excellent

NA = not available, IKDC = International Knee Documentation Committee, SANE = Single Assessment Numeric Evaluation.

teromedial and posterolateral rotatory instability, and Lachman and pivot-shift test results. If the evaluation under anesthesia confirms the preoperative diagnosis of an ACL tear, the graft is harvested before arthroscopy. If there is any uncertainty regarding the diagnosis, a diagnostic arthroscopy is done first. A well-padded tourniquet is applied to the proximal thigh of the surgical extremity, which is then placed in an arthroscopic leg holder. The foot of the table is lowered so the surgical knee can be hyperflexed to at least 120°. Prophylactic antibiotics are administered. The leg is then prepared and draped.

Graft Harvest

A 4-cm vertical incision is centered over the insertion of the gracilis and semitendinosus tendons, located approximately 2 cm distal and 2 cm medial to the tibial tubercle (**Figure 1**, *A*). Dissection is carried through the subcutaneous tissues with Metzenbaum scissors until the sartorial fascia is encountered. The overlying subcutaneous fat is cleared off with a laparotomy sponge. The gracilis and semitendinosus tendons are palpated directly (**Figure 1**, *B*). The sartorial fascia is incised in line with and just proximal to the gracilis tendon. A hemostat is then inserted underneath the fascia and tendons to protect the underlying medial collateral ligament (MCL) as the insertions of the gracilis and semitendinosus are sharply released from the tibia, creating an inverted L-shaped sartorial fascial flap (**Figure 1**, *C*). The tendons are more readily identified and separated on the undersurface of the fascial flap. A right-angle clamp is used to grasp the distal end of the gracilis tendon, and the tendon is separated from the fascia by blunt dissection. An attempt should be made to preserve the fascial layer for later closure. A No. 2 nonabsorbable suture is placed in the distal 25 mm of tendon in a whipstitch fashion. Before harvest, care is taken to ensure that all fascial bands connected to the tendon are released to decrease the risk of premature graft amputation (**Figure 1**, *D*). The gracilis tendon is harvested with a closed-end tendon stripper. The stripper is advanced parallel to the course of the tendon, aiming toward its insertion on the pubis, while tension is maintained on the grasping sutures (**Figure 1**, *E*). The semitendinosus tendon is harvested in a similar fashion. More extensive fascial connections to the medial head of the gas-

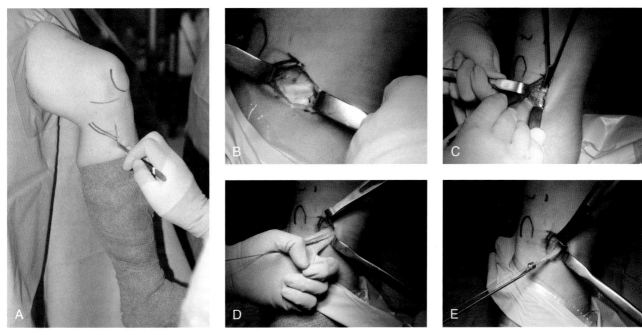

Figure 1 Harvesting the hamstring graft. **A,** An incision is made over the insertion of the hamstrings approximately 2 cm medial and 2 cm inferior to the tibial tubercle. **B,** After clearing off the overlying subcutaneous fat, the insertions of the gracilis and semitendinosus tendons are readily visible and palpable. **C,** A hemostat placed beneath the hamstring insertion protects the underlying medial collateral ligament as the tendons are released off the tibia. **D,** All fascial connections are released with a combination of sharp and blunt dissection before harvesting the graft. **E,** The tendon stripper is placed over the prepared tendon and advanced toward the origin of the tendon while tension is maintained on the sutures.

trocnemius are present and must be released for successful tendon harvest. If the skin overlying the gastrocnemius is seen to "pucker" when tension is placed on the semitendinosus tendon, these fascial bands have been inadequately released. When the tendon stripper is advanced over the freed semitendinosus, it should be aimed toward the ischial tuberosity to remain parallel to the tendon course.

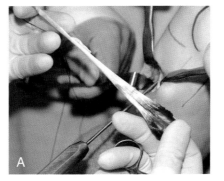 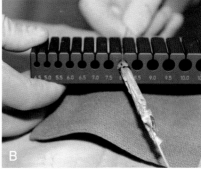

Figure 2 Hamstring graft preparation. **A,** The harvested semitendinosus tendon graft. **B,** The graft is placed in the sizing tube.

 66.1 Hamstring Harvest for ACL Reconstruction. Eugene M. Wolf, MD (3 min)

Graft Preparation

The harvested grafts are prepared on a back table. Muscle is stripped from the tendons with a #10 blade (**Figure 2, A**). The ends of the tendons are trimmed, and a running whipstich is passed with a No. 2 nonabsorbable suture in the proximal ends of the tendons. Each tendon is then looped over a heavy suture to create the quadruple-stranded graft for sizing purposes. The construct is passed through sizing tubes in 0.5-mm increments to determine the appropriate size of the tunnels for graft passage and seating (**Figure 2, B**).

Arthroscopy

An anterolateral portal is created adjacent to the lateral border of the patellar tendon. An anteromedial portal is created under direct visualization after localization with a spinal needle. Diagnostic arthroscopy is performed, and associated chondral or meniscal injuries are treated. If an inside-out meniscal repair is done, the sutures are tied after fixation of the graft. The

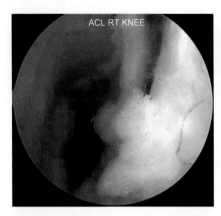

Figure 3 Appearance of the intercondylar notch after limited notchplasty.

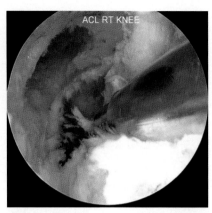

Figure 4 The femoral tunnel has been drilled. This tunnel is located slightly higher on the intercondylar wall than our current preference, in a more traditional location.

ACL remnant is identified and removed with arthroscopic scissors and a motorized shaver. Fibers of the ACL tibial footprint are preserved to later assist with proper tibial tunnel placement. The lateral wall and intercondylar notch roof lateral to the posterior cruciate ligament (PCL) are cleared of all soft tissue, and the over-the-top position is identified. A hooked probe is used to confirm the over-the-top position. Mistaking the more anterior "resident's ridge" for the over-the-top position leads to a too-anterior femoral tunnel. We prefer to perform a limited notchplasty to enhance visualization and limit potential graft impingement. A burr is used to remove a small amount of bone from the lateral wall and roof (**Figure 3**).

Tibial Tunnel Placement

Proper anatomic placement of the tibial and femoral tunnels is critical for the ACL reconstruction to resist anterior tibial translation and control rotational stability. With a transtibial technique, the location of the femoral tunnel is predetermined largely by the position of the tibial tunnel. Traditionally we have used the transtibial technique, but we have begun to transition to drilling the femoral tunnel independently of the tibial tunnel with the medial portal technique. With the transtibial technique, a tip ACL guide set at 50° is inserted into the joint

through the medial portal. The landmarks for the guidewire placement have been well described. We attempt to position our guidewire in the center of the preserved ACL footprint, which is located between the tibial spines at the level of the posterior edge of the anterior horn of the lateral meniscus. The coronal obliquity of the tibial tunnel is critical for proper anatomic placement of the femoral tunnel low on the lateral wall. Medial placement of the tibial starting point along the anterior edge of the MCL provides a proper tibial tunnel orientation. The guidewire is drilled through the tibia. The knee is brought into full extension to assess for impingement against the intercondylar roof. Although intraoperative fluoroscopy has been described by other authors as useful, we do not use it. We place a curet over the guide pin for stabilization during reaming. The guidewire is then over-reamed with a reamer sized 1 mm less than the measured quadrupled graft. The reamer and guidewire are then withdrawn, and water inflow is turned off. Next, the tibial tunnel is sequentially dilated in 0.5-mm increments to the size of the prepared graft, beginning with the size of the reamer used. The soft tissue around the tunnel entrance is cleared with the shaver.

Femoral Tunnel Placement

We use a femoral over-the-top position offset guide to place the guidewire at the desired location. The setting for the offset guide is chosen by adding 2 mm to the radius of the planned tunnel, to allow a posterior wall thickness of 2 mm. Therefore, for a 10-mm tunnel, we use a 7-mm offset guide (5 mm + 2 mm). The offset guide is inserted through the tibial tunnel into the notch. The tip of the guide is hooked into the over-the-top position and then rotated away from the PCL so the guidewire will enter the femur low on the lateral wall (approximately 10 o'clock for a right knee and 2 o'clock for a left knee). The appropriate guidewire is then drilled into the lateral femoral condyle and out through the soft tissues of the lateral thigh. The guide pin should exit the lateral thigh above the intermuscular septum. Next, we ream over the guide pin with the calibrated 4.5-mm EndoButton drill bit (Smith & Nephew, Andover, MA). This determines the overall femoral tunnel length from the tunnel entrance to the lateral femoral cortex and allows later passage of the EndoButton through the lateral femoral cortex. The EndoButton drill bit is then removed, and a closed-end femoral tunnel is drilled with the appropriately sized reamer as determined by the measured graft size for a line-to-line fit. We prefer to have at least 25 to 30 mm of graft residing in the femur. The depth of the femoral socket created must allow for this desired length plus an additional 8 mm for the EndoButton to clear the lateral femoral cortex and flip. The reamer and guide pin are then removed. Finally, the femoral tunnel is dilated to the desired depth with a dilator the size of the reamer used to create the tunnel (**Figure 4**).

Graft Preparation

The continuous-loop length for the EndoButton device must be calculated for final graft preparation. In general, we prefer to maximize the amount of graft residing in the femoral tunnel and use the smallest possible continuous loop. The two shortest continuous loops are 15 and 20 mm long. The length of the loop needed is determined by subtracting the desired length of graft in the tunnel from the overall femoral tunnel length, which is measured directly. For example, if the depth gauge reading is 45 mm for the overall femoral tunnel length and 30 mm of graft length is desired in the tunnel, a 15-mm continuous loop is selected (45 mm – 30 mm = 15 mm). Once the continuous-loop length is selected, the gracilis and semitendinosus tendons are passed through the loop and doubled over. The graft is then placed into the EndoButton holder with tension applied to the graft ends on the graft preparation board. No. 2 sutures of different colors are passed through the end holes of the EndoButton for graft passage and flipping of the EndoButton. The graft is marked with a pen at the dilated femoral tunnel length (**Figure 5**).

Graft Passage and Femoral Fixation

A Beath pin is passed through the tibial tunnel, into the joint, through the femoral tunnel, and out the anterolateral thigh. The sutures through the end holes of the EndoButton are passed through the eyelet of the Beath pin. The pin is then pulled, bringing the sutures out the thigh. One set of colored sutures is pulled, leading the EndoButton and graft into the knee joint and femoral tunnel. The other set is gently pulled to remove slack. If this second set of sutures is pulled too hard, the EndoButton will prematurely flip and prevent graft passage (**Figure 6**). The leading sutures are pulled until the previously made mark on the graft is seen to enter the femoral tunnel. At this point, the EndoButton should have passed the lateral femoral cortex and be able to be deployed. The flipping sutures are pulled, and the EndoButton should be felt to flip against the lateral femoral cortex. Gentle alternating pulls on the leading and flipping sutures will pro-

duce a rocking of the EndoButton against the lateral femoral cortex if properly deployed. If there is any concern about correct deployment, a mini C-arm fluoroscope can be brought in for verification.

Tibial Fixation

The hamstring graft is pulled distally to fully seat the EndoButton on the lateral femoral cortex. With manual tension applied to all four ends of the graft, we cycle the knee approximately 15 times. The arthroscope is then reinserted into the knee through the anterolateral portal. A nitinol guidewire

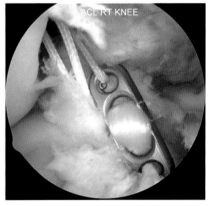

Figure 6 Passage of EndoButton sutures. The blue sutures are the leading sutures, which pull the graft into the femoral tunnel. After the EndoButton clears the lateral femoral cortex, the white sutures are pulled, flipping the EndoButton to seat against the cortex for secure graft fixation.

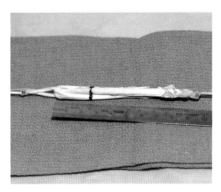

Figure 5 A prepared quadrupled graft with attached EndoButton. The depth of the femoral tunnel is marked.

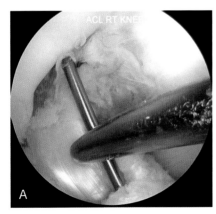
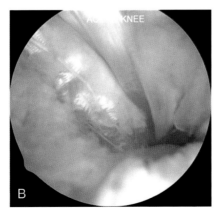
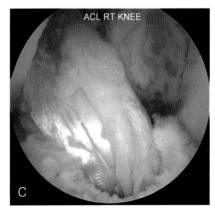

Figure 7 Tibial fixation. **A,** A nitinol wire is inserted anterior to the graft through the tibial tunnel and grasped with a hemostat. The interference screw will be inserted over the wire. **B,** Location of the interference screw anterior to the graft at the joint line. **C,** The completed ACL reconstruction.

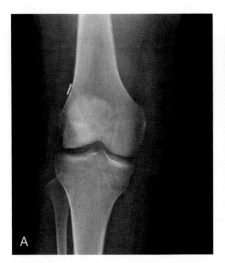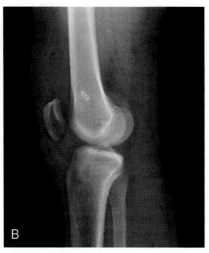

Figure 8 Postoperative AP (**A**) and lateral (**B**) radiographs of the completed reconstruction show the EndoButton fixation on the femur.

for the biointerference screw is inserted through the tibial tunnel anterior to the graft and into the joint. A hemostat is placed through the anteromedial portal to grasp the wire to prevent migration (**Figure 7, A**). A small notch is made at the tibial tunnel entrance for screw passage. The interference screw is then inserted over the wire. We typically use a 25-mm-long screw with a diameter equal to the size of the tunnel drilled. The arthroscope is withdrawn, and the knee is brought to full extension. An axial load is applied and, as constant tension is maintained on the graft, the screw is advanced over the wire. We attempt to place the screw as close to the joint line as possible (**Figure 7, B**), judging its position by feel as the screw passes through the hard tibial cortex, traverses the softer cancellous bone, and enters the second cortex at the joint line. The arthroscope is reinserted, and the hemostat is removed. A probe is used to palpate the graft at its entrance into the joint to ensure that the screw was not inserted too far. With fixation complete, the knee is tested for stability and range of motion (**Figure 7, C**).

Wound Closure

The passing sutures are pulled out of the lateral portion of the thigh. The sartorial fascial flap is closed with No. 0 Vicryl suture. The subcutaneous tissues are closed with interrupted 2.0 Vicryl sutures followed by a running subcuticular closure with 3.0 monocryl suture. Portal sites are closed with simple 3.0 nylon sutures. The knee is covered with a light dressing and placed in a hinged knee brace locked in full extension.

Rehabilitation

The patient is seen within the first week after surgery, and radiographs are taken (**Figure 8**). Weight bearing as tolerated is allowed immediately with the brace locked in full extension. The brace is typically worn for 4 weeks and unlocked for ambulation once good quadriceps control is established. Physical therapy is initiated within the first postoperative week. Emphasis is on achieving full extension initially with progression to flexion exercises. Patients progress to a stationary bike at 4 to 6 weeks and stair climbing at 6 to 8 weeks, followed by advancement of closed-chain strengthening and light jogging.

At 4 to 6 months after surgery, plyometrics and sport-specific exercises and drills are initiated. Patients gradually return to sports at 6 months after surgery.

Avoiding Pitfalls and Complications

Potential pitfalls related to harvest of the hamstrings primarily center around injury to the saphenous nerve and premature amputation of either the semitendinosus or gracilis tendon. Injury to the saphenous nerve can result in a painful neuroma. Flexion of the knee during harvest decreases tension on the nerve and may provide protection against injury during proximal dissection. Premature graft amputation can be prevented by careful release of all fascial band connections of the hamstring tendons to the gastrocnemius. If tension applied to the hamstrings before harvest results in puckering of the skin overlying the gastrocnemius, the fascial bands are not completely released.

Nonanatomic placement of the femoral tunnel can be avoided by correct placement of the tibial tunnel with proper coronal obliquity. If the femoral tunnel cannot be placed in the proper position with a transtibial technique, we drill the femoral tunnel with a medial portal technique with the knee hyperflexed.

Bibliography

Beynnon BD, Johnson RJ, Abate JA, Fleming BC, Nichols CE: Treatment of anterior cruciate ligament injuries, part 1. *Am J Sports Med* 2005;33:1579-1602.

Beynnon BD, Johnson RJ, Abate JA, Fleming BC, Nichols CE: Treatment of anterior cruciate ligament injuries, part 2. *Am J Sports Med* 2005;33:1751-1767.

Feller JA, Webster KE: A randomized comparison of patellar tension and hamstring tendon anterior cruciate ligament reconstruction. *Am J Sports Med* 2003;31:564-573.

Gobbi A, Tuy B, Mahajan S, Panuncialman I: Quadrupled bone-semitendinosus anterior cruciate ligament reconstruction: A clinical investigation in a group of athletes. *Arthroscopy* 2003;19:691-699.

Howell SM, Gittins ME, Gottlieb JE, Traina SM, Zoellner TM: The relationship between the angle of the tibial tunnel in the coronal plane and loss of flexion and anterior laxity after anterior cruciate ligament reconstruction. *Am J Sports Med* 2001;29:567-574.

Lidén M, Ejerhed L, Sernert N, Laxdal G, Kartus J: Patellar tendon or semitendinosus tendon autografts for anterior cruciate ligament reconstruction: A prospective, randomized study with a 7-year follow-up. *Am J Sports Med* 2007;35: 740-748.

Loh JC, Fukuda Y, Tsuda E, Steadman RJ, Fu FH, Woo SL: Knee stability and graft function following anterior cruciate ligament reconstruction: Comparison between 11 o'clock and 10 o'clock femoral tunnel placement. 2002 Richard O'Connor Award paper. *Arthroscopy* 2003;19:297-304.

Pagnani MJ, Warner JJ, O'Brien SJ, Warren RF: Anatomic considerations in harvesting the semitendinosus and gracilis tendons and a technique of harvest. *Am J Sports Med* 1993;21:565-571.

Pinczewski LA, Lyman J, Salmon LJ, Russell VJ, Roe J, Linklater J: A 10-year comparison of anterior cruciate ligament reconstruction with hamstring tendon and patellar tendon autograft: A controlled prospective trial. *Am J Sports Med* 2007; 35:564-574.

Prodromos CC, Fu FH, Howell SM, Johnson DH, Lawhorn K: Controversies in soft-tissue anterior cruciate ligament reconstruction: Grafts, bundles, tunnels, fixation, and harvest. *J Am Acad Orthop Surg* 2008;16:376-384.

Prodromos CC, Joyce BT, Shi K, Keller BL: A meta-analysis of stability after anterior cruciate ligament reconstruction as a function of hamstring versus patellar tendon graft and fixation type. *Arthroscopy* 2005;21:1202-1208.

Spindler KP, Kuhn JE, Freedman KB, Matthews CE, Dittus RS, Harrell FE Jr : Anterior cruciate ligament reconstruction autograft choice: Bone-tendon-bone versus hamstring: Does it really matter? A systematic review. *Am J Sports Med* 2004; 32:1986-1995.

Tashiro T, Kurosawa H, Kawakami A, Hikita A, Fukui N: Influence of medial hamstring tendon harvest on knee flexor strength after anterior cruciate ligament reconstruction: A detailed evaluation with comparison of single- and double-tendon harvest. *Am J Sports Med* 2003;31:522-529.

West RV, Harner CD: Graft selection in anterior cruciate ligament reconstruction. *J Am Acad Orthop Surg* 2005;13:197-207.

Video Reference

Wolf EM: *Hamstring Harvest for ACL Reconstruction*. Video clip from *Autogenous Hamstring ACL Reconstruction Using Cross-Pin Femoral Fixation*, in Johnson DJ, ed: *Surgical Techniques in Orthopaedics: Anterior Cruciate Ligament Reconstruction*. DVD. Rosemont, IL, American Academy of Orthopaedic Surgeons, 2002.

Coding

CPT Codes		Corresponding ICD-9 Codes	
Anterior Cruciate Ligament Repair			
29888	Arthroscopically aided anterior cruciate ligament repair/augmentation or reconstruction	717.83 717.84	717.84 844.2
Additional Procedures Referenced in Chapter			
29870	Arthroscopy, knee, diagnostic, with or without synovial biopsy (separate procedure)	715	733
20900	Bone graft, any donor area; minor or small (eg, dowel or button)	715	733
20902	Bone graft, any donor area; major or large	715	

CPT copyright © 2010 by the American Medical Association. All rights reserved.

Chapter 67

Quadriceps Tendon Autograft for Anterior Cruciate Ligament Reconstruction

Walter Shelton, MD

Indications

The quadriceps tendon is an excellent graft source for both primary and revision anterior cruciate ligament (ACL) reconstruction. A graft 10 to 12 mm wide and 7 to 8 mm thick with a length of 85 to 100 mm can be harvested in most adults. It can be used as a soft-tissue graft only, or it can be harvested with a 25-mm bone plug from the proximal patella. The quadriceps tendon is especially useful in skeletally immature patients in whom a soft-tissue graft is indicated; in small adults with hamstrings that may be inadequate in size; and in revision ACL surgery, when a bone–patellar tendon–bone or hamstring graft has already been harvested from the knee.

Contraindications

Substandard quality of the quadriceps tendon as a result of previous injury (eg, previous graft harvest, rupture, or partial or complete laceration) is a contraindication for use of this tissue

as an ACL graft. Patients with patellofemoral disease, such as arthritis, patella baja, patella alta, or recurrent dislocation of the patella, also may not be candidates for a quadriceps tendon autograft.

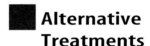

Alternative Treatments

Other grafts may be used instead of the quadriceps tendon autograft in patients in whom an ACL reconstruction is indicated. These include bone–patellar tendon–bone and hamstrings autografts. Allografts also are a popular alternative, and include bone–patellar tendon–bone, hamstrings, quadriceps tendon, Achilles, and posterior and anterior tibial tendon.

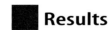

Results

The quadriceps tendon graft (64.4 ± 8.4 mm²) is larger than a bone–patellar tendon–bone graft (51.6 ± 6–9

mm²). This increased size translates into greater tensile strength: 1,953 N for a bone–patellar tendon–bone graft, 2,176 N for a quadriceps tendon graft, and 2,160 N for the normal ACL. Patient satisfaction and stability results with quadriceps tendon grafts are equal to those of bone–patellar tendon–bone grafts. An added bonus is a significant decrease in anterior knee pain and numbness compared with bone–patellar tendon–bone grafts. The quadriceps tendon graft can be harvested with a bone plug from the proximal patella, which can produce a longer graft but has not been shown to have any effect on postoperative results. A summary of the studies reporting results of ACL reconstruction using quadriceps tendon is provided in **Table 1**.

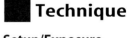

Technique

Setup/Exposure
A quadriceps tendon autograft can be harvested with the leg in a leg holder or draped free. Exposure is made through a short sagittal incision in the midline, just above the superior pole of the patella. As experience is gained in the harvest of this graft, the length of this incision can be decreased to approximately 2.5 cm.

Table 1 Results of Quadriceps Tendon Autograft for ACL Reconstruction

Author(s) (Year)	Number of Knees	Procedure or Approach	Mean Patient Age (Range)	Mean Follow-up (Range)	Results
Fulkerson et al (1998)	18	Central quadriceps free tendon	NA	NA	Morbidity less with quadriceps tendon than with BTB
Slullitel et al (2001)	40	Quadriceps tendon with bone block	NA	NA	40 stable knees
Noronha (2002)	240	Bone–quadriceps tendon graft	NA	NA	Quadriceps tendon ACL produced results equal to BTB with less morbidity.
Lee et al (2004)	67	Quadriceps tendon autograft	28 years (18-51)	41 months (27-49)	94% graded A and B (IKDC) Donor-site morbidity decreased
Geib et al (2008)	197	155 with bone plug 42 free quadriceps tendon	31 years (18-67)	56 months (24-137)	Quadriceps tendon stability equal to BTB, with less anterior knee pain and numbness and better extension

NA = not available, BTB = bone–patellar tendon–bone, IKDC = International Knee Documentation Committee.

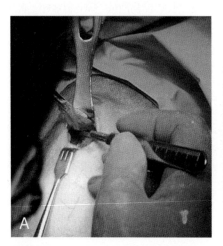 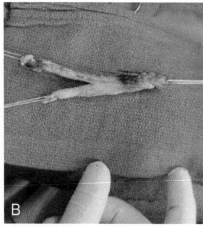

Figure 1 Harvesting a quadriceps tendon autograft. **A,** A No. 15 knife blade is used to dissect the quadriceps tendon from the patella. **B,** The interval between the vastus medialis and the rectus femoris tendons is dissected.

Instruments/Equipment Required

Instruments required to harvest a quadriceps tendon autograft are sharp No. 10 and No. 15 knife blades and standard retractors. A thin ruler also is helpful in gauging width, thickness, and length of the graft.

Procedure

The dorsum of the tendon is exposed, and subcutaneous fat is cleared away. A straight incision is made in the tendon adjacent to the vastus medialis obliquus and is carried for a length of 85 to 90 mm proximal to the patella, down to the bony insertion on the patella. It is very important to remain medial and adjacent to the vastus medialis obliquus as this is the thickest part of the quadriceps tendon. A second incision, 10 mm lateral and parallel to the first, is carried down to the patella. These two incisions are best accomplished with a No. 10 knife blade and are made to a depth of approximately 6 mm. A No. 15 knife blade is then used to begin removing the tendon from the superior pole of the patella to a depth of approximately 8 mm (**Figure 1**, *A*). A small fat pad at the superior attachment of the quadriceps tendon into the patella marks the level at which the dissection can be started proximally without entering the suprapatellar pouch. The dissection is carried approximately 35 mm proximally with a No. 15 knife blade, and a cylindrical sizer is used to determine the size of the graft in order to ream an appropriately sized femoral socket. Two whipstitches of No. 1 absorbable suture are placed in the dissected end of the quadriceps tendon and are used to place tension on the tendon as the remaining dissection is carried proximally with either scissors or the No. 15 knife blade, taking care to stay just above the suprapatellar pouch. At a level between 85 and 95 mm proximal to the patella, the quadriceps tendon is divided with a pair of scissors and removed from the incision. The defect in the tendon is then closed with a running No. 1 absorbable suture and any inadvertent penetration into the suprapatellar pouch is carefully closed. The

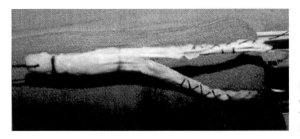

Figure 2 A quadriceps tendon autograft harvested with a bone plug from the superior patella.

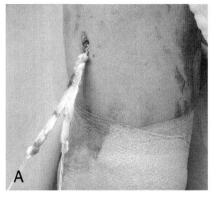

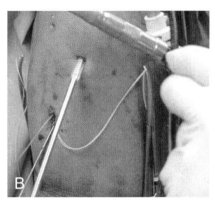

Figure 3 Placing the graft. **A,** The distal end of the graft is passed into the tibial tunnel. **B,** Insertion of the interference screw.

proximal end of the harvested tendon splits into the vastus medialis and the rectus femoris tendons, and this interval is dissected to within 50 mm of the distal end of the tendon graft (**Figure 1,** *B*). For a double-bundle ACL reconstruction, this dissection can be carried all the way to the end of the graft, dividing the graft into two parts. The larger rectus femoris is an excellent choice for the anteromedial bundle reconstruction of an ACL, and the smaller vastus intermedius can be used for the posterior lateral bundle. A layer of fat between these two tendons proximally is a constant finding and can be trimmed before sizing. A 25-mm bone plug from the superior patella can be harvested with the tendon if desired (**Figure 2**).

67.1 Quadriceps Tendon Graft Harvest for ACL Reconstruction. Walter R. Shelton, MD (3 min)

Following removal of the graft, both ends are sized. The preferred size of the graft is 9 mm for the distal 25 to 30 mm of the graft, which will be used in the femoral socket, and 10 to 11 mm for the remainder of the graft. After proper tunnels have been placed, the distal end of the graft is led into the tibial tunnel with the No. 1 absorbable sutures pulled out through the dorsal thigh, and the graft is seated into both the 9-mm femoral socket and the 10-mm tibial tunnel (**Figure 3,** *A*). The graft can be secured with either interference screws in both tunnels (**Figure 3,** *B*) or a cortical device on the femoral side and a screw and washer post on the tibial side, depending on the preference of the surgeon. If an interference screw is used on the tibial side, the two tails of the graft previously split are pulled tight, and the interference screw is introduced between them.

Wound Closure

The closure of the defect in the quadriceps tendon seals any inadvertent

puncture of the suprapatellar pouch. Comparison MRI studies at 1 year have shown the healed tendon to be thicker and wider than the normal side tendon. Closure is completed with subcutaneous sutures and adhesive strips.

Postoperative Regimen

For the first 48 to 72 hours, the leg is splinted, elevated, and iced. The splint is removed, the dressing is changed, and a rehabilitation program with rapid range of motion and crutch-protected weight bearing is instituted. For the first 3 weeks, patients are encouraged to bear weight as tolerated with two crutches. For weeks 3 through 6, they are graduated to one crutch under the opposite extremity with full weight on the surgical side. At 6 weeks, all crutches are discontinued. At 3 months, straight-line running is begun, and at 6 months, cutting and jumping sports are resumed.

Avoiding Pitfalls and Complications

Inadequate visualization of the quadriceps tendon during harvest can lead to surgeon frustration. Errors at this step include harvesting a graft that is too wide or too narrow, penetrating the suprapatellar pouch, or amputating the graft prematurely, resulting in a graft that is too short. Grafts that are too wide and bulky can be trimmed after harvest to the desired size. A graft that is too narrow can be augmented by harvesting an additional narrow strip and suturing the proximal ends together to obtain sufficient bulk. If the suprapatellar pouch is entered, careful side-to-side suturing of the defect allows healing of the tendon with minimal scarring to the synovium. In most cases, a graft length of 80 mm will be adequate, with 25 mm of graft in each tunnel and a 30-mm intra-articular ligament distance. When gaining experience with quadriceps tendon harvest, using a longer incision to provide greater visualization of the tendon helps prevent these complications. As the surgeon becomes more experienced in the procedure, the incision for harvesting a quadriceps graft can be reduced to 2.5 cm in length.

Bibliography

Fulkerson JP, McKeon BP, Donahue B, Tarinelli D: The central alternative in anterior cruciate ligament reconstruction: Techniques and recent observations. *Tech Orthop* 1998;13:367-374.

Geib TM, Shelton WR, Clark KL: Anterior cruciate ligament reconstruction using quadriceps tendon autograft: Intermediate term outcome. *Arthroscopy* 2009;25(12):1408-1414.

Lee S, Seong SC, Jo H, Park YK, Lee MC: Outcome of anterior cruciate ligament reconstruction using quadriceps tendon autograft. *Arthroscopy* 2004;20(8):795-802.

Noronha JC: Reconstruction of the anterior cruciate ligament with quadriceps tendon. *Arthroscopy* 2002;18(7):E37.

Schatzmann L, Brunner P, Stäubli HU: Effect of cyclic preconditioning on the tensile properties of human quadriceps tendons and patellar ligaments. *Knee Surg Sports Traumatol Arthrosc* 1998;6(Suppl 1):S56-S61.

Slullitel D Blasco A, Periotti G: Full-thickness quadriceps tendon: An easy cruciate reconstruction graft. *Arthroscopy* 2001;17(7):781-783.

Stäubli HU, Schatzmann L, Brunner P, Rincón L, Nolte LP: Quadriceps tendon and patellar ligament: Cryosectional anatomy and structural properties in young adults. *Knee Surg Sports Traumatol Arthrosc* 1996;4(2):100-110.

Woo SL, Hollis JM, Adams DJ, Lyon RM, Takai S: Tensile properties of the human femur-anterior cruciate ligament-tibia complex: The effects of specimen age and orientation. *Am J Sports Med* 1991;19(3):217-225.

Video Reference

Shelton WR: *Quadriceps Tendon Graft Harvest for ACL Reconstruction.* Video clip from Quadriceps Tendon Graft for ACL Reconstruction, in Johnson DJ, ed: *Surgical Techniques in Orthopaedics: Anterior Cruciate Ligament Reconstruction.* DVD. Rosemont, IL, American Academy of Orthopaedic Surgeons, 2002.

Coding

CPT Codes		Corresponding ICD-9 Codes	
Bone Graft Removal			
20900	Bone graft, any donor area; minor or small (eg, dowel or button)	715	733
20902	Bone graft, any donor area; major or large	715	733
Additional Procedures Referenced in This Chapter			
29888	Arthroscopically aided anterior cruciate ligament repair/augmentation or reconstruction	717.83 717.84	717.84 844.2
29889	Arthroscopically aided posterior cruciate ligament repair/augmentation or reconstruction	844.2	

CPT copyright © 2010 by the American Medical Association. All rights reserved.

Chapter 68

Double-Bundle Anterior Cruciate Ligament Reconstruction

Freddie H. Fu, MD, DSc (Hon), DPs (Hon)
Alexis Chiang Colvin, MD

■ Indications

Single-bundle anterior cruciate ligament (ACL) reconstruction is the current gold standard for restoring knee stability and enabling return to activity. Cadaver studies have shown, however, that single-bundle reconstructions may be inadequate in completely resisting both anterior tibial translation and rotational forces. Furthermore, patients with single-bundle ACL reconstruction also demonstrate abnormal rotational knee kinematics, which could potentially lead to long-term joint degeneration. An anatomic double-bundle reconstruction more closely reproduces knee kinematics, especially under rotatory loads.

Anatomic double-bundle ACL reconstruction is indicated for patients who have sustained an ACL rupture and have recurrent episodes of instability, would like to return to athletic activities, and have a repairable meniscal tear.

■ Contraindications

In our practice, we perform single-bundle ACL reconstruction in approximately 20% of patients. Indications for a single-bundle reconstruction include a small native ACL insertion site (less than 14 mm), open physes, severe arthritic changes, multiple injured ligaments, and a one-bundle tear (isolated anteromedial or posterolateral bundle).

■ Alternative Treatments

Nonsurgical treatment is considered in low-demand patients with no recurrent episodes of instability who do not wish to undergo ACL reconstruction. These patients are treated with functional bracing and rehabilitation.

■ Results

Anatomic double-bundle ACL reconstruction has been shown to restore knee stability and result in good patient-reported outcomes at midterm follow-up (**Table 1**). In several prospective, randomized studies comparing single-bundle and double-bundle ACL reconstruction, double-bundle reconstruction resulted in significantly better results on pivot-shift testing and better anterior stability as measured by Lachman and KT-1000 arthrometer (Medtronic, San Diego, CA) testing. No significant difference between the groups was seen on subjective testing, however, including International Knee Documentation Committee (IKDC), Lysholm, and Cincinnati scores.

A retrospective comparison of 135 knees with either single- or double-bundle ACL reconstruction found that patients with single-bundle reconstruction had significantly greater laxity on Lachman and KT-1000 arthrometer testing at 42- to 46-month follow-up; however, there was no difference in IKDC and Lysholm scores.

Dr. Fu or an immediate family member serves as a board member, owner, officer, or committee member of the Orthopaedic Research and Education Foundation, American Orthopaedic Society for Sports Medicine, International Society of Arthroscopy, and Knee Surgery and Orthopaedic Sports Medicine; serves as an unpaid consultant to Smith & Nephew; and has received research or institutional support from Breg, DePuy, Smith & Nephew, and Stryker. Neither Dr. Colvin nor any immediate family member has received anything of value from or owns stock in a commercial company or institution related directly or indirectly to the subject of this article.

Table 1 Results of Single-Bundle Versus Double-Bundle ACL Reconstructions

Author(s)/Year	Number of Knees	Procedure	Mean Patient Age (Range)	Mean Follow-up (Range)	Results	
					KT-1000 Side-to-Side Laxity	Pivot Shift
Järvelä (2007)	55	25 SB 30 DB	33 years (24-42)	14 months (12-20)	No significant difference	DB improved over SB, $P = 0.002$
Muneta et al (2007)	68	34 SB 34 DB	SB: 24 years (14-44) DB: 24 years (14-49)	SB: 25 months (18-41) DB: 25 months (18-40)	DB improved over SB, $P < 0.05$	DB improved over SB in males, $P = 0.05$
Siebold et al (2008)	70	35 SB 35 DB	SB: 29 years (17-42) DB: 29 years (17-45)	SB: 19 months (14-24) DB: 19 months (13-24)	DB improved over SB, $P = 0.054$	DB improved over SB, $P = 0.01$
Streich et al (2008)	49	25 SB 24 DB	SB: 29.2 years (16-36) DB: 30 years (17-37)	SB: 24.1 months (23-25) DB: 23.8 months (23-25)	No significant difference	No significant difference

SB = single bundle, DB = double bundle.

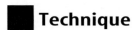

Technique

Setup/Exposure

The patient is positioned supine on the operating room table and examination under anesthesia is performed. The surgical leg is identified and a nonsterile tourniquet is placed on the proximal thigh. The leg is then placed in a leg holder. The nonsurgical leg is flexed and abducted. The foot of the table is dropped.

Instruments/Equipment/ Implants Required

Instruments used for anatomic double-bundle reconstruction that may not be standard on ACL reconstruction trays include an intra-articular ruler to measure the tibial and femoral insertion sites. Single-fluted femoral drills, usually sized 6, 7, and 8 mm, are necessary when the PL tibial tunnel approach is used to drill the anteromedial femoral tunnel. The purpose of the single-fluted drill is to drill the femoral tunnel without enlarging the tibial tunnel.

Our preference is to use two allografts, from the tibialis anterior, tibialis posterior, and/or semitendinosus. The grafts usually are 24 to 30 cm long, yielding 12- to 15-cm double-stranded grafts when doubled over. The diameters of the doubled allografts usually measure approximately 6 mm for the PL graft and 7 or 8 mm for the anteromedial graft. Hamstring autografts also can be used for the reconstruction, although the diameter of each graft tends to be smaller. The semitendinosus is doubled for the anteromedial graft, usually measuring 7 to 8 mm in diameter, and the doubled gracilis usually measures 5 to 6 mm in diameter for the posterolateral graft. For both allografts and autografts, a No. 2 nonabsorbable suture is used to whipstitch the ends of the graft for approximately 3 cm. An EndoButton CL (Smith & Nephew Endoscopy, Andover, MA) is used for graft fixation with size based on the measurement of the femoral tunnel. When the femoral tunnel is

short (which may occur when the anteromedial portal is used to drill the anteromedial femoral tunnel), the EndoButton Direct (Smith & Nephew Endoscopy) can be used to maximize the amount of graft in the tunnel.

Procedure

Three portals are used for an anatomic double-bundle ACL reconstruction—standard anterolateral and anteromedial portals and an accessory anteromedial (AAM) portal (**Figure 1**). The anterolateral portal is established high enough to provide visualization above the infrapatellar fat pad. The purpose of two portals on the medial side is that visualization of the femoral insertion of the ACL is better through the medial portal (**Figure 2**). All work on the femoral side is done with the arthroscope in the anteromedial portal. Diagnostic arthroscopy is done with attention to any cartilage or meniscal injury. The anteromedial portal is established with an 18-gauge spinal needle under direct visualization, close to

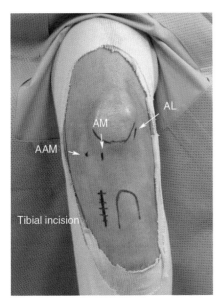

Figure 1 Photograph of a left knee with markings for portal placement for anatomic double-bundle ACL reconstruction. AAM = accessory anteromedial portal, AM = anteromedial portal, AL = anterolateral portal.

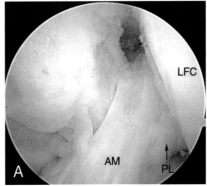

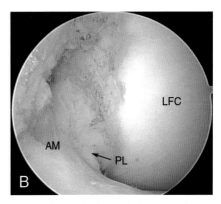

Figure 2 Arthroscopic views show the appearance of the ACL through the anterolateral portal **(A)** and anteromedial portal **(B)**. Note the improved visualization of the femoral insertion of the ACL through the anteromedial portal. AM = anteromedial bundle, PL = posterolateral bundle, LFC = lateral femoral condyle.

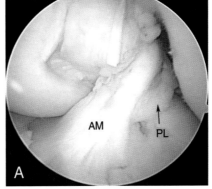

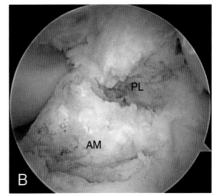

Figure 3 The anteromedial (AM) and posterolateral (PL) bundles are carefully dissected with a thermal probe **(A)**, and the tibial insertions are marked **(B)**.

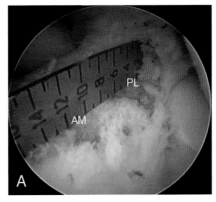

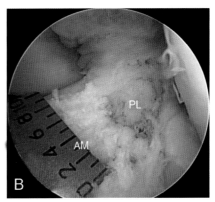

Figure 4 The length **(A)** and width **(B)** of the ACL tibial insertion are measured. AM = anteromedial bundle, PL = posterolateral bundle.

midline, ensuring that the needle follows the trajectory of the ACL. The fat pad is then débrided with a shaver. The AAM portal also is established with an 18-gauge spinal needle so that the portal is in the direction of the center of the posterolateral bundle of the ACL. Care is taken to make this portal above the medial meniscus and to avoid contact with the medial femoral condyle. Any necessary meniscal work is done at this time.

Attention is then turned to the intercondylar notch. The rupture pattern of the ACL is identified using a probe. A thermal device is used to carefully dissect the ruptured ACL and to mark the native tibial insertion sites of the anteromedial and posterolateral bundles (**Figure 3**). The posterolateral bundle insertion is posterolateral to the anteromedial bundle and adjacent to the lateral meniscal root. A ruler is used to measure the length and the width of the tibial insertion site (**Figure 4**). If the length is less than 14 mm, single-bundle reconstruction should be performed. Typically, the anteromedial bundle tunnel averages

7 or 8 mm in diameter and the posterolateral bundle averages 5 or 6 mm in diameter. Working through the AAM portal, the native femoral insertion sites of the anteromedial bundle and posterolateral bundle are marked

with a thermal device. The femoral insertion site length and width are measured (**Figure 5**).

A 45° microfracture awl is used to mark the center of the anteromedial and posterolateral bundles. A 3.2-mm guidewire is then tapped into the posterolateral bundle mark. The guidewire is tapped in with the knee in maximal flexion to avoid damage to the peroneal nerve and to maximize femoral tunnel length. The wire is then overdrilled to 20 mm with a 5-mm acorn drill or an acorn drill one size smaller than the target posterolateral tunnel size. The lateral cortex of the posterolateral tunnel is then broken through with a 4.5-mm EndoButton drill. The length of the posterolateral tunnel is measured, and the tunnel is dilated to the appropriate length for the EndoButton.

The tibial tunnels are then prepared. A 3- to 5-cm incision is centered on the tibia midway between the tibial tubercle and the posteromedial border of the tibia at the level of the tubercle. The arthroscope is then reintroduced into the anterolateral portal, and the tibial tunnels are drilled with the tip guide set to 45° for the posterolateral tunnel and 55° for the anteromedial tunnel. Care is taken to ensure that the guide is placed medial enough on the tibia when drilling the posterolateral tunnel so that there is an adequate bone bridge separating it from the more central anteromedial tunnel. The posterolateral tibial tunnel entry point is just anterior to the fibers of the superficial medial collateral ligament and distal to the entry point for the anteromedial tunnel. The tunnels are drilled one size smaller than the width measured and then dilated up to size. A curette should be placed over the guidewire while drilling to protect the femoral articular cartilage.

The arthroscope is then reintroduced into the anteromedial portal and a guidewire is used to determine the optimal portal to drill the anteromedial femoral tunnel. Our preference is to drill the anteromedial femoral tunnel through the anteromedial tibial tunnel. This can be accomplished 10% of the time; 60% of the time, the posterolateral tibial tunnel can be used. The anteromedial portal can be used to drill the anteromedial femoral tunnel 100% of the time; however, care must be taken not to violate the cartilage of the medial femoral condyle with the drill (**Figure 6**). The tunnel may also be shorter if made through the anteromedial portal. A different method of fixation, such as an EndoButton Direct, may be necessary to ensure at least 15 mm of graft in the tunnel. Once the approach is chosen, a 3.2-mm guidewire is tapped into the previously marked anteromedial site. This wire is overdrilled to 25 mm with a 5-mm acorn drill or an acorn drill one size smaller than the target anteromedial tunnel size. If the posterolateral tibial tunnel is used to approach the anteromedial femoral tunnel, a single-fluted drill is used to prevent further expansion of the posterolateral tunnel. The lateral cortex is broken

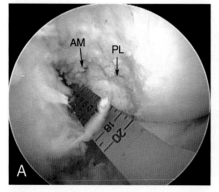
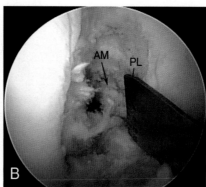

Figure 5 The length **(A)** and width **(B)** of the ACL femoral insertion are measured. AM = anteromedial bundle, PL = posterolateral bundle.

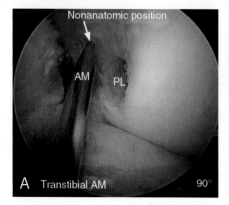
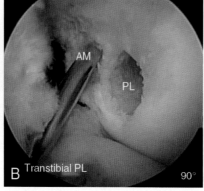
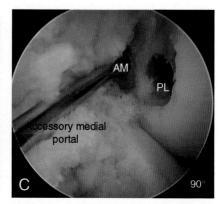

Figure 6 A guidewire is used to determine the best approach for the anteromedial femoral tunnel. The anteromedial femoral insertion can be reached 10% of the time using the anteromedial tibial tunnel **(A)**; 60% of the time, the PL tibial tunnel **(B)** can be used. Although the AAM portal **(C)** can always be used to drill the anteromedial femoral tunnel, care must be taken to not violate the cartilage of the medial femoral condyle with the drill. AM = anteromedial femoral tunnel, PL = posterolateral femoral tunnel.

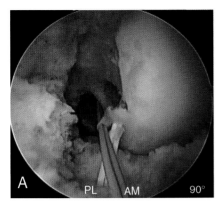

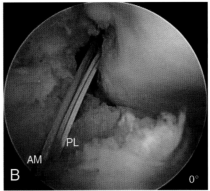

Figure 7 Correct position of the sutures. **A,** With the knee in 90° of flexion, the anteromedial suture (AM) should cross over the posterolateral suture (PL). **B,** With the knee at full extension, the anteromedial and posterolateral sutures should be parallel.

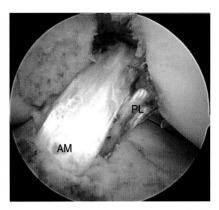

Figure 8 Arthroscopic appearance of the double-bundle ACL reconstruction with the knee in 90° of flexion. The anteromedial bundle (AM) should cross the posterolateral bundle (PL).

through with a 4.5-mm EndoButton drill, and the length of the tunnel is measured with the EndoButton ruler. The anteromedial femoral tunnel length and width are then increased appropriately with a dilator.

A Beath pin with a looped suture attached to the eyelet is then used to pass the grafts. The posterolateral graft is passed first, followed by the anteromedial graft. A Beath pin is introduced through the AAM portal, and a grasper is used to pull the suture loop into the posterolateral tibial tunnel. Another Beath pin with a looped suture is passed through the tunnel or portal that was used to create the anteromedial femoral tunnel, and a grasper is used to retrieve the suture loop into the anteromedial tibial tunnel. The suture loops can then be examined to ensure that they replicate the pattern of the anteromedial and posterolateral bundles. The anteromedial passing suture should cross the posterolateral passing suture with the knee at 90° of flexion (**Figure 7**). With the knee at full extension, the sutures should be parallel.

The posterolateral graft is passed using the suture loop, and the EndoButton is then flipped to secure the graft on the femoral side. The anteromedial graft is then passed using the suture loop, and the EndoButton is flipped to secure the femoral fixation. After the EndoButtons are successfully

flipped, the grafts are cycled approximately 20 times. The posterolateral bundle is fixed with a bioabsorbable interference screw on the tibial side with the knee in full extension. The anteromedial bundle is then fixed on the tibial side with the knee at 45° of flexion. The arthroscope is then reintroduced into the anterolateral portal, and the grafts are examined for correct position and tension (**Figure 8**). The knee is also taken through a full range of motion to document the absence of ACL or posterior cruciate ligament impingement. Radiographs are taken to confirm proper positioning of the EndoButtons.

 Video 68.1 Anatomic Double-Bundle ACL Reconstruction. Freddie Fu, MD; Carola F. vanEck, MD; Hector Mejia, MD; Verena M. Schreiber, MD; Alexis Chiang Colvin, MD (8 min)

Wound Closure

The tibial incision is closed with interrupted, buried No. 2-0 absorbable braided sutures for the subcutaneous tissue and a running subcuticular No. 4-0 absorbable monofilament suture. The portal sites are closed with simple No. 3-0 nylon sutures. A dry sterile dressing and cold therapy unit are

placed and the leg is placed in a postoperative brace with the knee in full extension.

————————∎

Postoperative Regimen

Postoperatively, the patient is allowed to bear weight as tolerated with crutches and is started on quadriceps sets, heel slides, and straight-leg raises. The crutches are discontinued once the patient has full knee extension and can perform a straight-leg raise without an extension lag, usually between 2 and 6 weeks. The leg is kept in a brace for 6 weeks, but the patient is allowed to unlock the brace for ambulating and can discontinue it at night after the first week. The use of a continuous passive motion (CPM) machine is started the first postoperative day for 2 hours, twice a day. Once the patient has 120° of flexion for 3 days, the CPM machine can be discontinued.

At 6 weeks postoperatively, closed kinetic chain exercises are initiated. Strengthening and proprioceptive activities are started at 2 months after surgery. Once the surgical extremity

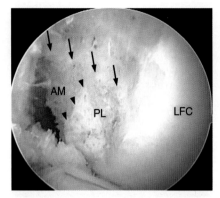

Figure 9 Arthroscopic view demonstrates the anatomy of the knee relevant to ACL reconstruction. With the knee in 90° of flexion, the lateral intercondylar ridge (arrows) marks the proximal border of the ACL insertion. The lateral bifurcate ridge (arrowheads) separates the anteromedial (AM) and posterolateral (PL) bundles. LFC = lateral femoral condyle.

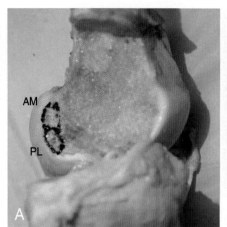

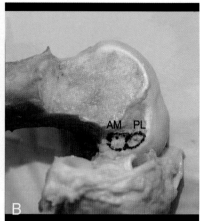

Figure 10 Photographs of a dissected cadaver knee demonstrate how the orientation of the femoral ACL insertion changes with knee flexion. **A,** With the knee in full extension, the anteromedial (AM) and posterolateral (PL) insertion sites on the femur are vertically oriented. **B,** With the knee in 90° of flexion, the usual position for surgery, the same insertion sites are horizontally oriented.

achieves 70% strength and proprioception of the uninvolved leg, the patient can progressively increase jogging speed, usually after 6 months. At 9 months, the patient is allowed to return to cutting and pivoting sports with a functional brace. The use of a functional brace is recommended for the first 1 to 2 years after surgery.

Avoiding Pitfalls and Complications

Portal Placement

The proper placement of the portals is critical to the success of the procedure. The AAM should be established using an 18-gauge spinal needle in the trajectory of the posterolateral femoral bundle. This portal is located medial and inferior to the anteromedial portal, and direct visualization should be used to prevent injury to the medial meniscus as well as to the articular surface of the medial femoral condyle.

The anteromedial portal should be used to visualize the femoral insertion site and the AAM used for a working portal. This avoids the necessity of a notchplasty.

Recognizing Insertion-Site Anatomy

The lateral intercondylar ridge is the proximal border of the ACL when the knee is in 90° of flexion and the anterior border when the knee is in full extension (**Figure 9**). The anteromedial and posterolateral femoral insertion sites are separated by the lateral bifurcate ridge.

Understanding the change in femoral insertion-site orientation with knee flexion is also important when performing an anatomic ACL reconstruction (**Figure 10**). When the knee is in full extension, the anteromedial and posterolateral femoral insertion sites are oriented vertically, with the anteromedial insertion site located proximal to the posterolateral femoral insertion site. When the knee is in 90° of flexion, the usual position for surgery, the femoral insertion sites are horizontally oriented, with the posterolateral femoral insertion site located anterior to the anteromedial femoral insertion site.

Bibliography

Anderson AF, Snyder RB, Lipscomb AB Jr: Anterior cruciate ligament reconstruction: A prospective randomized study of three surgical methods. *Am J Sports Med* 2001;29(3):272-279.

Fu FH, Shen W, Starman JS, Okeke N, Irrgang JJ: Primary anatomic double-bundle anterior cruciate ligament reconstruction: A preliminary 2-year prospective study. *Am J Sports Med* 2008;36:1263-1274.

Järvelä T: Double-bundle versus single-bundle anterior cruciate ligament reconstruction: A prospective, randomize clinical study. *Knee Surg Sports Traumatol Arthrosc* 2007;15(5):500-507.

Keays SL, Bullock-Saxton JE, Keays AC, Newcombe PA, Bullock MI: A 6-year follow-up of the effect of graft site on strength, stability, range of motion, function, and joint degeneration after anterior cruciate ligament reconstruction: Patellar tendon versus semitendinosus and gracilis tendon graft. *Am J Sports Med* 2007;35(5):729-739.

Loh JC, Fukuda Y, Tsuda E, Steadman RJ, Fu FH, Woo SL: Knee stability and graft function following anterior cruciate ligament reconstruction: Comparison between 11 o'clock and 10 o'clock femoral tunnel placement. 2002 Richard O'Connor Award paper. *Arthroscopy* 2003;19(3):297-304.

Muneta T, Koga H, Mochizuki T, et al: A prospective randomized study of 4-strand semitendinosus tendon anterior cruciate ligament reconstruction comparing single-bundle and double-bundle techniques. *Arthroscopy* 2007;23(6): 618-628.

Muneta T, Koga H, Morito T, Yagishita K, Sekiya I: A retrospective study of the midterm outcome of two-bundle anterior cruciate ligament reconstruction using quadrupled semitendinosus tendon in comparison with one-bundle reconstruction. *Arthroscopy* 2006;22(3):252-258.

Muneta T, Sekiya I, Yagishita K, Ogiuchi T, Yamamoto H, Shinomiya K: Two-bundle reconstruction of the anterior cruciate ligament using semitendinosus tendon with endobuttons: Operative technique and preliminary results. *Arthroscopy* 1999;15(6):618-624.

Siebold R, Dehler C, Ellert T: Prospective randomized comparison of double-bundle versus single-bundle anterior cruciate ligament reconstruction. *Arthroscopy* 2008;24(2):137-145.

Streich NA, Friedrich K, Gotterbarm T, Schmitt H: Reconstruction of the ACL with a semitendinosus tendon graft: A prospective randomized single blinded comparison of double-bundle versus single-bundle technique in male athletes. *Knee Surg Sports Traumatol Arthrosc* 2008;16(3):232-238.

Tashman S, Collon D, Anderson K, Kolowich P, Anderst W: Abnormal rotational knee motion during running after anterior cruciate ligament reconstruction. *Am J Sports Med* 2004;32(4):975-983.

Woo SL, Kanamori A, Zeminski J, Yagi M, Papageorgiou C, Fu FH: The effectiveness of reconstruction of the anterior cruciate ligament with hamstrings and patellar tendon: A cadaveric study comparing anterior tibial and rotational loads. *J Bone Joint Surg Am* 2002;84-A(6):907-914.

Yagi M, Wong EK, Kanamori A, Debski RE, Fu FH, Woo SL: Biomechanical analysis of an anatomic anterior cruciate ligament reconstruction. *Am J Sports Med* 2002;30(5):660-666.

Yamamoto Y, Hsu WH, Woo SL, Van Scyoc AH, Takakura Y, Debski RE: Knee stability and graft function after anterior cruciate ligament reconstruction: A comparison of a lateral and an anatomical femoral tunnel placement. *Am J Sports Med* 2004;32(8):1825-1832.

Yasuda K, Kondo E, Ichiyama H, et al: Anatomic reconstruction of the anteromedial and posterolateral bundles of the anterior cruciate ligament using hamstring tendon grafts. *Arthroscopy* 2004;20(10):1015-1025.

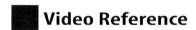

Video Reference

Fu FH, Colvin AC: Video. *Double-Bundle ACL Reconstruction*. Pittsburgh, PA, 2009.

Coding

CPT Codes		Corresponding ICD-9 Codes	
Anterior Cruciate Ligament Repair			
29888	Arthroscopically aided anterior cruciate ligament repair/augmentation or reconstruction	717.83 717.84	717.84 844.2
Additional Procedures Referenced in This Chapter			
29870	Arthroscopy, knee, diagnostic, with or without synovial biopsy (separate procedure)	715	
29880	Arthroscopy, knee, surgical; with meniscectomy (medial AND lateral, including any meniscal shaving)	836	717
29881	Arthroscopy, knee, surgical; with meniscectomy (medial OR lateral, including any meniscal shaving)	836	717
20900	Bone graft, any donor area; minor or small (eg, dowel or button)	715	733
20902	Bone graft, any donor area; major or large	715	733

CPT copyright © 2010 by the American Medical Association. All rights reserved.

Chapter 69
ACL Reconstruction in the Skeletally Immature Patient

Mininder S. Kocher, MD, MPH

 ## Indications

The prevalence of anterior cruciate ligament (ACL) injuries in children and adolescents has been increasing over the past decade. Numerous reconstructive procedures have been described for these injuries, but their management remains controversial. Nonsurgical treatment of complete ACL tears typically results in recurrent functional instability with a risk of injury to the menisci and articular cartilage, and conventional reconstruction techniques risk iatrogenic growth disturbance caused by physeal violation. One suggested solution has been to delay reconstruction in patients with significant growth remaining until they are closer to skeletal maturity so that the consequences of growth disturbance will be less severe. Recent studies have shown, however, that the risk of additional injury incurred when reconstruction is delayed (irreparable medial meniscal tears, lateral compartment injuries, patellotrochlear injuries) is significantly greater than the risk of significant growth disturbance when reconstruction is

performed in a skeletally immature patient.

ACL reconstruction generally is indicated for any patient who has functional instability with activities of daily living, refuses to comply with activity modification, or has a complete midsubstance ACL tear and a concomitant meniscal tear (the ACL+ knee). Surgical reconstruction also is indicated for any patient who develops symptoms of persistent instability (**Figure 1**) after an appropriate trial of nonsurgical treatment.

Contraindications

Surgery may be initially contraindicated for a prepubescent patient with an isolated ACL injury who is willing to comply with activity restrictions and brace wear. Reconstruction is contraindicated in a child who will not or cannot cooperate with postoperative rehabilitation. Primary repair rather than reconstruction may be indicated for proximal tears of the ACL, and distal tibial spine fractures should

be treated with arthroscopic reduction and internal fixation. Patients with associated medial collateral ligament injury may have decreased flexion that would impair rehabilitation, and flexion should be restored before surgery.

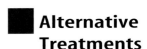

Alternative Treatments

Nonsurgical treatment consisting of rehabilitation, functional bracing, and avoidance of high-risk sports may be appropriate for the patient (and family) willing to accept the functional athletic limitations of an ACL-deficient knee, for the patient with a lower grade partial tear, and for the patient with a tear predominantly involving the anteromedial bundle. Nonsurgical treatment generally consists of three phases (**Table 1**), with the goal of preventing recurrent episodes of giving way that can lead to meniscal damage, intra-articular damage, and premature degenerative arthritis. Most reports of nonsurgical treatment have demonstrated poor results. Patients treated nonsurgically must be strongly discouraged from participating in high-risk sports that require cutting, pivoting, or jumping movements. The use of functional braces in skeletally immature athletes is controversial, and there is no clear

Dr. Kocher or an immediate family member has received royalties from Biomet; serves as a paid consultant to or is an employee of Biomet, CONMED Linvatec, Covidian, OrthoPediatrics, PediPed, Regen Biologics, and Smith & Nephew; has stock or stock options held in Pivot Medical; has received research or institutional support from CONMED Linvatec; and serves as a board member, owner, officer, or committee member of the American Academy of Orthopaedic Surgeons, the ACL Study Group, the American Orthopaedic Society of Sports Medicine, the Herodicus Society, the Pediatric Orthopaedic Society of North America, and the Steadman Hawkins Research Foundation.

consensus or scientific evidence to support their use.

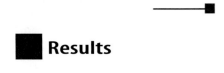

Results

Determining the overall success rate of surgical ACL reconstruction in skeletally immature patients is difficult if not impossible because of the variety of techniques and grafts used, the differing ages of the patients, and the criteria used to grade results (Table 2). In 18 studies in which the information was available, 323 (93%) of 349 patients returned to competitive sports at preinjury levels, and among 351 children and adolescents with surgical reconstruction, only one had a clinically significant growth disturbance (limb-length discrepancy of 2 cm). Reported Lysholm scores ranged from 93 to 99.

Techniques

Preoperative Planning

Techniques developed to treat ACL injuries in skeletally immature patients include primary ligament repair, extra-articular tenodesis, transphyseal reconstruction, partial transphyseal reconstruction, and physeal-sparing reconstruction. It is important to determine the best technique for each patient. Preoperative planning begins with determination of skeletal age as demonstrated on hand and wrist or knee radiographs with the use of skeletal atlases. Physiologic age is defined by the Tanner staging system. Informal Tanner staging is begun by questioning the patient in the office and is confirmed at the time of surgery. In addition to routine radiographs of the knee, MRI often is used to determine the presence of associated injuries, such as meniscal tears or chondral injuries. I prefer a procedure based on the physiologic age of the patient (**Figure 1**).

For prepubescent patients with associated chondral or repairable meniscal injuries or with functional instability after nonsurgical treatment, I perform a physeal-sparing, combined intra-articular and extra-articular reconstruction using an iliotibial band autograft. This technique can provide knee stability and improve function in prepubescent patients with complete intrasubstance ACL tears but does not

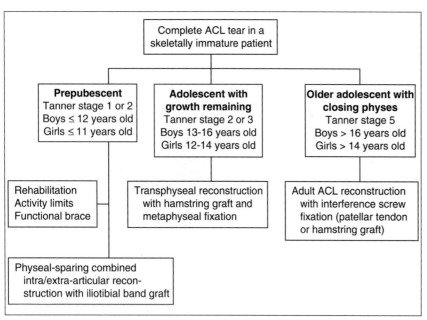

Figure 1 Algorithm for management of complete ACL injuries in skeletally immature patients. (Adapted with permission from Kocher MS: Anterior cruciate ligament reconstruction in the skeletally immature patient. *Op Tech Sports Med* 2006;14:124-134. Http://www.sciencedirect.com/science/journal/10601872.)

Table 1 Nonsurgical Rehabilitation Protocol for Anterior Cruciate Ligament Injuries in Skeletally Immature Patients

Phase	Time Frame	Activity
I	Time of injury to approximately 7-10 days	• Begin crutch-protected partial weight bearing. • Knee immobilizer used for comfort. Remove daily for active knee flexion exercises and passive knee extension exercises.
II	Begins when pain and discomfort have subsided; lasts approximately 6 weeks	• Primary goals: restore full range of motion and regain muscle balance and tone. • Crutch use is discontinued as strength returns. • Full passive knee extension is emphasized.
III	Begins when strength and stamina are equal to uninjured extremity	• Continue strength and range-of-motion activities. • Gradually return to low- or moderate-demand sports.

(Data from Stanitski CL: Anterior cruciate ligament injury in the skeletally immature patient: Diagnosis and treatment. *J Am Acad Orthop Surg* 1995;3:146-158.)

Table 2 Results of Anterior Cruciate Ligament Reconstruction in Skeletally Immature Patients

Author(s) (Year)	Number of Patients	Mean Age in Years (Range)	Graft Type	Mean Follow-up in Months (Range)	Results	Growth Disturbance
Transphyseal Procedures						
Lipscomb and Anderson (1986)	24	14 (12-15)	Hamstring autograft	51 (26-87)	16 had "normal" knee 8 had "improved" knee 15/24 returned to previous levels of sports	1 (2-cm LLD)
McCarroll et al (1994)	60	14 (13-17)	BPTB autograft	48 (24-84)	55/60 returned to previous levels of sports	None
Matava and Siegel (1997)	8	15	Hamstring autograft	32	All returned to preinjury sports levels	None
Aronowitz et al (2000)	19	13 (11-15)	Achilles allograft	25 (12-60)	All patients satisfied with results 16/19 returned to previous sports levels Lysholm 97	None
Edwards and Grana (2001)	19 (20 knees)	Girls: 13 (12-15) Boys: 14 (13-16)	Hamstring or BPTB autograft	34 (17-89)	19/20 returned to preinjury sports levels Lysholm 93	None
Fuchs et al (2002)	10	13 (9-15)	Patellar tendon autograft	40 (26-60)	9/10 returned to preinjury levels of sports Lysholm 95	None
Aichroth et al (2002)	45 (47 knees)	13 (11-15)	Hamstring autograft	49 (12-96)	75% satisfactory, 25% unsatisfactory (3 re-ruptures)	None
Shelbourne et al (2004)	16	15 (13-16)	Patellar tendon autograft	41 objective 67 subjective	All returned to competitive sports Average IKDC 95.4	None
Seon et al (2005)	11	15 (13-15)	Hamstring autograft	78 (45-131)	10/11 returned to pre-injury levels of sports Average Lysholm 97.8	None
McIntosh et al (2006)	16	14 (11-15)	Hamstring autograft	41 (24-112)	14/16 returned to previous levels of activity; 7 required reoperation	None
Kocher et al (2007)	59 (61 knees)	15 (12-17)	Hamstring autograft	43 (24-122)	2 required revision because of graft failure; Lysholm 91; all returned to cutting/pivoting sports	None
Bollen et al (2008)	5	13 (12-14)	Hamstring graft	35 (18-58)	All regained preinjury levels of activity, including 3 elite-level players	None

(continued on next page)

Table 2 (continued)

Author(s) (Year)	Number of Patients	Mean Age in Years (Range)	Graft Type	Mean Follow-up in Months (Range)	Results	Growth Disturbance
Partial Transphyseal Procedures						
Andrews et al (1994)	8	13 (10-15)	Fascia lata or Achilles tendon allograft	58 (22-94)	6 excellent, 1 good, 1 fair	None
Lo et al (1997)	5	13 (8-14)	Hamstring or quadriceps-patellar autograft	89 (54-119)	IKDC four grade A, one grade C (subsequent patellar dislocation)	None
Bisson et al (1998)	9	13 (10-15)	Hamstring autograft	39 (24-72)	7 excellent, 2 good 7/9 returned to previous sports Lysholm 99	None
Guzzanti et al (2003)	10	14 (13-14)	Hamstring autograft	40 (24-108)	All returned to high-level sports	None
Physeal-Sparing Procedures						
Parker et al (1994)	5	13 (10-14)	Hamstring autograft	33 (25-38)	4/5 returned to previous levels of sports Lysholm 95	None
Micheli et al (1999)	8	11 (2-14)	Iliotibial band autograft	66 (25-168)	All returned to previous sports Lysholm 97	None
Anderson (2003)	12	13 (11-16)	Hamstring autograft	48 (24-98)	8/12 able to participate in "very strenuous" activity, 4/12 in "strenuous" activity Average IKDC 96.5	None
Guzzanti et al (2003)	5	11 (10-12)	Hamstring autograft	69 (48-84)	All returned to vigorous sports and were asymptomatic	None
Kocher et al (2005)	44	10 (4-14)	Iliotibial band autograft	60 (24-180)	2/44 required repeat surgery because of graft failure; all returned to previous cutting/pivoting sports Average Lysholm 95.7, IKDC 96.7	None

LLD = limb-length discrepancy, BPTB = bone–patellar tendon–bone, IKDC = International Knee Documentation Committee.

risk iatrogenic growth disturbance because the distal femoral and proximal tibial physes are avoided. This reconstruction is nonanatomic, however, and patients and families are counseled that revision reconstruction may be needed if recurrent instability develops. As with nonsurgical treatment, this reconstruction may be a temporary solution, allowing further growth until more anatomic transphyseal reconstruction is possible.

For adolescent patients with growth remaining, initial nonsurgical treatment is not recommended because of the high risk of meniscal and chondral injury with an unstable knee and because the risks and consequences of growth disturbance from ACL reconstruction are less serious in these patients than in prepubescent patients. For these patients, an anatomic transphyseal reconstruction with hamstring tendon autograft and fixation away from the physes is recommended.

For older adolescents who are approaching skeletal maturity, conventional ACL reconstruction with patellar tendon or hamstring autograft and interference screw fixation is done, as in adults.

As in adult patients, acute ACL reconstruction is not done within the first 3 weeks after injury, to minimize the risk of arthrofibrosis. Preoperative rehabilitation is used to regain range of motion, decrease swelling, and resolve the reflex inhibition of the quadriceps muscle. If a displaced bucket-handle tear of the meniscus requires extensive repair, ACL reconstruction may be staged to protect the meniscal repair from the early mobilization needed after ACL reconstruction.

Procedure

PHYSEAL-SPARING
RECONSTRUCTION (FIGURE 2)

General anesthesia is used because local anesthesia with sedation may not be reliable in prepubescent children and has the potential for a paradoxical effect of sedation. The child is positioned supine on the operating table with a pneumatic tourniquet about the upper thigh, which is used routinely. Examination under anesthesia is done to confirm ACL insufficiency.

First, the iliotibial band graft is obtained. An approximately 6-cm incision is made obliquely from the lateral joint line to the superior border of the iliotibial band. Proximally, the iliotibial band is separated from the subcutaneous tissue with a periosteal elevator under the skin of the lateral thigh. The anterior and posterior borders of the iliotibial band are incised, and the incisions are carried proximally under the skin with curved meniscotomes (**Figure 3**, *A*). A curved meniscotome or open tendon stripper is used to detach the iliotibial band proximally (**Figure 3**, *B*). Alternatively, a second incision can be made at the upper thigh for release of the tendon. The

iliotibial band is left attached distally at the Gerdy tubercle (**Figure 3**, *C*). Dissection is done distally to separate the iliotibial band from the joint capsule and the patellar retinaculum. The free proximal end of the iliotibial band is then tubularized with a whip stitch using No. 5 Ethibond (Ethicon, Somerville, NJ) suture.

The knee joint is examined arthroscopically through standard anterolateral viewing and anteromedial working portals, and meniscal or chondral injuries are treated if necessary. The ACL remnant is excised. The over-the-top position on the femur and the over-the-front position under the intermeniscal ligament are identified. Minimal notchplasty is done to avoid injury to the perichondral ring of the distal femoral physis, which is in close proximity to the over-the-top position. The free end of the iliotibial band graft is brought through the over-the-top position with a full-length clamp (**Figure 3**, *D*) or a two-incision rear-entry guide and out the anteromedial portal.

A second incision of approximately 4.5 cm is made over the proximal medial tibia in the region of the insertion of the pes anserinus. Dissection is carried through the subcutaneous tissue to the periosteum. A curved clamp is placed from this incision into the joint under the intermeniscal ligament (**Figure 3**, *E*), and a curved rat-tail rasp is used to make a small groove in the anteromedial proximal tibia under the intermeniscal ligament to bring tibial graft placement more posterior. The free end of the graft is then brought through the joint (**Figure 3**, *F*), under the intermeniscal ligament in the anteromedial epiphyseal groove, and out the medial tibial incision. The graft is fixed on the femoral side through the lateral incision with the knee in 90° of flexion and 15° of external rotation. Mattress sutures are used to attach the graft to the lateral femoral condyle at the insertion of the lateral intermuscular septum to effect

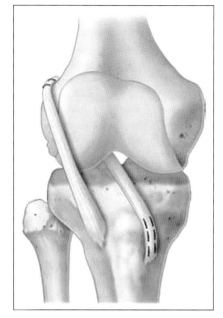

Figure 2 Drawing shows the intra-articular and extra-articular components of a completed physeal-sparing reconstruction. (Adapted with permission from Kocher MS: Anterior cruciate ligament reconstruction in the skeletally immature patient. *Op Tech Sports Med* 2006;14:124-134. Http://www-.sciencedirect.com/science/journal/10601872.)

an extra-articular reconstruction. The tibial side of the graft is then fixed through the medial incision with the knee flexed 20° and tension applied to the graft. A periosteal incision is made distal to the proximal tibial physis (verified by fluoroscopy), a trough is made in the proximal tibial medial metaphyseal cortex, and the graft is sutured to the periosteum at the rough margins with mattress sutures (**Figure 3**, *G*).

TRANSPHYSEAL
RECONSTRUCTION (FIGURE 4)

Usually general anesthesia is used, but local anesthesia can be used in emotionally mature adolescents. The patient is placed supine on the operating table, a pneumatic tourniquet is placed about the upper thigh (but not routinely used), and examination under anesthesia is done to confirm ACL insufficiency. If the diagnosis is in

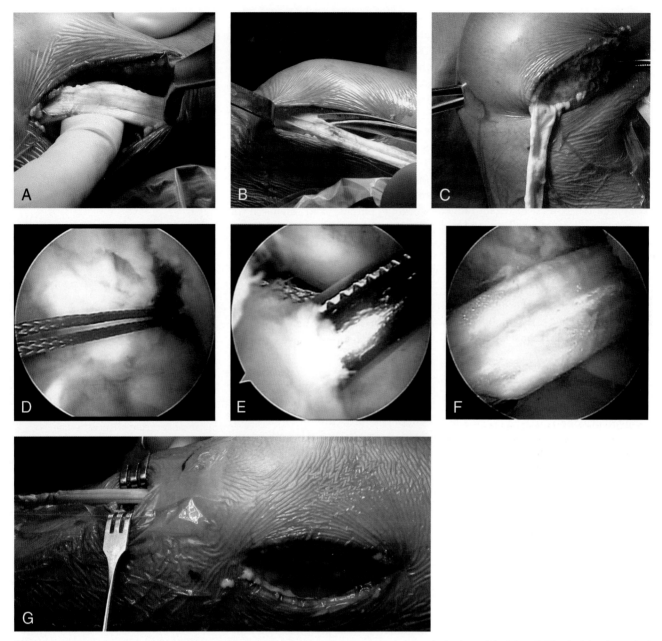

Figure 3 Physeal-sparing reconstruction. **A,** The iliotibial band graft is harvested through the lateral incision. **B,** The incision is carried proximally using a curved meniscotome. **C,** The graft is harvested free proximally and left attached to the Gerdy tubercle distally. **D,** The graft is brought through the knee in the over-the-top position using a full-length clamp. **E,** A curved clamp is placed under the intermeniscal ligament anteriorly. **F,** The graft is brought through the knee and under the intermeniscal ligament. **G,** The graft is brought out the medial tibial incision and fixed to a trough in the periosteum. (Adapted with permission from Kocher MS: Anterior cruciate ligament reconstruction in the skeletally immature patient. *Op Tech Sports Med* 2006;14:124-134. Http://www.sciencedirect.com/science/journal/10601872.)

doubt, arthroscopic examination can be done to confirm an ACL tear.

First, the hamstring tendons are harvested. A 4-cm incision is made over the palpable pes anserinus tendons on the medial side of the upper tibia (**Figure 5**, *A*). Dissection is carried through the skin to the sartorius fascia, with care taken to protect superficial sensory nerves. The sartorius tendon is incised longitudinally, and the gracilis and semitendinosus tendons are identified. The tendons are dissected free distally, and the free ends are whipstitched with No. 2 or No. 5 Ethibond sutures. The fibrous bands to the medial head of the gastrocnemius are sought and released. A closed tendon stripper is used to dissect the tendons free proximally. Alternatively, the tendons can be left attached distally and an open tendon stripper can be used to release them proximally. The free tendon graft is

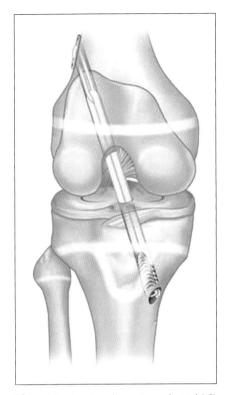

Figure 4 Drawing shows transphyseal ACL reconstruction using hamstring graft and metaphyseal fixation. (Adapted with permission from Kocher MS: Anterior cruciate ligament reconstruction in the skeletally immature patient. *Op Tech Sports Med* 2006;14:124-134. Http://www.sciencedirect.com/science/journal/10601872.)

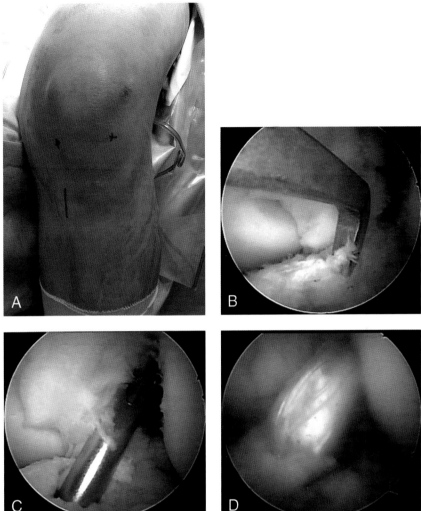

Figure 5 Transphyseal ACL reconstruction for adolescents with growth remaining. **A,** The gracilis and semitendinosus tendons are harvested through an incision over the proximal medial tibia (vertical line). **B,** The tibial guide is used to drill the tibial tunnel. **C,** The transtibial over-the-top offset guide is used to drill the femoral tunnel. **D,** Hamstring graft after fixation. (Adapted with permission from Kocher MS: Anterior cruciate ligament reconstruction in the skeletally immature patient. *Op Tech Sports Med* 2006;14:124-134. Http://www.sciencedirect-.com/science/journal/10601872.)

taken to a back table where excess muscle is removed and the remaining ends are whipstitched with No. 2 or No. 5 Ethibond sutures. The graft is folded over a closed-loop EndoButton (Smith & Nephew, Andover, MA), graft diameter is sized, and the graft is placed under tension.

Arthroscopic examination is done through standard portals. Any meniscal or chondral injuries are treated. The ACL remnant is excised, and the over-the-top position on the femur is identified. Minimal notchplasty is done to avoid injury to the perichondral ring of the distal femoral physis, which is close proximity to the over-the-top position.

A tibial tunnel guide set at 55° is placed through the anteromedial portal (**Figure 5,** *B*), and a guidewire is drilled through the graft harvest incision into the posterior aspect of the ACL tibial footprint. The guidewire entry point on the tibia should be kept medial to avoid injury to the tibial tubercle apophysis. The guidewire is reamed with the appropriate diameter reamer. Excess soft tissue at the tibial tunnel is excised to avoid arthrofibrosis. A transtibial over-the-top guide of the appropriate offset to ensure a 1- to 2-mm back wall is used to pass the femoral guide pin (**Figure 5,** *C*). The femoral guide pin is overdrilled with the EndoButton reamer and then both are removed to allow use of the depth gauge to measure femoral tunnel length. The guide pin is replaced and brought through the distal lateral thigh. The femoral tunnel is reamed to the appropriate depth, which is the length of the EndoButton plus 6 to 7 mm, to allow room to flip the Endobutton.

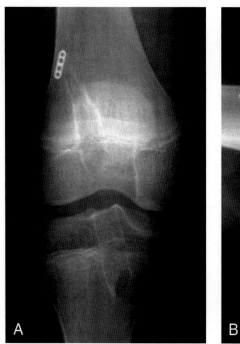
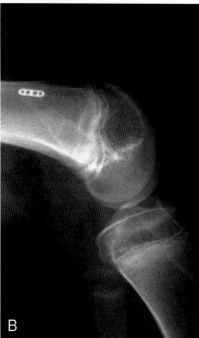
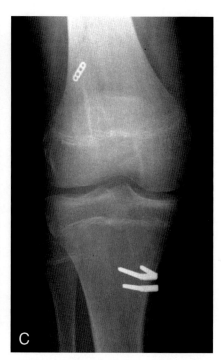

Figure 6 Postoperative AP (**A**) and lateral (**B**) radiographs show a knee after transphyseal reconstruction with autologous hamstrings for adolescents with growth remaining. **C,** AP radiograph shows alternate tibial fixation. (Adapted with permission from Kocher MS: Anterior cruciate ligament reconstruction in the skeletally immature patient. *Op Tech Sports Med* 2006;14:124-134. Http://www.sciencedirect.com/science/journal/10601872.)

The No. 5 Ethibond sutures on the EndoButton are placed in the slot of the guidewire and pulled through the tibial tunnel, through the femoral tunnel, and out the lateral thigh. These sutures are then pulled to bring the EndoButton and graft through the tibial tunnel and into the femoral tunnel. One set of sutures is used to "lead" the EndoButton, while the other set is used to "follow." Once the graft is fully seated in the femoral tunnel, the "follow" sutures are pulled to flip the Endobutton (**Figure 5**, *D*). The flip can be palpated in the thigh. Tension is applied to the graft to ensure that no graft slippage occurs. The knee is then extended to ensure there is no graft impingement, and then the knee is cycled approximately 10 times with tension applied to the graft. The graft is fixed on the tibial side with the knee in 20° to 30° of flexion, tension is applied to the graft, and a posterior force is placed on the tibia. The graft is fixed to the tibia with either a soft-tissue in-terference screw if there is adequate tunnel distance (at least 30 mm) below the physis to ensure metphyseal placement or with a post and spiked washer. Fluoroscopy can be used to ensure that fixation is away from the physis. Postoperative radiographs are shown in **Figure 6**.

━━━━━━━━■

■ Postoperative Regimen

Rehabilitation after ACL reconstruction in skeletally immature patients is essential to ensure a good outcome, allow a return to sports, and avoid re-injury, but it can be challenging, especially in prepubescent children. A therapist who is experienced in working with children can help monitor compliance with therapy and activity restrictions.

After physeal-sparing iliotibial band reconstruction in prepubescent patients, full weight bearing is not allowed for 6 weeks. After transphyseal hamstring reconstruction in adolescents, full weight bearing is not allowed for 2 weeks. A continuous passive motion (CPM) machine set at 0° to 90° and cryotherapy are used for 2 weeks postoperatively; a protective postoperative brace is used for 6 weeks.

Range of motion is limited from 0° to 90° for the first 2 weeks, followed by progression to full range of motion. This progression includes range-of-motion exercises, patellar mobilization, electrical stimulation, pool therapy, proprioception exercises, and closed-chain strengthening during the first 3 months after surgery. This is followed by straight-line jogging, plyometric exercises, sport-cord exercises, and sport-specific exercises. Return to full activity, including cutting and pivoting sports, usually is allowed at 6 months after surgery. A functional knee brace is used routinely during cutting and pivoting activities for the first 2 years after return to sports.

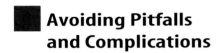

Avoiding Pitfalls and Complications

The most frequently cited potential complication of ACL reconstruction in skeletally immature patients is growth disturbance that can result in limb-length discrepancy or angular deformity; however, the actual occurrence of a clinically significant growth disturbance is rare. Rerupture has been reported in 3% to 15% of patients, all caused by trauma. Prolonged cast immobilization should be avoided because it can lead to postoperative stiffness.

Most complications of ACL reconstruction in skeletally immature patients can be avoided by careful attention to technical details during surgery: avoidance of fixation hardware across the lateral distal femoral physis, avoidance of injury to the vulnerable tibial tubercle apophysis, use of soft-tissue–only grafts (no bone block grafts), and avoidance of large tunnels. The 15 growth disturbances reported by the ACL Study Group and Herodicus Society all were associated with surgical errors such as malplacement of the proximal graft fixation, bone plugs across the physis, and staples over the tibial tubercle apophysis.

Pitfalls to avoid with the physeal-sparing iliotibial band reconstruction in prepubescent patients include harvesting a graft that is too short to reach the medial tibial incision and difficulty passing the graft through the posterior joint capsule or under the intermeniscal ligament. Care also should be taken to avoid dissection or notching around the posterolateral aspect of the physis during over-the-top femoral placement, to avoid injury to the perichondral ring that could cause subsequent deformity. Pitfalls to avoid with the transphyseal hamstring reconstruction in adolescents include amputation of the hamstring graft, poor tunnel placement, and graft impingement.

Acknowledgment

The author would like to acknowledge the assistance of Eric D. McFeely, BA, in preparing this chapter.

Bibliography

Aichroth PM, Patel DV, Zorrilla P: The natural history and treatment of rupture of the anterior cruciate ligament in children and adolescents: A prospective review. *J Bone Joint Surg Br* 2002;84(1):38-41.

Anderson AF: Transepiphyseal replacement of the anterior cruciate ligament in skeletally immature patients: A preliminary report. *J Bone Joint Surg Am* 2003;85-A(7):1255-1263.

Andrews M, Noyes FR, Barber-Westin SD: Anterior cruciate ligament allograft reconstruction in the skeletally immature athlete. *Am J Sports Med* 1994;22(1):48-54.

Aronowitz ER, Ganley TJ, Goode JR, Gregg JR, Meyer JS: Anterior cruciate ligament reconstruction in adolescents with open physes. *Am J Sports Med* 2000;28(2):168-175.

Bisson LJ, Wickiewicz T, Levinson M, Warren R: ACL reconstruction in children with open physes. *Orthopedics* 1998; 21(6):659-663.

Bollen S, Pease F, Ehrenraich A, Church S, Skinner J, Williams A: Changes in the four-strand hamstring graft in anterior cruciate ligament reconstruction in the skeletally-immature knee. *J Bone Joint Surg Br* 2008;90(4):455-459.

Edwards PH, Grana WA: Anterior cruciate ligament reconstruction in the immature athlete: Long-term results of intra-articular reconstruction. *Am J Knee Surg* 2001;14(4):232-237.

Fuchs R, Wheatley W, Uribe JW, Hechtman KS, Zvijac JE, Schurhoff MR: Intra-articular anterior cruciate ligament reconstruction using patellar tendon allograft in the skeletally immature patient. *Arthroscopy* 2002;18(8):824-828.

Guzzanti V, Falciglia F, Stanitski CL: Physeal-sparing intraarticular anterior cruciate ligament reconstruction in preadolescents. *Am J Sports Med* 2003;31(6):949-953.

Guzzanti V, Falciglia F, Stanitski CL: Preoperative evaluation and anterior cruciate ligament reconstruction technique for skeletally immature patients in Tanner stages 2 and 3. *Am J Sports Med* 2003;31(6):941-948.

Kocher MS, Garg S, Micheli LJ: Physeal sparing reconstruction of the anterior cruciate ligament in skeletally immature prepubescent children and adolescents. *J Bone Joint Surg Am* 2005;87(11):2371-2379.

Kocher MS, Smith JT, Zoric BJ, Lee B, Micheli LJ: Transphyseal anterior cruciate ligament reconstruction in skeletally immature pubescent adolescents. *J Bone Joint Surg Am* 2007;89(12):2632-2639.

Lipscomb AB, Anderson AF: Tears of the anterior cruciate ligament in adolescents. *J Bone Joint Surg Am* 1986;68(1):19-28.

Lo IK, Kirkley A, Fowler PJ, Miniaci A: The outcome of operatively treated anterior cruciate ligament disruptions in the skeletally immature child. *Arthroscopy* 1997;13(5):627-634.

Matava MJ, Siegel MG: Arthroscopic reconstruction of the ACL with semitendinosus-gracilis autograft in skeletally immature adolescent patients. *Am J Knee Surg* 1997;10(2):60-69.

McCarroll JR, Rettig AC, Shelbourne KD: Anterior cruciate ligament injuries in the young athlete with open physes. *Am J Sports Med* 1988;16(1):44-47.

McCarroll JR, Shelbourne KD, Porter DA, Rettig AC, Murray S: Patellar tendon graft reconstruction for midsubstance anterior cruciate ligament rupture in junior high school athletes: An algorithm for management. *Am J Sports Med* 1994;22(4):478-484.

McIntosh AL, Dahm DL, Stuart MJ: Anterior cruciate ligament reconstruction in the skeletally immature patient. *Arthroscopy* 2006;22(12):1325-1330.

Micheli LJ, Rask B, Gerberg L: Anterior cruciate ligament reconstruction in patients who are prepubescent. *Clin Orthop Relat Res* 1999;364:40-47.

Parker AW, Drez D Jr, Cooper JL: Anterior cruciate ligament injuries in patients with open physes. *Am J Sports Med* 1994;22(1):44-47.

Seon JK, Song EK, Yoon TR, Park SJ: Transphyseal reconstruction of the anterior cruciate ligament using hamstring autograft in skeletally immature adolescents. *J Korean Med Sci* 2005;20(6):1034-1038.

Shelbourne KD, Gray T, Wiley BV: Results of transphyseal anterior cruciate ligament reconstruction using patellar tendon autograft in tanner stage 3 or 4 adolescents with clearly open growth plates. *Am J Sports Med* 2004;32(5):1218-1222.

Stanitski CL: Anterior cruciate ligament injury in the skeletally immature patient: Diagnosis and treatment. *J Am Acad Orthop Surg* 1995;3(3):146-158.

Coding

CPT Code		Corresponding ICD-9 Codes	
29888	Arthroscopically aided anterior cruciate ligament repair/augmentation or reconstruction	717.83	844.2

Chapter 70

Anterior Cruciate Ligament Injuries With Bony Avulsion

Allen F. Anderson, MD
Christian N. Anderson, MD

Indications

Anterior cruciate ligament (ACL) injuries with bony avulsion most commonly involve the tibial attachment of the ACL, resulting in what is termed a tibial eminence or tibial spine avulsion fracture. The mechanisms of these fractures are similar to those of intrasubstance ACL tears, although biomechanical studies using animal models have shown that ACL avulsion fractures are more likely to occur at slower loading rates than intrasubstance ACL tears. Historically, ACL avulsion fractures were thought to occur almost exclusively in the pediatric population because of the relative weakness of the incompletely ossified tibial plateau. A review of the current literature, however, revealed that 45% of the reported ACL avulsion fractures occurred in adults.

ACL avulsion fractures vary considerably in fragment size, displacement, and comminution. The most commonly used classification system categorizes four fracture patterns, which are based on the degree of displacement of the tibial attachment of the ACL (**Figure 1**). A type I fracture is the least severe, having a nondisplaced or minimally displaced anterior margin and excellent bony apposition. In a type II fracture, the anterior one third to one half of the fragment is displaced, with an intact posterior hinge. Type III fractures are classified into two subcategories: type IIIA avulsion fractures involve complete separation of the fragment from the bony bed without apposition, whereas type IIIB fractures are displaced completely and rotated cephalad. Type IV fractures indicate comminution of the fragment.

A displaced tibial eminence fracture can result in instability of the knee and a mechanical block to knee extension. Consequently, the goals of treatment are to restore the continuity of the femur-ACL-tibia viscoelastic chain and prevent a mechanical block to extension. The methods of treatment that are used to achieve these goals depend on the characteristics of the fracture and on whether entrapment of soft tissue in the fracture prevents reduction.

Because type I fractures are nondisplaced, they are treated with cast immobilization. Treatment of type II fractures is more variable. They can be treated with closed reduction in extension and cast immobilization or with arthroscopic reduction and internal fixation (ARIF). We consider ARIF to be indicated if a type II fracture cannot be reduced in extension or if it converts to a type III in extension. Approximately half of type II fractures are irreducible; of these, 26% have entrapment of soft tissue within the fracture. ARIF also is advocated for all type II fractures in knees that have concurrent meniscal tears.

ARIF is recommended for all type III and IV fractures. Sixty-five percent of type III fractures contain entrapped soft tissue that must be retracted before fracture reduction (**Figure 2**). Arthroscopic examination is the best way to determine whether concomitant meniscal or chondral injuries are present and whether the tibial spine fracture is comminuted. Fractures that appear to be type III on radiographs can be discovered to be type IV when examined arthroscopically. An accurate assessment of the fracture size and degree of fragment comminution is important because the integrity of the fragment determines the type of internal fixation required. Cannulated screw fixation is more rigid than suture fixation, but it should be used only in noncomminuted fragments that are at least 3 times the width of the screw. Suture fixation is recommended if the

Dr. Allen Anderson or an immediate family member is a board member, owner, officer, or committee member for the American Orthopaedic Society for Sports Medicine and serves as a paid consultant to or is an employee of Genzyme. Neither Dr. Christian Anderson nor any immediate family member has received anything of value from or owns stock in a commercial company or institution related directly or indirectly to the subject of this chapter.

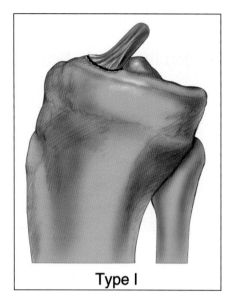

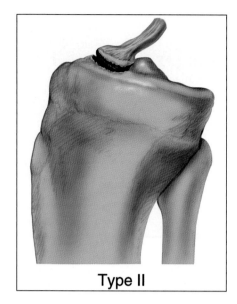

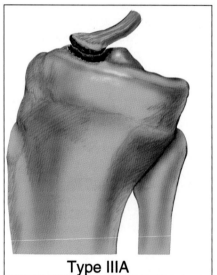

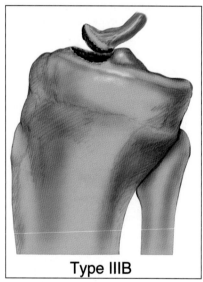

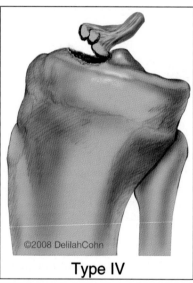

Figure 1 Classification system for tibial eminence fractures. Type I: nondisplaced or minimally displaced anterior margin. Type II: the anterior one third to one half of the fragment is displaced. Type IIIA: complete displacement of the fragment. Type IIIB: complete displacement and cephalad rotation of the fragment. Type IV: comminution of the fragment. (Illustrations ©2008 Delilah Cohn, Nashville, TN.)

tibial spine fragment is smaller than 1 cm in diameter or is comminuted.

Contraindications

Contraindications to ARIF as a treatment for tibial spine fractures in children and adolescents are rare. Active infection about the knee is an absolute contraindication to surgery. Failure to reduce the fragment arthroscopically is an indication to convert to open reduction of the fragment. A relative contraindication to arthroscopic surgery is a tibial spine fracture that has healed with a malunion. In this instance, open osteotomy and reduction of the fragment is technically easier than arthroscopic surgery.

The same conditions also are contraindications for ARIF in adults, as are certain medical comorbidities. Patients with significant rheumatoid arthritis, osteoarthritis, or limited functional demands are not candidates for this procedure. Concomitant injuries also may present a contraindication to arthroscopic surgery.

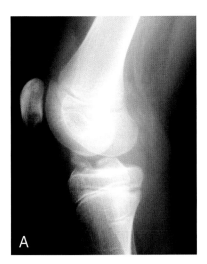
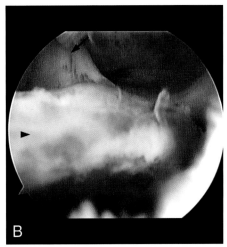

Figure 2 Images of a type IIIB tibial spine fracture in a 12-year-old boy. **A,** Lateral radiograph demonstrates a displaced fragment. **B,** Arthroscopic view shows the same type IIIB tibial spine fracture after the trapped intermeniscal ligament was retracted with a 2-0 monofilament suture. The arrow indicates the anterior cruciate ligament; the arrowhead indicates the fragment.

Alternative Treatments

Disagreement exists in the literature about whether it is best to treat type II injuries in children and adolescents with closed reduction and cast application or with ARIF. Residual problems with asymptomatic laxity, loss of extension, and less than optimal long-term outcomes have been reported with both closed reduction and ARIF. The reason for the controversy is the lack of clarity about the acceptable degree of anterior fragment elevation. It is reasonable to assume, however, that greater displacement of the fragment results in more laxity and greater potential for an extension block. Type II fractures that reduce after joint aspiration and extension should be followed closely for loss of reduction in the cast. If an acceptable reduction cannot be obtained or maintained, then surgical treatment is indicated.

Closed reduction and cast application is associated with poor outcomes in adults. Prolonged immobilization of the knee results in deleterious effects on the articular cartilage and the ligaments, which can lead to arthrofibrosis. Management of tibial spine fractures in adults should include anatomic reduction, rigid fixation, and early range-of-motion (ROM) therapy.

An alternative surgical option for adult patients is excision of the fragment and reconstruction of the ACL. Reattachment of the native ACL has the potential advantages of restoring normal joint kinematics and maintaining proprioception, but the outcome may be better after ACL reconstruction and aggressive rehabilitation than after poor fixation of an osteoporotic or comminuted fragment that limits postoperative therapy.

Open reduction and internal fixation through a small medial arthrotomy is a good alternative to ARIF. A variety of devices have been used to fix displaced fragments, including metal sutures, pins, threaded Kirschner wires, and staples. Nevertheless, arthroscopic fixation with cannulated screws for large fragments and suture fixation for comminuted fragments is now the standard of care.

Results

Because anterior tibial spine fractures occur infrequently, only case reports and small case series have been published, making it difficult to assess the results of treatment. The reported studies have investigated all four fracture types, some in children and some in adults, treated with a variety of methods and documented with different outcomes measures (**Table 1**). The limited data do appear to demonstrate, however, that the outcomes of the treatment of this injury are consistently different in children and in adults.

ARIF with sutures or cannulated screws provides excellent functional outcomes in children despite residual pathologic laxity. Persistent laxity may be the result of interstitial injury of the ACL at the time of fracture or of incomplete reduction. The use of epiphyseal screws avoids the proximal tibial physis, provides rigid fixation, and allows early ROM. Some surgeons have recommended suture fixation, which also can provide excellent results. Strong suture fixation permits early ROM and has the potential advantage that subsequent screw removal is not required. No comparative studies have been done to determine if the results of suture fixation are equivalent to those of screw fixation.

Some series report equally good results in adults as in children for the treatment of anterior tibial spine fractures. Other series have reported results in adults that were less satisfactory. The difference in outcomes between adults and children has been attributed to a higher number of associated injuries and the propensity for arthrofibrosis in adult patients. Emphasis should be placed on rigid fixation and early ROM therapy in this age group to minimize loss of motion.

Table 1 Results of Treatment of Tibial Eminence Fractures

Authors (Year)	Number of Knees/ Fracture Type	Procedure or Approach	Mean Patient Age in Years (Range)	Mean Follow-up (Range)	Results
Janarv et al(1995)	61 Type I: 8 Type II: 28 Type III: 25	Type I: cast only Type II: 21 cast only; 7 closed reduction Type III: 9 cast only; 3 reduction; 3 OR without IF; 10 ORIF with pins (1), wire (4), sutures (5).	All <16	16 years (10-39)	Pathologic knee laxity in 38% Lysholm score: 74% excellent, 13% good, 13% fair No correlation of age, displacement, or fixation type with outcome. Knee laxity had no effect on outcome except in type III with fixation.
Jung et al(1999)	16 Type II: 12 Type III: 4	ARIF with suture (polydioxane or polypropylene) fixation	31.8 (19-41)	27.3 months (12-59)	Muller score average: 88.3 IKDC: 4, A; 12, B Average ROM: 137° Telos device: all <4 mm anterior translation No cases of instability. All patients resumed normal activity.
Montgomery et al(2002)	17 Type II: 2 Type IIIA: 6 Type IIIB: 4 Type IV: 5	ARIF with suture fixation	36 (18-69)	5.4 years (2-9)	41% (7/17) had isolated injury. 47% had residual laxity after fixation. 53% had severe difficulty regaining motion. 24% required MUA to regain motion. An additional 24% required MUA plus arthroscopic débridement of anterior scar tissue impinging on the femoral notch. 75% of patients requiring >2 wks of immobilization developed motion problems. KT-1000: 12, <3 mm; 2, 3-5 mm; 1, >5 mm; 2 not reported 7/15 patients involved in sports returned to previous level.
Reynders et al (2002)	26 Type II: 16 Type III: 10	ARIF with antegrade cannulated screw and spiked washer fixation	Type II: 15 (13-17) Type III: 17 (16-18)	2-8 years	Type II group: 3, no laxity; 13, minor laxity Type III group: 10, positive anterior drawer test; 2, positive pivot-shift test (required ACL reconstruction), 4, elevation of the fragment Lysholm score average: 95.3 for type II group; 89.7 for type III group All returned to full activity except the 2 ACL reconstructions
Delcogliano et al (2003)	15 Type II: 6 Type III: 9	ARIF with suture fixation	22 (18-41)	18 months (15-57)	2 patients underwent arthrolysis at 2 months. IKDC: 5, A; 8, B; 2C KT-1000: all <5 mm All had radiographic union, 3 with increased tibial spine height. None had pain or activity limitation.
Kocher et al (2003)	80 Type II: 23 Type III: 57	ARIF: 71 ORIF: 5 Combined arthroscopic and open: 4	11.6 (5-16)	NA	Entrapment of AHMM, AHLM, or intermeniscal ligament: 26%, type II; 65%, type III Meniscal tear seen in 3.8%, all in type III injuries

Table 1 (continued)

Authors (Year)	Number of Knees/ Fracture Type	Procedure or Approach	Mean Patient Age in Years (Range)	Mean Follow-up (Range)	Results
Senekovic and Veselko (2003)	32 Type II: 8 Type III: 13 Type IV: 11	ARIF with cannulated screw fixation with use of toothed washer for small or comminuted fractures	22 (8-53)	37.5 months (16-69)	Lysholm score: 98.9 Lachman: negative in 26/28 KT-1000 average: 1.04 mm; no loss of motion Subjective evaluation: 27, normal; 1, nearly normal; 4 not reported Pediatric group decreased total treatment time; no growth disturbances
Hunter and Willis (2004)	17 Type II: 8 Type III: 9	Suture fixation: 7 Screw fixation: 10	26.6 (7.5-60.1)	32.6 months (14-51)	Best outcomes in younger patients Suture fixation, IKDC final score: 7, A; 1, B Screw fixation, IKDC final score: 2, A; 6, B; 1, C. No statistically significant difference for fixation types
Ahn and Yoo (2005)	14 Type IIIA: 4 Type IIIB: 3 Type IV: 3 Nonunion: 4	ARIF with suture fixation using 3 or more PDS sutures	26 (6-47)*	51 months (30-80)	All patients had full ROM Lachman: 13/14 negative Anterior drawer test: 13/14 negative KT-2000: 13/14 < 3mm Lysholm score average: 95.6 All patients returned to previous levels of activity. A 6-year-old patient had grade II Lachman and 5 mm KT-2000; she had 10° genu recurvatum and 1 cm increased leg length.
Zhao and Huangfu (2007)	18 All type III nonunions	ARIF with suture fixation	28.3 (19-39)	26 months (24-30)	IKDC: 17, normal; 1, nearly normal 15/18 returned to previous activity. No difference in preoperative and postoperative Tegner scores.

OR = open reduction, IF = internal fixation, ORIF = open reduction and internal fixation, ARIF = arthroscopic reduction and internal fixation, IKDC = International Knee Documentation Committee, ROM = range of motion, MUA = manipulation under anesthesia, ACL = anterior cruciate ligament, NA = not available, AHMM = anterior horn of the medial meniscus, AHLM = anterior horn of the lateral meniscus, PDS = polydioxanone.
*5 patients were 6-13 years old.

 # Technique

Setup
The injured limb is placed in an arthroscopic leg holder with the hip flexed 20° to facilitate C-arm fluoroscopic visualization of the knee in the lateral plane. The C-arm is positioned on the side of the table that is opposite the injured knee, and the monitor is placed at the head of the table. The tibial and femoral physes are viewed in both the anteroposterior and lateral planes before the limb is prepared and draped.

Instruments
The equipment necessary for ARIF includes a 4-mm 30° arthroscope, a shaver with a 3.5- or 4.5-mm synovectomy blade, and a standard video monitor. A fluid pump may be used, depending on the surgeon's preference. An arthroscopic probe or Freer elevator is used to reduce the fracture fragment. If screws are used for fixation, a wire driver and self-tapping cannulated 3.5-mm screws are necessary to secure the fragment. A curved suture passer and 2-0 monofilament suture may be necessary to pass a retraction suture if soft tissue is trapped in the fragment. A flexible suture passer is used to shuttle the suture through the tibial holes if suture fixation is used.

Procedure
SCREW FIXATION
The arthroscope is inserted into the anterolateral portal, and a probe is inserted through the anteromedial portal. The outflow cannula is inserted through the superolateral portal. The knee is lavaged, and intra-articular ex-

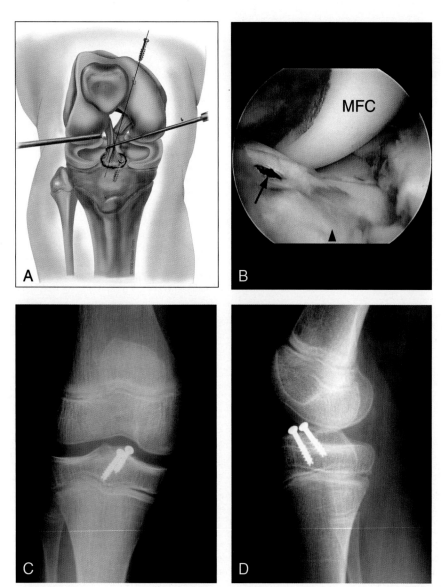

Figure 3 Arthroscopic reduction and internal fixation of a tibial spine avulsion fracture using screw fixation. **A**, Drawing demonstrates the positioning of the portals and instruments. With the knee flexed, a superomedial portal is established by first inserting an 18-gauge spinal needle at the level of the mid to upper patella at an angle that is as perpendicular as possible to the tibial plateau. After the fracture fragment is reduced and held in position by a probe inserted through the anteromedial portal, a 1.25-mm threaded guidewire is inserted into the fragment, the hole is drilled with C-arm visualization, and the appropriately sized 3.5-mm self-tapping cannulated cancellous screw is inserted. **B**, Arthroscopic view showing the fracture after fixation with two cannulated screws. The arrow indicates the cannulated screw; the arrowhead indicates the fragment. MFC = medial femoral condyle. AP (**C**) and lateral (**D**) radiographs demonstrate reduction of the fragment. (Part A ©2008 Delilah Cohn, Nashville, TN.)

amination is done systematically in the usual manner. If an unstable longitudinal-vertical meniscal tear is found, it is repaired. The ligamentum mucosum and part of the patellar fat pad can be removed with the shaver to improve visualization. The displaced tibial spine fragment is then elevated from the crater, and any interposed blood clot and debris in the fracture site are removed meticulously with a small curet and shaver. With the knee

flexed 45° to 60°, a superomedial portal is established by first inserting an 18-gauge spinal needle at the level of the mid to upper patella at an angle that is as perpendicular as possible to the tibial plateau (**Figure 3**, **A**).

If the anterior horn of the medial meniscus or the intermeniscal ligament has become trapped, it can be retracted with a probe placed through the superomedial portal. In some cases, it may be easier to use a 2-0 monofilament retraction suture inserted through the anteromedial portal with a 45° angle suture-passing instrument.

The probe or Freer elevator is inserted through the anteromedial portal to reduce the fragment. A 1.25-mm threaded guidewire is then inserted through the superomedial portal. The guidewire is inserted using real-time C-arm visualization to avoid crossing the tibial physis. It is important to avoid placing the guidewire in the posterior half of the fragment because doing so will cause the fragment to tilt anteriorly. If the fragment is large enough, the guidewire for the screw should be positioned so that there is room for an additional screw to be placed more laterally in the fragment. The guidewire should be inserted as vertically as possible through the fragment.

The measuring device is then placed over the guidewire, and the appropriately sized self-tapping 3.5-mm cannulated screw is chosen. A hole is drilled with the 2.7-mm cannulated drill bit using real-time C-arm visualization. The self-tapping screw is inserted. If the fragment is large enough, a second screw is inserted (**Figure 3**) and the knee is extended to determine whether the screw heads impinge on the femur.

SUTURE FIXATION

Suture fixation is indicated if the anterior tibial spine fracture is comminuted or has fragments that are too small to hold a screw (≤1 cm in diam-

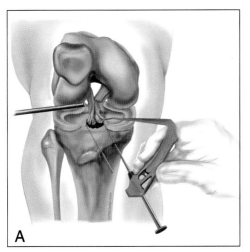
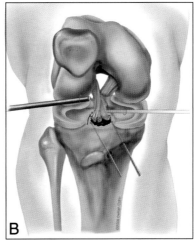
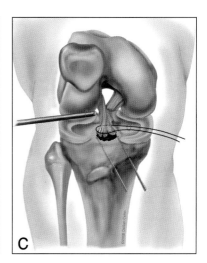
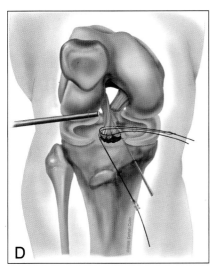
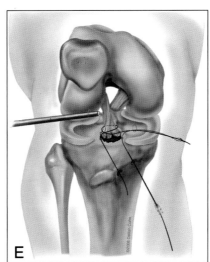
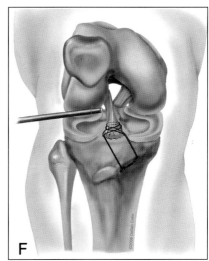

Figure 4 Arthroscopic reduction and internal fixation of a tibial spine avulsion fracture using suture fixation. **A**, An ACL drill guide, inserted through the anteromedial portal, is used to insert two 2.4-mm drill-tip guide pins that enter the joint at the lateral and medial edges of the fracture crater. **B**, A curved suture passer is used to pass a 2-0 monofilament suture or shuttle device through the posterior fibers of the ACL. **C**, A #2 nonabsorbable braided suture is shuttled through the ACL and pulled out the medial portal. **D**, The lateral guide pin is removed first and an 18-gauge spinal needle is placed in the drill hole. A flexible suture passer is inserted through the spinal needle and is pulled out through the medial portal. The braided suture limb on the medial side of the ACL is then loaded onto the flexible suture passer and pulled out through the lateral tibial drill hole. **E**, The medial drill-tip guide pin is then removed and, using the same technique, the lateral nonabsorbable braided suture limb is passed out through the medial hole creating a loop around the ACL and the fracture fragments. **F**, A second suture is then passed through the ACL fibers more anteriorly than the first and the limbs are passed through the same tibial drill holes as described above. (Illustrations ©2008 Delilah Cohn, Nashville, TN.)

eter). The arthroscopic preparation for suture fixation is similar to that for screw fixation. The anteromedial and anterolateral portals are established, the fat pad is débrided to improve visualization, any entrapped tissue is retracted, and the fracture crater is cleaned of clotted blood and debris.

An ACL drill guide is inserted through the anteromedial portal. The

entrance site for the pins on the anteromedial aspect of the tibia is determined by the point at which the drill guide encounters the skin. A short incision is made at that point and the periosteum is elevated. Two 2.4-mm drill-tip guide pins are inserted in the anteromedial aspect of the tibia 1 cm apart. One pin enters the joint at the medial side of the fracture crater and

the other at the lateral side (**Figure 4,** *A*). The drill guide is removed and a suture passer with a 90° tip is used to pass a 2-0 monofilament suture or shuttle device through the posterior fibers of the ACL, close to the bony fragment (**Figure 4,** *B*). A 5-mm cannula is then inserted through the anteromedial portal, and a grasper is used to retrieve both ends of the 2-0 monofilament suture. This suture is used to shuttle a #2 braided nonabsorbable suture through the ACL and out the cannula (**Figure 4,** *C*).

The lateral pin is then removed first and an 18-gauge spinal needle is placed in the drill hole. A closed-loop suture passer is then inserted in the spinal needle, and the suture passer is pulled out through the cannula in the medial portal. The #2 nonabsorbable braided suture limb on the medial side of the ACL is then loaded on the flexible suture passer and pulled out through the lateral tibial drill hole (**Figure 4,** *D*). The medial drill-tip guide pin is then removed and, using the same technique, the lateral #2 nonabsorbable braided suture limb is passed out through the medial hole, creating a loop around the ACL and the fracture fragments (**Figure 4,** *E*). A second suture is then passed through the ACL fibers more anteriorly than the first suture and the limbs of this suture are passed through the same tibial drill holes (**Figure 4,** *F*).

Most comminuted tibial spine fractures occur in adults. When suture fixation is necessary for pediatric patients in Tanner stage I, II, or III of sexual maturation, consideration should be given to drilling transepiphyseal holes. If the drill holes are made across the physis in patients in this age group, absorbable sutures should be used. Treatment for patients in Tanner stage IV of development is the same as for adults.

Postoperative Regimen

The postoperative protocol depends upon the security of the fracture fixation and on whether the patient is a child or an adult. Patients who have secure fixation of a large fragment using two screws can be treated with more aggressive rehabilitation. Adults should begin early ROM therapy because the most serious complication for adults is arthrofibrosis.

The rehabilitation process should be more cautious in a child or adolescent who has a tibial spine fracture that is secured with only one screw or with sutures. These patients are placed in a long-leg hinged brace locked at 30° of flexion for 4 weeks. They are encouraged to perform quadriceps contractions and leg raises. Passive ROM exercises and hamstring muscle stretching, done while the patient is prone, are started at 4 weeks after surgery. Six weeks after surgery, active ROM exercises are begun. The knee is fitted with a functional knee brace and partial weight bearing is begun, progressing to full weight bearing after 8 weeks. Exercises are introduced into the rehabilitation program in order of increasing difficulty. These exercises include hamstring and quadriceps muscle stretching, proprioception exercises, functional strengthening exercises, and aquatic strengthening exercises. The goal is to attain a full ROM equal to that of the contralateral, unaffected knee at 8 weeks after surgery.

In adults—and in children and adolescents whose fractures are fixed rigidly—rehabilitation can be more aggressive. These patients are placed in a long-leg hinged brace locked in extension. Quadriceps muscle contraction and straight-leg raises are encouraged. The day after surgery, passive ROM exercises and hamstring muscle stretches, done while the patient is prone, are started. Patients are allowed to walk with crutches using toe-touch weight bearing, progressing to full weight bearing after 6 weeks. Two weeks after surgery, the goal is to attain a ROM of 0° to 90° of flexion. Active ROM exercises, including terminal extension, are begun at 6 weeks, along with patellar mobilization. Patients are fitted with a functional knee brace, and full weight bearing is encouraged. Exercises are introduced in levels of increasing difficulty. Patients are allowed full participation in sports 4 to 6 months after surgery.

Avoiding Pitfalls and Complications

Loss of Motion

Loss of knee motion is the most common complication of a tibial spine fracture. This complication can result from arthrofibrosis, prominent hardware, or a fracture fragment that heals with a malunion. The development of arthrofibrosis following treatment of a tibial spine fracture has been attributed primarily to prolonged immobilization. The length of immobilization is dictated by the security of the fracture fixation, but the consensus is that early mobilization in adults is necessary to minimize the incidence of arthrofibrosis. An extension block caused by prominent hardware can be prevented by extending the knee under arthroscopic visualization to ensure that the screws do not impinge on the femur. Prominent screws can be countersunk, or a small notchplasty can be performed if necessary. A malunion can be prevented by proper fracture reduction.

Residual Laxity

Residual pathologic laxity following treatment of tibial spine fractures can result from either interstitial ACL failure before a tibial spine avulsion fracture or inadequate reduction of the fragment. Although it is a technically difficult procedure, countersinking the tibial spine fracture to prevent persistent laxity caused by interstitial injury is recommended by some authors.

Inadequate reduction or mild loss of reduction may cause the tibial spine to heal in an elevated position, resulting in permanent elongation of the femur-ACL-tibia viscoelastic chain. Better arthroscopic visualization with retraction of any interposed soft tissues will facilitate an anatomic reduction. Loss of reduction can be minimized by improving fixation or by tailoring the rehabilitation program to lower the intensity of the stress on the joint if the fracture fixation is weak. Overall, good functional outcomes can be achieved despite mild persistent laxity.

Inadequate Fracture Reduction
Interposition of the medial meniscus, intermeniscal ligament, or lateral meniscus has been found in 26% of type II fractures and 65% of type III fractures. Anatomic reduction of the fragment usually is impossible without retraction of the tissues with a probe or suture. If the entrapped intermeniscal ligament cannot be retracted, then it can be resected, or a small arthrotomy can be made to facilitate fracture reduction.

Fracture reduction can be difficult, even after the soft tissue has been retracted out of the way. A probe or small elevator inserted through the medial portal can be used to manipulate the fragment as the knee is rotated internally and externally and moved through a ROM of 35° to 75° of flexion. After reduction is obtained, the cannulated screw guidewire is inserted through the superomedial portal for provisional fixation.

ACL Interstitial Injury
The status of the ACL should always be evaluated to determine whether reduction of the tibial fragment will restore ACL continuity. Occasionally, an incomplete bony avulsion of the ACL (most commonly the anterior medial bundle) may occur, with the remainder of the ACL being torn from the tibia. ARIF of such tibial spine avulsion fractures will restore ACL function only partially. Consequently, ACL reconstruction may be the best method of treatment for these injuries.

———————————■

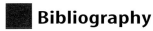

Bibliography

Ahn JH, Yoo JC: Clinical outcome of arthroscopic reduction and suture for displaced acute and chronic tibial spine fractures. *Knee Surg Sports Traumatol Arthrosc* 2005;13(2):116-121.

Binnet MS, Gürkan I, Yilmaz C, Karakas A, Cetin C: Arthroscopic fixation of intercondylar eminence fractures using a 4-portal technique. *Arthroscopy* 2001;17(5):450-460.

Delcogliano A, Chiossi S, Caporaso A, Menghi A, Rinonapoli G: Tibial intercondylar eminence fractures in adults: Arthroscopic treatment. *Knee Surg Sports Traumatol Arthrosc* 2003;11(4):255-259.

Doral MN, Atay OA, Leblebicioğlu G, Tetik O: Arthroscopic fixation of the fractures of the intercondylar eminence via transquadricipital tendinous portal. *Knee Surg Sports Traumatol Arthrosc* 2001;9(6):346-349.

Hunter RE, Willis JA: Arthroscopic fixation of avulsion fractures of the tibial eminence: Technique and outcome. *Arthroscopy* 2004;20(2):113-121.

Janarv PM, Westblad P, Johansson C, Hirsch G: Long-term follow-up of anterior tibial spine fractures in children. *J Pediatr Orthop* 1995;15(1):63-68.

Jung YB, Yum JK, Koo BH: A new method for arthroscopic treatment of tibial eminence fractures with eyed Steinmann pins. *Arthroscopy* 1999;15(6):672-675.

Kendall NS, Hsu SY, Chan KM: Fracture of the tibial spine in adults and children: A review of 31 cases. *J Bone Joint Surg Br* 1992;74(6):848-852.

Kocher MS, Micheli LJ, Gerbino P, Hresko MT: Tibial eminence fractures in children: Prevalence of meniscal entrapment. *Am J Sports Med* 2003;31(3):404-407.

Meyers MH, McKeever FM: Fracture of the intercondylar eminence of the tibia. *J Bone Joint Surg Am* 1959;41-A(2):209-222.

Montgomery KD, Cavanaugh J, Cohen S, Wickiewicz TL, Warren RF, Blevens F: Motion complications after arthroscopic repair of anterior cruciate ligament avulsion fractures in the adult. *Arthroscopy* 2002;18(2):171-176.

Reynders P, Reynders K, Broos P: Pediatric and adolescent tibial eminence fractures: Arthroscopic cannulated screw fixation. *J Trauma* 2002;53(1):49-54.

Senekovic V, Veselko M: Anterograde arthroscopic fixation of avulsion fractures of the tibial eminence with a cannulated screw: Five-year results. *Arthroscopy* 2003;19(1):54-61.

Wiley JJ, Baxter MP: Tibial spine fractures in children. *Clin Orthop Relat Res* 1990;255:54-60.

Zhao J, Huangfu X: Arthroscopic treatment of nonunited anterior cruciate ligament tibial avulsion fracture with figure-of-8 suture fixation technique. *Arthroscopy* 2007;23(4):405-410.

Coding

CPT Codes		Corresponding ICD-9 Codes	
Arthroscopic Reduction and Internal Fixation			
29855	Arthroscopically aided treatment of tibial fracture, proximal (plateau); unicondylar, includes internal fixation, when performed (includes arthroscopy)	823.00 823.10	823.02 823.12
29856	Arthroscopically aided treatment of tibial fracture, proximal (plateau); bicondylar, includes internal fixation, when performed (includes arthroscopy)	823.00 823.10	823.02 823.12

Chapter 71

Complications of Anterior Cruciate Ligament Reconstruction

Robert A. Arciero, MD
Drew Fehsenfeld, MD, PhD

Introduction

Despite a success rate better than 90%, approximately 1% of patients who undergo anterior cruciate ligament (ACL) reconstruction have poor results because of complications. Most complications can be prevented by avoiding common pitfalls in technique. When complications do occur, early recognition and intervention can reduce long-term morbidity.

Results

Four basic grafts are used in ACL reconstructions: bone–patellar tendon–bone (BPTB); quadrupled hamstring; Achilles, BPTB, and anterior tibialis allograft; and quadriceps tendon. Despite the numerous graft options and fixation methods, the results of these reconstructions are consistently good. Modern evaluation and outcomes assessment typically uses subjective and objective tools to determine effectiveness in ACL reconstruction. The Lysholm score, International Knee Documentation Committee (IKDC) score, laxity tests, instrumented arthrometer testing, Knee Injury and Osteoarthritis Outcome Score (KOOS), Short Form-36 (SF-36), and return to activity Tegner score typify a modern assessment of the ACL-reconstructed patient. Simply stated, no method or graft has consistently demonstrated superior outcomes (**Table 1**). The expectations are that approximately 90% of patients will be extremely satisfied with the outcome regardless of graft type or fixation. Generally speaking, the BPTB graft has been associated with greater anterior knee pain but better results on laxity testing and return to high level function. Soft-tissue grafts may be associated with modest increases in rerupture and tunnel widening but less knee pain. Therefore, it appears that the most critical factors in successful ACL reconstruction are proper anatomic tunnel preparation, graft placement, and avoiding complications.

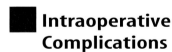

Intraoperative Complications

Graft Harvest
Studies support the efficacy of various graft choices for ACL reconstruction, with no graft type outperforming the others. Most ACL reconstructions performed in the United States use an autologous BPTB or hamstring graft, each of which is associated with unique complications that can occur during harvest and preparation. For years, the BPTB graft was the standard for ACL reconstruction, but several complications with the BPTB graft, including inadequate or fractured bone plug, graft tunnel mismatch, patellar fracture, patellar chondral injury, and postoperative anterior knee pain, have been reported in the literature. Although these complications are very rare (prevalence < 0.2%), their occurrence has led to the use of hamstring autograft as an alternative graft choice. Complications also have been associated with the use of hamstring autografts, however, including saphenous nerve neuroma, early truncation of the graft, and postoperative hamstring weakness. The most common and devastating complication is early truncation of the hamstring graft during harvest. Even though the risk of graft problems is small, preoperative planning should include a discussion of all graft options with the patient in case complications require the use of an alternative graft.

Short or Fractured Bone Plug
AVOIDING THE COMPLICATION
Short or fractured bone plugs most frequently occur when inappropriate

Dr. Arciero or an immediate family member is a member of speakers' bureau or has made paid presentations on behalf of Arthrex and has received research or institutional support from Arthrex. Neither Dr. Fehsenfeld nor any immediate family member has received anything of value from or owns stock in a commercial company or institution related directly or indirectly to the subject of this chapter.

Table 1 Results of Anterior Cruciate Ligament Reconstruction

Author(s)/ Year	Number of Patients or Knees	Type of Study	Procedure or Approach	Mean Patient Age in Years (Range)	Mean Follow-up (Range)	Results
Freedman et al (2003)	1,976 patients	Meta-analysis	1,348 BPTB 628 HSTG	22-45	24-96 months	BPTB had less re-rupture, less side-to-side difference on KT-1000, more anterior knee pain, greater patient satisfaction.
Aglietti et al (2004)	120 patients	PRCT	BPTB vs HSTG	25 (16-39)	Minimum 2 years	Visual analog, IKDC, KOOS, KT-1000, and Tegner were the same for both. Kneeling problems with BPTB. HSTG had greater tunnel widening.
Carey et al (2009)	746 knees	Meta-analysis	BPTB autograft vs BPTB allograft	(14-58)	49 months (24-99)	Lysholm score, instrumented laxity measurements, clinical failure rate same for both.
Taylor et al (2009)	64 knees	PRCT	BPTB vs HSTG	22 (17-45)	36 months (24-60)	Lysholm = 92 for both; Tegner, IKDC, SANE, KOOS, KT-2000 same for both.
Drogset et al (2009)	115 knees	PRCT	BPTB vs double HSTG	27 (18-50)	Minimum 2 years	Lysholm = 91 KT-1000: 1.5 for BPTB, 1.8 for HSTG

PRCT = prospective randomized clinical trial, BPTB = bone–patellar tendon–bone, HSTG = hamstring tendon graft, IKDC = International Knee Documentation Committee score, KOOS = Knee Injury and Osteoarthritis Outcome Score, SANE = Single Assessment Numeric Evaluation.

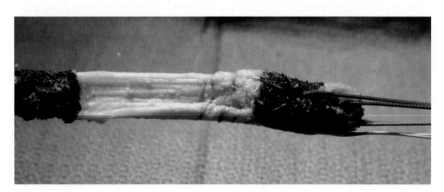

Figure 1 A fractured patellar bone plug can be salvaged by extending sutures to the tendon.

technique is used during harvest, especially when an osteotome is used to free the undersurface of the bone plug. If the osteotome is used to lever the bone rather than cut, the plug may fracture. Studies also have reported fracture of the bone plug during interference screw insertion because of high torque or divergence of the screw and tunnel. Ideally, bone plugs should be longer than 15 mm to provide adequate fixation with an interference screw. If a bone plug is shorter than 10 mm, an interference screw may not provide adequate stabilization of the graft, and alternative fixation should be considered.

MANAGING THE COMPLICATION

If the patellar bone plug fractures and a good tibial bone plug exists, the graft should be reversed. Using a Krakow stitch, two nonabsorbable sutures are placed in the patellar tendon approximately 1 cm from the end of the graft (**Figure 1**). A hole is drilled through the bone plug, and the sutures are shuttled through. The graft is shuttled into the knee, leading with the tibial bone plug, and an interference screw is used to secure the femoral side of the graft. The soft tissue is cleared 1 to 2 cm distal to the tibial tunnel with electrocautery or a Cobb elevator. A standard 2.5-mm hole is drilled in the prepared area from anteromedial to posterolateral. A 3.5- or 4.5-mm AO screw with a washer is placed, and the sutures securing the tibial side of the graft are tensioned and tied over the post with the knee in 20° of flexion. An interference screw can be added if desired.

Alternatively, a suspension cortical fixation or cortical button (EndoButton, Smith & Nephew, Mansfield, MA; or RetroButton, Arthrex, Naples, FL) can be used at the soft-tissue end.

POSTOPERATIVE REGIMEN

No modifications to the usual postoperative regimen are necessary. Protected weight bearing for 2 to 3 weeks with immediate active range of motion and quadriceps strengthening, as with a typical ACL reconstruction, is permitted.

Graft Tunnel Mismatch

AVOIDING THE COMPLICATION

If an autograft or allograft is too long, the bone block will protrude from the anterior tibia, which can compromise fixation on the tibial side by preventing adequate contact with an interference screw. Careful tibial tunnel planning can help avoid this complication. If preoperative lateral radiographs reveal patella alta, the tibial tunnel can be made steep and longer to accommodate the increased length. A prominent bone plug also may result from a short, shallowly angled tibial tunnel. Generally, the tibial tunnel angle should be between 45° and 55°, but the angle can be determined more accurately using the N + 10 rule, according to which the length of the tendinous portion of the graft (N) plus 10 equals the angle that will ensure that the bone plug is within the tibial tunnel. This can result in a vertical tibial tunnel, however, which does not allow proper placement of the femoral tunnel with a transtibial technique.

MANAGING THE COMPLICATION

If the tibial bone block is protruding, the graft should be removed and the guide pin replaced in the femoral tunnel. The femoral tunnel depth is increased by 5 to 10 mm and the bone plug is recessed in the tunnel. A curet is used to create a notch on the anterior aspect of the femoral tunnel. The notch should allow visualization of the recessed bone plug and the ligament. A guide pin is placed over the trabecular side of the recessed bone block, and the interference screw is inserted. Graft laceration is a risk,

and care should be taken to observe the interference screw as it passes anterior to the soft-tissue portion of the graft.

Alternatively, the femoral bone plug can be fixed using the standard technique with a soft-tissue bioabsorbable or biocomposite screw fixing the graft within the tibial tunnel, leaving the tibial bone plug prominent. A trough for the bone plug is cut in the inferior aspect of the tibial tunnel with a ¼-in osteotome. The graft is then further tensioned and the tibial bone block is secured in the trough with a 3.5-mm screw or staple.

The graft can be modified by shortening or removing the bone plug. The graft can be shortened using one of two techniques: the graft can be twisted on itself, or, if this does not adequately shorten the ligament, the bone plug can be rotated 180° and sutured to the tendon, shortening the working length of the graft by the length of the bone block. An interference screw is then inserted to secure the shortened graft. The bone block can be removed and the graft fixed with a suspensory technique. The tendon is prepared with two No. 0 nonabsorbable sutures using a running Krackow stitch. The graft is tensioned and secured on the tibial side over a post.

Video 71.1 Complications of ACL Reconstruction: Tunnel Lysis. Robert A. Arciero, MD (3 min)

POSTOPERATIVE REGIMEN

No modifications to the postoperative regimen are necessary.

Patellar Fracture

AVOIDING THE COMPLICATION

Patellar fractures, although rare, can occur intraoperatively and postoperatively in patients with a BPTB graft. Several poor harvest techniques have

been associated with these fractures, including excessive bone plug harvest, uneven cut depth, and overcutting at the corners. Each of these can create a stress riser that weakens the patella and may result in a fracture. Inappropriate hinging of the patella with an osteotome also can cause a fracture.

MANAGING THE COMPLICATION

Most of these patellar fractures are longitudinal, but transverse fractures that disrupt the extensor mechanism can occur. A fracture that occurs intraoperatively should be stabilized immediately to prevent displacement or propagation. Fractures that occur postoperatively because of a forceful eccentric contraction or direct blow should be managed according to standard principles. Nondisplaced longitudinal fractures can be managed with serial radiographic follow-up. If there is any question of stability of the fracture, interfragmentary fixation should be used so that rehabilitation is not compromised. Transverse fractures require surgical stabilization to restore the extensor mechanism and allow continued rehabilitation.

Fixation of simple transverse or longitudinal fractures is described here; management of more complex fractures is outside the scope of this chapter. The patient is positioned supine on a standard operating table, a tourniquet is placed high on the thigh, and the leg is prepared and draped free. The leg is then exsanguinated with a sterile Esmarch bandage, and the tourniquet is inflated to an appropriate level. The patella is approached through a longitudinal midline incision extending 1 cm above and below the patella. Medial and lateral skin flaps are created to expose the patella and retinaculum. The retinaculum often is disrupted and requires repair. The fracture edges are sharply exposed, and hematoma and soft tissue are cleaned from the fracture site. A large point-to-point reduction clamp

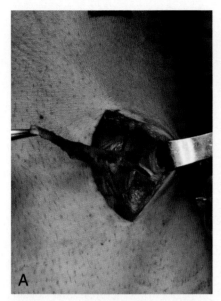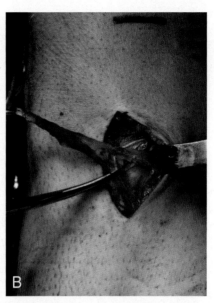

Figure 2 Hamstring graft harvest. **A,** Adequate visualization of the fascial bands to the hamstring tendons. **B,** Release with Mayo scissors.

is placed at the superior and inferior poles of the patella, and the fracture is reduced. Fluoroscopy and palpation of the joint surface through the disrupted retinaculum confirm adequate reduction of the articular surface.

Fixation can be obtained with tension band wires, cannulated screws with a tension band, or a tension band plate. Our technique is to place two 4.0-mm cannulated, partially threaded screws from distal to proximal. An 18-gauge tension band wire is passed through one screw and then woven over the patella and through the other screw to create a figure-of-8 configuration on the anterior aspect of the patella. The wire is then tensioned by twisting and lifting the free ends with a clamp. For longitudinal fractures, two 3.5-mm lag screws placed lateral to medial should provide adequate fixation. The wound is irrigated before closure. The retinaculum is closed with interrupted bioabsorbable sutures, the subcutaneous tissue is closed with a 2-0 bioabsorbable suture, and 3-0 prolene is used for the skin.

POSTOPERATIVE REGIMEN

The standard postoperative protocol after ACL reconstruction can be used with only slight modifications when a patellar fracture occurs. In patients with stable fixation, immediate active knee flexion and extension can be started. Early weight bearing in either a hinged knee brace locked in extension or a knee immobilizer is allowed for the first 4 to 6 weeks. If there is any question about the stability of fixation, rehabilitation should proceed more slowly and the patient should be monitored closely for loss of fixation. Symptoms or signs of hardware loosening or loss of reduction should signal a stop to any range-of-motion exercises.

Premature Hamstring Tendon Amputation

AVOIDING THE COMPLICATION

The most devastating complication during hamstring harvest is premature graft laceration or inadequate graft harvest. Graft laceration most often occurs when fascial bands to hamstring tendons remain when the tendon stripper is applied. The fascial bands force the stripper against the tendon, resulting in early truncation of the tendon. Increased resistance and failure to advance the tendon

stripper are early signs of unreleased fascial bands.

Several techniques help avoid early truncation of the hamstring grafts. Adequate exposure of the tendons will allow better identification of fascial bands to the gastrocnemius muscle. The tendons are palpated along their course to identify any obstructions to the tendon stripper. The fascial bands can be released with either blunt dissection or curved Mayo scissors (**Figure 2**). Additionally, if traction on the hamstring tendon causes dimpling of the popliteal fossa, a fascial band likely remains and must be identified and dissected free from the hamstrings. During harvest, the tendon stripper should be applied parallel to the tendon and traction maintained. If significant resistance is met, the tendon stripper should be removed and the hamstrings reexamined for remaining fascial bands.

MANAGING THE COMPLICATION

Even if amputation occurs, it may be possible to salvage the graft construct. Because the total graft length necessary is 7 cm (2 cm in each tunnel and 2.5 to 3.0 cm as the intra-articular portion), it may be possible to double the remaining properly harvested hamstring and sew the amputated graft together, resulting in a graft of the appropriate diameter. If a single tendon is truncated, adequate graft material may be obtained by harvesting a second hamstring tendon. Generally, the combined hamstrings should be at least 8 mm wide and 7 cm long (the articular portion of the ACL is 26 to 28 mm and, therefore, 2 cm of graft can reside in each tunnel). If inadequate graft is obtained, an alternative graft choice must be made.

POSTOPERATIVE REGIMEN

No modification to the postoperative regimen is necessary if the hamstring graft can be salvaged. If an alternative graft is used, the postoperative regimen should be modified based on the standard protocol associated with the graft used.

Graft Contamination

AVOIDING THE COMPLICATION

Contamination of the graft can occur in the process of graft preparation. Up to 60% of grafts dropped on the floor have been shown to have positive cultures. No standard protocol has been established for the management of graft contamination, but several options have been discussed in the literature, including cleaning and sterilization of the graft, harvesting an alternative graft, and using allograft. Harvesting an ipsilateral graft has been associated with extended rehabilitation and higher risk of motion deficits. Most important, the possibility of this situation should be discussed with the patient preoperatively because using an alternative graft requires patient consent.

MANAGING THE COMPLICATION

Methods for salvage of a contaminated graft include the use of sequential 15- to 20-minute soaks with 4% chlorohexidine gluconate, triple antibiotic solution, and sterile saline. This combination of solutions has been shown to result in consistently negative cultures. Historically, washing with a 10% povidone-iodine or triple antibiotic solution has been used with good results; however, some evidence suggests that graft contamination can persist with these procedures.

POSTOPERATIVE REGIMEN

When intraoperative graft contamination occurs, the patient should be monitored weekly for the first several postoperative weeks with a high index of suspicion for infection. The management of postoperative septic knee is discussed in more detail below.

Femoral Tunnel Posterior Wall Disruption

Posterior wall blowout occurs when the posterior femoral cortex is vio-

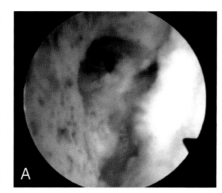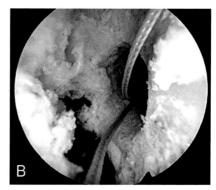

Figure 3 Arthroscopic views demonstrate femoral tunnel drilling. **A,** Femoral tunnel with posterior wall blowout. **B,** Femoral footprint confirming 1-mm posterior wall. (Part A reproduced with permission from Busam ML, Provencher MT, Bach BR Jr: Complications of anterior cruciate ligament reconstruction with bone-patellar tendon-bone constructs. *Am J Sports Med* 2008;36:387.)

lated during femoral tunnel drilling (**Figure 3**). Damage to the posterior cortex is most often caused by inadequate knee flexion or inaccurate placement of the femoral guide pin. It is important to recognize when this occurs by probing the posterior cortex after femoral tunnel drilling to confirm an intact 1-mm rim. If more than 5 mm of cortex is removed, the retrograde placement of an interference screw for fixation may not be possible. Errant placement of an interference screw will result in inadequate fixation and possible loss of the interference screw in the posterior fossa. Alternatives to femoral-side fixation of the graft should be considered, including suspensory fixation, antegrade placement of an interference screw using a two-incision technique, or tying sutures over a femoral screw or button.

AVOIDING THE COMPLICATION

Posterior wall blowout can be avoided by careful technique. The guide pin for the femoral tunnel is placed, and a probe is used to measure the distance between the pin and the posterior wall. The femoral tunnel is initially drilled for 5 mm, and a probe is used to evaluate the posterior cortex. If the orientation of the tunnel results in removal of posterior wall, the guide pin

can be redirected or the tunnel drilled at an increased knee flexion angle.

MANAGING THE COMPLICATION

If posterior wall blowout occurs, one technique for femoral fixation is to secure the graft over a femoral post. The femoral bone plug is prepared by passing two nonabsorbable sutures through 1-mm drill holes. A longitudinal incision is made on the lateral thigh over the femoral guide pin. The iliotibial band is identified and incised in line with the incision. The vastus lateralis is elevated anteriorly with a Cobb elevator to expose the lateral femur. The exit point for the femoral guide pin is identified, and the bone is exposed superior to the pin. A looped passing suture is placed using the guide pin, and the sutures securing the graft are shuttled through the femoral tunnel. A 2.5-mm hole is drilled from lateral to medial, and a 3.5-mm fully threaded cortical screw with a washer is placed. The screw is left slightly proud, and the graft sutures are tied over the post. The screw is then tightened to secure the graft.

Alternatively, the graft can be secured using a suspensory device such as an EndoButton or RetroButton. The femoral tunnel is prepared by advancing a 2.7-mm passing pin. The tunnel is then drilled to the depth of graft in-

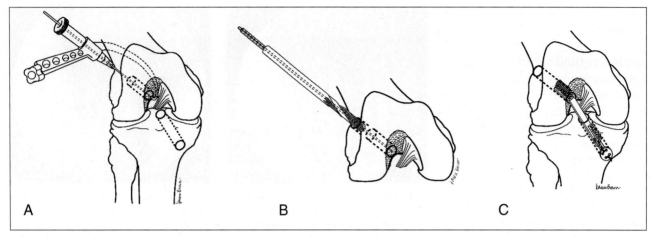

Figure 4 Technique for management of graft laceration. **A**, A rear-entry guide was used to position the guidewire from the lateral femur into the endoscopic tunnel. **B**, A 10-mm hole was created with a cannulated reamer. **C**, After the bony portion of the autograft was positioned flush with the intra-articular opening of the femoral tunnel, the free bony segment was placed into the tibial tunnel to eliminate dead space, and the graft was secured over a ligament button. (Reproduced with permission from Arciero RA: Endoscopic anterior cruciate ligament reconstruction: Complication of graft rupture and a method of salvage. *Am J Knee Surg* 1996;9(1):27-31.)

sertion plus 10 mm to allow flipping of the EndoButton. The bone block is prepared with two central holes using a 2.0-mm drill. Two No. 5 nonabsorbable sutures or 6-mm fiber tapes are passed through the bone tunnels and then through the central eyelets of the EndoButton. They are then tied at the appropriate length to accommodate the tunnel. The graft can be recessed in the femoral tunnel if the tibial bone plug protrudes from the tibial tunnel.

POSTOPERATIVE REGIMEN
No modifications in the postoperative regimen are necessary with stable fixation of the graft using alternative techniques.

Amputation of Bone Plug

AVOIDING THE COMPLICATION
Although uncommon, amputation of the bone plug can occur during insertion of an interference screw. Techniques to avoid this complication include painting the bone-tendon junction with a sterile marker to improve visualization, notching the anterior portion of the femoral tunnel, and positioning the graft with the cancellous bone anterior.

MANAGING THE COMPLICATION
If the graft is amputated at the femoral tunnel entrance, the interference screw and bone plug should be removed. An incision is made over the lateral femur, and the rear-entry guide is introduced into the joint (**Figure 4**). The guide is centered over the previously drilled femoral tunnel, and a reamer is used to extend the femoral tunnel to the lateral cortex. The amputated end of the graft is prepared with two No. 5 nonabsorbable sutures using a Krackow stitch. The graft is then reversed, with the intact bone plug inserted into the femoral tunnel flush with the intra-articular edge. The interference screw is then placed from outside-in to reduce the risk of graft laceration. The tibial side of the graft is tensioned and secured over a post or button. Alternatively, the soft-tissue end of the graft can be secured in the femoral tunnel with an interference screw if adequate graft tissue is present.

POSTOPERATIVE REGIMEN
No modifications in the postoperative regimen are necessary with stable fixation of the graft.

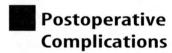

Postoperative Complications

Septic Knee
Septic arthritis occurs in less than 1% of patients following ACL reconstruction, but it is a potentially disastrous complication. Some reported risk factors for infection include previous knee surgery and a concomitant open procedure. Early studies suggested that infection was more likely to occur with allografts; however, more recent research shows similar rates of infection with autograft and allograft. Aggressive management of suspected infection is important because of the association with articular cartilage degradation and arthrofibrosis.

DIAGNOSIS
The diagnosis of septic arthritis in an ACL-reconstructed knee is difficult, and a delay in diagnosis is common. The presentation in the ACL-reconstructed knee can be more subtle than in an unoperated knee. Infections typically present in the first 2 to 4 weeks postoperatively; early signs and symptoms include mild pain, increased effusion, and loss of motion.

Initial diagnosis should consist of

blood work (erythrocyte sedimentation rate [ESR], C-reactive protein [CRP] level, white blood cell [WBC] count) and knee aspiration. In the early postsurgical period, the ESR and CRP level may remain elevated when infection is not present, making interpretation of elevated values difficult. However, multiple studies have shown these markers to have a high negative predictive value for joint infection. Knee aspirates have been reported to be the most reliably diagnostic of infection. Aspirates usually can show a variable WBC count from 25,000 to 100,000 with more than 90% neutrophils. Organisms frequently encountered include *Staphylococcus aureus* and *Staphylococcus epidermidis*. If findings support an infection, surgical irrigation and débridement of the knee joint are indicated. If cultures are negative and knee aspirates reveal a crystalline arthropathy, irrigation and débridement are not indicated, and standard management of gout or pseudogout is indicated.

MANAGING THE COMPLICATION

No consensus has been established for the management of septic arthritis after ACL reconstruction, but most authors agree that initial management of infection consists of arthroscopic or open irrigation and débridement followed by intravenous antibiotic therapy. In patients who are medically unstable and unable to undergo surgical intervention, bedside irrigation of the knee joint can be performed using two 18-gauge needles and a 100-mL syringe. The knee should be irrigated copiously with at least 10 L of fluid. This procedure can be repeated daily until symptoms improve or cultures are negative.

The goals of treatment are to prevent cartilage damage and restore motion. Graft retention versus removal remains controversial. Those favoring graft removal consider the graft material a focus for recurrent infection;

however, multiple studies have shown good success with retained grafts when the infection is eradicated using single or multiple irrigation and débridement procedures. With persistent infections, graft material and exposed hardware should be removed because these are a possible focus of infection. If the graft material is removed, successful revision reconstructions can be performed at 12 weeks if the infection has resolved. Outcomes of ACL reconstruction have been shown to be significantly worse following infection, with decreased Lysholm, Tegner activity, and KOOS ratings. However, knee stability based on KT-1000 measurement appears to be no different than after uncomplicated ACL reconstruction. Poor outcomes are thought to be caused mainly by articular cartilage injury and arthrofibrosis.

For surgical treatment, the patient is placed supine on the operating table and a tourniquet is applied to the proximal thigh. A lateral post is placed at the mid-level of the thigh to allow visualization of the medial compartment. The procedure can be done with general or regional anesthesia. Tourniquet use is not necessary, but if it is used, the leg should not be exsanguinated before inflation of the tourniquet because of the risk of bacteremia. Standard arthroscopic inferomedial and inferolateral portals are established. Samples of joint fluid are obtained and sent for Gram stain, culture, and crystal evaluation. Arthroscopic débridement removes fibrin clots, inflamed synovium, and scar tissue in the patellofemoral joint, medial and lateral gutters, medial and lateral compartments, and posterior fossa. The ACL graft is probed to test for competence, and lax grafts can be débrided. Standard equipment for an ACL reconstruction should be available in the event that the graft requires removal. A minimum of 15 L of saline should be used to irrigate the knee. Accessory parapatellar, posteromedial, and posterolateral por-

tals should be used freely to ensure thorough débridement.

POSTOPERATIVE REGIMEN

The knee is placed in a knee immobilizer to facilitate pain control and reduce inflammation. As symptoms resolve, the patient can be started on an aggressive range-of-motion program to prevent arthrofibrosis. Authors report various antibiotic regimens; however, most support 4 to 8 weeks of intravenous culture-specific antibiotics followed by oral antibiotics for a full 3 months. Infection can be monitored with serial measurements of the ESR and CRP level. Patients should be seen in clinic weekly for the first several weeks to monitor for recurrence of infection.

Loss of Motion

Loss of motion is the most common complication following ACL reconstruction, occurring in 4% to 10% of patients. The loss of terminal extension can produce strain on the quadriceps muscle and cause patellofemoral pain. Flexion loss is tolerated better than extension loss in activities of daily living but if extension is limited severely, to less than 90°, stair climbing or even sitting can be affected.

AVOIDING THE COMPLICATION

The etiology of postoperative stiffness is multifactorial. Surgical timing, graft malposition, formation of a cyclops lesion, and arthrofibrosis may contribute.

The influence of timing on outcome of ACL reconstruction is controversial. Several studies have shown that reconstruction at less than 3 weeks after injury, during the acute inflammatory period, results in an increased risk of motion loss. Other studies show no correlation between early surgery and stiffness. Most surgeons agree that the best results are obtained when motion is recovered, swelling is resolved, and quadriceps function is restored before surgery.

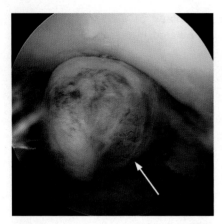

Figure 5 Arthroscopic view demonstrates a cyclops lesion located in the intercondylar notch.

The most common cause of motion loss after ACL reconstruction is graft malposition. A good understanding of the anatomic insertions of the ACL is key to avoiding this complication. The tibial tunnel should be centered 5 to 7 mm anterior to the PCL and parallel to the posterior border of the anterior horn of the lateral meniscus. If the tibial tunnel is placed too anteriorly, the graft will impinge on the intercondylar notch, resulting in loss of extension. Loss of extension causes anterior knee pain and impaired gait. The most frequently reported surgical error in ACL reconstruction is an anteriorly placed femoral tunnel. Confusing the over-the-top position with the "resident's ridge" can result in an anterior tunnel and loss of flexion. The femoral tunnel should be placed such that only a 1-mm rim of posterior cortex remains and the tunnel is 4 mm proximal to the distal articular surface. Malpositioning the tunnel too anteriorly also results in a nonisometric graft and increased strain that could cause graft failure.

The formation of a fibrous nodule, or cyclops lesion, in the anterior aspect of the intercondylar notch can cause a painful mechanical block to extension (**Figure 5**). Several theories have been suggested for the formation of these nodules, including inade-

quate débridement of the native ACL, anterior graft placement, and graft hypertrophy. Good outcomes have been reported with arthroscopic débridement of the nodule.

Arthrofibrosis is the formation of scar tissue within the knee, which can limit flexion and extension. Early rehabilitation protocols often included a period of immobilization, which contributed to the development of arthrofibrosis. Although the exact etiology is not well understood, a hyperinflammatory state is thought to cause scarring of the gutters and infrapatellar fat pad. Infrapatellar scarring draws the patella distally and posteriorly, resulting in pain and loss of flexion. The development of more accelerated rehabilitation protocols with immediate passive and active range of motion have decreased the occurrence of stiffness and improved patient outcomes; however, a small percentage of patients continue to develop arthrofibrosis. If rehabilitation does not adequately resolve motion deficits, surgical intervention for release of scar tissue may be necessary.

MANAGING THE COMPLICATION

A systematic approach is necessary to identify the etiology of motion loss and determine a plan for management. Initial evaluation should rule out infection because failure to recognize a septic knee will result in progressive, irreversible cartilage damage. In addition to determining the amount of extension and flexion loss, physical examination should focus on patellar mobility. Scarring of the anterior interval can be detected by increased pain in response to the Hoffa test and decreased superior excursion of the patella. Graft position should be determined with AP and lateral radiographs (**Figure 6**). The anterior edge of the tibial tunnel should be posterior to the Blumensaat line on the lateral radiograph, and the femoral tunnel should be on the posterior aspect of the condyle. Graft malposition alone

is not an indication for surgery, but it is predictive of a poor outcome for rehabilitation. Loss of motion with appropriate tunnel placement is caused by scar formation. MRI is useful for identifying other possible causes of motion loss, including a cyclops lesion (**Figure 7**), scarring of the gutters and fat pad, and meniscal tear. Loss of motion that does not respond to aggressive nonsurgical management is an indication for surgical intervention at 6 to 12 weeks postoperatively.

Early loss of motion in the first 2 to 3 weeks postoperatively should be managed with aggressive physical therapy, including quadriceps activation, rolling chair exercises, prone ankle hangs, towel rolls, patellar mobilization, and hemarthrosis management. Therapy may be augmented with hyperextension splints or cylinder casts. If motion deficits do not resolve with therapy, manipulation under anesthesia can be done from 4 to 6 weeks postoperatively. Late manipulation should be avoided because of the risk of fracture and chondral injury.

For surgery, the patient is positioned supine on the operating table. A tourniquet is placed high on the thigh, and the thigh is secured in a leg holder. The bed is slightly flexed and the leg is dropped to allow 90° of knee flexion. The leg is prepared and draped with sterile technique.

An examination under anesthesia is done to determine the baseline range of motion. Knee stability is assessed with the Lachman test, pivot-shift test, posterior drawer test, and varus/valgus stability test at 30° and 90° of flexion.

A vertical anterolateral portal is created adjacent to the patellar tendon and just inferior to the distal pole of the patella. Diagnostic arthroscopy is done to evaluate possible pathology, including cyclops lesion, scarring of the anterior interval and gutters, or other possible internal derangements. As the knee is extended, the interval between the fat pad and anterior tibia should move freely. Closure of the anterior interval can cause pain and decreased patellar mobility.

A standard anteromedial portal is established inferior to the distal pole of the patella and slightly medial to the patellar tendon. A 4.5- or 5.5-mm shaver or electrocautery device is introduced, and the scar tissue is débrided from the medial and lateral gutters and the suprapatellar pouch. The interval between the anterior tibia and fat pad is reestablished, and the intermeniscal ligament is mobilized from anterior scar tissue. The intercondylar notch is examined for a cyclops lesion: if present, it is débrided. The knee is ranged from flexion to extension and the clearance for the graft is evaluated. If the graft impinges on either the lateral femoral condyle or the superior notch, a notchplasty can be done to improve graft clearance. Graft position should be evaluated and documented.

If loss of extension is significant, a posterior release may be necessary. The Gillquist maneuver is helpful for evaluating the posterior aspect of the knee. This maneuver involves introducing the arthroscope through the intercondylar notch, under the posterior cruciate ligament, and directly over the insertion of the posterior horn of the medial meniscus. This provides a better view of the posteromedial compartment than the standard anterior view. A 70° arthroscope often is useful because of the limited arthroscope mobility in the posterior knee. An 18-gauge spinal needle is used to determine the optimal location for a posteromedial portal. An incision is made, and a switching stick is inserted into the posterior compartment. A working cannula is placed over the switching stick into the pos-

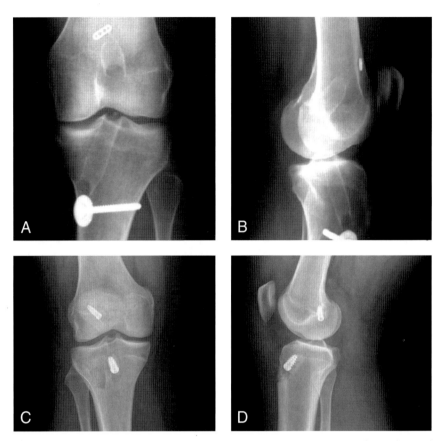

Figure 6 AP (**A**) and lateral (**B**) radiographs demonstrate a malpositioned femoral tunnel exiting vertically and anteriorly. AP (**C**) and lateral (**D**) views show appropriately placed femoral and tibial tunnels.

terior knee. The posterior capsule is released carefully with electrocautery or arthroscopic scissors. During posterior release, there is a risk of injury to the neurovascular structures.

POSTOPERATIVE REGIMEN
Immediate postoperative range of motion should be started with aggressive patellar mobilization. Special attention should be focused on obtaining and maintaining full extension. Therapy may include quadriceps activation, rolling chair exercises, prone ankle hangs, and towel rolls.

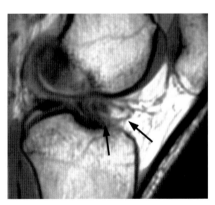

Figure 7 MRI of a knee with a cyclops lesion (arrows).

Bibliography

Aglietti P, Giron F, Buzzi R, Biddau F, Sasso F: Anterior cruciate ligament reconstruction: Bone-patellar tendon-bone compared with double semitendinosus and gracilis tendon grafts. A prospective, randomized clinical trial. *J Bone Joint Surg Am* 2004;86-A(10):2143-2155.

Almazán A, Miguel A, Odor A, Ibarra JC: Intraoperative incidents and complications in primary arthroscopic anterior cruciate ligament reconstruction. *Arthroscopy* 2006;22(11):1211-1217.

Arciero RA: Endoscopic anterior cruciate ligament reconstruction: Complication of graft rupture and a method of salvage. *Am J Knee Surg* 1996;9(1):27-31.

Busam ML, Provencher MT, Bach BR Jr: Complications of anterior cruciate ligament reconstruction with bone-patellar tendon-bone constructs: Care and prevention. *Am J Sports Med* 2008;36(2):379-394.

Carey JL, Dunn WR, Dahm DL, Zeger SL, Spindler KP: A systematic review of anterior cruciate ligament reconstruction with autograft compared with allograft. *J Bone Joint Surg Am* 2009;91(9):2242-2250.

Drogset JO, Strand T, Uppheim G, Odegård B, Bøe A, Grøntvedt T: Autologous patellar tendon and quadrupled hamstring grafts in anterior cruciate ligament reconstruction: A prospective randomized multicenter review of different fixation methods [published online ahead of print, December 3, 2009]. *Knee Surg Sports Traumatol Arthrosc.*

Freedman KB, D'Amato MJ, Nedeff DD, Kaz A, Bach BR Jr: Arthroscopic anterior cruciate ligament reconstruction: A metaanalysis comparing patellar tendon and hamstring tendon autografts. *Am J Sports Med* 2003;31(1):2-11.

Magit D, Wolff A, Sutton K, Medvecky MJ: Arthrofibrosis of the knee. *J Am Acad Orthop Surg* 2007;15(11):682-694.

McGuire DA, Hendricks S: Anterior cruciate ligament reconstruction graft harvesting: Pitfalls and tips. *Sports Med Arthrosc Rev* 2007;15:184-190.

Molina ME, Nonweiller DE, Evans JA, Delee JC: Contaminated anterior cruciate ligament grafts: The efficacy of 3 sterilization agents. *Arthroscopy* 2000;16(4):373-378.

Rue JP, Busam ML, Detterline AJ, Bach BR Jr: Posterior wall blowout in anterior cruciate ligament reconstruction: Avoidance, recognition, and salvage. *J Knee Surg* 2008;21(3):235-240.

Schollin-Borg M, Michaëlsson K, Rahme H: Presentation, outcome, and cause of septic arthritis after anterior cruciate ligament reconstruction: A case control study. *Arthroscopy* 2003;19(9):941-947.

Shelbourne KD, Wilckens JH, Mollabashy A, DeCarlo M: Arthrofibrosis in acute anterior cruciate ligament reconstruction: The effect of timing of reconstruction and rehabilitation. *Am J Sports Med* 1991;19(4):332-336.

Steadman JR, Dragoo JL, Hines SL, Briggs KK: Arthroscopic release for symptomatic scarring of the anterior interval of the knee. *Am J Sports Med* 2008;36(9):1763-1769.

Taylor DC, DeBerardino TM, Nelson BJ, et al: Patellar tendon versus hamstring tendon autografts for anterior cruciate ligament reconstruction: A randomized controlled trial using similar femoral and tibial fixation methods. *Am J Sports Med* 2009;37(10):1946-1957.

Video Reference

Arciero RA: Video. *Complications of ACL Reconstruction: Tunnel Lysis.* Farmington, CT, 2009.

Coding

CPT Codes		Corresponding ICD-9 Codes	
Bone Graft			
20900	Bone graft, any donor area; minor or small (eg, dowel or button)	820 821.10	820.9
20902	Bone graft, any donor area; major or large	820 821.10	820.9
Femoral Internal Fixation			
27514	Open treatment of femoral fracture, distal end, medial or lateral condyle, includes internal fixation, when performed	820 821.29	821.10 773.96
Patellar Internal Fixation			
27524	Open treatment of patellar fracture, with internal fixation and/or partial or complete patellectomy and soft tissue repair	820	821.10
Arthroscopic Meniscus Repair			
29822	Arthroscopy, knee, surgical; with meniscus repair (medial OR lateral)	717	717.6
29823	Arthroscopy, knee, surgical; with meniscus repair (medial AND lateral)	717	717.6
Arthroscopic Débridement of Loose or Foreign Bodies			
29874	Arthroscopy, knee, surgical; for removal of loose body or foreign body (eg, osteochondritis dissecans fragmentation, chondral fragmentation)	717	717.6

Chapter 72
Revision Anterior Cruciate Ligament Reconstruction

K. Donald Shelbourne, MD
Scott E. Urch, MD

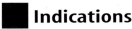 **Indications**

Anterior cruciate ligament (ACL) reconstruction is routinely performed in patients with active lifestyles who are unable to continue with their activities because of instability. When patients who have had ACL reconstruction reinjure the ACL-reconstructed knee or have recurrent instability from surgical failure or reinjury, the decision as to whether ACL revision surgery is in their best interest should be made with the same evaluation and consideration with which decisions about primary ACL reconstruction are made, with the understanding that postoperative goals may have changed.

The patient evaluation should include a thorough history to determine the following: first, did the previous ACL graft fail, or was the ACL reconstruction successful for establishing stability but then the patient suffered a reinjury? Second, does the patient have a lifestyle that requires a stable knee? If the patient is able and willing to modify his or her lifestyle, revision ACL reconstruction may not be required. Some patients, despite a relatively inactive lifestyle, may still experience giving way with everyday activities, and stability would help them. In these cases, a revision ACL reconstruction is considered.

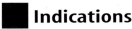 **Contraindications**

The most significant contraindication to revision ACL reconstruction is graft failure from infection. As with any significant joint infection, the infection should be treated completely, and revision surgery should be considered only after complete eradication of the infection. Significant bone loss from a previous surgery can be a cause for concern and occasionally will require staged bone grafting before revision ACL surgery.

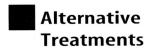 **Alternative Treatments**

The only true alternative to ACL revision surgery is modification of activities. Multiple graft choices and fixation choices are available for revision ACL reconstruction.

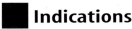 **Results**

The results of revision surgery for ACL reconstruction vary greatly (Table 1). A variety of graft sources have been used for revision surgery; current reports show a predominance of autograft tissue, including bone–patellar tendon–bone and hamstring grafts from the contralateral and ipsilateral knee and some reharvested grafts. Results indicate that good stability can be obtained with revision surgery, although the failure rates are not always reported. The general view is that results from revision ACL reconstruction are not as good as those of primary ACL reconstruction, but the variations in final result are most likely due to the same factors that affect the final result after primary ACL reconstruction: preoperative knee range of motion (good or poor), meniscal status (intact menisci or meniscectomy), articular cartilage integrity (normal or damaged), chronicity of the injury, and number of episodes of instability. Given the repeated instability episodes and high number of intra-articular injuries often found at revision surgery, the somewhat lower subjective scores are to be expected.

Dr. Shelbourne or an immediate family member has received royalties from DJ Orthopaedics; serves as an unpaid consultant for Kneebourne Therapeutics; owns stock or stock options in Abbott and Pfizer; and is a board member, owner, officer, or committee member for the American Orthopaedic Society for Sports Medicine. Neither Dr. Urch nor any immediate family member has received anything of value from or owns stock in a commercial company or institution related directly or indirectly to the subject of this chapter.

Table 1 Results of Revision Anterior Cruciate Ligament Reconstruction

Authors (Year)	Graft Choice (Number of Knees*)	Mean Age in Years (Range)	Mean Follow-up in Years (Range)	Results[†]
Uribe et al (1996)	BPTB allograft (19) IL HS autograft (2) CL BPTB autograft (16) IL BPTB autograft (17)	NR	2.7 (1.7-6.7)	Lysholm: 83.2 Tegner: 5.5 KT-1000 Autograft: 2.2 ± 1.3 Allograft: 3.3 ± 1.5
Kartus et al (1998)	CL BPTB autograft (12) IL BPTB autograft reharvested (12)	27 (23-33)	CL BPTB: 4.5 IL BPTB: 4.8	Lysholm CL BPTB: 84 IL BPTB: 62 Tegner CL BPTB: 6 IL BPTB: 5 KT-1000 IL BPTB: 3 CL BPTB: 2
Colosimo et al (2001)	IL BPTB autograft reharvested (13)	27.2	3.3	Lysholm: 77.6 Tegner: 5.8 KT-1000: 1.92
Noyes and Barber-Westin (2001)	IL BPTB autograft (39) IL BPTB autograft reharvested (11) CL BPTB autograft (5)	27 (14-48)	2.8 (2-6.2)	Cincinnati knee rating: 87 ± 11 Failure rate: 24%
Fox et al (2004)	BPTB allograft (32)	28 (16-57)	4.8 (2.1-12.1)	Tegner: 6.3 Lysholm: 75 Modified Cincinnati: 7.2 KT-1000: 1.9 ± 2.4 (27 patients < 3 mm, 3 patients 3-5 mm, 2 patients >5 mm)
Grossman et al (2005)	BPTB allograft (22) CL BPTB autograft (6) Achilles allograft (1)	30.2	5.6	Tegner: 11.86 Lysholm: 86.6 IKDC: 85.86 KT-1000 Autograft: 1.3 Allograft: 3.1
Shelbourne and Thomas (2005)	CL BPTB autograft (126)	24.7-27.5 (means among 3 groups)	4	IKDC: 71-85 (means among 3 groups) KT-1000: 2.1-2.8 (means among 3 groups)
Thomas et al (2005)	IL BPTB autograft (15) IL HS autograft (34)	35.4	6.2 (3-11)	IKDC: 61.2 ± 19.6 Westminster cruciometer, 89N force: 1.3 + 1.1
Ferretti et al (2006)	IL HS autograft	34 (21-39)	5	IKDC: 84 ± 12 Lysholm: 90 ± 10 KT-1000: 20 patients <3 mm, 6 patients 3-5 mm, 2 patients >5 mm Failure rate: 3/3%
Salmon et al (2006)	HS autograft (49) HS allograft (1)	27 (15-39)	7.4 (5-9)	Lysholm: 85 (range, 81-90) KT-1000: 2.5 (range, -1 to 4; failures excluded) Failure rate: 10%

Table 1 *(Continued)*

Authors (Year)	Graft Choice (Number of Knees*)	Mean Age inYears (Range)	Mean Follow-up in Years (Range)	Results†

Battaglia et al (2007)	Allograft (20) IL autograft (33) CL autograft (10)	31 (18-60)	6.1	IKDC
				  Good/excellent: 71%
				  Fair: 10%
				  Poor: 19%
				KT-1000 30-lb test:
				  30 (47.6%) <3 mm
				  20 (31.7%) 3-5 mm
				  10 (15.9%) >5 mm

Weiler et al (2007)	IL HS autograft	31 ± 8	2.5	Lysholm: 90 ± 9 KT-1000: 2.1 ± 1.6 Failure rate: 6.5%
Diamantopolous et al (2008)	BPTB autograft (41) HS autograft (45) Quad autograft (21)	38.8 ± 9.3	6.1 (2-8)	Lysholm: 88.5 ± 12.4 Tegner: 6.3 ± 1.8 KT-1000: 0.93 ± 1.15

BPTB = bone–patellar tendon–bone, IL = ipsilateral, HS = hamstring, CL = contralateral, NR = not reported, IKDC = International Knee Documentation Committee.

*Evaluated at follow-up.

† Subjective scores are mean ± SD. KT-1000 = mean manual maximum side-to-side difference measured on a KT-1000 arthrometer.

■ Technique

Setup/Exposure

After administration of general anesthesia and a bolus of 30 mg of ketorolac administered intravenously, the patient is positioned supine. A tourniquet is placed on the affected leg. If a patellar tendon graft from the contralateral knee is to be used in the revision, a tourniquet is placed on the opposite leg as well. After preparation and draping, the tourniquet is inflated to 300 mm Hg. An arthroscopic examination is done through a medial portal with a 0° arthroscope. The interior of the joint is evaluated, and any damage to the menisci is evaluated and treated. The remaining ACL graft, if present, is evaluated as well.

After the arthroscopic evaluation, the leg is re-prepared and a bump is placed under the affected leg to hold the knee at 30° of flexion. An incision is made along the medial border of the patellar tendon from the tip of the patella to the tibial tubercle. We make the incision along the scar from the previous ACL reconstruction if possible. An incision is then made with Bo-

vie electrocautery through the periosteum, parallel and just medial to the patellar tendon. A perpendicular incision is made approximately 4 cm below the joint surface, and a flap of the periosteum is elevated from the anterior tibia. At this point, any tibial fixation is identified and removed. The medial incision is carried proximally along the medial border of the patella to the level of the vastus medialis and then extended into the joint, creating a miniarthrotomy.

We use a two-incision technique, with the lateral incision centered over the thin region of the iliotibial band (ITB) approximately 3 to 4 cm above the patella to the joint line. The ITB is identified and split longitudinally just anterior to the thick part of the ITB. An index finger is then used to sweep the vastus lateralis from the lateral femur. A Slocum retractor is placed under the muscle for visualization. A longitudinal incision is made in the periosteum, and the periosteum is elevated to expose the lateral femur. If some type of lateral fixation was used in the previous surgery, it is removed at this time.

At this point, we prepare the interior of the joint. The soft tissue in the femoral notch lateral to the posterior cruciate ligament (PCL) is removed, and the lateral wall of the femur and posterior portion of the notch are cleared. If a femoral interference screw was used for the previous ACL reconstruction, it is removed at this time. We use a caliper to measure the distance between the PCL and the lateral wall of the femoral notch to ensure that at least 10 mm are available to accommodate a 10-mm graft. If not, a curet is used to remove just enough bone from the lateral wall to accommodate the graft.

Tunnel Placement

Once the exposure has been made and the previous hardware has been removed, the next step is to place the tunnels. This is a critical step, and the miniarthrotomy allows excellent visualization to achieve correct placement. A 3/32-inch guide pin is placed in the tibia into the approximate position of the tunnel about 4 cm below the joint line. The position of the tunnel starting point is moved either slightly me-

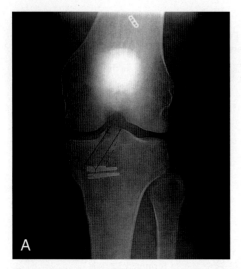
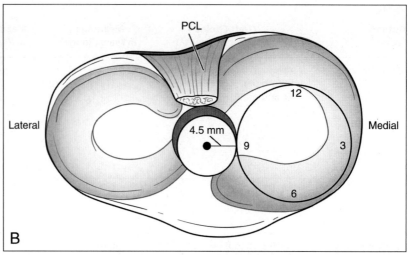

Figure 1 Tibial tunnel placement. **A,** AP radiograph shows where the previous tibial tunnel was placed (dotted lines). After the tibial hardware is removed, the entrance of the new tunnel is begun slightly medial to the old tunnel along a new path (solid line), making sure the exit is just medial to the tibial spine. **B,** Schematic shows a cross section of a right knee. If a clock face is superimposed on the medial tibial plateau, the tunnel is drilled so that the end point is directed just medial to the tibial spine and slightly anterior to where the tibial plateau drops off in the sagittal plane, at the 9-o'clock position in a right knee. A curette is used to place the tunnel into the exact position (shaded area). PCL = posterior cruciate ligament.

dial or lateral as necessary to avoid the previous tunnel (**Figure 1**, *A*). Because button fixation is used for both the femoral and tibial tunnel ends of the patellar tendon graft, it is unnecessary to create a completely new separate tunnel, although we attempt to make at least a partial new pathway for the tibial tunnel. The end point for the tibial tunnel is directed just medial to the tibial spine and just anterior to the point where the tibial plateau drops off in the sagittal plane. With the medial tibial plateau viewed as a clock face, the center of the tibial tunnel corresponds to the position just posterior to the 9-o'clock (right knee) or 3-o'clock (left knee) position (**Figure 1**, *B*). The guide pin is overreamed using a 9-mm cannulated reamer. The bone from the drilling is saved, to be used later to graft the site of the bone plugs. A curet is used to position the tunnel posterior and medial into the exact position.

The femoral tunnel is then drilled in a similar fashion. The knee is positioned in a figure-of-4 position. The intersection of the PCL and the posterior aspect of the notch roof are identified.

The guide pin should be placed so that it is in the center of a 10-mm circle. The circle should be such that the medial border is at the lateral aspect of the PCL and the posterior border is just anterior to the posterior cortex of the femur, leaving a thin shell of bone posterior on the femur (**Figure 2**, *A*). If the previous tunnel is in this position already, then the guide pin is placed within the tunnel and is redirected either proximal or distal, whichever is most appropriate in relation to the previous tunnel (**Figure 2**, *B*). Again, the position of the tunnel opening is most important, and, because button fixation is used laterally on the cortex of the femur, creating an entirely new tunnel is not necessary. It should, however, diverge from the previous tunnel to allow the bone plug to sit in freshly drilled bone. Once the guide pin is in the appropriate position, a 10-mm reamer is used to drill the tunnel. The bone created from the drilling is saved, separated from graft remnant, and used to bone-graft the patella and the tibia where the graft will be harvested. The femoral tunnel should exit approximately in the center of the lateral

incision, depending on the length of the patellar tendon graft.

Graft Harvest

Many graft sources are available for revision ACL reconstruction. Allografts have no donor-site morbidity, but the failure rate is higher than with other graft sources. Given that the patient has already had one graft failure, we choose to use a more reliable graft source. Hamstring tendons are another graft source, but they do not provide bone-to-bone healing, which is the most reliable for long-term stability. We use an autogenous patellar tendon graft for revision surgery, and the donor-site morbidity associated with the graft is minimized with appropriate rehabilitation before and after surgery.

Whether the patellar tendon graft is harvested from the ipsilateral or contralateral knee, the technique is the same. The subcutaneous tissue is carefully cleared to expose the patellar tendon from the patella superiorly to the tibial tubercle distally. The graft is then outlined with a blade so that it is 10 mm wide, with bone plugs measur-

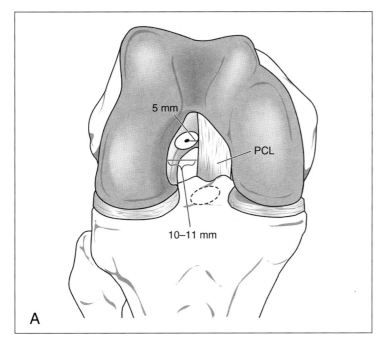
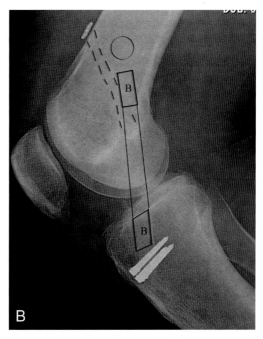

Figure 2 Femoral tunnel placement. **A,** Schematic shows placement of the new femoral tunnel. The tunnel is drilled so that the guide pin is placed 5 mm medial to the lateral border of the PCL and approximately 6 mm in front of the posterior cortex of the femur, leaving a thin shell of bone posterior on the femur. **B,** The dotted lines on this lateral radiograph show where the previous femoral tunnel was placed. The new femoral tunnel is begun at the entrance of the old tunnel, but the tunnel is directed slightly proximal and posterior, allowing the bone plug (B) to seat in fresh bone. The circle shows the exit of the femoral tunnel.

ing between 20 and 25 mm. A straight osteotome is used to score the proximal part of the patellar bone plug and the distal portion of the tibial bone plug. An oscillating saw is used to cut the medial and lateral borders of the patellar and tibial bone plugs. A curved osteotome is used to remove the patellar bone plug. The patellar bone plug, which will be used in the tibial tunnel, is shaped to fit through an 11-mm tunnel. Because the proximal portion of the tunnel was widened with a curet, this allows for a tighter fit. The tibial bone plug, which will be used in the femur, is shaped to fit in a 10-mm tunnel because the femoral tunnel was not modified after drilling (**Figure 3,** *A*). Three holes are drilled in each plug, and a No. 2 Ethibond suture (Ethicon, Johnson & Johnson, Somerville, NJ) is placed in each hole (**Figure 3,** *B*).

If a patellar tendon graft is being taken from a previously harvested tendon, a Merchant view radiograph and MRI scan are obtained preoperatively to confirm that the patella and patellar tendon are of good quality. The graft is obtained slightly medial or lateral to the original bone graft to ensure the best bone quality (**Figure 4**).

Graft Placement/Tensioning

Once the graft has been harvested and prepared, it is placed in position in the tunnels. A suture passer is passed through the tibial tunnel to retrieve the sutures of the patellar bone plug. The graft is brought into the tunnel from the inside of the joint and positioned so that the cancellous side of the bone plug is anterior and the tendon is posterior. The bone plug is positioned just below the tibial joint surface because this is the region of the best cancellous bone in the tibia (**Figure 5**).

The sutures are tied loosely over a 19-mm button covering the opening of the tunnel on the anterior surface of the tibia. The suture passer is used again to pass the suture through the femoral tunnel. The sutures are retrieved through the lateral incision. The proximal end of the graft is then positioned at the opening of the femoral tunnel and pulled into position from the lateral side. The bone plugs were sized before placement, but if either does not fit the tunnel, it is brought back into the knee and trimmed to allow it to fit into the tunnel. The knee is then positioned at 30° of flexion, and the femoral plug is tied over the lateral cortex of the femur with a 19-mm button. The button should lie flat against the cortex of the femur. Once secured, the tibial bone plug is pulled and seated as far distal in the tibial tunnel as possible. Observing the sutures on the femoral side will indicate when the tibial plug is seated. The sutures are then loosened on the tibial button and retied as tightly as possible with a sliding knot.

At this point, the knee is taken through a full range of motion from

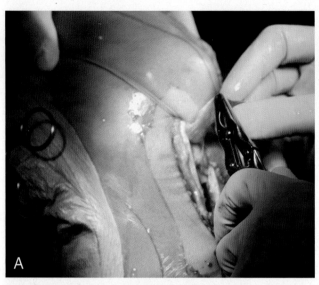 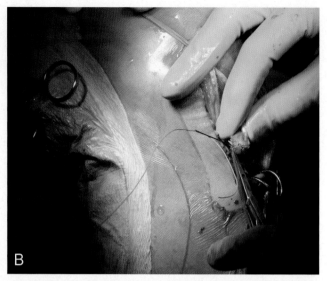

Figure 3 Intraoperative photographs show a bone–patellar tendon–bone graft being harvested. **A,** The tibial bone plug is shaped to fit a 10-mm tunnel. **B,** Three holes are drilled in each bone plug, and No. 2 Ethibond suture is placed in each hole so the sutures can be tied over buttons for fixation.

Figure 4 The dotted lines on this Merchant view show where the previous patellar tendon graft was harvested. A reharvested graft is obtained by moving slightly lateral of the previous graft harvest to ensure good bone quality.

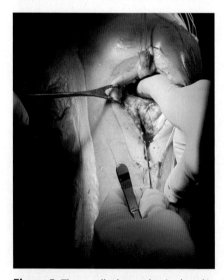

Figure 5 The patellar bone plug is placed in the tibial tunnel just below the tibial joint surface, where good cancellous bone is present.

hyperextension to complete flexion (**Figure 6**).

The tibial button is rechecked and, if it is seated snugly on the anterior tibia and will not lift from the femur, the procedure is completed. If the button has loosened, it is retied and the process is repeated until it is secured. This process allows the graft to seat into a position where it is not so tight as to restrict motion, but is tight enough to provide stability. If the tibial button continues to loosen, there most likely is impingement at the anterior edge of the femoral notch. If impingement is noted, a curet is used to widen the tunnel as needed. Once the impingement is removed, the button

is tightened, and the knee is taken through a full range of motion again until the button remains securely fastened to the anterior tibial cortex.

Wound Closure

After placement of the graft, the wounds are packed with a sponge and the tourniquet is deflated. All wounds are irrigated with saline solution, and bleeding is controlled with electrocautery. A drain is placed deep to the vastus lateralis in the lateral wound. The IT band is closed with No. 2-0 Vicryl (Ethicon), the skin edges are approximated with 3-0 Monocryl (Ethicon), and the skin is closed with 3-0 Prolene (Ethicon) in a subcuticular fashion.

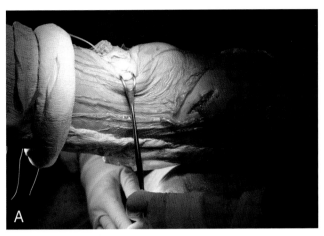 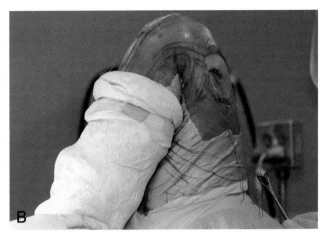

Figure 6 After button fixation, the knee is taken through a full range of motion, including full hyperextension **(A)** and full flexion **(B)**.

The patellar tendon defect is closed with No. 1 Vicryl incorporating the peritenon. The bone graft that was collected with tunnel drilling is placed in the patella and tibia. The peritenon is closed over both defects to keep the graft in position. If minimal bone graft is available, it is placed in the patellar defect. The miniarthrotomy is closed with No. 1 Vicryl in an interrupted fashion. A drain is placed subcutaneously, and the skin edges are approximated with 3-0 Monocryl. The skin is then closed with a 3-0 Prolene suture in a subcuticular fashion. If the contralateral patellar tendon was used, a drain is placed subcutaneously before closure. Adhesive strips and waterproof dressings are placed on all wounds. Antiembolism stockings are placed on both lower extremities. A cold/compression device is placed on the ACL-reconstructed knee. If a graft is used from the contralateral knee, an ice pack is placed over the harvest site.

Postoperative Regimen

A ketorolac drip is used for postoperative pain control (90 mg ketorolac in 1 L saline is run at 40 mL/h) as well as acetaminophen (1,000 mg) every 6 hours. Patients are kept overnight to control effusion and for patient education so the patient and caregiver can learn the regimen of care for the first 5 days postoperatively. The ACL-reconstructed knee is placed in a continuous passive motion (CPM) machine set to move from 0° to 30° of flexion continuously. The patient is kept in bed overnight with the knee elevated above the heart by the CPM machine. Patients begin gait training on the first postoperative day, but they continue to remain in bed with bathroom privileges only for the first week postoperatively; this routine of using cold/compression and elevation prevents a hemarthrosis from forming, improves patient comfort, and allows specific rehabilitation exercises. The patient begins active and passive range-of-motion exercises immediately postoperatively, including heel-prop and towel-stretch exercises to obtain full hyperextension and straight-leg–raise exercises for leg control. Exercises to obtain maximal flexion are done four times a day using a yardstick to measure progress. Patients continue this regimen for 5 days postoperatively. We have found that this rehabilitation protocol during the first 5 days is critical for minimizing postoperative complications.

Beginning at week 2, patients are allowed to begin to resume their daily activities. The focus is on maintaining knee hyperextension and advancing knee flexion as well. The basics of the primary ACL rehabilitation are not changed for patients with ACL revision, and patients are advanced through a progression of exercises and functional activities as their knees allow.

Avoiding Pitfalls and Complications

Preparation is the key to avoiding complications with ACL reconstruction. Ensuring that patients require and desire an ACL revision surgery is the first step. Next, it is important to obtain a thorough history and physical examination. It is important to obtain lateral, Merchant, and weight-bearing PA views of both knees to view the position of the tunnels and evaluate bone loss, the state of the previous graft site in the patella, and the previous fixation used.

It is helpful to obtain thorough surgical reports to determine what was done in the prior surgery and the type of hardware used. Because of the different manufacturers and types of hardware used for fixation, the appropriate equipment must be available to remove the hardware. Although existing hardware usually can be removed successfully, occasionally the hardware cannot be removed, and a plan must be in place for diverting the tunnel past the existing hardware while keeping the tunnel in the appropriate position. Because button fixation is used with this procedure, there is greater flexibility as to where the tunnels can be diverted.

Many of the complications and difficulties that are associated with revision ACL surgery can be related to the graft source and the method of doing

the surgery. Arthroscopic revision surgery can be technically demanding, because the exposure makes it difficult to have the flexibility needed to divert tunnels; this is less difficult with an open procedure. Fixation with interference screws or any fixation within the bone can be difficult when the tunnels are adjacent to each other, and bone grafting has been described as a staged procedure before ACL surgery. These difficulties are overcome with lateral fixation.

Positioning of the tunnels and the graft is key to both primary recon-

struction and revision surgery. The open technique allows excellent visualization and the ability to place the tunnels in the best position. Although patients sometimes do not like larger scars, in the setting of an ACL revision surgery, patients want a procedure they can count on. The open miniarthrotomy technique allows excellent and reliable graft placement, which allows the patient the best chance for a successful outcome.

———————■

■ Bibliography

Battaglia MJ II, Cordasco FA, Hannafin JA, et al: Results of revision anterior cruciate ligament surgery. *Am J Sports Med* 2007;35:2057-2066.

Colosimo AJ, Heidt RS Jr, Traub JA, Carlonas RL: Revision anterior cruciate ligament reconstruction with a reharvested ipsilateral patellar tendon. *Am J Sports Med* 2001;29:746-749.

Diamantopoulos AP, Lorbach O, Paessler HH: Anterior cruciate ligament revision reconstruction: Results in 107 patients. *Am J Sports Med* 2008;36:851-860.

Ferretti A, Conteduca F, Monaco E, De Carli A, D'Arrigo C: Revision anterior cruciate ligament reconstruction with doubled semitendinosus and gracilis tendons and lateral extra-articular reconstruction. *J Bone Joint Surg Am* 2006;88: 2373-2379.

Fox JA, Pierce M, Bojchuk J, Hayden J, Bush-Joseph CA, Bach BR: Revision anterior cruciate ligament reconstruction with nonirradiated fresh-frozen patellar tendon allograft. *Arthroscopy* 2004;20:787-794.

Grossman MG, ElAttrache NS, Shields CL, Glousman RE: Revision anterior cruciate ligament reconstruction: Three- to nine-year follow-up. *Arthroscopy* 2005;21:418-423.

Kartus J, Stener S, Lindahl S, Eriksson BI, Karlsson J: Ipsi- or contralateral patellar tendon graft in anterior cruciate ligament revision surgery: A comparison of two methods. *Am J Sports Med* 1998;26:499-504.

Noyes FR, Barber-Westin SD: Revision anterior cruciate surgery with use of bone-patellar tendon-bone autogenous grafts. *J Bone Joint Surg Am* 2001;83:1131-1143.

Salmon LJ, Pinczewski LA, Russell VJ, Refshauge K: Revision anterior cruciate ligament reconstruction with hamstring tendon autograft: 5- to 9-year follow-up. *Am J Sports Med* 2006;34:1604-1614.

Shelbourne KD, Thomas JA: Contralateral patellar tendon and the Shelbourne experience: Part II. Results of revision anterior cruciate ligament reconstruction. *Sports Med Arthrosc Rev* 2005;13:69-72.

Thomas NP, Kankate R, Wandless F, Pandit H: Revision anterior cruciate ligament reconstruction using a 2-stage technique with bone grafting of the tibial tunnel. *Am J Sports Med* 2005;33:1701-1709.

Uribe JW, Hechtman KS, Zvijac JE, Tjin-A-Tsoi EW: Revision anterior cruciate ligament surgery: Experience from Miami. *Clin Orthop Relat Res* 1996;325:91-99.

Weiler A, Schmeling A, Stöhr I, Kääb MJ, Wagner M: Primary versus single-stage revision anterior cruciate ligament reconstruction using autologous hamstring tendon grafts: A prospective matched-group analysis. *Am J Sports Med* 2007; 35:1643-1652.

Coding

CPT Code		Corresponding ICD-9 Codes	
29888-22*	Arthroscopically aided anterior cruciate ligament repair/augmentation or reconstruction	718.83	844.2

*Modifier 22 is appended to reflect the increased procedure services involved for revision.

Chapter 73

Posterior Cruciate Ligament Reconstruction: Overview

Frederick M. Azar, MD
Jack Conoley, MD

Introduction

The posterior cruciate ligament (PCL) has received much less attention than the anterior cruciate ligament (ACL), but it plays an important role in the stability and function of the knee joint, a fact that has become better understood over the last two decades. PCL injuries have been estimated to account for 3% to 20% of knee injuries, but the actual number may be considerably higher because acute tears often are not diagnosed. The most common mechanisms of PCL injury are (1) a posteriorly directed force applied to a flexed knee (such as a "dashboard" injury); (2) a fall onto a flexed knee with the foot plantar flexed, causing the tibial tubercle to strike the ground first, placing a posterior force on the proximal tibia; (3) hyperextension of the knee, which usually causes an avulsion injury; and (4) an anterior force applied to the anterior tibia with the knee hyperextended and the foot planted, which usually results in knee dislocation with multiple ligamentous injuries.

Most PCL injuries occur in association with other ligamentous injuries, including the posterolateral corner, lateral collateral ligament, ACL, medial collateral ligament, and posteromedial corner. Multiple ligamentous injuries may occur in an occult knee dislocation, and vascular examination should be done along with appropriate studies and monitoring. These combined injuries usually are the result of motor vehicle accidents or traumatic knee dislocations. Isolated PCL injuries are most frequent in athletes, and they usually result from a direct blow to the anterior tibia with the knee flexed 90°. Just over 50% of PCL injuries are partial tears, about 40% are complete tears, and only 5% to 7% are avulsion injuries. Acute isolated PCL injuries are associated with chondral injuries and meniscal injuries in 52% and 28% of patients, respectively.

Despite advances in the understanding of the complex anatomy and biomechanical functions of the PCL and a recognition of the frequency with which it is injured, controversy still exists about the natural history of the PCL-injured knee, indications for surgical treatment, techniques for reconstruction, and postoperative rehabilitation protocols.

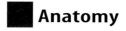

Anatomy

The PCL lies within the knee joint capsule, but it is considered an extra-articular structure because it is enclosed in its own synovial sheath. At its midpoint, the PCL has a cross-sectional area of 11 mm², and the ligament is 32 to 38 mm long. Like the ACL, the PCL can be divided into two functional bundles based on the relationship of the anatomic location of the femoral insertion to the tibial insertion. Some authors, however, have suggested that it is somewhat arbitrary to regard the PCL as comprising two bundles, a larger anterolateral (AL) bundle and a smaller posteromedial (PM) bundle, because the ligament is more accurately defined as a continuum of fibers comprising three or four or more bundles. Microsurgical dissection has identified four functionally distinct fiber regions based on their orientation and sites of bony insertion. Also considered part of the PCL complex are the meniscofemoral ligaments (ligament of Humphry, ligament of Wrisberg),

Dr. Azar or an immediate family member serves as a board member, owner, officer, or committee member for the American Orthopaedic Society for Sports Medicine. Neither Dr. Conoley nor any immediate family member has received anything of value from or owns stock in a commercial company or institution related directly or indirectly to the subject of this chapter.

Table 1 Classifications of Posterior Cruciate Ligament Injuries

Grade	Description
I	Posterior tibial subluxation <5 mm
II	Posterior tibial subluxation 5-10 mm
III	Posterior tibial subluxation >10 mm
I	Partial tear
II	Complete tear
III	Associated with other ligament injuries
Normal	No loss of tibial offset
A	Slight loss of tibial offset when posterior force is applied to tibia with knee flexed 90° (1+ posterior drawer)
B	Tibia is flush with femur (2+ posterior drawer)
C	Tibia can be displaced behind femur (3+ posterior drawer)
Undamaged secondary restraints	Posterior tibial subluxation <10 mm
Insufficient	Posterior tibial subluxation >10 mm

although these structures generally are not considered in PCL reconstruction techniques.

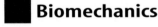

Biomechanics

The PCL provides the primary restraint to posterior tibial translation and is a secondary restraint to external rotation of the tibia. The PCL was once believed to have twice the tensile strength of the ACL, but more recent studies have shown that the load to failure of the PCL is only marginally greater than that of the ACL. The stiffness and ultimate load of the PCL also have been shown to be highly dependent on the portion of the ligament tested. The mean ultimate load for the AL bundle is 1,120 N, whereas the mean ultimate load for the PM bundle is less than half that (419 N); the mean stiffness of the AL bundle is 120 N/mm, compared with 57 N/mm for the PM bundle. A biomechanical study demonstrated nearly normal knee kinematics when the PM bundle was sectioned and the AL bundle was intact, confirming that the AL bundle provides the primary restraint to posterior tibial translation. Other sectioning studies have shown that the meniscofemoral ligaments contribute 28% to the total force resisting posterior translation.

Evaluation

The hallmark test for diagnosis of PCL injury is the posterior drawer test with the knee in 90° of flexion. The severity of the PCL injury can be graded in various ways (**Table 1**). The most common grading system is based on the amount of posterior tibial subluxation identified with posterior drawer testing. Posterior tibial subluxation also can be measured with an arthrometer, kneeling or gravity stress radiographs, or a stress radiograph device. Because of the subjectivity of the posterior drawer test, some authors have suggested that PCL injuries should be categorized by the competence of the remaining ligament or ligament remnant and should be designated as either undamaged (<10 mm of posterior tibial displacement) or insufficient (>10 mm of posterior tibial displacement). Changing the rotation of the foot during the posterior drawer test can help assess different structures. With the foot in internal rotation, the posterior drawer will decrease if the medial collateral ligament and posterior oblique ligament are intact; with the foot in external rotation, the posterolateral corner can be assessed.

Other clinical testing should be done to identify associated injuries. Generally, if there is a grade III injury to the PCL, other ligaments also have been injured, most commonly the posterolateral corner structures. The dial test done with the knee at 90° and 30° of flexion helps identify posterolateral corner injury; more pronounced external rotation compared to the normal knee at 30° of flexion is indicative of an injury to the posterolateral corner structures. Increased external rotation at both 30° and 90° of flexion indicates combined injuries.

Plain radiographs and, occasionally, three-dimensional CT are needed to rule out tibial spine avulsions and tibial plateau fractures, but plain radiographs may be negative with acute injuries. Stress radiographs are useful for quantifying the amount of laxity compared with the unaffected knee, and a recent study found that more than 12 mm of difference was an indication of posterolateral corner injury. MRI can confirm acute injury to the PCL and other ligaments and evaluate the menisci, but is of little benefit in chronic injuries because the ligament may appear to be healed but remain functionally deficient.

Nonsurgical Treatment

Most isolated grade I or II tears of the PCL can be treated nonsurgically, with generally good short-term subjective results. Nonsurgical treatment typically involves reducing inflammation, reestablishing knee motion, and emphasizing quadriceps strengthening. Increased quadriceps strength has been associated with higher knee scores in some series. Although many patients with isolated PCL tears have only a few functional limitations, as many as 25% report a feeling of residual instability, and results tend to worsen with time. Biomechanical and clinical studies have shown that PCL deficiency can result in not only persistent symptoms but also premature osteoarthritis of the medial compartment, followed by osteoarthritis of the patellofemoral compartment.

Reconstruction Techniques

With increased understanding of the importance of the PCL has come an increased use of surgical reconstruction to restore anterior-posterior stability. Reconstruction is recommended for combined ligamentous injuries; posterolateral corner injuries; and persistent pain, instability, and disability after appropriate nonsurgical treatment. Grade III injuries require reconstruction, especially in young, athletic individuals. Reconstruction typically improves laxity by at least one grade, and reconstruction of acute injuries is more successful than that of chronic injuries.

Several techniques have been developed for PCL reconstruction, including transtibial single- and double-bundle and tibial inlay techniques using a variety of autografts and allografts and fixation methods. The relative advantages and disadvantages of these techniques continue to be a matter of considerable debate; no one technique has been shown to be clearly superior to the others. Controversy currently is centered on the optimal location of tibial fixation, the number of graft bundles, the best placement of the femoral tunnel or tunnels, and appropriate graft tensioning during reconstruction.

Historically, the most commonly used technique for PCL reconstruction has been the transtibial single-bundle technique. With this technique, the graft passes proximally and posteriorly through the tibia and makes a 90° turn (the "killer turn") around the superior edge of the posterior aperture of the tibial tunnel before entering the knee joint. This sharp bend in the graft has been suggested to lead to graft elongation and failure. To avoid the killer turn, a tibial inlay technique was developed in which the femoral tunnel or tunnels are placed arthroscopically and an open technique is used for creation of a trough in the posterior tibia to allow the graft to be secured to the anatomic tibial attachment site of the PCL, which provides a more direct route to the femoral tunnel and avoids the killer turn associated with the transtibial tunnel, although this can still be present at the femoral tunnel. However, this technique requires changing the position of the patient during surgery, the additional incision in the popliteal fossa increases surgical time, and the posterior approach may place the neurovascular structures at risk of injury. More recently, arthroscopic techniques have been developed for both single- and double-bundle tibial inlay reconstructions. These techniques use a reverse reamer through the tibia to create the bone block, and the inlay is secured with sutures and a button. Comparison studies of transtibial and tibial inlay techniques have shown no significant differences in laxity or short-term clinical outcomes. Biomechanical comparisons have shown superiority of the inlay technique in some studies and equivocal results in others.

Another area of controversy is the necessity of reconstructing the PM bundle of the PCL. Most reconstruction techniques have focused on the AL bundle because it is the larger and stronger of the two. Biomechanical studies that confirm the importance of the PM bundle in providing a restraint to posterior tibial translation throughout knee flexion have increased interest in double-bundle reconstruction techniques. Although some biomechanical studies described statistically significant improvements in anterior-posterior stability and rotation with double-bundle reconstruction, other studies showed no significant differences in stability between single- and double-bundle PCL reconstructions, and still others found improvement only when double-bundle PCL reconstructions were done for combined PCL and posterolateral corner injuries. Contradictory results also have been reported from biomechanical studies of graft tension with the two techniques, with some authors reporting improved in situ graft forces with double-bundle techniques and others reporting no difference between the two techniques. Clinical studies also have not shown a definite advantage for double-bundle reconstruction (**Table 2**).

Table 2 Results of Treatment of Posterior Cruciate Ligament Injuries

Authors (Year)	Number of Patients	Technique	Mean Patient Age in Years (Range)	Mean Follow-up	Results
Nyland et al (2002)	19	Double-bundle, allografts	"Athletically active"	2 years	Lysholm scores: 63% excellent, 27% good, 5% fair, 5% poor; Final knee-ligament evaluation: 47% normal, 42% nearly normal, 5% abnormal, 5% severely abnormal
Chen et al (2002)	49	Single-bundle transtibial, quadriceps (22), and hamstring (27) autografts	29 (19-54)	28 months (range, 24-36)	Excellent/good results in 86% with quadriceps graft, 89% with hamstrings; No significant difference in activity level, ligamentous laxity, or final rating
Deehan et al (2003)	27	Single-bundle, 4-strand hamstring autograft	27 (18-57)	Median 40 months (range, 24-64)	93% rated knee as normal or near normal; 63% participated in moderate or strenuous activity
Wang, Weng, et al (2004)	35	Double- and single-bundle, hamstring tendons	29	41 months for single-bundle; 28 months for double-bundle	No significant difference in function, laxity, radiographic changes; Overall satisfaction comparable
Houe and Jorgensen (2004)	16	Double-bundle, hamstring tendons Single-bundle, BPTB	31 (19-46)	35 months (range, 25-51)	Good clinical outcomes in both groups, no major differences
Wang, Chan, et al (2004)	55	Single- and double-bundle, hamstring autografts (32) and allografts (23)	30 (16-64)	34 months	Comparable functional results and clinical outcomes; No difference in ligament laxity or radiographic changes; Complications more frequent with autografts.
Sekiya et al (2005)	21	Arthroscopic single-bundle	38 (20-62)	6 years (range, 3-11)	57% with normal or near normal knee; 62% with normal or near normal activity level; All had improvement in laxity of at least one grade
Garofalo et al (2006)	15	Double-bundle, patellar tendon-bone-semitendinosus autograft	28 (17-43)	3 years (range, 2-5)	Lysholm score: excellent 13%, good 87%; Results appear to be no better than those of single-bundle PCL reconstructions
Hatayama et al (2006)	20	Double- and single-bundle, hamstring tendons	32 (17-57)	Minimum 2 years	KT-2000 difference 3.4 mm with single bundle, 4.9 mm with double bundle; No difference in short-term stability
Seon and Song (2006)	43	21 transtibial 22 tibial inlay	29	34 months (range, 24-80)	Both produced relatively good clinical and stress radiography results; No significant differences between the two techniques
MacGillivray et al (2006)	20	Transtibial and tibial inlay	29 (17-49)	5.5 years (range, 2-15)	No significant differences in posterior drawer, KT-1000, or functional testing or in Lysholm, Tegner, or AAOS knee scores; Neither technique consistently restored AP stability to original state

Table 2 *(Continued)*

Authors (Year)	Number of Patients	Technique	Mean Patient Age in Years (Range)	Mean Follow-up	Results
Chan et al (2006)	20	Arthroscopic single-bundle, quadruple hamstring tendon allograft	29 (20-57)	40 months (range, 36-50)	18 (90%) of 20 had excellent or good results; 17 (85%) normal or near normal
Wu et al (2007)	22	Arthroscopic single-bundle, quadriceps autograft	27 (18-49)	66 months (range, 60-76)	19 (86%) had good or excellent results; 82% of knees rated as normal or nearly normal
Jackson et al (2008)	26	Endoscopically assisted single-bundle, hamstring tendons	28 (18-57)	Minimum 10 years (range, 10-12)	IKDC score 87; Lysholm score improved from 64 to 90; 23/26 participated in moderate to strenuous activities
Zhao et al (2008)	18	Double-bundle, "sandwich style" reconstruction, hamstring tendons	34 (19-42)	24 months (range, 24-26)	16 knees graded as normal, 2 as nearly normal; IKDC scores increased from 64 to 96; Lysholm scores increased from 59 to 95
Fanelli et al (2008) (abstract only)	90	Arthroscopic single- and double-bundle; Achilles and anterior tibial allografts	NR	15-72 months	Both techniques provided excellent results; Results did not indicate that one technique was clearly superior to the other; data complicated by inclusion of multiligament-injured knees
Kim et al (2009)	29	8 transtibial single-bundle 11 arthroscopic inlay single-bundle 10 arthroscopic inlay double-bundle	33	37 months	Mean side-to-side difference differed significantly between arthroscopic tibial inlay double-bundle group (3.6) and transtibial single-bundle group 5.6); No significant difference between arthroscopic inlay single-bundle (4.7) and transtibial group; Mean ROM and Lysholm scores similar
Wong et al (2009)	55	Arthroscopic single-bundle, hamstring autografts	30 (16-60)	46 months	Significant improvements in pain and function; Normal or near-normal knees in 67.5%; No significant differences between anteromedial and anterolateral approaches
Hermans et al (2009)	22	Single-bundle (AL); BPTB, STG autografts; 1 Achilles autograft	31 (17-52)	9 years (range, 6-12)	IKDC, Lysholm, VAS scores fair to good, significantly better than preoperative scores; Final Tegner score significantly lower than preinjury score; Patients who had surgery within 1 year of injury had significantly better results than those who waited longer.
Lim et al (2010)	22	Double-bundle, tibial double cross-pin fixation	36 (18-59)	33 months (range, 24-60)	20 (88%) normal or nearly normal, 2 (12%) abnormal; KT-2000 arthrometer difference 11 mm preop, 3 mm postop; No complications

AAOS = American Academy of Orthopaedic Surgeons; AP = anterior-posterior; AL = anterolateral; IKDC = International Knee Documentation Committee; ROM = range of motion; VAS = visual analog scale; BPTB = bone–patellar tendon–bone; STG = semitendinosus and gracilis tendon; NR = not reported.

Table 3   Causes of Failure of Posterior Cruciate Ligament Reconstruction

Biologic reasons

Graft incorporation or remodeling (allograft)

Tunnel erosion

Tunnel expansion

Technical reasons

Failure of fixation

Bone-plug breakage

Loss of interference fixation

Creep or graft slippage (soft tissue)

High internal graft stress

Nonisometric behavior of the anterolateral bundle

Internal stress at tunnel edges ("killer turn")

Surgical decision making

Failure to treat associated instability patterns

Primary repair versus reconstruction

Inappropriate rehabilitation

Early continous passive motion or aggressive range of motion

Early hamstring resistance exercises

Early weight bearing in patients with combined ligamentous injuries

Adapted with permission from Cooper DE, Stewart D: Posterior cruciate ligament reconstruction using single-bundle patella tendon graft with tibial inlay fixation: 2- to 10-year follow-up. *Am J Sports Med* 2004;32:346-360.

In general, reconstruction of isolated PCL injuries has produced good to excellent results in about 80% to 90% of patients (**Table 2**), regardless of the technique used.

Nondisplaced bony avulsions of the PCL from the femur or tibia can be treated with immobilization. Displaced avulsions should be treated with repair of the avulsed bony fragment; even avulsion injuries diagnosed late can be repaired with screw fixation if the PCL substance is sufficient. A careful examination for associated injuries, such as popliteal artery disruption, should precede any treatment of a PCL avulsion fracture because the fracture may be part of a knee dislocation with injuries of multiple structures. Because of the risk of injury to neurovascular injuries in the popliteal space with posterior approaches, modifications of the open technique have been developed. A "safe" posteromedial approach that exposes the avulsion fracture by splitting the fibers of the medial gastrocnemius and preserving the lateral half of the fibers was reported to protect the neurovascular elements in the popliteal space while facilitating placement of a lag screw. Arthroscopic fixation of avulsion fractures has been described, but few clinical studies are available to evaluate results. A biomechanical comparison of open screw fixation and arthroscopic suture fixation found no difference in tibial displacement or stiffness.

Rehabilitation

In general, the rehabilitation protocol after PCL reconstruction takes longer than that for isolated ACL reconstruction. Supervised physical therapy is necessary for about 6 months after surgery, with return to sports (especially contact sports) often delayed for 9 to 12 months. A hinged knee brace is kept in extension for the first week after surgery, then unlocked for range-of-motion exercises; crutches are used for ambulation during the first 6 to 8 weeks. Quadriceps strengthening is the initial focus of rehabilitation, and quadriceps sets and straight-leg raises are begun on the first postoperative day. Active hamstring exercises are avoided because of the potential for posterior tibial subluxation that would stress the reconstruction. The crutches and brace are discontinued at about 8 weeks if good quadriceps strength and control, full knee extension, knee flexion of 90° to 100°, and a normal gait pattern have been regained. Exercises are progressed to include stationary biking, pool therapy, balance and proprioception exercises, treadmill walking, and eventually sport-specific exercises.

Complications

Failure of PCL reconstruction can be related to biologic reasons, technical errors, or rehabilitation errors (**Table 3**). Complications related to nonsurgical treatment include residual laxity, stiffness, knee pain, and degenerative joint disease. In addition to these, complications related to surgical treatment may include neurovascular injuries, osteonecrosis of the medial femoral condyle, compartment syndrome, and tourniquet complications. Failure to recognize and treat associated ligamentous and meniscal injuries is a primary cause of failure of PCL reconstruction. Complications of PCL reconstruction are discussed in detail in chapter 78.

■ Bibliography

Chan YS, Yang SC, Chang CH, et al: Arthroscopic reconstruction of the posterior cruciate ligament with use of a quadruple hamstring tendon graft with 3- to 5-year follow-up. *Arthroscopy* 2006;22(7):762-770.

Chen CH, Chen WJ, Shih CH: Arthroscopic reconstruction of the posterior cruciate ligament: A comparison of quadriceps tendon autograft and quadruple hamstring tendon graft. *Arthroscopy* 2002;18(6):603-612.

Deehan DJ, Salmon LJ, Russell VJ, Pinczewski LA: Endoscopic single-bundle posterior cruciate ligament reconstruction: Results at minimum 2-year follow-up. *Arthroscopy* 2003;19(9):955-962.

Fanelli GC, Edson CJ, Reinheimer KN, Beck J: Arthroscopic single-bundle versus double-bundle posterior cruciate ligament reconstruction. *Arthroscopy* 2008;24(6 supplement 1):e26.

Garofalo R, Jolles BM, Moretti B, Siegrist O: Double-bundle transtibial posterior cruciate ligament reconstruction with a tendon-patellar bone-semitendinosus tendon autograft: Clinical results with a minimum of 2 years' follow-up. *Arthroscopy* 2006;22(12):1331-1338, e1.

Hatayama K, Higuchi H, Kimura M, Kobayashi Y, Asagumo H, Takagishi K: A comparison of arthroscopic single- and double-bundle posterior cruciate ligament reconstruction: Review of 20 cases. *Am J Orthop (Belle Mead NJ)* 2006;35(12):568-571.

Hermans S, Corten K, Bellemans J: Long-term results of isolated anterolateral bundle reconstructions of the posterior cruciate ligament: A 6- to 12-year follow-up study. *Am J Sports Med* 2009;37(8):1499-1507.

Houe T, Jørgensen U: Arthroscopic posterior cruciate ligament reconstruction: One- vs. two-tunnel technique. *Scand J Med Sci Sports* 2004;14(2):107-111.

Jackson WF, van der Tempel WM, Salmon LJ, Williams HA, Pinczewski LA: Endoscopically-assisted single-bundle posterior cruciate ligament reconstruction: Results at minimum ten-year follow-up. *J Bone Joint Surg Br* 2008;90(10):1328-1333.

Kim SJ, Kim TE, Jo SB, Kung YP: Comparison of the clinical results of three posterior cruciate ligament reconstruction techniques. *J Bone Joint Surg Am* 2009;91(11):2543-2549.

Lim HC, Bae JH, Wang JH, et al: Double-bundle PCL reconstruction using tibial double cross-pin fixation. *Knee Surg Sports Traumatol Arthrosc* 2010;18(1):117-122.

MacGillivray JD, Stein BE, Park M, Allen AA, Wickiewicz TL, Warren RF: Comparison of tibial inlay versus transtibial techniques for isolated posterior cruciate ligament reconstruction: Minimum 2-year follow-up. *Arthroscopy* 2006;22(3):320-328.

Nyland J, Hester P, Caborn DN: Double-bundle posterior cruciate ligament reconstruction with allograft tissue: 2-year postoperative outcomes. *Knee Surg Sports Traumatol Arthrosc* 2002;10(5):274-279.

Sekiya JK, West RV, Ong BC, Irrgang JJ, Fu FH, Harner CD: Clinical outcomes after isolated arthroscopic single-bundle posterior cruciate ligament reconstruction. *Arthroscopy* 2005;21(9):1042-1050.

Seon JK, Song EK: Reconstruction of isolated posterior cruciate ligament injuries: A clinical comparison of the transtibial and tibial inlay techniques. *Arthroscopy* 2006;22(1):27-32.

Wang CJ, Chan YS, Weng LH, Yuan LJ, Chen HS: Comparison of autogenous and allogenous posterior cruciate ligament reconstructions of the knee. *Injury* 2004;35(12):1279-1285.

Wang CJ, Weng LH, Hsu CC, Chan YS: Arthroscopic single- versus double-bundle posterior cruciate ligament reconstructions using hamstring autograft. *Injury* 2004;35(12):1293-1299.

Wong T, Wang CJ, Weng LH, et al: Functional outcomes of arthroscopic posterior cruciate ligament reconstruction: Comparison of anteromedial and anterolateral trans-tibia approach. *Arch Orthop Trauma Surg* 2009;129(3):315-321.

Wu CH, Chen AC, Yuan LJ, et al: Arthroscopic reconstruction of the posterior cruciate ligament by using a quadriceps tendon autograft: A minimum 5-year follow-up. *Arthroscopy* 2007;23(4):420-427.

Zhao J, Xiaoqiao H, He Y, Yang X, Liu C, Lu Z: Sandwich-style posterior cruciate ligament reconstruction. *Arthroscopy* 2008;24(6):650-659.

Transtibial Single-Bundle PCL Reconstruction

Gregory C. Fanelli, MD

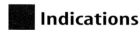 Indications

Single-bundle, single femoral tunnel, transtibial tunnel posterior cruciate ligament (PCL) reconstruction is an anatomic reconstruction of the anterolateral bundle of the PCL. The anterolateral bundle tightens in flexion, and although this reconstruction reproduces that biomechanical function, it cannot reproduce the broad anatomic insertion site of the normal PCL.

The indications for surgical treatment of acute PCL injuries include insertion site avulsions, a tibial step-off that has decreased 6 mm or more, and PCL tears combined with other structural injuries. The primary indication for surgical treatment of chronic PCL injuries is an isolated PCL tear that becomes symptomatic, as demonstrated by progressive functional instability.

Contraindications

There are no specific contraindications to transtibial single-bundle PCL reconstruction. Most surgeons do not recommend any reconstruction of isolated grade I or II PCL injuries.

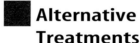 Alternative Treatments

In addition to nonsurgical treatment, alternative treatments include reconstruction using arthroscopic double-bundle techniques and open and arthroscopic-assisted tibial inlay procedures, as well as combinations of these procedures using various graft materials.

Results

Single-bundle reconstruction of PCL injuries, whether isolated or concomitant with other ligamentous injuries, obtains good results in up to 90% of patients (**Table 1**). These results are comparable to those reported with double-bundle reconstructions. Improvements in function and activity level and high levels of patient satisfaction are reported with various graft choices and with both transtibial and tibial inlay techniques.

 Technique

The patient is positioned supine, and both knees are examined after administration of general or regional anesthesia. A tourniquet is applied to the surgical extremity, and the leg is prepared and draped in a sterile fashion. Allograft tissue is prepared before the surgical procedure. The arthroscopic instruments are inserted with the inflow through the superolateral patellar portal, the arthroscope in the inferolateral patellar portal, and the instruments in the inferomedial patellar portal. The portals are interchanged as necessary. The joint and the PCL are evaluated thoroughly arthroscopically, the PCL tear is identified, and the residual stump of the PCL is débrided with hand tools and a synovial shaver. The PCL anatomic insertion sites are retained for anatomic reference points.

Incision

An extracapsular posteromedial safety incision approximately 1.5 to 2.0 cm long is made (**Figure 1**, *A*). The crural fascia is incised longitudinally, taking precautions to protect the neurovascular structures. The interval is developed between the medial head of the gastrocnemius muscle and the posterior capsule of the knee joint, which is anterior. The surgeon's gloved finger is positioned so that the neurovascular structures are posterior to the finger

Dr. Fanelli or an immediate family member has received royalties from Arthrotek.

Table 1 Results of Posterior Cruciate Ligament Reconstruction

Authors (Year)	Technique	Number of Patients	Mean Age in Years (Range)	Mean Follow-up (Range)	Results
Fanelli et al (2004)	Single-bundle Achilles tendon allograft, arthroscopic transtibial tunnel	41	NR	2 to 10 years	Normal posterior drawer and tibial step-off 70% for overall group Normal posterior drawer and tibial step-off 91.7% with mechanical graft tensioning Statistically significant improvement with KT 1000, HSS, Tegner, Lysholm, and stress radiography ($P \leq 0.05$).
Cooper and Stewart (2004)	Single-bundle BPTB (allograft or autograft), tibial inlay fixation	41	28	40 months	IKDC: 28 normal/near normal, 11 abnormal, 2 severely abnormal Mean 4° flexion loss, no extension loss All patients satisfied with outcomes
Wang et al (2004)	Double- and single-bundle hamstring tendons	35	29	Single-bundle: 41 months Double-bundle: 28 months	No significant difference in function, laxity, radiographic changes Overall satisfaction comparable
Sekiya et al (2005)	Single-bundle Achilles tendon allograft	21	38 (20-62)	6 years (3-11)	IKDC: 57% normal/near normal function, 62% normal/near normal activity level All patients had improved laxity of at least 1 grade.
MacGillivray et al (2006)	Tibial inlay (7) Endoscopic transtibial (13)	20	29 (17-49)	6 years (2-15)	90% of patients satisfied No significant differences between techniques
Fanelli et al (2008)	45 single-bundle Achilles tendon allograft 45 double-bundle Achilles tendon allograft and tibialis anterior allograft Arthroscopic transtibial tunnel	90	NR	(24 to 72 months)	No statistically significant difference in single-bundle versus double-bundle PCL reconstruction in PCL-based, multiple-ligament–injured knees Mean side-to-side differences < 3 mm in each group
Hermans et al (2009)	Single-bundle (AL) BPTB graft	25	31 (17-52)	9 years (6-12)	IKDC, Lysholm, functional VAS significantly better than preoperative scores All patients satisfied with outcomes IKDC (22 patients): 1 normal, 8 nearly normal, 13 abnormal, 0 severely abnormal
Wong et al (2009)	Single-bundle transtibial AM vs AL hamstring autograft	55	30 (16-60)	48 months	No significant difference between techniques IKDC normal/near normal in 68% Two thirds had normal posterior laxity

NR = not reported, BPTB = bone–patellar tendon–bone, PCL = posterior cruciate ligament, IKDC = International Knee Documentation Committee, VAS = visual analog scale, AM = anteromedial, AL = anterolateral.

and the posterior aspect of the joint capsule is anterior. This positioning allows monitoring of the surgical instruments, including the over-the-top PCL instruments and the PCL/ACL drill guide, as they are positioned in the posterior aspect of the knee, and confirms accurate placement of the guidewire before tibial tunnel drilling in the medial-lateral and proximal-distal directions (**Figure 1**, *B*). This anatomic surgical interval is the same as that used in the tibial inlay posterior approach.

Positioning the Drill Guide
The curved over-the-top PCL instruments are used to elevate the posterior

knee joint capsule away from the tibial ridge on the posterior aspect of the tibia. This capsular elevation enhances correct drill guide and tibial tunnel placement (**Figure 2**, *A*). The arm of the PCL/ACL drill guide is inserted into the knee through the inferomedial patellar portal and positioned in the PCL fossa on the posterior tibia (**Figure 2**, *B*). The bullet portion of the drill guide contacts the anteromedial aspect of the proximal tibia approximately 1 cm below the tibial tubercle, at a point midway between the tibial crest anteriorly and the posteromedial border of the tibia. This positioning creates a tibial tunnel that is relatively vertically oriented and has its posterior exit point in the inferior and lateral aspect of the PCL tibial anatomic insertion site. This positioning creates an angle of graft orientation that causes the graft to turn two very smooth 45° angles on the posterior aspect of the tibia, eliminating the "killer turn" of 90° (**Figure 2**, *C*).

Drilling the Tibial Tunnel

The surgeon confirms that the tip of the guide is in the posterior aspect of the tibia by placing a finger through the extracapsular posteromedial safe-ty incision. Intraoperative AP and lateral radiographs and arthroscopic observation also can be used to confirm drill guide and guide pin placement. A blunt spade-tipped guidewire is drilled from anterior to posterior. The appropriately sized standard cannulated reamer is used to create the tibial tunnel. The surgeon's finger in the posteromedial safety incision protects the neurovascular structures and confirms the accuracy of the tibial tunnel placement. The standard cannulated drill is advanced to the posterior cortex of the tibia. The drill chuck is then disengaged from the drill and the tibial tunnel reaming is completed by hand, which provides an additional margin of safety.

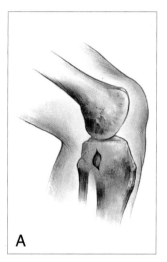
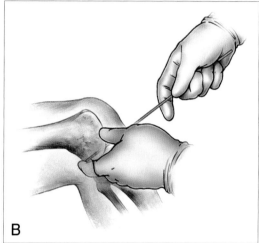

Figure 1 **A,** A posteromedial safety incision is used to protect the neurovascular structures, confirm the accuracy of the tibial tunnel placement, and facilitate the flow of the surgery. **B,** The positioning of the drill guide is monitored by the surgeon's gloved finger to ensure accuracy of placement and avoidance of neurovascular structures. (Adapted with permission from Fanelli GC: *Rationale and Surgical Technique for PCL and Multiple Knee Ligament Reconstruction,* ed 2. Warsaw, IN, Biomet Sports Medicine, 2008, pp 1-8.)

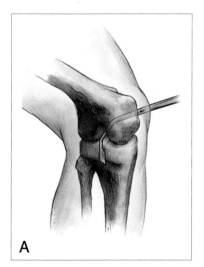
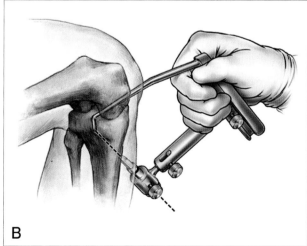
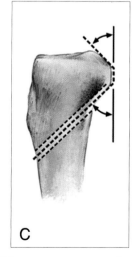

Figure 2 Positioning the drill guide. **A,** The posterior capsule is elevated from the proximal tibia with curved PCL instruments to prepare for tibial tunnel creation. **B,** The PCL drill guide is positioned for creation of the tibial tunnel. **C,** The tibial tunnel is oriented to eliminate acute graft angle turns around the posterior tibia. (Adapted with permission from Fanelli GC: *Rationale and Surgical Technique for PCL and Multiple Knee Ligament Reconstruction,* ed 2. Warsaw, IN, Biomet Sports Medicine, 2008, pp 1-8.)

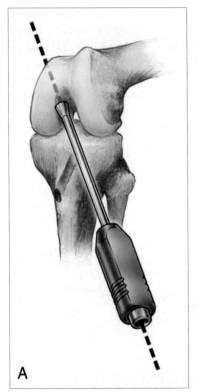

A

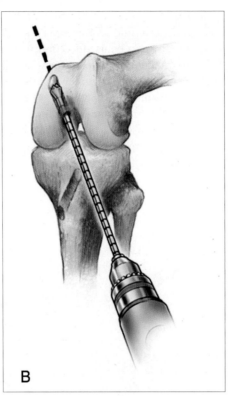

B

Figure 3 Drilling the femoral tunnel. **A,** The femoral aimer is positioned through a low anterolateral portal to position a guidewire in the PCL anterolateral bundle footprint. **B,** An endoscopic reamer is used to create the PCL anterolateral bundle femoral tunnel from inside out. (Adapted with permission from Fanelli GC: *Rationale and Surgical Technique for PCL and Multiple Knee Ligament Reconstruction,* ed 2. Warsaw, IN, Biomet Sports Medicine, 2008, pp 1-8.)

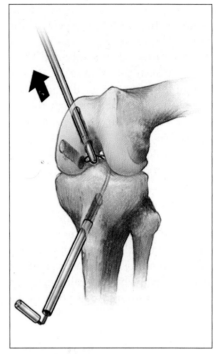

Figure 4 A suture passing device is used to assist with graft passage. (Adapted with permission from Fanelli GC: *Rationale and Surgical Technique for PCL and Multiple Knee Ligament Reconstruction,* ed 2. Warsaw, IN, Biomet Sports Medicine, 2008, pp 1-8.)

Drilling the Femoral Tunnel

The PCL femoral tunnel is made from the inside out using a handheld aimer. Insertion of the appropriately sized aimer through a low anterolateral patellar portal creates the PCL femoral tunnel. The aimer is positioned directly on the footprint of the PCL femoral insertion site (**Figure 3,** *A*). The appropriately sized guidewire is drilled through the aimer, through the bone, and out a small skin incision. Care is taken to ensure that no compromise of the articular surface occurs. The single-bundle aimer is removed, and an acorn reamer is used to drill the anterior lateral PCL femoral tunnel endoscopically from the inside out (**Figure 3,** *B*).

Graft Passage

A suture-passing device is introduced through the tibial tunnel and into the knee joint and is retrieved through the femoral tunnel with an arthroscopic grasping tool. The traction sutures of the graft material are attached to the loop of the suture-passing device, and the PCL graft material is pulled into position (**Figure 4**).

Graft Fixation

Fixation of the PCL graft is accomplished with primary and backup fixation on both the femoral and tibial sides. Our preferred graft source for single-bundle PCL reconstruction is an Achilles tendon allograft. Femoral fixation is accomplished with cortical suspensory backup fixation using polyethylene ligament fixation buttons and aperture opening fixation with bioabsorbable interference screws. A tensioning boot is applied to the traction sutures of the graft material on its distal end and set for 20 pounds, and

the knee is cycled through 25 full flexion-extension cycles for graft pretensioning and settling (**Figure 5**). The graft is tensioned in approximately 70° of knee flexion. Graft fixation is achieved with primary aperture opening fixation with bioabsorbable interference screws and backup fixation with a ligament fixation button, a screw and post, or a screw and spiked ligament washer assembly.

When multiple ligament surgeries are done during the same surgical session, the PCL reconstruction is done first, followed by the ACL reconstruction and then the collateral ligament surgery.

Wound Closure

At the completion of the procedure, the tourniquet is deflated and the wounds are irrigated. The incisions are closed in the standard fashion.

———————————■

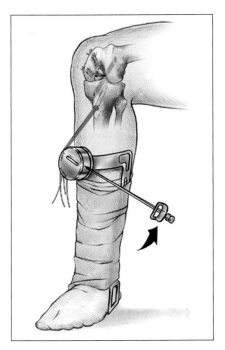

Figure 5 Graft fixation. A mechanical graft tensioning boot is used for pre-tensioning and tensioning the PCL graft during final fixation. This device can be used with single- and double-bundle PCL reconstruction surgical techniques. (Adapted with permission from Fanelli GC: *Rationale and Surgical Technique for PCL and Multiple Knee Ligament Reconstruction,* ed 2. Warsaw, IN, Biomet Sports Medicine, 2008.)

Postoperative Regimen

The knee is immobilized in a long-leg brace with the knee in full extension for 5 weeks, and the patient is instructed to be non–weight-bearing on crutches. Progressive range of motion and progressive weight bearing occur during weeks 6 through 10. The crutches are discontinued at the end of postoperative week 10. Progressive strength training begins and range-of-motion exercises are continued. Return to sports and heavy labor occurs 6 to 9 months after surgery, when sufficient strength, range of motion, and proprioceptive skills have returned.

Avoiding Pitfalls and Complications

Factors contributing to the success of arthroscopically assisted single-bundle transtibial PCL reconstruction include identification and treatment of all pathology (especially posterolateral and posteromedial instability), accurate tunnel placement, placement of strong graft material at anatomic graft insertion sites, minimization of graft bending, use of a mechanical graft tensioning device, final graft tensioning at 70° to 90° of knee flexion using primary and backup fixation, and appropriate postoperative rehabilitation.

Reconstruction of the PCL is technically demanding, however. Complications include failure to recognize associated ligament injuries, neurovascular complications, persistent posterior sag, osteonecrosis, knee motion loss, anterior knee pain, and fractures. A comprehensive preoperative evaluation, including an accurate diagnosis, a well-planned and carefully executed surgical procedure, and a supervised postoperative rehabilitation program will help to reduce the incidence of such complications.

Bibliography

Cooper DE, Stewart D: Posterior cruciate ligament reconstruction using single-bundle patella tendon graft with tibial inlay fixation: 2- to 10-year follow-up. *Am J Sports Med* 2004;32(2):346-360.

Fanelli GC: Arthroscopic PCL reconstruction: Transtibial technique, in Fanelli GC, ed: *Posterior Cruciate Ligament Injuries. A Guide To Practical Management.* Springer-Verlag, New York, 2001.

Fanelli GC, Edson CJ: Combined posterior cruciate ligament-posterolateral reconstructions with Achilles tendon allograft and biceps femoris tendon tenodesis: 2- to 10-year follow-up. *Arthroscopy* 2004;20(4):339-345.

Fanelli GC, Edson CJ, Reinheimer KN, Beck J: Arthroscopic single bundle v double bundle posterior cruciate ligament reconstruction. *Arthroscopy* 2008;24(Suppl):e26.

Fanelli GC, Monahan TJ: Complications in posterior cruciate ligament and posterolateral corner surgery. *Oper Tech Sports Med* 2001;9(2):96-99.

Hermans S, Corten K, Bellemans J: Long-term results of isolated anterolateral bundle reconstructions of the posterior cruciate ligament: A 6- to 12-year follow-up study. *Am J Sports Med* 2009;37(8):1499-1507.

MacGillivray JD, Stein BE, Park M, Allen AA, Wickiewicz TL, Warren RF: Comparison of tibial inlay versus transtibial techniques for isolated posterior cruciate ligament reconstruction: Minimum 2-year follow-up. *Arthroscopy* 2006;22(3): 320-328.

Miller MD, Cooper DE, Fanelli GC, Harner CD, LaPrade RF: Posterior cruciate ligament: current concepts. *Instr Course Lect* 2002;51:347-351.

Sekiya JK, West RV, Ong BC, Irrgang JJ, Fu FH, Harner CD: Clinical outcomes after isolated arthroscopic single-bundle posterior cruciate ligament reconstruction. *Arthroscopy* 2005;21(9):1042-1050.

Wang CJ, Weng LH, Hsu CC, Chan YS: Arthroscopic single- versus double-bundle posterior cruciate ligament reconstructions using hamstring autograft. *Injury* 2004;35(12):1293-1299.

Wong T, Wang CJ, Weng LH, et al: Functional outcomes of arthroscopic posterior cruciate ligament reconstruction: Comparison of anteromedial and anterolateral trans-tibia approach. *Arch Orthop Trauma Surg* 2009;129(3):315-321.

Coding

CPT Code		Corresponding ICD-9 Codes	
29889	Arthroscopically aided posterior cruciate ligament repair/augmentation or reconstruction	717.84	844.2

Chapter 75

Double-Bundle Posterior Cruciate Ligament Reconstruction

Christopher D. Harner, MD
Samuel P. Robinson, MD
James R. Romanowski, MD

Indications

Most isolated grade I and II posterior cruciate ligament (PCL) injuries do well with nonsurgical management that includes a rehabilitation program focusing on quadriceps strengthening. Reconstruction of grade II PCL injuries is indicated when nonsurgical treatment fails. Usually, single-bundle augmentation or reconstruction is sufficient to restore stability, but patients with severe instability (both translational and rotational) are good candidates for double-bundle PCL reconstruction. This anatomic reconstruction corrects laxity by reconstructing both the anterolateral and posteromedial bundles to reduce both posterior tibial translation and external rotation.

Contraindications

Double-bundle PCL reconstruction is not indicated for low-grade PCL injuries that can be treated successfully with nonsurgical methods. In addition, patients with abnormal limb alignment, mechanical axis abnormalities, and visual gait disturbances should not be treated with isolated double-bundle PCL reconstruction. Long-term successful treatment of these problems may require more than an isolated soft-tissue reconstruction. Revision reconstructions require adequate bone stock to support tunnels and facilitate bone-tendon healing. Additional procedures can be done either concurrently with double-bundle PCL reconstruction or as staged procedures.

Alternative Treatments

Examination under anesthesia (EUA) is a critical factor in deciding between single- and double-bundle transtibial PCL reconstruction. An EUA not only helps determine the degree of laxity in posterior tibial translation and external rotation, but it also helps evaluate for associated ligamentous injuries to the posterolateral corner (PLC), lateral collateral ligament, and/or medial collateral ligament. In patients with a grade II PCL injury with an associated grade II or III PLC injury, a single-bundle augmentation or single-bundle PCL reconstruction with PLC repair or reconstruction is typically done. If the EUA reveals an isolated grade II or III PCL injury in a young patient or a chronic grade III PCL injury with an associated grade II or III PLC, lateral collateral ligament, or medial collateral ligament injury, a double-bundle PCL reconstruction is indicated, with appropriate surgical correction of the associated injuries.

Once the decision has been made regarding the PCL surgical plan, diagnostic arthroscopy is performed to evaluate the exact injury patterns of the anterolateral and posteromedial bundles of the PCL. If either of the PCL bundles is intact, an augmentation procedure is done to reconstruct the deficient bundle. Every effort is made to preserve native tissue if possible. If no structurally significant portions of the PCL remain, a double-bundle reconstruction is done.

Another alternative is a tibial inlay approach for PCL reconstruction rather than the transtibial technique described in this chapter. We believe that there are significant disadvantages

Dr. Harner or an immediate family member serves as a board member, owner, officer, or committee member of the Musculoskeletal Transplant Foundation and serves as a paid consultant to or is an employee of Smith & Nephew. Neither of the following authors or any immediate family members has received anything of value from or owns stock in a commercial company or institution related directly or indirectly to the subject of this article: Dr. Robinson and Dr. Romanowski.

Table 1 Results of Double-Bundle Posterior Cruciate Ligament Reconstruction

Authors (Year)	Number of Patients	Technique	Mean Patient Age in Years (Range)	Mean Follow-up (Range)	Results
Nyland et al (2002)	19 "athletically active"	Double-bundle, allografts	36 (25-47)	27 months (25-29)	Lysholm scores: 63% excellent, 27% good, 5% fair, 5% poor Final knee ligament evaluation: 47% normal, 42% nearly normal, 5% abnormal, 5% severely abnormal
Houe and Jorgensen (2004)	16	Double-bundle, hamstring tendons Single-bundle, BPTB	31 (19-46)	35 months (25-51)	Good clinical outcomes in both groups, no major differences
Wang et al (2004)	35	Double- and single-bundle, hamstring tendons	29	Single-bundle: 41 months (28-54) Double-bundle: 28 months (24-32)	No significant difference in function, laxity, radiographic changes Overall satisfaction comparable
Hatayama et al (2006)	20	Double- and single-bundle, hamstring tendons	32 (17-57)	2 years minimum	KT-2000 arthrometer difference 3.4 mm with single-bundle, 4.9 mm with double-bundle No difference in short-term stability
Garofalo et al (2006)	15	Double-bundle, patellar tendon–bone–semi-tendinosus autograft	28 (17-43)	3 years (2-5)	Lysholm scores: 13% excellent, 87% good Results appear to be no better than those of single-bundle PCL reconstructions
Lim et al (2009)	22	Double-bundle, tibial double cross-pin fixation	36 (18-59)	33 months (24-60)	20 (88%) normal or nearly normal, 2 (12%) abnormal KT-2000 arthrometer difference: 11 mm preoperatively, 3 mm postoperatively No complications

BPTB = bone–patellar tendon–bone; PCL = posterior cruciate ligament.

to this technique, the most important being the need to dissect around the neurovascular structures in the posterior aspect of the knee. We use a transtibial technique because it is less difficult and less dangerous and takes less time.

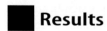

Results

Although there are no long-term evaluations of transtibial double-bundle PCL reconstruction, preliminary results are promising (**Table 1**). Biomechanical testing in cadaver models has

shown a reduction in both posterior tibial translation and external rotation as well as more normal knee kinematics. Of 19 patients who had double-bundle PCL reconstruction using a transtibial technique with a tibialis anterior allograft, 17 (89%) were rated as normal or near normal, and posterior tibial translation with respect to the femur averaged 2.4 mm at 2-year follow-up. Knee stability was greater in patients who had double-bundle reconstruction than in those who underwent a single-bundle procedure. Other clinical studies comparing double-bundle to single-bundle PCL reconstruction found no significant

difference in Lysholm score, activity level, or graft laxity. Further study is needed to confirm early findings, show long-term clinical success, and help resolve unanswered questions concerning PCL reconstruction technique, graft type, fixation techniques, timing of reconstruction, and treatment of associated injuries.

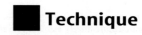

Technique

Setup
The patient is placed supine on the operating table with a bump beneath

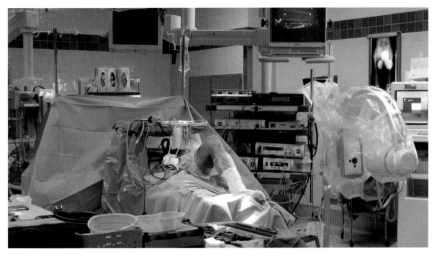

Figure 1 Setup and patient positioning for double-bundle PCL reconstruction.

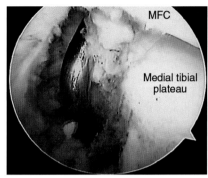

Figure 2 Arthroscopic view of the PCL curet placed through the anteromedial portal, as seen through the posteromedial portal. MFC = medial femoral condyle.

the hip of the surgical lower extremity (**Figure 1**). We use no tourniquet or leg holder. A sandbag is attached to the table distally in a position in which flexing the knee to 90° will keep the foot secure. A post is placed laterally to assist with rotational control of the lower extremity. Fluoroscopy is readily available in the operating room.

Examination Under Anesthesia

An EUA is done on all patients; it is critical in the determination of the surgical plan. Although all potential treatment options should be discussed at length with the patient as part of informed consent and appropriate equipment and grafts need to be obtained preoperatively, it is important to reserve final treatment decisions until the information obtained from the EUA is available. Once the decision to proceed with double-bundle PCL reconstruction has been made, the incisions are marked and injected with 0.25% bupivacaine with epinephrine, and the lower extremity is prepared and draped sterilely.

Portal Placement

Four portals are used: anterolateral, anteromedial, superolateral outflow, and posteromedial. The first three are part of our routine knee arthroscopy.

The posteromedial portal is established after the diagnostic arthroscopy with the use of a spinal needle under arthroscopic observation with a 70° arthroscope placed through the anterolateral portal, medial to the cruciate ligaments in the femoral notch, and into the posterior aspect of the knee (Gillquist view).

Diagnostic Arthroscopy

Diagnostic arthroscopic examination is done to confirm the findings, investigate the pattern of PCL bundle injury, evaluate associated ligamentous injury, and evaluate capsular, meniscal, or cartilage injury. Using a shaver and arthroscopic cautery, the femoral insertions of the anterolateral and posteromedial bundles of the PCL are identified and cleared. Care should be taken to preserve any native PCL tissue that remains intact. An anterior drawer force is placed on the knee to keep tension on the ACL and avoid incidental débridement of its lax fibers.

Procedure

TIBIAL TUNNELS

A PCL curet is placed through the anteromedial portal, through the notch, and into the posterior aspect of the proximal tibia. Careful dissection is done to clear the tissue anteriorly to

provide a space for viewing. The 70° arthroscope is then placed through the notch to examine the posterior aspect of the tibia, as well as the posterior tibial space. An arthroscopic shaver can be inserted through the posteromedial portal to assist in débriding scar tissue and ligamentous remnants from the area of the PCL insertion. Care must be taken to keep the shaver blades facing anteriorly to avoid injury to the posterior neurovascular structures. Adequate débridement requires repositioning of the arthroscope in the posteromedial portal and the PCL curet in the anteromedial portal (**Figure 2**). When débridement is complete, the PCL insertion site should be visible at least 2 to 3 cm distal to the posterior tibial joint line.

The position of the anterolateral tibial tunnel is determined first. The arthroscope is placed in the posteromedial portal and the PCL guide is placed in the anterolateral portal. The tip of the guide is placed in the distal and lateral aspect of the tibial PCL footprint. A lateral fluoroscopic view of the knee is used to confirm the position of the guide in the anterolateral tibial insertion site. An oblique incision is made over the anterolateral aspect of the tibia to establish a starting point for the anterolateral tibial guidewire. The dissection is carried down to the anterior compartment, which is then elevated off the anterolateral as-

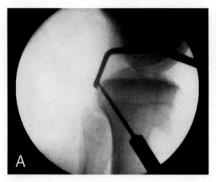
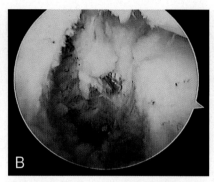

Figure 3 Anterolateral tibial guidewire placement. **A,** Fluoroscopic view. **B,** Arthroscopic view via posteromedial portal.

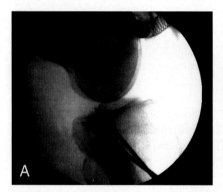
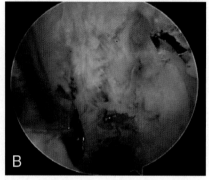

Figure 4 Posteromedial tibial guidewire placement. **A,** Fluoroscopic view. **B,** Arthroscopic view via the posteromedial portal.

pect of the proximal tibia. If the PLC is being repaired or reconstructed concurrently, we use an extended approach that incorporates the anterolateral incision. The PCL guide is set between 45° and 50° as needed to avoid reaming the posterior tibial cortex distal to the PCL insertion. A guidewire is then advanced to the cortex of the posterior tibia under fluoroscopic guidance (**Figure 3**). Care is taken to avoid injuring the posterior neurovascular structures.

The posteromedial tibial tunnel is then prepared using a similar technique. The tip of the PCL guide is placed in an anatomic location in the proximal and medial aspect of the PCL footprint. This position is confirmed using lateral fluoroscopic imaging. An oblique incision is made over the anteromedial tibia to establish a starting point for the posteromedial tibial guidewire just distal to the tibial flare.

The PCL guide is set between 45° to 50° as needed to avoid reaming the posterior cortex of the tibia distal to the PCL insertion. Under fluoroscopic guidance, the posteromedial guidewire is advanced to the posterior tibial cortex (**Figure 4**).

Once the anterolateral and posteromedial tibial guidewires are appropriately placed, the tunnels are drilled and dilated. Typically, the anterolateral bundle requires a graft diameter of 8 to 9 mm and the posteromedial bundle requires a graft diameter of 6 to 7 mm. Cannulated compaction drills are undersized by 1 to 2 mm. Care is taken while drilling to protect the posterior neurovascular structures by placing the arthroscope in the posteromedial portal and the PCL curet over the tip of the guidewire (**Figure 5,** *A* and *B*). Penetration of the posterior cortex should be completed with a hand reamer. Once the tunnels are

drilled, they can be dilated to the appropriate size (**Figure 5,** *C* and *D*).

FEMORAL TUNNELS

With a 30° arthroscope in the anteromedial portal, a Steadman awl is used to mark the center of the anterolateral and posteromedial bundles (**Figure 6**). Once these insertion sites are marked, the knee is flexed to 120°. A guidewire is placed through the anterolateral portal to the marked center of the anterolateral femoral tunnel. The guidewire is tapped into place with a mallet and an acorn reamer is used to drill the tunnel to a depth of 30 to 40 mm (**Figure 7**). Care is taken when inserting the acorn reamer to avoid the articular surface of the medial femoral condyle. Once the correct diameter of the tunnel is reached, an EndoButton (Smith & Nephew Endoscopy, Andover, MA) drill bit is used to penetrate the medial femoral cortex and the total length of the tunnel is measured.

The posteromedial femoral tunnel is created in a similar fashion. The knee is flexed to 110°, a guidewire is tapped into place with a mallet, and an acorn reamer is used to drill the tunnel to a depth of 25 mm. Similar precautions apply with regard to the articular surface of the medial femoral condyle.

GRAFT PREPARATION

Our graft of choice is an anterior tibial tendon allograft because it is readily available, its mechanical properties roughly match the demands required of a native PCL, it works well with our preferred fixation technique, and we have been pleased with the outcomes using this technique. Graft selection ultimately depends, however, on the timing and extent of the injury, the availability of graft options, the experience of the surgeon, and the preferences of the patient. Other allograft options include the posterior tibial, hamstring, and Achilles tendons. Autograft options also are available, in-

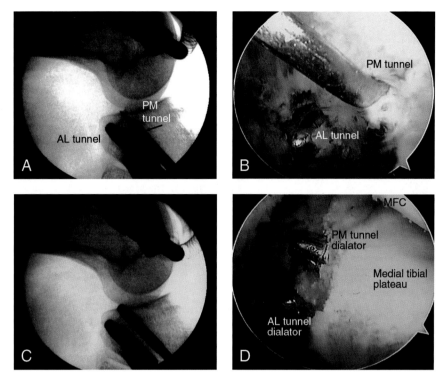

Figure 5 Drilling and dilating the tibial tunnels. **A,** Fluoroscopic lateral view shows guide pin placement and reaming of the posteromedial tunnel. **B,** Arthroscopic view from the posteromedial portal with the PCL curet over the tip of the posteromedial guidewire. **C,** Intraoperative fluoroscopy shows the two tibial dilators. **D,** Arthroscopic view. AL = anterolateral, PM = posteromedial.

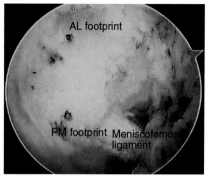

Figure 6 Arthroscopic view of the PCL footprint. The femoral insertions of the anterolateral and posteromedial bundles are marked with a pilot hole for guide pin placement. Note that the meniscofemoral ligaments are preserved. AL = anterolateral, PM = posteromedial.

GRAFT PASSAGE

Historically, graft passage has been the most difficult part of PCL surgery using a transtibial technique; however, our technique allows safe, relatively simple graft passage. We first place two 8-French pediatric feeding tubes in a retrograde fashion through each tibial tunnel. With the help of a grasper in the posteromedial portal, we advance the feeding tubes into the notch and then retrieve them out the anterolateral portal. If the meniscofemoral ligaments remain intact, it is important to pass the feeding tubes below these structures. A suture then is advanced inside each pediatric feeding tube and the feeding tubes are pulled out the tibial tunnel to advance the suture shuttles.

The anterolateral graft is passed first, by tying the anterolateral suture shuttle to the free ends of the suture tails of the whipstitched end that are exiting the anterolateral portal. The graft is advanced into the knee through the anterolateral portal and out the tibial tunnel. The femoral side of the graft (with the loop) is then passed into the femoral tunnel using a Beath pin through the corresponding anterolateral femoral tunnel. The posteromedial graft is then passed in the

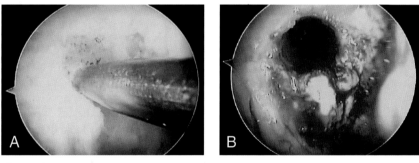

Figure 7 Drilling the femoral tunnels. **A,** The anterolateral guidewire is in place and ready to be used to drill the anterolateral tunnel. **B,** The drilled anterolateral femoral tunnel.

cluding the patellar, quadriceps, and hamstring tendons.

Graft preparation depends on the type of fixation preferred by the surgeon. Because we use post fixation, the graft for each bundle is prepared using a single anterior tibial allograft looped through a continuous synthetic loop to be used on the femoral post. The anterolateral bundle graft

usually requires a 40-mm loop, whereas the posteromedial graft generally requires a 50-mm loop. The free ends are whipstitched and left free to tie over the tibial post. The intraarticular portions of the graft are marked at both ends so the lines can be seen arthroscopically at the mouth of the femoral and tibial tunnels (**Figure 8**).

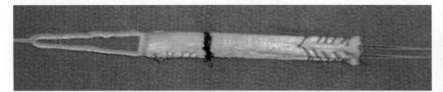

Figure 8 A tibialis anterior allograft is prepared and ready for passage.

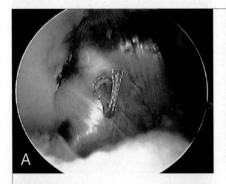

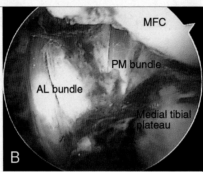

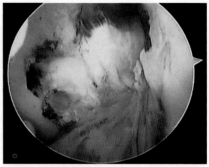

Figure 9 The posteromedial graft is passed after the anterolateral graft has been passed.

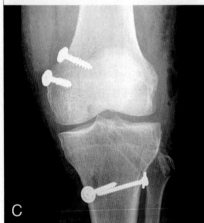

Figure 10 Double-bundle PCL reconstruction. **A,** View from the anterolateral portal. **B,** View from the posteromedial portal. **C,** Postoperative AP radiograph. AL = anterolateral, PM = posteromedial, MFC = medial femoral condyle.

same fashion using the appropriate suture shuttle (**Figure 9**).

GRAFT TENSIONING AND FIXATION

Once the grafts are passed, they are fixed on the femoral side with two AO 6.5-mm cancellous screws with washers. Although several fixation options exist, we have found cancellous screws to provide excellent fixation, easy removal if needed, and minimal cost. An oblique incision is made in the superomedial aspect of the knee along the Langer lines. The dissection is carried down over the vastus medialis obliquus, which is then bluntly split in line with its fibers. Once the

femoral side has been appropriately fixed, PLC or collateral ligament reconstruction or repair is done. When these associated procedures are completed, the PCL grafts can be tensioned and fixed on the tibial side. The knee is then cycled, keeping manual tension on the two PCL bundles. Two AO 4.5-mm bicortical screws with washers are placed approximately 1 cm distal to each tibial tunnel. The anterolateral graft is tensioned first, with the knee at 90° of flexion, and an anterior drawer force is applied. The posteromedial graft is tensioned next, with the knee at 30° of flexion, and an anterior drawer force is ap-

plied. **Figure 10** shows a completed reconstruction.

Wound Closure

Wounds are copiously irrigated and débrided of bone dust and other debris. Deep and fascial layers are closed with interrupted heavy absorbable sutures, superficial subcutaneous layers are closed with interrupted chromic gut sutures, and the skin is closed with an absorbable running stitch.

■ Postoperative Regimen

Immediately after surgery, patients are placed in a brace that is worn for 8 weeks. The brace is locked in extension for the first week and then unlocked only for physical therapy. At 4 to 6 weeks, the brace is unlocked for ambulation. Patients are allowed weight bearing as tolerated but use crutches for a full 8 weeks to prevent limping and the development of a flexion contracture. Patients are cautioned against posterior tibial translation, and no continuous passive motion is used. Formal physical therapy begins immediately after surgery, and no open-chain hamstring work is allowed. Patients are expected to progress through a multiphase rehabilitation program that focuses on quadriceps strengthening, range of motion, and gait training. At approximately 3 months after surgery, functional strengthening and proprioception work using closed kinetic chain exercises is begun. Patients can usually return to heavy-duty work at 9 months and to sports at 1 year.

———■

Avoiding Pitfalls and Complications

Neurovascular Injury

The most devastating complication of PCL surgery is iatrogenic injury to the posterior neurovascular structures. For this reason, PCL reconstruction should not be done at an ambulatory surgery center, and a vascular surgeon should always be available in case of emergency. There are a few key techniques to keep in mind to protect these structures from inadvertent injury:

- When working in the posterior aspect of the knee, always keep the shaver blade directed anteriorly.
- Use fluoroscopy when drilling tibial tunnels to ensure that the guidewire does not advance. Placing a PCL curet over the tip of the guidewire also will help limit the guidewire from advancing inadvertently.

- The penetration of the posterior cortex of the tibia should be done under arthroscopic observation with the reamer in hand (not on power).
- Avoid the use of a tourniquet so injury can be identified immediately.

Intra-articular Injury

Although not as devastating as injury to the posterior neurovascular structures, iatrogenic injury to other intra-articular structures can lead to poor outcomes. Techniques to avoid inadvertent injury include the following:

- Keep an anterior drawer force on the knee while using the shaver in the notch. Tension across the ACL will prevent its fibers from inadvertently being débrided by the shaver.
- When drilling the femoral tunnels over a guidewire, be aware of the articular cartilage of the medial femoral condyle. If there is insufficient room to pass the reamer, use a smaller reamer over the guidewire. Dilators and acorn reamers can be used after the guidewire has been removed to increase the tunnel diameter to the appropriate size.

Graft Passage

Historically, graft passage has been the most difficult part of transtibial PCL

reconstruction techniques. The technique described here, which uses an 8-French pediatric feeding tube, simplifies graft passage and enables the graft to be passed without significant difficulty.

Tunnel Placement and Fixation

As with any ligament reconstruction, the procedure is successful only if the graft is in the correct position and secure fixation is maintained. The following techniques can minimize the risk of errors in tunnel placement or tunnel fixation:

- Take time for a careful débridement and identification of the PCL insertion sites. Correct tunnel placement is critical, so landmarks and residual PCL tissue should be used to ensure that the tunnel locations are anatomic.
- Fluoroscopy should be used to confirm anatomic guidewire placement to the insertion sites and prevent damage to the posterior tibial cortex distally.
- Avoid stacking the tibial tunnels on the medial side of the knee. We have found that this has simplified tibial tunnel preparation, enabled easier graft passage, allowed for more secure tibial fixation, and prevented tunnel coalescence.

———■

Bibliography

Berg EE: Posterior cruciate ligament tibial inlay reconstruction. *Arthroscopy* 1995;11:69-76.

Boynton MD, Tietjens BR: Long-term follow-up of the untreated isolated posterior cruciate ligament-deficient knee. *Am J Sports Med* 1996;24:306-310.

Garofalo R, Jolles BM, Moretti B, Siegrist O: Double-bundle transtibial posterior cruciate ligament reconstruction with a tendon-patellar bone-semitendinosus tendon autograft: Clinical results with a minimum 2 years' follow-up. *Arthroscopy* 2006;22:1331-1338.

Harner CD, Höher J: Evaluation and treatment of posterior cruciate ligament injuiries. *Am J Sports Med* 1998;26:471-482.

Harner CD, Janaushek MA, Kanamori A, Yagi M, Vogrin TM, Woo SL: Biomechanical analysis of a double-bundle posterior cruciate ligament reconstruction. *Am J Sports Med* 2000;28:144-151.

Hatayama K, Higuchi H, Kimura M, et al: A comparison of arthroscopic single- and double-bundle posterior cruciate ligament reconstruction: Review of 20 cases. *Am J Orthop* 2006;35:568-571.

Houe T, Jorgensen U: Arthroscopic posterior cruciate ligament reconstruction: One- vs. two-tunnel technique. *Scand J Med Sci Sports* 2004;14:107-111.

Jakob RP, Ruegsegger M: Therapy of posterior and posterolateral knee instability. *Orthopade* 1993;22:405-413.

Klimkiewicz JJ, Harner CD, Fu FH: Single bundle posterior cruciate ligament reconstruction: University of Pittsburgh approach. *Oper Tech Sports Med* 1999;7:105-109.

Lim HC, Bae JH, Wang JH, et al: Double-bundle PCL reconstruction using tibial double cross-pin fixation. *Knee Surg Sports Traumatol Arthrosc* 2009 Apr 28 [Epub ahead of print].

Mannor DA, Shearn JT, Grood ES, Noyes FR, Levy MS: Two-Bundle posterior cruciate ligament reconstruction: An in vitro analysis of graft placement and tension. *Am J Sports Med* 2000;28:833-845.

Markolf KL, Feeley BT, Jackson SR, McAllister DR: Biomechanical studies of double- bundle posterior cruciate ligament reconstructions. *J Bone Joint Surg Am* 2006;88:1788-1794.

Nyland J, Hester P, Caborn DN: Double-bundle posterior cruciate ligament reconstruction with allograft tissue: 2-year postoperative outcomes. *Knee Surg Sports Traumatol Arthrosc* 2002;10:274-279.

Race A, Amis AA: PCL reconstruction: In vitro biomechanical comparison of 'isometric' versus single and double-bundled 'anatomic' grafts. *J Bone Joint Surg Br* 1998;80:173-179.

Shelbourne K, Davis T, Patel D: The natural history of acute, isolated nonoperatively treated posterior cruciate ligament injuries: A prospective study. *Am J Sports Med* 1999;27:276-283.

Torg JS, Barton TM, Pavlov H, Stine R: Natural history of the posterior cruciate ligament-deficient knee. *Clin Orthop Relat Res* 1989;246:208-216.

Wang CJ, Weng LH, Hsu CC, Chan YS: Arthroscopic single- versus double-bundle posterior cruciate ligament recon-structions using hamstring autograft. *Injury* 2004;35:1293-1299.

Coding			
CPT Code		**Corresponding ICD-9 Codes**	
Arthroscopic PCL Repair			
29889	Arthroscopically aided posterior cruciate ligament repair/augmentation or reconstruction	717.84	844.2

Chapter 76

Tibial Inlay Technique

Richard D. Parker, MD
Sam Akhavan, MD

■ Indications

Most acute posterior cruciate ligament (PCL) injuries (**Figure 1**) can be successfully treated nonsurgically with a course of rest and physical therapy concentrating on quadriceps rehabilitation; surgical intervention is reserved for grade III injuries in young, high-level athletes, peel-off injuries, or high-energy ruptures associated with other ligamentous injuries. In a small percentage of patients, however, late instability and pain will develop, as well as degenerative changes involving the medial and patellofemoral compartments. Surgical treatment generally is indicated for patients with chronic, isolated grade III abnormal laxity of the PCL for which nonsurgical treatment has been unsuccessful. Patients with chronic PCL tears (**Figure 2**) should be evaluated for additional ligamentous injuries. If combined injuries are found, the PCL should be reconstructed along with the other ligamentous injuries. Another indication for reconstruction is

an isolated tear that causes continued pain and instability not responsive to nonsurgical management; however, it is important to note that reconstruction of isolated PCL tears has yielded inconsistent results.

Suggested indications for the tibial inlay technique include high-performance athletes; revision procedures when the tibial tunnel is too wide or too proximal; and patients with osteopenia from disuse, fracture, or previous osteotomy to prevent proximal graft migration in the tibial tunnel (windshield-wiper effect).

■ Contraindications

In general, PCL reconstruction is contraindicated in the patient with an acute grade I or II isolated tear that produces mild posterior (< 10 mm) and rotatory (< 5°) laxity and no significant varus or valgus laxity. Reconstruction also is contraindicated in the patient with a knee dislocation

that involves arterial or venous injury that compromises limb viability. There are no contraindications specific to the tibial inlay reconstruction technique.

■ Alternative Treatments

The initial treatment of an isolated acute grade I or II PCL injury is nonsurgical, with the goals of reducing inflammation, reestablishing knee motion, and emphasizing quadriceps strengthening. Gradual return to activity usually is possible within 3 to 6 weeks, depending on the severity of the injury and the demands of the patient's sport or occupation. Surgical reconstruction generally is required for more severe PCL injuries and those associated with additional injury to the posterolateral corner.

Several techniques, both open and arthroscopic, have been described for the reconstruction of isolated PCL injuries. The most commonly used is an arthroscopic transtibial tunnel reconstruction. This technique restores PCL stability but requires the graft to curve around the posterior aspect of the proximal tibia (the "killer turn"), which can cause PCL laxity, friction, abrasion, and ultimately graft failure.

Dr. Parker or an immediate family member is a member of a speakers' bureau or has made paid presentations on behalf of the Musculoskeletal Transplant Foundation, Sanofi-Aventis, and Smith & Nephew; is a paid consultant for or is an employee of Sanofi-Aventis and Smith & Nephew; and has received research or institutional support from Aircast, Arthrex, Biomet, Breg, DePuy, DJ Orthopaedics, Johnson & Johnson, National Institutes of Health, Orthopaedic Scientific Research Foundation, Sanofi-Aventis, Smith & Nephew, Stryker, and Zimmer. Neither Dr. Akhavan nor any immediate family member has received anything of value from or owns stock in a commercial company or institutiion related diretly or indirectly to the subject of this chapter.

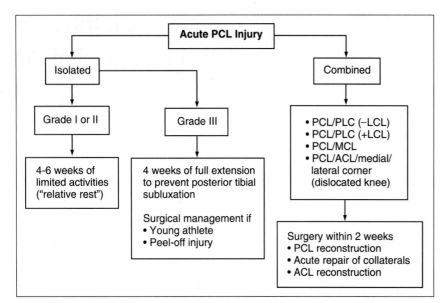

Figure 1 Treatment algorithm for acute PCL injuries. PCL = posterior cruciate ligament, PLC = posterolateral corner, MCL = medial collateral ligament, ACL = anterior cruciate ligament.

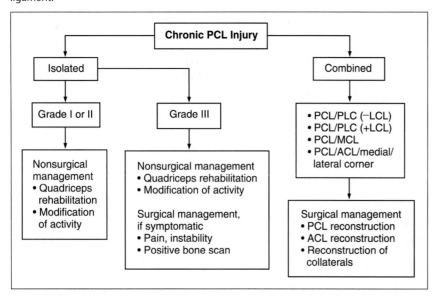

Figure 2 Treatment algorithm for chronic PCL injuries. PCL = posterior cruciate ligament, PLC = posterolateral corner, LCL = lateral collateral ligament, MCL = medial collateral ligament, ACL = anterior cruciate ligament. .

Biomechanical studies have demonstrated failure at this location before completion of cyclic loading to 2,000 cycles.

The tibial inlay technique places the bone block of the graft anatomically in the sulcus on the posterior tibial plateau at the site of the PCL anatomic insertion, avoiding the killer turn and resulting in less posterior translation and graft abrasion. Both the transtibial and tibial inlay techniques provide immediate stability, and we continue to perform transtibial PCL reconstruction in select patients. The tibial inlay technique, however, is currently the preferred technique at our institution, for several reasons: (1) it more closely duplicates the normal PCL anatomy, (2) it avoids the killer turn, and (3) it is easier and safer, although it is not an all-arthroscopic technique.

Graft Options

Graft options for PCL reconstruction are similar to those for anterior cruciate ligament (ACL) reconstruction and include commonly used autografts such as bone–patellar tendon–bone, hamstring, and quadriceps. Disadvantages of these grafts include donor-site morbidity and increased surgical time. Achilles, patellar, and posterior and anterior tibial tendon allografts often are used for multiple ligament reconstructions. Although allografts avoid problems with donor-site morbidity and can decrease surgical time, they carry a risk of viral transmission, and graft incorporation is slower than with autografts. Notwithstanding these limitations, an Achilles tendon allograft obtained from a reputable bone bank is the graft we currently prefer for PCL reconstruction.

Single-Bundle or Double-Bundle Reconstruction

Historically, the anterolateral bundle has been the focus of single-bundle PCL reconstructions because it is larger and stronger than the posteromedial bundle; however, the interest in double-bundle ACL reconstruction has brought a renewed interest in reconstructing both bundles of the PCL. Although some biomechanical studies have suggested that double-bundle techniques restore normal knee kinematics more effectively than single-bundle techniques, others have found no difference in tibial translation between the two techniques. A recent evaluation of transtibial single-bundle, arthroscopic inlay single-bundle, and arthroscopic inlay double-bundle techniques found no significant difference in posterior tibial translation between the transtibial and arthroscopic inlay single-bundle techniques, but posterior tibial

Table 1 Results of Tibial Inlay Technique

Authors (Year)	Procedure	Number of Patients or Procedures	Mean Follow-up (Range)	Results
Cooper and Stewart (2004)	Tibial inlay, single-bundle	41 patients	39 months	All patients rated knee as improved or greatly improved. Posterior drawer improved from 3+ preoperatively in all patients to normal in 9 patients, 1+ in 25 patients, and 2+ in 7 patients at follow-up. IKDC ratings improved from D in all patients preoperatively to follow-up ratings of A in 4 patients, B in 24 patients, C in 11 patients, and D in 2 patients.
Noyes and Barber-Westin (2005)	Tibial inlay	19 patients	35 months	18 out of 19 patients rated their knee as improved 11 patients returned to low-impact sports, 2 patients participated in strenuous sports without problems.
Jung et al (2005)	Modified tibial inlay	12 patients	2 years minimum	Good clinical results in 11 of 12 patients
Seon and Song (2006)	Transtibial Tibial inlay	21 knees 22 knees	32 months 36 months	Improvements in activity levels, Lysholm scores, posterior drawer testing, and KT-1000 in both groups No significant differences in clinical or radiographic results
Mariani and Margheritini (2006)	Tibial inlay	9 patients	15 months	ROM and effusion IKDC rating of D in all patients preoperatively, rating of A in all patients postoperatively Overall postoperative IKDC ratings normal in 5 patients, B in 3 patients, C in 1 patient
MacGillivray et al (2006)	Arthroscopic transtibial Tibial inlay	13 procedures 7 procedures	6 years (2-15)	No significant differences in posterior drawer, KT-1000, and functional testing or Lysholm, Tegner, or AAOS scores
Kim et al (2009)	Arthroscopic tibial inlay, single-bundle Arthroscopic tibial inlay, double-bundle Transtibial single-bundle	11 patients 10 patients 8 patients	36 months 29 months 46 months	Mean ROM and Lysholm scores similar among the three groups of patients Arthroscopic inlay double-bundle reconstruction produced better posterior stability than transtibial single-bundle reconstruction
Shon et al (2010)	Single-bundle Double-bundle	14 patients 16 patients	90 months 64 months	No significant differences in clinical or radiographic results

ROM = range of motion, KT-1000 Knee Ligament Arthrometer (MedMetric, San Diego, CA), AAOS = American Academy of Orthopaedic Surgeons, IKDC = International Knee Documentation Committee.

translation was significantly less with the arthroscopic inlay double-bundle technique. No clear-cut indications currently exist for a double-bundle reconstruction, except perhaps chronic PCL laxity.

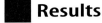

▪ Results

Given the relative infrequency of PCL reconstruction in the sports-injured patient, it is difficult to conduct a randomized prospective study with sufficient power to definitively determine the optimal mode of reconstruction. Some comparisons of the inlay technique with the all-arthroscopic technique found no difference in outcomes. Our decision to use the inlay technique has been based on basic science research that has shown that

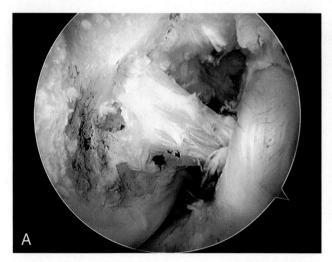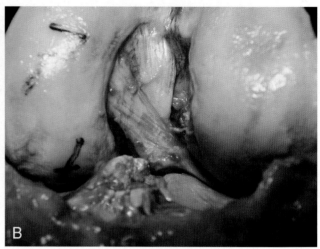

Figure 3 The femoral anatomic attachment site (FAAS) of the PCL. **A,** Arthroscopic view of the FAAS in a left knee after débridement. Note the intact meniscofemoral ligament of Wrisberg. **B,** Intraoperative view of the FAAS of the PCL in a left knee.

avoidance of the killer turn can lead to decreased laxity at follow-up. Current outcomes of PCL reconstruction rely primarily on retrospective studies and control groups (**Table 1**). Two studies of the inlay technique with at least 2-year follow-up have shown satisfactory outcomes with significantly less posterior laxity at final follow-up. Biomechanical studies identify concerns regarding the long-term viability of the implanted graft, the failure of which could result in long-term instability and arthrosis.

Technique

Setup/Exposure

The inlay technique requires two changes of position, from supine to prone and back to supine, so we typically use two operating tables to make these transitions easier. In addition, because the tibial insertion of the PCL extends below the tibial shelf, the use of a 70° arthroscope along with the traditional 30° arthroscope can improve visualization of this site. We also use a sterile tourniquet, although we inflate it only during the prone approach to the tibial insertion. Addi-

tional equipment includes a PCL femoral drill guide, a graft passer, osteotomes, a standard 6.5-mm stainless steel cancellous screw with washer, and blunt-tipped PCL (vaginal) retractors with differential angles of retraction.

PATIENT POSITIONING

The surgery begins with the patient supine on the operating table. After induction of general anesthesia, both knees are examined to identify any associated capsuloligamentous injuries and to determine the presence or absence of injury to the posterolateral and posteromedial structures in the operative extremity. Before preparation and draping, the involved knee joint is injected with 0.25% bupivicaine with 1:400,000 epinephrine and 2 mg of morphine sulfate. The opposite lower extremity is placed in a padded gynecologic stirrup that is widely abducted away from the surgical extremity, and a sterile cover is placed over it. The surgical extremity is allowed to hang free so that full knee flexion can be obtained during surgery. A lateral post is used during the arthroscopic treatment of associated intra-articular pathology.

Procedure

ARTHROSCOPIC EVALUATION AND DÉBRIDEMENT

Without inflation of the tourniquet, the surgeon completes a diagnostic arthroscopic examination, treats articular cartilage and meniscal pathology, and documents the PCL injury and the status of the ACL and meniscofemoral ligaments. The ACL typically appears lax because of the posterior tibial subluxation, but an anterior drawer maneuver will restore its normal appearance. With care taken to preserve the intact meniscofemoral ligament (**Figure 3,** *A*), the PCL remnant on the medial wall of the intercondylar notch is débrided arthroscopically to allow identification of the femoral anatomic attachment site (FAAS) of the PCL complex, which comprises the PCL and the anterior and posterior meniscofemoral ligaments of Humphrey and Wrisberg, respectively. The FAAS is located anterior and distal in the notch, approximately 8 to 10 mm from the articular margin at the 11-o'clock position in a left knee and the 1-o'clock position in a right knee (**Figure 3,** *B*). Remnants of the PCL are left at the femoral footprint to provide an anatomic landmark for placement of the femoral tunnel guidewire, and a curet is used to score the desired femoral tunnel site. Although the FAAS is marked at this stage, it will be rechecked later through a small medial arthrotomy before guide pin placement. If concomitant ACL surgery is planned, the ACL femoral and tibial anatomic attachment sites are identified and drilled at this time.

GRAFT PREPARATION

If an Achilles tendon allograft is used (**Figure 4, A**), the calcaneal bone plug—ideally, 10 mm wide, 20 mm long, and approximately 5 mm thick—is prepared for implantation in the posterior tibial trough. The tendinous end of the Achilles tendon graft is rolled into a tube and held with Krackow-type sutures so that it will pass easily through the femoral tunnel (**Figure 4, B**). If a bone–patellar tendon–bone autograft is used, the patellar bone plug usually is 10 mm wide and 30 mm long, whereas the tibial bone plug is 10 mm wide, 20 mm long, and approximately 5 mm thick. The patellar bone plug is contoured to fit in the femoral tunnel and should pass easily through a 9-mm sizer. The tibial bone plug is contoured to fit in a trough made at the tibial attachment site of the PCL.

Once the bone plugs are contoured, a 2-mm drill is used to make two holes in the patellar bone plug, one 5 mm and one 15 mm from the distal tip. A No. 5 nonabsorbable suture is passed through each hole for later graft passage and tensioning. For either graft choice, a hole is drilled with a 3.2-mm drill bit through the center of the bone plug. To avoid the screw angling toward the joint, the hole should be angled slightly distally to make up for the slope of the posterior tibia; the surgeon should drill from the cancellous side to avoid injury to the soft-tissue portion of the graft. The hole is then overdrilled with a 4.5-mm drill and tapped accordingly. A 35-mm-long, partially threaded, 6.5-mm screw and

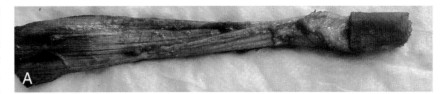
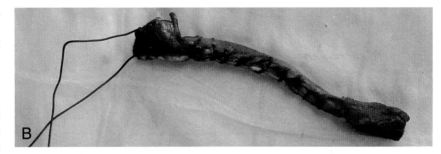
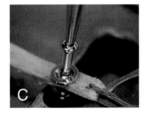
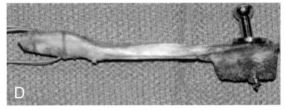

Figure 4 Preparation of the PCL graft. **A**, Achilles tendon allograft before preparation. The bone plug will ultimately be placed in the posterior trough on the tibia. **B**, A Krackow stitch is passed through the tendinous end of the Achilles tendon allograft and the graft is tubularized. **C**, A 6.5-mm cancellous screw is inserted in the bone plug with a washer. This will be used to fix the plug onto the tibia. **D**, If a bone–patellar tendon–bone graft is used, the larger plug is prepared for the tibia and two sutures are passed through 2-mm drill holes in the femoral bone plug.

washer are inserted until the screw protrudes approximately 5 mm past the cancellous surface (**Figure 4, C and D**). Alternatively, two small-fragment cancellous screws can be used to fix the posterior bone plug. A cadaver study showed no difference in pull-out strength between the two techniques.

FEMORAL TUNNEL CREATION

If an autograft is used, the femoral tunnel can be made through the same incision used for graft harvest. If an allograft is used, a small medial arthrotomy is made adjacent to the patellar tendon, extending to the vastus medialis obliquus at the level of the adductor tubercle. The arthrotomy extends posteriorly along the inferior aspect of the muscle, which is elevated anteriorly to expose the medial femoral condyle. The intercondylar notch

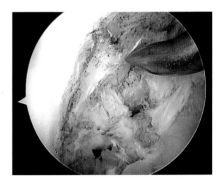

Figure 5 Arthroscopic view of the FAAS following débridement. The eventual site of the femoral tunnel is marked with a punch.

is exposed by retracting the patella laterally. The previously marked FAAS is identified and checked for accurate placement. The PCL femoral guide tip is placed through the arthrotomy at the FAAS, approximately 8 mm proximal to the articular margin. This should leave the edge of the tunnel 2

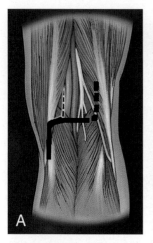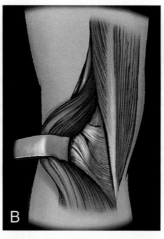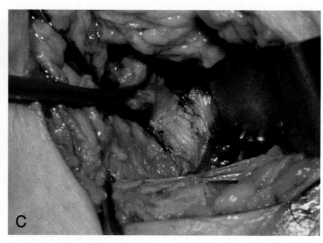

Figure 6 Exposure of the PCL tibial attachment. **A,** Modified Burke incision for the posterior approach. **B,** Exposure is performed between the medial head of the gastrocnemius and the semimembranosus tendon. The neurovascular structures are located lateral to the medial head of the gastrocnemius. **C,** Remnants of the tibial attachment of the PCL are identified and excised. (Parts A and B reproduced with permission from the Cleveland Clinic Center for Medical Art & Photography, Cleveland, OH.)

to 3 mm from the articular edge after drilling (**Figure 5**).

The femoral tunnel should be angled proximally and posteriorly to decrease the obliquity, which decreases the stress on the graft as it enters the tunnel. Using the aiming guide, the femoral guide pin is drilled from the outside in to reproduce the normal PCL tracking angle of approximately 85°, which is difficult to do with an inside-out technique. To replicate the anatomic position of the anterolateral bundle of the PCL, the guide pin should enter the intercondylar notch at the 11- or 1-o'clock position approximately 8 to 10 mm proximal to the articular surface of the medial femoral condyle and should be directed laterally, posteriorly, and proximally. The diameter of the femoral tunnel is determined by adding 1 mm to the size of the femoral tendinous portion of the Achilles allograft, which usually is 9 mm, resulting in a tunnel size of 10 mm. The edges of the tunnel are chamfered and smoothed with a rasp. A suture passing device is placed within the tunnel, and an 18-gauge wire loop or commercially available graft passer is placed through the tunnel and directed posteriorly into the notch to be used for later graft passage

through the posterior approach. Alternatively, the femoral tunnel can be drilled arthroscopically through the lateral portal with a commercially available flexible drill system. The wound is loosely approximated, and the tourniquet is deflated if used. A sterile circumferential dressing is placed, and the entire leg is covered in a sterile bag that is overwrapped with a long elastic wrap.

APPROACH TO THE POSTERIOR TIBIA

A second operating room table is positioned beside the patient and, under the direction of the surgeon and anesthetist, the patient is turned prone onto the second table. The first operating table is cleaned and prepared for the patient to be placed supine after posterior dissection and graft placement. All bony prominences are padded, and the sterile dressing is removed. If there is any question of a break in sterile technique, the entire leg is prepared and draped again. Without inflating the tourniquet, a modified Burke approach to the posterior tibia is made with a horizontal limb near the flexion crease of the knee and the vertical limb over the medial aspect of the gastrocnemius muscle (**Figure 6, A**).

The landmarks for the incision are the medial border of the medial head of the gastrocnemius, the lateral border of the semitendinosus, the popliteal crease, and the midline of the distal thigh. The skin is incised and the fascia is exposed with care to avoid the medial sural cutaneous nerve, which is vulnerable near the midline at this level. The fascia is incised, and the interval between the medial head of the gastrocnemius and semitendinosus is developed (**Figure 6, B**). The fascia over the proximal popliteus muscle near the distal portion of the insertion of the PCL is incised to allow distal retraction of the popliteus muscle if necessary. A broad, blunt retractor is placed in this interval, and the medial head of the gastrocnemius is retracted laterally, with care taken to protect the neurovascular bundle. A portion of the medial gastrocnemius origin can be released if more exposure is needed, but typically this is not necessary. The inferior medial geniculate artery and vein are ligated as necessary. The capsule is incised longitudinally and reflected medially and laterally to expose the tibial insertion of the PCL (**Figure 6, C**). The remaining scar tissue and PCL remnants are excised with care to avoid the menis-

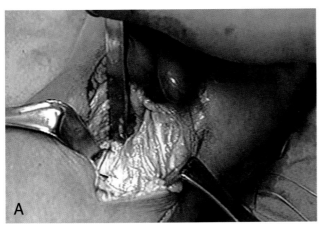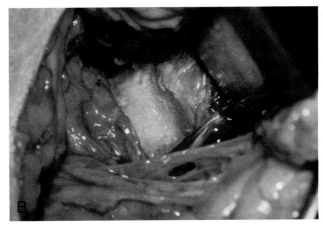

Figure 7 Creation of the bone trough. **A,** An osteotome is used to decorticate the posterior tibia and create a bony trough the size of the bone plug, which is placed posteriorly. **B,** Bony trough for the graft bone plug.

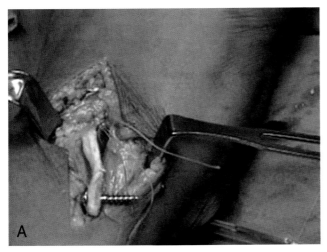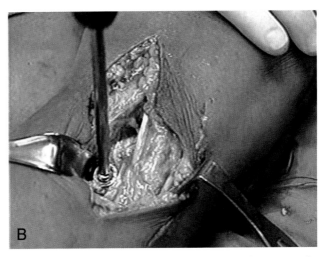

Figure 8 Final graft positioning and fixation. **A,** The graft is brought back into the surgical field by sliding it through the graft passer. **B,** The screw is tightened to fix the bone plug. The angle should be directed slightly distally.

cofemoral ligaments. Flexing the knee 15° to 20° and externally rotating the tibia will increase exposure.

TIBIAL GRAFT FIXATION

The graft insertion site on the posterior tibia is marked, and an approximately 11 × 20–mm cortical window is made with an osteotome to correspond to the prepared bone plug (Figure 7). The graft is brought into the surgical field (Figure 8, *A*), and the previously placed graft passer is used to pass the femoral plug through the intercondylar notch and into the femoral tunnel. The tibial bone plug is fit-

ted into the prepared trough on the back of the tibia, and a 6.5-mm screw is used to secure the bone plug to the posterior tibia (Figure 8, *B*). Tension is placed on the femoral end of the graft to ensure adequate fixation, and correct screw placement is confirmed with radiographs. The capsule and fascia are closed with No. 1 nonabsorbable suture, the subcutaneous tissue is closed with 2-0 absorbable suture, and the skin is closed with a subcuticular closure. The leg is again covered with a sterile cover, and the patient is placed supine on the first operating table.

FEMORAL GRAFT FIXATION

The sterile cover is removed. If there is any concern about a break in sterile technique, the leg is prepared and draped once more. The knee is flexed to 80° in neutral rotation, an anterior drawer is applied to the proximal tibia, and the graft in the femoral tunnel is tensioned by pulling on the sutures in the femoral bone plug. If using a bone–patellar tendon–bone graft, the amount of bone within the femoral tunnel must be determined to help choose the appropriate screw size and fixation method. If 20 to 25 mm of bone is in the femoral tunnel, the graft is fixed with a 9 × 20–mm interference screw placed proximally to secure the bone plug distally in the tunnel (closest to the articular surface). If less than 20 mm of bone plug is within the femoral tunnel or an Achilles tendon allograft is being used, a trough is made in the medial femoral condyle and the graft is fixed with either two spiked staples or by tying the sutures to a 6.5-mm post in the medial femoral condyle. Alternatively, an interference screw can be used within the femoral tunnel with backup staple fixation. After fixation, the knee is flexed and extended to ensure an adequate range of motion. A gentle posterior drawer test performed with the knee in 90° of flexion can be used to ensure that the anterior tibial step-off has been restored.

Wound Closure

Once stability is satisfactory, the wounds are irrigated and closed in layers, and a cryotherapy pad and compressive stocking are applied with the knee immobilized in full extension.

Postoperative Regimen

The leg is immobilized for 4 weeks in a cast or brace, with care not to allow posterior sag. If a cast is used, it is changed at 1 week and 2 weeks after surgery; at 4 weeks, the cast is removed and a brace is applied. At 4 weeks after surgery, the patient should begin gentle range-of-motion exercises. Once the patient achieves 90° of motion, the knee immobilizer is discontinued and a posterior stabilizing knee brace is applied. The brace is worn for all activities for the first 2 months, but only for new activities thereafter. Isotonic quadriceps, extension, and closed-chain exercises are used to strengthen the hamstring muscles, but isotonic hamstring mus-

cle exercises are not allowed. At approximately 3 months after surgery, if the patient is walking well with no pain and good balance and strength, a slideboard activity is begun, followed by agility drills and sport-specific activities. Most athletes return to sports approximately 9 to 10 months after surgery.

Avoiding Pitfalls and Complications

Technique Tips

When a bone–patellar tendon–bone graft is used, careful attention should be paid to the tibial fixation site because the graft is a fixed length. Once the graft is fixed on the posterior tibia, it is tensioned on the femoral side, and the position of the bone plug in the femoral tunnel is assessed. If 25 mm or more of the bone plug is within the femoral tunnel at this point, the tibial attachment site is accepted. If less than 25 mm of bone is within the femoral tunnel, the tibial attachment site can be adjusted distally. The tibial attachment site can be moved distally up to 10 mm without affecting the mechanical properties of the reconstruction. If more than 10 mm of distal placement is needed, the tibial attachment site should not be moved, and the femoral end should be fixed in a trough as described.

It may be necessary to divide a portion of the upper (proximal) aspect of the popliteus muscle to gain good exposure of the posterior tibia. When placing the 6.5-mm screw in the tibial bone plug, it is helpful to angle the screw slightly distally to avoid having the screw angle toward the articular surface when the graft is placed on the posterior slope of the tibia.

To determine the anatomic insertion site of the PCL on the femur 8 to 10 mm from the articular margin, the tip of an angled curet is placed at the articular margin, and a thumb is

placed on the curet 8 to 10 mm from the edge of the skin where the curet enters the medial portal. Advancing the curet until the thumb touches the skin places the curet tip 8 to 10 mm off the articular margin, and this spot can be marked.

Complications

If an ACL reconstruction is performed in conjunction with a PCL reconstruction, the tibial tunnel for the ACL graft can be damaged during the inlay procedure if the 6.5-mm screw securing the bone plug to the tibia is directed into the ACL tibial tunnel. This can be avoided by directing the screw slightly laterally. Because the starting points for the ACL and PCL tibial tunnels are close, care must be taken that these do not intersect. Leaving a drill in one tunnel while the other is being drilled can avoid this complication.

The posterior neurovascular structures can be injured by excessive penetration with a guide pin during drilling of a tibial tunnel. This can be avoided by locking the pin into the drill 1 cm shorter than the distance required to reach the guide tip and advancing it slowly the rest of the way by hand. Also, a curet can be placed through the posteromedial portal over the tip of the pin to stop advancement of the pin during reaming. The proximity of the popliteal artery makes it vulnerable to injury during screw placement. However, a cadaver study found that in knees in which the posteromedial approach was used, no screw was within 21 mm of the popliteal artery.

Any surgical procedure carries a risk of infection, and the process of repositioning the patient twice for this surgery increases the opportunity for contamination. The use of a sterile tourniquet and strict attention to detail by the surgeon and staff minimizes this risk.

Bibliography

Campbell RB, Jordan SS, Sekiya JK: Arthroscopic tibial inlay for posterior cruciate ligament reconstruction. *Arthroscopy* 2007;23(12):1356, e1-e4.

Cooper DE, Stewart D: Posterior cruciate ligament reconstruction using single-bundle patella tendon graft with tibial inlay fixation: 2- to 10-year follow-up. *Am J Sports Med* 2004;32(2):346-360.

Cosgarea AJ, Jay PR: Posterior cruciate ligament injuries: Evaluation and management. *J Am Acad Orthop Surg* 2001;9(5): 297-307.

Jung YB, Jung HJ, Tae SK, Lee YS, Lee KH: Reconstruction of the posterior cruciate ligament with a mid-third patellar tendon graft with use of a modified tibial inlay method. *J Bone Joint Surg Am* 2005;87(2, Suppl 1):247-263.

Kim SJ, Kim TE, Jo SB, Kung YP: Comparison of the clinical results of three posterior cruciate ligament reconstruction techniques. *J Bone Joint Surg Am* 2009;91(11):2543-2549.

MacGillivray JD, Stein BE, Park M, Allen AA, Wickiewicz TL, Warren RF: Comparison of tibial inlay versus transtibial techniques for isolated posterior cruciate ligament reconstruction: Minimum 2-year follow-up. *Arthroscopy* 2006;22(3): 320-328.

Mariani PP, Margheritini F: Full arthroscopic inlay reconstruction of posterior cruciate ligament. *Knee Surg Sports Traumatol Arthrosc* 2006;14(11):1038-1044.

Matava MJ, Ellis E, Gruber B: Surgical treatment of posterior cruciate ligament tears: An evolving technique. *J Am Acad Orthop Surg* 2009;17(7):435-446.

McAllister DR, Miller MD, Sekiya JK, Wojtys EM: Posterior cruciate ligament biomechanics and options for surgical treatment. *Instr Course Lect* 2009;58:377-388.

Noyes FR, Barber-Westin S: Posterior cruciate ligament replacement with a two-strand quadriceps tendon-patellar bone autograft and a tibial inlay technique. *J Bone Joint Surg Am* 2005;87(6):1241-1252.

Oliviero J, Miller MD: Posterior cruciate ligament reconstruction: Tibial inlay technique. *Tech Knee Surg* 2003;2(1):63-72.

Papalia R, Osti L, Del Buono A, Denaro V, Maffulli N: Tibial inlay for posterior cruciate ligament reconstruction: A systematic review. *Knee* 2010;17(4):264-269.

Seon JK, Song EK: Reconstruction of isolated posterior cruciate ligament injuries: A clinical comparison of the transtibial and tibial inlay techniques. *Arthroscopy* 2006;22(1):27-32.

Shon OJ, Lee DC, Park CH, Kim WH, Jung KA: A comparison of arthroscopically assisted single and double bundle tibial inlay reconstruction for isolated posterior cruciate ligament injury. *Clin Orthop Surg* 2010;2(2):76-84.

Whiddon DR, Zehms CT, Miller MD, Quinby JS, Montgomery SL, Sekiya JK: Double compared with single-bundle open inlay posterior cruciate ligament reconstruction in a cadaver model. *J Bone Joint Surg Am* 2008;90(9):1820-1829.

Wind WM Jr, Bergfeld JA, Parker RD: Evaluation and treatment of posterior cruciate ligament injuries: Revisited. *Am J Sports Med* 2004;32(7):1765-1775.

Coding

CPT Code		Corresponding ICD-9 Codes	
29889	Arthroscopically aided posterior cruciate ligament repair/augmentation or reconstruction	717.84	844.2

Chapter 77

Posterior Cruciate Ligament Injury: Bony Avulsion

Marc R. Safran, MD
David C. Hay, MD

■ Indications

The posterior cruciate ligament (PCL) is a principal static stabilizer of the knee. Although sports and noncontact injuries to the PCL are less common than injuries to the anterior cruciate ligament (ACL), PCL ruptures are present in 3% to 37% of traumatic knee injuries. Bony avulsions, primarily from the tibial insertion, represent a small but important subset of PCL injuries.

Although isolated PCL injuries are often well tolerated by patients following rehabilitation, if nonsurgical management fails, PCL reconstruction may be required. PCL reconstruction can restore normal posterior translation and laxity intraoperatively, but these are rarely maintained at follow-up of longer than 1 year. It is generally accepted that current surgical techniques are unable to clinically restore normal knee mechanics.

Bony PCL avulsions are particularly important because reattachment of the PCL and its bony attachment may be an easy way to facilitate long-term restoration of normal PCL function and more normal knee kinemat-ics. Bony PCL avulsions usually can be easily identified on initial injury radiographs without reliance on MRI, although MRI may help identify these and associated injuries. Additionally, MRI can augment the physical examination, because identification of an injured PCL may be particularly difficult in a patient with multiple injuries about the knee. MRI also helps to evaluate concomitant injuries commonly associated with PCL rupture or bony avulsion.

The mechanism of injury to the knee that results in the different types of PCL injuries—an intrasubstance PCL injury, a soft-tissue avulsion from bone, or a bony avulsion fracture—has not been studied; however, it likely is related to the rate of loading during the injury. The most common mechanism for these injuries is a direct blow to the anterior aspect of the tibia or forced knee hyperextension. Dashboard injury (impact of a flexed knee into the dashboard of a car during a motor vehicle accident) is common. Forceful landing or falling on a plantar flexed foot may cause a PCL injury. The posteriorly directed force to the proximal tibia may injure the PCL, either within its substance or as a bony avulsion. Any direct contact to the knee causing posterior translation of the tibia or hyperextension of the knee in high-energy situations should raise suspicion for ligamentous knee injury.

On examination, patients usually have significant posterior laxity, a positive posterior drawer sign, and a posterior sag, where the medial femoral condyle is positioned at or posterior to the medial tibial plateau. Thorough orthopaedic, neurologic, and vascular examinations should be done to rule out other associated injuries. When posterior laxity is identified, care should be taken to examine the medial collateral ligament and posteromedial corner, as well as the posterolateral corner, lateral collateral ligament, and ACL, because any of these structures may be injured in conjunction with the PCL itself.

PCL tibial bony avulsions can be identified on initial radiographs, usually the lateral view. The tibial avulsion is seen as an ovoid avulsed fragment of bone visible at the proximal posterior tibia, just distal and posterior to the joint line.

Displacement of more than 2 mm or displacement seen on posterior stress radiographs is an indication for fixation, particularly if the fragment is more than 7 mm in diameter. If there is any doubt about a bony avulsion frac-

Dr. Safran or an immediate family member serves as an unpaid consultant to Cool Systems, has received research or institutional support from Smith & Nephew and DJ Orthopaedics, and owns stock or stock options in Cool Systems. Neither Dr. Hay nor any immediate family member has received anything of value from or owns stock in a commercial company or institution related directly or indirectly to the subject of this chapter.

ture or about the size of the fracture, a CT scan can be helpful.

The results of PCL reconstruction, either acute or delayed, are suboptimal with regard to restoring knee kinematics because the reconstructed graft stretches out postoperatively and the complex anatomy is rarely replicated. Internal fixation of a bony avulsion of the PCL, however, where the integrity and anatomy of the PCL are maintained, can reliably restore normal function of the PCL once the bone is healed. Furthermore, clinical follow-up series show better outcomes with early rather than delayed fixation, and this is our rationale for acute intervention.

Anatomic fixation of an acute PCL bony avulsion can be done easily and safely, and the bone will heal reliably in this metaphyseal region if fixation is rigid. Early intervention can reliably and reproducibly restore PCL function with low morbidity.

Alternatively, if fixation is delayed long enough that the bony fragment may become osteopenic or resorb completely, rigid internal fixation may be difficult if not impossible. The PCL may then atrophy, shortening to such a degree that anatomic repair is not possible. Delayed internal fixation of a PCL tibial avulsion therefore is not ideal; however, good results were described in a single patient treated 4.5 years after injury. Thus, fixation of a chronically displaced bony avulsion can be considered as long as bone is present for fixation.

Contraindications

Surgical fixation of the bony avulsion is contraindicated in patients whose acute medical condition, age, infection, or medical comorbidities preclude surgery. Additionally, patients unwilling or unable to comply with postoperative protection and rehabili-

tation are not candidates for surgical intervention.

Nonsurgical management can be considered for patients with acceptable anterior-posterior stability and nondisplaced avulsion fractures or negative stress radiographs; however, internal fixation will allow more aggressive rehabilitation.

Alternative Treatments

Nondisplaced fractures treated closed will heal with good results, but treatment of displaced bony avulsions with immobilization has yielded only fair results. Patients develop significant knee stiffness. Long-term outcomes are similar to those of patients with grade II or III PCL ruptures, depending on the amount of displacement and resultant PCL laxity.

Newly described arthroscopically assisted and all-arthroscopic techniques have been proposed to treat displaced bony avulsions of the PCL. These techniques aim to avoid dissection about the posterior structures of the knee; however, they require a great deal of arthroscopic skill to efficiently and safely achieve good reduction and fixation. Currently, these techniques have been used by expert arthroscopists in small cohorts with good results. Our technique limits the risk to the posterior neurovascular structures and can be done by the typical orthopaedist, who may lack the arthroscopic skills for an all-arthroscopic repair. We continue to advocate open reduction and internal fixation as the gold standard to achieve the best result in bony avulsion injuries of the PCL.

Results

Good to excellent results have been uniformly achieved with open anatomic reduction and internal fixation of tibial bony PCL avulsion fractures (**Table 1**). Small or comminuted fragments that cannot support screw fixation have less predictable outcomes. Regardless, if stable anatomic reduction can be obtained, restored PCL biomechanics and good to excellent outcomes can be expected.

Techniques

Setup/Exposure
The patient is placed prone on the operating table with chest rolls and a thigh tourniquet in place but not inflated. The genitals are protected, and padding is placed under the bony prominences of the lower extremity. The affected lower extremity is draped free to allow manipulation. An impervious stocking is used to isolate the foot.

A modified Burks approach is used for safe access to the PCL insertion. The skin incision is based over the horizontal flexor crease of the knee and then gently curved longitudinally down the medial border of the gastrocnemius (**Figure 1**, *A*). Dissection is carried through the subcutaneous tissue with the goal of developing the medial border of the medial head of the gastrocnemius muscle (**Figure 1**, *B*). Care should be taken to avoid the saphenous vein, although this usually is medial and distal to the dissection at this location. The medial sural cutaneous nerve also may be encountered; however, this is typically encountered more distally and laterally.

Procedure
The deep fascia overlying the medial gastrocnemius is incised longitudinally, and the interval between the

Table 1 Results of Treatment for Bony Posterior Cruciate Ligament Avulsion

Author(s) (Year)	Number of Knees	Approach	Mean Patient Age in Years (Range)	Mean Follow-up in Months (Range)	Results
Meyers (1975)	14 (12 acute, 2 chronic)	8 posterior open approach (6 acute injury, 2 chronic) 6 cast treatment	(14-48)	NR	6 cast treatment 1 union 5 nonunion (4 with positive posterior drawer test) 8 surgical 6 acute injury (5 union, 5 "excellent" function) 2 chronic injury (2 union, "good functional capacity")
Safran et al (1999)	18	Untreated	32 (19-51)	29 (1-234)	15 positive posterior drawer grade II, 3 positive posterior drawer grade III 13 "some pain" 10 "some instability" 9 "instability going up and down stairs" 4 "instability with activities of daily living 9 returned to previous level activity (4 college/professional athletes) Statistically significant differences in kinesthesia and proprioception at 45° and 110°, respectively, in PCL-injured knees
Kim et al (2001)	14 (11 acute, 3 delayed)	Arthroscopic	35 (17-57)	39 (24-72)	No nonunions 11 acute 9 no instability (IKDC grade: 5 A, 4 B; KT-2000 side-to-side difference 1.1 mm) 2 arthrofibrosis (IKDC grade B, KT-2000 side-to-side difference 1.8 mm) 3 delayed (IKDC grade C, KT-2000 side-to-side difference 3.7 mm)
Yang et al (2003)	16 (14 acute, 2 chronic)	Modified open posterior	28 (14-51)	36 (24-58)	Hughston criteria Subjective: 69% good, 31% fair, 0% poor Functional: 75% good, 25% fair, 0% poor Objective: 69% good, 31% fair, 0% poor
Zhao et al (2006)	29 (all acute)	Arthroscopic suture Endoscopically placed titanium button	32 (21-47)	32 (24-41)	No nonunions KT-1000: side-to-side difference <2 mm (mean 0.6 ± 0.4 mm) in 28 knees; 4 mm in 1 knee IKDC subjective knee score: mean 97.1 (range, 91-100) Lysholm score: mean 97.4 (range, 93-100) All patients satisfied
Nicandri et al (2008)	10	Modified open posterior	33 (14-62)	28 (12-48)	No nonunions 8 knees: grade I laxity postoperatively 2 knees: grade II laxity postoperatively No side-to-side extension difference greater than 2° No side-to-side flexion difference greater than 10°

IKDC = International Knee Documentation Committee, PCL = posterior cruciate ligament.

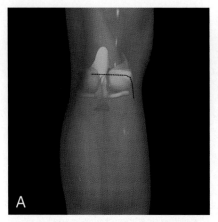 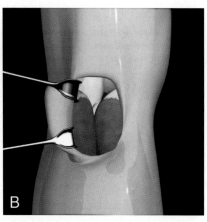

Figure 1 Skin incision and musculofascial exposure for PCL reconstruction. **A,** The skin incision is carried horizontally along the popliteal crease and then curved distally at the medial head of the gastrocnemius. **B,** The deep fascia overlying the medial gastrocnemius is incised longitudinally. The interval between the semimembranosus and the medial head of the gastrocnemius is then developed.

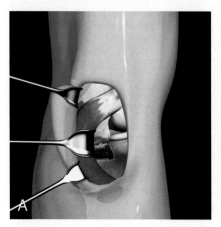 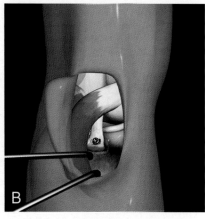

Figure 2 Exposure for PCL reconstruction. **A,** The medial head of the gastrocnemius muscle is retracted laterally, past the midline. **B,** Two Steinmann pins can be placed in the proximal tibia to assist in retraction during surgery.

semimembranosus and the medial head of the gastrocnemius is developed. This not a true internervous plane because both muscles are innervated by tibial branches of the sciatic nerve, but the plane usually can be developed without difficulty with blunt finger dissection. This interval should be developed until good exposure to the posterior joint capsule is obtained.

The medial head of the gastrocnemius then is retracted laterally to gain exposure to the posterior knee while allowing safe mobilization and protection of the popliteal neurovascular bundle (**Figure 2,** *A*). Retraction can be accomplished either manually by an assistant or with one or more 5/64-in Steinmann pins inserted into the posterior tibia lateral to midline, from posterior to anterior, and bent laterally to help maintain muscle retraction (**Figure 2,** *B*). The motor branch to the medial head of the gastrocnemius branches from the tibial division of the sciatic nerve in the popliteal fossa, innervating the medial gastrocnemius from its lateral side; thus, this nerve and the innervation of the muscle are not at risk. The thick muscle belly protects the motor branch and the popliteal neurovascu-

lar structures from all but the most vigorous retraction.

To aid exposure, the knee can be flexed and the ankle plantar flexed to relax the gastrocnemius and allow better access to the posterior capsule. If necessary, a portion of the tendinous origin of the medial head of the gastrocnemius can be released to provide more exposure.

With the posterior capsule well exposed, the posterior bony landmarks of the proximal tibia and distal femur should be palpated to localize the joint line and orient the surgeon. The medial geniculate artery runs along the midposterior capsule at this level and can be ligated if necessary. A vertical incision is then made in the posterior capsule. The capsulotomy is centered over the PCL insertion, taking into consideration eventual screw placement. Care should be taken to avoid transection of the meniscofemoral ligament, if present.

The avulsed bony fragment is identified and the ligament is inspected. Hematoma and fibrinous tissue are mechanically débrided from the fragment and recipient bed, and the joint is irrigated. The bony bed of the PCL insertion is prepared, and the ligament is freed from the surrounding tissue to allow anatomic reduction. The fragment is inspected carefully to determine what type of fixation is most appropriate. Preliminary reduction is held with one or more Kirschner wires. A cannulated screw is then placed through the fragment to secure it (**Figure 2,** *B*). Depending on the fragment size, one or two 6.5-mm, 4.5-mm, or 3.5-mm screws are used, angled anteriorly, distally, and slightly medially (**Figure 3**). A washer usually is used, particularly if the fragment is thin. The goal is stable anatomic reduction of the fragment, and this is essential to achieve good outcomes. If there is tension on the repair during attempted reduction, flexing the knee will relieve some tension from the PCL, allowing for easier reduction.

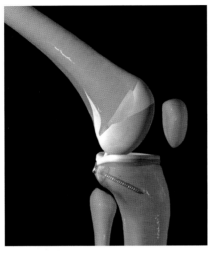

Figure 3 A repaired bony avulsion of the PCL from the tibia viewed from the side. The screw is angled anteriorly, distally, and slightly medially.

Wound Closure

The posterior joint capsule is then closed with 0 braided absorbable sutures. The gastrocnemius is allowed to settle back into position, and its fascia is closed with 2-0 braided absorbable sutures. Subcutaneous layers are approximated, and the skin is closed in routine fashion.

Postoperative Regimen

The knee is placed in a brace. Weight bearing is based on the fixation strength. Generally, patients are non–weight bearing for the first 3 weeks postoperatively, but straight-leg raises and quadriceps setting exercises are allowed in the brace. A continuous passive motion machine is used for 4 to 6 hours a day, with no limit on range of motion. At 3 weeks, patients can begin partial weight bearing with the leg in full extension, and by 6 weeks, the brace and crutches can be discontinued.

Avoiding Pitfalls and Complications

The most common complication of bony avulsions of the PCL is missed or delayed diagnosis of other injuries of the knee. It is imperative that a thorough and systematic physical examination be done, with detailed capsuloligamentous, motor, sensory, and vascular examinations. Additionally, a full imaging workup, including radiographs and MRI, should be obtained. Reported series are small, but they show that complex injuries are more common than isolated PCL avulsion fractures. Femoral fractures, tibial fractures (shaft and plateau), and patellar fractures are all commonly associated bony injuries. ACL, lateral collateral ligament, medial collateral ligament, and posterolateral corner injuries are commonly associated capsuloligamentous injuries.

Our preferred surgical approach significantly reduces risk to the neurovascular structures of the posterior knee, but injury to these structures still can occur, either as a result of overly zealous retraction or dissection lateral to the medial head of the gastrocnemius.

The avulsed fragment should be débrided and the PCL freed to allow reduction; flexion of the knee can help with reduction. The fragment should be examined carefully to determine the best method of fixation. If the fragment is large enough, 6.5-mm cannulated screws are effective; however, if the fragment is less than 1 cm in diameter, a screw this size may comminute the bony fragment. In small, comminuted, or osteopenic pieces, screw fixation is not advised, and alternative fixation should be considered, such as suture anchor fixation or suture–bone tunnel fixation to allow stable reduction of bony fragments to the bone bed.

Arthrofibrosis, loss of motion, and flexion contracture may complicate the postoperative course. A monitored postoperative rehabilitation protocol using early, protected range of motion can minimize this problem. If rigid internal fixation is achieved and intraoperative assessment reveals that there is no excessive tension on the repair when the knee is extended, then full extension is recommended, provided this does not negatively influence the healing of concomitant injuries. Patellar mobilization techniques also may help reduce the risk of loss of knee flexion. Additionally, timing of surgical reconstructions in a multiligament-injured knee to allow coordination of rehabilitation protocols can help to avoid loss of motion.

Hardware failure and nonunions are infrequent, but progressive images should be obtained as rehabilitation is advanced. The decision to revise fixation should be made based on symptoms and bone stock remaining for revision.

Bibliography

Burks RT, Schaffer JJ: A simplified approach to the tibial attachment of the posterior cruciate ligament. *Clin Orthop Relat Res* 1990;254:216-219.

Griffith JF, Antonio GE, Tong CW, Ming KM: Cruciate ligament avulsion fractures. *Arthroscopy* 2004;20:803-812.

Kim SJ, Shin SJ, Choi NH, Cho SK: Arthroscopically assisted treatment of avulsion fractures of the posterior cruciate ligament from the tibia. *J Bone Joint Surg Am* 2001;83:698-708.

Meyers MH: Isolated avulsion of the tibial attachment of the posterior cruciate ligament of the knee. *J Bone Joint Surg Am* 1975;57:669-672.

Nicandri GT, Klineberg EO, Wahl CJ, Mills WJ: Treatment of posterior cruciate ligament tibial avulsion fractures through a modified open posterior approach: Operative technique and 12- to 48-month outcomes. *J Orthop Trauma* 2008;22:317-324.

Safran MR, Allen AA, Lephart SM, Borsa PA, Fu FH, Harner CD: Proprioception in the posterior cruciate ligament deficient knee. *Knee Surg Sports Traumatol Arthrosc* 1999;7:310-317.

Yang CK, Wu CD, Chih CJ, Wei KY, Su CC, Tsuang YH: Surgical treatment of avulsion fracture of the posterior cruciate ligament and postoperative management. *J Trauma* 2003;54:516-519.

Zhao J, He Y, Wang J: Arthroscopic treatment of acute tibial avulsion fracture of the posterior cruciate ligament with suture fixation technique through Y-shaped bone tunnels. *Arthroscopy* 2006;22:172-181.

Coding

CPT Codes		Corresponding ICD-9 Codes	
Arthroscopic Posterior Cruciate Ligament Repair			
29889	Arthroscopically aided posterior cruciate ligament repair/augmentation or reconstruction	717.84	844.2

CPT copyright © 2010 by the American Medical Association. All rights reserved.

Chapter 78

Complications of Posterior Cruciate Ligament Reconstruction

David R. McAllister, MD
Tony Quach, MD

Indications

Posterior cruciate ligament (PCL) tears that require surgical reconstruction are relatively uncommon. There is no consensus regarding indications for surgery, especially for isolated PCL injuries, or preferred surgical technique. The anatomic insertion of the PCL on the tibia and its complex surrounding neurovascular structures make anatomic reconstruction more challenging. Avoiding complications requires meticulous preoperative planning, precise surgical technique, and appropriate postoperative rehabilitation.

Results

Failures can be broadly classified into primary and secondary failures. Primary failures involve technical errors such as improper tunnel placement, inadequate graft fixation, and failure to recognize and treat associated ligamentous or meniscal pathologies. Secondary failures are attributed to poor graft incorporation caused by inap-

propriate postoperative rehabilitation, repeat traumatic event, or noncompliance with postoperative protocols. Many authors have reported on failed anterior cruciate ligament (ACL) reconstructions, but few published studies have investigated the causes of failure after PCL reconstruction. In one large series of failed PCL surgeries, however, a single factor was identified in 44% of the failures. The most common causes of failure were associated posterolateral ligament deficiency (40%), improper graft tunnel placement (33%), and varus malalignment (31%); 71% of patients had moderate to severe pain with activities of daily living, 49% rated the knee as poor, and none rated the knee as good or normal. Significant functional limitations were found with walking (49%) and squatting (90%).

Intraoperative Complications

Neurovascular Injuries
Neurovascular injuries are not the most common complications of PCL

reconstruction, but they are certainly the most devastating. The PCL inserts approximately 1 cm below the tibial articular margin in a depression between the medial and lateral portions of the tibial plateau posteriorly. When recreating the tibial insertion with either a transtibial or tibial inlay technique, the popliteal artery and vein and the tibial nerve are at immediate risk. One author described laceration of the popliteal artery during a transtibial arthroscopic PCL reconstruction; emergency revascularization was done with an interposition saphenous vein graft.

Neurovascular injury can occur with aberrant guidewire placement, inadvertent guidewire advancement, and overreaming with the drill bit or winding up of the soft tissues surrounding the neurovascular structures. A thorough understanding of PCL anatomy and the surrounding structures is crucial **(Figure 1)**. The popliteal artery is lateral to the central axis of the knee in 94% of individuals. The artery is central in 6% of knees, and it is never medial to the central axis. With a transtibial technique, the average distance from the guide pin to the popliteal artery is 4.2 mm in the sagittal plane and 1.6 mm in the coronal plane. With an inlay technique, the average distance between the center of the tibial screw to the closest

Dr. McAllister or an immediate family member serves as a board member, owner, officer, or committee member of the Musculoskeletal Transplant Foundation and is a paid consultant to or an employee of the Musculoskeletal Transplant Foundation. Neither Dr. Quach nor any immediate family member has received anything of value from or owns stock in a commercial company or institution related directly or indirectly to the subject of this chapter.

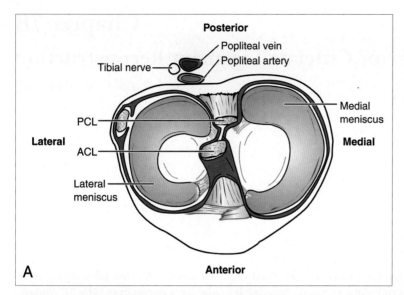
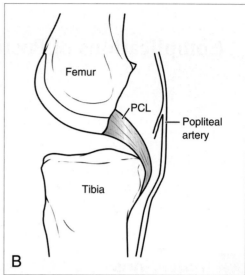

Figure 1   Drawings illustrate the anatomic relationship between the popliteal artery and the PCL in the axial (**A**) and sagittal (**B**) planes. (Adapted with permission from Matava MJ, Sethi NS, Totty WG: Proximity of the posterior cruciate ligament insertion to the popliteal artery as a function of the knee flexion angle: Implications for posterior cruciate ligament reconstruction. *Arthroscopy* 2000;16(8):796-804, pp 797-799.)

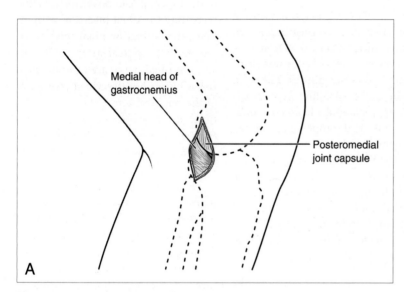
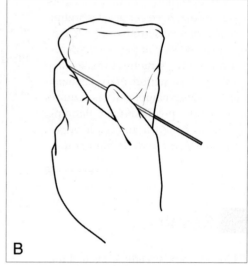

Figure 2   Drawings illustrate a posteromedial safety incision, which can be used to minimize the risk of neurovascular injury. **A,** Extra-articular posteromedial safety incision. **B,** A finger or an instrument can be inserted through the safety incision and used to protect the neurovascular bundle.

point of the popliteal artery is 21.1 mm.

Several methods of minimizing the risk of neurovascular injury during the creation of the transtibial tunnel have been described. A posteromedial safety incision has been suggested to protect the neurovascular structures. The approach is a 2-cm incision just

inferior to the posteromedial joint line between the posterior capsule and the medial head of the gastrocnemius muscle (**Figure 2**). Various accessory portals, including the posteromedial portal, transpatellar tendon portal, and posterior transseptal portal, can be used to improve viewing of the PCL insertion. An accessory portal through

the femoral tunnel can be used to view the posterior slope for tibial tunnel creation (**Figure 3**).

The distance between the PCL and the neurovascular structures can be increased by increasing knee flexion and performing a limited arthroscopic posterior capsular release. The distance from the PCL to the popliteal artery is increased from 5.9 mm to 7.8 mm when knee flexion increases from full extension to 90° of flexion, and a limited posterior capsular release can increase the distance of the popliteal artery to the PCL insertion from 4.4 mm to 14.7 mm. Other methods of minimizing the risk of iatrogenic neurovascular injury are the use of an oscillating drill and hand reaming of the posterior cortex. Intraoperative radiographs or fluoroscopy can be used to help confirm guidewire placement and monitor drill advancement.

Besides direct trauma, neurovascular injuries can be caused by popliteal artery occlusion and neurapraxia. PCL reconstructions generally are longer surgeries than other arthroscopic procedures, and it is crucial to ensure safe positioning and adequate padding around all bony prominences and superficial neurovascular structures. In addition, tourniquet times should be minimized as much as possible, and deflation of the tourniquet should be followed by close inspection of the posterior wounds to be sure hemostasis has been achieved. If significant bleeding is encountered, intraoperative vascular surgery consultation should be obtained.

Residual Laxity

Residual posterior laxity measured by instrumented and objective testing often is present postoperatively and can lead to suboptimal results. Although the causes of residual posterior laxity following isolated PCL reconstruction are not fully understood, one cause is failure to recognize and treat other ligamentous injuries. A thorough history and physical examination are the best screening tools for evaluating concomitant injuries. A grade 3 posterior drawer test or knee instability to varus/valgus loading in full knee extension suggests multiple ligamentous injuries. When the physical examination is equivocal, MRI or an

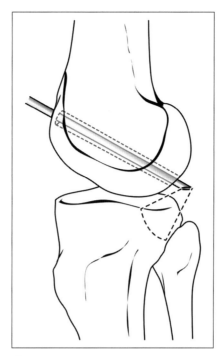

Figure 3 Drawing shows the PCL insertion region as seen through a femoral tunnel accessory portal. (Adapted with permission from Bach BR Jr, Aadalen KJ, Mazzocca AD: An accessory portal for posterior cruciate ligament tibial insertion visualization. *Arthroscopy* 2004;20(suppl 2):155-158.)

examination under anesthesia may be helpful.

Another cause of residual posterior sag is improper tunnel placement. There is no consensus in the literature regarding the optimal technique for PCL reconstruction. Surgical options include single- and double-bundle as well as transtibial and tibial inlay reconstructions. In single-bundle reconstruction, the femoral tunnel should be positioned to replicate the anterolateral bundle of the PCL in the anterior and distal portion of the native PCL femoral footprint. Some surgeons prefer a double-bundle technique for PCL reconstruction, although clinical studies to date have shown no advantage of this technique when compared with single-bundle PCL reconstruction. For this technique of PCL reconstruction, the femoral tunnels should be placed anatomically within the centers of the footprints for the anterolat-

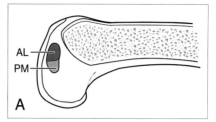
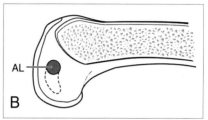
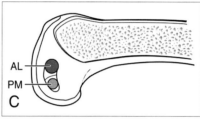

Figure 4 Drawings illustrate femoral tunnel positions for single- and double-bundle PCL reconstruction. **A,** Femoral footprint for the PCL. **B,** Optimal femoral tunnel position for single-bundle PCL reconstruction. **C,** Optimal femoral tunnel position for double-bundle PCL reconstruction. AL = anterolateral, PM = posteromedial. (Adapted with permission from Miller MD, Harner CD, Koshiwaguchi S: Acute posterior cruciate ligament injuries, in Fu FH, Harner CD, Vince KG, eds: *Knee Surgery*. Baltimore, MD, Williams & Wilkins, 1994, p 753.)

eral and posteromedial footprints of the native PCL (**Figure 4**). It is important to control the location and size of the tunnels to ensure that both tunnels are adequately spaced to prevent fracture between the tunnels.

There is considerable debate about the respective advantages of the transtibial and tibial inlay techniques for PCL reconstruction. Biomechanical studies have shown that the tibial inlay technique better resists cyclic loading, with less graft thinning and stretch-out compared with the transtibial technique. Clinical studies, however, have not been conclusive. If a transtibial technique is used, the

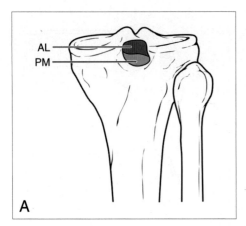
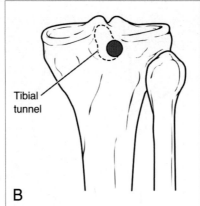
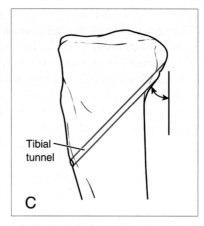

Figure 5 Drawings illustrate tibial tunnel position for PCL reconstruction. **A,** Tibial footprint for the PCL. Optimal tibial tunnel position as seen from the front (**B**) and side (**C**). AL = anterolateral, PM = posteromedial. (Parts A and B are adapted with permission from Miller MD, Harner CD, Koshiwaguchi S: Acute posterior cruciate ligament injuries, in Fu FH, Harner CD, Vince KG, eds: *Knee Surgery*. Baltimore, MD, Lippincott Williams & Wilkins, 1994, p 753. Part C is adapted with permission from Fanelli GC, Edson CJ, Reinheimer KN, Garofalo R: Posterior cruciate ligament and posterolateral corner reconstruction. *Sports Med Arthrosc* 2007;15(4):168-175.)

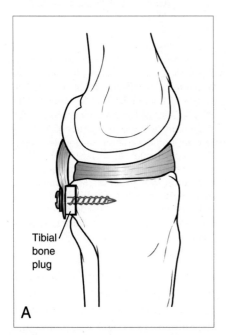
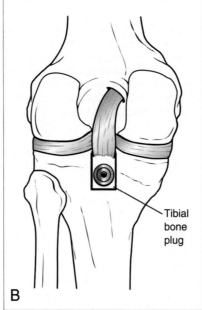

Figure 6 Drawings show the optimal graft position for the tibial inlay technique as seen from the side (**A**) and from the front (**B**). (Adapted with permission from Wind WM Jr, Bergfeld JA, Parker RD: Evaluation and treatment of posterior cruciate ligament injuries: Revisited. *Am J Sports Med* 2004;32(7):1765-1775.)

guide pin should be positioned as steeply as possible (**Figure 5**). This will decrease graft bending at the "killer turn," which is necessary for the graft to reach the femoral tunnel. For the tibial inlay technique, the graft needs to be positioned anatomically between the medial and lateral prom-inences in the posterior tibia (**Figure 6**). In both techniques, it is important to prevent graft kinking and hang-up as the graft is passed through the tun-nels, because this can lead to residual laxity. This can be achieved by direct palpation for the tibial inlay technique and by arthroscopic confirmation of graft tension throughout the knee range of motion.

Other causes of residual posterior laxity include improper graft tension-ing, inadequate graft fixation, poor graft tissue, and overly aggressive postoperative rehabilitation. In both single- and double-bundle reconstruc-tions, the graft should be tensioned with the knee flexed 70° to 90°. Ten-sioning of the graft with the knee in extension will result in increased graft tension with knee flexion, which can cause a decrease in knee range of mo-tion or graft failure. Commercially available mechanical tensioning de-vices can restore anatomic tibial step-off. Adequate graft fixation provides mechanical support while the graft in-corporates biologically. Fixation de-vices include interference screws, but-tons, staples, and screws and washers. Graft fixation is adequate if the physi-ologic forces acting on the graft do not exceed the pull-out strength of the fix-ation. The mean peak force on the PCL during walking is 330 N; this can increase to 1,860 N during full squats and closed-chain leg presses. Because the PCL experiences considerable forces after reconstruction, it is impor-tant to follow a slow and deliberate rehabilitation program. Early knee flexion beyond 90° and isolated open-chain hamstring-strengthening exercises must be avoided to prevent increasing the forces on the PCL graft. Table 1 describes a typical PCL postoperative rehabilitation program.

Compartment Syndrome

Some PCL tears occur in combination with other ligamentous injuries and are usually a result of high-energy trauma. As a result, it is possible to have capsular tears, and extravasation of irrigation fluid during arthroscopic surgery may cause compartment syndrome. This can be especially problematic when an arthroscopic fluid pump is used in the setting of an acute injury. In these cases, it is necessary to monitor the thigh and calf compartments during and after surgery to look for signs of impending compartment syndrome. Compartment syndrome also can occur from postoperative bleeding. Deflating the tourniquet before wound closure helps to minimize this risk. Gluteal compartment syndrome after PCL reconstruction has been described and is likely a result of patient positioning.

Perioperative Fractures

Perioperative fractures can occur as a result of tunnel convergence. For combined ACL and PCL reconstructions, the tibial tunnels must diverge to minimize the risk of tibial fracture. For double-bundle PCL reconstruction, there must be adequate spacing between the anterolateral and posteromedial tunnels to prevent a bone bridge fracture. Fractures also can occur in the patella after bone–patellar tendon–bone graft harvesting.

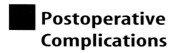

Postoperative Complications

Loss of Motion

Loss of motion after PCL reconstruction seems to occur much less fre-

Table 1 Postoperative Rehabilitation Following Posterior Cruciate Ligament Reconstruction

Postoperative Period	Activity/Physical Therapy
0 to 3 weeks	Hinged knee brace locked in 10° of flexion, ice and elevation, non–weight bearing with crutches
3 to 6 weeks	Brace unlocked from 0° to 90° of flexion for active knee extension and passive flexion Patella mobilization exercises Progressive weight bearing with knee brace locked in extension No hamstring exercises
6 to 16 weeks	Discontinue knee brace Continue active knee extension and passive flexion Squats/wall slides to assist with regaining flexion Progressive range of motion including prone hang and aquatic therapy Start proprioceptive training Quadriceps strengthening including straight-leg raises, quadriceps sets, and leg extensions. Closed-chain kinetic exercises including leg presses and resistance stationary bicycle No hamstring exercises
16 to 24 weeks	Continue quadriceps strengthening and add hamstring/quadriceps co-contraction exercises Start light jogging and endurance training No isolated hamstring exercises
24 to 36 weeks	Progress to running and sprinting Continue open- and closed-chain quadriceps strengthening Start isolated low-resistance hamstring exercises Start sport-specific rehabilitation
36 to 52 weeks	Progress to return to full sports activity

quently than after ACL reconstruction, and it usually does not result in any functional impairment. Loss of flexion is more common, but extension also can be affected. Loss of motion can be caused by postoperative adhesions, improper graft tensioning, inadequate postoperative rehabilitation, and heterotopic ossification. Postoperative adhesions can be minimized by limiting extensive dissections and usually can be treated successfully with arthroscopic lysis of adhesions or manipulation under anesthesia. Postoperative rehabilitation needs to be slow and cautious to prevent graft failure. In particular, deep knee flexion and isolated hamstring contractions should be avoided be-

cause these activities subject the PCL graft to high forces. However, knee range-of-motion exercises need to be emphasized after 3 weeks postoperatively to prevent arthrofibrosis.

Osteonecrosis

Osteonecrosis of the medial femoral condyle is a rare complication after PCL reconstruction. It is hypothesized that drilling the femoral tunnel too close to the articular surface compromises the vascular supply. It is currently unknown whether double-bundle PCL reconstruction with the creation of two femoral tunnels predisposes to this problem. The femoral tunnel should be 8 to 10 mm proximal to the articular margin, and excessive soft-tissue dissection over the medial femoral condyle should be avoided. Patients with this problem usually present with persistent medial femoral condylar pain. Treatment includes protected weight bearing, and in some cases bone grafting of the tunnel may help alleviate symptoms.

Other Complications

Less common complications following PCL reconstruction include deep vein thrombosis, infection, and wound complications. PCL reconstructions usually are longer surgeries compared with other arthroscopic procedures, and it is important to minimize tourniquet time to decrease the risk of deep vein thrombosis. Treatment usually is anticoagulation, if the patient does not have any contraindications to antico-

agulation medications. Postoperative infection and wound complications can be minimized with perioperative antibiotics and meticulous sterile technique. Longitudinal incisions in the flexion crease posteriorly should be avoided to decrease the risk of wound breakdown.

Revision PCL Reconstruction

Only a few published studies discuss treatment options for failed PCL reconstruction. The first step in planning a revision PCL reconstruction is identifying the cause of failure of the previous operation, but that is not al-

ways possible. A thorough history and physical examination, as well as a review of previous surgical reports and current radiographs, may help identify the cause of failure. It is important to note any previous neurovascular injuries. Technical considerations include choice of graft, femoral tunnel placement, and a choice of a transtibial or tibial inlay technique. A two-stage revision with tunnel bone grafting may be needed if previous tunnels show excessive bone resorption. High tibial osteotomy should be considered for any significant varus malalignment. Contraindications to revision PCL reconstruction include severe degenerative arthritis, fixed posterior drawer, and active infection.

Bibliography

Ahn JH, Wang JH, Lee SH, Yoo JC, Jeon WJ: Increasing the distance between the posterior cruciate ligament and the popliteal neurovascular bundle by a limited posterior capsular release during arthroscopic transtibial posterior cruciate ligament reconstruction: A cadaveric angiographic study. *Am J Sports Med* 2007;35(5):787-792.

Athanasian EA, Wickiewicz TL, Warren RF: Osteonecrosis of the femoral condyle after arthroscopic reconstruction of a cruciate ligament: Report of two cases. *J Bone Joint Surg Am* 1995;77(9):1418-1422.

Bach BR Jr, Aadalen KJ, Mazzocca AD: An accessory portal for posterior cruciate ligament tibial insertion visualization. *Arthroscopy* 2004;20(suppl 2):155-158.

Cohen SB, Boyd L, Miller MD: Vascular risk associated with posterior cruciate ligament reconstruction using the arthroscopic transtibial tunnel technique. *J Knee Surg* 2004;17(4):211-213.

Fanelli GC, Orcutt DR: Complications of posterior cruciate ligament reconstruction. *Sports Med Arthrosc Rev* 2004;12(3): 196-201.

Houe T, Jørgensen U: Arthroscopic posterior cruciate ligament reconstruction: One- vs. two-tunnel technique. *Scand J Med Sci Sports* 2004;14(2):107-111.

Johnson DH, Fanelli GC, Miller MD: PCL 2002: Indications, double-bundle versus inlay technique and revision surgery. *Arthroscopy* 2002;18(9 suppl 2):40-52.

Keser S, Savranlar A, Bayar A, Ulukent SC, Ozer T, Tuncay I: Anatomic localization of the popliteal artery at the level of the knee joint: A magnetic resonance imaging study. *Arthroscopy* 2006;22(6):656-659.

Krysa J, Lofthouse R, Kavanagh G: Gluteal compartment syndrome following posterior cruciate ligament repair. *Injury* 2002;33(9):835-838.

Makino A, Costa-Paz M, Aponte-Tinao L, Ayerza MA, Muscolo DL: Popliteal artery laceration during arthroscopic posterior cruciate ligament reconstruction. *Arthroscopy* 2005;21(11):1396.

Markolf KL, Feeley BT, Jackson SR, McAllister DR: Where should the femoral tunnel of a posterior cruciate ligament reconstruction be placed to best restore anteroposterior laxity and ligament forces? *Am J Sports Med* 2006;34(4):604-611.

Markolf KL, Zemanovic JR, McAllister DR: Cyclic loading of posterior cruciate ligament replacements fixed with tibial tunnel and tibial inlay methods. *J Bone Joint Surg Am* 2002;84(4):518-524.

Matava MJ, Sethi NS, Totty WG: Proximity of the posterior cruciate ligament insertion to the popliteal artery as a function of the knee flexion angle: Implications for posterior cruciate ligament reconstruction. *Arthroscopy* 2000;16(8):796-804.

Miller MD, Kline AJ, Gonzales J, Beach WR: Vascular risk associated with a posterior approach for posterior cruciate ligament reconstruction using the tibial inlay technique. *J Knee Surg* 2002;15(3):137-140.

Noyes FR, Barber-Westin SD, Albright JC: An analysis of the causes of failure in 57 consecutive posterolateral operative procedures. *Am J Sports Med* 2006;34(9):1419-1430.

Oakes DA, Markolf KL, McWilliams J, Young CR, McAllister DR: Biomechanical comparison of tibial inlay and tibial tunnel techniques for reconstruction of the posterior cruciate ligament: Analysis of graft forces. *J Bone Joint Surg Am* 2002; 84(6):938-944.

Ogata K, McCarthy JA: Measurements of length and tension patterns during reconstruction of the posterior cruciate ligament. *Am J Sports Med* 1992;20(3):351-355.

Wang CJ, Weng LH, Hsu CC, Chan YS: Arthroscopic single- versus double-bundle posterior cruciate ligament reconstructions using hamstring autograft. *Injury* 2004;35(12):1293-1299.

Coding

CPT Codes		Corresponding ICD-9 Codes	
	Arthroscopic Posterior Cruciate Ligament Repair		
29889	Arthroscopically aided posterior cruciate ligament repair/augmentation or reconstruction	717.84	844.2

Chapter 79

Collateral Ligament Reconstruction: Overview

Frederick M. Azar, MD

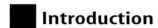

Introduction

The medial collateral ligament (MCL) is the most frequently injured ligament of the knee, although the anterior cruciate ligament (ACL) is the most frequently "torn" ligament and the ligament for which surgical treatment is most often required. Injuries involving the lateral and posterolateral aspect of the knee are much less common than injuries to the medial structures. One study reported only 12 (1.6%) isolated lateral collateral ligament (LCL) injuries in 735 patients with knee ligament injuries; 32 (4.4%) had posterolateral injuries associated with cruciate ligament injuries. Review of the records of 1,833 patients with acute knee injuries identified 819 (45%) with ligament injuries; of these, 319 (39%) had isolated grade I collateral ligament tears, and 306 (96%) of these were MCL injuries. More recently, MRI evaluation of 331 consecutive patients with knee injuries and a hemarthrosis identified 126 with isolated ligament injuries; of these, 83 (66%) had isolated ACL injuries, 28 (22%) had isolated superficial MCL tears, 11 (9%) had isolated posterior cruciate ligament tears, and

4 (3%) had isolated posterolateral corner tears.

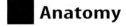

Anatomy

The MCL is a strong, broad ligament that originates from the medial femoral epicondyle, runs distally approximately 10 to 12 cm, and inserts on the medial tibial metaphysis 4 to 5 cm below the joint line. Beneath the superficial MCL, the capsule of the knee joint thickens and forms a set of short, vertically oriented bands known as the deep MCL or medial capsular ligament. Biomechanical studies have shown that the MCL is the primary medial stabilizer of the knee that resists valgus loading. With the knee in 25° of flexion, the MCL provides almost 80% of the restraint to valgus stress. The superficial MCL also plays a secondary role in resisting external rotation and anterior-posterior translation, and the deep MCL acts as a secondary stabilizer against valgus stress. In biomechanical studies, transection of the MCL has been shown to result in 2° to 5° of laxity or 3 to 5 mm of joint opening when a valgus stress is applied.

The LCL is a round, cordlike ligament that averages almost 70 mm in length. Its origin is on the lateral femoral epicondyle and its insertion is on the lateral aspect of the fibular head. The LCL is the primary static stabilizer against varus stress. Along with the popliteus tendon and the popliteofibular ligament, the LCL also serves as a secondary restraint against external rotation and posterior displacement.

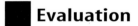

Evaluation

Evaluation of a patient with a suspected knee ligament injury begins with the history; it is important to determine the mechanism of injury. Injuries to the MCL typically are caused by a valgus load to a partially flexed knee or an external rotation force on the tibia in relation to the femur. The most frequent cause of LCL injury is a blow to the anteromedial side of the fully extended knee; lateral knee injuries also can occur with hyperextension of the knee or external tibial rotation. A patient with an MCL injury may report feeling a "pop" in the medial knee at the time of injury. Physical examination also can help identify the injured structures (**Tables 1** and **2**). Pain well localized to the medial side of the knee with local soft-tissue swelling is indicative of MCL injury

Dr. Azar or an immediate family member serves as a board member, owner, officer, or committee member of the American Board of Orthopaedic Surgery, the American Orthopaedic Society for Sports Medicine, the Arthroscopy Association of North America, and the American Academy of Orthopaedic Surgeons and has received research or institutional support from DePuy and Synthes.

Table 1 Physical Examination of the Medial Collateral Ligament

Test	Technique	Result	Significance
Valgus stress test at 0° and 30°	Valgus force is applied to the tibia while stabilizing the femur (with knee in 0° and 30° of flexion). The opposite leg is compared.	Grade I: 0-5 mm opening, firm end point Grade II: 5-10 mm opening, firm end point Grade III: 10-15 mm opening, soft end point	Opening at 30° indicates isolated MCL injury; opening at 0° indicates other ligament tears (ACL, PCL, posterior oblique ligament).
Slocum modified anterior drawer test	Valgus force is applied with the knee in 15° of external rotation and 80° of flexion.	Test is positive if there is a noticeably increased prominence of the medial condyle compared with the other side.	A positive test indicates disruption of the deep MCL; such disruption allows the meniscus to move freely and allows the medial tibial plateau to rotate anteriorly, leading to increased prominence of the medial tibial condyle.
Anterior drawer test in external rotation	The anterior drawer test is done with knee in 90° of flexion with external rotation applied to proximal tibia.	Test is positive if there is a noticeably increased anterior translation of the medial condyle.	Isolated disruption of the MCL should not lead to increased anteromedial translation; it usually indicates involvement of posteromedial structures.

MCL = medial collateral ligament, ACL = anterior cruciate ligament, PCL = posterior cruciate ligament.

Adapted with permission from Singhal M, Patel J, Johnson D: Medial collateral ligament injuries in adults, in DeLee JC, Drez D Jr, Miller MD, eds: *Orthopaedic Sports Medicine: Principles and Practice*, ed 3. Philadelphia, PA, Elsevier, 2010, p 1630.

rather than ACL injury, which usually produces a vague localization of pain and a large knee effusion. LCL injuries result in pain at the lateral joint line and possibly swelling in this area, and the knee may feel unstable in full extension. Palpation of all ligaments and bony structures will identify any point tenderness, which has been reported to accurately determine the location of the injury in nearly 80% of patients.

For patients with MCL injuries, plain radiographs are helpful to rule out an avulsion fracture or a Pellegrini-Stieda lesion (calcification of the MCL from a previous injury). When the physical examination results are equivocal, MRI is useful to determine the severity of the MCL sprain, identify the exact location of the injury, and evaluate for injuries to other structures (such as meniscal tear, ACL injury). In patients with LCL injuries, AP, lateral, and patellofemoral views should be obtained to rule out a fracture (arcuate fracture, Segond fracture, or posterolateral corner avulsion fracture) or other bony

abnormality. When physical and radiographic examinations are inclusive, MRI is effective in evaluating the structures of the posterolateral corner; it has been reported to be 100% accurate in identifying the LCL and 85% to 95% accurate in defining the iliotibial band, the meniscotibial fibers of the lateral capsular ligament, the popliteus, and the fabellofibular ligament.

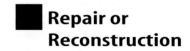

Classification

Acute injuries of both collateral ligaments are classified as follows: grade I—ligament fibers are torn but not completely disrupted and there is no instability; grade II—fibers are partially torn, allowing 3 to 5 mm of laxity, but the ligament remains in continuity; grade III—the ligament is completely disrupted, as is the posterior oblique ligament. A more complex classification system has been developed, but its validity and reliability

have not been established. Although treatment recommendations often are based on the grade of injury, a more important factor in treatment decision making is whether the MCL or LCL injury is isolated or combined with other pathologies. Suggested criteria for diagnosis of an isolated MCL injury include: (1) up to grade II laxity with a firm end point in flexion, (2) no instability to valgus stress in extension, (3) no significant rotatory or anterior-posterior subluxation, (4) no significant effusion, and (5) normal stress radiographs.

Repair or Reconstruction

Indications and Contraindications

The primary treatment of most isolated MCL injuries continues to be nonsurgical, with an emphasis on early rehabilitation. The MCL is an ex-

Table 2 Physical Examination of the Lateral Collateral Ligament

Test	Technique	Result	Significance
External rotation recurvatum	With the patient supine and the knees and hips fully extended, the great toe and foot of both extremities are lifted simultaneously.	Test is positive if the knee falls into a position of recurvatum and varus. Increase in external rotation can be seen by lateral rotation of tibial tubercle.	Usually indicates combined cruciate and posterolateral injury Sensitivity is variable—33% to 94%.
Varus stress test at 0° and 30° of flexion	Valgus force is applied to the tibia while stabilizing the femur (with knee in 0° and 30° of flexion). The opposite leg is compared.	Opening at 0° is often indicative of injury to the LCL, lateral capsule, popliteus tendon, and possibly the superficial layer of the iliotibial band. Increased laxity at 30° indicates a complete tear of the LCL and possibly other posterolateral structures.	LCL is the primary restraint to varus stress, and biomechanical sectioning studies demonstrate that increases in varus opening are not present unless there is concurrent injury to the LCL.
Posterolateral rotation (dial) test	With the patient supine or prone, the femur is stabilized while the tibia, ankle, and foot are rotated with the knee in 30° and 90° of flexion.	Increased external rotation (as noted by the position of the tibial tubercle) compared with the uninvolved leg is a positive test.	An increase of 10° to 15° of external rotation at 30° of flexion indicates injury to the PLC. With knee in 90° of flexion, decreased external rotation indicates isolated injury to the PLC; increased rotation indicates injury to the PLC and PCL.
Posterolateral drawer test	With the knee flexed to 80° and the hip to 45° and the foot stabilized by the examiner, the posterior drawer test is performed in external, neutral, and internal rotation.	Test is positive if posterior translation is increased compared with the opposite knee.	Increased posterior translation in external rotation indicates injury to the PLC and popliteus complex. Increased translation in neutral or internal rotation indicates injury to the PCL.

LCL = lateral collateral ligament, PLC = posterolateral corner, PCL = posterior cruciate ligament.

Adapted with permission from Schorfhaar AJ, Mair JJ, Fetzer GB, Wolters BW, LaPrade RF: Lateral and posterolateral injuries of the knee, in DeLee JC, Drez D Jr, Miller MD eds: *Orthopaedic Sports Medicine: Principles and Practice*, ed 3. Philadelphia, PA, Elsevier, 2010, pp 1725-1728.

tracapsular structure and has an ability to heal with little or no valgus laxity when the torn ends of the ligament are closely apposed. In one series of high school football players with MCL injuries treated nonsurgically, those with grade I injuries returned to play in about 11 days; those with grade II injuries returned to play in about 20 days. In a prospective study of 38 patients with grade I or II MCL injuries treated nonsurgically, 74% returned to preinjury activity levels and 95% returned to work at 3 months after injury; only mild decreases in Lysholm scores and activity levels were noted at 10-year follow-up. Nonsurgical treatment of grade III isolated MCL injuries remains controversial. While one report noted "poor and unacceptable" outcomes at 9-year follow-up after

nonsurgical treatment and another found residual valgus instability in two high school football players, most series have reported outcomes of nonsurgical treatment that were equal to or better than those of surgical treatment. In general, grade III MCL injuries can be treated nonsurgically, but only after careful exclusion of any associated injuries that may require surgical treatment such as cruciate ligament injury, meniscal tear requiring repair, or entrapment of the MCL. In knees with multiligament injuries, delayed reconstruction of the cruciate injuries after the MCL injury has had adequate time to heal (4 to 8 weeks) should be considered. However, a recent prospective randomized study of 47 patients with combined knee ligament injuries compared outcomes in

23 patients who had early (<23 days) ACL reconstruction and MCL repair with those in 24 patients who had early ACL reconstruction and nonsurgical treatment of the MCL injury. At an average follow-up of 27 months, no differences in knee function, stability, range of motion, strength, or return to activity were reported. Nonsurgical treatment of the torn MCL allowed faster restoration of flexion and quadriceps muscle power, leading the authors to recommend early ACL reconstruction followed by 6 weeks of hinged knee bracing to protect the healing ligaments from large valgus forces.

Several indications have been cited for surgical repair of acute isolated MCL tears. They include MRI identification of a complete avulsion of the superficial and deep MCL from the tibia with disruption of the posterior oblique ligament and meniscal coronary ligament in an athlete, an associated tibial plateau fracture, and valgus instability with the knee in 0° of flexion.

Isolated acute grade I and II LCL ligament injuries also are almost always treated nonsurgically. The knee is placed in an unlocked hinged brace with immediate institution of a functional rehabilitation program that emphasizes endurance exercises and quadriceps strengthening but avoids aggressive hamstring strengthening exercises. Grade III LCL injuries are less likely to heal with nonsurgical treatment, so surgical treatment often is recommended. Acute repair of posterolateral corner injuries has been shown by some to produce better outcomes than later reconstructive procedures, whereas others have reported better results with reconstruction. In knees with multiligament injuries, failure to treat the LCL injury results in increased failure rates of cruciate ligament reconstruction and poorer outcomes.

General Principles of Reconstruction

Chronic instability of the medial or lateral compartment is rarely a single-plane laxity. Instability sufficient to justify reconstruction generally involves multiligament injuries, and combinations of procedures frequently are necessary.

Principles of reconstruction of the medial side of the knee are (1) repair and retention of the medial meniscus, if possible; (2) reconstruction of the capsular structures, especially the posterior capsule; (3) restoration of the meniscotibial or meniscofemoral ligament; (4) reconstruction of the posterior oblique ligament at the deep posterior corner; (5) reestablishment of the influence of the semimembranosus unit to the posterior oblique ligament, medial meniscus, and posterior capsule; and (6) reconstruction of the MCL. Basic principles of reconstruction of the lateral side of the knee include (1) restoration of normal tension of the capsular and collateral ligamentous structures from the midlateral axis of the tibia to the midline posteriorly, (2) reinforcement of the structures by fascial suture when tissue quality is poor, (3) meniscal retention if reparable, and (4) reinforcement of the reconstructed tissues with dynamic transfers.

———■

■ Prophylactic Knee Bracing

Two large epidemiologic studies demonstrated consistent trends of decreased risk of MCL injury in football players wearing braces, and a biomechanical study suggested that rigid knee braces provide up to 30% greater MCL resistance to valgus stress. Despite these findings, the use of bracing has been discouraged because of the perception that braces compromise athletic performance; one study of college football players, however, found that selected knee braces did not significantly reduce speed or agility. No consensus currently exists as to the benefits of brace wear by participants in contact sports, but it does appear that braces provide some protection to the MCL.

———■

Bibliography

Azar FM: Evaluation and treatment of chronic medial collateral ligament injuries of the knee. *Sports Med Arthrosc* 2006; 14:84-90.

Battaglia MJ II, Lenhoff MW, Ehteshami JR, et al: Medial collateral ligament injuries and subsequent load on the anterior cruciate ligament: A biomechanical evaluation in a cadaveric model. *Am J Sports Med* 2009;37(2):305-311.

Bradley J, Honkamp NJ, Jost P, West R, Norwig J, Kaplan LD: Incidence and variance of knee injuries in elite college football players. *Am J Orthop* 2008;37(6):310-314.

Chen L, Kim PD, Ahmad CS, Levine WN: Medial collateral ligament injuries of the knee: Current treatment concepts. *Curr Rev Musculoskelet Med* 2008;1(2):108-113.

DeLee JC, Riley MB, Rockwood CA Jr: Acute posterolateral rotatory instability of the knee. *Am J Sports Med* 1983;11(4): 199-207.

Fanelli GC, Edson CJ, Reinheimer KN: Evaluation and treatment of the multiligament-injured knee. *Instr Course Lect* 2009;58:389-395.

Hughston JC, Andrews JR, Cross MJ, Moschi A: Classification of knee ligament instabilities: Part I. The medial compartment and cruciate ligaments. *J Bone Joint Surg Am* 1976;58(2):159-172.

Hughston JC, Andrews JR, Cross MJ, Moschi A: Classification of knee ligament instabilities: Part II. The lateral compartment. *J Bone Joint Surg Am* 1976;58(2):173-179.

Jones L, Bismil Q, Alyas F, Connell D, Bell J: Persistent symptoms following non operative management in low grade MCL injury of the knee: The role of the deep MCL. *Knee* 2009;16(1):64-68.

LaPrade RF, Heikes C, Bakker AJ, Jakobsen RB: The reproducibility and repeatability of varus stress radiographs in the assessment of isolated fibular collateral ligament and grade-III posterolateral knee injuries: An in vitro biomechanical study. *J Bone Joint Surg Am* 2008;90(10):2069-2076.

Miyamoto RG, Bosco JA, Sherman OH: Treatment of medial collateral ligament injuries. *J Am Acad Orthop Surg* 2009;17(3):152-161.

Murphy KP, Helgeson MD, Lehman RA Jr: Surgical treatment of acute lateral collateral ligament and posterolateral corner injuries. *Sports Med Arthrosc* 2006;14(1):23-27.

Najibi S, Albright JP: The use of knee braces: Part 1. Prophylactic knee braces in contact sports. *Am J Sports Med* 2005;33(4):602-611.

Pietrini SD, LaPrade RF, Griffith CJ, Wijdicks CA, Ziegler CG: Radiographic identification of the primary posterolateral knee structures. *Am J Sports Med* 2009;37(3):542-551.

Pietrosimone BG, Grindstaff TL, Linens SW, Uczekaj E, Hertel J: A systematic review of prophylactic braces in the prevention of knee ligament injuries in collegiate football players. *J Athl Train* 2008;43(4):409-415.

Robinson JR, Bull AM, Thomas RR, Amis AA: The role of the medial collateral ligament and posteromedial capsule in controlling knee laxity. *Am J Sports Med* 2006;34(11):1815-1823.

Warren LF, Marshall JL: The supporting structures and layers on the medial side of the knee: An anatomical analysis. *J Bone Joint Surg Am* 1979;61(1):56-62.

Wijdicks CA, Griffith CJ, LaPrade RF, et al: Radiographic identification of the primary medial knee structures. *J Bone Joint Surg Am* 2009;91(3):521-529.

Chapter 80

Treatment of Acute and Chronic Posterolateral Corner Injuries

Robert F. LaPrade, MD, PhD

■ Indications

The fact that grade III posterolateral corner injuries do not heal is well documented in the orthopaedic literature. Because of the instability that can result if these injuries are not treated, repair or reconstruction of posterolateral corner injuries within 2 to 3 weeks of injury is recommended. The timing of surgery is important because the results of early repair and reconstruction have been reported to be better than those of late reconstruction.

Limb alignment must be evaluated and any varus malalignment corrected before any soft-tissue reconstruction of the posterolateral corner structures is undertaken because of the high risk that the reconstruction will stretch out if alignment is not corrected first. In patients who have normal or corrected alignment, a posterolateral reconstruction is necessary to correct any resultant varus, external or internal rotation, or posterolateral rotation instability.

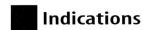

■ Contraindications

Relative contraindications to acute repairs include infection, open wounds, tibial nerve injuries, and patients for whom surgery may not be recommended because of their overall health. In addition, repair of any associated popliteal artery injuries may take priority over immediate posterolateral reconstructions.

For patients with chronic posterolateral corner injuries, contraindications include advanced arthritic changes of the knee, poor vascular supply, and concerns about compliance with the postoperative rehabilitation protocol.

■ Alternative Treatments

For patients with acute injuries in whom surgery is not possible, a program of casting followed by early range of motion may be successful, but these patients must be followed closely to assess for any residual instability because casting has been shown to maintain the amount of instability and not improve it. In patients who

may be poor candidates for surgery because of an inability to comply with the rehabilitation protocol, associated comorbidities, or advanced age, a medial compartment unloader brace can be used to control the side-to-side instability that can result from untreated posterolateral corner injuries.

■ Results

The results of acute repairs of posterolateral corner injuries are generally good if they are done within the first 2 to 3 weeks after injury and the tissue quality is good (**Table 1**). Midsubstance tears of the popliteal tendon and fibular collateral ligament (FCL; also called the lateral collateral ligament) should be augmented or reconstructed for best results. Early surgical treatment has been shown to yield better results than cast immobilization in several studies; the amount of increased varus opening is not improved with casting.

The results of reconstruction of chronic posterolateral corner injuries are variable (**Table 1**). Treatment of varus instability in chronic injuries remains problematic, with most reports indicating 60% to 75% of patients have increased varus translation postoperatively. In most circumstances, the reconstructions for which results have been reported are nonanatomic or

Dr. LaPrade or an immediate family member has received royalties from Arthrex, serves as a paid consultant to or is an employee of iBalance, and has received research or institutional support from Linvatec and Arthrex.

Table 1 Results of Posterolateral Corner Surgery

Authors (Year)	Number of Knees	Injury Type	Mean Patient Age in Years (Range)	Mean Follow-up in Years	Outcomes
Noyes and Barber-Westin (1995)	20	Chronic	24 (14-43)	3.5	76% success rate
Latimer et al (1998)	10	Chronic	32	2.3	Varus restored in 6 of 10
Krukhaug et al (1998)	25 (7 nonsurgical)	Acute	25.5 (16-75)	7.5	Early surgical treatment better than casting; 2+ and 3+ varus instability not improved by casting
Ross et al (2004)	13	Acute	NR	2.5	IKDC: 3 normal, 6 nearly normal

NR = not reported, IKDC = International Knee Documentation Committee.

sling procedures rather than anatomic reconstructions. Outcomes studies on anatomic posterolateral corner reconstructions are still pending.

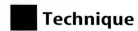

Technique

Setup/Exposure

A sandbag usually is taped to the foot of the operating table to allow the knee to be positioned in approximately 70° of flexion for the surgical approach. In addition, a bump is placed under the ipsilateral hip to ensure that the knee can be positioned without the need for an assistant to hold it in place during the procedure. The initial exposure usually is done without a tourniquet. The standard posterolateral surgical approach is a lateral-based hockey stick–shaped incision starting proximally, centered over the posterior border of the iliotibial band, and extending distally over the Gerdy tubercle and the proximal aspect of the anterior compartment of the leg. The incision is made through the skin and the underlying subcutaneous tissues to identify the superficial layer of the iliotibial band. A posteriorly based skin flap is developed by sharp dissection along the superficial layer of the iliotibial band, toward the short and long heads of the biceps

femoris. Sharp dissection is preferred to minimize skin flaps and provide better exposure of anatomic structures. In the rare situation in which the iliotibial band is torn, a more proximal dissection may be necessary to follow it distally and meticulously dissect it out from scar tissue for later repair.

Once the long head of the biceps has been identified, a fine-point hemostat is used for further dissection. Neurolysis of the common peroneal nerve is done by fine dissection posterior to the long head of the biceps, with care to avoid injury to the nerve. The nerve itself usually is identified 1.5 to 2 cm distal to the fibular head, where it crosses the lateral aspect of the fibula. An approximately 6-cm neurolysis is done. Once the neurolysis is completed, the nerve can be gently retracted; blunt dissection between the soleus and lateral gastrocnemius muscles allows identification of the popliteofibular ligament attachment on the fibular head and the posterior capsule.

A horizontal splitting incision is now made through the anterior arm of the long biceps into the biceps bursa to identify the FCL. A traction stitch is placed into the substance of the FCL or its remnant (**Figure 1**). Pulling on the stitch helps determine the course

of the remaining FCL and allows identification of its femoral attachment site if it is still intact.

In acute injuries where the biceps femoris has been torn off the fibular head, the biceps femoris should be carefully dissected from the surrounding scar tissue and a stout retraction stitch placed into its main substance. When the posterolateral corner injury is more than 10 to 14 days old, it is important to dissect out the biceps femoris and place the knee in full extension to verify that the avulsed biceps tendon can be approximated back to the fibular head. Often, a proximal release of the long head of the biceps is necessary to release any scar tissue so that it can be reattached to its fibular attachment with the knee fully extended.

Palpation of the lateral epicondyle and popliteal sulcus allows identification of the femoral attachments of the main posterolateral structures. An iliotibial band–splitting incision is then made directly over these two anatomic landmarks. Careful dissection along the undersurface of the superficial area of the iliotibial band will preserve the deeper lateral capsular ligament. A small incision over the lateral epicondyle, which can be more easily identified by putting tension on the retraction stitch placed in the FCL, allows identification of the FCL femoral at-

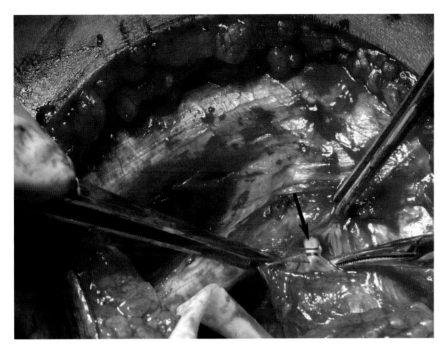

Figure 1 Lateral view of a right knee. A horizontal splitting incision has been made through the anterior arm of the long biceps to expose the FCL. A traction stitch has been placed in the FCL remnant (arrow) to allow identification of its course.

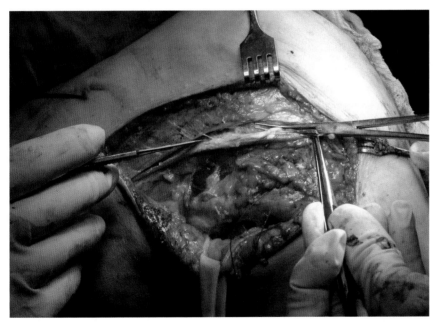

Figure 2 Lateral view of a right knee. A splitting incision through the superficial layer of the iliotibial band allows identification of the femoral attachments of the FCL and popliteus tendon. Care must be taken to avoid injury to the meniscofemoral portion of the middle third of the lateral capsular ligament.

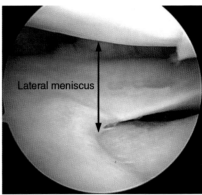

Figure 3 Arthroscopic view of the lateral compartment of a right knee. Note the arthroscopic "drive-through" sign (double-headed arrow), indicating severe lateral compartment gapping.

identification of its femoral attachment site and determine whether it is still intact. Placing a finger on the musculotendinous junction of the popliteus can verify that no musculotendinous junction avulsion injury has occurred. Further retraction of the lateral capsule also helps determine if there has been a tear of the popliteomeniscal fascicles.

With an isolated posterolateral corner injury, an arthroscopic examination of the knee is done to verify that the anterior cruciate ligament (ACL) and posterior cruciate ligament are intact and determine if any other intra-articular pathology needs to be treated. The amount of lateral compartment gapping can be verified, and injuries to the coronary ligament of the posterior horn of the lateral meniscus and other posterolateral structures can be identified (**Figure 3**).

After the arthroscopic examination is completed and any intra-articular pathology is treated, repair or reconstruction of the posterolateral corner structures can be undertaken.

Instruments/Equipment/Implants Required

Fine dissection often is necessary for the posterolateral corner approach, and a curved, fine-point hemostat is useful. In addition, cruciate ligament

tachment site (**Figure 2**). Once the FCL attachment site on the femur has been identified, a vertical incision is made 1 cm anterior to this location

through the lateral capsule, to identify the popliteal tendon femoral attachment. A hemostat placed under the popliteal tendon will assist in the

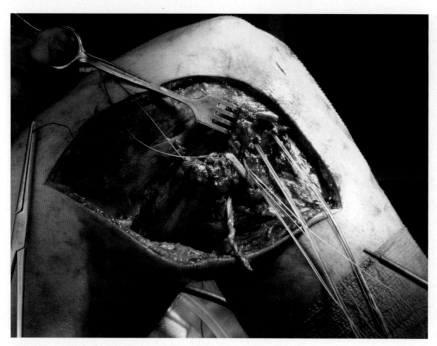

Figure 4 Lateral view of a right knee. The surgical rake is retracting the meniscotibial portion of the middle third of the lateral capsular ligament. The three suture anchors are in the proximal metaphyseal bone of the tibia. (Note that an FCL graft is coursing through the tunnel in the fibular head.)

reconstruction guides are useful to place guide pins for reaming of reconstruction tunnels. An appropriate suture-anchor system should be available if structures need to be repaired directly back to bone. Nonabsorbable sutures and surgical buttons may be required for recess procedures, and cannulated bioabsorbable or metal interference screws may be necessary for fixation.

Procedure

ACUTE REPAIRS

For avulsions of the FCL and popliteal tendon directly off the femur, suture anchors have not been found to be effective in restoring stability and allowing early range of motion. In these circumstances, a recess procedure is recommended. A recess procedure is accomplished by placing an eyelet pin through the attachment site of the avulsed structure, exiting anteromedially on the femur. A 5-mm reamer is used to ream over the pin to a depth of approximately 1 cm. A nonabsorbable

suture is placed in the end of the avulsed tendon or ligament and the end of the suture is passed into the eyelet pin and pulled medially across the femur to recess the torn ligament into the bone tunnel. The sutures can then be tied over a surgical button placed deep to the vastus medialis obliquus muscle while the knee is in full extension.

Structures that are acutely avulsed off the fibular head, such as the popliteofibular ligament, biceps femoris tendon, fabellofibular ligament, and the FCL, usually can be repaired with suture anchors placed directly at their anatomic attachment sites.

For structures torn off the tibia, either a direct suture repair into the metaphyseal bone of the tibia or a suture anchor repair of the avulsed structures can be done. This most commonly involves a direct repair of the lateral meniscus and its avulsed capsule back to the lateral tibia (**Figure 4**).

Intrasubstance tears of some of the posterolateral structures can be re-

paired with direct end-to-end suture, including the popliteomeniscal fascicles to the lateral meniscus, the coronary ligament of the posterior horn of the lateral meniscus, and other capsular structures. Direct end-to-end repairs of the FCL and popliteal tendon have been reported to have a much lower chance of success than reconstruction, and augmented repair or acute reconstruction of these structures should be considered.

Midsubstance tears of the FCL can be reconstructed with a distally based strip of the biceps, which can be reattached to both the fibular head and the femoral attachment site with anchors or sutures. These types of augmented repairs may be more appropriate for patients with open physes in whom drilling a reconstruction tunnel may not be advisable.

Anatomic reconstruction of the FCL may be indicated in older patients. The use of an autologous or allograft semitendinosus tendon has been described, with tunnels drilled at the anatomic attachment sites of the femoral attachment and through the fibular head. With the foot in neutral rotation and the knee flexed slightly, the graft is tightened with a valgus force to reduce any lateral compartment gapping. An examination under anesthesia should be done to verify that the varus instability has been eliminated after the graft is fixed.

ANATOMIC POSTEROLATERAL CORNER RECONSTRUCTIONS

In patients with severe, acute midsubstance posterolateral corner injuries or chronic posterolateral injuries, anatomic reconstruction can be undertaken if alignment is normal or has been corrected. The skin incision is the same as that used for acute repair. A standard posteriorly based skin flap is dissected out, and neurolysis of the common peroneal nerve is done. After identification of the FCL through a horizontal incision into the long head of the biceps to enter the biceps bursa, the anterior aspect of the biceps femoris is taken down off the fibular head and the FCL attachment site on the lateral aspect of the fibular head is identified. Blunt dissection between the soleus muscle and the lateral gastrocnemius muscle exposes the attachment site of the popliteofibular ligament on the posteromedial aspect of the fibular head. A periosteal elevator is used to clean the soleus muscle off this location and to identify the posteromedial downslope of the fibular styloid where the popliteofibular ligament attachment is located. A guide pin is drilled between these two attachment sites from lateral to medial, with a retractor placed medially to protect the neurovascular structures (**Figure 5**). When guide pin position and adequate bone to support a reconstruction tunnel have been verified, a 6- or 7-mm reamer is used to create the tunnel (**Figure 6**).

The tibial tunnel is made between the flat spot just distal and medial to the Gerdy tubercle, anterior to the musculotendinous junction of the popliteus posteriorly. The musculotendinous junction of the popliteus can be identified by elevating the remnant of the popliteus and palpating for a small sulcus of bone at this location along the posterior aspect of the tibia. Dissection just distal and medial to the Gerdy tubercle identifies a flat spot into which an anterior-based guide pin is drilled. An ACL aiming device is used to drill the guide pin from anterior to posterior, exiting at the musculotendinous junction of the popliteus (**Figure 7**). This guide pin should exit the tibia approximately 1 cm medial and proximal to the exit site of the fibular head tunnel for the popliteofibular ligament graft. A blunt probe placed through the fibular head tunnel can help verify that this guide pin is in the correct location. When the position is verified, a 9-mm reamer is placed over the guide pin and the tibial tunnel is reamed from anterior to posterior.

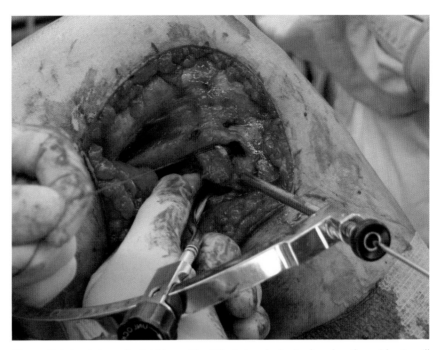

Figure 5 Lateral view of a right knee. The ACL aiming device is placed so the guide pin will pass between the FCL attachment on the fibular head laterally and the popliteofibular ligament attachment on the posteromedial aspect of the fibular styloid medially.

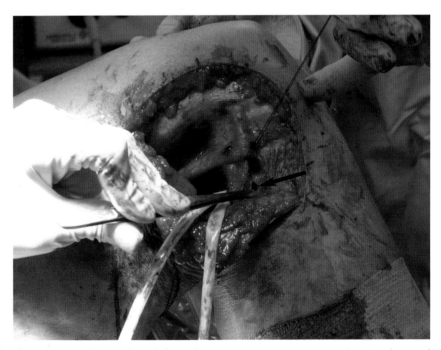

Figure 6 Lateral view of a right knee demonstrates a 7-mm reconstruction tunnel reamed through the fibular head (arrow). The FCL remnant is being tensioned with a traction stitch.

For creation of femoral tunnels, the femoral attachment sites of the popliteus and FCL are identified through the iliotibial band–splitting incision.

Sharp dissection is carried down to the lateral epicondyle, and the attachment site of the FCL, which is just proximal and posterior to the lateral epicon-

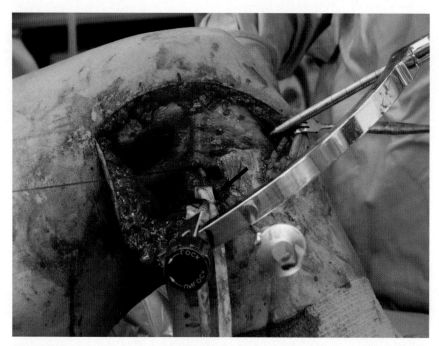

Figure 7 Lateral view of a right knee. An ACL aiming device is being used to drill a guide pin from the flat spot just distal and medial to the Gerdy tubercle to the musculotendinous junction of the popliteus. Note the blunt obturator placed in the fibular head tunnel (arrow) to assist with identification of the correct position of the musculotendinous junction of the popliteus.

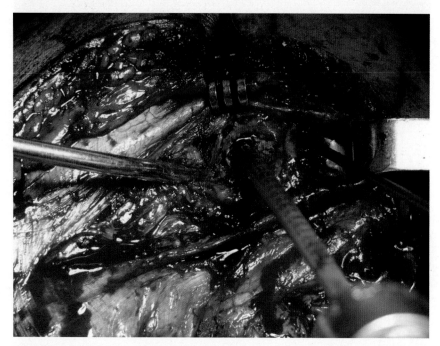

Figure 8 Lateral view of a right knee. Two eyelet-passing pins have been placed through the attachment sites of the popliteal tendon (to the right) and FCL. After verification of the average 18.5-mm distance between the centers of these two attachment points, the tunnels for the reconstruction grafts are reamed with a 9-mm reamer. This shows reaming being done for the FCL tunnel on the femur.

dyle, is identified. An ACL aiming guide opened to 90° is used to drill an eyelet-passing pin through the attachment site, exiting over the anteromedial aspect of the thigh, proximal to the adductor tubercle. After this eyelet pin is placed, a second passing pin is placed directly through the popliteal tendon attachment on the popliteal sulcus, exiting the anteromedial aspect of the thigh parallel to the first pin. It is important to measure between the two eyelet pins before reaming the femoral tunnels to verify that they are approximately 18.5 mm apart (**Figure 8**). If necessary, the correct anatomic attachment sites can be verified by identification of the femoral attachment site of the gastrocnemius tendon, which is usually located 13.8 mm from the FCL femoral attachment. Once the two femoral attachment sites have been verified, a 9-mm reamer is used to create tunnels 25 mm deep at each site, and the guide pins are removed.

Once other intra-articular reconstruction has been completed, such as fixation of any cruciate ligament grafts in the femoral tunnels, the posterolateral corner reconstruction grafts are placed.

An Achilles tendon graft with 9 × 20–mm bone plugs is split lengthwise and tubularized. Passing sutures are placed into the bone plugs (**Figure 9**).

The eyelet pins are placed back into their respective tunnels, and the passing sutures are placed into the guide pins. The bone plugs are pulled into the femoral tunnels and fixed in place with cannulated interference screws. When good purchase of the bone plugs in the respective tunnels is verified, the grafts are placed along their anatomic courses (**Figure 10**). The FCL graft is passed under the superficial layer of the iliotibial band and the lateral aponeurosis of the long head of the biceps femoris, then through the fibular head tunnel. While traction is applied to the graft to tighten it, it is fixed in the fibular head tunnel with the knee in 20° of flexion, a lateral force applied to the knee to reduce any lateral compartment gapping, and the foot in neutral rotation. It is important to verify at this time that varus stability has been restored to the knee. The popliteal tendon graft is then passed down the popliteal hiatus, exiting posteriorly at the knee along the popliteal musculotendinous junction. The graft that has been passed and fixed through the fibular head now becomes the popliteofibular ligament graft along its medial course. The popliteofibular ligament and popliteal tendon grafts are then simultaneously passed out anteriorly through the respective tibial tunnels. Each individual graft must be tightened to verify that all slack is removed from the grafts. They are then fixed in their respective tibial tunnels with cannulated interference screws while the knee is flexed to approximately 60°, distal traction is placed on the grafts, and the foot is in neutral rotation (**Figure 11**).

Examination under anesthesia should verify that all varus and posterolateral rotation has been eliminated.

Wound Closure

Wound closure is similar for both acute and chronic posterolateral corner injuries. The horizontal splitting incision through the biceps femoris bursa is repaired. The lateral capsular incision to the popliteus is repaired with horizontal mattress sutures, as is the iliotibial band–splitting incision. The deep tissues are closed with 0 and 2-0 absorbable sutures. A subcuticular stitch is used to close the skin incision. A sterile dressing is applied, a cold compression device is placed over the knee, and a knee immobilizer is applied to keep the knee in full extension.

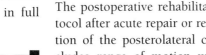

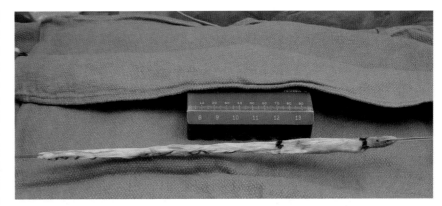

Figure 9 A prepared FCL reconstruction graft from a split Achilles tendon. Passing sutures are placed in the 9-mm-diameter bone plug with the distal aspect of the graft tubularized. Note that the first 70-mm section of the graft is slightly larger, to match the average length of the FCL, while the more distal aspect of the graft is slightly smaller, to allow for passing it through the reconstruction tunnels.

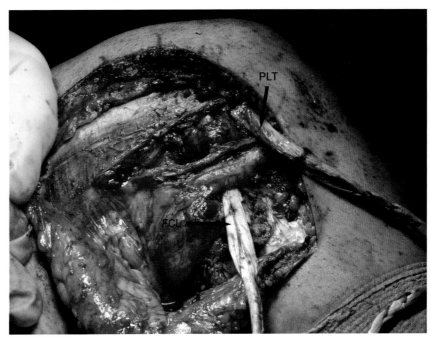

Figure 10 Lateral view of a right knee. The two grafts used to reconstruct the popliteus tendon and FCL have been fixed in femoral tunnels. Note that the FCL graft has been placed along its anatomic course under the superficial layer of the iliotibial band. The popliteal tendon (PLT) graft is to the right.

Postoperative Regimen

The postoperative rehabilitation protocol after acute repair or reconstruction of the posterolateral corner includes range of motion within the "safe zone" that was determined intra- operatively. Range-of-motion exercise is started immediately after surgery within this safe zone for the first 2 weeks and then is slowly increased as tolerated. Patients are kept non–weight bearing for 6 weeks and then slowly weaned off crutches when they can walk without a limp. A progressive strengthening program is initi-

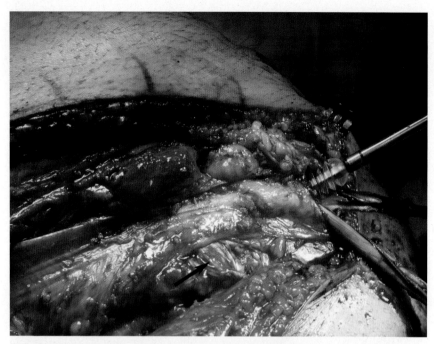

Figure 11 The popliteal tendon and popliteofibular ligament grafts have been passed from posterior in the knee to the anterior aspect. While traction is applied to the grafts, they are fixed in the tibial tunnel with bioabsorbable screws. Note the FCL graft (arrow) as it passes through its fibular head tunnel.

ated at 6 weeks, including the use of a stationary bike, gentle leg presses, and further progression of activities as tolerated.

After reconstruction of chronic posterolateral corner injuries, patients are allowed to undertake full knee range of motion as tolerated, depending on other concurrent ligament reconstructions. They should work on range of motion out of the knee immobilizer several times daily. Straight-leg raises should be done in the knee immobilizer until they can be done without an extension sag. Partial protected weight bearing can begin at 6 weeks postoperatively, and crutches can be discontinued when the patient can walk without a limp. Activities are slowly progressed, and open-chain hamstring exercises are avoided for the first 4 months postoperatively. If there are no other associated arthritic changes of the knee or other limitations because of concurrent surgeries, a jogging program can begin at 4 months and activities can be increased as tolerated.

Avoiding Pitfalls and Complications

One important pitfall to avoid is an inadequate release of the fascia during neurolysis of the common peroneal nerve, especially in acute injuries, because this could lead to a foot-drop deformity. It is important to release the peroneus longus fascia, which is lateral to the common peroneal nerve, to minimize the risk of a foot drop postoperatively. Another pitfall to avoid is failure to verify that bone around the guide pin for the fibular head tunnel is adequate to hold a fixation screw after the tunnel is reamed.

It is especially important not to mistake pseudolaxity of the ACL caused by a posterolateral corner injury for a torn ACL. An arthroscopic examination may be necessary if the integrity of the ACL is in doubt.

Bibliography

Arthur A, LaPrade RF, Agel J: Proximal tibial opening wedge osteotomy as the initial treatment for chronic posterolateral corner deficiency in the varus knee: A prospective clinical study. *Am J Sports Med* 2007;35(11):1844-1850.

Coobs BR, LaPrade RF, Griffith CJ, Nelson BJ: Biomechanical analysis of an isolated fibular (lateral) collateral ligament reconstruction using an autogenous semitendinosus graft. *Am J Sports Med* 2007;35(9):1521-1527.

Gollehon DL, Torzilli PA, Warren RF: The role of the posterolateral and cruciate ligaments in the stability of the human knee: A biomechanical study. *J Bone Joint Surg Am* 1987;69(2):233-242.

Harner CD, Vogrin TM, Höher J, Ma CB, Woo SL: Biomechanical analysis of a posterior cruciate ligament reconstruction: Deficiency of the posterolateral structures as a cause of graft failure. *Am J Sports Med* 2000;28(1):32-39.

Krukhaug Y, Molster A, Rodt A, Strand T: Lateral ligament injuries of the knee: *Knee Surg Sports Traumatol Arthrosc* 1998; 6:21-25.

LaPrade RF: Arthroscopic evaluation of the lateral compartment of knees with grade 3 posterolateral knee complex injuries. *Am J Sports Med* 1997;25(5):596-602.

LaPrade RF, Gilbert TJ, Bollom TS, Wentorf F, Chaljub G: The magnetic resonance imaging appearance of individual structures of the posterolateral knee: A prospective study of normal knees and knees with surgically verified grade III injuries. *Am J Sports Med* 2000;28(2):191-199.

LaPrade RF, Johansen S, Wentorf FA, Engebretsen L, Esterberg JL, Tso A: An analysis of an anatomical posterolateral knee reconstruction: An in vitro biomechanical study and development of a surgical technique. *Am J Sports Med* 2004;32(6):1405-1414.

LaPrade RF, Ly TV, Wentorf FA, Engebretsen L: The posterolateral attachments of the knee: A qualitative and quantitative morphologic analysis of the fibular collateral ligament, popliteus tendon, popliteofibular ligament, and lateral gastrocnemius tendon. *Am J Sports Med* 2003;31(6):854-860.

LaPrade RF, Muench C, Wentorf F, Lewis JL: The effect of injury to the posterolateral structures of the knee on force in a posterior cruciate ligament graft: A biomechanical study. *Am J Sports Med* 2002;30(2):233-238.

LaPrade RF, Resig S, Wentorf F, Lewis JL: The effects of grade III posterolateral knee complex injuries on anterior cruciate ligament graft force: A biomechanical analysis. *Am J Sports Med* 1999;27(4):469-475.

Latimer HA, Tibone JE, ElAttrache NS, McMahon PJ: Reconstruction of the lateral collateral ligament of the knee with patellar tendon allograft: Report of a new technique in combined ligament injuries. *Am J Sports Med* 1998;26(5):656-662.

Noyes FR, Barber-Westin SD: Surgical reconstruction of severe chronic posterolateral complex injuries of the knee using allograft tissues. *Am J Sports Med* 1995;23(1):2-12.

Noyes FR, Barber-Westin SD, Albright JC: An analysis of the causes of failure in 57 consecutive posterolateral operative procedures. *Am J Sports Med* 2006;34(9):1419-1430.

Ross G, DeConciliis GP, Choi K, Scheller AD: Evaluation and treatment of acute posterolateral corner/anterior cruciate ligament injuries of the knee. *J Bone Joint Surg Am* 2004;86(Suppl 2):2-7.

Terry GC, LaPrade RF: The posterolateral aspect of the knee: Anatomy and surgical approach. *Am J Sports Med* 1996;24(6):732-739.

Veltri DM, Deng XH, Torzilli PA, Maynard MJ, Warren RF: The role of the popliteofibular ligament in stability of the human knee: A biomechanical study. *Am J Sports Med* 1996;24(1):19-27.

Coding

CPT Codes		Corresponding ICD-9 Codes	
Ligament Reconstruction/Augmentation			
27428	Ligamentous reconstruction (augmentation), knee; intra-articular (open)	717.81 844.2	717.9
27429	Ligamentous reconstruction (augmentation), knee; intra-articular (open) and extra-articular	717.84	844.2
Arthroscopic Posterior Cruciate Ligament Repair			
29889	Arthroscopically aided posterior cruciate ligament repair/augmentation or reconstruction	717.84	844.2
Casting			
29345	Application of long leg cast (thigh to toes);	717.81 844.2	717.9
29358	Application of long leg cast brace	717.81 844.2	717.9
29365	Application of cylinder cast (thigh to ankle)	717.81 844.2	717.9
29405	Application of short leg cast (below knee to toes);	717.81 844.2	717.9
29425	Application of short leg cast (below knee to toes); walking or ambulatory type	717.81 844.2	717.9
29435	Application of patellar tendon bearing (PTB) cast	717.81 844.2	717.9

CPT copyright © 2010 by the American Medical Association. All rights reserved.

Chapter 81

Treatment of Acute and Chronic Medial-Side Injuries

Christopher Kaeding, MD
David C. Flanigan, MD

 Acute Injuries

Indications

The decision whether to treat an acute medial collateral ligament (MCL) injury surgically or nonsurgically depends on the injury classification. Injuries to the MCL have traditionally been classified as grade I, II, or III injuries (**Table 1**). In grade I injuries, functional integrity is maintained, with no increased laxity on valgus stress testing; grade II injuries have partial loss of structural function, with increased laxity but an end point observed on stress testing; and grade III injuries are characterized by complete disruption of the MCL, with wide opening and no clear end point on stress testing.

Valgus stress testing is done with the knee in 30° of flexion to isolate the MCL. Knees with grade I or II MCL injuries are stable to stress testing in full extension. All grade III injuries should have an assessment of valgus stability in full extension as well as at 30°. Increased opening to valgus stress in full extension implies that the posteromedial corner is disrupted as well.

ACUTE ISOLATED INJURIES

Isolated grade I and II MCL injuries do not require surgical treatment; numerous studies have demonstrated consistently excellent results with nonsurgical treatment. Since the 1980s, most isolated grade III MCL injuries have been treated nonsurgically as well. Surgical repair might be considered for a grade III isolated MCL injury if it is torn from the tibia and disruption of the posteromedial capsule is present. Grade III injuries in which the ligament is torn at its tibial insertion are believed to not heal as well as those that occur on the femoral side. If the medial side of the knee opens widely to valgus stress in full extension as well as at 30° of flexion, the posteromedial capsule and posterior oblique ligament are disrupted as well. Another finding that indicates posteromedial corner injury is increased internal rotation with the knee in full extension. A very high percentage of grade III MCL injuries have associated ligament injuries, often the anterior cruciate ligament (ACL) or posterior cruciate ligament (PCL).

ACUTE COMBINED MCL/ACL INJURIES

The ligament most commonly injured with the MCL is the ACL. Fortunately, because most of these combined injuries involve only a grade I or II MCL injury, the consensus is to reconstruct the ACL in the standard fashion and treat the MCL nonsurgically. In this situation, one must be aware of the MCL injury during the arthroscopy and ACL reconstruction so as to not place too much valgus stress on the knee, especially while viewing the medial compartment, to avoid worsening the compromised medial structures. During the postoperative phase, care also must be taken to minimize valgus stress to the knee until the MCL has healed. Treatment of a grade III MCL injury combined with an ACL tear remains somewhat controversial. Historically, both were treated surgically; more recently, most surgeons treat the grade III MCL nonsurgically and reconstruct the ACL. A full range of motion must be restored before reconstruction of the ACL. Primary surgical repair of the medial complex in a combined MCL/ACL grade III injury may be considered, where the posteromedial corner also is torn. In combined MCL/PCL injuries, if the knee is lax in full extension, primary repair of the medial structures may be indicated.

Dr. Kaeding or an immediate family member serves as a paid consultant to or is an employee of Biomet and has received research or institutional support from DJ Orthopaedics. Neither Dr. Flanigan nor any immediate family member has received anything of value from or owns stock in a commercial company or institution related directly or indirectly to the subject of this chapter.

Table 1 Classification of Medial Collateral Ligament Injuries

Grade	Examination Findings		Implications	Treatment
	0°	30°		
I	No laxity	No laxity	Stable	Nonsurgical
II	No laxity	Laxity with end point	Posteromedial corner intact	Nonsurgical
III	Laxity	Laxity without end point	Posteromedial injury	Consider surgical

ACUTE MULTILIGAMENT INJURIES

Primary repair or reconstruction is currently recommended for acute grade III medial-side injuries in dislocated knees. Most experienced surgeons dealing with knee dislocations recommend reestablishing the function of the cruciate ligaments combined with primary repair or reconstruction of the medial and lateral complexes. The indications for reconstruction or repair of the multiligament-injured knee are discussed in the chapters on knee dislocation.

When the decision is made to surgically treat a medial-side knee injury, anatomic repair is much easier if the surgery can be done within 14 days of the injury. Thereafter, scar formation greatly impedes the delineation of the anatomy.

Contraindications

Contraindications to surgical repair of an acute isolated MCL injury include a nonambulatory patient, an active local infection, grade I or II injury, a low-demand patient, and a patient with significant increased risk for anesthesia and surgery.

Alternative Treatments

For an isolated grade III medial-side knee injury with posteromedial corner involvement or disruption of the tibial insertion of the MCL, a common alternative to surgical treatment is protecting the injured structures with bracing for 6 to 12 weeks and non-weight bearing for as long as the patient has pain or a sense of instability with weight bearing. This is followed

by progressive weight bearing. Physical therapy focuses on strength, motion, gait training, and proprioception training.

For a grade III MCL injury combined with an ACL or PCL injury requiring reconstruction, an alternative to surgical repair is to allow the MCL to heal without treatment and reevaluate medial stability before cruciate ligament reconstruction.

Results

The literature published since 1990 regarding isolated medial-side knee injuries has emphasized that nonsurgical management of isolated MCL injuries produces good results (**Table 2**). Results of primary repair of medial-side injuries in multiligament-injured knees are discussed in the chapters on knee dislocation.

Technique

SETUP/EXPOSURE

If no arthroscopic procedure is planned, the patient is positioned supine with the lower extremity prepared and draped below the hip to allow manipulation of the extremity. The hip is then abducted and externally rotated. The leg is then placed in a modified figure-of-4 position to allow exposure of the medial knee while also placing the knee in varus. If arthroscopy is planned, the extremity can be placed in a traditional thigh holder or an arthroscopy post can be used, with care taken to allow exposure of the distal 6 to 8 inches of the medial thigh. Bony landmarks are palpated, and the joint

line, medial femoral epicondyle, and pes anserinus tendon insertion are identified and marked with a surgical pen (**Figure 1**). The incision extends from just proximal to the medial femoral epicondyle to 1 cm distal to the pes anserinus tendon insertion site. Often in acute injuries, once the sartorial fascia has been identified with blunt dissection of the subcutaneous fat, the ecchymotic injured tissues can be readily identified. If not already disrupted, the deep fascia is incised in line with the incision, and blunt dissection with a finger typically reveals the disrupted tissues. Some scissor dissection to identify the superficial MCL may be needed to fully delineate the pathology.

INSTRUMENTS/EQUIPMENT/IMPLANTS REQUIRED

For primary repair of acute medial-side knee injuries, standard soft-tissue instruments are sufficient. Although intraoperative fluoroscopy is not routinely needed, having it available is prudent. The surgeon's preferred suture anchors should be available, as well as No. 0 and No. 2 sutures for ligament and capsular repair. Postoperatively, the repair should be protected by a splint, knee immobilizer, or brace.

PROCEDURE

The superficial MCL, deep MCL, posterior oblique ligament (POL), and posteromedial capsule should be examined. Once the torn structures have been identified, their anatomic attachment sites are determined. The superficial MCL may be torn distally, prox-

Table 2 Results of Treatment of Medial Collateral Ligament Injuries

Author(s) (Year)	Number of Knees	Condition Treated	Mean Patient Age (Range)	Mean Follow-up (Range)	Results
Ellsasser et al (1974)	74	Acute isolated MCL injuries	NA	Study conducted over 13 professional football seasons	93% success rate in nonsurgically treated cases Nonsurgical recovery ranged from ≤3 weeks to 8 weeks
Holden et al (1983)	46	Acute isolated MCL injuries	"College-age"	8-year study period	80% of injuries responded successfully to nonsurgical treatment program Average time for return to competition ≤3 weeks to 8 weeks
Indelicato (1983)	36	Acute isolated MCL injuries	19.4 years (17-38)	Surgical group: 3.1 years (2.8-4.3) Nonsurgical group: 2.4 years (1.9-3.0)	85% good/excellent results in nonsurgical group compared with 94% in surgical group Nonsurgical group regained strength in significantly less time (*P* < 0.001)
Jones et al (1986)	24	Acute isolated MCL injuries	16.5 years (14-18)	6 months	Stable knee achieved in 22 cases Average recovery time 29 days Mean time to return to competitive sports 34 days
Indelicato et al (1990)	28	Acute isolated MCL injuries	"College-age"	46 months (18-72)	20 subjects had good/excellent results Average time for return to full contact after injury, 9.2 weeks
Andersson and Gillquist (1992)	107	Combined ACL and MCL injuries	NA	52 ± 8 months (35-74)	In subjects who underwent ACL repair, there was no difference in prognosis between those with isolated lesions and those with combined lesions
Reider et al (1994)	35	Acute isolated MCL injuries	20.1 years (14-36)	5.3 years (2.5-8)	All subjects achieved good/excellent ratings on HSS scale
Hillard-Sembell et al (1996)	66	Combined ACL and MCL injuries	35 years (16-63)	45 months (21-108)	No relationship detected between valgus instability and the method of treatment of ligament tears (*P* > 0.4)
Millett et al (2004)	18	Combined ACL and MCL injuries	NA	Minimum 2-year follow-up	Clinical and functional outcomes were good with low motion complication rates No ACL graft failure or valgus instability found at follow-up
Yoshiya et al (2005)	27	Reconstruction of chronic MCL laxity	NA	27 months (24-48)	Postoperative medial stability and range of motion graded normal or nearly normal according to the IKDC evaluation system
Halinen et al (2006)	27	Combined ACL and MCL injuries	NA	27 months (20-37)	No statistically significant difference between groups treated surgically and nonsurgically for MCL injury
Hara et al (2008)	53	Combined ACL and MCL injuries	NA	Minimum 24-month follow-up	No clinically significant differences in laxity as measured by KT-1000 arthrometer No clinically significant difference between 90% of patients who underwent only ACL reconstruction versus those with combined valgus laxity

MCL = medial collateral ligament, NA = not available, ACL = anterior cruciate ligament, HSS = Hospital for Special Surgery, IKDC = International Knee Documentation Committee.

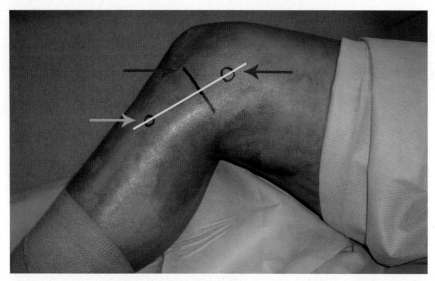

Figure 1 Anatomic landmarks are marked prior to repair of a medial-side injury. Features marked are the tibial attachment site under the pes anserinus tendons (green arrow), the femoral attachment site (blue arrow), the joint line (red arrow), and the skin incision (yellow line).

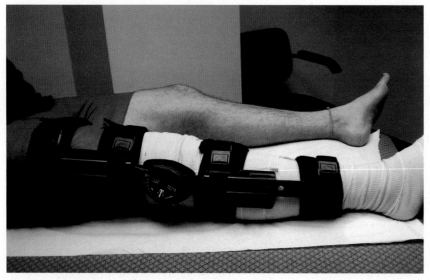

Figure 2 A range-of-motion brace is used postoperatively.

imally, or in its midsubstance. The posteromedial structures are defined and injuries are noted. Most acute medial-side soft-tissue injuries can be repaired with sutures or suture anchors. The deep MCL is treated first, followed by the superficial MCL, and finally the POL and posteromedial capsule. Reattachments to bone are done with suture anchors, and soft-tissue–to–soft-tissue repairs are done with sutures. These repairs are done with the knee in a varus position. Once the repairs have been made, the knee is moved through a range of motion to assess satisfactory strength of the repair as well as any possible overtightening.

WOUND CLOSURE

Once satisfactory repair has been achieved, the sartorial fascia is repaired with resorbable 0 suture, and the subcutaneous tissue and skin are closed in the surgeon's preferred fashion. At our institution, we close the subcutaneous tissue with 2-0 Vicryl (Ethicon, Somerville, NJ) to approximate skin edges and then a running subcuticular 3-0 Prolene (Ethicon, Somerville, NJ) stitch with one or two escape loops every 4 to 5 cm. A sterile dressing is applied, followed by a splint, knee immobilizer, or postoperative range-of-motion brace (**Figure 2**).

Postoperative Regimen

The postoperative regimen described here is used after primary repair of an isolated injury; however, the protocol may be modified if there are associated injuries or additional procedures were performed. The medial repair typically is treated with a short period of immobilization (1 to 2 weeks), followed by use of a postoperative range-of-motion brace to protect the repair from valgus stress. The patient is kept non–weight bearing for 4 to 8 weeks, depending on the natural alignment of the lower extremity. The more valgus the alignment of the knee, the longer the repair is protected from weight bearing. Quadriceps sets and straight-leg raises are started immediately after surgery. A stationary bike can be used around 4 weeks after surgery. After weight bearing has been progressed, the patient continues brace use until 12 weeks postoperatively. Controlling pain and swelling, minimizing quadriceps atrophy, attaining full range of motion, and protecting the repair from valgus stress are the primary goals during the first 6 weeks after surgery.

Avoiding Pitfalls and Complications

All patients should receive prophylactic antibiotics to minimize the risk of surgical-site infection. The saphenous nerve should be identified as it exits the adductor canal and travels along the posterior border of the pes anserinus tendons to avoid injury. If the superficial MCL is avulsed from the tibia, the pes anserinus tendon insertion can be used as a guide to its natural attachment site. A retractor should be used to pull the pes anserinus tendons posterior and inferior to reveal the superficial MCL native insertion site under the gracilis and semitendinosus tendons, just before they attach to the tibia. If the superficial MCL is avulsed from the femur and its native attachment is unclear, intraoperative fluoroscopy can be used to identify the adductor tubercle and medial epicondyle. Multimodal postoperative pain management can minimize the risk of a postoperative pain syndrome. This can include regional block with or without a catheter, cold therapy, nonsteroidal anti-inflammatory drugs, and narcotic analgesics.

Chronic Injuries

Indications

Any residual laxity after an isolated grade III MCL injury usually is minor and not a clinical problem. Although most isolated MCL injuries treated nonsurgically do well, chronic, clinically significant laxity develops in a small number of patients. This is more likely to occur when the injured knee continues to be subjected to valgus stress, resulting in the torn medial structures healing in an elongated position. Chronic laxity is more likely to be clinically significant in patients who have a biomechanical valgus thrust during stance and gait.

A patient with clinically significant symptoms of instability caused by isolated chronic medial laxity that does not respond to physical therapy and a brace or medial heel wedge is a candidate for surgical reconstruction. A failure of nonsurgical modalities for several months should be documented. Patients with persistent, clinically significant medial laxity after ACL recon-

struction and rehabilitation also are surgical candidates.

Contraindications

Chronic laxity alone without clinical symptoms of instability is not an indication for reconstruction. Pathologic anatomic valgus alignment may be a relative contraindication to reconstruction because the construct may stretch and fail due to the high loads imposed. Active infection and low-demand patients also are contraindications.

Alternative Treatments

Chronic medial knee laxity with clinical instability may be treated with a strengthening program and a knee brace. A medial heel wedge also may decrease valgus instability symptoms. If significant valgus anatomic alignment exists, a corrective osteotomy may be considered. Once a more neutral alignment is achieved, the valgus instability symptoms may resolve.

Results

Few studies have reported the clinical results of isolated medial-side knee reconstruction. The results of medial reconstruction as part of a multiligament-reconstructed knee are reported in the chapters on knee dislocation.

Technique

SETUP/EXPOSURE

Setup and exposure are the same as for reconstruction of an acute injury.

INSTRUMENTS/EQUIPMENT/IMPLANTS REQUIRED

Autograft tissue such as gracilis and semitendinosus tendons can be used, but more commonly an allograft is used to reconstruct the superficial MCL. An Achilles tendon allograft is a common choice. Guide pins with eyelets and cannulated drill bits are used to create tunnels at the attachment sites. Sizing sleeves are used to assess

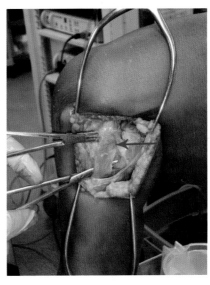

Figure 3 Superficial dissection of the MCL (arrow). Hemostats are placed under the ligament on either side of the joint line.

the graft diameter. Cannulated interference screws are used to secure the graft in the tunnels. Intraoperative fluoroscopy should be available.

PROCEDURE

The skin incision extends from proximal to the medial femoral epicondyle to just distal to the pes anserinus tendon insertion site. The deep fascia is exposed and incised in line with the skin incision to expose the native MCL from the medial epicondyle to the pes anserinus tendon insertion (**Figure 3**). Care must be taken to protect the gracilis and semitendinosus tendons during incision of the deep fascia. The native MCL often can be well delineated where it was not originally damaged, and the condition of the native superficial MCL should be evaluated. It is mobilized as much as possible to facilitate the plication of the underlying deep MCL and a vest-over-pants plication of the superficial MCL. If laxity of the POL is to be corrected, its attachment to the posterior border of the native MCL must be identified and mobilized so that it can be advanced over the allograft MCL reconstruction. After plication of the native deep and superficial MCLs, an

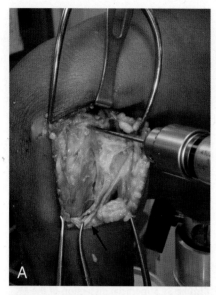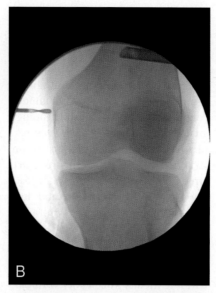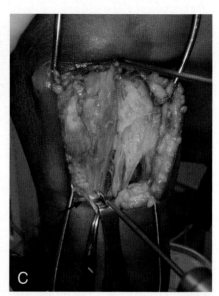

Figure 4 Placing the guide pins for repair of a chronic MCL injury. **A,** The femoral guide pin is placed. The arrow indicates a clamp that is pulling the distal pes anserinus tendons inferiorly to expose the MCL tibial attachment site. **B,** Fluoroscopic image shows the eyelet guide pin placed at the femoral attachment site. **C,** Placement of the tibial guide pin with the pes anserinus tendons being retracted. The arrow indicates a clamp that is pulling the distal pes anserinus tendons inferiorly to expose the MCL tibial attachment site.

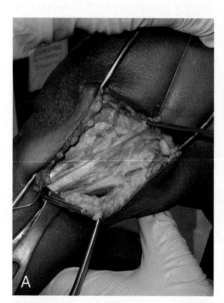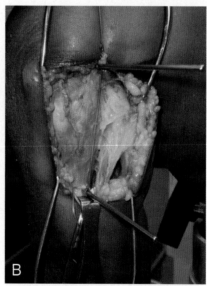

Figure 5 A suture is tied to one guide pin and looped around the other to assess isometry with the knee in extension (**A**) and in flexion (**B**).

eyelet guide pin is drilled into the native femoral attachment site of the superficial MCL and advanced across the distal femur (**Figure 4,** *A*). The placement of the femoral attachment site guide pin in the medial epicondyle just anterior to the adductor tubercle should be confirmed by intraoperative fluoroscopy (**Figure 4,** *B*). The land-

mark for the tibial tunnel is the pes anserinus tendon insertion site. The gracilis and semitendinosus tendons are retracted posteriorly and inferiorly to reveal the native attachment site. A second eyelet guide pin is drilled into the tibial attachment site of the superficial MCL and advanced across the tibia (**Figure 4,** *C*). A suture tied to one

guide pin and looped over the other can be used to assess the isometry of the pin placements as the knee is moved through a range of motion (**Figure 5**).

The allograft is tagged on each end with a resorbable No. 2 suture, sized with a sizing sleeve, and soaked in antibiotic irrigation solution. The appropriately sized drill bit is placed over the tibial pin, and a 30-mm–deep tunnel is created. The drill is then removed while the eyelet guide pin is left in place. The tag sutures from one end of the allograft are placed through the eyelet of the tibial guide pin and the guide pin is pulled through the tibia, thus passing the tag sutures through the tibial tunnel and out through the other side of the tibia (**Figure 6,** *A*). Pulling on the sutures will seat the graft into the tibial tunnel. A cannulated interference screw is then passed over a guide pin to secure the graft in the tibial tunnel (**Figure 6,** *B*). After fixation of the graft is confirmed, the absorbable tag suture that extends beyond the skin is then cut short and allowed to retract beneath the skin. Alternatively, one or two

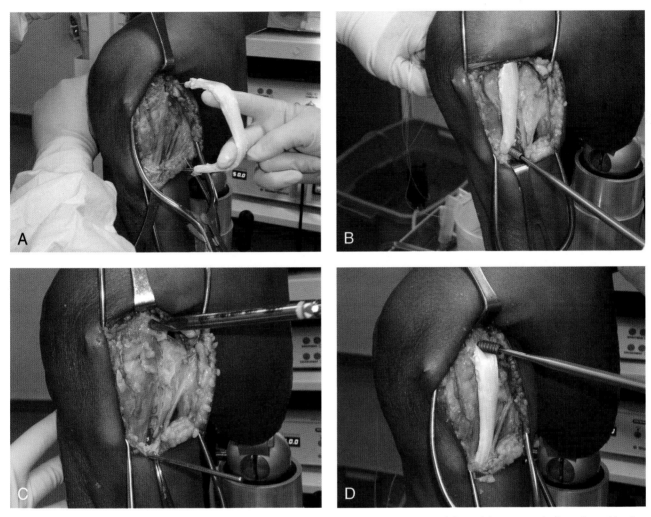

Figure 6 Placing and fixing the graft for repair of a chronic MCL injury. **A,** Tag sutures are passed through bone tunnels via eyelet guide pins. **B,** A tibial interference screw is placed. **C,** The femoral tunnel is drilled over the guide pin. **D,** The graft is fixed in the femoral tunnel with an interference screw over the femoral guide pin.

4.5-mm bicortical screws with large spiked washers can be used on the tibial side. The appropriately sized cannulated drill is then placed over the femoral attachment site eyelet guide pin and used to drill a tunnel across the distal femur (**Figure 6,** *C*). The guide pin should be left in place as the drill bit is removed. The absorbable tag sutures on the other end of the graft are passed through the eyelet of the femoral guide pin. The pin is pulled through the femur, and the sutures are then used to pull the graft into the femoral tunnel. The surgeon needs to make sure that the graft is not so long that it bottoms out against the bottom of the tunnel, thus preventing proper tensioning of the graft. This can be corrected by either deepening the tunnel or shortening the graft. Once the graft has been pulled into the femoral tunnel, the knee is flexed 30° and placed in varus stress. With the knee held in this position, the graft is placed under moderate manual tension and is fixed in the femoral tunnel with a cannulated interference screw placed over a guide pin (**Figure 6,** *D*). The knee is then moved through a range of motion to assess isometry (**Figure 7**). Probing and a very gentle valgus stress can be used to assess integrity of the reconstruction. If the posteromedial structures are to be tightened, they are advanced over the MCL graft and secured with sutures.

WOUND CLOSURE
After the wound is irrigated, the deep fascia can be closed with absorbable sutures. Subcutaneous tissue and skin are closed in a standard manner. After application of a sterile dressing, the reconstruction is protected from valgus stress by a splint, knee immobilizer, or postoperative brace (**Figure 2**).

Postoperative Regimen
Early range of motion is encouraged, with the knee protected from valgus

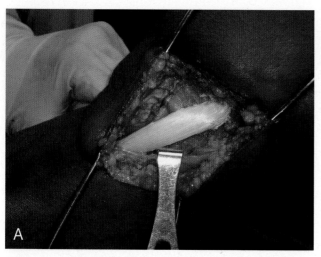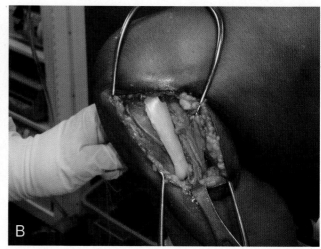

Figure 7 Isometry of the MCL reconstruction is assessed with the knee in extension (**A**) and in flexion (**B**).

stress for 6 to 8 weeks with protected weight bearing and a hinged postoperative brace. The more valgus the alignment of the extremity, the longer the period of protection. Quadriceps-stimulating exercises are initiated immediately postoperatively. During the first 6 weeks, emphasis is placed on protecting the reconstruction while increasing range of motion, controlling swelling, and minimizing quadriceps atrophy. At around 6 weeks, the patient is weaned from crutches, and progressive resistance exercises and proprioceptive training are emphasized. The patient continues to use a brace until at least 12 weeks after surgery for activities of daily living and for 1 year for more vigorous activities. Controlled cutting drills can be added at 3 to 4 months, with return to play at around 6 months. The progression after the first 12 weeks may vary according to the individual's condition and situation.

Avoiding Pitfalls and Complications

In any grade III MCL injury, associated ligament injuries should be suspected, and posteromedial laxity should be evaluated. The posteromedial corner should be reconstructed at the time of the MCL reconstruction if posteromedial laxity exists. The course of the saphenous nerve along the posterior border of the pes should be kept in mind to avoid injuring it. Intraoperative fluoroscopy is used to check isometry and to ensure proper attachment sites of the superficial MCL graft. Early motion with patellar mobilization is important to avoid postoperative contractures.

———————————————— ■

■ Bibliography

Andersson C, Gillquist J: Treatment of acute isolated and combined ruptures of the anterior cruciate ligament: A long-term follow-up study. *Am J Sports Med* 1992;20:7-12.

American Medical Association. Subcommittee on Classification of Sports Injuries: *Standard Nomenclature of Athletic Injuries.* Chicago, IL, American Medical Association, 1966.

Ellsasser JC, Reynolds FC, Omohundro JR: The non-operative treatment of collateral ligament injuries of the knee in professional football players: An analysis of seventy-four injuries treated non-operatively and twenty-four injuries treated surgically. *J Bone Joint Surg Am* 1974;56(6):1185-1190.

Halinen J, Lindahl J, Hirvensalo E, Santavirta S: Operative and nonoperative treatments of medial collateral ligament rupture with early anterior cruciate ligament reconstruction: A prospective randomized study. *Am J Sports Med* 2006; 34(7):1134-1140.

Hara K, Niga S, Ikeda H, Cho S, Muneta T: Isolated anterior cruciate ligament reconstruction in patients with chronic anterior cruciate ligament insufficiency combined with grade II valgus laxity. *Am J Sports Med* 2008;36(2):333-339.

Hillard-Sembell D, Daniel DM, Stone ML, Dobson BE, Fifthian DC: Combined injuries of the anterior cruciate and medial collateral ligaments of knee: Effect of treatment on stability and function of the joint. *J Bone Joint Surg Am* 1996;78: 169-176.

Holden DL, Eggert AW, Butler JE: The nonoperative treatment of grade I and II medial collateral ligament injuries to the knee. *Am J Sports Med* 1983;11(5):340-344.

Indelicato PA: Non-operative treatment of complete tears of the medial collateral ligament of the knee. *J Bone Joint Surg Am* 1983;65(3):323-329.

Indelicato PA, Hermansdorfer J, Huegel M: Nonoperative management of complete tears of the medial collateral ligament of the knee in intercollegiate football players. *Clin Orthop Relat Res* 1990;256(256):174-177.

Jones RE, Henley MB, Francis P: Nonoperative management of isolated grade III collateral ligament injury in high school football players. *Clin Orthop Relat Res* 1986;213:137-140.

Millett PJ, Pennock AT, Sterett WI, Steadman JR: Early ACL reconstruction in combined ACL-MCL injuries. *J Knee Surg* 2004;17(2):94-98.

Reider B, Sathy MR, Talkington J, Blyznak N, Kollias S: Treatment of isolated medial collateral ligament injuries in athletes with early functional rehabilitation: A five-year follow-up study. *Am J Sports Med* 1994;22:470-477.

Yoshiya S, Kuroda R, Mizuno K, Yamamoto T, Kurosaka M: Medial collateral ligament reconstruction using autogenous hamstring tendons: Technique and results in initial cases. *Am J Sports Med* 2005;33(9):1380-1385.

Coding

CPT Codes		Corresponding ICD-9 Codes	
	Ligament Repair		
27427	Ligamentous reconstruction (augmentation), knee; extra-articular	844.1 905.7	717.82
27428	Ligamentous reconstruction (augmentation), knee; intra-articular (open)	844.1 905.7	717.82
27429	Ligamentous reconstruction (augmentation), knee; intra-articular (open) and extra-articular	844.1 905.7	717.82

CPT copyright © 2010 by the American Medical Association. All rights reserved.

Chapter 82

Knee Dislocation: Overview and Strategies

Michael J. Stuart, MD
Bruce A. Levy, MD

Introduction

Knee dislocation is a limb-threatening injury with potentially devastating outcomes. Optimal treatment strategies remain controversial, and currently there is a paucity of data in the literature to help guide decision making. Neurovascular structures at risk include, but are not limited to, the popliteal artery and peroneal nerve. Injury patterns typically involve at least three of the four major knee ligaments. The dislocated knee may not be initially recognized because of a spontaneous reduction.

Primary treatment consists of closed reduction and treatment of vascular compromise. Surgical management of all damaged ligamentous structures is preferred for most patients who have satisfactory vascular supply, skin coverage, rehabilitation potential, and anticipated future activity demands. Injury classification based on the specific ligamentous structures involved guides the surgical technique. The timing and extent of surgery remain controversial because of concerns about knee arthrofibrosis. Newer and improved surgical tech-

niques, the use of allogeneic graft sources, and controlled postoperative knee range of motion have reduced the risk of knee stiffness. Surgical reconstruction and/or repair of the knee ligaments and associated structures followed by early rehabilitation protocols provides the highest level of function.

High-velocity knee dislocations are caused by motor vehicle accidents, industrial or farm trauma, and falls from more than 5 feet. These patients may present with polytrauma, including injuries to other organ systems, neurovascular involvement, open dislocations, and fractures. On the other end of the spectrum, low-velocity knee dislocations result from athletic injuries, stepping in a hole, and falls from less than 5 feet. This type of dislocation has a better prognosis because of fewer vascular injuries, reduced meniscal damage, and fewer osteochondral fractures. Ultra-low–velocity dislocations occur during activities of daily living in morbidly obese patients. This patient population presents unique treatment challenges because of body habitus.

Classification

Classification schemes for the dislocated knee can direct management, predict the risk of associated injuries, and shed light on the prognosis. The anatomic classification described by Schenck and associates is the most useful in organizing a treatment plan (**Table 1**).

Evaluation

A dislocation should be suspected in any knee with multidirectional instability. The neurovascular status of the limb must be evaluated promptly because of the devastating consequences of ischemia. Immediate surgical exploration or further vascular imaging is done as indicated. The knee is reduced and splinted near full extension, and the neurovascular status is reevaluated. The ligament injury pattern and associated injuries are determined by physical examination, stress radiographs, and MRI.

Initial Evaluation

It is imperative to immediately evaluate the neurovascular status of the limb and determine if the injury is open or closed, if the joint is reducible

Dr. Stuart or an immediate family member serves as a paid consultant to or is an employee of Stryker and Fios and has received research or institutional support from DePuy, Biomet, Stryker, and Zimmer. Dr. Levy or an immediate family member serves as a paid consultant to or is an employee of Valpo Orthotec.

Table 1 Anatomic Knee Dislocation Classification System

Classification	Injury Description
KD I	PCL-intact KD with a functioning PCL and variable collateral ligament involvement (usually lateral)
KD II	Complete bicruciate injury with both collateral ligaments intact (uncommon)
KD III	An injury to both cruciate ligaments and one collateral ligament, either medial (M) or lateral (L) structures
KD IV	An injury to both cruciate ligaments and both collateral ligaments
KD V	A KD with periarticular fracture

KD = knee dislocation, PCL = posterior collateral ligament.

Appending a C to these classifications indicates circulatory injury; an N denotes neurologic damage. For example, KD III-MC implies tearing of both cruciate ligaments and the medial collateral ligament, with an associated popliteal artery injury.

Adapted from Schenck RC Jr, Hunter RE, Ostrum RF, Perry CR: Knee dislocations. *Instr Course Lect* 1999;48:515-522.

or irreducible, and if any associated fractures are present.

Neurovascular Assessment

A thorough neurovascular examination of the entire lower extremity is imperative not only to rule out injury to the peroneal nerve, but also to assess for signs of compartment syndrome. The manual muscle strength of the anterior tibial, peroneal, and extensor hallucis longus muscles and the gastrocnemius-soleus complex are tested, as are skin sensation to light touch in the superficial, deep peroneal, and tibial nerve distributions.

The popliteal artery can be injured when the knee dislocates because it is tethered between the adductor hiatus proximally and the soleus arch distally. Careful physical examination is crucial to rule out arterial injury. The dorsalis pedis and posterior tibial pulses should be palpated in both feet and compared. Repeated examinations are required as vessel spasm, thrombosis, or progression of an intimal tear may cause delayed ischemia. The neurovascular examination should be repeated before and after any manipulation of the extremity.

Soft-Tissue Assessment

First, the leg is inspected for skin color and temperature, capillary refill, and popliteal swelling. Adequate perfusion is determined, as well as whether the knee joint is open or closed, dislocated, subluxated, or reduced. Compartment syndrome is assessed by palpation of the lower leg compartments for firmness and tenderness as well as pain with passive stretch.

Assessment of Joint Reduction

If the joint is dislocated, it is promptly reduced by applying longitudinal traction. The position of the tibia relative to the femur provides a clue to the mechanism of injury and helps guide the reduction technique. It is important to recognize that posterolateral knee dislocations may be irreducible by closed means. This "irreducible dislocation" is indicated by puckering of the medial skin, the posterolateral position of the tibia relative to the femur, persistent medial joint-space widening, and lateral tibial subluxation. Joint reduction is blocked because the medial femoral condyle protrudes through the soft tissues and the medial retinaculum is displaced into the notch.

The optimal position for maintenance of joint reduction is in extension or slight flexion. If the joint maintains reduction, a knee brace or splint is applied. If joint reduction is not achieved or maintained, surgical management is required for reduction and possible application of a knee-spanning external fixator.

Vascular Status/Imaging

Pulses in the affected extremity should be palpated. The assessment of a pulse is subjective, with pulses described as normal, diminished, or absent. After lower extremity trauma, the most helpful sign is an absent or diminished pulse because it will lead to further evaluation. If obvious signs of limb ischemia are present, such as absent pulses, an expanding hematoma, or an audible bruit, an emergency vascular surgery consult is needed. The vascular surgeon will typically proceed with an angiogram in the operating room to locate the zone of injury, followed by immediate exploration, repair, or bypass grafting of the popliteal artery. If the patient does not have an ischemic limb, the treatment algorithm for vascular assessment includes serial examination of pedal pulses and measurement of the ankle-brachial index (ABI), which equals the Doppler systolic arterial pressure in the injured lower extremity divided by the Doppler systolic arterial pressure in the uninjured upper extremity (**Figure 1**).

Ankle-Brachial Index

The ABI, also known as the ankle pressure index or ankle-arm index, is a noninvasive screening tool for patients who have sustained lower extremity trauma and suspected vascular injury. Determining the ABI is relatively fast, inexpensive, and safe and requires only a blood pressure cuff and Doppler machine. With the patient supine, a blood pressure cuff is applied to the ankle of the injured lower extremity, the cuff is inflated, then slowly deflated, and a Doppler probe is used to determine the systolic pressure. The probe can be placed over the posterior tibial artery or the dorsalis pedis artery (**Figure 2**). The systolic pressure of the injured extremity is then compared with the systolic pressure of an uninjured upper extremity, typically from the ipsilateral side.

Understanding the limitations of any examination is essential. The ABI may not detect injury to vessels such as the profunda femoris or the peroneal arteries. Nonobstructive lesions, such as intimal flaps, can go unrecognized. Limb alignment should be restored before obtaining an ABI to reduce false-negative or false-positive results. False-positive results can be caused by hypovolemic shock and peripheral vascular disease.

An ABI greater than 0.9 has been shown to have a 100% negative predictive value for vascular injury. In other words, patients with an ABI of greater than 0.9 are essentially at a 0% risk of having a major arterial lesion. If the ABI is less than 0.9, however, then the patient is at risk for vascular injury, and further vascular assessment with either duplex ultrasonography or conventional or CT angiogram is recommended.

Duplex Ultrasonography

Duplex ultrasonography has been proven to be an excellent noninvasive diagnostic imaging tool. This modality can detect blood flow velocities and wave-form characteristics, allowing the surgeon to understand the hemodynamic severity of an injury (**Figure 3**). The examination is portable and does not expose the patient to contrast material or require intravascular access, allowing for evaluation in the emergency department, intensive care unit, or operating room. Duplex ultrasonography also is one tenth the cost of conventional arteriography.

Duplex ultrasonography has been shown to be highly sensitive and spe-

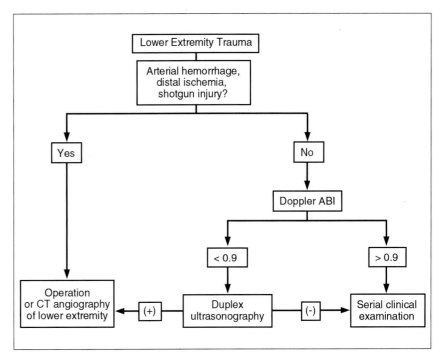

Figure 1 Treatment algorithm for vascular assessment in lower extremity trauma. ABI = ankle-brachial index. (Adapted with permission from Redmond JM, Levy BA, Dajani KA, Cass JR, Cole PA: Detecting vascular injury in lower-extremity orthopedic trauma: The role of CT angiogram. *Orthopedics* 2008;31:761-767.)

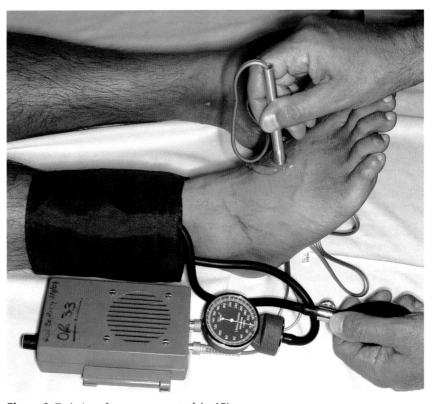

Figure 2 Technique for measurement of the ABI.

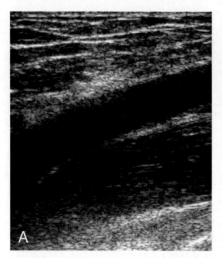
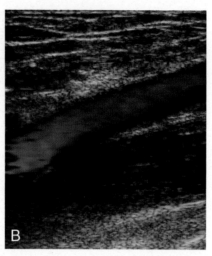

Figure 3 Duplex ultrasonography without (**A**) and with (**B**) Doppler flow. (Reproduced with permission from Redmond JM, Levy BA, Dajani KA, Cass JR, Cole PA: Detecting vascular injury in lower-extremity orthopedic trauma: The role of CT angiogram. *Orthopedics* 2008;31:761-767.)

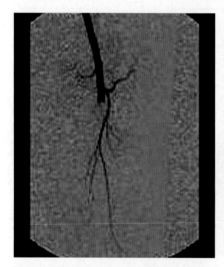

Figure 4 Conventional angiography demonstrates popliteal artery thrombosis.

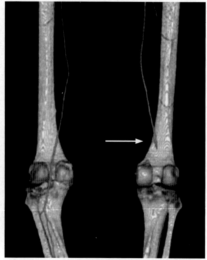

Figure 5 CT angiography demonstrates popliteal artery thrombosis (arrow). (Reproduced with permission from Redmond JM, Levy BA, Dajani KA, Cass JR, Cole PA: Detecting vascular injury in lower-extremity orthopedic trauma: The role of CT angiogram. *Orthopedics* 2008;31:761-767.)

With a sensitivity reported to be 95% to 100% and a specificity of 90% to 98%, arteriography is often ordered to rule out an injury when physical examination is believed to be inadequate for detecting arterial injury; this practice is termed exclusion arteriography.

Potential complications of conventional arteriography include contrast nephropathy, puncture-site problems, allergic reactions, and distal ischemia. Contrast nephropathy varies in incidence from 1% in the general population to 92% in patients with diabetes or renal insufficiency. Hematoma, pseudoaneurysm, arteriovenous fistula, hemorrhage, thrombosis, and femoral neuralgia are clinically significant local complications occurring in 1.7% to 3.6% of patients. Severe anaphylactic reactions or reactions that cause respiratory compromise are rare, occurring in less than 1% of cases.

Conventional arteriography has other drawbacks aside from the medical complications. Cost is an issue because arteriography is significantly more expensive than all other diagnostic examinations, ranging from $3,000 to $6,000. In addition, a trained radiologist or surgeon needs to be available 24 hours a day for femoral artery cannulation and contrast administration.

CT Angiography

CT angiography (CTA) has recently been shown to be relatively noninvasive, sensitive, and specific (**Figure 5**). Most trauma centers now have multidetector-row CT scanners readily available, making CTA an attractive option.

Unlike conventional arteriography, CTA of the lower extremity is obtained by gaining access to the peripheral venous system and injecting contrast material via the antecubital vein. A CT scan of the lower extremities is then obtained while the arteries fill with contrast. The image is then reformatted to visualize the appropriate vessels. Contrast extravasation, pseudo-

cific for the detection of arterial injury as confirmed by either conventional arteriography or surgical findings. In a series of 86 patients with penetrating trauma, no patient with negative results on duplex ultrasonography developed signs or symptoms of a vascular injury, whereas all four patients with positive results on duplex ultrasonography had vascular injuries that were confirmed with conventional arteriography.

Duplex ultrasonography does have limitations. Its accuracy depends on

the technical ability of the ultrasound technician, and it requires the availability of a qualified ultrasonography team 24 hours a day.

Arteriography

Conventional angiography has been considered the gold standard for evaluating arterial injuries (**Figure 4**).

aneurysm formation, abrupt narrowing of an artery, loss of opacification of an arterial segment, and arteriovenous fistula formation all suggest arterial injury.

CTA has several advantages over conventional arteriography: (1) the avoidance of arterial cannulation, (2) decreased cost, (3) decreased contrast load, and (4) less reliance on a specialized team of surgeons and interventional radiologists.

Despite its significant advantages, CTA is not free from potential sequelae. Extravasation of intravenous contrast can cause tissue damage and lead to compartment syndrome in rare cases. Contrast nephropathy has been reported to be as high as 4% in patients undergoing CTA in settings other than trauma with similar contrast load.

Ligmentous Examination

AWAKE EXAMINATION

The integrity of the ligamentous structures should be assessed by means of a careful and meticulous physical examination. To determine if the extensor mechanism is intact, the patient is asked to lift the leg and extend the knee against gravity. Assessment of anterior cruciate ligament integrity is done with a Lachman test at 30° of flexion. Posterior cruciate ligament integrity is determined with posterior sag and drawer tests at 90° of flexion. Posterolateral corner integrity is evaluated with a dial test at 30° and 90° of flexion. Asymmetric external rotation (more than 10° to 15°) at 30° of flexion is consistent with an isolated injury, whereas asymmetric rotation at 30° and 90° of flexion is consistent with an injury to both the posterolateral corner and posterior cruciate ligament. Medial collateral ligament and lateral collateral ligament integrity is evaluated by applying a varus and valgus stress at 0° and 30° of flexion. Increased medial or lateral joint space opening with the knee in full extension is indicative of a combined cruciate and collateral ligament injury. Increased medial and lateral joint space opening at 30° of flexion is consistent with medial and lateral collateral disruption, respectively. Comparison examination of the uninjured knee will help differentiate ligament instability patterns, especially in a patient with generalized ligamentous laxity.

EXAMINATION UNDER ANESTHESIA

Examination under anesthesia may be helpful to further define the pattern and the extent of the damaged ligaments and capsular structures. Fluoroscopic comparison views while applying varus/valgus or anterior/posterior translation stress may help determine the extent of ligamentous damage or identify a physeal injury in a skeletally immature patient.

Diagnostic Imaging

RADIOGRAPHS

For an acute injury, AP, lateral, oblique, and patellar views are obtained to determine if the joint is dislocated, subluxated, or reduced (**Figure 6**). After a spontaneous reduction, slight joint space widening may be the only clue to a knee dislocation. Radiographs also are helpful to identify periarticular and osteochondral fractures. Careful evaluation for avulsion fractures will provide clues to specific ligament involvement and guide surgical technique. For example, lateral collateral ligament, popliteofibular ligament, and biceps femoris insertion avulsions all may be attached to an avulsed fibular head fragment. If initial radiographs demonstrate the knee in a dislocated or subluxated position, then repeat films are necessary after reduction to verify satisfactory position.

STRESS RADIOGRAPHS

Comparison views while applying varus/valgus or anterior/posterior translation stress may help determine the extent of ligamentous damage or identify a physeal injury in a skeletally immature patient.

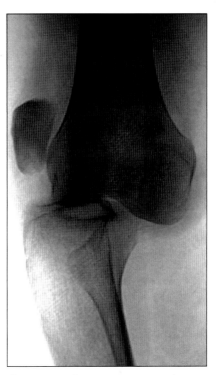

Figure 6 AP fluoroscopic image of a posterolateral dislocation with an associated lateral patellar dislocation. (Reproduced with permission from Stuart MJ: Evaluation and treatment principles of knee dislocations. *Op Tech Sports Med* 2001;9:91-95.)

MAGNETIC RESONANCE IMAGING

MRI is an excellent imaging modality that will not only assist in or confirm the clinical diagnosis, but usually will help with developing a treatment plan. Physical examination alone can be limited because of pain, muscle spasm, swelling, ipsilateral fractures, vascular injuries, bilateral injuries, or polytrauma. For example, a positive valgus stress test at 30° may be consistent with a medial collateral ligament injury, but the MRI will define exactly where the ligament is torn and thus has treatment implications. MRI is also essential in the assessment of associated intra- and extra-articular injuries that are difficult to diagnose clinically, such as meniscal tears, intraosseous contusions, occult fractures, capsular disruptions, and muscle strains. MRI is invaluable in planning specific procedures required (reattachment or reconstruction), the

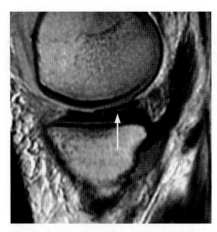

Figure 7 A sagittal T1-weighted MRI of a dislocated knee following attempted reduction of an "irreducible dislocation." Note the interposed medial retinacular tissue within the medial compartment (arrow). (Reproduced with permission from Stuart MJ: Evaluation and treatment principles of knee dislocations. *Op Tech Sports Med* 2001;9:91-95.)

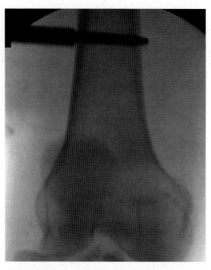

Figure 8 Fluoroscopic image demonstrates placement of the distal femoral pin above the patella to avoid penetration into the suprapatellar pouch.

number and types of grafts needed, and the order of repair and reconstruction. The complexity of the injury and the magnitude of the treatment justify this valuable and cost-effective resource. The sagittal MRI in **Figure 7** shows an irreducible dislocation, recognized by the lateral subluxation of the tibia caused by an interposed medial retinacular tissue.

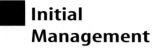

Initial Management

After a knee dislocation is reduced, either spontaneously or by manual closed reduction, the neurovascular status of the extremity is immediately reassessed. Our current protocol for thromboembolic prophylaxis is to initiate low-molecular-weight heparin and mechanical measures immediately after the vascular assessment is complete and continue treatment until definitive surgical management. Examination under anesthesia and comparison fluoroscopic stress radiographs are used to determine the ex-

tent of ligamentous injury. If necessary, a joint-spanning external fixator is applied. At the appropriate time, MRI of the knee is obtained to further define the injury pattern.

External Brace
A posterior-based splint or knee brace can be applied for a knee dislocation that has spontaneously reduced or one that has been manually reduced and has maintained reduction.

External Fixation
Indications for the use of initial knee-spanning external fixation include a vascular injury requiring repair, gross instability in the AP (coronal) plane with failure to maintain reduction, inability to tolerate immobilization in a knee brace alone, and open knee dislocation with soft-tissue compromise.

Spanning external fixation is applied in the operating room under anesthesia with the use of fluoroscopy. The patient is placed supine, and sterile preparation and draping are done. Extreme care is taken to hold the limb and prevent redislocation during this time. The limb is elevated slightly above the opposite side to allow ade-

quate visualization in the sagittal plane (lateral view) for pin placement. Care is taken to not overdistract the joint because this may cause injury to the neurovascular structures.

Two 5- or 6-mm threaded half pins are placed in the femur on the anterolateral surface, at an angle of approximately 45° relative to the coronal plane. The distal pin is inserted approximately 5 to 10 cm proximal to the patella to avoid intra-articular penetration at the suprapatellar pouch (**Figure 8**). Two more pins are placed in the tibia on the anteromedial surface, at an angle of approximately 30° relative to the coronal plane. The proximal pin is inserted approximately 10 cm below the level of the joint to avoid proximity to future posterior cruciate ligament tunnels. Each pair of pins should be spaced adequately apart to improve stability based on the design characteristics of the spanning fixator utilized, and if possible, should be placed out of the path of potential future surgical incisions. The simplest stable connection that can be made with available frame components is used to bridge the knee. Using MRI-compatible, radiolucent connecting rods and placing metal clamps away from the knee will facilitate imaging. Traction and realignment are achieved manually, and the frame clamps are tightened. After sterile dressings are applied, alignment and stability are confirmed (**Figure 9**).

Definitive Management

The skin is suitable for surgical intervention when the swelling has subsided and the abrasions are healed. Our current protocol is to perform definitive repair/reconstruction of all ligamentous structures at 3 to 4 weeks after injury. This allows time for soft-

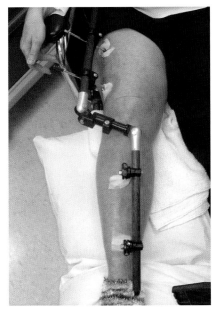

Figure 9 Photograph of knee-spanning external fixation with anterolateral femoral and anteromedial tibial pin placement.

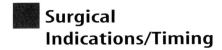

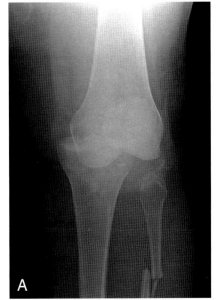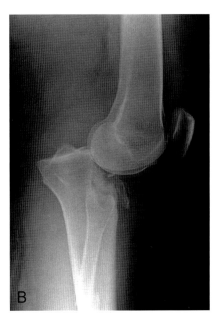

Figure 10 AP (**A**) and lateral (**B**) radiographs demonstrate a knee fracture-dislocation.

tissue healing and recovery from inflammation and is a short enough interval to avoid extensive fibrosis.

Surgical Indications/Timing

Surgical management, in particular early surgical reconstruction and repair, currently is favored. Absolute indications for surgery include irreducible dislocations, dysvascular limbs, and open injuries. Associated fractures or avulsion-type injuries often do better with early repair within 2 to 3 weeks of injury, because anatomic dissection is easier in the absence of scar tissue, and the tissues are robust enough to accommodate suture repair. In patients with vascular injury requiring surgical revascularization, and in some patients who are morbidly obese or who have ligamentous hypermobility or extensive soft-tissue loss requiring grafting, a period of immobilization followed by delayed reconstruction may be indicated.

Open Dislocation
An open knee dislocation is an absolute indication for surgery, which typically is done in an urgent fashion as for any open musculoskeletal injury. If there is significant soft-tissue injury that may require multiple débridement procedures and plastic surgery intervention, we typically place a knee-spanning external fixator. Definitive multiligament knee reconstruction is delayed until complete resolution of the soft-tissue envelope and absence of infection have been achieved.

Irreducible Dislocation
Irreducible dislocations present with the classic medial-side skin puckering from a posterolateral knee dislocation and are an absolute indication for immediate surgical intervention.

Fracture-Dislocation
Knee dislocations may be associated with avulsion-type injuries, rim fractures, tibial plateau fractures, distal femoral fractures, and even floating knee injuries. These are typically grossly unstable injuries that often require a staged approach. As a gen-

eral rule, fracture treatment is first, followed by knee ligament reconstruction, depending on the specific injury pattern. For example, in a complex bicondylar tibial plateau fracture with associated anterior cruciate ligament/posterior cruciate ligament/posterolateral corner injury, it is important to restore normal bony architecture first with open reduction and internal fixation, achieve bony union, and then perform a delayed multiligament knee reconstruction once adequate rehabilitation has been completed. This would allow for proper length-tension ratios of each of the ligamentous structures. However, in the case of an anterior cruciate/posterior cruciate ligament injury with a large fibular head avulsion, single-staged multiligament knee reconstruction and open reduction and internal fixation of the fibular head may be performed at the same time. An example of a high-energy fracture-dislocation of the knee is shown in **Figure 10**. This injury resulted in a dislocation of both the tibiofemoral and proximal tibiofibular joints.

■ Bibliography

Berkseth RO, Kjellstrand CM: Radiologic contrast-induced nephropathy. *Med Clin North Am* 1984;68(2):351-370.

Brautigan B, Johnson DL: The epidemiology of knee dislocations. *Clin Sports Med* 2000;19(3):387-397.

Dubberley J, Burnell C, Longstaffe A, MacDonald PB: Irreducible knee dislocation treated by arthroscopic debridement. *Arthroscopy* 2001;17(3):316-319.

Green NE, Allen BL: Vascular injuries associated with dislocation of the knee. *J Bone Joint Surg Am* 1977;59(2):236-239.

Hessel SJ, Adams DF, Abrams HL: Complications of angiography. *Radiology* 1981;138(2):273-281.

Huang FS, Simonian PT, Chansky HA: Irreducible posterolateral dislocation of the knee. *Arthroscopy* 2000;16(3):323-327.

Inaba K, Potzman J, Munera F, et al: Multi-slice CT angiography for arterial evaluation in the injured lower extremity. *J Trauma* 2006;60(3):502-506, discussion 506-507.

Knudson MM, Lewis FR, Atkinson K, Neuhaus A: The role of duplex ultrasound arterial imaging in patients with penetrating extremity trauma. *Arch Surg* 1993;128(9):1033-1037, discussion 1037-1038.

Levy BA, Zlowodzki MP, Graves M, Cole PA: Screening for extremity arterial injury with the arterial pressure index. *Am J Emerg Med* 2005;23(5):689-695.

Mills WJ, Barei DP, McNair P: The value of the ankle-brachial index for diagnosing arterial injury after knee dislocation: A prospective study. *J Trauma* 2004;56(6):1261-1265.

Redmond JM, Levy BA, Dajani KA, Cass JR, Cole PA: Detecting vascular injury in lower-extremity orthopedic trauma: The role of CT angiography. *Orthopedics* 2008;31(8):761-767.

Schenck RC Jr, Hunter RE, Ostrum RF, Perry CR: Knee dislocations. *Instr Course Lect* 1999;48:515-522.

Shelbourne KD, Klootwyk TE: Low-velocity knee dislocation with sports injuries: Treatment principles. *Clin Sports Med* 2000;19(3):443-456.

Shelbourne KD, Porter DA, Clingman JA, McCarroll JR, Rettig AC: Low-velocity knee dislocation. *Orthop Rev* 1991;20(11):995-1004.

Wascher DC: High-velocity knee dislocation with vascular injury: Treatment principles. *Clin Sports Med* 2000;19(3):457-477.

Chapter 83
Surgical Treatment of Knee Dislocation

Eric C. McCarty, MD
Brett Gibson, MD

■ Indications

Traumatic knee dislocations represent complex injuries involving disruption of at least one cruciate ligament with associated collateral ligament injury. Most commonly, both cruciate ligaments and the medial collateral ligament (MCL) or both cruciate ligaments and the lateral collateral ligament (LCL) and/or posterolateral corner are involved. Injury to the posterior cruciate ligament (PCL) may involve a complete or partial tear with varying degrees of instability. The role of nonsurgical management is limited in a true knee dislocation, regardless of the specific constellation of injury. The absence of an established treatment algorithm presents a unique challenge to the orthopaedic surgeon given the variable injury patterns and potential complicating factors involved.

The ideal timing of surgery remains a topic of debate. Various factors should be considered in deciding when to proceed with definitive treatment. In the past, concern for arthro-

fibrosis prevented early treatment of ligament injuries in most patients. More recent evidence suggests that this complication may be prevented by an aggressive postoperative rehabilitation program focusing on early range-of-motion exercises. In the presence of associated fractures, osteochondral defects, meniscal injury, or extensor mechanism injury, early treatment may be desirable to allow definitive management of all injuries under a single anesthesia. Often, intra-articular or periarticular fractures, including intercondylar eminence fractures and tibial PCL avulsions, should be allowed to heal completely before any necessary ligament reconstructions are performed. Extensive surgery during the early postinjury period poses a significant risk to the integrity of the soft-tissue envelope. In patients with combined anterior cruciate ligament (ACL) and MCL injuries and mild PCL laxity, delayed treatment may offer an advantage over early treatment by allowing the MCL and PCL to scar in before isolated ACL reconstruction is done at

a later date. Ultimately, the exact timing of reconstruction remains a matter of surgeon preference.

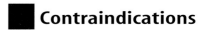

■ Contraindications

Patients with knee dislocations often present with multiple other injuries, some of which may be life- or limb-threatening. Standard trauma assessment followed by treatment of any life-threatening comorbidities should precede treatment of any knee dislocation. Limb-threatening conditions such as vascular injury or soft-tissue compromise occur frequently with knee dislocations and take precedence over definitive management of any ligamentous injuries.

The prevalence of injury to the popliteal artery in the setting of knee dislocation ranges from 10% to 65%. Even patients with low-energy mechanisms of dislocation or a knee that has spontaneously reduced should be evaluated for vascular injury because of the significant displacement that occurs at the time of injury. Nearly 20% of patients who present to a Level 1 trauma center with a dysvascular limb have been shown to require amputation, with prolonged warm ischemia time representing a significant risk factor for amputation. If immediate vascular intervention is required,

Dr. McCarty or an immediate family member serves as a board member, owner, officer, or committee member of the American Orthopaedic Society for Sports Medicine and the International Society of Arthroscopy, Knee Surgery and Orthopaedic Sports Medicine; has received royalties from DJ Orthopaedics; is a member of a speakers' bureau or has made paid presentations on behalf of the Musculoskeletal Transplant Foundation; and has received research or institutional support from Stryker. Neither Dr. Gibson nor any immediate family member has received anything of value from or owns stock in a commercial company or institution related directly or indirectly to the subject of this chapter.

treatment of all ligament injuries should be delayed to allow for healing of the vascular repair and to ensure that proper revascularization occurs.

Rarely, posterolateral dislocations are irreducible because the medial femoral condyle becomes incarcerated in a disrupted anteromedial capsule. When this occurs, immediate open reduction is indicated to avoid prolonged traction on the neurovascular structures. This involves repair of any injured structures that are accessible through the same incision. Unnecessary surgical dissection should be avoided to prevent soft-tissue complications, and treatment of the ligamentous injuries should be delayed.

Open injuries often are a contraindication to acute repair, depending on the size of the injury and surrounding soft-tissue disruption. The degree of injury to the soft tissue often is extensive, regardless of the size of any open wounds. Degloving injuries may occur because of the high-energy nature of many knee dislocations. Surgical exposure should be limited to avoid any further compromise of the soft-tissue envelope; definitive procedures should be delayed until the soft-tissue integrity has been fully restored. Multiple débridements often are necessary for significant soft-tissue injury, and flap coverage may be necessary. Temporary joint-spanning external fixation often is required to stabilize the joint as the soft tissues recover. Compartment syndrome following knee dislocation is treated with urgent fasciotomy and delayed reconstruction.

Other contraindications to surgical treatment are less absolute. They include elderly or sedentary patients with low functional demands and those with significant comorbidities or severe preexisting degenerative changes. The decision to proceed with surgery should be made only after a thorough discussion with the patient of the risks and benefits involved.

Alternative Treatments

Considerable variability exists regarding the surgical management of knee dislocations. Reconstruction of the cruciate ligaments can be done arthroscopically or through an open incision. Arthroscopic reconstruction is minimally invasive and, in addition to minimizing the burden on the soft-tissue envelope, may allow patients to participate in postoperative rehabilitation sooner. Although the cruciate ligaments typically require reconstruction, collateral ligament and posterolateral corner injuries can be treated with either open repair or reconstruction. Primary repair beyond the early postinjury period often is prohibitively difficult because of abundant scar formation, and reconstruction may be necessary in this situation. Depending on the degree of residual instability present after cruciate ligament reconstruction, the MCL may be managed nonsurgically. The PCL is reconstructed using either a single-bundle or double-bundle configuration. Although double-bundle PCL reconstruction is more anatomic, the additional surgery required may not be justified in this setting. If the posteromedial bundle of the PCL remains intact, this can be preserved, and single-bundle reconstruction of the anterolateral bundle can be undertaken. The use of autograft for multiligament knee reconstruction may require additional incisions, resulting in increased postoperative pain and potential donor-site morbidity, but no graft option has shown a clear advantage over the others. Postoperative management varies from immediate rehabilitation in some type of protective brace to a period of immobilization up to 6 weeks after surgery. Previous reports suggest that PCL laxity is increased without a period of immobilization; however, the risk of arthrofibrosis must be considered. Data are lacking regarding the optimal surgical technique; ultimately, surgeon preference dictates the specific strategy used.

Results

Published studies of the surgical treatment of knee dislocation consist mostly of small retrospective case series (**Table 1**). Considerable variability exists in the literature regarding injury pattern and treatment protocol. Surgical treatment has demonstrated significantly better outcomes than nonsurgical treatment. Cruciate stability after reconstruction has been shown to be superior to that after repair, although one study reported acceptable function in spite of residual laxity when repair was done in the acute setting. Acceptable results have been reported for both allografts and autografts, although no study has compared the two directly. Staged reconstruction has shown no significant advantage over simultaneous reconstruction, although a significant percentage of patients in one series did not require reconstruction of the cruciate ligaments when a staged approach was used. In combined ACL and PCL reconstructions, the PCL graft has demonstrated a tendency for increased laxity on instrumented testing compared with the ACL graft. Rehabilitation protocols in recent studies have been inconsistent, but they typically involve early range-of-motion exercises with a period of protected weight bearing. Most patients achieve full range of motion, but some require manipulation under anesthesia. Several studies have reported favorable functional results, but patients rarely rated the reconstructed knee as normal on subjective evaluation. Return to sports has been shown to be more common when injuries are treated acutely, but overall, postoperative activity level is unpredictable.

Technique

Setup/Exposure

Before the patient is taken to the operating room, the availability of a vascular surgeon should be confirmed; blood should be made available by the blood bank in case of intraoperative vascular injury. The choice of anesthesia depends on multiple factors, including comorbidities, anesthesia history, and patient preference. General anesthesia is preferred, but epidural anesthesia with sedation also can be used. A femoral or sciatic nerve block also can be used for postoperative pain control at the discretion of the patient, surgeon, and anesthesiologist. A Foley catheter is placed to facilitate fluid management during the procedure.

The patient is placed supine with a thigh tourniquet in place. Inflation of the tourniquet may not be necessary unless an open procedure is planned or excess bleeding is encountered during arthroscopy. A sandbag or bump is secured to the table as a heel rest to allow the knee to be positioned in 90° of flexion. A lateral post is applied for valgus stress and to prevent the hip from externally rotating while the knee is flexed 90°. Examination of the knee under anesthesia is done with the knee at 0°, 30°, and 90° of flexion to assess the stability of the cruciate and collateral ligaments and the posterolateral corner (**Figure 1**). MRI evaluation at the time of surgery is helpful for correlation with examination findings. The extremity to be operated on is confirmed before the incision is made.

An arthroscopic technique is used for both ACL and PCL reconstructions. Before the incision is made, the joint is injected with a combination of 25 mL of sterile saline and 25 mL of a 1:1 mixture of 1% lidocaine and 0.25% bupivacaine, both with epinephrine. The portal sites and any open incisions are marked and also injected with a 1:1 mixture of 1% lidocaine and 0.25% bupivacaine with epinephrine.

The epinephrine causes vasoconstriction that limits bleeding during the arthroscopic procedure and thus improves visualization. The anterolateral arthroscopy portal is established along the lateral border of the patellar tendon at the midpoint between the patella and the lateral joint line. The anteromedial portal is established under direct vision with the use of a spinal needle, approximately 1 cm from the medial border of the patellar tendon. If a PCL reconstruction is done, a posteromedial portal also is established under direct visualization. The spinal needle is placed in the soft spot along the joint line, posterior to the MCL and anterior to the hamstring tendons. A cannula can be used for the posteromedial portal if desired to facilitate the passage of instruments. An incision is created at the anteromedial tibia at the midpoint between the tibial tubercle and the medial flare of the tibial metaphysis. The incision starts superiorly at the level of the tibial tubercle, approximately 2 cm inferior to the joint line. Both the ACL and the PCL tunnels are accessible through this incision. A small subvastus incision is made near the medial border of the trochlear articular surface to provide access to the femoral PCL tunnel. If MCL repair or reconstruction is necessary, the subvastus and anteromedial tibial incisions can be connected with a curvilinear incision. To provide access to the lateral structures, a curvilinear incision is made from the posterior aspect of the lateral epicondyle to the midpoint between the Gerdy tubercle and the fibular head.

Instruments/Equipment/Implants Required

A 30° arthroscope is used for most cruciate ligament reconstructions. A 70° arthroscope is useful for viewing the posterior tibia during preparation and drilling of the PCL tunnel. Gravity inflow is used to prevent excess fluid extravasation into the soft tissues.

Fluoroscopy is essential during PCL tibial tunnel preparation for passage of the guide pin and reamer to avoid overpenetration and allow anatomic tunnel placement.

Several graft options are available for ligament reconstruction. Use of an allograft minimizes donor-site morbidity and avoids additional incisions required for autograft harvest. An anterior or posterior tibial tendon allograft is preferred for ACL reconstruction, and an Achilles tendon allograft is used for reconstruction of the PCL. Both Achilles tendon and soft-tissue allografts can be used for posterolateral corner reconstructions. A tibial tendon allograft is used to reconstruct the MCL if repair or imbrication is not possible. A double-armed No. 2 high-strength nonabsorbable braided suture is passed through the soft-tissue grafts. For Achilles tendon allografts, the soft-tissue portion is tubularized during suture passage to facilitate passage of the graft, and two No. 5 high-strength nonabsorbable braided sutures are passed through small drill holes in the bone block.

For PCL reconstructions, a metal interference screw is used to secure the bone block portion of the Achilles tendon allograft on the femoral side. The tibial side is fixed with a bioabsorbable interference screw. A flip-button device secures the ACL graft on the femoral side, and a bioabsorbable interference screw is used on the tibial side. For both ACL and PCL grafts, tibial fixation can be augmented with staples or a post (4.5-mm fully threaded cortical screw and washer) if desired. Collateral ligament reconstructions can be done with either a flip button or interference screw fixation.

Diagnostic arthroscopy is done initially to assess the quality of the articular cartilage surfaces, identify any meniscal pathology, and confirm cruciate ligament injury. Articular cartilage defects and meniscal tears are treated appropriately at this time. Mi-

Table 1 Results of Combined Cruciate Ligament Repair or Reconstruction

Authors (Year)	Number of Knees	Procedure	Mean Patient Age in Years (Range)
Shapiro and Freedman (1995)	7	Combined ACL/PCL reconstruction (allograft)	26.3 (15-35)
Noyes and Barber-Westin (1997)	11 (7 acute, 4 chronic)	Combined ACL/PCL reconstruction 6 MCL repair or reconstruction 6 PLC reconstruction	26.5 (17-42)
Wascher et al (1999)	13 (9 acute, 4 chronic)	Combined ACL/PCL reconstruction (allograft) 7 MCL injuries 6 PLC injuries	27.5 (14-51)
Mariani et al (2001)	15	Combined ACL/PCL reconstruction (autograft)	25.1 (18-35)
Dedmond and Almekinders (2001)	206 (132 surgical, 74 nonsurgical)	Meta-analysis comparing surgical and nonsurgical treatment	NA
Fanelli and Edson (2002)	35 (19 acute, 16 chronic)	Combined ACL/PCL reconstruction (autograft or allograft) 15 MCL injuries (brace) 25 PLC repair	NA
Harner et al (2004)	31 (19 acute, 12 chronic)	Combined ACL/PCL reconstruction (allograft)	28.4 (16-51)
Strobel et al (2006)	17	Combined ACL/PCL/PLC reconstruction (autograft)	30.7 (15.5-58.2)
Bin and Nam (2007)	15	Stage 1: MCL (10 knees) or PLC (8 knees) repaired or reconstructed within 2 weeks Stage 2: ACL (3 knees) or PCL (7 knees) reconstructed at 3 to 6 months if unstable	30.4 (20-51)
Ibrahim et al (2008)	20	Combined ACL/PCL/PLC reconstruction (autograft) Collateral ligaments reconstructed with artificial LARS (ligament and augmentation system) ligament (J.K. Orthomedic, Dollard-des-Ormeaux, Quebec, Canada)	27.3 (17-45)

ACL = anterior cruciate ligament, PCL = posterior cruciate ligament, PLC = posterolateral corner; NA = not available; IKDC = International Knee Documentation Committee; HSS = Hospital for Special Surgery.

crofracture is the preferred first-line method of treatment of cartilage defects during multiligament reconstruction if the characteristics of the defect allow, and inside-out meniscal repair is preferred for tears in the red or red-white zone greater than 1 cm in length, with partial meniscectomy reserved for irreparable meniscal tears. The meniscal sutures can be tied as they are placed or after the ligament reconstruction is complete to avoid any undue tension on the repair during the reconstructive procedure.

Procedure

After diagnostic arthroscopy, the cruciate ligaments are reconstructed. A single-bundle reconstruction is recommended for both the ACL and PCL. The priority is to establish all necessary tunnels before placing any grafts. The tunnels are drilled first for the PCL and then for the ACL.

POSTERIOR CRUCIATE LIGAMENT

The tibial remnant of the PCL is débrided from the posterior tibia with a 4.0-mm full-radius resector. Care is taken to avoid the posterior capsule because the distance between the popliteal artery and the tibial insertion of the PCL has been shown to be 7 to 10 mm with the knee distended, depending on the degree of knee flexion. A soft-tissue elevator can be used to elevate any remaining ligament from the tibia. Alternating between the an-

Table 1 (Continued)

Mean Follow-up (Range)	Results
51.4 months (39-63)	All knees treated a mean of 9.6 days after injury; average flexion arc 118°; 4 had arthrofibrosis requiring manipulation; 6 with functional rating good or excellent
4.8 years (2.5-9)	10 had <3 mm instrumented laxity at 20°; 9 had <3 mm instrumented laxity at 70°; 9 had full range of motion at follow-up; 5 had arthrofibrosis requiring additional procedures; return to sports more favorable after early treatment; failure: 18% PCL, 9% ACL, 18% PLC
38 months (24-54)	Mean laxity 4.5 mm at 20°, 5.0 mm at 70°; average extension loss 3°, flexion loss 5°; 2 had arthrofibrosis requiring manipulation; IKDC: A 8%, B 46%, C 38%, D 8%; Lysholm score 88; 6 returned to unrestricted sports, 4 to modified sports
36 months (24-56)	IKDC: A 20%, B 47%, C 20%, D 7%; Lysholm score 95.1; HSS score 89.6; Tegner activity score 5.5; 7 returned to preinjury activity level
NA	Range of motion 123° surgical, 108° nonsurgical; Flexion contracture 0.5° surgical, 3.5° nonsurgical; Lysholm score 85.2 surgical, 66.5 nonsurgical; No significant difference in stability or return to preinjury activity level
(24-120 months)	94% normal Lachman and pivot-shift; 46% normal posterior drawer; All had <3 mm instrumented laxity; Lysholm score 91.2; HSS score 86.8; Tegner activity score 5.3
3.7 years (2-6)	Average extension loss 1°, flexion loss 12°; 4 acute cases had arthrofibrosis requiring manipulation; laxity improved more predictably after acute surgery; IKDC: A 0%, B 35%, C 39%, D 26%; Lysholm score 87; return to work or sports less predictable
41.3 months (24.0-66.3)	Average time to surgery 70.2 months after injury; mean instrumented laxity 2 mm; IKDC: A 0%, B 29%, C 59%, D 12%; subjective stability improved significantly
88.9 months (35-110)	5 did not require ACL or PCL reconstruction; 4 had grade 2 PCL instability; Lysholm score 87.6
53 months (36-96)	Mean extension loss 0°-2°; mean flexion loss 10°-15°; IKDC: A 0%, B 45%, C 45%, D 10%; Lysholm score 91

terolateral and posteromedial portals with the 30° and 70° arthroscopes will optimize viewing, as will use of a posteromedial portal.

After adequate débridement of the tibial remnant, a 15-mm offset PCL guide is set between 50° and 55° and inserted through the anteromedial portal. Ideally, the guide pin should exit at the distal and lateral aspect of the native PCL insertion. The posterior root of the medial meniscus serves as an additional anatomic landmark

for tibial tunnel placement. Under fluoroscopic guidance and with the knee in 90° of flexion, the guide pin is placed through an incision on the anteromedial proximal tibia. The scope is positioned to allow constant observation of the target site on the posterior tibia. After satisfactory placement of the guide pin in an anatomic position, the tibial tunnel is drilled according to the measured diameter of the soft-tissue portion of the Achilles tendon allograft. A curet is inserted

through the anteromedial portal and used to cover the guide pin during reaming to prevent advancement into the posterior capsule. The reamer is advanced to the posterior tibial cortex using power and then breached by hand to allow greater control and prevent overpenetration.

Attention is then turned to the femoral tunnel. With the knee still flexed at 90°, a femoral PCL guide is placed at the anterior aspect of the native PCL footprint, which lies approximately 5

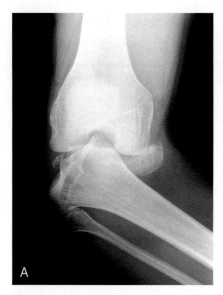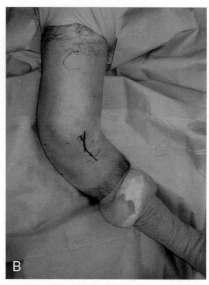

Figure 1 Knee dislocation. **A,** Preoperative AP view of a knee in extreme varus angulation. **B,** Clinical examination of an unstable knee in the operating room demonstrates gross lateral laxity with position of knee similar to that demonstrated in part A.

to 6 mm posterior to the medial femoral condyle articular margin. The guide pin is passed in a retrograde fashion through a small subvastus incision. The starting point is close to the medial trochlear cartilage, and care must be taken to avoid penetrating the articular cartilage during pin placement. The final diameter of the reamer must be accounted for during pin placement to prevent violation of the articular cartilage during drilling. After the guide pin is advanced into the joint, the tunnel is drilled to a diameter determined by the bone block of the Achilles allograft, which is typically 9 or 10 mm in diameter. Dilators can be used to ensure that the PCL graft will pass easily through both the femoral and tibial tunnels. Overdilation of the tunnels should be avoided.

ANTERIOR CRUCIATE LIGAMENT

The next step is the preparation of the ACL tunnels and then any collateral tunnels, followed by passage of the grafts. The ACL is fixed on the femoral side. The first step in establishing the ACL tunnels is removal of the soft tissue from the lateral wall with a shaver or curet to facilitate identification of

its posterior extent. Any remaining femoral or tibial ACL remnant is débrided using a 4.0- or 5.5-mm full-radius resector. Violation of the patellar fat pad with the shaver is avoided unless necessary for visualization, because this may result in increased scarring that could limit range of motion or cause pain postoperatively. The minimal notchplasty required to provide a clear view of the posterior aspect of the lateral wall of the femur is then made. If the PCL has been reconstructed, placement of the tibial guide pin must be referenced off the anterior root of the lateral meniscus and the center of the tibial spine. The center of the native ACL footprint also can be used. The tibial tunnels for both ACL and PCL reconstruction are accessed through the same anteromedial incision on the proximal tibia. The pin is advanced using a commercially available elbow or tip guide with the knee flexed 90°, allowing for a 1- to 2-cm bone bridge between tunnels on the anteromedial tibia. Again, the final reamer size must be taken into account during passage of the guide pin to leave a sufficient bone bridge. The ACL tibial tunnel is located proximal

and medial on the tibia relative to the PCL tunnel. After passage of the guide pin into the joint, the tibial tunnel is drilled according to the measured diameter of the tibial tendon allograft, which is typically between 7.5 and 8.5 mm.

The knee is then hyperflexed to 110°, and the femoral offset guide is inserted through the anteromedial portal. Proper positioning of the offset guide on the lateral wall is difficult to achieve with a transtibial approach. A small curet can be used to mark the desired orientation of the tunnel on the lateral wall before hyperflexion and placement of the offset guide to help confirm the correct starting point for the guide pin. For a right knee, the tunnel should be placed at the 10 to 11 o'clock position on the lateral wall. The opposite cortex of the femur is engaged but not penetrated by the guide pin, and a flip-button reamer is then advanced over the pin and through the cortex. The guide pin is removed, and a depth gauge is used to measure the length of the tunnel. To determine how far to drill the tunnel, the size of the flip button (15 mm recommended) is subtracted from the length of the femoral tunnel, and 8 mm is added to allow for flipping of the flip-button device. The femoral tunnel typically is drilled to a length of 25 to 30 mm.

For the PCL reconstruction, a malleable wire suture passer is advanced through the tibial tunnel and retrieved through the anteromedial portal. A suture relay is then passed in antegrade fashion through the tibial tunnel. The intra-articular portion of the suture relay is retrieved through the femoral tunnel with an arthroscopic loop grasper. The soft-tissue portion of the PCL graft is passed first through the femoral tunnel and then through the tibial tunnel so that the bone block rests firmly within the femoral tunnel. The graft is fixed on the femoral side with a 7 × 20-mm metal interference screw with the knee still flexed at 90°.

Tensioning of the graft and fixation on the tibial side is not done until after the ACL graft is secured on the femoral side and any other collateral grafts have been passed. An anterior drawer is applied so that the medial tibial plateau rests 10 mm anterior to the medial femoral condyle, which is the normal anatomic relationship. The graft is tensioned with the knee flexed 90°, and a bioabsorbable interference screw equal in diameter to the soft-tissue portion of the graft is then placed for tibial fixation. This can be reinforced with a staple or post at the surgeon's discretion.

After the PCL graft is fixed on the femoral side, the ACL is fixed on the femoral side. For placement of the ACL graft, a Beath pin is placed through the anteromedial portal through the femoral tunnel. A suture is then passed through the femoral tunnel and out the lateral thigh, and then a loop is retrieved through the tibial tunnel. The graft is then secured to the flip-button device and passed with the suture relay through the tibial tunnel and into the femoral tunnel with the knee flexed 90°. After the flip button is flipped, securing the graft on the femoral side, the PCL graft can be tensioned as described. The ACL graft is then tensioned with the knee in full extension with a bump under the knee and fixed using a bioabsorbable interference screw. Tibial fixation of the ACL graft can be reinforced with a staple or a post if desired.

LCL AND POSTEROLATERAL CORNER
Repair or reconstruction of the lateral structures is done after cruciate reconstruction, again noting that all of the preparation, including incisions, tunnels, and graft passage, has been done before tensioning of the cruciate ligaments. A curvilinear incision is made between the posterior edge of the iliotibial band and the biceps femoris tendon. The iliotibial band can be partially released at the Gerdy tubercle to improve exposure if necessary. The

peroneal nerve is identified posterior to the short head of the biceps tendon proximally and followed distally as it courses along the fibular neck. The nerve is protected and tagged with a vessel loop for easy identification during the lateral reconstruction (**Figure 2, A**). The LCL and popliteofibular ligament are then identified. For acute injuries (within 3 weeks), these structures can be repaired through drill holes in the fibular head with No. 2 high-strength nonabsorbable braided suture. The lateral and posterolateral capsular structures can be fixed with suture anchors into the proximal tibia because this is the area that typically avulses off in a posterolateral knee dislocation (**Figure 2, B**). Fibular head avulsions can be fixed with a screw and washer. If treatment is delayed, reconstruction usually is necessary. Anatomic reconstruction of the LCL and popliteofibular ligament is preferred. The LCL is reconstructed with an Achilles tendon allograft, with the bone block oriented horizontally in the femur placed at the native origin of the LCL just proximal and posterior to the femoral epicondyle. The graft is fixed in the tunnel with a 7 × 20-mm metal interference screw. The soft-tissue portion of the graft is tubularized with No. 2 heavy duty nonabsorbable suture. This is passed through the fibular head through an oblique drill hole, starting from posterior through the head just under the attachment of the biceps femoris and advancing anteroinferiorly (**Figure 2, C**). This graft is then fixed with an interference screw in the fibular head with the knee in approximately 30° of flexion and with a slight valgus force. The end of the graft is then brought up superiorly and tied to itself, thus reconstructing the LCL and approximating the popliteofibular ligament (**Figure 2, D**). An additional Achilles tendon graft is then used to reconstruct the popliteus tendon and is passed under the reconstructed LCL. The femoral drill hole for the poplit-

eus tendon is then made at its attachment at the top part of the sulcus. The bone block of the Achilles tendon graft is fixed with an interference screw. The soft-tissue graft is passed under the LCL and through a tunnel drilled in the tibia that starts posterolateral in the popliteal tibial sulcus and advances to the anterolateral tibia along the distal medial aspect of the Gerdy tubercle. This graft is fixed with an interference screw with the knee in approximately 30° of flexion with a valgus stress and internal rotation of the tibia. Both soft-tissue tunnels for the Achilles tendon grafts are approximately 7 to 8 mm in diameter.

MEDIAL COLLATERAL LIGAMENT
If MCL repair or reconstruction is planned, a curvilinear incision is made along the medial aspect of the knee. The infrapatellar branch of the saphenous nerve is identified and protected. Acute disruptions of the MCL can be repaired with No. 2 nonabsorbable braided suture or with suture anchors for femoral or tibial avulsions. Imbrication can be done if the ligament remains intact but is incompetent. For a chronic injury, the MCL should be reconstructed only if the ligament is completely disrupted and there is residual valgus laxity in full extension following cruciate reconstruction. The posterior oblique ligament can be identified along the posterior border of the superficial MCL and advanced anteriorly. The ligament is then sutured to the superficial MCL in a pants-over-vest fashion with 0 nonabsorbable braided suture with the knee in full extension. A tibial tendon allograft is used for MCL reconstruction. The femoral attachment is identified with a Kirschner wire in its location, which is at the medial epicondyle about 1 cm distal and anterior to the adductor tubercle. The isometry of this point can be checked with the graft placed around the wire and then brought down along the tibia to an area of attachment of the superficial

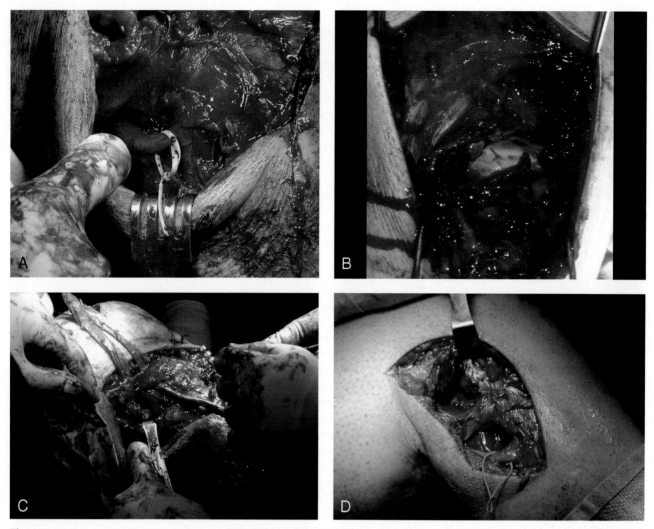

Figure 2 Intraoperative photographs demonstrate lateral reconstruction following knee dislocation. **A,** Identification and protection of the peroneal nerve. Note the blue vessel loop around the nerve to allow for identification during entire procedure. **B,** The lateral side of the joint demonstrates gross disruption of the capsule and ligamentous structures with exposed joint visible. **C,** The Achilles tendon allograft tissue strand is passed under the iliotibial band before passing it through the fibular head. **D,** The completed reconstruction of the LCL, with the iliotibial band retracted anteriorly and superiorly.

MCL just above the pes anserinus tendons. Once the appropriate area is identified, the femoral tunnel is drilled and either an interference screw or a flip-button device is passed through the lateral side for fixation. The doubled graft is then brought down and spread over the tibia and stapled into place with the knee in 30° of flexion and a varus force applied.

Wound Closure

After securing all grafts, the knee is moved through a range of motion and reexamined to ensure that the knee is stable. The wounds are copiously irrigated with antibiotic saline solution. The deep layer is closed with 0 braided absorbable suture, and the subcutaneous layer is closed with 2-0 braided absorbable suture. The skin is closed with a running subcuticular 3-0 monofilament suture, and adhesive strips are applied. Arthroscopy portals are closed with 3-0 nylon suture. The dorsalis pedis pulse is palpated to assess limb perfusion, and all compartments are palpated before application of a dressing. The wound is dressed with sterile adaptic, 4 × 4 gauze, and soft dressings and secured with a sterile cotton roll and a 6-in elastic bandage. Cryotherapy is used to reduce swelling, and the knee is placed in a hinged knee brace locked at 0° of extension.

━━━━━━━━━━━━■

Postoperative Regimen

After surgery, the patient is admitted overnight to the orthopaedic floor for observation. Deep vein thrombosis prophylaxis is reserved for high-risk patients. Initial rehabilitation goals focus on pain and edema control measures until sufficient wound healing has occurred. For the first 2 weeks after surgery, the knee remains in the hinged knee brace locked in extension. Initial range-of-motion goals focus on achieving full passive extension to 0°. Hyperextension is avoided in patients with PCL or posterolateral corner repair or reconstruction. Isometric quadriceps sets and straight-leg raises are permitted to promote firing of the quadriceps.

At 2 weeks postoperatively, passive range of motion is progressed to 90°. This represents a compromise between maintaining optimal tension of the grafts and avoiding arthrofibrosis. Active knee flexion is avoided for at least 6 weeks after surgery to prevent posteriorly directed forces on the tibia and thus protect the PCL graft, which has the greatest tendency to develop laxity in the early postoperative period. Patients with sedentary jobs are allowed to return to work at 2 weeks if desired.

Full weight bearing with crutches is allowed at 4 weeks after surgery. The brace is unlocked at 4 to 6 weeks postoperatively and discontinued by 6 to 8 weeks. The patient is weaned from crutches once full extension and at least 90° of knee flexion are achieved. Balance and proprioceptive training can then be initiated. Active-assisted range-of-motion exercises are started at 6 to 8 weeks to promote additional knee flexion. Strengthening at this point consists of closed-chain quadriceps and hamstring exercises and open-chain short-arc quadriceps exercises from 60° to 75° of flexion. Open-chain hamstring exercises are avoided for a total of 12 weeks.

Full symmetric knee flexion should be achieved by 3 months after surgery. Failure to achieve 90° of flex-ion at 3 months is an indication for manipulation under anesthesia. Return to low-impact activities such as cycling is allowed at about 6 to 8 weeks postoperatively. The patient may start a running program by 4 to 6 months if 80% quadriceps strength is achieved on functional testing. Manual laborers should not return to work for at least 6 months after surgery. Athletes may resume cutting or pivoting sports activity between 9 and 12 months.

Avoiding Pitfalls and Complications

Compromise of the soft-tissue envelope is common after traumatic knee dislocation. Surgical techniques that preserve the vascularity of the skin should be used whenever possible. Minimally invasive techniques, including arthroscopic and mini-open approaches, should be used. The use of allografts avoids any additional skin incisions required for graft harvesting. If an open approach is necessary, careful planning of incision placement is required to ensure that viable skin bridges are maintained. All arthroscopic procedures should be done under gravity inflow to prevent excess fluid extravasation that may result in a compartment syndrome of the leg or thigh. Compartments should be palpated periodically during any arthroscopic procedures. A tourniquet rarely is used because of the length of the procedure and potential vascular compromise that may already be present.

Neurovascular injury is common with knee dislocation. Injury to the popliteal artery or peroneal nerve may occur either at the time of dislocation or intraoperatively. Careful assessment and documentation of neurovas-cular status both pre- and postoperatively allow the injuries to be treated in a timely fashion and avoid any confusion about the timing of the neurovascular injury. The peroneal nerve is identified and protected during posterolateral corner repair or reconstruction, and the saphenous nerve is protected during the medial approach to the knee. Preparation of the tibial tunnel for PCL reconstruction presents a significant risk of popliteal artery injury. The use of fluoroscopy is essential during tunnel preparation to avoid arterial injury by overpenetration of the guide pin or reamer. A posteromedial arthroscopy portal and a 70° arthroscope are used to further aid in visualization of the posterior tibia. The use of PCL-specific guides or a curet is recommended to protect the posterior capsule during tunnel preparation. As an additional safeguard, the reamer can be advanced through the posterior tibial cortex by hand.

Proper graft tensioning is critical to minimize residual laxity after multiligament knee reconstruction. The PCL graft is tensioned first, with the knee in 90° of flexion. An anterior drawer maneuver is done during tensioning of the PCL graft so that the anteromedial border of the tibia is 10 mm anterior to the medial femoral condyle, thus recreating the anatomic tibiofemoral relationship. Next, the knee is brought into full extension to tension the ACL graft. The medial and lateral structures are tensioned last. Application of an internal rotation force on the tibia with the knee at 30° of flexion reduces the posterolateral corner before tensioning of the graft. The MCL graft is tensioned at 30° of flexion under a gentle varus stress. The knee is then moved through a range of motion and reexamined to confirm that all grafts are adequately fixed and appropriately tensioned.

■ Bibliography

Bin SI, Nam TS: Surgical outcome of 2-stage management of multiple knee ligament injuries after knee dislocation. *Arthroscopy* 2007;23(10):1066-1072.

Dedmond BT, Almekinders LC: Operative versus nonoperative treatment of knee dislocations: A meta-analysis. *Am J Knee Surg* 2001;14(1):33-38.

Fanelli GC, Edson CJ: Arthroscopically assisted combined anterior and posterior cruciate ligament reconstruction in the multiple ligament injured knee: 2- to 10-year follow-up. *Arthroscopy* 2002;18(7):703-714.

Goitz RJ, Tomaino MM: Management of peroneal nerve injuries associated with knee dislocations. *Am J Orthop* 2003; 32(1):14-16.

Harner CD, Waltrip RL, Bennett CH, Francis KA, Cole B, Irrgang JJ: Surgical management of knee dislocations. *J Bone Joint Surg Am* 2004;86(2):262-273.

Ibrahim SA, Ahmad FH, Salah M, Al Misfer AR, Ghaffer SA, Khirat S: Surgical management of traumatic knee dislocation. *Arthroscopy* 2008;24(2):178-187.

Mariani PP, Margheritini F, Camillieri G: One-stage arthroscopically assisted anterior and posterior cruciate ligament reconstruction. *Arthroscopy* 2001;17(7):700-707.

Mariani PP, Santoriello P, Iannone S, Condello V, Adriani E: Comparison of surgical treatments for knee dislocation. *Am J Knee Surg* 1999;12(4):214-221.

Mills WJ, Barei DP, McNair P: The value of the ankle-brachial index for diagnosing arterial injury after knee dislocation: A prospective study. *J Trauma* 2004;56(6):1261-1265.

Miranda FE, Dennis JW, Veldenz HC, Dovgan PS, Frykberg ER: Confirmation of the safety and accuracy of physical examination in the evaluation of knee dislocation for injury of the popliteal artery: A prospective study. *J Trauma* 2002;52(2):247-251, discussion 251-252.

Noyes FR, Barber-Westin SD: Reconstruction of the anterior and posterior cruciate ligaments after knee dislocation: Use of early protected postoperative motion to decrease arthrofibrosis. *Am J Sports Med* 1997;25(6):769-778.

Patterson BM, Agel J, Swiontkowski MF, Mackenzie EJ, Bosse MJ; LEAP Study Group: Knee dislocations with vascular injury: Outcomes in the Lower Extremity Assessment Project (LEAP) Study. *J Trauma* 2007;63(4):855-858.

Schenck RC Jr, Hunter RE, Ostrum RF, Perry CR: Knee dislocations. *Instr Course Lect* 1999;48:515-522.

Shapiro MS, Freedman EL: Allograft reconstruction of the anterior and posterior cruciate ligaments after traumatic knee dislocation. *Am J Sports Med* 1995;23(5):580-587.

Stannard JP, Sheils TM, Lopez-Ben RR, McGwin G Jr, Robinson JT, Volgas DA: Vascular injuries in knee dislocations: The role of physical examination in determining the need for arteriography. *J Bone Joint Surg Am* 2004;86-A(5):910-915.

Strobel MJ, Schulz MS, Petersen WJ, Eichhorn HJ: Combined anterior cruciate ligament, posterior cruciate ligament, and posterolateral corner reconstruction with autogenous hamstring grafts in chronic instabilities. *Arthroscopy* 2006;22(2): 182-192.

Wascher DC, Becker JR, Dexter JG, Blevins FT: Reconstruction of the anterior and posterior cruciate ligaments after knee dislocation: Results using fresh-frozen nonirradiated allografts. *Am J Sports Med* 1999;27(2):189-196.

Coding

CPT Codes		Corresponding ICD-9 Codes	
Open Fixation of Knee Dislocation			
27556	Open treatment of knee dislocation, includes internal fixation, when performed; without primary ligamentous repair or augmentation/reconstruction	717.81 84.2 836.0 996.42	717.9 836.50 905.6
27557	Open treatment of knee dislocation, includes internal fixation, when performed; with primary ligamentous repair	717.81 844.2 836.60 996.42	717.9 836.50 905.6
27558	Open treatment of knee dislocation, includes internal fixation, when performed; with primary ligamentous repair, with augmentation/reconstruction	717.81 844.2 836.60 996.42	717.9 836.50 905.6
Arthroscopic Posterior Cruciate Ligament Repair			
29889	Arthroscopically aided posterior cruciate ligament repair/augmentation or reconstruction	717.81 844.2 836.60 996.42	717.9 836.50 905.6
Arthroscopic Anterior Cruciate Ligament Repair			
29888	Arthroscopically aided anterior cruciate ligament repair/augmentation or reconstruction	717.81 844.2 836.60 996.42	717.9 836.50 905.6

Chapter 84
Complications of Knee Dislocations

Claude T. Moorman III, MD
Gregg T. Nicandri, MD

 Introduction

A traumatic knee dislocation is a rare event, accounting for less than 0.5% of joint dislocations and less than 0.02% of all orthopaedic injuries. The complications that result from either the injury itself or from the treatment of the injury can be quite devastating. Knee dislocations occur from a variety of mechanisms that can result in numerous patterns of bony, cartilaginous, capsular, and ligamentous disruption and often are associated with other severe injuries. Treatment therefore depends on the particular injuries involved.

Vascular Injury

The popliteal artery is tethered proximally by the adductor hiatus and distally by the soleus arch. A knee dislocation places this artery in a particularly vulnerable position. The incidence of popliteal artery injury following knee dislocation has been estimated to be as high as 32%. Delayed recognition (beyond 8 hours) of an occlusive injury is likely to result in an above-the-knee amputation, so timely recognition of this injury is of vital importance. Vascular injury should be suspected in a patient with multiligament knee injuries as a result of high-velocity trauma or in a morbidly obese patient (regardless of mechanism) because the incidence of vascular injury in these patients is estimated at 30% and 41%, respectively. Popliteal artery injury also can occur in a significant number of low-velocity injuries; therefore, the vascular status of the limb in every patient with known or suspected knee dislocation should be thoroughly evaluated.

A vascular evaluation protocol should approximate the algorithm shown in **Figure 1**. First, the pedal, posterior tibial, and popliteal pulses are palpated. Patients with hard physical signs of vascular injury (expanding hematoma, absent pulses, hemorrhage, or bruit) are taken to the operating room for immediate vascular repair. In some instances, the vascular surgeon may require an immediate on-table angiogram. It is important that arteriography be done on the operating table in these patients because the average time for formal study may delay management of the popliteal injury by as much as 3 hours. If the patient has no hard physical signs but does have a normal, symmetric pulse examination, ankle-brachial indices (ABIs) are determined. ABIs are important to obtain when evaluating the vascular status of the limb because significant vascular injury has been documented in the presence of palpable peripheral pulses. Patients who have asymmetric pulses or ABIs less than 0.90 should have immediate angiography to evaluate for vascular compromise. A conscious patient without hard signs of vascular injury, with normal pulse examination, and with ABIs greater than 0.90 can be observed for 24 hours. If surgical intervention on the extremity is anticipated, duplex ultrasound arteriography is used to confirm arterial patency and normal flow velocities.

If vascular injury is recognized, consultation and coordination with the vascular surgery team are indicated. The vascular and the orthopaedic surgical teams must work together to expedite and ensure protection of the vascular repair during multiligament knee reconstruction and rehabilitation. In stable patients, concurrent ligament repair or reconstruction can

Dr. Moorman or an immediate family member serves as a board member, owner, officer, or committee member of the Southern Orthopaedic Association; is a member of a speakers' bureau or has made paid presentations on behalf of Nutramax; has received research or institutional support from Histogenics, Stryker, Breg, and Mitek; and holds stock or stock options in Healthsport. Neither Dr. Nicandri nor any immediate family member has received anything of value from or owns stock in a commercial company or institution related directly or indirectly to the subject of this chapter.

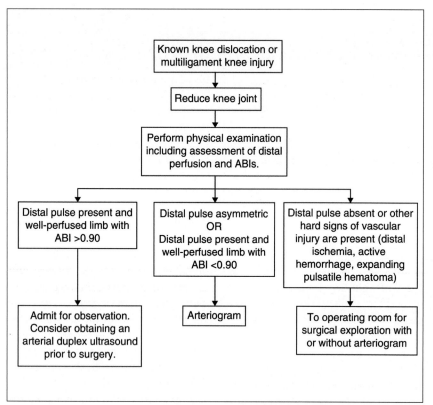

Figure 1 Algorithm used at Duke University Medical Center for the diagnosis of vascular injury following multiligament knee injuries. ABI = ankle-brachial index.

be considered at the time of the vascular repair. Regardless of when ligament reconstruction is done, the orthopaedic surgeon must avoid putting excessive tension on the vascular repair when manipulating the knee. After the orthopaedic procedure, the stability of the knee should be assessed; if concern exists that any remaining instability may compromise the vascular repair, external fixation should be considered. We recommend that the vascular surgeon who repaired the vascular injury be available at the time of ligamentous reconstruction to advise the orthopaedic surgeon about the anatomy of the vascular anastamosis, to assist should the vascular repair be compromised, and to assess the status of the vascular repair after the completion of the orthopaedic procedure.

Occlusion of the popliteal artery occasionally has been identified immediately after ligament reconstruction. This is thought to be the result of an unrecognized non–flow-limiting intimal tear that occurs at the time of the injury and that either progresses to a flow-limiting tear or results in thrombosis. The stasis that results from the use of a tourniquet can further increase the risk of occlusion when an unrecognized intimal tear is present or in patients who have had previous vascular reconstruction. For this reason, every effort is made to avoid the use of a tourniquet when operating on patients with multiligament knee injuries. Preoperative arteriography is recommended when the use of a tourniquet is considered a possibility.

Neurologic Injury

The peroneal nerve is at great risk for stretch injury at the time of knee dislocation because of its approximation to the neck of the fibula. Common peroneal nerve injury occurs most frequently with anterior and anteromedial dislocations that result in disruption of both cruciate ligaments and the posterolateral structures of the knee. The prevalence of this injury in association with knee dislocation is reported to be as high as 40%. The severity of the neurologic injury can vary from neurapraxia to complete disruption. Most often the injury is a result of traction, which leads to axonotmesis over a large segment of the nerve. In this case, the prognosis for full neural recovery is poor. A clinical examination must be performed at the time of injury to carefully document any sensory and motor deficits so that new injury or a progression of injury that occurs at the time of surgery can be differentiated from injury resulting from the initial trauma. Recovery also is compared with this initial clinical examination.

Most patients with peroneal nerve injuries require posterolateral corner repair or reconstruction. A complete neurolysis is done at the time of surgery to examine the extent of nerve injury. In acute injuries, the nerve can be difficult to identify because of the severe injury to the tissues surrounding the nerve. In chronic injuries, the nerve can be difficult to identify because of the significant scar tissue that encases the injured area. In either case, the nerve trunk is identified either proximally—outside the zone of injury, as it courses under the long head of the biceps femoris—or distally, just posterior to the origin of the peroneus longus from the fibular shaft. Once the nerve is identified, dissection proceeds slowly into the zone of injury until either both ends of a completely lacerated nerve are identi-

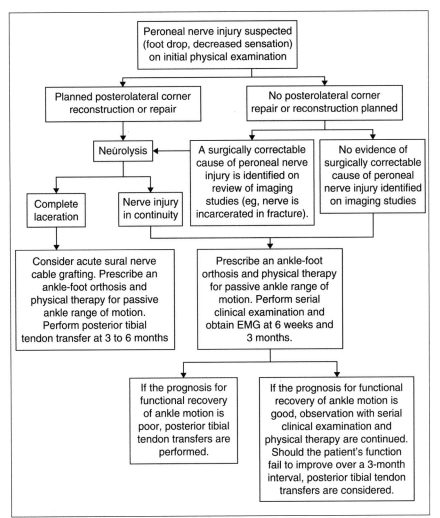

Figure 2 Algorithm used at Duke University Medical Center for the management of peroneal nerve injury following knee dislocation. EMG = electromyography.

For nerve injuries in continuity, which are more common than complete lacerations, we do not routinely perform nerve grafting. The extent of the injury and all sensory and motor deficits are carefully documented in the surgical report. Electromyographic evaluation generally is obtained at 6 weeks and 3 months after injury. If there is no evidence of recovery, either by clinical examination or electromyography, a posterior tibialis tendon transfer is considered. Although the potential for nerve recovery exists for up to 2 years after injury, the poor prognosis for complete functional recovery without surgery and the ankle flexibility and freedom that tendon transfers provide warrant consideration of early surgical intervention. If other injuries preclude a posterior tibial tendon transfer, the foot drop is managed with an ankle-foot orthosis.

In the rare cases where no posterolateral corner reconstruction is done despite the presence of a common peroneal nerve injury, a protocol similar to that for nerve injuries in continuity is followed. The nerve is not explored unless decompression is believed to increase the likelihood of functional recovery (eg, the nerve is incarcerated in a fracture). A treatment algorithm for managing peroneal nerve injury associated with knee dislocation is presented in **Figure 2**.

fied or the nerve is completely decompressed and freed of all attachments.

If the nerve is completely lacerated, an intraoperative consultation is obtained from a foot and ankle or hand specialist with expertise in nerve repair or grafting. Because these injuries often result from high-velocity trauma and traction, simple repair rarely is an option and sural nerve cable grafting is considered. Functional recovery has been reported in some series following this procedure, but this has not often been our experience. For this reason, we begin discussions with a foot and ankle specialist relatively early in the postoperative period for consideration of posterior tibial tendon transfer. In addition, some authors believe that the severe equinovarus deformity that often occurs after this injury presents a significant obstacle to reinnervation and that early correction of these forces may improve the chance of nerve recovery. The tendon transfer usually is done 3 to 6 months after the original ligament reconstruction. Following the tendon transfer, most of our patients eventually are able to ambulate with a nearly normal gait pattern without the assistance of an ankle-foot orthosis.

Deep Vein Thrombosis

Deep vein thrombosis (DVT) is a serious concern because of the severity of these injuries. In addition, knee dislocation patients are generally non–weight bearing for at least 6 weeks because of associated injuries. Our typical prophylactic protocol, based on the American Academy of Orthopaedic Surgeons' clinical guidelines for total knee arthroplasty, involves instructing patients to wear a compressive stocking and take 325 mg of enteric-coated aspirin twice daily for the entire period of restricted weight bearing. During the pre- and postoperative periods, if there is any suspicion of a DVT (eg, a report of calf pain or swelling), the patient is referred to the emergency department and undergoes a venous duplex ultrasound of the lower extremities.

If a DVT has been detected, we work with either the inpatient medical service or the patient's primary physician to ensure that the patient is appropriately treated. For further discussion about the diagnosis and treatment of DVT in patients who have knee surgery, see chapter 37.

Wound Breakdown and Infection

Knee dislocations are high-energy injuries that result in significant damage to the soft-tissue envelope surrounding the knee, increasing the patient's susceptibility to wound breakdown and infection. When evidence of severe cutaneous injury exists, surgery should be delayed until swelling decreases and blisters have resolved, indicating that the soft tissues have had time to begin healing. Incisions for multiligament knee reconstruction must be carefully planned to avoid incisions through significantly damaged tissue, multiple incisions that leave inadequate skin bridges, dissection that includes undermining of skin flaps, and closure resulting in excessive tension on the wound, all of which may increase the likelihood of breakdown. Postoperative infection is decreased with perioperative antibiotic coverage. Prophylactic intravenous antibiotic therapy is recommended before surgery and for 24 hours postopera-

tively. We generally use a weight-based dose of cefazolin, substituting clindamycin or vancomycin in patients who have allergies to cephalosporins.

When infection is suspected because of the presence of fever, swelling, warmth, or increased knee pain, laboratory studies (white blood cell count, erythrocyte sedimentation rate, and C-reactive protein level) are obtained. If the results of these tests and the clinical examination are contradictory or equivocal, an arthrocentesis is done and the joint fluid is sent to the laboratory for culture, cell count, and crystal analysis. When infection is identified, the patient is brought to the operating room immediately for open or arthroscopic débridement and lavage and then is treated postoperatively with culture-specific antibiotics as directed by consultation with the infectious disease team. With superficial and acute deep infections, we attempt to treat the infection with retention of the hardware and grafts. Should the infection be chronic or refractory to multiple attempts at irrigation and débridement, hardware and reconstructed ligaments are removed and treatment is individualized based on the severity of the infection, the condition of the soft tissues, the functional goals of the patient, and the recommendations of the infectious disease consultants.

Compartment Syndrome

Ischemic reperfusion injury after a vascular repair is a common cause of acute compartment syndrome in patients with knee dislocations. This complication is well known, and when ischemic time is thought to have exceeded 6 hours, prophylactic fasciotomies are done on all four compartments. In addition, knee disloca-

tions often are associated with significant capsular and fascial defects that, during arthroscopy, may result in fluid extravasation into the soft tissues, leading to compartment syndrome. To limit the likelihood of compartment syndrome, surgery should be delayed until the soft tissues have had an opportunity to heal, and the amount of time the joint is distended should be limited by using "dry scope" or open techniques and by avoiding high pump pressures.

Symptoms suggestive of compartment syndrome include a tense compartment, pain out of proportion to findings from the physical examination, an increasing narcotic requirement, and pain during passive extension of the toes or ankle dorsiflexion. If the clinical examination is equivocal or a patient is not responsive, direct measurement of intracompartmental pressures is indicated. Compartment pressures within 20 mm Hg of diastolic pressure are considered diagnostic of compartment syndrome, and fasciotomy is required. We typically use a single-incision fasciotomy.

Loss of Motion

For most activities of daily living, the functional range of knee motion is believed to be from 10° to 125°, and loss of this motion can be quite debilitating. Knee stiffness is a frequent complication after both nonsurgical and surgical treatment of knee dislocations. Manipulation under anesthesia or arthroscopic lysis of adhesions can be necessary for these patients to achieve adequate motion. The cause of stiffness generally is multifactorial and can be related to scarring—from the injury itself, surgery, or immobilization—as well as from inappropriately tensioned or malpositioned grafts. The type of reconstruction, the timing of surgery, and the graft choice all may play a role in the development of postoperative knee stiffness; however, this remains controversial. In general, we prefer early (within 3 weeks) reconstruction of all injured ligaments using autologous tissues when possible.

To prevent this complication, an individualized rehabilitation protocol must be formulated. The challenge of designing these programs is balancing the importance of restoring mobility of the knee joint with maintenance of the integrity of the reconstructed ligaments. Because of the complexity of the rehabilitation program, we always advise our patients preoperatively that participating in supervised physical therapy is essential for a successful outcome. Frequent visits to a physical therapist are necessary for at least the first 3 months postoperatively; a program that consists solely of at-home physical therapy is strongly discouraged. Initially, we focus on patient education to ensure that patients have an understanding of their limitations. The primary goal of physical therapy is to achieve full extension. The focus on extension is based on evidence that extension loss is poorly tolerated and tends to be more difficult to manage than loss of flexion; as little as 5° of extension loss can produce a noticeable limp and increase strain on the patellofemoral joint. Early range of motion is begun under the direction of a physical therapist with specific care to prevent posterior tibial sagging in patients who have undergone posterior cruciate ligament (PCL) reconstruction. Once patients have a complete understanding of their restrictions and can perform their exercises correctly in the presence of the therapist, they are instructed to continue passive range-of-motion exercises at home while wearing a hinged brace. Continuous passive motion (CPM) is not recommended in the hospital or at home in the immediate postoperative period because it may result in uncontrolled varus, valgus,

rotary, or posterior stresses to the reconstructed tissues.

In a patient with stiffness, tunnel malposition must be considered. AP and lateral radiographs are obtained, and when routine radiographs are inadequate, a CT or MRI scan is ordered. Newer MRI techniques are able to limit the artifact from hardware while allowing assessment of the soft tissues and other possible causes of stiffness.

If by 6 weeks the patient continues to have significant stiffness (defined as the inability to attain full knee extension or more than 90° of flexion despite the use of physical therapy), we consider examination under anesthesia and manipulation. After manipulation, these patients are hospitalized with an indwelling epidural catheter, and we use a dynamic extension splint to regain full knee extension or CPM to maintain the flexion obtained at the time of manipulation. Unlike in the immediate postoperative period, in the already stiff knee any uncontrolled forces that may occur as the result of CPM use will be unlikely to result in recurrent laxity, and the benefit of maintaining a functional knee range of motion outweighs this risk.

When stiffness persists despite previous manipulation or persists 3 months beyond the initial operation, we think that manipulation alone has a low likelihood of success and may cause further injury, such as chondral damage, periarticular fractures, and patellar or quadriceps tendon rupture. For these patients, arthroscopic lysis of adhesions and arthroscopic or open posterior capsular release are considered. The surgical treatment should include débridement of scar tissue from within the suprapatellar pouch and the medial and lateral gutters and an anterior interval release. If reduced or asymmetric patellar mobility persists, a lateral retinacular release or, rarely, a medial release, may be required. The intracondylar notch must be evaluated for notch stenosis or the possibility of a cyclops lesion. Signifi-

cant scar tissue or bony nodules that are identified in the notch should be removed, and an open or arthroscopic posterior release is done if significant extension loss persists despite arthroscopic lysis of adhesions (**Figure 3**).

―――――■

■ Recurrent Laxity or Instability

Recurrent laxity, particularly in association with PCL and posterolateral corner injuries, remains a problem in patients who have multiligament knee reconstruction. We believe that the best approach to these problems is prevention.

Protection of the reconstructed PCL is accomplished by preventing posterior tibial translation. To accomplish this, a towel or pad should be placed behind the proximal tibia in gravity-dependent positions, and passive knee flexion exercises should be done prone. All patients who undergo PCL reconstruction are restricted from active hamstring activation for the first 8 weeks, and resistive hamstring exercises are avoided until 12 weeks postoperatively.

Protection of the reconstructed posterolateral corner necessitates prevention of hyperextension, varus, and external rotation stresses. To accomplish this, the period of non–weight bearing is increased to 12 weeks, with particular attention paid to avoiding a varus thrust during gait training. For patients who have a neutral or varus alignment, a medial unloader brace is considered for up to 1 year postoperatively.

In a patient with graft laxity or failure, it is entirely possible that an injury was missed. Failure to treat combined injuries at the time of reconstruction increases the stress on the reconstructed ligament. If it is determined that a cruciate or collateral ligament injury was not treated appropriately at

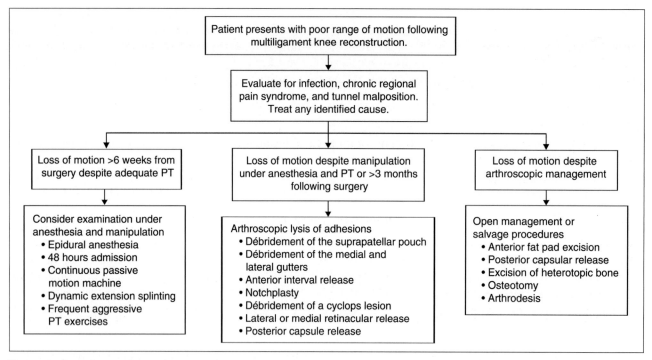

Figure 3 Algorithm used at Duke University Medical Center for the management of stiffness following multiligament knee surgery. PT = physical therapy.

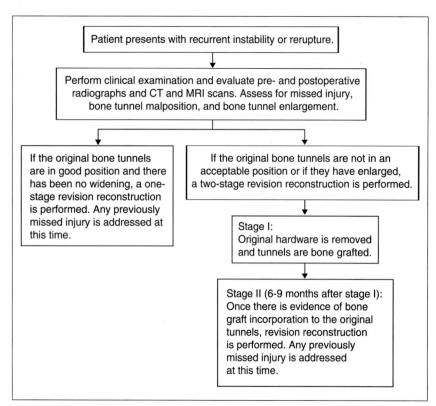

Figure 4 Algorithm used at Duke University Medical Center for the management of instability following multiligament knee reconstruction.

the time of initial reconstruction, it should be reconstructed at the time of revision surgery. Revision surgery can be done as a one- or two-stage procedure. In general, if previous tunnel position is adequate and no significant osteolysis has occurred, a one-stage procedure is done. If the original tunnels are not adequate for revision, the hardware should be removed and the previous tunnels débrided, and bone grafting is recommended. The second stage of reconstruction is done once the bone graft has been incorporated into the original tunnels, usually between 6 and 9 months after the first stage.

Occasionally, a patient sustains recurrent trauma to the previously affected knee and ruptures one or more of the reconstructed ligaments. The same evaluation is done as for the original injury, again ensuring adequate tunnel placement and no evidence of osteolysis before attempting a one-stage revision reconstruction **(Figure 4)**.

■ Bibliography

Carlisle JC, Parker RD, Matava MJ: Technical considerations in revision anterior cruciate ligament surgery. *J Knee Surg* 2007;20(4):312-322.

Cole BJ, Harner CD: The multiple ligament injured knee. *Clin Sports Med* 1999;18(1):241-262.

Ferraresi S, Garozzo D, Buffatti P: Common peroneal nerve injuries: Results with one-stage nerve repair and tendon transfer. *Neurosurg Rev* 2003;26(3):175-179.

Hegyes MS, Richardson MW, Miller MD: Knee dislocation: Complications of nonoperative and operative management. *Clin Sports Med* 2000;19(3):519-543.

LaPrade RF, Pedtke AC, Roethle ST: Arthroscopic posteromedial capsular release for knee flexion contractures. *Knee Surg Sports Traumatol Arthrosc* 2008;16(5):469-475.

Magit D, Wolff A, Sutton K, Medvecky MJ: Arthrofibrosis of the knee. *J Am Acad Orthop Surg* 2007;15(11):682-694.

Maheshwari R, Taitsman LA, Barei DP: Single-incision fasciotomy for compartmental syndrome of the leg in patients with diaphyseal tibial fractures. *J Orthop Trauma* 2008;22(10):723-730.

Medvecky MJ, Zazulak BT, Hewett TE: A multidisciplinary approach to the evaluation, reconstruction and rehabilitation of the multi-ligament injured athlete. *Sports Med* 2007;37(2):169-187.

Mills WJ, Barei DP, McNair P: The value of the ankle-brachial index for diagnosing arterial injury after knee dislocation: A prospective study. *J Trauma* 2004;56(6):1261-1265.

Niall DM, Nutton RW, Keating JF: Palsy of the common peroneal nerve after traumatic dislocation of the knee. *J Bone Joint Surg Br* 2005;87(5):664-667.

Patterson BM, Agel J, Swiontkowski MF, Mackenzie EJ, Bosse MJ, LEAP Study Group: Knee dislocations with vascular injury: Outcomes in the Lower Extremity Assessment Project (LEAP) Study. *J Trauma* 2007;63(4):855-858.

Seroyer ST, Musahl V, Harner CD: Management of the acute knee dislocation: The Pittsburgh experience. *Injury* 2008; 39(7):710-718.

Shelbourne KD, Porter DA, Clingman JA, McCarroll JR, Rettig AC: Low-velocity knee dislocation. *Orthop Rev* 1991; 20(11):995-1004.

Steadman JR, Dragoo JL, Hines SL, Briggs KK: Arthroscopic release for symptomatic scarring of the anterior interval of the knee. *Am J Sports Med* 2008;36(9):1763-1769.

Coding

CPT Codes		Corresponding ICD-9 Codes	
Knee Dislocation Repair/Reconstruction			
27420	Reconstruction of dislocating patella; (eg, Hauser type procedure)	836.5 905.6	836.6
27422	Reconstruction of dislocating patella; with extensor realignment and/or muscle advancement or release (eg, Campbell, Goldwaite type procedure)	836.5 905.6	836.6
27424	Reconstruction of dislocating patella; with patellectomy	836.5 905.6	836.6
27556	Open treatment of knee dislocation, includes internal fixation, when performed; without primary ligamentous repair or augmentation/reconstruction	836.5 905.6	836.6
27557	Open treatment of knee dislocation, includes internal fixation, when performed; with primary ligamentous repair	836.5 905.6	836.6
27558	Open treatment of knee dislocation, includes internal fixation, when performed; with primary ligamentous repair, with augmentation/reconstruction	836.5 905.6	836.6
Peroneal Nerve Repair			
64856	Suture of major peripheral nerve, arm or leg, except sciatic; including transposition	956.3	
64857	Suture of major peripheral nerve, arm or leg, except sciatic; without transposition	956.3	
Peroneal Tendon Repair			
27675	Repair, dislocating peroneal tendons; without fibular osteotomy	905.8	
27676	Repair, dislocating peroneal tendons; with fibular osteotomy	905.8	
Knee Manipulation			
27570	Manipulation of knee joint under general anesthesia (includes application of traction or other fixation devices)	836.5 905.6	836.6
Capsular Release, Open			
27435	Capsulotomy, posterior capsular release, knee	905.6	
Capsular Release, Arthroscopic			
29873	Arthroscopy, knee, surgical; with lateral release	905.6	
Arthroscopic Lysis of Adhesions			
29884	Arthroscopy, knee, surgical; with lysis of adhesions, with or without manipulation (separate procedure)	905.6	

CPT copyright © 2010 by the American Medical Association. All rights reserved.

Chapter 85

Meniscal Injuries: Overview and Management Strategies

Scott A. Rodeo, MD

 Introduction

Meniscal injuries are one of the most common types of injury seen by orthopaedic surgeons. The central principle in treating meniscal injuries is to preserve meniscal structure and function. This overview chapter reviews some general principles that apply to the management of meniscal injuries and provides "pearls" that may assist the clinician in treating these injuries.

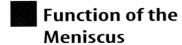

Function of the Meniscus

The primary function of the meniscus is load transmission across the tibiofemoral joint, which serves to decrease the contact stresses on articular cartilage. The viscoelastic properties of the meniscus, which result from swelling pressure afforded by proteoglycan and water in the matrix, give the meniscus the ability to act as a shock absorber. The lateral meniscus transmits approximately 70% of the load in the lateral compartment, and the medial meniscus transmits approximately 50% of the load in the

Dr. Rodeo or an immediate family member serves as a paid consultant to or is an employee of Wyeth; has received research or institutional support from Wyeth; and owns stock or stock options in Cayenne Medical.

medial compartment. A recent biomechanical study demonstrated a proportional increase in articular contact stress and decrease in contact area as more of the meniscus was excised. In a cadaver model using pressure-sensitive film, partial meniscectomy led to a 10% decrease in contact area and a 65% increase in peak local contact stresses. After total meniscectomy, contact areas decreased approximately 75%, and peak local contact stresses increased approximately 235%.

Another important function of the meniscus that is not as commonly recognized is its role in joint stability. The medial meniscus acts as a secondary restraint to anterior tibial translation in the anterior cruciate ligament (ACL)-deficient knee. The medial meniscus also contributes to valgus stability in the ACL-deficient knee. Other important functions of the meniscus include its role in articular cartilage lubrication, as well as proprioception via mechanoreceptors at the meniscocapsular attachments.

Clinical studies of patients following meniscectomy support these basic functions of the meniscus, with progressive degenerative joint disease. Degenerative changes progress more rapidly following total meniscectomy

than following partial meniscectomy. Also, degenerative changes progress more rapidly following lateral meniscectomy than following medial meniscectomy. Rapid development of lateral compartment arthrosis has been observed in particular following lateral meniscectomy in young patients with valgus alignment. These data provide a rationale for aggressive attempts to preserve the meniscus, especially on the lateral side.

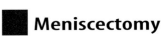

Meniscectomy

Excision of a torn meniscus is a very common orthopaedic surgical procedure. The primary factor that determines patient outcome is the degree of concomitant arthrosis. Clinical studies demonstrate successful outcomes in approximately 90% of patients with acute meniscal injury and/or minimal degenerative changes, whereas a successful outcome is seen in only approximately 60% to 70% of patients with degenerative meniscal tears. The primary goal in performing meniscectomy is to satisfactorily resect the torn meniscal segment while avoiding any damage to the articular surface. The surgeon should use the smallest instruments and shavers that allow efficient removal of the torn meniscus. Use of thermal devices is not recommended because of the

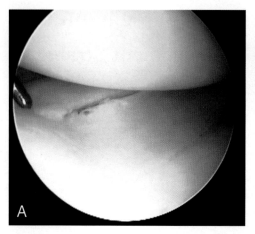

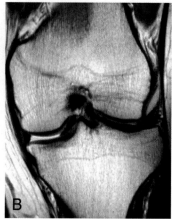

Figure 1 Arthroscopic view (**A**) and proton density–weighted MRI (**B**) demonstrate a vertical longitudinal tear in the vascular periphery of the meniscus. This type of tear is repairable.

Figure 2 Arthroscopic view of a radial tear that extends all the way to the capsule, disrupting the circumferential collagen fiber architecture of the meniscus.

risk of thermal injury to articular chondrocytes.

Types of Meniscal Tears

Accurate identification of the tear pattern provides information about the etiology of a tear, guides treatment, and even helps predict the outcome. For example, a vertical longitudinal tear pattern is commonly associated with ACL insufficiency and is typically repairable (**Figure 1**). A horizontal cleavage tear indicates degenerative meniscal tissue, which is not amenable to repair. A radial split tear often occurs in the lateral meniscus in young patients, and this pattern is tantamount to total meniscectomy if the tear extends all the way to the capsule, because it disrupts the circumferential collagen fiber architecture of the meniscus (**Figure 2**). Accordingly, attempts should be made to repair the inner vascular portion of a radial tear. A meniscal cyst is typically seen in a degenerative meniscal tear, and treatment requires complete decompression of the cyst with communication into the cyst cavity.

Meniscal Repair

Technique
Several suture techniques and implants are available for meniscal repair. Although specific repair techniques may be preferred for certain tear patterns and locations, any of the various techniques can be used to successfully repair a meniscus, and the choice of technique is often made based on surgeon preference and comfort with a specific device or technique. Regardless of the specific repair technique that is chosen, the most important factor is adherence to the basic principles of tear recognition, assessment of vascularity, preparation of the tissue for repair, and stable implant or suture placement. It is important to identify factors such as knee instability and malalignment that may adversely affect healing of the meniscus.

The meniscal tear should first be prepared by removal of any fibrinous material covering the torn meniscus, with abrasion of the adjacent synovium and capsule to stimulate a healing response. I prefer to use small rasps for this, taking care not to penetrate or damage the capsule to which the meniscus will be repaired. Whether sutures or an implant is used, the device should be placed so that it is perpendicular to the tear. A vertical mattress suture pattern is

stronger than a horizontal suture because the vertical mattress pattern better captures the circumferential collagen fiber bundles. Use of permanent suture is recommended for tears with poorer healing potential, such as tears with marginal vascularity or in older patients.

Other options include use of an exogenous fibrin clot or use of the commercially available techniques for isolating platelet-rich plasma (PRP) to provide serum-derived cytokines that may stimulate healing. A fibrin clot may be prepared by stirring whole blood with a glass rod with a roughened surface to which the clot will adhere (**Figure 3**). The clot has the consistency of chewing gum, allowing it to be secured to the meniscus with a suture. More recently, I have been using a platelet-rich fibrin matrix (PRFM) for isolated meniscus repair (**Figure 4**). This material isolates and concentrates platelets with their associated cytokines. The proprietary techniques for preparation of the PRFM or PRP avoid premature platelet activation and subsequent degranulation, thus allowing sustained release of higher concentrations of platelet-derived cytokines than a simple exogenous fibrin clot produced by stirring whole blood. The fibrin clot or PRP material can be attached to a suture at the tear site or simply inserted

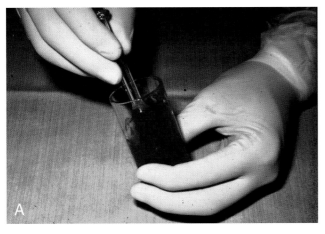

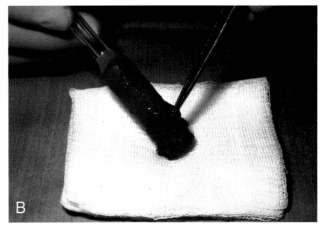

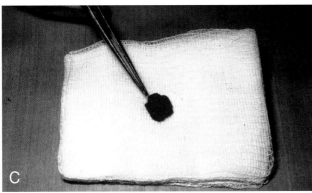

Figure 3 Preparation of a fibrin clot for meniscal repair. **A,** Whole blood is stirred using a glass rod with a rough surface. **B,** The fibrin clot adheres to the glass rod. **C,** The fibrin clot is ready for implantation at the meniscus repair site.

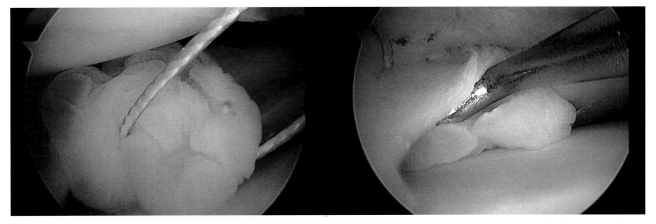

Figure 4 Arthroscopic views of platelet-rich fibrin matrix (PRFM) being placed at the meniscus repair site to augment healing.

beneath the meniscus at the repair site. I recommend attachment to a suture to secure the material at the repair site.

Special Tear Patterns

Several uncommon tear types require special consideration. A discoid lateral meniscus may be unstable because capsular attachments are absent. Although the traditional literature indicates that the attachment to the posterior capsule is usually deficient, I (and others) have seen anterior capsular detachments. Direct repair is recommended. The inner aspect of the meniscus is trimmed to restore more normal meniscal shape (saucerization) (**Figure 5**). A horizontal cleavage plane is often present within the discoid meniscus. The unstable tibial-side flap of meniscus may be resected in this setting.

Disruption of the popliteomeniscal fascicles that attach to the lateral meniscus can result in an unstable meniscus (**Figure 6**). This tear pattern is sometimes missed on MRI because the body of the meniscus will appear normal; however, the meniscus can be unstable and the patient may have mechanical symptoms. A formal repair of the posterior horn to the posterior capsule should be performed.

An uncommon tear is complete avulsion of the posterior horn from its tibial attachment. This tear should be repaired directly to bone with sutures through a drill hole (**Figure 7**).

Complications

One of the most significant complications that can occur with meniscal repair is nerve entrapment by suture or direct nerve injury by the passing needles. The saphenous nerve is at risk on the medial side. The outside-in technique is often used for repair of a tear in the mid-aspect of the medial meniscus, and at this level the saphenous nerve runs near the medial joint line. Furthermore, the outside-in technique is often done with just a small incision down to the capsule, which increases the risk to the saphenous nerve.

The peroneal nerve is at risk on the lateral side. Injury to the peroneal nerve can be avoided by maintaining the knee in flexion during needle passage across the meniscus, as flexion allows the peroneal nerve to fall posteriorly. It is also important to always stay anterior to the biceps tendon to avoid peroneal nerve injury. Careful placement of the posterior retractor when using the inside-out technique for lateral meniscus repair is critical for safe suture passage.

Although all-inside techniques have the advantage of less risk of nerve injury, there is still potential for injury to posterior neurovascular structures. All-inside techniques are typically used for far posterior tears, and needles passed across the posterior meniscus may pass close to the popliteal artery and vein. The depth of needle penetration needs to be controlled to avoid injury to the posterior neurovascular structures.

Articular cartilage injury is a potential complication that is most commonly related to abrasive damage from all-inside implants. Some of the available implants are composed of relatively rigid materials such as polylactic acid and can thus cause direct injury to the overlying articular surface. I prefer to use suture-based materials for meniscal repair for this rea-

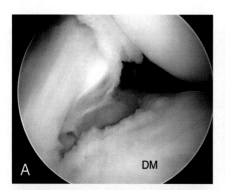

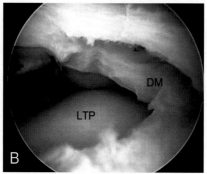

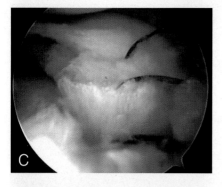

Figure 5 **A,** A complete discoid lateral meniscus. **B,** The lateral meniscus after saucerization. Note the horizontal cleavage tear within the meniscus. **C,** The discoid meniscus repaired to the capsule. DM = discoid meniscus, LTP = lateral tibial plateau.

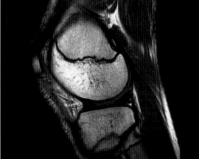

Figure 6 Sagittal proton density–weighted MRI demonstrates injury to the popliteomeniscal fascicle.

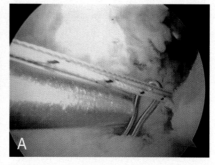

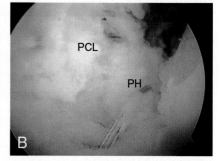

Figure 7 **A,** A passing wire is passed through a small drill hole in the tibial plateau to retrieve sutures passed through the avulsed posterior horn of the lateral meniscus. **B,** Posterior horn sutures in the drill hole in the tibia. PH = posterior horn lateral meniscus, PCL = posterior cruciate ligament.

son. To avoid articular cartilage injury, rigid implants should not be left excessively proud on the femoral surface of the meniscus (**Figure 8**).

Another potential complication is entrapment of the posterior capsule, resulting in a flexion contracture. This can occur if sutures are passed such that they capture and shorten the posterior capsule. The sutures should be tied with the knee near full extension to avoid this complication.

Rehabilitation

Information is lacking regarding the effect of mechanical load (magnitude and types of load) on the biology of meniscal healing. I typically prescribe partial weight bearing for the first 4 weeks following meniscal repair to protect the healing meniscus from excessive loads; however, I believe that the postoperative regimen can be modified for the specific type of meniscal tear. For example, with a vertical longitudinal tear, it may well be safe to bear weight after repair because compressive axial loads may coapt the tear. In contrast, with a radial tear, axial loads from weight bearing may cause distraction of the tear. I especially recommend a conservative rehabilitation regimen following repair of a complex tear or tears with poorer healing potential (eg, older patient age, chronic tears, or tears with marginal vascularity). Further studies are required to define the safe magnitudes

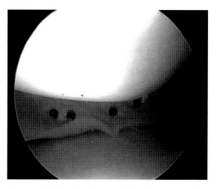

Figure 8 Meniscal repair implants on the femoral surface of the repaired meniscus. Such implants may damage the overlying femoral articular surface if they are left proud on the meniscus.

and types of load that will optimize meniscal healing.

Bibliography

Baratz ME, Fu FH, Mengato RL: Meniscal tears: The effect of meniscectomy and of repair on intraarticular contact areas and stress in the human knee. A preliminary report. *Am J Sports Med* 1986;14:270-275.

Cohen SB, Boyd L, Miller MD: Vascular risk associated with meniscal repair using Rapidloc versus FasT-Fix: Comparison of two all-inside meniscal devices. *J Knee Surg* 2007;20(3):235-240.

Good CR, Green DW, Griffith MH, Valen AW, Widmann RF, Rodeo SA: Arthroscopic treatment of symptomatic discoid meniscus in children: Classification, technique, and results. *Arthroscopy* 2007;23(2):157-163.

Lee SJ, Aadalen KJ, Malaviya P, et al: Tibiofemoral contact mechanics after serial medial meniscectomies in the human cadaveric knee. *Am J Sports Med* 2006;34(8):1334-1344.

Levy IM, Torzilli PA, Warren RF: The effect of medial meniscectomy on anterior-posterior motion of the knee. *J Bone Joint Surg Am* 1982;64(6):883-888.

Schimmer RC, Brülhart KB, Duff C, Glinz W: Arthroscopic partial meniscectomy: A 12-year follow-up and two-step evaluation of the long-term course. *Arthroscopy* 1998;14(2):136-142.

Yocum LA, Kerlan RK, Jobe FW, et al: Isolated lateral meniscectomy: A study of twenty-six patients with isolated tears. *J Bone Joint Surg Am* 1979;61(3):338-342.

Chapter 86

Arthroscopic Meniscectomy

Frederick M. Azar, MD
Robert H. Miller III, MD
Seth Rosenzweig, MD

Overview

Meniscal injuries are among the most common injuries treated by orthopaedic surgeons. Approximately 850,000 meniscal surgeries are done in the United States each year. Although many of these injuries occur in athletes, with an estimated rate of 61 injuries per 100,000 athletes annually, one large study that included more than 1,000 patients found that approximately 32% of meniscal injuries occurred with non-sports activities, 39% were sports related, and 29% of patients could not identify any specific event or incident for their injuries. In the past, meniscal tears were treated with complete meniscectomy because menisci were thought to be useless embryologic remnants. As evidence accumulated, however, regarding the important multiple functions of the menisci, meniscal preservation became a priority, and treatment advanced from open total meniscectomy to open partial meniscectomy and, ultimately, to arthroscopic partial meniscectomy.

Indications

Indications for arthroscopic treatment of meniscal injuries include (1) symptoms that affect activities of daily living, work, or sports activities (instability, locking, swelling, pain); (2) positive physical findings of joint line tenderness, joint effusion, limitation of motion, and provocative signs (pain with squatting, positive pinch test, positive McMurray test); (3) failure of nonsurgical treatment—including activity modification, medication, and physical therapy—to resolve or improve symptoms; and (4) exclusion of other causes of knee pain by patient history, physical examination, and imaging studies. Subtotal or total meniscectomy is justified only when the meniscus is irreparably torn, and the meniscal rim should be preserved if at all possible.

Contraindications

The few contraindications to arthroscopic mensicectomy include asymptomatic tears, local or remote infection, serious medical cormorbidities, and lack of appropriate equipment or experience. Relative contraindications include significant osteoarthritis and severe knee malalignment. Advanced age and excess weight or obesity have not been shown to be significant factors in determining the outcome of arthroscopic meniscectomy, and so they generally are not considered contraindications.

Alternative Treatments

Not all meniscal lesions require surgical treatment. Nonsurgical management, especially in older patients with minimal or no symptoms, includes activity modification, nonsteroidal anti-inflammatory drugs (NSAIDs), and

Dr. Azar or an immediate family member serves as a board member, owner, officer, or committee member of the American Board of Orthopaedic Surgery, the American Orthopaedic Society for Sports Medicine, the Arthroscopy Association of North America, and the American Academy of Orthopaedic Surgeons and has received research or institutional support from DePuy and Synthes. Neither of the following authors nor any immediate family member has received anything of value from or owns stock in a commercial company or institution related directly or indirectly to the subject of this chapter: Dr. Miller and Dr. Rosenzweig.

physical therapy. In an early study of nonsurgical treatment, only 6 of 52 patients with stable tears ultimately required surgery. A more recent study comparing surgical and nonsurgical treatment of degenerative meniscal tears in 26 patients with an average age of 48 years found that a significant percentage of patients improved enough with a 4-week course of NSAIDs to avoid meniscectomy. Although the Lysholm scores at 3-year follow-up were significantly better in the surgical group, the activities of daily living scores were not significantly better. In a prospective randomized study that included 90 patients 45 to 64 years of age with degenerative meniscal tears, arthroscopic partial medial meniscectomy combined with exercise did not produce greater improvement in symptoms than exercise alone. Several studies of meniscal tears in conjunction with anterior cruciate ligament injuries have documented good results with nonsurgical treatment of the meniscal lesions. However, a study of 58 recreational athletes with MRI-documented meniscal tears treated nonsurgically found at 2-year follow-up that 36 (62%) had undergone surgical treatment because of persistent symptoms; 26 (84%) of 31 patients treated surgically who were available for follow-up were able to resume sports at their preinjury level, compared with 15 (68%) of the 22 who underwent nonsurgical treatment.

Another alternative to meniscectomy is meniscal repair. The most common criteria for meniscal repair include (1) a vertical longitudinal tear more than 1 cm long located within the vascular zone, (2) a tear that is unstable and displaceable into the joint, (3) an informed and cooperative patient who is active and younger than 40 years, (4) a knee that either is stable or can be stabilized with a simultaneous ligamentous reconstruction, and (5) a bucket-handle portion and

remaining meniscal rim that are in good condition. If repair is not possible, meniscectomy is indicated.

———————■

Results

Subjective results of arthroscopic partial meniscectomy have been consistently favorable, ranging from about 80% to 95% good to excellent results (**Table 1**); objective results have not been as good. Some reports also have noted that osteoarthritic changes develop or accelerate in knee joints after meniscectomy; however, the radiographic changes reported after arthroscopic partial meniscectomy appear to be minimal in most patients and to have little effect on patient function or satisfaction. No correlation has been proven between the development or worsening of osteoarthritis and age, sex, or body mass index of the patient. Some studies have found worse outcomes after medial partial meniscectomy than after lateral meniscectomy, whereas others have noted no significant differences. ACL-deficient knees have been cited as being associated with worse results than ACL-stable knees.

Partial meniscectomy has long been considered to be superior to total meniscectomy because it may result in less degeneration of the knee joint. However, a prospective, randomized study involving 182 patients found no significant difference at 8-year follow-up between the functional results of those with partial meniscectomy and those with total meniscectomy, although those with partial meniscectomy had significantly higher Lysholm scores. Also, no significant radiographic differences between the two groups were observed at either 6- or 10-year follow-up. A more recent comparison of partial and total meniscectomy in 36 patients found no difference in knee function at 14-year follow-up, but radiographic

changes were more common after total meniscectomy (13 of 18 patients) than after partial meniscectomy (6 of 18 patients).

———————■

Technique

Preoperative Planning

The goal of the meniscectomy is to leave an intact, balanced, peripheral rim of meniscus. This can increase the stability of the joint and protect the articular surface by its load-bearing functions. The amount of meniscectomy can be classified as partial, subtotal, or total.

Partial meniscectomy involves excision of only the loose, unstable meniscal fragments, such as the displaceable inner edge in bucket-handle tears or the flaps in flap tears or in oblique tears. In partial meniscectomies, a stable and balanced peripheral rim of healthy meniscal tissue is preserved.

Subtotal meniscectomy is most commonly required for complex or degenerative tears of the posterior horn of either meniscus. Resection of the involved portion by necessity extends out to and includes the peripheral rim of the meniscus. Generally, most of the anterior horn and a portion of the middle third of the meniscus are not resected.

Total meniscectomy is required when the meniscus is detached from its peripheral meniscosynovial attachment, and intrameniscal damage and tears are extensive. If the body of the peripherally detached meniscus is salvageable, total meniscectomy is not warranted, and meniscal repair should be considered.

Procedure

LATERAL MENISCAL TEARS

Most lateral meniscal excisions or repairs are done with the knee in the figure-of-4 position (**Figure 1**) or the crossed-leg sitting position. The foot of the table can be flexed or extended.

Table 1 Results of Arthroscopic Meniscectomy

Authors (Year)	Number of Knees	Procedure	Mean Patient Age in Years (Range)	Mean Follow-up (Range)	Results
Osti et al (1994)	41 (athletes)	Arthroscopic partial lateral meniscectomy	26 years (17-40)	3 years (2-5)	85% excellent/good results 98% of athletes returned to full sports activities at average of 55 days.
Burks et al (1997)	146	Arthroscopic partial meniscectomy (medial/lateral)	36 years	15 years (14-16)	88% (97/111) good results in ACL-stable knees 58% (17/35) good results in ACL-deficient knees
Higuchi et al (2000)	67	Arthroscopic partial meniscectomy (medial/lateral)	27 years (8-52)	12 years (10-16)	79% (53) satisfactory, 21% (14) unsatisfactory 55% able to return to same level of activity, 8% at higher level, 37% at lower level "Mild" radiographic deterioration in 48%
Chatain et al (2001)	317	Arthroscopic medial meniscectomy	38 years (11-66)	11.5 years (10-15)	91% regarded knee as normal or nearly normal. 96% very satisfied or satisfied with results IKDC scores: 60% pain-free, 87% could perform moderate activities with no pain
Hoser et al (2001)	31	Arthroscopic partial lateral meniscectomy	43 years	10 years (9-12)	Lysholm scores excellent/good in 18 (58%), fair in 5 (16%), poor in 8 (26%) High rate of degenerative changes and frequent reoperation (29%)
Hulet et al (2001)	74 ("stable" knees)	Arthroscopic medial meniscectomy	36 years	12 years	95% satisfied or very satisfied 57% had grade A function and 43% had grade B. At 5 years, 53% had returned to sporting activities.
Scheller et al (2001)	75	Arthroscopic partial lateral meniscectomy	41 years	10 years (5-15)	Lysholm scores excellent/good in 77% Radiographic changes in 78%
Bonneux and Vandekerckhove (2002)	31	Arthroscopic partial lateral meniscectomy	25 years	8 years	IKDC scores excellent/good in 48% Lysholm scores excellent/good in 65% Tegner scores dropped from 7.2 to 5.7. Fairbank changes noted in 93%.
Camanho et al (2006)	435	Arthroscopic meniscectomy	59 years	4 years	Good results in 363 (84%), poor results in 71 (16%) Results worse with degenerative tears than with traumatic injuries
Herrlin et al (2007)	90	Arthroscopic partial medial meniscectomy (47) or supervised exercise (43)	56 years	6 months	Both groups had decreased knee pain, improved knee function, and high satisfaction rates. Meniscectomy did not produce improved results over exercise alone.
Bin et al (2008)	68 (with grade IV OA)	Arthroscopic medial meniscectomy	63 years (51-77)	52 months (37-83)	Mean VAS decreased from 7 to 3. Mean Lysholm score increased from 66 to 83. 4 (6%) required TKA at average of 50 (range, 20-75) months.

ACL = anterior cruciate ligament, IKDC = International Knee Documentation Committee, OA = osteoarthritis, VAS = visual analog scale, TKA = total knee arthroplasty.

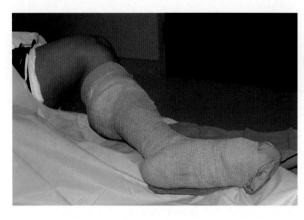

Figure 1 Photograph shows the figure-of-4 position, used to apply varus force to the flexed knee to widen the lateral compartment. (Reproduced with permission from Phillips BB: Arthroscopy of the lower extremity, in Canale ST, Beaty JH, eds: *Campbell's Operative Orthopaedics*, ed 11. Philadelphia, PA, Elsevier, 2008, pp 2811-2922.)

The hip is slightly flexed, abducted, and externally rotated, while the knee is flexed to 30° to 90° and the tibia is internally rotated. The figure-of-4 position also can reduce overall joint distention by collapsing the suprapatellar pouch, making viewing and the use of suction and motorized cutters and trimmers in the lateral compartment more difficult. Inflow through the arthroscopic sheath allows the best visualization.

BUCKET-HANDLE TEARS

A probe or a blunt trocar can be used to reduce the meniscal fragment to its normal position (**Figure 2**). With the fragment back in its anatomic position, the small remaining attachments can be assessed much more accurately. Beginning posteriorly, the meniscal fragment is almost completely detached with basket forceps, scissors, a shaver, or an arthroscopic knife. This cut should not be done blindly, to avoid harm to the normal meniscus, articular cartilage, or both. Exposure can be aided by passing the arthroscope through the intercondylar notch to look down onto the posterior horn of the meniscus while cutting, or a posteromedial portal can be made if necessary to look directly down onto the meniscus for visualization or to pass through the posterior compartment for cutting of the meniscus (**Figure 3**). A small tag of meniscal tissue is left intact posteriorly to prevent the meniscus from floating freely in the posterior compartment after anterior release. The anterior horn attachment is divided with angled scissors, basket forceps, or an arthroscopic knife.

The release of the anterior attachment should be flush with the intact anterior rim so that no stump remains. If the approach is difficult from the ipsilateral portal, changing portal sites and approaching from the contralateral portal with the operating instrument often facilitates making this cut. A hemostat is used to dilate the capsular incision before attempting menis-

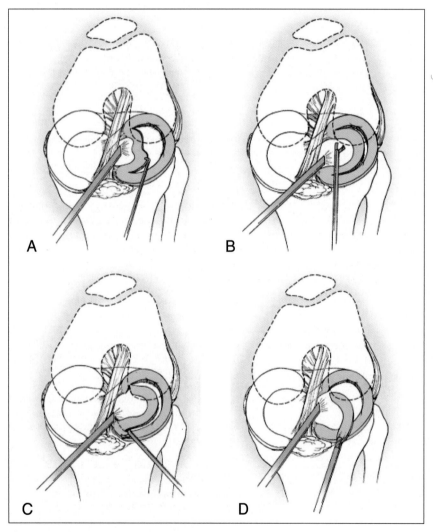

Figure 2 Drawings show the two-portal technique for arthroscopic partial meniscectomy for a bucket-handle tear of the lateral meniscus. **A,** The tear is probed. **B,** After reduction of the tear, the posterior attachment is partially released with scissors. **C,** The anterior attachment is released with scissors. **D,** The tenuous remaining posterior attachment is avulsed with a grasper and extracted. (Reproduced with permission from Phillips BB: Arthroscopy of the lower extremity, in Canale ST, Beaty JH, eds: *Campbell's Operative Orthopaedics*, ed 11. Philadelphia, PA, Elsevier, 2008, pp 2811-2922.)

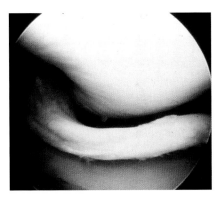

Figure 3 Arthroscopic view of a bucket-handle meniscal tear.

cal removal. A grasping clamp is inserted through the ipsilateral portal to grasp the meniscal fragment as close to its remaining posterior attachment as possible. With the meniscal fragment in view, the grasping forceps are twisted and rotated at least two revolutions while traction is applied to avulse the small bridge previously created. If the meniscal fragment does not come loose as planned, a grasper can be used through the lateral portal for traction on the meniscus, and arthroscopic scissors can be passed through the same portal to complete the resection posteriorly. If it is still difficult with this technique, an accessory portal can be made 1 cm medial to the anteromedial portal using the spinal needle. The other option is to make an accessory midpatellar portal for the arthroscope, using the two anterior portals for instrumentation. The fragment should be observed as it exits the joint to ensure complete removal. Occasionally, the fragment is so large that it lodges within the subcutaneous tissues. In these circumstances, the skin incision may have to be enlarged to deliver the fragment.

If there are no additional tears, a motorized meniscal shaver is used to smooth the remaining rim. Before the procedure is completed, the posterior compartment should be examined with either a 30° or 70° arthroscope inserted through the intercondylar notch, or a 30° oblique arthroscope inserted through the corresponding posterior portal.

LONGITUDINAL INCOMPLETE INTRAMENISCAL TEARS

Longitudinal incomplete intrameniscal tears may extend from the superior surface into the body of the meniscus or may enter from the inferior surface. These often are extremely difficult to view and treat. This type of tear is commonly located in the posterior horn of the meniscus and may be only a few millimeters long. By the time such a tear extends more than 1 or 2 cm, it usually becomes complete and often displaceable. Usually, a significant amount of stress must be applied to the knee to open up the appropriate compartment to view small tears. The first sign of such a tear may be a wrinkled or buckled inner meniscal border. If the incomplete tear begins from the superior surface, the probe tip passes into it, but not through to the inferior surface. Inferior incomplete tears are even more difficult to view and explore, especially in a tight knee. The tip of the probe passes into the inferior tear, but not through to the superior surface of the meniscus. Vigorous attempts to hook the probe into an unseen inferior tear should be avoided because of the danger of extending the tear. If such a tear exists, gentle probing can make the inner border of the meniscus buckle and evert.

The technique for resecting this tear is similar to that for bucket-handle tears. A 15° up-biting low-profile basket can facilitate removal of a posterior horn tear. The resection is performed through the ipsilateral portal, trimming back to a stable contoured peripheral rim (**Figure 4**).

HORIZONTAL, OBLIQUE, RADIAL, AND COMPLEX TEARS

When resecting horizontal, oblique, radial, and complex tears, it is imperative to evaluate and remove only damaged tissue and maintain functional, healthy meniscal tissue (**Figure 5**). With horizontal tears of long-term duration, a meniscal cyst may be present; this usually is evident on preoperative MRI. Generally, the superior and the inferior leaves are resected back to relatively normal stable tissue (**Figure 6**). The cleft should be probed. If a meniscal cyst is present, a small curved curet, placed through the cleft and aimed toward the surgeon's finger on the exterior extent of the meniscal cyst, can be used to open the cyst and drain it into the knee. A shaver or suction also can be used to open and decompress the cyst. A spinal needle placed exteriorly to enter the cyst is helpful for localizing the cyst.

With flap tears, the flap often is rolled up under the normal portion of the meniscus, and its size and contour are not apparent. Some flaps are posterior to the femoral condyle; careful examination of the posterior compartments is necessary to fully evaluate these tears (**Figure 7**). Resection of a flap tear or a complex tear generally is accomplished with a basket forceps to morcellize the tear and careful probing to ensure that the meniscal tissue remaining is of relatively normal contour with a smooth transition at its edges.

Radial tears can be partial or complete. A partial-depth radial tear of the meniscus is treated with saucerization, balancing, and contouring of the edges. Complete radial tears that go to the meniscosynovial junction are difficult problems. Some authors recommend horizontal mattress repair of the peripheral portion of the meniscus because resection would result in loss of the functional protective mechanism of the meniscus.

PARTIAL EXCISION OF DISCOID MENISCUS

The objective of partial excision of a discoid meniscus is to remove the central portion, leaving a balanced rim of meniscus about the width of the normal lateral meniscus. The width is dic-

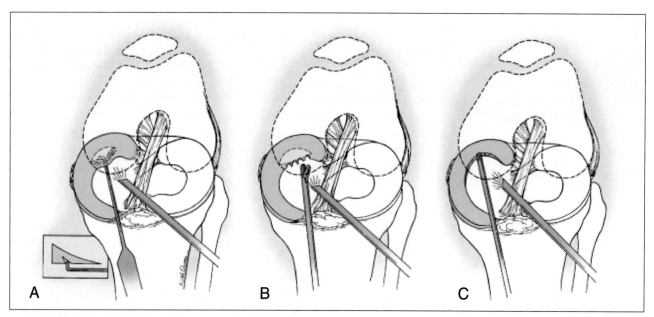

Figure 4 Drawings show the technique for arthroscopic partial meniscectomy for a longitudinal incomplete intrameniscal tear. **A,** The tear is probed. **B,** Fragment is removed bit by bit with basket forceps. **C,** The rim is smoothed and contoured with a motorized trimmer. (Reproduced with permission from Phillips BB: Arthroscopy of the lower extremity, in Canale ST, Beaty JH, eds: *Campbell's Operative Orthopaedics*, ed 11. Philadelphia, PA, Elsevier, 2008, pp 2811-2922.)

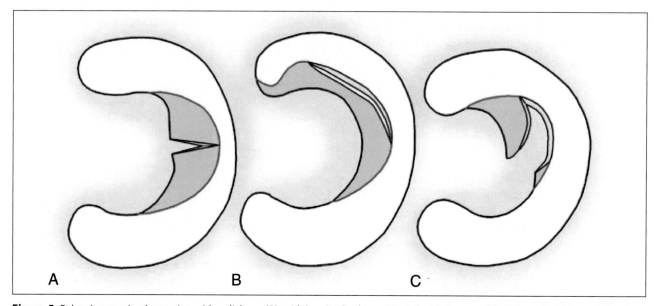

Figure 5 Balancing meniscal resection with radial tear (**A**), with longitudinal tear (**B**), and with flap tear (**C**). (Adapted with permission from Newman AP, Daniels AU, Burks RT: Principles and decision making in meniscal surgery. *Arthroscopy* 1993;9:33-51.)

tated, however, by the location and extent of the tear within the meniscus. If the free inner edge of the meniscus is not noted in the systematic diagnostic arthroscopy of the lateral compartment, a discoid lateral meniscus may be responsible. The tibial plateau may be completely covered by the meniscus, and the lateral compartment may appear to be devoid of a lateral meniscus; alternatively, varying portions may be covered (**Figure** 8). If a discoid meniscus is suspected, exploration should be focused more centrally in the lateral compartment or near the intercondylar eminence to search for a free meniscal edge (**Figure** 9).

Postoperative Regimen

Several postoperative rehabilitation protocols have been described for patients with arthroscopic meniscectomy, but all have the same primary objectives: decreasing inflammation, restoring motion, increasing strength, and facilitating a safe return to activity. Basic principles of rehabilitation include no range-of-motion restrictions

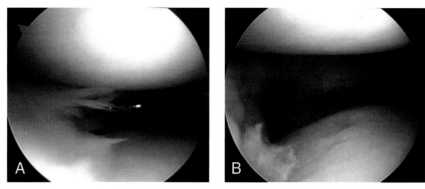

Figure 6 Arthroscopic views of a horizontal cleavage tear before (**A**) and after (**B**) partial meniscectomy.

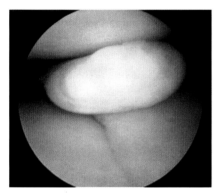

Figure 7 Arthroscopic view of a radial flap tear of the meniscus.

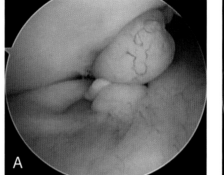
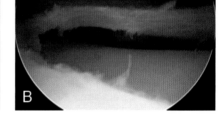

Figure 8 Arthroscopic views of a discoid meniscus before (**A**) and after (**B**) partial meniscectomy.

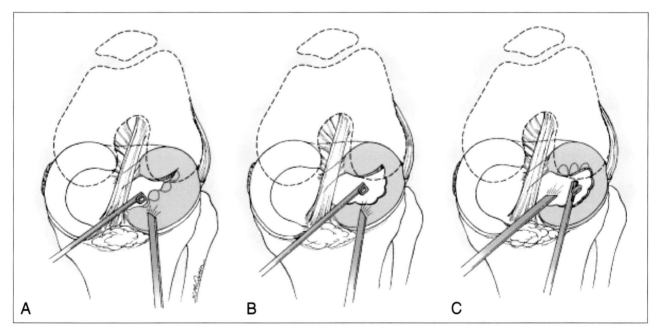

Figure 9 Drawings show the technique for excision of discoid lateral meniscus. **A,** The anterior portion of discoid lateral meniscus is removed with rotary basket forceps. **B,** The anterior rim is contoured with a 90° rotary basket forceps. **C,** The posterior discoid fragment is removed with a basket forceps. (Reproduced with permission from Phillips BB: Arthroscopy of the lower extremity, in Canale ST, Beaty JH, eds: *Campbell's Operative Orthopaedics*, ed 11. Philadelphia, PA, Elsevier, 2008, pp 2811-2922.)

or bracing; immediate, full weight bearing with crutches as needed; icing of the knee for 20 minutes every 2 to 3 hours while awake; NSAIDs at 2 weeks if not contraindicated; and active, passive, and active-assisted range-of-motion exercises and straight-leg raising exercises immediately postoperatively. Return to sports is allowed when the following are achieved: full range of motion, no effusion, and 80% strength compared with the uninjured leg. This usually occurs at 4 to 6 weeks after surgery.

Avoiding Pitfalls and Complications

Early reports of knee arthroscopy documented complication rates as high as 1.4%, primarily from fluid extrasavation; improved instrumentation and techniques have made this type of complication rare. Other reported complications include infection; deep vein thrombosis, with or without pulmonary embolism; recurrent effusions; synovial-cutaneous and arteriovenous fistulas; osteonecrosis; and nerve injury. These generally are isolated case reports, and the frequency of these complications is very low (<0.1%).

Most complications of arthroscopic meniscectomy can be avoided by careful attention to detail. Preserving the meniscal rim and avoiding aggressive resection of the meniscal capsule will help prevent hemarthrosis. Avoiding the use of a tourniquet also is helpful because then sources of excessive bleeding are apparent during the procedure, allowing the use of a coagulation device to stop intra-articular bleeding before the surgery is completed. The popliteal artery is at risk during meniscectomy when intercondylar attachments are cut using a posteromedial or posterolateral portal.

Nerve injuries can be caused by direct trauma from a scalpel or sharp trocar, mechanical compression or compression from fluid extravasation, or prolonged ischemia from excessive tourniquet use. Many complications can be avoided by marking portals appropriately, making sure the scalpel penetrates the skin only, using a hemostat to spread down to the joint capsule in proximity to a nerve, and routinely using blunt trocars. Maintaining proper joint distention and distraction, padding nerve and bony prominences, and proper patient positioning also greatly reduce the chances of nerve complications.

Thromboembolic complications have been associated with prolonged tourniquet times (> 60 minutes), duration of surgery, patients older than 50 years, and a history of deep vein thrombosis. Minimizing surgical and tourniquet times, avoiding postoperative immobilization, and using thrombophylaxis may be beneficial in patients at risk of thromboembolic complications.

The use of prophylactic antibiotics is still controversial. A retrospective review of 3,231 arthroscopic knee surgeries, of which 2,780 were arthroscopic meniscectomies, found infection rates of 0.15% in those who received antibiotics and 0.16% in those who did not. Prophylactic antibiotics may be appropriate for reducing the risk of infection in high-risk patients such as those with diabetes, immune problems, and skin disorders; nevertheless, they are still used routinely in most meniscectomies.

Herniation of small fat globules and synovial tissue may occur through any arthroscopic portal; generally, the larger the portal, the greater likelihood of this complication. Synovial fistulas are rare, but they can follow suture reactions or stitch abscesses. Portals should be sutured routinely rather than closed with adhesive strips. If a synovial fistula develops, the patient should receive antibiotics and the knee should be immobilized for to 7 to 10 days to allow the fistula to close spontaneously.

Bibliography

Andersson-Molina H, Karlsson H, Rockborn P: Arthroscopic partial and total meniscectomy: A long-term follow-up study with matched controls. *Arthroscopy* 2002;18(2):183-189.

Bin SI, Lee SH, Kim CW, Kim TH, Lee DH: Results of arthroscopic medial meniscectomy in patients with grade IV osteoarthritis of the medial compartment. *Arthroscopy* 2008;24(3):264-268.

Bonneux I, Vandekerckhove B: Arthroscopic partial lateral meniscectomy long-term results in athletes. *Acta Orthop Belg* 2002;68(4):356-361.

Burks RT, Metcalf MH, Metcalf RW: Fifteen-year follow-up of arthroscopic partial meniscectomy. *Arthroscopy* 1997; 13(6):673-679.

Camanho GL, Hernandez AJ, Bitar AC, Demange MK, Camanho LF: Results of meniscectomy for treatment of isolated meniscal injuries: Correlation between results and etiology of injury. *Clinics (Sao Paulo)* 2006;61(2):133-138.

Chatain F, Robinson AH, Adeleine P, Chambat P, Neyret P: The natural history of the knee following arthroscopic medial meniscectomy. *Knee Surg Sports Traumatol Arthrosc* 2001;9(1):15-18.

Hede A, Larsen E, Sandberg H: Partial versus total meniscectomy: A prospective, randomised study with long-term follow-up. *J Bone Joint Surg Br* 1992;74(1):118-121.

Herrlin S, Hållander M, Wange P, Weidenhielm L, Werner S: Arthroscopic or conservative treatment of degenerative medial meniscal tears: A prospective randomised trial. *Knee Surg Sports Traumatol Arthrosc* 2007;15(4):393-401.

Higuchi H, Kimura M, Shirakura K, Terauchi M, Takagishi K: Factors affecting long-term results after arthroscopic partial meniscectomy. *Clin Orthop Relat Res* 2000;377:161-168.

Hoser C, Fink C, Brown C, Reichkendler M, Hackl W, Bartlett J: Long-term results of arthroscopic partial lateral meniscectomy in knees without associated damage. *J Bone Joint Surg Br* 2001;83(4):513-516.

Hulet CH, Locker BG, Schiltz D, Texier A, Tallier E, Vielpeau CH: Arthroscopic medial meniscectomy on stable knees. *J Bone Joint Surg Br* 2001;83(1):29-32.

Marder RA, Moehring HD: Nonoperative treatment of MRI-documented meniscal tears in recreational athletes. *Clin J Sports Med* 1994;4:151-216.

McNicholas MJ, Rowley DI, McGurty D, et al: Total meniscectomy in adolescence: A thirty-year follow-up. *J Bone Joint Surg Br* 2000;82(2):217-221.

Osti L, Liu SH, Raskin A, Merlo F, Bocchi L: Partial lateral meniscectomy in athletes. *Arthroscopy* 1994;10(4):424-430.

Pearse EO, Craig DM: Partial meniscectomy in the presence of severe osteoarthritis does not hasten the symptomatic progression of osteoarthritis. *Arthroscopy* 2003;19(9):963-968.

Reigstad O, Grimsgaard C: Complications in knee arthroscopy. *Knee Surg Sports Traumatol Arthrosc* 2006;14(5):473-477.

Rimington T, Mallik K, Evans D, Mroczek K, Reider B: A prospective study of the nonoperative treatment of degenerative meniscus tears. *Orthopedics* 2009;32(8):pii http://www.orthosupersite.com/view.aspx?rid=41915.

Scheller G, Sobau C, Bülow JU: Arthroscopic partial lateral meniscectomy in an otherwise normal knee: Clinical, functional, and radiographic results of a long-term follow-up study. *Arthroscopy* 2001;17(9):946-952.

Weiss CB, Lundberg M, Hamberg P, DeHaven KE, Gillquist J: Non-operative treatment of meniscal tears. *J Bone Joint Surg Am* 1989;71(6):811-822.

Coding

CPT Codes		Corresponding ICD-9 Codes	
Arthroscopic Meniscectomy			
29880	Arthroscopy, knee, surgical; with meniscectomy (medial AND lateral, including any meniscal shaving)	836.0 836.2	836.1
29881	Arthroscopy, knee, surgical; with meniscectomy (medial OR lateral, including any meniscal shaving)	836.0 836.2	836.1
Arthroscopic Meniscal Repair			
29882	Arthroscopy, knee, surgical; with meniscus repair (medial OR lateral)	836.0 836.2	836.1
29883	Arthroscopy, knee, surgical; with meniscus repair (medial AND lateral)	836.0 836.2	836.1

CPT copyright © 2010 by the American Medical Association. All rights reserved.

Chapter 87
Meniscal Repair: All-Inside Technique

Annunziato Amendola, MD
Davide Edoardo Bonasia, MD

Overview

In 1991, Morgan described the first all-inside technique for the treatment of posterior horn meniscal tears. This method used a hook passer and a monofilament absorbable suture that could be tied with an arthroscopic knot technique. Because the indications were limited and the technique was demanding, it did not become popular. With the increasing emphasis on preservation of the meniscus and the development of new meniscal repair devices over the past several years, the all-inside technique has now become a widely performed procedure. Clinical studies have demonstrated satisfactory healing rates when all-inside techniques are used with the appropriate indications. The most commonly used all-inside devices can be described as sutureless devices, hybrid suture devices, and suture devices.

Sutureless devices include staples, cross-bar devices, screws, and barbed devices of different shapes and sizes.

All of them are bioabsorbable and most are made of polylactic acid (PLA). The newest sutureless devices have a low-profile design that allows them to be completely covered by meniscal tissue, which reduces the risk of chondral damage.

Hybrid suture devices were designed to reproduce fixation similar to horizontal and vertical sutures, the latter long considered to be the strongest meniscal fixation method. The hybrid devices are made of absorbable or nonabsorbable pre-tied sliding sutures connected at the edges with bioabsorbable bars or caps. Because they are pre-tied, they do not require arthroscopic knot-tying techniques during surgery.

Suture devices are all-suture devices. Some come with pre-tied knots; others require an arthroscopic knot-tying technique.

Currently the most widely used devices are the hybrid sutures and some low-profile sutureless devices.

———————■

Indications

Management of meniscal tears usually requires a three-step decision process. The first step is to determine whether a surgical or nonsurgical method of treatment is appropriate. Meniscal tears usually are treated surgically when the knee is painful or swollen, catching or locking is present, and clinical and MRI findings are positive for a meniscal tear.

Once surgery is indicated, the next step is deciding between meniscectomy and repair. The choice depends primarily on the suitability of the tear for repair (eg, type and location of the meniscal tear), but also on the patient's age, activity level, and associated knee pathologies. Repair is generally indicated when (1) the patient is younger than 40 years, active, and compliant; (2) the knee is stable and has neutral axial alignment; (3) the tear pattern is acute, nondegenerative, and vertical-longitudinal; (4) a full-thickness tear longer than 10 mm is present; and (5) the tear is located in the vascular meniscal zone (red-red or red-white).

These indications are relative. Some partial-thickness tears or tears in patients older than 40 years can be repaired.

The last step is to choose an all-inside technique, an inside-out or outside-in technique, or a hybrid

Dr. Amendola or an immediate family member serves as a board member, owner, officer, or committee member of the Arthroscopy Association of North America and the International Society of Arthroscopy, Knee Surgery and Orthopaedic Sports Medicine; has received royalties from Arthrex; is a member of a speakers' bureau or has made paid presentations on behalf of Genzyme and the Musculoskeletal Transplant Foundation; serves as a paid consultant to or is an employee of Arthrex, Arthrosurface, and Link Orthopaedics; has received research or institutional support from Arthrosurface; and owns stock or stock options in Arthrosurface. Neither Dr. Bonasia nor an immediate family member has received anything of value from or owns stock in a commercial company or institution related directly or indirectly to the subject of this chapter.

approach. The ideal indications for all-inside suture repair, because of lower neurovascular injury risks, are posterior horn and some midportion meniscal tears. Tears must be reducible, and healthy meniscal tissue should be present on either side of the tear to allow fixation.

Contraindications

Meniscal surgery is generally not indicated for older patients with arthritis unless they engage in high-demand activities or have persistent mechanical pain unresponsive to physical therapy; asymptomatic patients with positive MRI findings, but without provocative signs (painless squatting or negative McMurray and Apley grind tests); short (<10 mm), stable vertical-longitudinal tears (in stable knees, they may heal spontaneously), especially in the presence of anterior cruciate ligament (ACL) reconstruction; and stable partial-thickness (<50%) tears (in stable knees they may heal spontaneously).

In an athlete, however, the indications are somewhat different. It may be prudent to enhance healing of partial tears or small tears with synovial abrasion or multiple punctures and to repair with all-inside suturing so that the tear will not propagate when sports activities are resumed.

When surgery for meniscal pathology is required, repair is generally contraindicated if the patient is older than 40 years or is not compliant; tears have a chronic or degenerative pattern; the knee is unstable and a simultaneous ligament reconstruction is not planned; the tear pattern is oblique, radial, or horizontal (although repairs of radial and oblique tears have been described, the outcomes are controversial); or the tear is located in the avascular white-white zone (>5 mm from the periphery).

If meniscal repair is required, an all-inside technique is contraindicated when tears are located in the anterior horn of the meniscus. Although techniques have been described for all-inside anterior horn repair, the lower neurovascular injury risk makes the outside-in technique preferable for these tears.

Alternative Treatments

When surgery is contraindicated, treatment may include cryotherapy, rest, nonsteroidal anti-inflammatory medication, and physical therapy, mainly based on muscle stretching and strengthening and knee proprioception.

Partial meniscectomy is still performed frequently in spite of the fact that altered knee biomechanical function and an increased risk of chondral deterioration are associated with this procedure. Even if a meniscal repair is feasible, partial meniscectomy may be preferable in certain situations when a quicker recovery is desired.

Total meniscectomy, open or arthroscopic, is currently an obsolete technique. Open meniscal repair also is uncommon, but it may be indicated if an arthrotomy of the knee is required for treatment of associated pathology (eg, tibial plateau fractures or multiple knee ligament injuries) or for anterior or posterior meniscal root avulsions.

Results

Both biomechanical and clinical results should be considered for all-inside meniscal repair techniques. These two issues are closely related,

because the higher the strength of fixation, the higher the clinical success rates. Many biomechanical multi-device studies have been reported in the literature. A few of them are summarized in **Table 1**. Although these studies attempted to identify the strongest fixation devices, they are not comprehensive, and it is difficult to compare results because each study uses a different type of testing protocol. What can be inferred from them, however, is that the latest generation devices have fixation strengths equal to or greater than vertical mattress sutures, which are considered the gold standard for meniscal repair.

What is still concerning about all-inside techniques is the clinical outcome. Clinical studies report failure rates ranging from 0% to 43.5% (**Table 2**). These failure rates range widely for most devices, however, and no randomized controlled trials or long-term follow-up series are available. Furthermore, studies have different methods of follow-up evaluation—clinical findings, MRI, and second-look arthroscopy. Second-look arthroscopy is probably the only reliable method for assessing healing or failure in a meniscal repair. MRI does not always show small unhealed tears, and physical examination can be negative with a failed repair. Another limitation of these studies is the different rates of associated ACL reconstruction. It has been shown that ACL reconstruction combined with meniscal repair increases meniscal healing rates, so results may be biased by different rates of concomitant ACL procedures. Advantages of the all-inside technique include shorter surgical time, easy device insertion, better cosmetic result, and a lower risk of neurovascular injury than with the inside-out technique.

Reported complications related to meniscal devices include implant migration (predominantly with the Meniscus Arrow, Clearfix Screws, and

Table 1 Results of Biomechanical Studies of All-Inside Meniscal Repair

Authors (Year)	Type of Test	Results*
Barber and Herbert (2000)	Failure strength (porcine model)	Double vertical suture: 113 N (2-0 Mersilene): 113 N Single vertical suture: (2-0 Mersilene): 80 N BioStinger: 57 N Horizontal mattress suture (2-0 Mersilene): 56 N T-Fix: 50 N Meniscus Arrow: 33 N Clearfix Screw: 32 N SDsorb Meniscal Staple: 31 N Mitek Meniscal Repair System: 30 N Biomet Meniscal Staple: 27 N
Bellemans et al (2002)	Cyclic loading (human fresh frozen menisci model)	Horizontal mattress suture (PDS-1): 53 N Vertical loop suture (PDS-1): 46 N T-Fix: 48 N Meniscus Arrow (16 mm): 39 N Meniscus Arrow (13 mm): 33 N Mitek Meniscal Repair System: 18 N Meniscus Arrow (10 mm): 19 N Arthrex Meniscal Dart: 11 N SDsorb Meniscal Staple: 4.3 N
Zantop et al (2005)	Failure strength after 1,000 cycles (bovine model)	Vertical FasT-Fix: 94 N Horizontal FasT-Fix: 81 N Vertical suture (2-0 Ethibond): 71 N Horizontal suture (2-0 Ethibond): 50 N RapidLoc: 30 N
Chang et al (2005)	Load-to-failure and cyclic testing (porcine model)	Vertical FasT-Fix: 146 N Vertical mattress suture (VMS 0): 133 N Meniscal Viper Repair System: 111 N

*Manufacturer information: Mersilene, PDS, Ethibond, and VMS: Ethicon, Somerville, NJ; Bio-Stinger: Linvatec, Largo, FL; T-Fix: Acufex Microsurgical, Inc, Mansfield, MA; Meniscus Arrow: Bionx Implants, Malvern, PA; Clearfix screw: Innovasive Devices, Marlborough, MA; SDsorb meniscal staple: Surgical Dynamics, Norwalk, CT; Mitek meniscal repair system: Mitek, Westwood, MA; Biomet meniscal staple: Biomet, Warsaw, IN; Arthrex Meniscal Dart: Arthrex Inc., Naples, FL; FasT-Fix: Smith & Nephew, Inc., Andover, MA; RapidLoc: DePuy Mitek, Raynham, MA; Meniscal Viper Repair System: Arthrex, Naples, FL.

BioStinger tacks), chondral injuries due to device migration or failed resorption (Arrow, RapidLoc, Bio-Stinger, Mitek Fastener, and Clearfix Screw), broken devices, foreign body reactions, penetration through superficial structures (skin, iliotibial band, medial collateral ligament), and inflammatory reaction to PLA. The last issue worth considering is the higher cost of all-inside implants compared to classic sutures.

Given the mechanical strength of the construct and the higher healing rates described in the literature, the inside-out vertical mattress suture appears to be the best method for meniscal repair; however, all-inside techniques, particularly the hybrid approach, may be more appropriate for very posterior tears because of the proximity of these tears to neurovascular structures.

▪ Techniques

Setup/Patient Positioning
The patient is placed supine with the affected leg in a leg holder. Regional or general anesthesia provides better muscle relaxation and is preferable to local anesthesia. Avoiding tourniquet use reduces the risk of deep vein thrombosis, allows earlier quadriceps recovery, and allows evaluation of tear vascularity during the procedure. A standard arthroscopic surgical field is prepared. Gravity flow is safer and inexpensive, but sometimes a constant flow and pressure pump are helpful to better visualize structures.

Instruments/Equipment/ Implants Required
A standard arthroscopic instrument set, 30° and 70° arthroscopes, and a motorized shaver are needed. A standard anterolateral portal is made 1 cm above the lateral joint line, and a standard anteromedial portal is made 1 cm above the medial joint line and medial to the edge of the patellar tendon. A diagnostic arthroscopic examination of the entire knee is done, and then the meniscal tear is carefully evaluated and probed (**Figure 1**). The arthroscope should be placed through the ipsilateral portal and the instruments through the contralateral one. For tears extending near the posterior horn root, access with instruments is easier through the ipsilateral portal. The knee should be held in slight flexion with valgus stress to better view the medial meniscus and in 90° of flexion with varus stress (Cabot or figure-of-4 position) for viewing the lateral meniscus.

Meniscal Bed Preparation
Before fixation, meniscal bed preparation is mandatory. A small shaver can be used to débride the loose edge and the synovium above the tear to produce bleeding down onto the tear. A meniscal rasp also can be used to prepare the peripheral rim. Trephination

Table 2 Clinical Results for Commonly Used Meniscal Repair Devices

Author(s)/Year	Device*	No. of Meniscal Repairs	Mean Patient Age (Years)	Mean Follow-up (Months)	Failure Rate
Venkatachalam et al (2001)	T-Fix	7	28	21	42.9%
	Meniscus Arrow (Bionx)	23	28	21	43.5%
Jones et al (2002)	Meniscus Arrow (Bionx)	39	29.9	29.7	5.1%
Laprell et al (2002)	Mitek Meniscal Repair System	37	27.3	12	13.5%
Kocabey et al 2004	T-Fix	55	26.7	10.3	1.8%
Barber et al (2005)	BioStinger	47	27	26.5	9%
Frosch et al (2005)	Meniscus Screws (Clearfix)	40	27.7	17.6	10%
Haas et al (2005)	FasT-Fix	37	27	24.3	14%
Hantes et al (2005)	Meniscus Screws (Clearfix)	48	32.7	19	25%
Oberlander and Chisar (2005)	Polysorb Meniscal Stapler XLS	11	35.6	30	0%
Barber and Coons (2006)	BioStinger	41	29.8	38.6	4.9%
Hantes et al (2006)	RapidLoc	20	25	22	35%
Kotsovolos et al (2006)	FasT-Fix	61	32.6	18	9.8%
Quinby et al (2006)	RapidLoc	54	24	34.8	9.3%

*Manufacturer information: Polysorb Meniscal Stapler XLS: USS Sports Medicine, Norwalk, CT; BioStinger: Linvatec, Largo, FL; FasT-Fix: Smith & Nephew, Andover, MA; Mitek Meniscal Repair System: Mitek, Westwood, MA; Clearfix screw: Innovasive Devices, Marlborough, MA; RapidLoc: DePuy Mitek, Raynham, MA; T-Fix: Acufex Microsurgical, Mansfield, MA; Meniscus Arrow: Bionx Implants, Malvern, PA.

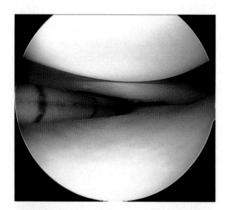

Figure 1 Measurement of the tear and its distance from the meniscal periphery with a calipered probe.

should be used to improve blood supply and fibrovascular tissue ingrowth in less vascularized zones to promote meniscal tear healing (**Figure 2**). This technique consists of making small perpendicular perforations with a large spinal needle or a small trephine from the tear site to the peripheral, vascularized zone of the meniscus.

Other techniques have been described to improve healing and meniscal cartilage ingrowth in more central and unstable tears: fibrin clot and exogenous fibrin glue placement, synovial abrasion, bone marrow stimula-

tion (eg, microfractures in the intercondylar notch, mesenchymal cells), and use of growth factors. After meniscal bed preparation is completed, the meniscal tear is repaired.

Repair

Techniques differ substantially depending on the device used for the repair, but some general principles are applicable to all. First, if associated ligamentous surgery is needed, we prefer to repair the meniscus first. A cannula, usually provided with the specific instrument set, should always

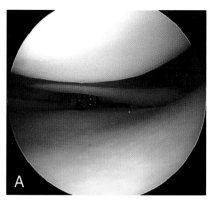
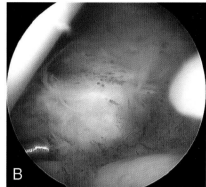
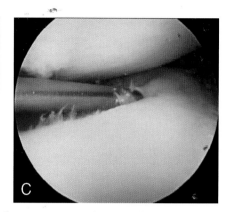

Figure 2 Preparation of the meniscal bed. **A,** Rasping of the edges of the tear. **B,** Bleeding after rasping. **C,** Trephination of the edges of the tear with a spinal needle.

be used to avoid entrapment of the device or its delivery system in the soft tissues and to prevent the early delivery of the device itself.

When using a tack, the correct size of the device should be determined first by measuring the distance from the capsule to the tear with a calipered probe and deciding the entrance point for the repair. This can prevent the tack from being too prominent inside the joint or outside the capsule (**Figure 3**). To protect the articular cartilage and reduce the risk of chondral damage, the device should be placed parallel to the tibial plateau and the tack should be completely covered by meniscal tissue before the delivery system is removed when this is allowed by the specific surgical technique.

When using a hybrid suture device, the distance between the periphery of the meniscus and the entry point selected should be measured (**Figure 1**). Most devices have a depth limiter on the handle or as a separate cannula that should be set before starting the repair. If the device chosen has an intra-articular rigid component (eg, Mitek RapidLoc), this should be well sunk in meniscal tissue and parallel to the tibial surface to reduce the risk of chondral injury. When placing a vertical suture, it is easier to place the first anchor superior and the second inferior. When a bar is released in the cap-

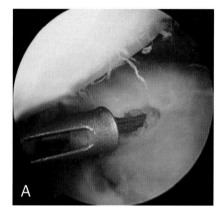
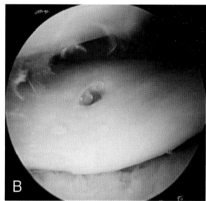

Figure 3 Insertion of a tack device. **A,** The tack is inserted. **B,** The head of the tack device is slightly proud to the articular surface.

sular tissue, the strength of the fixation should always be tested by pulling on the suture. Finally, it is important not to cut the sutures before all implants are placed, so that tension can be adjusted as needed.

Special Situations

Unusual or unexpected situations, such as the avulsion of a meniscal root, may require more demanding techniques (**Figure 4**). For a vertical meniscal tear extending from the anterior to the posterior root of the meniscus, a hybrid technique can be useful (**Figure 5**).

■ **Postoperative Regimen**

Rehabilitation protocols vary widely. Although in the past rehabilitation programs were cautious, with immobilization and non–weight bearing for 4 to 6 weeks, accelerated rehabilitation is now preferred. Active motion in a hinged brace (0° to 90°) is allowed immediately. Full weight bearing and muscular strengthening are permitted as soon as tolerated. At 4 weeks, the brace usually is removed and unrestricted range of motion is started. Running is permitted at 2 to 3 months, and return to sport activities is usually allowed 4 to 5 months after surgery,

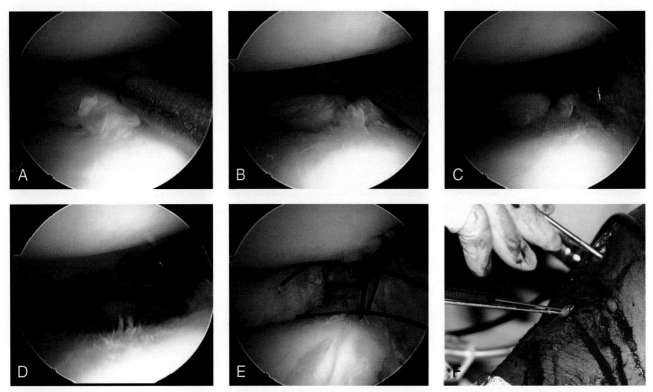

Figure 4 Technique for repair of posterior meniscal root avulsion. **A,** The lateral compartment reveals a complete avulsion of the posterior root. **B,** An ACL guide is used to make two drill holes from the anteromedial tibia into the posterior root insertion area. **C,** The drill tip is shown entering the joint in the desired position. **D,** A Caspari suture punch is used to place two sutures through the posterior root of the meniscus. **E,** Each meniscal suture is passed in its respective tibial tunnel with a Houston suture passer. **F,** Leading sutures are tied together on the anteromedial tibia.

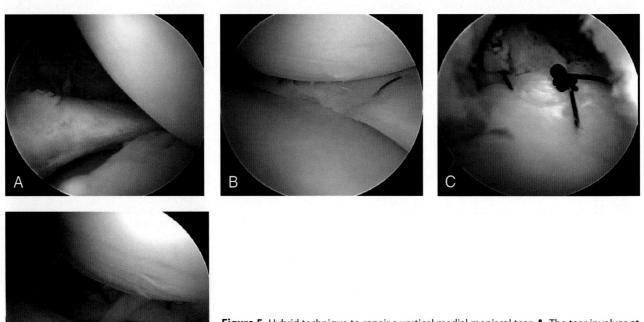

Figure 5 Hybrid technique to repair a vertical medial meniscal tear. **A,** The tear involves at least two thirds of the meniscus. **B,** A posteromedial approach is made, the neurovascular structures are protected with a spoon retractor, and vertical mattress sutures are placed with an inside-out technique. **C,** The most posterior part of the tear is fixed with an all-inside technique. In this case, two 2-0 polydioxanone (PDS) sutures were placed with a hooked suture passer. **D,** Once all sutures are placed, they can be tied.

when proprioception of the affected limb is equal to that of the contralateral limb. Accelerated programs have not demonstrated lower healing rates than more cautious ones.

Rehabilitation programs should be individualized for each patient. The protocol used depends on the type, location, and stability of the tear; fixation; tissue quality; and patient activity level. After repair of a very unstable tear (eg, a bucket-handle tear), a hinged knee brace in full extension is worn for 2 weeks with full weight bearing. Range of motion is increased to 0° to 90° at 2 weeks after surgery. At 6 weeks, 0° to 120° of motion is allowed. At 3 months, full motion, bicycling, and running are permitted. At 6 months, the patient can return to pivoting sports.

If the meniscal tear is stable, a different rehabilitation program is followed. Early motion from 0° to 90° and crutch-protected weight bearing are allowed for the first 6 weeks and then progressed to 0° to 120° of motion with full weight bearing until the third month. At 3 months, free motion, bicycling, and running are permitted. At 6 months, the patient can return to pivoting sports.

More accelerated programs are designed for professional athletes with particular demands.

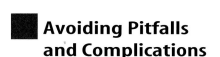

Avoiding Pitfalls and Complications

In addition to device-specific principles, some general guidelines are helpful to avoid problems with all-inside techniques. As in every surgical procedure, the indications should be clear. Reparability, thickness, location, and stability of the tear should be assessed arthroscopically before starting the repair. Probing and measurement of the meniscal tissue are important, especially when the implant size must be decided or when an insertion limiter should be adjusted according to the device chosen. Correct placement of the portals is mandatory, as well as skill in using accessory portals if necessary. Finally, careful preparation of the meniscal bed is necessary before fixing the meniscus.

Bibliography

Barber FA, Click SD: Meniscus repair rehabilitation with concurrent anterior cruciate reconstruction. *Arthroscopy* 1997; 13(4):433-437.

Barber FA, Coons DA: Midterm results of meniscal repair using the BioStinger meniscal repair device. *Arthroscopy* 2006;22(4):400-405.

Barber FA, Herbert MA: Meniscal repair devices. *Arthroscopy* 2000;16(6):613-618.

Barber FA, Johnson DH, Halbrecht JL: Arthroscopic meniscal repair using the BioStinger. *Arthroscopy* 2005;21(6):744-750.

Barber FA, McGarry JE: Meniscal repair techniques. *Sports Med Arthrosc* 2007;15(4):199-207.

Bellemans J, Vandenneucker H, Labey L, Van Audekercke R: Fixation strength of meniscal repair devices. *Knee* 2002;9(1): 11-14.

Bryant D, Dill J, Litchfield R, et al: Effectiveness of bioabsorbable arrows compared with inside-out suturing for vertical, reparable meniscal lesions: A randomized clinical trial. *Am J Sports Med* 2007;35(6):889-896.

Carter TR: Meniscus repair in 2007. *Tech Knee Surg* 2007;6(4):233-241.

Chang HC, Nyland J, Caborn DN, Burden R: Biomechanical evaluation of meniscal repair systems: A comparison of the Meniscal Viper Repair System, the vertical mattress FasT-Fix Device, and vertical mattress ethibond sutures. *Am J Sports Med* 2005;33(12):1846-1852.

Frosch KH, Fuchs M, Losch A, Stürmer KM: Repair of meniscal tears with the absorbable Clearfix screw: Results after 1-3 years. *Arch Orthop Trauma Surg* 2005;125(9):585-591.

Haas AL, Schepsis AA, Hornstein J, Edgar CM: Meniscal repair using the FasT-Fix all-inside meniscal repair device. *Arthroscopy* 2005;21(2):167-175.

Hantes ME, Kotsovolos ES, Mastrokalos DS, Ammenwerth J, Paessler HH: Arthroscopic meniscal repair with an absorbable screw: Results and surgical technique. *Knee Surg Sports Traumatol Arthrosc* 2005;13(4):273-279.

Hantes ME, Zachos VC, Varitimidis SE, Dailiana ZH, Karachalios T, Malizos KN: Arthroscopic meniscal repair: A comparative study between three different surgical techniques. *Knee Surg Sports Traumatol Arthrosc* 2006;14(12):1232-1237.

Harris B, Miller MD: Biomedical devices in meniscal repair. *Sports Med Arthrosc* 2006;14(3):120-128.

Jones HP, Lemos MJ, Wilk RM, Smiley PM, Gutierrez R, Schepsis AA: Two-year follow-up of meniscal repair using a bioabsorbable arrow. *Arthroscopy* 2002;18(1):64-69.

Kocabey Y, Nyland J, Isbell WM, Caborn DN: Patient outcomes following T-Fix meniscal repair and a modifiable, progressive rehabilitation program, a retrospective study. *Arch Orthop Trauma Surg* 2004;124(9):592-596.

Kotsovolos ES, Hantes ME, Mastrokalos DS, Lorbach O, Paessler HH: Results of all-inside meniscal repair with the FasT-Fix meniscal repair system. *Arthroscopy* 2006;22(1):3-9.

Laprell H, Stein V, Petersen W: Arthroscopic all-inside meniscus repair using a new refixation device: A prospective study. *Arthroscopy* 2002;18(4):387-393.

Lee CK, Suh JT, Yoo CI, Cho HL: Arthroscopic all-inside repair techniques of lateral meniscus anterior horn tear: A technical note. *Knee Surg Sports Traumatol Arthrosc* 2007;15(11):1335-1339.

Lozano J, Ma CB, Cannon WD: All-inside meniscus repair: A systematic review. *Clin Orthop Relat Res* 2007;455:134-141.

Morgan CD: The "all-inside" meniscus repair. *Arthroscopy* 1991;7(1):120-125.

Oberlander MA, Chisar MA: Meniscal repair using the Polysorb Meniscal Stapler XLS. *Arthroscopy* 2005;21(9):1148.

Quinby JS, Golish SR, Hart JA, Diduch DR: All-inside meniscal repair using a new flexible, tensionable device. *Am J Sports Med* 2006;34(8):1281-1286.

Venkatachalam S, Godsiff SP, Harding ML: Review of the clinical results of arthroscopic meniscal repair. *Knee* 2001;8(2):129-133.

Zantop T, Eggers AK, Musahl V, Weimann A, Petersen W: Cyclic testing of flexible all-inside meniscus suture anchors: Biomechanical analysis. *Am J Sports Med* 2005;33(3):388-394.

Coding

CPT Codes		Corresponding ICD-9 Codes	
Arthroscopic Meniscal Repair			
29882	Arthroscopy, knee, surgical; with meniscus repair (medial OR lateral)	717.1 717.42 836.0	717.2 717.43 836.1
29883	Arthroscopy, knee, surgical; with meniscus repair (medial AND lateral)	717.1 717.42 836.0	717.2 717.43 836.1

Chapter 88

Meniscal Repair: Outside-In Technique

Thomas Carter, MD

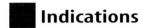

Indications

In the outside-in technique, suture material is passed from outside the knee across the meniscus tear to secure the ends of the tear. Although the outside-in technique has been described for the repair of tears in all regions of the meniscus, it is considered the procedure of choice for repair of anterior horn tears and also is effective for middle horn tears. The technique carries minimal risk of neurovascular injury when treating these tears, and incisions are small.

Tears in the anterior meniscal body and anterior horn (such as the anterior extension of a bucket-handle tear) often are difficult or impossible to access with inside-out or all-inside techniques through standard anterior portals, and the outside-in method is useful in this situation. Outside-in techniques minimize risk to neurovascular structures by starting at a safe anatomic interval adjacent to the joint line and passing away from the neurovascular structures into the joint cavity under direct arthroscopic observation.

Contraindications

The outside-in technique is generally not appropriate for tears in the posterior horn because of the difficulty of orienting the needle and suture perpendicular to the meniscal tear. The amount of soft tissue in the posterior region of the joint makes it difficult to localize the joint line and place the needle into the joint. If needles are passed blindly, there is a risk of articular cartilage damage.

Alternative Treatments

Most meniscal tears are not suitable for repair, and excision is the most common alternative treatment. If a tear is thought to be repairable, inside-out and all-inside techniques are alternatives to outside-in. As the name implies, the inside-out method is basically the reverse of the outside-in technique. It typically involves making a 2- to 3-cm skin incision correlating to the area of the tear and dissecting to the capsule. Sutures are then

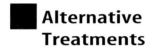

placed into the knee and across the meniscus, and then retrieved and tied outside the capsule.

The all-inside technique secures the tear completely by arthroscopic methods. The goals of the all-inside method are to decrease surgical time and limit tissue trauma as compared to the other techniques. The procedure is very appealing, but there are still many pitfalls to overcome despite continued improvement in surgical instruments.

The surgeon should not think of the three methods as mutually exclusive, but rather as complementary to one another. As noted above, outside-in is considered the method of choice for anterior horn tears. Although the other techniques can in theory be used for anterior tears, the sharp curve required to place anterior fixation can be very difficult or, with some fixation devices, impossible. Conversely, the outside-in technique has limited use in posterior repairs. Because of the typically oblique orientation of the needles when passed, it can be difficult to place the sutures perpendicular across the tear and fully appose the tissue. All three methods are well suited for middle horn tears. Inside-out and all-inside techniques are preferred for posterior horn tears. All-inside techniques are particularly well suited for tears in proximity to the meniscal root, where inside-out sutures may be hard to retrieve and

Dr. Carter or an immediate family member has received royalties from Arthrex; is a member of a speakers' bureau or has made paid presentations on behalf of Arthrex, Musculoskeletal Transplant Foundation, and Regeneration Technologies; serves as a paid consultant for or is an employee of Arthrex and Regeneration Technologies; and holds stock or stock options in Regeneration Technologies.

Table 1 Results of Outside-In Meniscus Repair

Authors (Year)	Number of Knees	Mean Patient Age (Range)	Mean Follow-up (Range)	Assessment Method	Success Rate
Morgan et al (1991)	74	NR	8.5 months	Second-look arthroscopy	84% (62 of 74)
Rodeo and Warren (1996)	90	NR	Minimum 3 years (36-89 months)	CT/arthrography	87% (78 of 90)
van Trommel et al (1998)	51	28 (14-50)	15 months (3-80)	Arthroscopy, CT/arthrography, MRI, or combination	76% (39 of 51)

NR = not reported.

carry a greater risk of neurovascular injury.

Meniscal allografts are an option when a meniscus is not repairable and is subsequently completely excised. The indications for meniscal allograft are very narrow, however, and long-term benefits are still unknown.

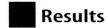

Results

Only a few published series have included only outside-in techniques. Most reports of meniscal repair using the outside-in method also involve inside-out or all-inside methods, with successful outcomes typically in the 80% to 85% range. The results of three series using only outside-in repair are listed in **Table 1**. Of 74 outside-in repairs evaluated with second-look arthroscopy, 62 (84%) were successful. All 12 failed repairs (16%) were in knees with delayed anterior cruciate ligament reconstructions, and 11 of the 12 recurrent tears occurred in the posterior horn. In another report, 90 patients with outside-in repairs were evaluated. Ligament stability also had a profound effect on success in this study. Of the 13 repairs in unstable knees, 5 (38%) failed. Conversely, only 5 (15%) of the 33 repairs in stable knees and 2 (5%) of the 38 repairs in knees with concomitant anterior cruciate ligament reconstructions failed.

Healing rates by meniscal region were evaluated in 51 repairs. Healing rates were significantly lower in tears that involved the posterior horn of the medial meniscus because of the difficulty in placing sutures perpendicular to tears in this region, resulting in suboptimal tear apposition. As a result, this technique was not recommended as the primary method for repairing these tears.

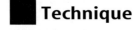

Technique

Setup/Exposure

The leg is prepared in the standard arthroscopic setup. It is important that the position allows knee flexion of at least 90° to facilitate suture retrieval, in particular from the lateral side.

The tear surfaces are prepared to stimulate bleeding, usually with shaver débridement and rasping of the edges; however, too aggressive an approach can damage the meniscus, and care must be taken to avoid articular cartilage injury. Suturing clotted blood into the tear in conjunction with the repair is beneficial but is technically challenging. Trephination with a spinal needle into the outer border can be used for vascular channel access, but it may not provide sufficient uniform bleeding.

Because hemarthrosis is associated with better healing rates, several

methods have been described to produce diffuse bleeding. Débriding the fat pad with its excellent vascular supply is one means to initiate a hemarthrosis. Anterior fibrosis is a concern with this method, and aggressive patellar mobilization is vital to prevent it. Removing bone from the intercondylar notch, similar to a notchplasty, is another way to initiate a hemarthrosis.

Procedure

The outside-in technique was initially described using a polydioxanone suture (PDS) placed through a spinal needle across the tear, then retrieved and pulled out of the knee. A "mulberry knot" was then placed and the suture passed back into the knee. When the suture was pulled back, it reduced the inner fragment of the tear against the peripheral component (**Figure 1**). With the initial suture used to stabilize the tear, a second suture was placed in similar fashion. The two strands of suture were then tied together outside the capsule to secure the tear. The method has a proven success rate, but the fixation strength and intra-articular prominence of the knots have been concerns.

Since the original description, numerous modifications of the technique have been described and instruments developed in an effort to improve outside-in repairs. Nevertheless, several basic steps apply to all. The starting point for entry of the nee-

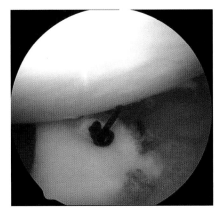

Figure 1 Arthroscopic view of a mulberry knot secured across a meniscal tear.

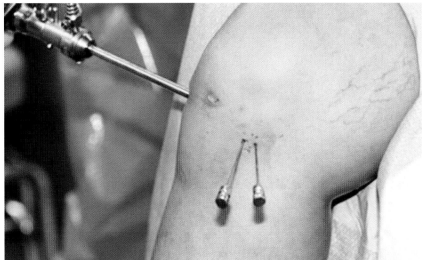

Figure 2 Spinal needles being placed from outside in.

dle is located by palpating the skin at the joint line while arthroscopically observing for capsule indentation. Transillumination with the arthroscope can be helpful in determining this location, as well as for identifying subcutaneous vessels and nerves to limit injury.

The needle can be inserted directly through the skin or through a stab incision (**Figure 2**). The benefit of placing a needle through the skin is that needle placement can be easily changed and corrections made before any incision is made; the drawback is the neurovascular risk. Conversely, a puncture incision has less chance of neurovascular insult. On the medial side in particular, a more conservative approach is appropriate because of the several branches of the saphenous nerve. A more extensive skin incision is made only rarely, except in the posterolateral corner, where it is required to avoid peroneal nerve injury.

The sutures can be passed into the knee using various means, with the type of suture playing a role. Most commonly used are 18- or 19-gauge spinal needles and No. 2 absorbable monofilament suture. If looped sutures are used, 16-gauge spinal needles are used (**Figure 3**). More sophisticated commercially available instruments can be used, but they carry an increased cost. For repair of a posterior horn tear, however, the com-

mercial devices with curved needles and cannulas often are preferred. Because nonabsorbable suture is difficult to advance through spinal needles, it has historically not been the suture of choice with the outside-in method; however, nonabsorbable suture can be used with newer surgical instruments.

As with any meniscal repair, the needle can be passed through either the superior (femoral) or inferior (tibial) surface, but it is common practice to secure the superior surface first because of the ease of seeing tear apposition. If the meniscus is difficult to stabilize when passing the initial needle, a probe or similar instrument can be used to steady the tear. A second needle is then passed adjacent to the first needle. Although vertical sutures have the greatest pull-out strength, the initial suture should be placed to provide optimal stability of the tear regardless of orientation.

With the tear secured with the needles, the suture is passed and retrieved (**Figure 4**). The most basic method is the mulberry knot technique. A variation of this is to bring the ends of the two passed sutures out of the knee and tie them together. The sutures are then pulled back into the knee. One strand of the suture is pulled firmly to pull

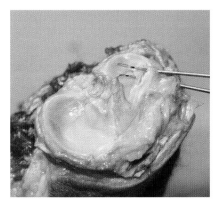

Figure 3 Cadaver specimen showing the position of the needles across the tear, with suture looped through them.

the knot through the meniscus and outside the capsule. The knot is cut, and the end of the suture is brought out farther. In the process, it becomes a single suture with both free ends outside the knee. The suture is then tied, avoiding the concerns about strength and knot abrasion. However, this technique carries its own set of problems. The main problem is that when the knot is passed through the meniscus, additional damage can occur. Furthermore, tissue may become trapped when the tied sutures are brought back into the knee; this can be avoided by retrieving the sutures out of the knee through a cannula.

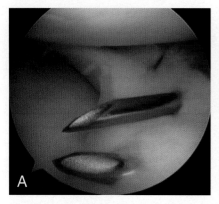
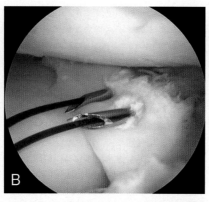

Figure 4 Arthroscopic view of the outside-in technique. **A,** Spinal needles have been placed from outside in. **B,** Suture has been passed through the needles.

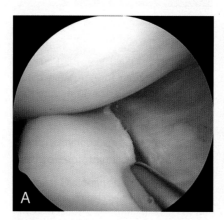

Figure 5 A looped wire is placed through a needle and used to retrieve the suture.

The next advancement of the technique was the suture loop method, which involves placing a looped absorbable monofilament suture through the needle and into the knee. In the original technique, the loop is pulled out of the knee and a suture, either absorbable or nonabsorbable, is placed through the loop. The loop is then pulled back into the knee, across the tear, and outside the capsule. The loop is then passed through the second needle and the same technique is used to place the other arm of the suture across the tear and out the knee to be tied. A wire cable loop can be used instead of the absorbable monofilament suture to ease passage through the knee and limit the risk of the loop breaking (**Figure 5**); however, the wire loop is more costly and can abrade the articular cartilage.

At present, the suture loop method is most often used, but the suture is passed arthroscopically rather than by pulling the loop out of the knee. Typically, a grasper or similar device holding the suture is passed through the loop along with the suture. The grasper is released and the suture is retrieved on the other side of the loop. This can be technically challenging if the loop does not open sufficiently to pass the suture. If needed, a probe or needle can be used to open the loop. Another option is to place a third spi-

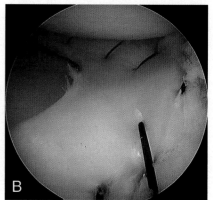

Figure 6 Arthroscopic views of a meniscal tear before (**A**) and after (**B**) outside-in repair.

nal needle oriented so that it goes through the loop. The suture is then passed through the needle and, in the process, through the loop.

More recently, several companies have developed disposable open-ended retrievers that can pass through the needle and bypass the need for a loop. A suture is placed into the knee, delivered to the retriever, and pulled outside the capsule. With this technique, the cost of the disposable instrument must be weighed against its convenience.

When repairing the anterior horn of a tear, the suture often can be retrieved directly through the anterior portal. The suture is passed in standard fashion using spinal needles, but a grasper can be used to retrieve the suture just above the meniscus and

through the capsule, which has already been penetrated during portal insertion. Care must be taken to avoid trapping the capsule with this technique. Using a knot pusher placed through a cannula avoids this complication and allows direct visualization of the knots as they are tied.

To complete the repair, as with any of the meniscal repair techniques, the sutures are placed at 3- to 5-mm intervals (**Figure 6**). Although vertical sutures may be preferred because of their greater pull-out strength, horizontal sutures should be used as needed to correctly appose the torn edges. In addition, the tibial surface of the meniscus should be thoroughly inspected during the repair. With large tears, often the inferior aspect of the meniscus is not fully secured; sutures should be placed inferiorly if there is any question of this.

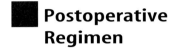 Postoperative Regimen

Published protocols for rehabilitation following meniscal repair vary widely. At one end of the spectrum, the knee is immobilized with no weight bearing for 4 to 6 weeks. At the opposite end, full weight bearing is allowed and knee motion is unrestricted. Most rehabilitation programs fall between these two extremes.

Most protocols permit protected weight bearing, with a range of motion from 0° to 90° for the initial 4 weeks. Running typically is permitted at 3 to 4 months and full activities at 4 to 6 months. It should be remembered that these are general guidelines. For example, rehabilitation after repair of an acute red-red zone tear can be progressed faster than after repair of a chronic tear in a less vascular area. Concurrent procedures, such as an anterior cruciate ligament reconstruction, need to be considered in postoperative treatment.

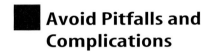 Avoid Pitfalls and Complications

The most common pitfall of any meniscal repair is failure to heal requiring additional surgery. With proper patient selection and attention to surgical technique, the success rates of repair are typically 80% to 85%.

The major pitfall of the outside-in method compared to inside-out and all-inside techniques involves repair of posterior horn tears. Optimally, the sutures should pass through the meniscus at 90° across the tear to fully appose the torn edges. Posterior passage of the sutures from outside in typically places the sutures in the meniscus at an oblique angle and decreases the rate of complete apposition of the tear. In addition, blind passage of needles in this area carries an increased risk of articular damage. As a result, it is preferable to use other methods for repairing posterior horn tears.

As with any arthroscopic meniscal repair, neurovascular injury is the most common complication reported. On the lateral side, the peroneal nerve is at risk; staying in front of the biceps femoris attachment on the fibular head avoids the nerve. Saphenous nerve injury can occur with medial repairs. Transillumination with the arthroscope can be helpful when trying to locate the nerve and its branches. In addition, after making the skin incision, blunt dissection to the capsule can minimize injury. With anterior horn repairs, the risk of entrapment of the capsule and fat pad can be limited by dissecting down to the capsule when tying the sutures and by initiating immediate patellar mobilization exercises.

Bibliography

Arnoczky SP, Warren RF: Microvasculature of the human meniscus. *Am J Sports Med* 1982;10(2):90-95.

Bach BR Jr, Dennis M, Balin J, Hayden J: Arthroscopic meniscal repair: Analysis of treatment failures. *J Knee Surg* 2005;18(4):278-284.

Becker R, Stärke C, Heymann M, Nebelung W: Biomechanical properties under cyclic loading of seven meniscus repair techniques. *Clin Orthop Relat Res* 2002;400(400):236-245.

Cooper DE, Arnoczky SP, Warren RF: Meniscal repair. *Clin Sports Med* 1991;10(3):529-548.

DeHaven KE: Meniscus repair. *Am J Sports Med* 1999;27(2):242-250.

Eggli S, Wegmüller H, Kosina J, Huckell C, Jakob RP: Long-term results of arthroscopic meniscal repair: An analysis of isolated tears. *Am J Sports Med* 1995;23(6):715-720.

Greis PE, Holmstrom MC, Bardana DD, Burks RT: Meniscal injury: II. Management. *J Am Acad Orthop Surg* 2002;10(3):177-187.

Johnson MJ, Lucas GL, Dusek JK, Henning CE: Isolated arthroscopic meniscal repair: A long-term outcome study (more than 10 years). *Am J Sports Med* 1999;27(1):44-49.

McCarty EC, Marx RG, DeHaven KE: Meniscus repair: Considerations in treatment and update of clinical results. *Clin Orthop Relat Res* 2002;402:122-134.

Morgan CD, Wojtys EM, Casscells CD, Casscells SW: Arthroscopic meniscal repair evaluated by second-look arthroscopy. *Am J Sports Med* 1991;19(6):632-637, discussion 637-638.

Rodeo SA, Warren RF: Meniscal repair using the outside-to-inside technique. *Clin Sports Med* 1996;15(3):469-481.

van Trommel MF, Simonian PT, Potter HG, Wickiewicz TL: Different regional healing rates with the outside-in technique for meniscal repair. *Am J Sports Med* 1998;26(3):446-452.

Wojtys EM, Chan DB: Meniscus structure and function. *Instr Course Lect* 2005;54:323-330.

Coding

CPT Codes		Corresponding ICD-9 Codes	
Arthroscopic Meniscal Repair			
29882	Arthroscopy, knee, surgical; with meniscus repair (medial OR lateral)	717.1 717.42 836.0	717.2 717.43 836.1
29883	Arthroscopy, knee, surgical; with meniscus repair (medial AND lateral)	717.1 717.42 836.0	717.2 717.43 836.1

CPT copyright © 2010 by the American Medical Association. All rights reserved.

Chapter 89

Meniscal Repair: Inside-Out Technique

Jason L. Koh, MD
Dukhwan Ko, MD

Indications

Inside-out meniscal repairs are the gold standard for meniscal repair and should be considered whenever the indications exist for meniscal repair in general. Meniscal repair typically is indicated for tears longer than 7 mm that are not degenerative and that involve minimal damage or deformity of the fragment. Specific indications for the inside-out technique are tears in the middle to posterior half of the meniscus and radial tears of the meniscus. Because inside-out repairs have been demonstrated to have superior biomechanical stability, this technique also is indicated when additional biomechanical security of the repair is desired. Good results have been reported for repairs in the avascular zone in young patients.

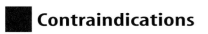

Contraindications

Degenerative, irreducible, or irreparable meniscal tears are contraindica-

tions to meniscal repair. Horizontal cleavage, flap, complex, and other degenerative tears are not suitable for repair and can be best treated by partial meniscectomy. Meniscal repairs in the unstable knee also have a higher chance of failure, although success can be improved by concurrent ligament reconstruction. Some authors have suggested that small, incomplete, stable tears less than 7 mm in length do not need repair. Repair is generally not recommended in elderly, less active patients and those not willing to comply with the postoperative rehabilitation.

Alternative Treatments

Partial meniscectomy can be done for the tears that are not appropriate for repair. Anterior meniscal tears generally are repaired by outside-in or mini-open techniques. Many posterior meniscal tears can be repaired by all-inside techniques; however, the all-

inside devices have certain risks of complications such as implant breakage or migration, cartilage wear, and damage to neurovascular structures. They also have been noted to have inferior results with longer-term follow-up. Hybrid repairs using a combination of all-inside and outside-in suturing techniques also can be used.

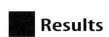

Results

Various methods have been used to assess the success of meniscal repair, including clinical examination, arthrography, MRI, and second-look arthroscopy. When evaluating reported results, therefore, the criteria used for evaluation must be clearly identified. Even considering the fact that success rates vary depending on the criteria selected to evaluate the surgical result, however, the inside-out meniscal repairs have shown overall good to excellent results, ranging from 73% to 93% (**Table 1**).

Several factors have been found to influence the results of inside-out meniscal repair, including location of tear (rim width), tear length, chronicity of tear, concomitant anterior cruciate ligament (ACL) insufficiency, and whether the tear is medial or lateral.

Dr. Koh or an immediate family member serves as a board member, owner, officer, or committee member of the Illinois Association of Orthopaedic Surgeons; is a member of a speakers' bureau or has made paid presentations on behalf of Aesculap/B. Braun and Arthrex; and has received research or institutional support form Aesculap/B. Braun, Arthrex, and Enturia. Neither Dr. Ko nor any immediate family member has received anything of value from or owns stock in a commercial company or institution related directly or indirectly to the subject of this chapter.

Table 1 Results of Inside-Out Meniscal Repair

Authors (Year)	Number of Repairs	Status of ACL	Evaluation Criteria	Mean Follow-up (Range)	Results
Buseck and Noyes (1991)	66	Reconstructed	Arthroscopy	1 year (6-25 months)	80% healed completely 14% healed partially 6% failed Results better with repairs in outer 1/3 rim width
Cannon and Vittori (1992)	90	22 stable 68 reconstructed	Arthroscopy or arthrogram	7 months for stable knees 10 months for reconstructed knees (3-33 months)	50% healed (stable) 93% healed (reconstructed) Results better with lateral meniscus, small rim width
Tenuta and Arciero (1994)	54	14 stable 40 reconstructed	Arthroscopy	11 months (4-30 months)	57% healed (stable) 90% healed (reconstructed) Results better with age <30 years, early repair Results worse with rim width >4 mm
Eggli et al (1995)	54	Stable	Clinical ± MRI	7.5 years ± 0.8 years (23-116 months)	73% success Results better with acute injury (<8 weeks), age <30 years, tear length <2.5 cm Results worse with rim width >3 mm, absorbable sutures.
Rubman et al (1998)	198	70 stable 126 reconstructed 2 not reconstructed concurrently or after	Clinical in all knees Arthroscopy in 91 knees	42 months (clinical) 18 months (arthroscopy) (2-81 months)	Clinical (198): 80% asymptomatic Arthroscopy (91): 23 completely healed, 35 partially healed, 33 failed Results better with lateral meniscus, acute injury (<10 weeks)
Johnson et al (1999)	38	Stable	Clinical	10.8 years (8.1-13.3 years)	76% success Results worse with increased rim width

ACL = anterior cruciate ligament.

Tears with a rim width less than 3 mm or in the outer third of the rim can be expected to have a greater potential for healing, but even for tears extending into the avascular zone, acceptable results have been reported, with no symptoms reported in 80% to 87% of patients. With regard to tear length, failure rates increased to 59% if the tear was more than 4 cm long. In contrast, repairs of tears less than 2 cm long had a 15% failure rate, and repairs of tears between 2.0 and 3.9 cm had a 20% failure rate. Acute tears (those repaired within 8 weeks of the injury) had a better success rate than tears repaired after 8 weeks. Concom-

itant ACL insufficiency is an important factor in meniscal healing. It is now well accepted that meniscal repairs performed at the time of ACL reconstruction have a higher healing rate (83% to 93%) than isolated repairs (50% to 75%), most likely due to the enhanced healing environment from the blood from the bone tunnels. Medial meniscal repairs, particularly of the posterior horn, showed a higher failure rate than repairs of the lateral meniscus. A study of 51 lateral meniscal repairs reported a failure rate of 16%, whereas a study of 66 medial meniscal repairs reported a 30% failure rate. Suture choice also has been

shown to have an effect on the success rates of meniscal repair, with nonabsorbable sutures performing better. Some studies have reported that patients younger than 30 years showed better healing, but others have shown no statistical significance for patient age in predicting successful outcome.

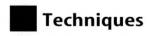

■ Techniques

Setup/Patient Positioning

The patient is placed supine on a standard operating table, and a tourniquet is applied to the upper thigh. The leg is prepared and draped to allow adequate circumferential exposure around the posteromedial and posterolateral aspects of the knee.

Diagnostic Arthroscopy and Preparation for Repair

A complete diagnostic arthroscopy is done to identify any pathology in the knee, and lesions such as ACL tears or articular cartilage defects are treated at the time of meniscal repair. Any associated ACL deficiency should be treated at the time of the meniscal repair because the rate of successful repair is much higher in ACL-reconstructed knees.

In the inside-out technique, the location of working portals is very important and should be determined by the location of the tear. For medial meniscal tears, the medial portal should be made at the medial border of the patellar tendon if possible, to allow the appropriate (vertical) orientation of suture needles to the tear site. For tears in the posterior horn of the lateral meniscus, the medial portal should be placed slightly more proximally and adjacent to the patellar tendon for access above the tibial spines. An arthroscopic probe is inserted into the joint, and the tear is assessed for its repairability (ie, whether it can be reduced and would heal). Once the tear is determined suitable for repair, it is prepared with meniscal rasps or arthroscopic shavers to stimulate bleeding within the tear (**Figure 1**).

Medial Exposure

A 3- to 4-cm longitudinal incision is made over the palpated arthroscopic probe at the posteromedial aspect of the joint line with the knee flexed 60°. Transillumination of the joint line at the area of the tear is helpful (**Figure 2**, *A*). The subcutaneous tissue is carefully dissected down to the sartorius fascia or superficial medial collateral ligament with Metzenbaum scissors. The saphenous nerve typically lies

posterior to the incision; however, the anatomy is variable and branches may pass across the incision (**Figure 2**, *B*). If the incision is posterior, the anterior border of the sartorial fascia is incised, and the pes anserines are retracted posteriorly. Blunt dissection with the fingers is used posterior to the medial collateral ligament and anterior to the pes anserines, and the medial head of the gastrocnemius and the semimembranosus can be easily palpated. A popliteal retractor, spoon, or speculum can be placed against the posterior aspect of the capsule, anterior to the medial head of gastrocnemius, and superior to the semimembranosus tendon (**Figure 2**, *C*).

Lateral Exposure

A similar 3- to 4-cm longitudinal incision is made at the posterolateral aspect of the joint line with the knee flexed 90° so that the peroneal nerve lies posterior. The subcutaneous tissue is dissected down to the iliotibial tract and biceps fascia. The interval between the iliotibial tract and biceps tendon is identified, and an incision is made at the anterior border of the biceps tendon. If the incision and tear are more anterior, a small longitudinal split in the iliotibial band will allow exposure of the capsule. The peroneal nerve courses posterior to the biceps tendon and around the fibular neck. After the biceps tendon is retracted posteriorly, the lateral collateral ligament and lateral head of the gastrocnemius are identified. The interval between the posterolateral capsule and gastrocnemius is made with blunt dissection with a finger or blunt-tipped scissors, and the popliteal retractor is placed into the posterior aspect of the capsule, anterior to the lateral gastrocnemius (**Figure 3**).

Suturing of the Tear

After appropriate exposure of the capsule, the meniscal tear fragment is reduced with a probe. We prefer to use

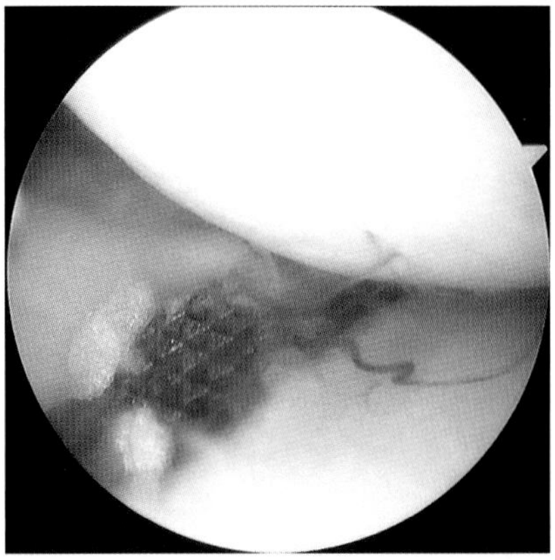

Figure 1 Arthroscopic view shows a tear being rasped at the posteromedial corner at the meniscocapsular junction. This is done before meniscal repair to increase healing potential.

zone-specific single cannulas and double-armed No. 2-0 nonabsorbable braided sutures, although monofilament sutures can be used. Single cannulas have a lower profile than double cannulas and create less risk of scuffing the adjacent articular cartilage. In addition, they allow for a wider range of suture positioning. We prefer to use nonabsorbable sutures because of the lengthy healing period required after meniscal repair. For medial meniscal tears, viewing typically starts from the lateral portal, and the zone-specific cannula with the suture needle is placed through the medial portal. The viewing and working portals can be switched according to the location of the tear, however, and often it is safer to direct the needle from across the joint. The specific amount of curvature of the cannula can be chosen with the incision and tear configuration in mind; if the tip of the cannula can be palpated through the incision, there is a high likelihood that the suture needle will be able to be seen and retrieved safely from within the incision. With the knee flexed 20°, valgus force applied, and the tear reduced, the first suture needle is passed through the meniscus and capsule. Often, the needle can be partially de-

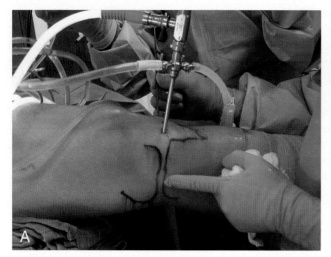

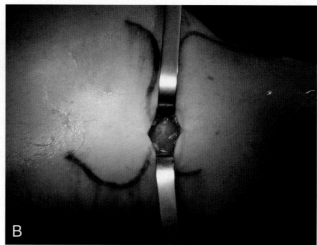

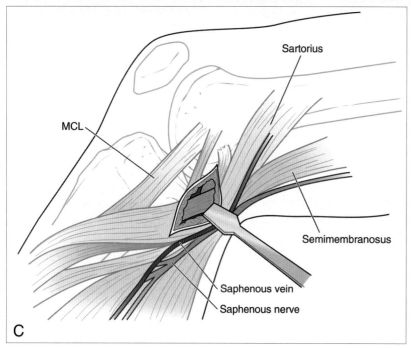

Figure 2 Medial exposure for inside-out meniscal repair. **A,** Intraoperative photograph shows transillumination of the joint line in preparation for a medial exposure. **B,** Intraoperative photograph shows a branch of the saphenous nerve crossing from lower left to right in the incision for the medial approach. **C,** Drawing of the knee shows the relevant anatomic structures for a posteromedial incision. MCL = medial collateral ligament.

ployed into the fragment and used as a joystick to help reduce the tear. The assistant retrieves the suture needle through the open incision and cuts the needle off the suture for safety. If the needle cannot be easily seen, the cannula tip can be palpated after withdrawing the needle. The light source from the arthroscope can be used to illuminate the incision. It is often easier to see the sutures passed through the most anterior portion of the tear first before trying to identify the more posterior stitches. After the first needle is passed, the cannula is repositioned, the second needle is passed and delivered to form a mattress stitch, and the two arms of suture are held with a clamp for later tying. Vertical mattress sutures provide better pullout strength than horizontal mattress sutures. Ideally, vertical mattress sutures should be placed at 3- to 5-mm intervals at alternating superior and inferior surfaces of the meniscus. This can be difficult, however, and oblique suturing can provide similar pullout strength. All the sutures are tied sequentially to the capsule with appropriate tension (**Figure 4**).

For a lateral meniscal repair, the knee is placed in the figure-of-4 position with a varus force applied. The arthroscope is placed in the lateral portal, and the zone-specific cannula and suture needle are placed through

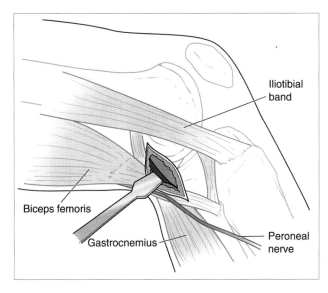

Figure 3 Drawing of the knee shows relevant anatomic structures for a posterolateral incision. ITB = iliotibial band.

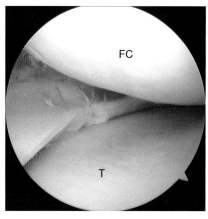

Figure 4 Arthroscopic view shows an inside-out vertical mattress repair of a longitudinal tear of the medial meniscus. FC = femoral condyle, T = tibial plateau.

the medial portal. Sutures are passed through the meniscus under direct arthroscopic vision and are retrieved at the posterolateral incision, with appropriate protection of the posterior neurovascular structures. The sutures should be tied over the capsule with the knee extended to avoid capturing the posterior capsule in flexion.

Postoperative Regimen

Early motion does not seem to adversely affect the result of meniscal repair; however, high degrees of flexion are associated with increased pressure and shear forces on the meniscus. Extreme knee flexion actually can cause subluxation of the posterior horn of the lateral meniscus off the posterior tibial plateau. Therefore, early motion is permitted but is limited to an arc of flexion from 0° to 70° for the first 4 weeks. For most tears, partial weight bearing is allowed for 4 to 6 weeks and full weight bearing after 6 weeks. Some authors have suggested allowing full weight bearing in extension if the tear is stable, as the joint forces may actually provide compression across the tear site. With radial tears,

however, touch-down weight bearing only is permitted for a full 6 weeks because the hoop stresses will tend to separate the meniscal fragments. When meniscal repair has been done with ACL reconstruction, a typical postoperative ACL protocol can be followed with no adverse affects. When there is no effusion and full flexion to 135° is possible, jogging is permitted at 3 months postoperatively and full sports activity at 6 months.

Avoiding Pitfalls and Complications

Complications of inside-out meniscal repairs are similar to those of general arthroscopic knee surgeries and include hemarthrosis, infection, postoperative stiffness, and deep vein thrombosis. Complications specific to this procedure are neurovascular injury and failure of meniscal healing. Overall, a 2.5% rate of complications has been reported, with 1.0% saphenous nerve injury, 0.2% peroneal nerve injury, and 0.1% vascular injury.

Medially, the saphenous nerve is at risk; therefore, medial repairs are riskier than lateral repairs. The saphenous nerve can be injured by needle passage

or during posteromedial exposure for the repair of the medial meniscal tear. Damage to the saphenous nerve can cause postoperative paresthesia or persistent medial joint pain. When this is recognized in the recovery room, immediate return to the operating room for exploration of the wound should be considered because the results of late treatment are often less than satisfactory. The neurovascular structures around the knee are dynamic; their positions change with varying degrees of flexion. Most authors recommend that medial meniscal repairs be done with the knee in 10° to 30° of flexion. Peroneal nerve injuries have been reported in lateral meniscal repair. Lateral meniscal repairs should be done with the knee in about 90° of flexion. In this position, the peroneal nerve drops posteriorly, minimizing the risk of injury. Popliteal artery injury has also been reported. Attention to anatomic detail, knee positioning, careful surgical dissection, placement of a deep retractor anterior to major neurovascular structures, and proper needle placement will prevent these neurovascular complications.

Arthrofibrosis remains a problem after meniscal repair. A high proportion of meniscal repairs are done in

ACL-deficient knees undergoing concomitant ACL reconstruction. The more accelerated rehabilitation protocol currently used after ACL reconstruction has decreased the incidence of arthrofibrosis. Postoperative knee flexion contracture can develop if the sutures are tied with the knee flexed because they can capture or tether the posterior capsule. Therefore, the knee should be extended when the sutures are tied.

Failure of healing is a possible complication because healing potential is decreased in isolated tears without ACL reconstruction or in degenerative, old, or avascular tears. Several healing enhancement techniques can be used in these circumstances to improve the success rate.

Synovial abrasion can stimulate bleeding and synovial proliferation at the edge of the tear. Trephination by multiple spinal needle perforations at the rim of tear also can create a bleeding response at the tear site. Another technique that can be considered is microfracture of the intercondylar notch wall to increase bleeding and allow interosseous mesenchymal stem cells access to the tear site.

Fibrin clot interposition is a well-known technique to enhance meniscal healing. The fibrin clot appears to act as a chemotactic and mitogenic stimulus for reparative cells and to provide a scaffold for the reparative process. To prepare the clot, approximately 20 to 30 mL of peripheral blood is sterilely withdrawn from the patient by venipuncture. The blood is placed in a small metal cup and a ground-glass syringe plunger (usually obtained from an epidural spinal kit) is used to stir the blood until a ring-shaped, gel-like clot is formed on the plunger; the clot is gently scraped off the glass and, if necessary, is cut to create a more linear shape. Absorbable suture is used to capture the clot, and an eyed meniscal repair needle can be used to help deliver the clot into the tear location through an open cannula. Delivery of the clot to and around the site may be easier before all suturing is complete. The inflow may need to be turned off before delivery of the clot.

 Bibliography

Austin KS, Sherman OH: Complications of arthroscopic meniscal repair. *Am J Sports Med* 1993;21(6):864-868, discussion 868-869.

Barber FA, McGarry JE: Meniscal repair techniques. *Sports Med Arthrosc* 2007;15(4):199-207.

Barrett GR, Richardson K, Ruff CG, Jones A: The effect of suture type on meniscus repair: A clinical analysis. *Am J Knee Surg* 1997;10(1):2-9.

Boyd KT, Myers PT: Meniscus preservation: Rationale, repair techniques and results. *Knee* 2003;10(1):1-11.

Buseck MS, Noyes FR: Arthroscopic evaluation of meniscal repairs after anterior cruciate ligament reconstruction and immediate motion. *Am J Sports Med* 1991;19(5):489-494.

Cannon WD Jr: Arthroscopic meniscal repair, in McGinty JB, Caspari RB, Jackson RW, Poehling GG, eds: *Operative Arthroscopy*, ed 2. Philadelphia, PA, Lippincott-Raven, 1996, pp 299-315.

Cannon WD Jr, Vittori JM: The incidence of healing in arthroscopic meniscal repairs in anterior cruciate ligament-reconstructed knees versus stable knees. *Am J Sports Med* 1992;20(2):176-181.

Eggli S, Wegmüller H, Kosina J, Huckell C, Jakob RP: Long-term results of arthroscopic meniscal repair: An analysis of isolated tears. *Am J Sports Med* 1995;23(6):715-720.

Greis PE, Holmstrom MC, Bardana DD, Burks RT: Meniscal injury: II. Management. *J Am Acad Orthop Surg* 2002;10(3):177-187.

Henning CE, Clark JR, Lynch MA, Stallbaumer R, Yearout KM, Vequist SW: Arthroscopic meniscus repair with a posterior incision. *Instr Course Lect* 1988;37:209-221.

Hunter LY, Louis DS, Ricciardi JR, O'Connor GA: The saphenous nerve: Its course and importance in medial arthrotomy. *Am J Sports Med* 1979;7(4):227-230.

Johnson MJ, Lucas GL, Dusek JK, Henning CE: Isolated arthroscopic meniscal repair: A long-term outcome study (more than 10 years). *Am J Sports Med* 1999;27(1):44-49.

Medvecky MJ, Noyes FR: Surgical approaches to the posteromedial and posterolateral aspects of the knee. *J Am Acad Orthop Surg* 2005;13(2):121-128.

Morgan CD, Casscells SW: Arthroscopic meniscus repair: A safe approach to the posterior horns. *Arthroscopy* 1986;2(1): 3-12.

Naqui SZ, Thiryayi WA, Hopgood P, Ryan WG: A biomechanical comparison of the Mitek RapidLoc, Mitek Meniscal repair system, clearfix screws and vertical PDS and Ti-Cron sutures. *Knee* 2006;13(2):151-157.

Noyes FR, Barber-Westin SD: Arthroscopic repair of meniscus tears extending into the avascular zone with or without anterior cruciate ligament reconstruction in patients 40 years of age and older. *Arthroscopy* 2000;16(8):822-829.

Rubman MH, Noyes FR, Barber-Westin SD: Arthroscopic repair of meniscal tears that extend into the avascular zone: A review of 198 single and complex tears. *Am J Sports Med* 1998;26(1):87-95.

Small NC: Complications in arthroscopic meniscal surgery. *Clin Sports Med* 1990;9(3):609-617.

Tenuta JJ, Arciero RA: Arthroscopic evaluation of meniscal repairs: Factors that effect healing. *Am J Sports Med* 1994; 22(6):797-802.

Williams RJ III, Kadrmas WR: Arthroscopic meniscus repair: Inside-out technique, in Cole BJ, Sekiya JK, eds: *Surgical Techniques of the Shoulder, Elbow, and Knee in Sports Medicine.* Philadelphia, PA, Elsevier/Saunders, 2008, pp 427-434.

Coding

CPT Codes		Corresponding ICD-9 Codes	
	Arthroscopic Meniscal Repair		
29882	Arthroscopy, knee, surgical; with meniscus repair (medial OR lateral)	717.1 717.42 836.0	717.2 717.43 836.1
29883	Arthroscopy, knee, surgical; with meniscus repair (medial AND lateral)	717.1 717.42 836.0	717.2 717.43 836.1

CPT copyright © 2010 by the American Medical Association. All rights reserved.

Chapter 90
Discoid Meniscus

Sherwin S. W. Ho, MD
Joshua T. Snyder, MD

▮ Indications

The menisci are two crescent-shaped fibrocartilage structures that normally serve to deepen the articular surface between the femoral condyles and the medial and lateral tibial plateaus. The menisci are thicker at the perimeter and cover the peripheral two thirds of the tibial plateau. Variations from this typical form have been described for more than 100 years; discoid menisci were first described in an anatomic study in 1889. Discoid menisci occasionally require surgical intervention.

Discoid menisci are the most common meniscal variants. Both the medial and lateral menisci can be affected, but the lateral meniscus is affected much more frequently. Discoid medial menisci occur in less than 1% of the population, whereas discoid lateral menisci (DLMs) are found in 1% to 15% of knees in arthroscopic studies. A much higher incidence of DLM is found in certain races, such as Asian populations. Cadaver studies have described an incidence in the midrange of arthroscopic studies; therefore, it is reasonable to suggest an incidence of approximately 5% in the United States, with a slightly higher incidence in Asian populations. Patients with a symptomatic DLM commonly have a discoid meniscus in the contralateral knee as well, either symptomatic or asymptomatic.

The most commonly used classification system for DLM is that of Watanabe and associates (**Figure 1**). This classification describes three types, based on the size and degree of peripheral attachment. Type I discoid menisci (incomplete) have an intact meniscocapsular rim and incompletely cover the lateral tibial plateau. Type II discoid menisci (complete) have an intact meniscocapsular rim, but the entire tibial plateau is covered by meniscal tissue. The type III, or Wrisberg variant, can be either complete or incomplete. It is distinguished by a lack of complete posterior capsular attachment to the meniscus; the only posterior attachment is the ligament of Wrisberg (posterior meniscofemoral ligament). Type III discoid menisci are therefore more mobile and often considered to be the cause of the classic "snapping knee syndrome." Wrisberg variants account for approximately 33% of all discoid menisci.

A more recent classification by Jordan and associates may be better at determining the need for surgical treatment because it includes clinical symptoms and meniscal tears and focuses more on peripheral stability. This system, like the Watanabe classification, defines three subtypes (**Figure 2** and **Table 1**).

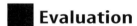

▮ Evaluation

A high level of suspicion is needed to diagnose a discoid meniscus. The symptoms can be quite variable, depending on the type of discoid meniscus present. A discoid medial meniscus usually causes symptoms similar to those of a DLM but with symptoms on the medial instead of the lateral side. Stable DLMs usually are asymptomatic. Symptoms of an unstable or torn DLM include mechanical block to flexion or extension, pain, effusion, catching, joint line tenderness, and locking. Extension block is the most common symptom with symptomatic DLM. The so-called snapping knee syndrome (when reduction of the subluxated meniscus, most commonly during knee extension, produces an audible and sometimes palpable snap) occurs with unstable Wrisberg variants. There are no specific provocative

Dr. Ho or an immediate family member is a member of a speakers' bureau or has made paid presentations on behalf of Biomet; has received research or institutional support from DJ Orthopaedics and Breg; and has stock or stock options held in DJ Orthopaedics. Neither Dr. Snyder nor any immediate family member has received anything of value from or owns stock in a commercial company or institution related directly or indirectly to the subject of this chapter.

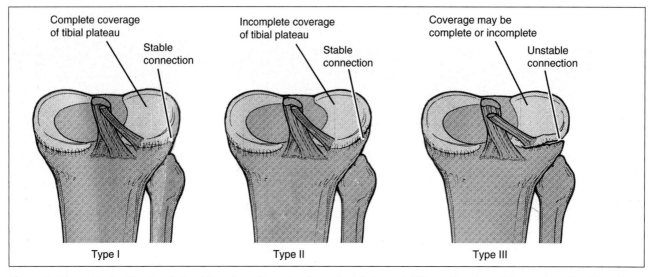

Figure 1 Watanabe classification of discoid meniscus. Posterior views of a right knee are shown. Type I—stable complete discoid meniscus; type II—stable incomplete discoid meniscus; type III—unstable discoid meniscus secondary to lack of complete meniscotibial ligament. (Adapted with permission from Watanabe M: Arthroscopy of the knee joint, in Helfet AJ, ed: *Disorders of the Knee*. Philadelphia, PA, Lippincott, 1974, p 45.)

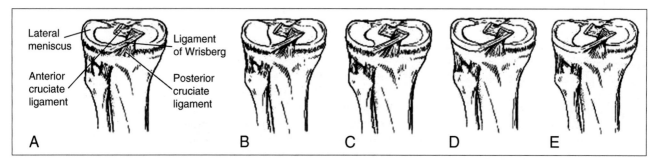

Figure 2 Posterior views of lateral meniscal variants in a left knee. **A,** Normal lateral meniscus. Note the normal shape and posterior tibial attachment. The presence or absence of a meniscofemoral ligament is variable. **B,** Complete discoid lateral meniscus (DLM). **C,** Incomplete DLM. Note the intact posterior tibial attachments in both the complete and incomplete discoid types. **D,** Wrisberg-type meniscal variant with near-normal shape. **E,** Wrisberg variant with discoid shape. In Wrisberg variants, the posterior tibial attachment is lacking, leaving the Wrisberg ligament as the only posterior attachment. (Reproduced from Jordan MR, Duncan J, Bertrand S: Lateral meniscal variants: Evaluation and treatment. *J Am Acad Orthop Surg* 1996;4:191-200.)

Table 1 Proposed Classification of Discoid Menisci

Classification	Correlation*	Tear†	Symptoms†
Stable	Complete/incomplete	Yes/no	Yes/no
Unstable with discoid shape	Wrisberg type	Yes/no	Yes/no
Unstable with normal shape	Wrisberg variant	Yes/no	Yes/no

*Watanabe originally depicted the Wrisberg "type" as normal in shape; however, Jordan and associates believe that the unstable type with a normal shape is more a Wrisberg "variant" than a true discoid meniscus.
†Stable and unstable types can be further subclassified on the basis of whether there is a tear and whether there are symptoms.
Adapted with permission from Jordan MR, Duncan JB, Bertrand SL: Discoid lateral meniscus: A review. *South Orthop J* 1993;2:239-253.

maneuvers to diagnose a discoid meniscus; however, the McMurray test may be positive if a tear is present.

Radiographic and MRI evaluations often are helpful to aid in diagnosis. Changes on plain radiographs usually are subtle, and MRI is more accurate. Standard plain radiographs of both knees including weight-bearing AP view, weight-bearing skier's view, and lateral and Merchant views should be obtained. A widened lateral joint space is the most common finding. Other findings are related to the type of lesion and duration of symptoms.

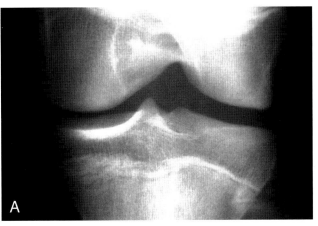
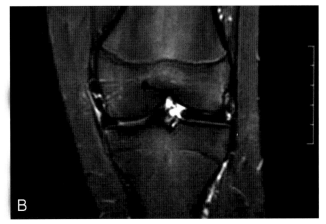

Figure 3 Images of the left knee of a 16-year-old female athlete with a DLM demonstrate a flattened lateral femoral condyle. **A,** AP radiograph. **B,** Coronal T2-weighted MRI. Note the increased transverse diameter of the meniscus.

These include cupping of the lateral tibial plateau, lateral joint lipping, flattening of the lateral femoral condyle (**Figure 3,** *A*), calcification of the meniscus, obliquity of the joint space, elevated fibular head, and degenerative changes. In a therapeutic case series of 128 symptomatic DLMs, no evidence was found on plain radiographs.

MRI typically is diagnostic when a DLM is suspected. The diagnosis is made when the meniscus is seen on three or more successive 5-mm sagittal slices with a connection between the anterior and posterior horns (the "bow-tie configuration"), which normally is seen on only two consecutive slices. Additional findings include a transverse meniscal diameter of more than 15 mm or more than 20% of the tibial width on coronal images (**Figure 3,** *B*). Increased height (thickness) of the meniscus on coronal slices either in the posterior or anterior horn also is suggestive of discoid meniscus. Complete discoid menisci are easier to diagnose on MRI than Wrisberg or unstable types. MRI findings may be subtle or even absent. If symptoms persist, an arthroscopic evaluation may be warranted to confirm the diagnosis of a DLM.

Alternative Treatments

In the case of a discoid meniscus without a tear, a trial of nonsurgical treatment consisting of observation and activity restrictions can be viewed as an alternative treatment. If symptoms persist, however, arthroscopic evaluation is indicated.

When an asymptomatic discoid meniscus is encountered in the course of arthroscopic knee surgery for other diagnoses, we typically recommend saucerization to create a more normal meniscal shape and thereby decrease the risk of tearing. An alternate option is to leave the discoid meniscus alone and follow the patient for the development of any symptoms.

Results

Until the last 15 to 20 years, the typical treatment of symptomatic discoid meniscus was a complete meniscectomy; therefore, long-term outcomes have been poor. More recent studies regarding the current treatment of discoid meniscus are now being published, and short-term follow-up studies are positive (**Table 2**). A study of 125 symptomatic complete or incomplete DLMs without significant articular erosions found that in the short term (less than 5-year follow-up) for complete DLMs, total meniscectomy had better clinical results than partial meniscectomy. Beyond 5 years of follow-up, however, the patients with partial meniscectomy had better clinical results. There were no differences radiographically between complete or partial meniscectomy of complete discoid menisci. Partial meniscectomy of incomplete DLMs produced better results at both short- and long-term follow-up. Radiographic results also were better over the long term when incomplete DLMs were treated with partial meniscectomy. Overall, partial meniscectomy was better than complete meniscectomy. Another recent study has shown that partial repair with partial meniscectomy also can give good results.

Technique

The goal of treating a discoid meniscus is to produce a stable meniscus that approximates the shape and size of a normal, nondiscoid meniscus. The surgeon must, therefore, have a clear idea of what the footprint of a

Table 2 Results of Surgical Treatment of Discoid Meniscus

Authors (Date)	Number of Knees	Mean Patient Age in Years (Range)	Mean Follow-up (Range)	Results
Bellier et al (1989)	19	10.5	≤ 3 years	Excellent results with complete meniscectomy in 18 of 19 knees. No complications.
Kim et al (2007)	125	NR	>5 years	74 complete DLM total meniscectomy had better clinical results before 5 years but no difference from partial meniscetomy after 5 years. Partial meniscectomy had better radiographic outcomes after 5 years. 51 incomplete DLM did better with partial meniscectomy regardless of time.
Good et al (2007)	30	10.1 (3-20)	37.4 months (12-77)	All patients had full ROM to 135° of flexion; 3 patients had residual knee pain, and 4 had intermittent mechanical symptoms. Two patients had limited activity at final follow-up.
Ahn et al (2008)	28	9 (4-15)	60.9 months (24-94)	All returned to previous lifestyle. No reoperations performed. Lysholm Score improved from 75 to 95.5; HSS score increased from 80.3 to 95.9.

DLM = discoid lateral meniscus, NR = not reported, ROM = range of motion, HSS = Hospital for Special Surgery.

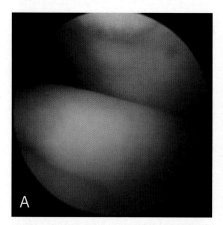 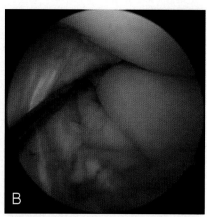

Figure 4 Arthroscopic images of a DLM in the left knee of a 16-year-old female athlete. **A,** On initial viewing, the large discoid meniscus protrudes into the intercondylar notch and can be mistaken for a bucket-handle meniscus fragment. **B,** On further examination with a probe, the typical appearance of a DLM is better appreciated.

normal meniscus looks like arthroscopically based on common intra-articular landmarks, such as the insertion point of the anterior cruciate ligament, intermeniscal ligaments, the meniscofemoral ligaments of Wrisberg and Humphrey, the tibial spine, and the popliteus and popliteal hiatus. The arthroscopic appearance of a typical discoid meniscus can be confusing because the excess meniscal tissue may look like a displaced bucket-handle meniscal fragment (**Figure 4**).

Instruments/Equipment Required

Wide basket punches (biters) with straight, angled, and rounded ends and angled, side-biting (90°), and reverse-biting punches (**Figure 5**) are helpful for the saucerization procedure.

Procedure

Arthroscopic treatment begins with removing the excess, central portion of the discoid meniscus, or "saucerizing" it, using a variety of punches. In some cases, an accessory medial portal created 2 cm medial to the standard anteromedial portal is helpful for viewing and trimming the anterior horn from the medial side (**Figure 6**).

Besides creating a more normal "footprint" of meniscal tissue as viewed in the axial plane, the surgery must address the coronal and sagittal profile of the meniscus as well. The discoid meniscus is thicker centrally than a normal meniscus and does not have a normal tapered cross section (**Figure 7, A** through **C**). The cut edge of the meniscus must be tapered by angling the biter to re-create a more normal wedge-shaped cross-sectional contour of the meniscus to match the curved contour of the femoral condyles. This will help prevent a prominent free edge or stress riser that might

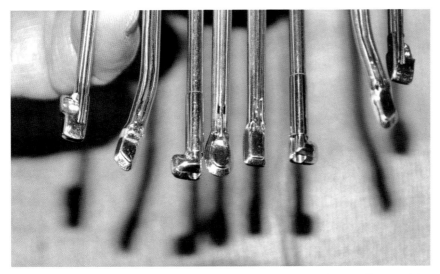

Figure 5 Photograph shows a variety of arthroscopic biters and punches used in saucerizing a discoid meniscus. From left to right: reverse right, curved/angled right, 90° right, oval, straight duck-bill, 90° left, curved/angled left, and reverse left.

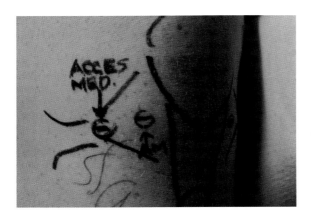

Figure 6 An accessory medial portal may be used in conjunction with the standard anteromedial (AM) portal when trimming the anterior horn of a DLM in a left knee.

niques using an 18-gauge spinal needle as a suture passer are useful for anterior horn tears (**Figure 8**). Shoulder arthroscopy instruments (cannulas, suture passers, suture shuttles, knot pushers, etc) are helpful for side-to-side and all-inside repairs of radial and flap tears.

Complex tear patterns with tears in more than one direction are approached individually and with some creativity. In most cases, one portion of the tear can be trimmed to create a simple tear pattern, which then can be repaired (**Figure 9**). For tears other than vertical tears in the vascular zone, augmentation of the repair with platelet-rich plasma or other biologic agents to stimulate a better healing response is currently being explored in an attempt to improve healing rates in tears not typically repaired.

Even after careful saucerization of a discoid meniscus, with or without meniscal repair, the remaining meniscal rim is not normal and is at greater risk for a recurrent tear than a normal native meniscus, although long-term follow-up studies are still needed.

Postoperative Regimen

Following saucerization of a discoid meniscus, patients are allowed to bear weight as tolerated. Physical therapy is needed only if a patient has difficulty regaining motion or strength. Most patients recover with a home exercise program and can return to normal activities within 1 to 3 weeks and to most sports activities within 3 to 6 weeks.

Following repair of a torn discoid meniscus, patients are kept in a long-leg, hinged postoperative brace, as we would prescribe for any meniscal repair. During the first 3 weeks following surgery, we keep the patient non–weight-bearing with the brace

catch or not glide smoothly against the adjacent condyle.

Given that it is typically younger patients who present with symptomatic torn discoid menisci, any tears remaining after saucerization should be repaired if at all possible. All Wrisberg variants require stabilization by meniscocapsular suturing. Careful rasping of the capsule is important for stimulating a better healing response. Because there is no peripheral rim of meniscus to repair to (**Figure 7, D**), suture repair of the meniscus to the capsule (inside-out technique) is recommended.

Any vertical tears in the vascular zone should be repaired, and in teenage patients it is reasonable to attempt repair of horizontal cleavage tears (the most common tear pattern), large flap tears, and deep radial tears in which resection would leave behind little or no functioning meniscal tissue. Horizontal cleavage tears can be repaired with standard horizontal and vertical mattress sutures. For radial and flap tears, it is helpful to use a combination of repair techniques, instrumentation, and accessory incisions, always mindful of the location of the saphenous and peroneal nerves. Outside-in tech-

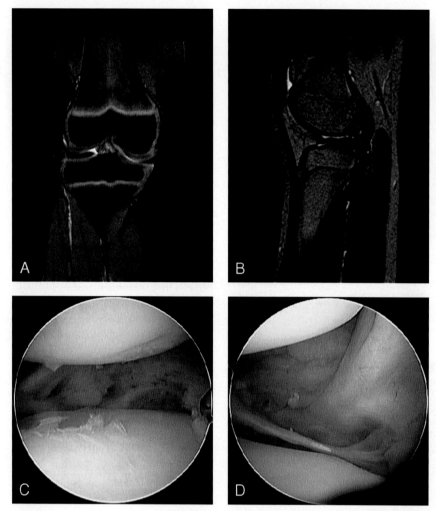

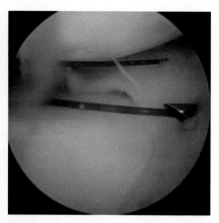

Figure 8 Outside-in technique for repair of anterior horn in a nondiscoid meniscus tear using 0 polypropylene suture shuttle.

Figure 7 Images of a Watanabe type III DLM in the right knee of a 7-year-old girl who presented with locking episodes. Coronal (**A**) and sagittal (**B**) T2-weighted MRIs demonstrate the lack of tapering of the discoid meniscus as compared with the more normal tapering of the medial meniscus. **C,** Arthroscopic appearance of the capsular rim. **D,** Close-up arthroscopic view of the lateral compartment shows the popliteus tendon and a thin wisp of remaining meniscal tissue comprising the popliteal hiatus, leaving little or no meniscal rim to repair to.

unlocked from 0° to 90° and allow partial weight bearing with the brace locked in extension. During weeks 4 through 6 we allow 0° to 90° with weight bearing as tolerated and full knee motion without weight. The brace is discontinued after 6 weeks, and the patient is allowed to resume normal daily activities. Jumping, squatting, twisting, cutting, and similar activities that are known to stress meniscal repairs are restricted for 6 months.

Avoiding Pitfalls and Complications

One of the main pitfalls to avoid in resecting or saucerizing a discoid meniscus is taking too much meniscal tissue and leaving behind an inadequate amount of meniscus. Conversely, leaving too much meniscal tissue behind risks continued symptoms or tearing the remaining rim. Re-creating a normal, tapered, crescent-shaped meniscus is much more difficult than performing a routine meniscectomy,

particularly when reshaping the anterior horn of the lateral meniscus. One reason is that anterior horn tears are much less common than posterior horn tears, so the surgeon usually has less experience working on the anterior horn. Also, because the arthroscopic portals typically are placed directly over the anterior horns, it is technically more challenging to visualize and work on the anterior half of the meniscus. Visualization also is difficult because of the limited space, as the excess meniscal tissue and thickened anterior horn of a discoid meniscus take up much of the joint space. It is therefore helpful to place the initial portal on the contralateral side (medial or opposite the discoid meniscus) and then place the lateral (discoid) portal under direct arthroscopic visualization using a 25- or 22-gauge 1.5-in needle to find the best angle and position from which to work on the central portion of the meniscus.

It may be helpful to briefly review the normal crescent shape of the lateral (or medial) meniscus, to better visualize how much of the central portion of the discoid meniscus you will need to remove to achieve your goal. The angle of each bite of the meniscus becomes more important as the surgeon attempts to re-create the normal curvature of the inner edge of the me-

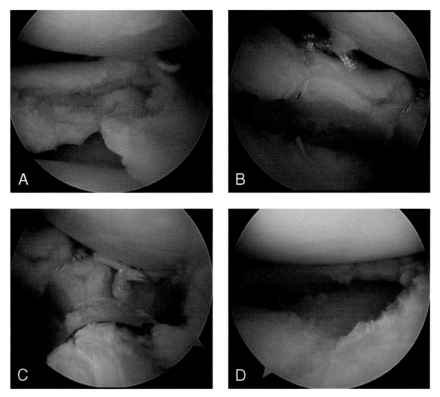

Figure 9 Repair of a complex tear. **A,** A complex tear (horizontal and central radial tears) in a DLM in the left knee of a 20-year-old man. **B,** Posterior horn repair of the horizontal tear after saucerization of the central radial tear with vertical sutures. **C,** Anterior horn repair with vertical sutures. **D,** The completed DLM saucerization and repair.

not wandering too far from or too close to the meniscosynovial junction.

For work on the anterior horn of the meniscus, it is helpful to use an accessory (second) medial portal, which allows the surgeon to both view and work on the anterior horn at the same time. Alternatively, a reverse-biting basket forceps can be used to trim the anterior horn; however, these forceps typically have a relatively small bite, and the instrument itself can block visualization of the portion of the meniscus being trimmed.

When there is damage to the undersurface of the anterior horn of the meniscus, it is helpful to create an inframeniscal portal. This is done by inserting an 18-gauge spinal needle through the same skin portal. The spinal needle is redirected beneath the anterior horn of the meniscus. Then the undersurface of the needle shaft is followed with a No. 11 blade scalpel to create the inframeniscal portal. This allows direct access to the undersurface tear without the shaver blade blocking visualization.

niscus. Marking the cut line by lightly pinching the meniscus with the biter or punch before actually making a cut helps avoid a too-deep or too-shallow bite.

It is helpful to switch the angle of the arthroscope frequently as well as to switch portals and reevaluate the angle and curve of the resection every few bites to make sure the cut line is

Bibliography

Ahn JH, Lee SH, Yoo JC, Lee YS, Ha HC: Arthroscopic partial meniscectomy with repair of the peripheral tear for symptomatic discoid lateral meniscus in children: Results of minimum 2 years of follow-up. *Arthroscopy* 2008;24(8):888-898.

Bellier G, Dupont JY, Larrain M, Caudron C, Carlioz H: Lateral discoid menisci in children. *Arthroscopy* 1989;5(1):52-56.

Dickhaut SC, DeLee JC: The discoid lateral-meniscus syndrome. *J Bone Joint Surg Am* 1982;64(7):1068-1073.

Good CR, Green DW, Griffith MH, Valen AW, Widmann RF, Rodeo SA: Arthroscopic treatment of symptomatic discoid meniscus in children: Classification, technique, and results. *Arthroscopy* 2007;23(2):157-163.

Jordan MR, Duncan J, Bertrand S: Lateral meniscal variants: Evaluation and treatment. *J Am Acad Orthop Surg* 1996;4(4):191-200.

Kim SJ, Chun YM, Jeong JH, Ryu SW, Oh KS, Lubis AM: Effects of arthroscopic meniscectomy on the long-term prognosis for the discoid lateral meniscus. *Knee Surg Sports Traumatol Arthrosc* 2007;15(11):1315-1320.

Watanabe M, Takada S, Ikeuchi H: *Atlas of Arthroscopy*. Tokyo, Igaku-Shoin, 1969.

Woods JH, Whelan JM: Discoid meniscus. *Clin Sports Med* 1990;9:695-706.

Young RB: *Memoirs and Memoranda in Anatomy*. London, Williams and Norgate, 1889.

Coding

CPT Codes		Corresponding ICD-9 Codes	
Arthroscopic Meniscal Repair			
29880	Arthroscopy, knee, surgical; with meniscectomy (medial AND lateral, including any meniscal shaving)	717.4 717.9	717.5
29881	Arthroscopy, knee, surgical; with meniscectomy (medial OR lateral, including any meniscal shaving)	717.4 717.9	717.5
Radiologic Examination, Knee			
73560	Radiologic examination, knee; one or two views	717.4 717.9	717.5
73562	Radiologic examination, knee; three views	717.4 717.9	717.5
73564	Radiologic examination, knee; complete, four or more views	717.4 717.9	717.5
73565	Radiologic examination, knee; both knees, standing, anteroposterior	717.4 717.9	717.5
73721	Magnetic resonance (eg, proton) imaging, any joint of lower extremity; without contrast material	717.4 717.9	717.5
73722	Magnetic resonance (eg, proton) imaging, any joint of lower extremity; with contrast material(s)	717.4 717.9	717.5
73723	Magnetic resonance (eg, proton) imaging, any joint of lower extremity; without contrast material(s), followed by contrast material(s) and further sequences	717.4 717.9	717.5

Chapter 91
Patellofemoral Injuries: Overview and Strategies

Kurt P. Spindler, MD
Joseph P. DeAngelis, MD

■ Introduction

Injuries that affect the balance of forces about the patella or disrupt the extensor mechanism are common in athletes. Patellar instability and disruptions of the extensor mechanism are sources of considerable disability because of their profound effect on lower extremity function. A systematic approach to diagnosis can be used to understand the pathophysiology of patellar dysfunction. With a good understanding of normal patellofemoral function and the etiology of the injury, a well-founded approach to treatment can produce good outcomes.

The patella is a triangular sesamoid bone that functions as a fulcrum to maximize leg strength during flexion and extension of the knee. For a given quadriceps force, the patella increases the length of the moment arm about the knee to increase the torque responsible for knee flexion and extension. At the same time, the patella also acts as a pulley, changing the direction of the quadriceps muscle force as it passes over the knee to affect the tibia.

In its capacity as a fulcrum and a pulley, the patella must absorb all the normal (joint reaction) forces of the patellofemoral joint and is subject to several times the body weight during activity.

The cartilage of the patellofemoral joint experiences an impressive range of compressive force, ranging from one-half body weight to seven to eight times body weight with deep squatting, jogging, and jumping (**Table 1**). The variation in load across the joint helps maintain cartilage health by facilitating the diffusion of nutrients and improving perfusion.

Because of the need to transmit such sizable loads, the cartilage on the articular surface of the patella is the thickest in the human body and is contoured with multiple facets unique to each individual. Although the contour of the articular surface contributes to the stability of the patellofemoral joint, many passive and dynamic forces influence the position of the patella in the femoral sulcus. Of these restraints, the medial patellofemoral ligament (MPFL) is the primary source of ligamentous stability, and

Table 1 Force Across the Patellofemoral Joint With Activity

Activity	Force
Walking	0.5 × BW
Stair climbing	3 to 4 × BW
Deep squatting (120°)	7 to 8 × BW
Jogging	7 × BW
Deceleration/jumping	7 to 8 × BW

BW = body weight.

the vastus medialis obliquus (VMO) is the primary dynamic stabilizer.

———————■

■ Diagnosis

To aid in the diagnosis of patellofemoral injuries in athletes, it is helpful to distinguish between patellar instability and disruption of the extensor mechanism (**Table 2**). To make this distinction, the presenting signs and symptoms should be reviewed carefully to determine if the problem is directly related to patellar motion rather than to an inability to extend the lower extremity. Patellar instability can present as a complete dislocation requiring intervention (reduction) or

Dr. Spindler or an immediate family member has received royalties from Connective Orthopaedics; serves as a consultant for or is an employee of Connective Orthopaedics; owns stock or stock options in Connective Orthopaedics; received research or institutional support from Smith & Nephew; and is a board member, owner, officer, or committee member for the Orthopaedic Research and Education Foundation and the Southern Orthopaedic Association. Dr. DeAngelis or an immediate family member serves as a paid consultant to or is an employee of Connective Orthopaedics.

Table 2 Diagnosis of Patellar Injuries in Athletes

	Patellar Instability (Distinguish subluxation versus dislocation)	Disruption of the Extensor Mechanism (Distinguish quadriceps tendon versus patellar tendon)
History and physical examination	Acute versus chronic Crepitus Tracking Q angle Apprehension	Ability to actively extend Ability to maintain extension Palpable defect Gap size
Radiographs	Loose body Osteochondral defect	Tendon calcification Osteophytes
MRI	Bone bruising Focal articular defects Osteochondral fragments Medial patellofemoral ligament integrity	Tissue quality Gap size

as a more subtle subluxation of the patella within the trochlea. Similarly, injuries to the extensor mechanism can affect any part of the extensor chain and can include partial tendon tears as well as complete disruptions.

———————■

 Patellar Instability

Patients with patellar instability may report an acute or recurrent (chronic) event that may or may not be related to trauma. The injury or its associated sequelae may contribute to the clinical course, and, ultimately, based on the complete clinical presentation including the history, physical examination, and radiographic evaluation, surgical intervention may facilitate the athlete's return to competition.

Patellofemoral dislocations are infrequent. The most common type is a lateral dislocation, which typically results from indirect injury. Often, contraction of the quadriceps is combined with rotation of the limb in a flexed position. This position produces internal rotation of the femur combined with external rotation of the tibia around a valgus knee. The patella dislocates laterally and is easily reduced with knee extension. This injury is seen in athletes who participate in soccer, gymnastics, and ice hockey. Interestingly, in describing the events surrounding a lateral patellar dislocation, patients may report a medial dislocation because of the prominence of an uncovered medial femoral condyle.

Medial dislocations, on the other hand, often are iatrogenic, resulting from an overzealous lateral release or excessive medialization of the tibial tubercle. Superior dislocations are rare. They occur in the elderly when the patella's descent during knee hyperextension becomes obstructed by a superior femoral osteophyte. Rarely, an intra-articular, or horizontal, dislocation occurs when the quadriceps tendon detaches from the superior pole of the patella and the patella becomes incarcerated within the intercondylar notch.

Epidemiology

The overall incidence of primary patellar dislocation is approximately 6 per 100,000, but the frequency is 29 per 100,000 in individuals aged 10 to 17 years. Acute patellar dislocations account for 2% to 3% of all knee injuries and are the second most common cause of traumatic knee hemarthrosis, after anterior cruciate ligament injuries. Girls between 10 and 17 years of age are at highest risk for patellar dislocation, and the risk of patellar dislocation among girls with previous patellofemoral symptoms is three times higher than for boys of the same age with previous subluxation or dislocation. More than 50% of all primary patellar dislocations occur during sports activities, and up to 55% of patients fail to return to sports activity after a primary patellar dislocation.

Recurrence rates range from 15% to 44% after nonsurgical treatment of acute dislocation. If the patient has a subsequent patellar dislocation, there is a 50% chance of recurrent episodes. Several studies have shown that younger patients have higher redislocation rates than older patients.

Factors contributing to patellar instability include osseous abnormalities such as patella alta, a distance of more than 20 mm between the tibial tubercle and the trochlear groove, trochlear dysplasia, and soft-tissue abnormalities such as a torn MPFL or a weak VMO.

Degenerative changes have been reported to be uncommon after patellar dislocation, and one study found that degenerative changes were less frequent among patients with occasional recurrent dislocations than among those with stable patellae. When significant degenerative changes occur as a result of patellar dislocations, they generally do not become apparent until more than 5 years after the injury.

Evaluation

In evaluating patellar instability, the physical examination often reveals a hypermobile patella with well-localized discomfort. Tenderness can result from injuries sustained during the dislocation (MPFL, medial epicondyle, lateral trochlea, medial patellar facet) or during reduction (lateral aspect of the lateral femoral condyle, medial trochlea). Patellar motion, tilt, and tracking need to be quantified and

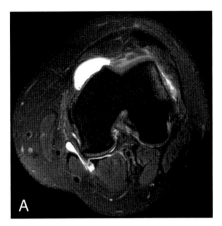 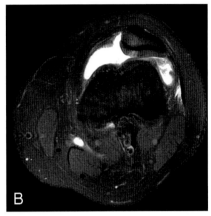

Figure 1 Posttraumatic T2-weighted MRIs demonstrate the bone bruise pattern following patellar dislocation. Marrow edema can be seen on the lateral aspect of the lateral femoral condyle (**A**) and on the posteromedial patella (**B**).

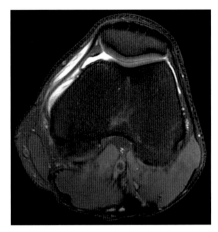

Figure 2 T2-weighted MRI demonstrates normal MPFL anatomy.

compared with the contralateral extremity to best understand the patient's native anatomy. Crepitus and catching often accompany an injury to the articular surface of the patella, whereas apprehension is the most telling clinical sign following an acute dislocation. Careful palpation of the patellar facets and the margins of the trochlea may aid in localizing an articular injury, and a deliberate, systematic examination may reveal a loose body.

The entire lower extremity should be examined carefully, including observing the overall limb alignment (including the foot-thigh and Q angles), assessing the patient's ability to complete a single-leg squat, and evaluating proprioception. These elements of the examination will provide a thorough understanding of the kinetic chain and may reveal associated deficiencies that contribute to patellar instability.

All patients should have a radiographic examination that includes AP, lateral, and axial (Merchant) projections of the affected side. These views allow the identification of any gross malalignment, subluxation or dislocation, or fracture. Intra-articular loose bodies also may be seen on radiographs, but the absence of loose bodies on a radiograph should not be regarded as definitive; fewer than one

half of osteochondral loose bodies are identified radiographically. A study of knee dislocations in adolescents found that only about one third of articular injuries and loose bodies were identified on radiographs. When appropriate, comparison radiographs can reveal important side-to-side differences.

Plain radiographs tend to underestimate the presence and size of articular lesions, so MRI should be considered if a cartilage injury is suspected. Chondral injury to the lateral femoral condyle is estimated to occur in 31% to 40% of individuals with knee dislocations and 5% to 12% of individuals with injuries to the lateral trochlear groove. MRI also may show a characteristic pattern of bone bruising unique to patellar dislocations. After an acute dislocation, marrow edema can be seen on the lateral aspect of the lateral femoral condyle and the posteromedial patella (**Figure 1**). Increased signal intensity is not present in the distal end of the lateral femoral condyle near the sulcus terminalis or in the lateral tibial plateau, because the injury is associated with an acute tear of the anterior cruciate ligament. As an additional benefit, MRI provides precise characterization of the chondral surfaces and can identify defects on both sides of the patellofemoral joint. Careful interpretation of the im-

ages also can identify loose osteochondral injuries and injuries to the MPFL and VMO. **Figure 2** demonstrates a normal MPFL.

Treatment

Many patients with patellar instability benefit from nonsurgical management; however, there are several well-defined surgical indications, for which intervention will improve patient outcomes. **Figure 3** illustrates indications for nonsurgical versus surgical treatment.

NONSURGICAL TREATMENT

At the time of presentation, it is important to confirm that a patient is able to complete a straight-leg raise after the patella has been reduced. This test will evaluate the integrity of the extensor mechanism and confirm the adequacy of the reduction. Radiographs need to be scrutinized carefully for intra-articular fragments, and MRI should be ordered when clinically indicated. Generally, postreduction immobilization should be limited to no more than 3 days to prevent loss of motion in the affected knee. Early rehabilitation in the form of quadriceps activation exercises (quadriceps sets and straight-leg exercises) will help overcome the quadriceps inhibition that accompanies the acute event.

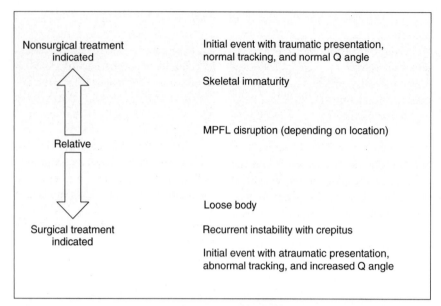

Figure 3 A relative approach to the treatment of patellar instability.

Therapeutic modalities for reducing pain and swelling may facilitate a return of function and patient satisfaction. When indicated, aspiration of an intra-articular effusion may prove beneficial, because all patients should be encouraged to resume full weight bearing on the affected extremity as soon as tolerated. When necessary, crutches may be used for safety while the patient's confidence and comfort return to normal. After the acute period of injury, supportive orthoses and closed-chain exercises can aid in the return of function.

SURGICAL TREATMENT

In certain situations, surgical intervention following a patellar dislocation is indicated (**Figure 3**). If there is a high degree of suspicion for intra-articular loose bodies, prompt removal of the loose fragments will benefit the patient's recovery. These fragments may come in the form of a focal chondral injury or a larger osteochondral defect identified on plain radiographs or MRI. Even if the diagnostic imaging is equivocal, however, the tracking and alignment of the patella need to be examined closely. If patellar tracking is asymmetric or reveals a sig-

nificant increase in patellar tilt or subluxation, early surgical management is warranted.

When surgical intervention is indicated, a complete arthroscopic examination of the knee should be done, at the same time as the excision of loose fragments. Internal fixation of loose osteochondral fragments is beneficial in the long term. A lateral release may be necessary when abnormal patellar tilt or subluxation is present. For persistent patellar subluxation or tilt, repair or reconstruction of the MPFL should be considered. From the preoperative MRI, it is possible to identify the location of the MPFL and determine if it has been disrupted (**Figure 2**). When the MPFL is torn, these images also can help plan for a primary repair if the tissue is of good quality or if it is avulsed from either its origin or insertion. Preoperative planning also can help determine if the injured ligament is too attenuated to allow for repair and a reconstruction is needed. However, a recent systematic review of MPFL reconstruction and a prospective randomized trial of MPFL reconstruction for all acute patellar dislocations concluded that there was no

significant benefit to surgical intervention.

For an evidence-based approach, a literature search for the best surgical techniques for treating patellar instability reveals that most studies examine outcomes for a particular surgical technique (or combination of techniques). Few articles compare two or more techniques, and much of the literature on this topic is older and focused on case series with small patient populations. The result is a mix of retrospective and prospective reports, with little use of controls or randomization to aid in the validation of one methodology or another.

In addition to these techniques for surgical management, other reconstructive options should be considered for continued or recurrent instability. A lateral retinacular release is the least invasive way to affect the forces about the patella and can be used in limited circumstances. When a lateral release does not suffice, a proximal or distal realignment may be necessary. For instability that occurs between full extension and 30° of knee flexion, a proximal realignment often is most appropriate. Conversely, if patellar instability is present with the knee flexed (more than 30°), distal procedures usually are more effective. These interventions include distal soft-tissue realignment and transfer of the tibial tubercle.

━━━━━━━━■

■ Disruptions of the Extensor Mechanism

Injuries to the extensor mechanism are rare. They affect males eight times as often as females. Unlike patellar tendon injuries, which usually occur in a younger population, quadriceps tendon ruptures are most common after the age of 40 years, with a peak incidence in the sixth decade of life.

The youngest reported patient with a midsubstance patellar tendon rupture is an otherwise healthy 9-year-old who had repeat rupture at age 10 years.

When patients present to the emergency department, these injuries often are overlooked, resulting in a misdiagnosis rate of 39% to 67% reported in past studies. With an acute rupture, a delay in diagnosis places the athlete at a considerable disadvantage, potentially compromising the quality of the repair and further delaying return to activity. To further complicate the diagnosis, unusual presentations are possible, including simultaneous rupture of both the quadriceps and patellar tendons as well as bilateral tendon ruptures.

In the absence of a well-defined traumatic etiology, a thorough examination should attempt to identify the underlying pathology that predisposed the individual to a spontaneous tendon rupture. Conditions commonly associated with spontaneous tendon rupture include diabetes mellitus, systemic lupus erythematosus, rheumatoid arthritis, gout, systemic steroid use, hyperparathyroidism, end-stage renal disease, and the use of fluoroquinolone antibiotics.

As with other spontaneous tendon ruptures, patients often report a sudden onset of debilitating pain, described as being "shot" or "stabbed," followed by a rapid loss of function. The tendon rupture may be audible; this is often best appreciated by witnesses. The failure of the tendon typically occurs with eccentric loading of the muscle during explosive athletic performance. In some instances, an antecedent discomfort may be revealed on questioning, suggesting a prodromal tendinosis or tendinitis

that culminated in the spontaneous tendon failure.

Partial and chronic tears of the extensor mechanism have a less dramatic and often unusual presentation, making the diagnosis more challenging. With partial tears of the quadriceps or patellar tendon, the extremity often maintains much of its function, and the patient is able to extend the knee once the pain or the weight of gravity is avoided. Also, there may be no palpable defect in the extensor mechanism, further confounding the diagnosis. With a chronic tear, the patient may have accommodated to a long-standing disability and then sustained an acute rupture, resulting in a timeline for the injury that is inconsistent with the clinical examination on presentation.

With any injury to the extensor mechanism, a complete history should be taken, followed by a thorough physical examination. Close inspection and palpation of the quadriceps and patellar tendons may reveal a defect, or gap, in the tissue that may be tender on examination. The inability to complete a straight-leg raise in the supine position is a common sign of a disruption of the entire extensor chain (including the medial and lateral retinacula). The inability to extend a flexed knee against resistance while seated demonstrates a patellar or quadriceps tendon disruption; however, because the medial and lateral retinacula of the knee are part of the extensor mechanism, in a patient with a tendon injury and intact retinacula, the ability to maintain an extended position, perform a straight-leg raise, or actively extend the knee without resistance may be preserved.

Strength testing should be performed. For completeness, extensor function should be tested with and

without both manual resistance and gravity. The ability to extend the knee while seated or supine (against gravity) should be compared with the ability to extend the knee while in the lateral decubitus position (affected side up, without gravity). This method may help elucidate subtle differences.

All patients with suspected extensor injuries should have a complete radiographic examination to evaluate the relative position of the patella and to exclude fracture or dislocation. With quadriceps tendon ruptures, the patella migrates distally (patella baja), unchecked by the pull of the quadriceps. Conversely, when the patellar tendon is disrupted, a high-riding patella (patella alta) can be seen on lateral radiographs. In patients with chronic disruptions, lateral radiographs of the injured and uninjured knees, flexed to 30°, can be compared to determine the length of the repair or reconstruction. Also, the presence of calcification in the soft tissues or prominent osteophytes may help to better explain the etiology and chronicity of the tear.

The role of MRI in acute tendon injuries depends on the level of clinical suspicion. When a complete disruption is present, additional imaging may not provide additional benefit; however, when there is uncertainty about the clinical diagnosis, an MRI of the knee may help identify a partial tear, a complete tear with intact retinacula, or other injuries that indirectly affect the patient's ability to extend the knee.

When a chronic tendon injury is identified, MRI can help characterize the quality of the remaining soft tissue, determine the size of the residual tissue gap, and plan for the reconstruction, with or without augmentation.

———————◾

■ Bibliography

Arendt EA, Fithian DC, Cohen E: Current concepts of lateral patella dislocation. *Clin Sports Med* 2002;21(3):499-519.

Atkin DM, Fithian DC, Marangi KS, Stone ML, Dobson BE, Mendelsohn C: Characteristics of patients with primary acute lateral patellar dislocation and their recovery within the first 6 months of injury. *Am J Sports Med* 2000;28(4):472-479.

Buchner M, Baudendistel B, Sabo D, Schmitt H: Acute traumatic primary patellar dislocation: Long-term results comparing conservative and surgical treatment. *Clin J Sports Med* 2005;15(2):62-66.

Casey MT Jr, Tietjens BR: Neglected ruptures of the patellar tendon: A case series of four patients. *Am J Sports Med* 2001; 29(4):457-460.

Christiansen SE, Jakobsen BW, Lund B, Lind M: Isolated repair of the medial patellofemoral ligament in primary dislocation of the patella: A prospective randomized study. *Arthroscopy* 2008;24(8):881-887.

Colvin AC, West RV: Patellar instability. *J Bone Joint Surg Am* 2008;90(12):2751-2762.

Dath R, Chakravarthy J, Porter KM: Patella dislocations. *Trauma* 2006;8:5-11.

Dedmond BT, Patterson L, McBryde A Jr, Kirol BG: Repeat patellar tendon rupture in a child. *Am J Orthop* 2005;34(10): 501-504.

Elias DA, White LM, Fithian DC: Acute lateral patellar dislocation at MR imaging: Injury patterns of medial patellar soft-tissue restraints and osteochondral injuries of the inferomedial patella. *Radiology* 2002;225(3):736-743.

Fithian DC, Paxton EW, Stone ML, et al: Epidemiology and natural history of acute patellar dislocation. *Am J Sports Med* 2004;32(5):1114-1121.

Mäenpää H, Lehto MU: Patellar dislocation: The long-term results of nonoperative management in 100 patients. *Am J Sports Med* 1997;25(2):213-217.

Nomura E, Inoue M, Kurimura M: Chondral and osteochondral injuries associated with acute patellar dislocation. *Arthroscopy* 2003;19(7):717-721.

Sanders TG, Paruchuri NB, Zlatkin MB: MRI of osteochondral defects of the lateral femoral condyle: Incidence and pattern of injury after transient lateral dislocation of the patella. *AJR Am J Roentgenol* 2006;187(5):1332-1337.

Smith TO, Walker J, Russell N: Outcomes of medial patellofemoral ligament reconstruction for patellar instability: A systematic review. *Knee Surg Sports Traumatol Arthrosc* 2007;15(11):1301-1314.

Stanitski CL, Paletta GA Jr: Articular cartilage injury with acute patellar dislocation in adolescents: Arthroscopic and radiographic correlation. *Am J Sports Med* 1998;26(1):52-55.

Stefancin JJ, Parker RD: First-time traumatic patellar dislocation: A systematic review. *Clin Orthop Relat Res* 2007;455: 93-101.

Chapter 92

Medial Patellofemoral Ligament Repair for Acute Patellar Instability

Keith Kenter, MD

Introduction

Acute patellar dislocations are among the most common acute knee injuries in children and adolescents. Predisposing factors that have been associated with patellar dislocations include patellofemoral dysplasia, patella alta, a family history of patellar dislocation, and female sex. Reported risk factors for recurrent patellar dislocations include dysplasia of the patellofemoral joint, young age at the time of the first patellar dislocation, and female sex.

Indications

As with any acutely dislocated joint, immediate reduction is considered the standard of care. After reduction, non-surgical treatment traditionally has been the treatment of choice. A systematic review of the literature in 2007 recommended initial nonsurgical management of first-time traumatic patellar dislocation, except in specific circumstances: presence of an osteochondral fracture, substantial disruption of the medial patellar stabilizers, lateral subluxation of the patella, and failure to improve with appropriate rehabilitation. This recommendation has been challenged because of high recurrence rates, and primary repair of the medial soft tissues has become popular. More recently, repair and reconstruction of the medial patellofemoral ligament (MPFL) have been recognized as the surgical treatments of choice for acute patellar dislocation. Prospective studies comparing treatments suggest surgical treatment to provide faster return to activity and to reduce the risk of recurrence. Despite efforts to identify which patients with acute patellar dislocations are prone to reinjury or late disability, the population at risk has not yet been clearly defined.

Absolute indications for surgical treatment of an acute patellar instability are an irreducible patella, an open patellar dislocation, significant articular chondral injury, complete disruption of the medial soft-tissue structures, and a history of patellar instability. Immediate surgical intervention also should be considered for a first-time patellar dislocation in a young athlete.

Contraindications

Contraindications to immediate surgical treatment of acute patellar instability are an active knee infection, a compromised soft-tissue envelope, and a medically high-risk patient. A relative contraindication is a low-demand elderly patient. I do not repair or reconstruct the MPFL in patients with acute knee dislocations because of concerns about postoperative knee stiffness.

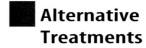

Alternative Treatments

Surgical treatment of acute patellar instability has been directed toward the medial soft-tissue structures. Classically, the medial retinaculum and vastus medialis obliquus (VMO) muscle are plicated or advanced near the medial patellar border. This technique is thought to stabilize the patella more medially with the dynamic force of the medial quadriceps musculature. This may be true except when the injury is off the femur. Biomechanical, radio-

---

Dr. Kenter or an immediate family member serves as a board member, owner, officer, or committee member for the American Orthopaedic Association and the American Orthopaedic Society for Sports Medicine and has received research or institutional support from Stryker and the National Institutes of Health.

Table 1 Results of Immediate Repair for Acute Patellar Instability

Author (Year)	Number of Knees	Mean Patient Age in Years (Range)	Mean Follow-up (Range)	Outcomes
Vainionpää et al (1990)	55	21 (14-54)	≥ 2 years	9% redislocation 80% satisfactory
Sallay et al (1996)	12	25 (14-46)	34 months (24-60)	No redislocations 58% good/excellent 42% fair
Ahmad et al (2000)	8	32 (16-56)	3 years (minimum 1.5)	No redislocations 96% satisfactory
Nam and Karzel (2005)	23	23 (12-65)	4.4 years (1.4-14)	1 redislocation 1 subluxation 91% good/excellent 9% fair
Miller et al (2007)	25	25 (13-54)	61 months (24-120)	No redislocations 96% satisfactory

graphic, and surgical exploration studies have suggested that the most frequent site of injury on the medial aspect is near the level of the femoral epicondyle, and MPFL avulsion at the femoral attachment in primary traumatic patellar dislocations has been shown to be predictive of subsequent patellar instability.

Along with medial soft-tissue advancement and repair, lateral retinacular release has been recommended in the belief that the tight lateral structures pull the patella and act as a predisposing factor for recurrence. Most clinical and cadaver studies have demonstrated little or no benefit to patellar stability from this procedure; however, most authors recommend that lateral retinacular release be reserved for residual decrease in patellar tilt.

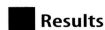

Results

The MPFL is considered the most important restraining structure against lateral patellar displacement. Direct repair of this ligament to its bony attachment has demonstrated excellent results in patients with acute patellar instability (**Table 1**). MPFL reconstruction using the semitendinosus tendon, gracilis tendon, adductor magnus tendon, fascia lata, and quadriceps tendon also has been described. Most of these studies are in patients with recurrent patellar instability. No study has compared the outcomes of direct repair and reconstruction of the MPFL in patients with acute patellar instability.

Comparisons of nonsurgical and surgical treatment of acute patellar instability have shown conflicting results. One prospective randomized study of 40 young adults found a significantly lower rate of redislocation in those treated surgically, although no clear benefits could be determined at long-term follow-up. A large retrospective study of 126 patients found no significant differences between surgical and nonsurgical treatment in redislocation rates, activity levels, or functional and subjective outcomes.

Technique

Setup/Exposure

Preoperative planning is important when surgery is done for acute patellar instability. Diagnostic imaging can help determine the type and location of the pathoanatomy. Typical radiographs include standard AP, lateral, and Merchant axial views. MRI can provide information about the location of the injury (**Figure 1**), which is important in planning skin incisions, and identify intra-articular injuries that may require special equipment; for example, articular cartilage fixation devices may be needed for severe chondral injuries. All patients receive preoperative antibiotics.

Patients are placed supine with the knee positioned at the bend in the table in case flexion of the knee is needed. General or regional anesthesia can be used. A tourniquet can be used if desired, but this is not mandatory. A complete diagnostic arthroscopic evaluation of the knee is done to assess any intra-articular injuries, which can be treated at this time (**Figure 2**).

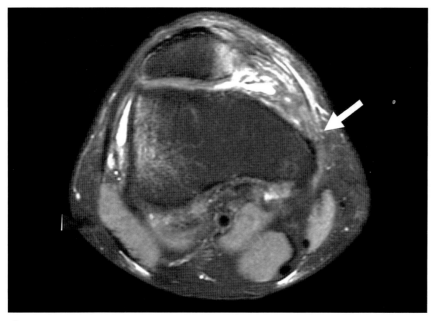

Figure 1 T2-weighted axial MRI demonstrates common findings with acute patellar dislocations. Note bone bruising on the medial patella and lateral femoral condyle. The area of low signal intensity (arrow) indicates disruption of the MPFL from the medial femoral epicondyle.

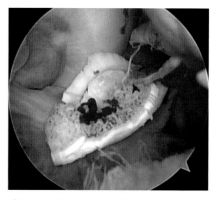

Figure 2 Arthroscopic view of a loose osteochondral fragment from the lateral femoral condyle following acute patellar dislocation.

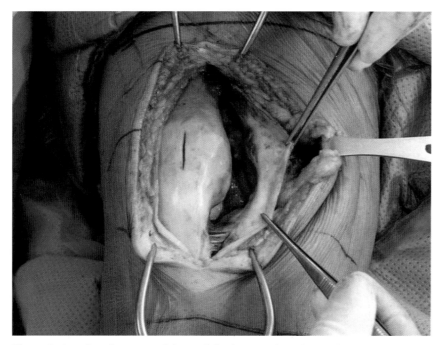

Figure 3 Complete disruption of the medial soft tissues from the patella in a patient with a 3-week history of patellar instability. A defect is seen at the medial edge of the patella.

Procedure

After the intra-articular pathoanatomy has been treated arthroscopically, the knee is placed at 30° to 40° of flexion with the patella sitting in the trochlear groove of the femur. If the injury pattern is localized to the medial patella, then a midline knee incision is made. Dissection is carried toward the medial epicondyle to create a skin flap to allow a more functional incision. Muscle fibers of the VMO and the medial retinaculum are identified and the defect can be seen (**Figure 3**). The bone at the medial edge of the patella can be roughened to create bleeding to help with the biologic process of soft-tissue healing to bone. Either suture anchors or transosseous tunnels can be placed on the medial edge of the patella (**Figure 4**, *A*). The medial soft tissues then are repaired with permanent sutures to their anatomic positions on the patella, closing the defect anatomically (**Figure 4**, *B*).

More commonly, however, the MPFL will have been avulsed off the medial femoral epicondyle. An incision is made between the patella and the medial femoral epicondyle to expose the VMO muscle fibers, which are retracted superiorly to expose the injured tissue underneath. At times an incision parallel to the inferior border of the muscle fibers is needed to help with VMO retraction. The injured medial retinaculum can be lifted to see the avulsed MPFL edge (**Figure 5**, *A* and *B*). The origin of the MPFL on the medial femur is roughened to help with the reparative process. Typically, a suture anchor is placed and the MPFL is repaired with permanent suture (**Figure 5**, *C*). The medial retinaculum is then repaired with permanent sutures, and the edge of the VMO is repaired, if needed.

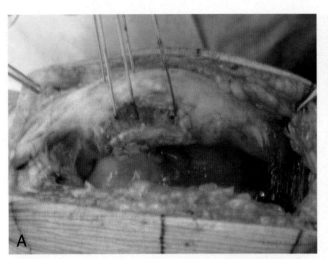
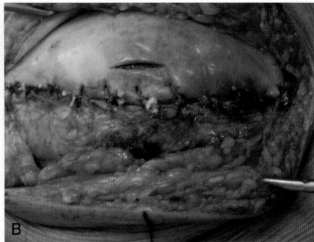

Figure 4 Intraoperative photographs shows repair of avulsion of the MPFL from the medial patella. **A,** Medial edge of patella with permanent sutures placed in a transosseous fashion. **B,** Closure of medial soft-tissue defect with permanent sutures.

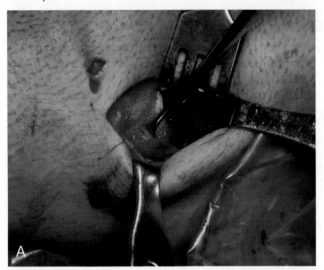
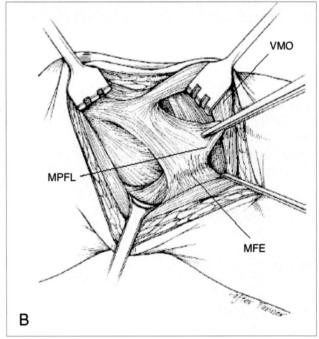
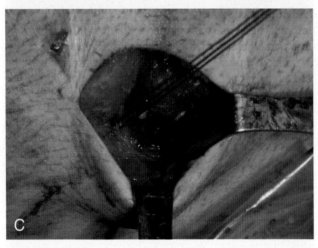

Figure 5 Repair of avulsion of the MPFL from the medial femoral epicondyle. **A,** Intraoperative photograph shows exposure. Note that the clamp is around the edge of the MPFL. **B,** Drawing demonstrates the anatomy of the MPFL. VMO = vastus medialis obliquus; MFE = medial femoral epicondyle. **C,** Intraoperative photograph shows the MPFL after repair with suture anchor and permanent suture. (Part B reproduced from Boden BP, Pearsall AW, Garrett WE Jr, Feagin JA Jr: Patellofemoral instability: Evaluation and management. *J Am Acad Orthop Surg* 1997;5:47-57.)

Patellar mobility and tilt are assessed after the repairs. If there is a concern about decreased patellar tilt, a lateral retinacular release can be done (**Figure 6**).

Wound Closure

The wounds are irrigated and hemostasis is maintained. The subcutaneous tissue and skin are closed with absorbable sutures, and the wound is secured with adhesive strips. Typically there is no need for drain placement. The arthroscopic portals are closed with nylon sutures. The wounds are cleaned and dressed, and an ice-pack machine, if wanted, and a knee brace locked at 0° are applied in the operating room.

———■

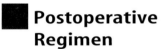

Postoperative Regimen

The postoperative protocol begins with pain management using regional blocks, ice packs, and oral medications. Patients return for wound check and suture removal 7 days postoperatively. Physical therapy is started with weight bearing in the brace as tolerated. Active and active-assisted range-of-motion exercises are begun out of the brace, and quadriceps activation is started with electrical stimulation techniques. Once quadriceps independence and good gait mechanics are demonstrated, patients are allowed to discontinue the brace, usually at about 2 weeks. Range-of-motion exer-

cises are continued to achieve full active motion by 4 to 6 weeks. Closed kinetic chain exercises to increase quadriceps strength are continued and increased after full knee motion has been reached. Cardiovascular exercises that protect the surgical lower extremity also are developed during this time. Functional sport exercises and plyometrics are initiated at about 3 months. From 4 to 6 months, patients increase their sporting activities in controlled environments and continue to work on quadriceps strength and endurance. Other lower extremity and core muscle strengthening exercises are continued during this time. Patients typically are released for unlimited activity at 4 to 6 months. Typically, a functional brace is not prescribed to use for sports. If articular cartilage repair was done, a continuous passive motion machine is used and weight-bearing status is modified based on the specific articular cartilage repair techniques.

———■

Avoiding Pitfalls and Complications

Complications of surgical intervention in patients with acute patellar instability can be minimized by understanding the goals of the patient, careful preoperative planning, and good surgical techniques, including arthroscopic treatment of intra-articular pathology. Most arthroscopic setups use a fluid pump system, which

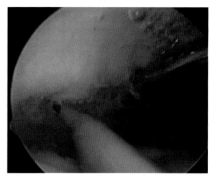

Figure 6 Arthroscopic view through the anteromedial portal of lateral retinacular release with intra-articular cautery. The cannula is seen in the superolateral portal.

can help in the evacuation of hematomas and improve vision of acute injuries. It is important to monitor the intra-articular pressure to avoid fluid extravasation into the soft tissues, which can produce significant soft-tissue swelling and pain and slow the postoperative course. Postoperative knee stiffness is the most common complication following immediate repair for acute patellar instability. Minimizing postoperative swelling, maximizing postoperative pain relief, and avoiding overtightening of the medial structures will help prevent this complication. Repair of the MPFL is done with the knee flexed 30° to 40° with the patella sitting in the trochlear groove of the femur. Increased contact forces on the medial patellar facet have been demonstrated in biomechanical studies, but these mostly are associated with MPFL reconstructions.

———■

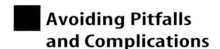

Bibliography

Ahmad CS, Stein BE, Matuz D, Henry JH: Immediate surgical repair of the medial patellar stabilizers for acute patellar dislocation: A review of eight cases. *Am J Sports Med* 2000;28(6):804-810.

Arendt EA, Fithian DC, Cohen E: Current concepts of lateral patella dislocation. *Clin Sports Med* 2002;21(3):499-519.

Boden BP, Pearsall AW, Garrett WE Jr, Feagin JA Jr: Patellofemoral instability: Evaluation and management. *J Am Acad Orthop Surg* 1997;5(1):47-57.

Buchner M, Baudendistel B, Sabo D, Schmitt H: Acute traumatic primary patellar dislocation: Long-term results comparing conservative and surgical treatment. *Clin J Sports Med* 2005;15(2):62-66.

Davis DK, Fithian DC: Techniques of medial retinacular repair and reconstruction. *Clin Orthop Relat Res* 2002;402:38-52.

Elias DA, White LM, Fithian DC: Acute lateral patellar dislocation at MR imaging: Injury patterns of medial patellar soft-tissue restraints and osteochondral injuries of the inferomedial patella. *Radiology* 2002;225(3):736-743.

Fithian DC, Paxton EW, Stone ML, et al: Epidemiology and natural history of acute patellar dislocation. *Am J Sports Med* 2004;32(5):1114-1121.

Miller JR, Adamson GJ, Pink MM, Fraipont MJ, Durand P Jr: Arthroscopically assisted medial reefing without routine lateral release for patellar instability. *Am J Sports Med* 2007;35(4):622-629.

Nam EK, Karzel RP: Mini-open medial reefing and arthroscopic lateral release for the treatment of recurrent patellar dislocation: A medium-term follow-up. *Am J Sports Med* 2005;33(2):220-230.

Nikku R, Nietosvaara Y, Aalto K, Kallio PE: Operative treatment of primary patellar dislocation does not improve medium-term outcome: A 7-year follow-up report and risk analysis of 127 randomized patients. *Acta Orthop* 2005;76(5):699-704.

Palmu S, Kallio PE, Donell ST, Helenius I, Nietosvaara Y: Acute patellar dislocation in children and adolescents: A randomized clinical trial. *J Bone Joint Surg Am* 2008;90(3):463-470.

Sallay PI, Poggi J, Speer KP, Garrett WE: Acute dislocation of the patella: A correlative pathoanatomic study. *Am J Sports Med* 1996;24(1):52-60.

Sillanpää PJ, Mattila VM, Mäenpää H, Kiuru M, Visuri T, Pihlajamäki H: Treatment with and without initial stabilizing surgery for primary traumatic patellar dislocation: A prospective randomized study. *J Bone Joint Surg Am* 2009;91(2):263-273.

Sillanpää PJ, Peltola E, Mattila VM, Kiuru M, Visuri T, Pihlajamäki H: Femoral avulsion of the medial patellofemoral ligament after primary traumatic patellar dislocation predicts subsequent instability in men: A mean 7-year nonoperative follow-up study. *Am J Sports Med* 2009;37(8):1513-1521.

Stefancin JJ, Parker RD: First-time traumatic patellar dislocation: A systematic review. *Clin Orthop Relat Res* 2007;445:93-101.

Vainionpää S, Laasonen E, Silvennoinen T, Vasenius J, Rokkanen P: Acute dislocation of the patella: A prospective review of operative treatment. *J Bone Joint Surg Br* 1990;72(3):366-369.

Coding

CPT Codes		Corresponding ICD-9 Codes	
Ligament Reconstruction/Augmentation			
27428	Ligamentous reconstruction (augmentation), knee; intra-articular (open)	717.81 844.2	717.9
27429	Ligamentous reconstruction (augmentation), knee; intra-articular (open) and extra-articular	717.84	844.2

Chapter 93

Chronic Patellar Instability

John P. Fulkerson, MD

◼ Indications

Recurrent patellar instability is disabling, particularly for individuals who wish to participate in vigorous activities. Chronic or recurrent patellar instability is related to extensor mechanism imbalance, either as a result of an underlying disorder of alignment or secondary to disruption of supportive structures around the patella and extensor mechanism. To reestablish stability and prevent instability events, accurate identification of the underlying cause of instability is required so that treatment can be designed to correct or compensate for this imbalance.

Recurrent instability, particularly when it involves dislocation of the patella, is damaging to the patellar articular surface and may lead to serious, permanent articular loss, particularly on the distal medial aspect of the patella. Excessive shear stress on the patella with pressure on the distal aspect of the patella in early knee flexion can also produce painful, soft, distal patellar articular cartilage that is symptomatic even in the absence of instability events (**Figure 1**). Consequently, indications for surgical treatment of recurrent patellar instability include pain resulting from distal or medial patellar injury secondary to instability, disabling recurrent instability, recurrent dislocation, functional daily instability, and limitation of athletic or work activity because of extensor mechanism instability.

Indications for specific surgical procedures are somewhat complicated and should be based on careful identification of both the underlying causes of instability and any anatomic deficiencies that perpetuate instability, such as medial patellofemoral ligament disruption. The primary structural considerations are abnormality of the relationship between the femoral trochlea and the tibial tuberosity (TT-TG index), disruption of the medial patellofemoral ligament (MPFL), flattening or deficiency of the trochlea, excessive femoral anteversion, poor lower extremity core stability and balance, and presence of articular lesions secondary to recurrent overload and imbalance. Secondary adaptive tightness of the lateral retinaculum also should be considered, but it is not generally believed to be a primary cause of instability.

◼ Contraindications

The primary contraindication to patellar instability surgery is a lack of adequate information or understanding to design an accurate surgical plan. Stabilization of the extensor mechanism should be done only with a full understanding of the underlying causes of instability and how best to correct them. No one operation is appropriate for all patients.

Gross obesity and smoking are relative contraindications to any tubercle transfer surgery. Tibial tubercle surgery should be used with caution and combined with careful management of diabetes or metabolic disorders when present.

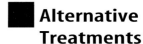

◼ Alternative Treatments

In milder cases, modification of activities, bracing, strengthening of the quadriceps and hamstrings, and rehabilitation of lower extremity balance

Dr. Fulkerson or an immediate family member serves as a board member, owner, officer, or committee member of the American Board of Orthopaedic Surgery; the American Orthopaedic Association; the American Orthopaedic Society for Sports Medicine; the Arthroscopy Association of North America; the International Society of Arthroscopy, Knee Surgery and Orthopaedic Sports Medicine; and the Orthopaedic Research and Education Foundation. In addition, Dr. Fulkerson or an immediate family member has received royalties from Arthrex and DJ Orthopaedics, serves as an unpaid consultant to DJ Orthopaedics and the Musculoskeletal Transplant Foundation, and owns stock or stock options in DJ Orthopaedics.

(core stability) may be sufficient to control instability events.

Results

Results of several studies are summarized in **Table 1**. Acute repair of a torn

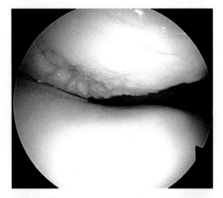

Figure 1 Arthroscopic view demonstrates a distal patella articular injury. (Photo courtesy of John P. Fulkerson, Farmington, CT.)

medial retinaculum and/or MPFL is generally not effective; healing should be allowed for later restoration if needed. Medial imbrication alone can be effective as a treatment for recurrent instability but is more likely to be successful when minimal or no trochlear dysplasia or malalignment is present. Procedures that address recurrent instability in the presence of more serious dysplasia and malalignment include MPFL tendon graft reconstruction (to restore medial support), tibial tubercle transfer (to correct an abnormally high TT-TG index or patella alta and balance patellar tracking) and trochleoplasty (to capture the patella into a deeper femoral sulcus). All of these procedures are effective for controlling instability in appropriately selected patients, but pain, arthrofibrosis, and less satisfactory objective results have been reported following trochleoplasty. Anteromedial tibial tubercle transfer has been reported to

yield a 97% return to sport, unload a distal or lateral articular lesion, and correct lateral tracking related to an abnormally high TT-TG index and Q angle, and the procedure can be modified to reduce patella alta. The procedure or combination of procedures used should be customized to the individual patient.

Evaluation

Although deficiency of the MPFL is a constant component of patellar instability, simply reconstructing the ligament does not compensate for serious malalignment of the extensor mechanism. In a patient with evidence of ongoing symptomatic subluxation and evidence of chronic lateral facet overload, predisposing factors may range from overall lower extremity balance to fixed incongruity between

Table 1 Results of Surgical Treatment for Patellar Dislocation

Authors (Year)	Number of Knees	Procedure or Approach	Mean Patient Age in Years (Range)	Mean Follow-up (Range)	Results
Carney et al (2005)	18	Medial tibial tubercle transfer	NR	26 years	7% recurrent dislocation 54% good/excellent
Nam and Karzel (2005)	23	Mini open medial reefing and lateral release	23 (12-65)	4.4 years (1.4-14)	91% good or excellent 4% redislocation
Verdonk et al (2005)	12	Trochleoplasty	27	18 months (8-34)	Subjective: 77% good or very good Objective: 23% good/excellent
Schöttle et al (2006)	48	Arthroscopic medial retinacular repair	NR	1 year	Medial repair effective at 1 year in patients with minimal or no trochlear dysplasia
Steiner et al (2006)	34	MPFL reconstruction	27	66.5 months (24-130)	85% good results (Kujala) No redislocation
Sillanpää et al (2008)	61	Nonsurgical treatment vs repair of acute MPFL tear	20 (19-22)	7.5 years (6-11)	No improvement of stability with acute arthroscopic repair
Tjoumakaris et al (2010)	41	Anteromedial tibial tubercle transfer	20	46 months (22-71)	IKDC 95% normal or near normal 97% return to sports

IKDC = International Knee Documentation Committee; MFPL = medial patellofemoral ligament; NR = not reported.

the tibial tubercle (TT) and the central trochlear groove (TG). Trochlear dysplasia also is common in people with chronic instability and is probably adaptive to chronic lateral patellar tracking, much as a shallow acetabulum is adaptive to chronic lateral hip subluxation and anatomic deficiency. In many patients, restoration of balance through proper rehabilitation or surgical compensation for imbalances to permit central, optimal tracking of the patella offers the best hope of normalizing articular loads in the patellofemoral joint while creating a stable configuration to allow proper retinaculum-ligament balancing. Often, rehabilitation and surgical balancing go hand-in-hand.

In patients with traumatic disruption of the MPFL or with minimal or no evidence of extensor mechanism dysplasia or malalignment, proximal rebalancing of the patellofemoral joint alone through release of the adaptively tight lateral retinaculum and restoration (imbrication or advancement) of the healed, elongated MPFL may be all that is needed.

As instability becomes more profound and recurrent dislocation is more frequent because of trochlear dysplasia caused by chronic extensor mechanism imbalance, compensatory surgery becomes more important to establish central tracking of the patella before restoring support on the medial side. Radiographs (including a Merchant view), CT, and MRI can be helpful for identifying structural deficiencies and abnormal distances between the central trochlea and the tibial tubercle. In general, patients with more severe lateral patellar subluxation, particularly when bilateral and structural (TT-TG distance > 15-20 mm), require medialization of the tibial tubercle to compensate for the structural incongruities. For instance, in some patients, excessive femoral anteversion may contribute to chronic lateral patellar tracking. In these patients, rather than derotat-ing the hip, the structural problem can be compensated for by moving the tibial tubercle. This brings the patella back into a reasonable balance with the central trochlea, which is structurally and functionally internally rotated relative to the lower leg because of the femoral anteversion. Medial transfer of the tibial tubercle results in central patellar tracking, reduced susceptibility to instability including dislocation, and improved quality of life. Although tibial tubercle transfer does not correct the underlying pathology, it can be an effective and relatively benign compensatory approach compared to derotating the hip. This is particularly true when there is a disparity between the central trochlea and the tibial tuberosity, when patella alta is present, and when compensation for other factors such as trochlear dysplasia are considerations.

Physical Examination

The physical examination should establish the degree of deficiency in both the medial and lateral support around the patella. In patients who have had previous surgery of the extensor mechanism, it is particularly important to eliminate the possibility of medial patellar subluxation by doing a provocative medial displacement of the patella with the knee in extension, followed by prompt flexion of the knee to determine if entry of the patella into the trochlea from medial to lateral causes symptoms. Similarly, the examiner should test to see if the patella enters the trochlea in a *J* configuration (exaggerated translation of the patella from too far lateral into the trochlea with flexion of the knee). The examiner should determine the extent of MPFL deficiency by displacing the patella laterally with the knee in extension and then slowly flexing the knee to see if the MPFL is doing its cardinal job of delivering the patella from a slightly lateralized position to the central trochlea in the first degrees of knee flexion. With more flexion, normally the trochlea deepens and controls patellar stability, making the medial capsule less important. With severe trochlear deficiency, however, the patella may slide out farther into flexion with tensioning of the extensor mechanism. Deficiencies of this degree require more extensive stabilization of the extensor mechanism and are most often a reflection of a chronically lateralized extensor mechanism, which will likely require medial transfer of the tibial tubercle as part of the solution. Less commonly, in severe cases, trochleoplasty or MPFL reconstruction or both also may be necessary to achieve long-term stability.

Watching the patient do a single-leg knee bend permits the examiner to assess the extent to which excessive static and functional internal rotation at the hip complicates the patient's difficulty with lateral patellar instability. To the extent that this is problematic, the examiner should emphasize core stability affecting the lower extremity function, particularly hip abductors and external rotators, before considering surgery.

Imaging

Radiographic studies are imperative. A standard axial view, taken in 45° of knee flexion (Merchant view), will give a good overview of patellar tracking. In short, if the patella stays lateralized with the knee at 45° of flexion, the lateral tracking vector is substantial and will require medialization. Midpatellar transverse CT cuts obtained at 0°, 15°, 30°, and 45° of knee flexion will more specifically document the nature of patellar entry into the trochlea in early knee flexion. The patella should be centralized in the trochlea by placing the knee in 10° to 15° of flexion.

Surgical Treatment Options

The more severe the lateralization of the extensor mechanism and secondary lateral trochlear dysplasia, the more likely the patient is to require medialization of the tibial tuberosity as part of the corrective surgery. Medialization of the tibial tuberosity compensates for alignment factors that cause lateral tracking of the patella and balances patellar tracking in the central trochlea before soft-tissue restoration is done around the patella.

MPFL Imbrication or Advancement

In patients with a TT-TG index less than 15 (less than 15 mm between the tibial tubercle and the central trochlear groove in the medial-lateral plane), and with a normal or mildly elevated congruence angle or Q angle, imbrication or advancement of the healed elongated MPFL, with lateral release as necessary to mobilize the lateral side, may be all that is necessary, particularly when the trochlea is normal or nearly normal. It is important to recognize that the MPFL generally heals after an initial dislocation, which explains why medial imbrications, such as the Insall procedure, have worked traditionally. Medial imbrication or advancement of the medial patellofemoral structures, however, has inherent risk the more the extensor mechanism is lateralized, because medial imbrication can create a posteromedially oriented tether on the medial patellofemoral joint, resulting in overload of the medial patella exactly where the patella often is injured during patellar dislocation. This is true also of MPFL reconstruction used to "realign" the extensor mechanism. Thus, the concept should be to balance the extensor mechanism tracking first, then restore medial support to establish proper initial entry of the patella into the trochlea in early

knee flexion (normal MPFL function). I do not support the routine use of an MPFL tendon graft to pull the patella from a fixed lateral tracking pattern. Examining the contralateral uninjured knee, as originally recommended by Hawkins, is helpful in understanding the patient's underlying imbalance.

Tibial Tubercle Transfer

With a TT-TG ratio greater than 20 or with lateralizing forces on the extensor mechanism, including lateral trochlear dysplasia, medial tibial tubercle transfer to create balance is advisable before doing any secondary soft-tissue reconstruction. Once the tibial tubercle is moved to stabilize the extensor mechanism in the trochlea, the medial retinacular structures can be advanced through a mini-open approach or arthroscopically to reestablish MPFL function (the MPFL fails at approximately 200 N). A normal tracking pattern should be observed arthroscopically at the end of the reconstruction (the patella entering the trochlea from a slightly lateralized position into the central trochlea in early flexion, without overmedialization and without excessive posteromedial force on the patellar articular surface), particularly if an articular lesion is present on the medial patella.

MPFL Reconstruction

MPFL reconstruction is important when medial patellar support is seriously deficient and when a secure tether for the patella is needed medially. This becomes more important with more serious dysplasia and often is used in combination with medial transfer of the tibial tuberosity, using the tibial tuberosity transfer to correct the tracking vector and an MPFL tendon graft reconstruction to produce a more secure than normal medial support. Tendon graft reconstruction of the MPFL creates strong support for the patella medially, but it should not be used to force the patella from a lat-

eralized position into the central trochlea, because this will create abnormally elevated articular pressure on the patella and likely cause eventual patellofemoral arthrosis. Tendon graft reconstruction of the MPFL, therefore, is most often indicated in patients with medial patellofemoral capsuloligamentous loss and as a supplement to medial tibial tubercle transfer in patients with severe extensor mechanism lateralization and dysplasia.

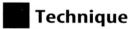

Technique

Before the procedure begins, the surgeon should have a clear idea of the underlying problems and a sense of the degree of dysplasia and lateral tracking.

Procedure

The surgeon generally begins with an arthroscopic evaluation to identify the location and extent of articular injuries. Lateral release usually is accomplished arthroscopically when indicated for any component of tilt and lateral tether. Articular lesions can be débrided arthroscopically, with care taken to remove all unstable articular cartilage flaps. The extent of lateral tracking and lateral patellofemoral joint degeneration, as well as the extent of injury to the medial patella following dislocation, are pertinent in determining the appropriate corrective procedure.

LATERAL RELEASE

In patients with minimal dysplasia and minimal lateralization, particularly if there is a component of patellar tilt from adaptive lateral shortening, some limited lateral release may be indicated to help balance the extensor mechanism. Lateral release, of course, should only be done such that true release of a lateral tether and tilt may be

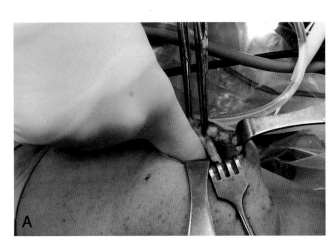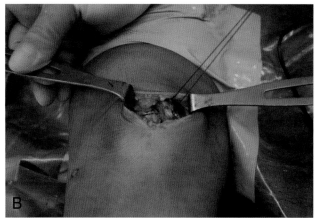

Figure 2 Open medial imbrication. **A,** The healed MPFL is palpated. **B,** The tendon is imbricated only enough to normalize tracking. (Photo courtesy of John P. Fulkerson, Farmington, CT.)

documented. In other words, no "release" should be done unless an overtight, tilting deformity is documented.

MEDIAL IMBRICATION OR ADVANCEMENT

At this point, in a patient with limited dysplasia and lateral tracking and if at least 3 months have passed since the last instability event, simple advancement of the MPFL may be sufficient. In general, all that may be needed is a short medial incision, release of the vastus medialis obliquus (VMO) tendon from the patella, palpation of the MPFL (healed) from its deep side to establish that the structure is intact (**Figure 2**, *A*) but elongated, and then retensioning or advancement of the healed MPFL to create a medial tether (**Figure 2**, *B*). This is particularly attractive after a traumatic dislocation of the patella in which there are no dysplastic factors and when the patient simply needs to have medial support reestablished to normal. At the end of the procedure, the patella should track normally without evidence of abnormal articular loading. Arthroscopic imbrication also can be done in patients with minimal dysplasia and a healed MPFL (**Figure 3**). Postoperatively, patients are kept in a knee immobilizer for 6 weeks but start a single arc of knee flexion daily after

10 to 14 days, gaining 90° of flexion by 4 weeks after surgery.

MPFL RECONSTRUCTION

In patients with a grossly deficient MPFL, a tendon graft (allograft or autograft) is necessary to achieve medial stabilization (**Figure 4**, *A*). I prefer to avoid drilling the patella and therefore stabilize the graft by passing it deep to the VMO and then through a small slot in the VMO tendon and suturing it securely onto the quadriceps tendon on the patellar side (**Figure 4**, *B*). On the femoral side, I have been using a technique in which the tendon graft is passed distal to the adductor tubercle, then back under the adductor insertion so that the graft loops back and can be sutured to the adductor tendon insertion and to itself. The graft must be anatomically well situated at the normal MPFL femoral origin between the adductor tubercle and the medial epicondyle. This area is abraded to bleeding bone, and a staple or suture anchors are placed in this region to hold the MPFL tendon graft in proper alignment. This procedure provides a secure reconstruction without drilling into the patella, thereby eliminating this added risk of patellar fracture; however, it is indicated strictly to restore normal MPFL structure and stability, not to pull the patella from an abnormal tracking pattern. Postopera-

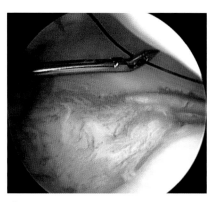

Figure 3 Arthroscopic medial imbrication. (Photo courtesy of John P. Fulkerson, Farmington, CT.)

tive treatment is the same as after MPFL advancement or imbrication.

TIBIAL TUBERCLE TRANSFER

Tibial tubercle transfer is a powerful procedure for patellofemoral stabilization but must be used only when lateral tracking is related to fixed dysplasia, malalignment, or incongruity of the TT-TG index. In practice, this is fairly common among patients with recurrent patellar instability. When it is apparent that the patella is chronically lateralized, the TT-TG index is greater than 15 to 20, and the lateral trochlea is flattened, medialization of the tibial tubercle is indicated. When the distal medial patellar cartilage is

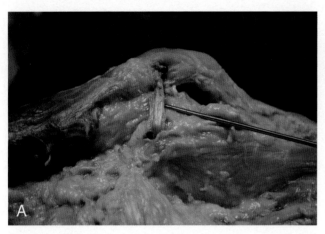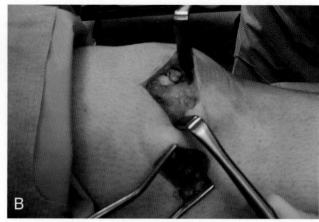

Figure 4 MPFL reconstruction. **A,** The MPFL originates just distal and anterior to the adductor tubercle and attaches to the deep vastus medial obliquus (VMO) tendon at the proximal patella. A tendon graft reconstruction (simulated here in a cadaver knee) should reproduce this structure accurately. **B,** Intraoperative photograph shows the completed reconstruction. The MPFL tendon graft is attached to the deep VMO tendon and then sutured into the distal medial quadriceps tendon to avoid drilling into the patella. (Photos courtesy of John P. Fulkerson, Farmington, CT.)

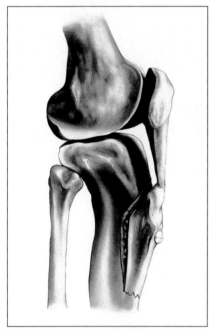

Figure 5 Drawing of an anteromedial tibial tubercle transfer. (Illustration courtesy of John P. Fulkerson, Farmington, CT.)

damaged, anteromedial tibial tubercle transfer is preferable.

After adequate exposure, and arthroscopic lateral release if needed, the anterior tibialis muscle is reflected posteriorly, the patellar tendon is isolated, and a cut is made deep to the tibial tuberosity with an oscillating saw. The osteotomy should taper anteriorly at its distal extent. Then an osteotome cut (½-inch osteotome) is made above the patellar tendon insertion to allow medial rotation of the tibial tuberosity through a greenstick fracture at its distal extent. The tuberosity can then be rotated to a position that allows central tracking of the patella, being sure not to overmedialize, as viewed with an arthroscope. Usually, this is about 1 cm of medialization. The osteotomized bone pedicle is then held securely in place with two cortical lag screws into the posterior tibial cortex, hemostasis is achieved, and early motion is started. Often the medial capsule and MPFL are imbricated to restore normal length, but without attempting to pull the patella with the medial structure. Again, every attempt should be made to avoid adding load to an articular lesion.

ANTEROMEDIAL TIBIAL TUBERCLE TRANSFER
When a symptomatic distal lesion is present, anteromedial tibial tubercle transfer is preferable (**Figure 5**). This procedure unloads the injured distal medial patella and will restore a normal TT-TG relationship, Q angle, and central patellar tracking. An oblique osteotomy is made distally, tapered anteriorly at its distal extent, and the tubercle osteotomy bone pedicle is rotated anteromedially. Stabilization and rehabilitation are the same as after straight medial transfer of the tibial tubercle. With the anterior transfer component, load to the distal medial "dislocation lesion" is minimized. Anteromedial tibial tubercle transfer returns 97% of patients with patellar instability to athletics.

MEDIAL PATELLAR INSTABILITY
In a patient who has had previous patellofemoral surgery, medial patellar instability should be suspected when the patient reports sudden shifting, giving way, or collapsing of the knee. This usually is distinctly different and more disabling than lateral instability. It can be elicited by pushing the patella medially with the knee extended and then suddenly flexing the knee. If this reproduces the symptoms, the patient probably has a medial patellar subluxation problem and requires repair or reconstruction of the lateral retinaculum (**Figure 6**). If there is insufficient lateral retinaculum to repair, the lateral 7 mm of patellar tendon can be released at the tibial tubercle level, left attached to the patella, and then

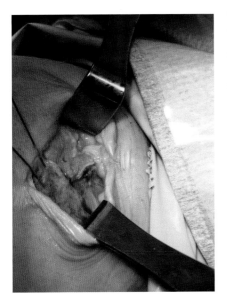

Figure 6 Intraoperative photograph shows lateral repair to control medial patellar subluxation. (Photo courtesy of John P. Fulkerson, Farmington, CT.)

sewn back on itself through the iliotibial band, so that it tethers the patella laterally and prevents medial subluxation.

Avoiding Pitfalls and Complications

If medial capsule reconstruction is done to stabilize the patella, any imbricating or tightening that will add load to a symptomatic or potentially symptomatic medial articular lesion (common after patella dislocation) should be avoided. Reconstruction of the MPFL should not be used as a means of relocating or transferring the patella, but rather as a restorative procedure for medial support when alignment and abnormal tracking of the patella have been corrected or are not believed to be major contributing factors to the instability. Pulling the patella medially to central tracking from a fixed lateral tracking pattern, neglecting to correct underlying malalignment, and overloading a medial articular lesion may cause pain and are contraindicated.

The goal of surgery should be to minimize morbidity and create stable tracking of the patella without adding abnormal load to the joint. Pitfalls involved in extensor mechanism realignment surgery include adding excessive load to the patella, thereby adding a risk of eventual articular breakdown (using medial reconstruction to realign the patella instead of using it to reestablish normal medial support); moving the extensor mechanism too far and creating a medial subluxation; overreleasing laterally, thereby making the patient prone to medial subluxation; and advancing the healed MPFL to support the extensor mechanism medially when the underlying dysplasia and malalignment will overcome this potentially vulnerable medial support. Other pitfalls include failing to adequately mobilize the knee after extensor mechanism surgery, excessive immobilization, and surgery that restricts knee range of motion (inaccurate capsuloligamentous surgery); failing to recognize medial patellar subluxation (in which the patella enters the trochlea from too far medial to the trochlea, thereby moving laterally in early knee flexion, simulating lateral patellar displacement) and worsening the patient's condition by further medializing the extensor mechanism; imbricating or advancing an incompetent MPFL and expecting it to provide adequate support; or improper placement of MPFL fixation. In addition, patellar fracture can occur as a complication of drilling of the patella for MPFL reconstruction, and tibial tubercle or tibial fracture can occur if the tubercle osteotomy is not tapered anteriorly at its distal extent.

Bibliography

Amis AA, Firer P, Mountney J, Senavongse W, Thomas NP: Anatomy and biomechanics of the medial patellofemoral ligament. *Knee* 2003;10(3):215-220.

Arendt EA, Fithian DC, Cohen E: Current concepts of lateral patella dislocation. *Clin Sports Med* 2002;21(3):499-519.

Bicos J, Fulkerson JP, Amis A: Current concepts review: The medial patellofemoral ligament. *Am J Sports Med* 2007;35(3):484-492.

Carney JR, Mologne TS, Muldoon M, Cox JS: Long-term evaluation of the Roux-Elmslie-Trillat procedure for patellar instability: A 26-year follow-up. *Am J Sports Med* 2005;33(8):1220-1223.

Dejour H, Walch G, Neyret P, Adeleine P: [Dysplasia of the femoral trochlea]. *Rev Chir Orthop Reparatrice Appar Mot* 1990;76(1):45-54.

Elias JJ, Cosgarea AJ: Technical errors during medial patellofemoral ligament reconstruction could overload medial patellofemoral cartilage: A computational analysis. *Am J Sports Med* 2006;34(9):1478-1485.

Farr J, Schepsis A, Cole B, Fulkerson J, Lewis P: Anteromedialization: Review and technique. *J Knee Surg* 2007;20(2): 120-128.

Fithian DC, Paxton EW, Post WR, Panni AS; International Patellofemoral Study Group: Lateral retinacular release: A survey of the International Patellofemoral Study Group. *Arthroscopy* 2004;20(5):463-468.

Fulkerson JP: Anteromedial tibial tubercle transfer, in Jackson DW, ed: *Master Techniques in Orthopaedic Surgery: Reconstructive Knee Surgery*. Philadelphia, PA, Lippincott Williams & Wilkins, 2003, pp 13-25.

Fulkerson JP, Becker GJ, Meaney JA, Miranda M, Folcik MA: Anteromedial tibial tubercle transfer without bone graft. *Am J Sports Med* 1990;18(5):490-496, discussion 496-497.

Fulkerson JP, Schutzer SF, Ramsby GR, Bernstein RA: Computerized tomography of the patellofemoral joint before and after lateral release or realignment. *Arthroscopy* 1987;3(1):19-24.

Goutallier D, Bernageau J, Lecudonnec B: [The measurement of the tibial tuberosity. Patella groove distanced technique and results (author's transl)]. *Rev Chir Orthop Reparatrice Appar Mot* 1978;64(5):423-428.

Grelsamer RP: Patellar malalignment. *J Bone Joint Surg Am* 2000;82-A(11):1639-1650.

Halbrecht JL: Arthroscopic patella realignment: An all-inside technique. *Arthroscopy* 2001;17(9):940-945.

Merchant AC, Mercer RL, Jacobsen RH, Cool CR: Roentgenographic analysis of patellofemoral congruence. *J Bone Joint Surg Am* 1974;56(7):1391-1396.

Nam EK, Karzel RP: Mini-open medial reefing and arthroscopic lateral release for the treatment of recurrent patellar dislocation: A medium-term follow-up. *Am J Sports Med* 2005;33(2):220-230.

Nomura E, Horiuchi Y, Kihara M: Medial patellofemoral ligament restraint in lateral patellar translation and reconstruction. *Knee* 2000;7(2):121-127.

Pidoriano AJ, Weinstein RN, Buuck DA, Fulkerson JP: Correlation of patellar articular lesions with results from anteromedial tibial tubercle transfer. *Am J Sports Med* 1997;25(4):533-537.

Post WR: Clinical evaluation of patients with patellofemoral disorders. *Arthroscopy* 1999;15(8):841-851.

Schöttle PB, Scheffler SU, Schwarck A, Weiler A: Arthroscopic medial retinacular repair after patellar dislocation with and without underlying trochlear dysplasia: A preliminary report. *Arthroscopy* 2006;22(11):1192-1198.

Schutzer SF, Ramsby GR, Fulkerson JP: The evaluation of patellofemoral pain using computerized tomography: A preliminary study. *Clin Orthop Relat Res* 1986;204:286-293.

Sillanpää PJ, Mäenpää HM, Mattila VM, Visuri T, Pihlajamäki H: Arthroscopic surgery for primary traumatic patellar dislocation: A prospective, nonrandomized study comparing patients treated with and without acute arthroscopic stabilization with a median 7-year follow-up. *Am J Sports Med* 2008;36(12):2301-2309.

Steiner TM, Torga-Spak R, Teitge RA: Medial patellofemoral ligament reconstruction in patients with lateral patellar instability and trochlear dysplasia. *Am J Sports Med* 2006;34(8):1254-1261.

Tjoumakaris FP, Forsythe B, Bradley JP: Patellofemoral instability in athletes: Treatment via modified Fulkerson osteotomy and lateral release. *Am J Sports Med* 2010;38(5):992-999.

Tom A, Fulkerson JP: Restoration of native medial patellofemoral ligament support after patella dislocation. *Sports Med Arthrosc* 2007;15(2):68-71.

Verdonk R, Jansegers E, Stuyts B: Trochleoplasty in dysplastic knee trochlea. *Knee Surg Sports Traumatol Arthrosc* 2005;13(7):529-533.

Coding

CPT Codes		Corresponding ICD-9 Codes	
Patellar Dislocation Reconstruction			
27420	Reconstruction of dislocating patella (eg, Hauser type procedure)	718.26 905.6	836.3 717.9
27422	Reconstruction of dislocating patella; with extensor realignment and/or muscle advancement or release (eg, Campbell, Goldwaite type procedure)	718.26 905.6	836.3 717.9
Lateral Reticulum Release, Open			
27425	Suture of infrapatellar tendon; primary	718.26 905.6	836.3 717.9
Lateral Reticulum Release, Arthroscopic			
29873	Suture of infrapatellar tendon; primary	718.26 905.6	836.3 717.9
Ligament Reconstruction			
27428	Ligamentous reconstruction (augmentation), knee; intra-articular (open)	718.26 905.6 717.9	836.3 717.89
27429	Ligamentous reconstruction (augmentation), knee; intra-articular (open) and extra-articular	718.26 905.6 717.9	836.3 717.89

Chapter 94

Rupture of the Extensor Mechanism

Thomas M. DeBerardino, MD

Indications

The extensor mechanism of the knee is composed of the patellar tendon and quadriceps tendon. Rupture of either tendon is a rare but significant injury requiring prompt diagnosis and treatment. Quadriceps tendon ruptures are more common in patients older than 40 years and often are associated with underlying medical conditions. Galen is credited with the first report of a rupture of the quadriceps tendon in a wrestler, nearly 2,000 years ago. A combination of acute pain, inability to actively extend the knee, and a suprapatellar gap are all typical clinical findings (**Figure 1**). Quadriceps tendon rupture may result from either indirect or direct mechanisms. Various imaging modalities, including plain radiographs, ultrasonography, and MRI, can be used to evaluate quadriceps tendon injury.

Complete tendon rupture requires surgical repair for optimal results; several techniques have been described. Early repair of the ruptured extensor mechanism provides the best chance for full functional recovery. One study of 20 patients suggested that repair should be done within 2 or 3 days of injury to achieve a successful outcome and that late repair led to unsatisfactory recovery. The natural history of an untreated extensor mechanism rupture is complete extensor mechanism dysfunction. Untreated acute ruptures result in chronic injuries that are more difficult to manage surgically, often requiring complex reconstructive procedures. Good results have been reported in some series, however.

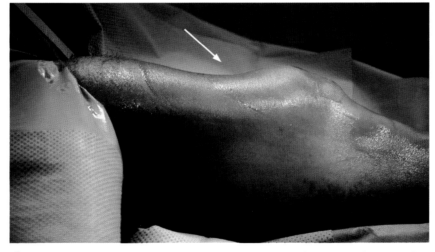

Figure 1 Lateral photograph of a knee with an acute rupture of a right quadriceps tendon. Note the suprapatellar gap (arrow).

Dr. DeBerardino or an immediate family member serves as a board member, owner, officer, or committee member of the American Orthopaedic Society for Sports Medicine and the American Board of Orthopaedic Surgery; is a member of a speakers' bureau or has made paid presentations on behalf of Arthrex, Genzyme, and the Musculoskeletal Transplant Foundation; serves as an unpaid consultant to Arthrex; and has received research or institutional support from Arthrex, Genzyme, DJ Orthopaedics, the Musculoskeletal Transplant Foundation, and Histogenics.

Contraindications

There are relatively few contraindications to repair or reconstruction of a rupture of the extensor mechanism. Certainly, a planned knee fusion would negate the need to repair or reconstruct the ruptured extensor mechanism. Compromised general health status or associated injuries are relative contraindications for acute repair. Additionally, a compromised local soft-tissue environment, from either a contaminated open wound or a wound lacking adequate skin coverage for closure over the repair site, is a contraindication for acute repair. In these cases, it is prudent to wait until

Table 1 Results of Extensor Mechanism Repair

Authors (Year)	Portion of Extensor Mechanism	Number of Injuries (Number of Patients)	Mean Patient Age in Years (Range)	Mean Follow-up in Months (Range)	Results
Rasul and Fischer (1993)	Quadriceps tendon	19 (19) 17 acute, 2 chronic	47 (16-72)	NR	Acute: all excellent Chronic: both good
Rougraff et al (1996)	Quadriceps tendon	53 (44) Acute vs chronic NR	59 (13-85)	67.2 (24-155)	All excellent/good
Kasten et al (2001)	Patellar tendon	29 (27) All acute	NR	98 (12-192)	26 excellent/good 3 fair
Bushnell et al (2008)	Patellar tendon	14 (14) All acute	35 (25-50)	29 (3-112)	11 excellent 3 poor (failures)

NR = not reported.

the soft-tissue envelope about the knee extensor mechanism and knee joint is cleared of infection and affords adequate skin for secure wound closure.

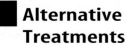

Alternative Treatments

The gold standard for managing acute quadriceps or patellar tendon ruptures depends on the type of tear. For midsubstance tears, a direct repair is used; the standard repair for the more common tendon avulsion injuries uses sutures passed through patellar bone tunnels. Several authors have studied the use of suture anchors as an alternative repair technique for acute quadriceps and patellar tendon ruptures. Suture anchors have the advantage of not requiring exposure of the opposite end of the patella. They also decrease surgical morbidity and potential problems with knots placed in the area of the patellar tunnel end points. However, suture anchors represent an additional cost compared with bone tunnels.

Chronic ruptures of the extensor mechanism can be reconstructed or augmented with several allograft options. Reports in the literature have

shown good functional results using an Achilles tendon allograft for either the quadriceps or patellar tendon. Soft-tissue options such as allograft or autograft hamstring tendons or allograft tibialis also can be used to augment these chronic injuries.

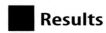

Results

The long-term results of repairs after rupture of the extensor mechanism are appropriately divided into studies that focus on the quadriceps tendon rupture and those that focus on the patellar tendon rupture. In general, the results reported are better with acute repairs than with chronic augmentations and reconstructions (Table 1).

A review of reported series indicates that all described surgical techniques are effective as long as postoperative therapy is started expeditiously. Regaining range of motion comparable to the uninjured side was not a problem in most series. One series noted a preponderance of midsubstance quadriceps ruptures in a slightly younger cohort (<40 years), whereas ruptures off the patella occurred predominantly in the older cohort (>40 years). In general, patient age, sex, mechanism of in-

jury, site of rupture, and type of repair did not affect the outcome of treatment.

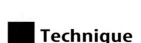

Technique

Setup/Exposure
The exposure for the repair of both the quadriceps tendon and patellar tendon is a direct approach through a midline incision (**Figure 2**).

Instruments/Equipment/ Implants Required
With the patient supine and the well leg adequately protected and padded, a routine extremity drape is placed over the surgically prepared knee to the upper thigh to expose the entire lower extremity. A tourniquet is not routinely applied to avoid capturing the proximally retracted extensor mechanism. Having a sterile tourniquet available is prudent, however. A basic orthopaedic surgical setup is needed for both quadriceps and patellar tendon repairs.

Procedure
In the case of an avulsion off the proximal pole of the patella, the quadriceps tendon is freed of any investing scar tissue. In chronic repairs, this allows

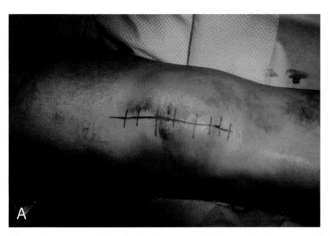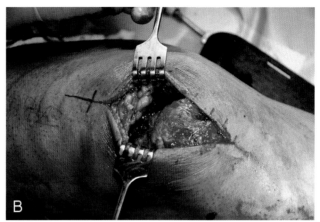

Figure 2 Incision (**A**) and initial exposure (**B**) for repair of a ruptured right knee quadriceps tendon.

easy advancement and trial reduction of the tissue onto the proximal pole of the patella (**Figure 3**, *A* and *B*). My preferred technique for placing the permanent repair sutures within the torn edge of the tendon uses two deep medial and lateral Krackow sutures (No. 2 or No. 5 double-armed permanent suture). These Krackow sutures are started about 3 cm proximal to the shorter posterior aspect of the free end of the tendon and exit within the posterior half of the free edge of the tendon. A Beath pin is used to drill the transpatellar holes. Alternatively, a standard 2.5-mm AO drill can be used to drill the three holes, and a Hewson suture passer to deliver the permanent repair sutures through the tunnels for the final repair. The four suture limbs are passed through the patellar drill holes from proximal to distal. The more medial and lateral suture arms traverse the medial and lateral patellar tunnels. The more central arms of each Krackow suture are combined to traverse the central patellar tunnel (**Figure 3**, *C* through *F*). Because the quadriceps tendon has such a significant anteroposterior thickness, an additional set of more superficial and distal Krackow sutures are commonly placed in the anterior half of the tendon. These two sutures begin about 2 to 3 cm proximal to the longer anterior aspect of the free end of the ten-

don and exit within the anterior half of the free edge of the tendon (**Figure 3**, *G* through *I*). These sutures are secured to the patella using suture anchors. Alternatively, they can be sutured to the distal free edge of stout tissue overlying the lower portion of the patella if the tissue is adequate to hold these important sutures. This repair technique provides an anatomic reattachment of the broad posterior and more distal anterior aspect of the quadriceps tendon insertion on the patella through a double-row repair similar to the repair commonly done with arthroscopic rotator cuff repairs.

A patellar tendon rupture from the inferior pole of the patella is repaired in a similar fashion using two or three No. 2 double-armed permanent sutures passed cephalad up through patellar drill holes. Retinacular sutures often are needed to repair the torn medial and lateral retinacula and capsular tissue. When the quality of the tendon tissue is questionable, I recommend augmenting the repair with a cerclage wire or additional No. 2 double-armed permanent suture passed through a transverse drill hole in the distal patella and the tibial tubercle.

Patellar tendon ruptures that avulse off the tibial tubercle can be challenging. The footprint of the patellar tendon insertion is broader on

the tibial tubercle than is the footprint of the origin on the distal pole of the patella (**Figure 4**, *A*). The free end of the tendon and tibial tubercle are freshened with a rongeur (**Figure 4**, *B*). I recommend a corresponding broad reattachment technique that uses four No. 2 double-armed permanent sutures, which allow an anatomic repair to the tubercle similar to the common arthroscopic double-row repair of a torn rotator cuff. The oblique cross section of the distal tendon is divided into four virtual quadrants: deep medial, deep lateral, superficial medial, and superficial lateral (**Figure 4**, *A*). A Krackow stitch is placed to control each section. The deep medial and lateral Krackow sutures are passed using preplaced looped passing sutures in a criss-crossed fashion through oblique drill holes in the proximal aspect of the tibial tubercle from deep medial to superficial lateral and from deep lateral to superficial medial (**Figure 4**, *C* and *D*). The superficial sutures are combined with the exiting deep suture tails and secured in the more distal aspect of the tubercle using suture anchors (**Figure 4**, *E* and *F*). This double-row fixation method provides a theoretically improved reestablishment of the broad insertion footprint of the tendon onto the tubercle.

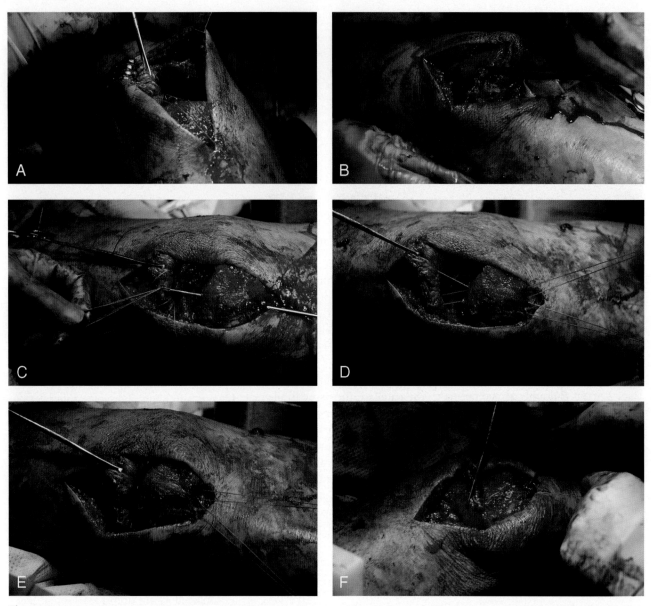

Figure 3 Sequential intraoperative photographs of a repair of a ruptured quadriceps tendon. **A,** The quadriceps tendon is freed of any investing scar tissue. **B,** An adequate trial reduction is confirmed. **C,** Three small parallel tunnels are drilled along the long axis of the patella. **D,** The four sutures are passed up through the three drill holes with one arm from each pair of sutures joining to pass through the central drill hole. **E,** The original suture limbs are paired as they exit the drill holes. **F,** A low-tension anatomic reduction is confirmed with the aid of a clamp as the sutures are tied so the knots are juxtaposed to the patellar tendon edges distally.

Wound Closure

Before closure, the wound is irrigated. The subcutaneous tissue is closed with absorbable suture in layers, and nylon sutures or staples are used for the skin closure. A suction drain can be placed for 1 to 2 days postoperatively because hemarthrosis is common.

Postoperative Regimen

The postoperative protocol after extensor mechanism repair includes a multimodal pain management program. Standard pain medications often are supplemented with diazepam to treat the muscle spasms. These can be significant, especially with chronic repairs when the retracted myotendinous unit is suddenly brought back to a normal resting length from a shortened position. A knee immobilizer is worn for the first 6 weeks, and weight bearing is allowed and encouraged as tolerated with the assistance of crutches until adequate quadriceps function returns, usually by the sec-

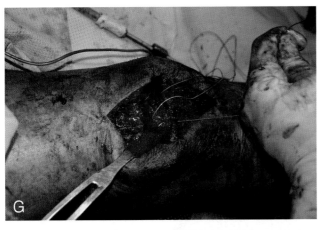

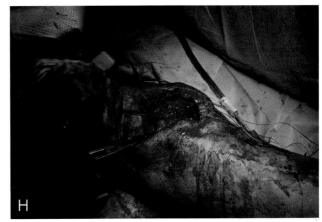

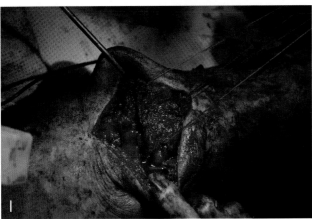

Figure 3 (continued) G, Absorbable sutures are placed as needed to secure any residual loose tendon edges and the repair site. **H,** The final repair of the quadriceps tendon is checked. **I,** Additional absorbable sutures are added as needed to close the concomitant tears in the retinacular tissue medial and lateral to the repair.

ond or third week. Deep vein thrombosis prophylaxis is based on a surgical time of less than one hour, early ambulation on the first postoperative day, mechanical compression with sequential compression stockings, and/or foot pumps (while in bed). Most patients leave the hospital after the first physical therapy session on the day after the surgery. Motion is allowed immediately in a supervised therapy setting, with knee motion from 0° to 45° for the first 3 weeks, then from 0° to 90° for the next 3 weeks unless otherwise limited to less flexion because of a difficult repair or reconstruction. Straight-leg raises (in the brace for the first 4 to 6 weeks) also are encouraged. Strengthening exercises should be initiated at week 7. Sports activities can be resumed gradually after 3 months. No resisted strengthening is allowed until 10 to 12 weeks postoperatively.

■ **Avoiding Pitfalls and Complications**

Over- or undertightening of the extensor mechanism repair is a pitfall that must be avoided. For chronic ruptures, I recommend having both extremities prepared and visible in the surgical field to allow the surgeon to directly compare the final patellar position before the repair is secured. Frozen allograft tissue also should be readily available, especially with chronic ruptures for which a repair may not be feasible and an extensor mechanism reconstruction technique must be used. Several reconstruction techniques have been described. Many use an Achilles tendon allograft, which is versatile and can be used for both chronic quadriceps and patellar tendon reconstructions. The bone plug can be secured in a trough made in the tibial tubercle for patellar tendon reconstruction or in a trough in the patella for quadriceps tendon reconstruction. Care also must be taken to handle thick skin and subcutaneous wound edges gently to prevent wound complications.

A recent study reported associated injuries in patients with ruptures of the knee extensor mechanism who required surgical repair over a 10-year period. Thirty-three patients with patellar tendon ruptures and 31 patients with quadriceps tendon ruptures were reviewed. Almost one third of patients with patellar tendon ruptures had an

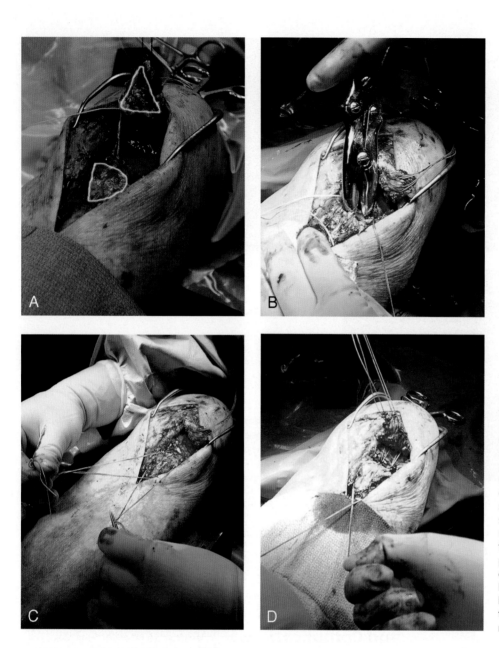

Figure 4 Sequential intraoperative photographs of a double-row repair of an avulsed patellar tendon. **A,** With the Krackow sutures in place, a trial reduction of the matched triangular footprints (yellow lines) of the patellar tendon and tibial tubercle insertion site is confirmed. **B,** The bony insertion site is prepared with a rongeur to provide a bleeding bed for healing. **C,** Two drill holes are placed obliquely across the tubercle, and the two deep sets of Krackow sutures criss-cross the tubercle as they are passed through the drill holes. **D,** An anatomic trial reduction is confirmed.

associated intra-articular knee injury, and 10% of patients with quadriceps tendon ruptures had an associated intra-articular knee injury. The most common associated injuries in patients with patellar tendon ruptures were tears of the anterior cruciate ligament (18%) and medial meniscus (18%). A high index of suspicion for associated injuries is required. The authors recommended MRI or diagnostic arthroscopy in patients with patellar tendon ruptures, especially those with high-

energy direct-impact mechanisms of injury.

Loss of knee motion is one of the most common complications after extensor mechanism repair. Full knee flexion is more difficult to obtain than full extension, in large part because of a delay in allowing flexion in some rehabilitation protocols. Extensor weakness is another complication associated with repair of the extensor mechanism. The quadriceps muscle atrophies, leading to an extensor lag.

Appropriate rehabilitation that allows motion as healing progresses helps to avoid these complications.

Other potential surgical complications include wound infection and skin dehiscence, which often are associated with the subcutaneous positioning of wires and nonabsorbable sutures used for the repair. Avoidance of suture placement directly in line with the incision will help to prevent wound complications.

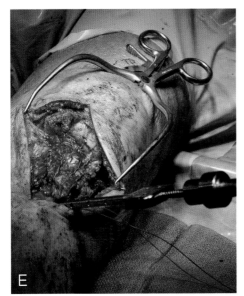

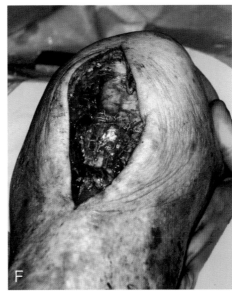

Figure 4 (continued) **E,** The superficial sutures are combined with the paired deep sutures distally and secured with suture anchors. **F,** The safe arc of passive motion providing maintenance of an anatomic reduction of the final repair is confirmed prior to wound closure.

Use of a postoperative closed suction drain is recommended to avoid hemarthrosis. Cerclage wires can break eventually, necessitating removal because of potential wire extrusion and skin irritation. Patella alta or baja (infera) or patellar incongruity also can occur and lead to subsequent patellofemoral arthritis. Accordingly, close attention should be paid to reestablishing the correct patellofemoral alignment when repairing the extensor mechanism. Draping both legs into the surgical field allows direct comparison of patellar height. Finally, rerupture of the repaired tendon may occur, requiring revision surgery.

Bibliography

Bushnell BD, Tennant JN, Rubright JH, Creighton RA: Repair of patellar tendon rupture using suture anchors. *J Knee Surg* 2008;21(2):122-129.

Greis PE, Lahav A, Holmstrom MC: Surgical treatment options for patella tendon rupture. Part II: Chronic. *Orthopedics* 2005;28(8):765-769, quiz 770-771.

Hardy JR, Chimutengwende-Gordon M, Bakar I: Rupture of the quadriceps tendon: An association with a patellar spur. *J Bone Joint Surg Br* 2005;87(10):1361-1363.

Ilan DI, Tejwani N, Keschner M, Leibman M: Quadriceps tendon rupture. *J Am Acad Orthop Surg* 2003;11(3):192-200.

Kasten P, Schewe B, Maurer F, Gösling T, Krettek C, Weise K: Rupture of the patellar tendon: A review of 68 cases and a retrospective study of 29 ruptures comparing two methods of augmentation. *Arch Orthop Trauma Surg* 2001;121(10): 578-582.

Kerin C, Hopgood P, Banks AJ: Delayed repair of the quadriceps using the Mitek anchor system: A case report and review of the literature. *Knee* 2006;13(2):161-163.

Konrath GA, Chen D, Lock T, et al: Outcomes following repair of quadriceps tendon ruptures. *J Orthop Trauma* 1998; 12(4):273-279.

Larsen E, Lund PM: Ruptures of the extensor mechanism of the knee joint: Clinical results and patellofemoral articulation. *Clin Orthop Relat Res* 1986;213:150-153.

McKinney B, Cherney S, Penna J: Intra-articular knee injuries in patients with knee extensor mechanism ruptures. *Knee Surg Sports Traumatol Arthrosc* 2008;16(7):633-638.

Park SS, Kubiak EN, Wasserman B, Sathappan SS, Di Cesare PE: Management of extensor mechanism disruptions occurring after total knee arthroplasty. *Am J Orthop (Belle Mead NJ)* 2005;34(8):365-372.

Pocock CA, Trikha SP, Bell JS: Delayed reconstruction of a quadriceps tendon. *Clin Orthop Relat Res* 2008;466(1): 221-224.

Rasul AT Jr, Fischer DA: Primary repair of quadriceps tendon ruptures: Results of treatment. *Clin Orthop Relat Res* 1993; 289:205-207.

Ravalin RV, Mazzocca AD, Grady-Benson JC, Nissen CW, Adams DJ: Biomechanical comparison of patellar tendon repairs in a cadaver model: An evaluation of gap formation at the repair site with cyclic loading. *Am J Sports Med* 2002; 30(4):469-473.

Rougraff BT, Reeck CC, Essenmacher J: Complete quadriceps tendon ruptures. *Orthopedics* 1996;19(6):509-514.

Schmidle G, Smekal V: Transpatellar refixation of acute quadriceps tendon ruptures close to the proximal patella pole using FiberWire. *Oper Orthop Traumatol* 2008;20(1):65-74.

Coding

CPT Codes		Corresponding ICD-9 Codes	
	Extensor Mechanism Rupture Repair		
27380	Suture of infrapatellar tendon; primary	727.65	727.66
27381	Suture of infrapatellar tendon; secondary reconstruction, including fascial or tendon graft	727.65	727.66

CPT copyright © 2010 by the American Medical Association. All rights reserved.

Index

A

Reticulum, 801
Retinacular release, 275
Rod, intramedullary, 169

S

Short Form-36 (SF-36), 149–150
Simultaneous bilateral total knee arthroplasty (SBTKA)
(*see* Arthroplasty, total knee)
Skeletally immature patients, 593–601
Skin problems, 303–310
Split-thickness skin graft (*see* Grafts)
Stems
cemented, 411–413
uncemented, 408–411
STSG (*see* Grafts)
Surgical Care Improvement Project (SCIP), 327
Synovectomy, 488
Synovial impingement, 124
Synovitis, 296

T

Templating
acetate, 64–70
and complex TKA, 158–159
digital, 64–69
and revision TKA, 335
stemmed implants, 70–71
valgus knee, 227
Tendinitis, 296
Tendon
infrapatellar, 801, 810
peroneal, 734
THA (*see* Arthroplasty, total hip)
Thrombosis, deep vein (*see* Deep vein thrombosis)
Tibial inlay
alternative treatments
graft options, 657–658
single- vs double-bundle, 658
complications, 664
contraindications, 657
indications, 657
patient positioning, 660
postoperative regimen, 664
procedure
arthroscopic evaluation, 660
débridement, 660

femoral graft fixation, 663–664
femoral tunnel creation, 661–662
graft preparation, 660–661
posterior tibia, 662
tibial graft fixation, 662–663
results, 658–659
setup/exposure, 660
wound closure, 664
Tibiofemoral instability, 348–351
TKA (*see* Arthroplasty, total knee)
Total hip arthroplasty (*see* Arthroplasty, total hip)
Total knee arthroplasty (TKA) (*see* Arthroplasty, total knee)
TT-TG index, 793–798

U

UHMWPE (*see* Polyethylene)
Ultrasonography, 709–710
Unicompartmental knee arthroplasty (UKA)
(*see* Arthroplasty, unicompartmental knee)
Uniplane, application, 266

V

Valgus knee, 223–232
Varus knee, 235–241
Varus-valgus constraint (VVC), 441–444
Vastus medialis obliquus (VMO)
and minimally invasive surgery (MIS), 23–28
MPFL repair, 787, 789
patellar instability, 797
patellofemoral injuries, 781–783
and primary TKA, 4–5, 33–35
Venous foot pumps (VFP), 329
Venous thromboembolism (VTE), 321–324
Vitamin E, 58

W

Western Ontario and McMaster University Osteoarthritis
Index (WOMAC), 149–151, 513

Z

Zirconium-niobium alloy, 58